Experimental Designs

THE PRACTICE OF Nursing Research THIRD EDITION

Conduct, Critique, & Utilization

Nancy Burns, PhD, RN, FAAN

Professor and Director
Center for Nursing Research
University of Texas at Arlington
Arlington, Texas

Susan K. Grove, PhD, RN, ANP, GNP

Professor and Assistant Dean
University of Texas at Arlington
Arlington, Texas

W. B. SAUNDERS COMPANY
A Division of Harcourt Brace & Company
Philadelphia London Toronto Montreal Sydney Tokyo

W. B. SAUNDERS COMPANY
A Division of Harcourt Brace & Company

The Curtis Center
Independence Square West
Philadelphia, Pennsylvania 19106

Library of Congress Cataloging-in-Publication Data

Burns, Nancy, Ph. D.
    The practice of nursing research : conduct, critique & utilization
/ Nancy Burns, Susan K. Grove. — 3rd ed.
        p.   cm.
    Includes bibliographical references and index.
    ISBN 0-7216-3054-5
    1. Nursing—Research—Methodology.   I. Grove, Susan K.
II. Title.
    [DNLM: 1. Nursing Research.   WY 20.5 B967p 1997]
RT81.5.B86   1997
610.73′072—dc20
DNLM/DLC
                                                                96-20036

THE PRACTICE OF NURSING RESEARCH   ISBN 0–7216–3054–5

Printed in the United States of America.

Last digit is the print number: 9   8   7   6   5   4

To Barbara Carper and Peggy Chinn,
Who so willingly shared their knowledge with us during our
doctoral education and carefully cultivated our understanding of
theory and research

To nurses,
who care enough to seek better ways to provide excellent
nursing care through research

Preface

Research is a major force in the nursing profession and is being used to change practice, education, and health policy. Our aim in developing the third edition of *The Practice of Nursing Research* is to increase the excitement about research and to facilitate the quest for knowledge through research. The depth and breadth of content presented in this edition reflect the increase in research activities and the growth in research knowledge since the last edition. Nursing research is an integral part of baccalaureate education, graduate education, and clinical practice. An increasing number of nurses are involved in research activities such as critiquing research, utilizing research findings in practice, and conducting sophisticated quantitative and qualitative studies.

The third edition of our text provides comprehensive coverage of nursing research and is focused on the learning needs and styles of today's nursing student. We have retained the sequencing of the content from the second edition, which has facilitated ease in reading and understanding. The major strengths of this book through three editions have been:

- A clear, direct writing style that facilitates student learning;
- A nursing perspective and framework that links research to the rest of nursing;
- Balanced and detailed coverage of both quantitative and qualitative research techniques;
- Rich and frequent illustration of major points and concepts from the most current nursing research literature; and
- Exciting coverage of research utilization, a topic of vital and growing importance in a health care arena where intense emphasis is being placed on improving both the quality and the cost-effectiveness of patient care.

Almost all examples have been updated to clearly illustrate points under discussion and to demonstrate the direct connection between research and clinical practice. The book continues to be based on a strong conceptual framework that links nursing research with practice, theory, knowledge, and philosophy.

Our text provides a comprehensive introduction to nursing research for undergraduate, graduate, and practicing nurses. At the master's and doctoral level, the text provides not only substantive content related to research but also practical applications based on the authors' experiences in conducting various types of nursing research, familiarity with the research literature, and experience in teaching nursing research at various educational levels. In a baccalaureate program, in which research is a separate course at the upper division or senior level, this text can be used to direct students' study of the entire field of nursing research (critique, utilization, and conduct). The text can also be used in a course that focuses primarily on critique and utilization. In addition, the book will be a valuable resource for practicing nurses.

The third edition of our text is organized into 4 units, containing 27 chapters. Unit I introduces the reader to the world of nursing research. The content and presentation of this unit have been designed to assist the reader in overcoming the barriers frequently experienced in understanding the language used in nursing research. The unit also includes a classification system for types of quantitative and qualitative research and introduces the reader to these types of research.

Unit II provides an in-depth presentation of the research process for both quantitative and qualitative research. As with previous editions, this text provides extensive coverage of the many types of qualitative research: phenomenology, grounded theory, ethnography, historical analysis, philosophical inquiry, and critical social theory. Content on quantitative methodologies remains strong as well, with new material added on the development and implementation of interventions, and expanded information on physiologic studies. Chapter 21 is a completely new chapter in this edition and addresses the exciting new area of outcomes research. With the growing emphasis in health care on results and cost-effectiveness, all health care providers, and most especially nurses, will have to scrutinize and evaluate the outcomes of the services and interventions they provide. The methodology described in this chapter provides the tools for that scrutiny and will help the clinician document the effectiveness of health care from the standpoint of the system, the provider, and the patient. Also found in this unit is the most extensive coverage in any comparable text on ethics and research. Included are current federal guidelines for approving studies and an extensive discussion of scientific misconduct in the execution and publication of research studies.

Unit III addresses the implications of research for the discipline and profession of nursing. Content is provided to direct the student in critiquing both quantitative and qualitative research. Critical inquiry is directed not only toward the examination of a study's methodology, but also its importance to the body of knowledge in nursing. Specific steps are provided to direct nurses in using research findings to improve practice.

Unit IV addresses seeking support for research. Readers are given direction for developing quantitative and qualitative research proposals and seeking funding for their research.

An *Instructor's Manual* is available to those who teach from this text. It includes learning activities, evaluation strategies (including test questions), and transparency masters for overhead projection. New with this edition is a *Study Guide* that focuses the student's learning on relevant terms, key ideas, making connections, and exercises in critique and critical thinking. A study disk is included that helps students evaluate their own learning with feedback that directs them to specific sections of the textbook when their understanding requires expansion.

The changes in the third edition of this text reflect the advances in nursing research and also incorporate comments from outside reviewers, colleagues, and students. Our desire to promote the continuing development of the profession of nursing was the incentive for investing the time and energy required to develop this third edition.

Nancy Burns, PhD, RN, FAAN
Susan K. Grove, PhD, RN, ANP, GNP

Acknowledgments

Writing the third edition of this textbook has allowed us the opportunity to examine and revise the content of the previous edition based on input from the literature and a number of scholarly colleagues. A textbook such as this requires the composite of the ideas of many. We have attempted to extract from the nursing literature the essence of nursing knowledge related to the conduct of nursing research. Thus, we would like to thank those nursing scholars who shared their knowledge with those of us in the nursing discipline and made this knowledge accessible for inclusion in the textbook.

The ideas from the literature were synthesized and discussed with our colleagues to determine their contribution to the third edition. Thus, we would like to express our appreciation to the Dean and faculty of the School of Nursing at The University of Texas at Arlington for their support during the long and sometimes arduous experiences that are inevitable in developing a book of this magnitude. We would like to extend a special thanks to Dr. Dorothy J. Stuppy for her scholarly input and willingness to share expertise during the development of this text. We would also like to express gratitude to our students for the questions they raised regarding the content of this text.

We would also like to recognize the excellent reviews of the colleagues who helped us make important revisions in this text; a list of their names appears on p. ix.

A special thanks is extended to the people at the W. B. Saunders Company, who have been extremely helpful to us in producing an attractive, appealing text. The people most instrumental in the development and production of this book include Thomas Eoyang, Vice President & Editor-in-Chief, Nursing Books, and Melanie Nordlinger, Editorial Assistant.

On a personal note, development of this text would not be possible without the constant support and stimulating discussion with our husbands Jerry Burns and Jack R. Suggs. We appreciate their positive attitude and endurance during the times of intense work.

Reviewers

Ellen Russell Beatty, EdD, RN
Southern Connecticut State University
New Haven, Connecticut

Mary E. Burman, PhD, RN
University of Wyoming
Laramie, Wyoming

Karin Kirchhoff, PhD, RN, FAAN
University of Utah
Salt Lake City, Utah

Cecil Lengacher, PhD, RN, ARNP
University of South Florida
Tampa, Florida

Geri B. Neuberger, EdD, MN, RN, ARNP
University of Kansas
Kansas City, Kansas

Olive Santavenere, PhD, MS, RN
Southern Connecticut State University
New Haven, Connecticut

Karen Soeken, PhD
University of Maryland
Baltimore, Maryland

Contents

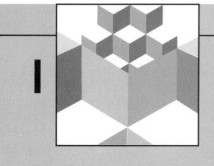

Introduction to Nursing Research

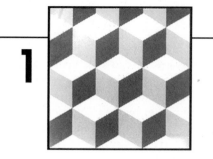

1

Discovery of the World of Nursing Research

Welcome to the world of nursing research. You might think it is strange to consider research a "world," but it is truly a new way of experiencing reality. Entering a new world requires learning a unique language, incorporating new rules, and using new experiences to learn how to interact effectively within that world. As you become a part of this new world, your perceptions and methods of reasoning will be modified and expanded. To many nurses, research is a relatively new world, and we believe this textbook can facilitate entry into this world.

The purpose of this chapter is to explain broadly the world to be explored. A definition of nursing research is provided and the significance of research to nursing is addressed. The chapter concludes with the presentation of a framework that connects nursing research to the rest of nursing. This framework introduces concepts and relationships that are further developed throughout the text.

DEFINITION OF NURSING RESEARCH

The root meaning of the word *research* is to search again or to examine carefully. More specifically, research is diligent, systematic inquiry or investigation to validate and refine existing knowledge and generate new knowledge. The concepts *systematic* and *diligent* are critical to the meaning of research because they imply planning, organization, and persistence. Systematic, diligent inquiry

is necessary for researchers to address the following questions: What needs to be known? What research methods are needed to generate this knowledge? How might a phenomenon be described? What methods of measurement should be used? How can other elements of the world be prevented from interfering with measurement? What meaning can be extracted from these measurements?

Many disciplines conduct research, so a question often raised is "What distinguishes nursing research from research in other disciplines?" This question has been debated among nurses and with members of other disciplines. In some ways, there is no difference because the knowledge and skills required for research do not vary from one discipline to another. However, looking at a different dimension of research, there are distinctions.

The research within any discipline must be consistent with the philosophy of that discipline. Thus, nursing's philosophical orientation, theories, and existing body of knowledge provide a basis for identifying the gaps in the knowledge base and determining what needs to be known. The focus of nursing's unique body of knowledge includes the responses of the holistic person to health and illness as the person interacts with an ever-changing environment. Nursing acts are implemented to promote the holistic person's health and to facilitate the person's growth toward his or her potential within the environment (Keller, 1981). Thus, nursing studies focus on understanding human needs and the use of nursing interventions to promote health, prevent illness, and effectively treat illness. From a holistic perspective, people are considered to be greater than the sum of their parts and studying the parts can never completely explain the whole. Therefore, the holistic perspective influences the development and implementation of nursing research and the interpretation of study findings (Stevenson, 1988).

Defining nursing research also requires examining differing views about what is relevant knowledge for nursing. One view is that nursing research should focus on the general knowledge that is directly useful in clinical practice. This view is evident in the American Nurses Association's (1981, p. 2) definition of nursing research as "the development of knowledge about health and the promotion of health over the full lifespan, care of persons with health problems and disabilities, and nursing actions to enhance the ability of individuals to respond effectively to actual or potential health problems." This view was strongly supported in the 1980s and continues to have a strong impact on the research conducted in the 1990s.

Another view is that nursing research includes studies of nursing education, nursing administration, health services, and characteristics of nurses and the nursing role as well as clinical situations. Those who support this view argue that findings from these studies indirectly influence nursing practice and thus add to nursing's body of knowledge. Educational research is necessary to provide an efficient, effective educational background. Nursing administration and health services studies are necessary to promote quality in the health care system. Management studies influence the organization and provision of nursing care.

We believe nursing research encompasses both of these views. Therefore, in this text, *nursing research* is defined as a scientific process that validates and refines existing knowledge and generates new knowledge that directly and indirectly influences nursing practice.

SIGNIFICANCE OF NURSING RESEARCH

The primary goal of nursing research is to develop a scientific knowledge base for nursing practice.

Broadly, nursing is accountable to society for providing quality, cost-effective care and for seeking ways to improve that care. More specifically, nurses are accountable to their patients. A solid research base will provide evidence of the nursing actions that are effective in promoting positive patient outcomes (Hegyvary, 1991). If nursing actions have limited scientific predictability, nurses have inadequate rationale for taking or not taking a specific action in a situation. Although nursing practice will always involve a degree of uncertainty, research can greatly reduce this.

Nursing's scientific knowledge base is derived from the focus or unique perspective of the discipline and provides an organizing framework for nursing practice (McMurrey, 1982). Currently, this body of knowledge is relatively limited (Bednar, 1993) but is constantly expanding with the generation of new information using a variety of research methods. The knowledge generated through research is essential for description, explanation, prediction, and control of nursing phenomena.

DESCRIPTION

Description involves identifying the nature and attributes of nursing phenomena and sometimes the relationships among these phenomena (Chinn & Kramer, 1995). Through research, nurses are able to describe what exists in nursing practice, discover new information, or classify information for use in the discipline. For example, studies might focus on describing the problems of drug use in society, such as discovering information about how pregnant crack cocaine users perceive their problems and respond to them (Kearney, Murphy, Irwin, & Rosenbaum, 1995). Research focused on description is essential groundwork for studies that will provide explanation, prediction, and control of nursing phenomena.

EXPLANATION

In *explanation,* the relationships among phenomena are clarified and the reasons why certain events occur are identified. For example, the etiologies and criteria of nursing diagnoses identified through descriptive research require explanatory research to test the proposed relationships between the etiologies and criteria for each diagnosis (Carlson-Catalano & Lunney, 1995). These relationships are proposed based on clinical experience and theoretical works. Linking nursing interventions with patient outcomes is also an area of explanatory research. Through research, the patient outcome of pain relief has been linked to positioning, massage, and distraction. Identifying relationships among nursing phenomena provides a basis for conducting research for prediction and control.

PREDICTION

Through *prediction,* one can estimate the probability of a specific outcome in a given situation (Chinn & Kramer, 1995). However, predicting an outcome does not necessarily enable one to modify or control the outcome. With predictive knowledge, nurses could anticipate the effects that nursing interventions would have on patients and families. For example, predictive research on immobility could provide nurses with the knowledge to estimate the effects of prolonged bed rest on the hospitalized patient's recovery. Currently, health promotion research is being conducted to predict the effects of health behaviors, such as regular exercise, balanced diet, and no smoking, on health status and longevity (U.S. Department of Health and Human Services, 1994).

CONTROL

If one can predict the outcome of a situation, the next step is to control or manipulate the situation to produce the desired outcome. Dickoff, James, and Wiedenbach (1968) described control as the ability to write a prescription to produce the desired results. Nurses could prescribe certain interventions to help patients and families achieve their goals. They might prescribe an exercise to increase a patient's activity tolerance or an interven-

tion of therapeutic communication and touch to help a patient and family cope with their fears. Few studies have developed knowledge that is useful for prediction and control in nursing practice. However, the extensive clinical studies conducted in the last two decades have expanded the scientific knowledge needed for description, explanation, prediction, and control of phenomena within nursing.

FRAMEWORK LINKING NURSING RESEARCH TO THE WORLD OF NURSING

In exploring nursing research, a framework is helpful to establish connections between research and the various elements of nursing. A framework linking nursing research to the world of nursing is presented in the following pages and is used as an organizing model for this textbook. In the framework model (see Figure 1–1), nursing research is not an entity disconnected from the rest of nursing but rather is influenced by and influences all other nursing elements. The concepts in this model are pictured on a continuum from concrete to abstract. The discussion of this model introduces this continuum and progresses from the concrete concept of the empirical world to the most abstract concept of nursing philosophy.

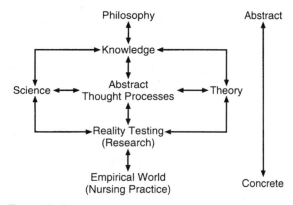

Figure 1–1
Framework linking nursing research to the world of nursing.

CONCRETE–ABSTRACT CONTINUUM

Figure 1–1 presents the components of nursing on a concrete–abstract continuum. This continuum demonstrates that nursing thought flows from both concrete to abstract thinking and from abstract to concrete thinking. *Concrete thinking* is oriented toward and limited by tangible things or events that are observed and experienced in reality. The focus of concrete thinking is immediate events that are limited by time and space. In the past, nursing was seen as a doing profession rather than as a thinking profession. The nurse was expected to do the work, not to ask why. Therefore, nurses tended to be concrete, "practical" thinkers. This type of thinking and behavior was valued and rewarded. Problem solving was considered important only if the effect was immediate. The rudiments of these values are still present to some extent in nursing education and practice.

Abstract thinking is oriented toward the development of an idea without application to, or association with, a particular instance. Abstract thinkers tend to look for meaning, patterns, relationships, and philosophical implications. This type of thinking is independent of time and space. In the past, nurses who were able to think in abstract ways were often considered dreamers, with their heads in the clouds. Their behaviors were considered impractical, and their skills in problem solving and decision making were discouraged. Currently, abstract thinking is fostered in graduate education and is an essential skill for developing theory and research. Abstract thinking is also evolving as a valuable skill in responding to problem situations in clinical practice. For example, nurse practitioners must explore *why* patients are experiencing symptoms, examine the patients' perceptions of their symptoms, and determine patterns among these symptoms before they can accurately diagnose and treat their patients.

Nursing research requires skills in both concrete and abstract thinking. Abstract thought is required to identify researchable problems, design studies, and interpret findings. Concrete thought is necessary in both planning and implementing the detailed steps of data collection and analysis. This back-and-forth flow between abstract and concrete thought may be one reason why nursing research seems foreign and complex.

EMPIRICAL WORLD

The *empirical world* is experienced through our senses and is the concrete portion of our existence. It is what is often called reality, and "doing" kinds of activities are part of this world. There is a sense of certainty about the empirical or real world; it seems understandable, predictable, controllable. This world also appears to have more substance to it than do ideas, and it feels safe and secure. Concrete thinking is focused on the empirical world and words associated with this thinking include practical, down to earth, solid, and factual. Concrete thinkers want facts. Whatever they know must be immediately applicable to the current situation.

The practice of nursing takes place in the empirical world, as demonstrated in Figure 1–1. Some components of the research process also take place in the empirical world. For example, research ideas, which are developed into research problems, are primarily derived from the empirical world. Data collection involves actually measuring some aspect of the empirical world (measurement of reality). In a study, a blood pressure cuff or weight scale might be used to measure reality or reality might be measured with an interview and observation. The findings generated through research are used in clinical practice, which is within the empirical world.

REALITY TESTING

People tend to validate or test the reality of their existence through their senses. In everyday activities, they constantly check out the messages received from their senses. For example, they might ask, "Am I really seeing what I think I am seeing?" Sometimes their senses can play tricks on them. This is why instruments have been developed to record sensory experiences more accurately. For example, does the patient just feel hot or does he have a fever? Thermometers were developed to test this sensory perception accurately.

Research is a way of validating reality. This measurement of reality is done in terms of the researcher's perception. For example, the researcher might ask, "Do patients consume more oxygen when they use a bedside commode than when they use a bedpan?" Our senses would tell us that getting up on a bedside commode would use more oxygen, but nursing research indicates that this is not accurate (Winslow, Lane, & Gaffney, 1984). Thus, nursing research is a way of testing reality—a way of understanding what really goes on in the empirical world.

ABSTRACT THOUGHT PROCESSES

Abstract thought processes influence every element of the nursing world. In a sense, they link all the elements together. Without skills in abstract thought, a person is trapped in a flat existence in the empirical world, an existence in which that world can be experienced but not understood (Abbott, 1952). Through abstract thinking, theories (which explain the nursing world) can be tested and included in the body of scientific knowledge. Abstract thinking also allows scientific findings to be developed into theories. Abstract thought allows both science and theories to be blended into a cohesive body of knowledge, guided by a philosophical framework, and applied in clinical practice. Abstract thinking is actually more useful in clinical practice than one might think. For example, an abstract thinker is often the one who will recognize patterns in the incidence of infection in patients receiving a specific treatment and who will contemplate ideas about the relationships between the infection and other elements of the patient's care.

Three major abstract thought processes—introspection, intuition, and reasoning—are important in nursing (Silva, 1977). These thought processes are used in practicing nursing, developing and evaluating theory, critiquing and using scientific findings, planning and implementing research, and building a body of knowledge.

Introspection

Introspection is the process of turning your attention inward toward your own thoughts. It occurs at two levels. At the more surface level, you are aware of the thoughts you are experiencing. You have an increased awareness of the flow and interplay of feelings and ideas that occur in constantly changing patterns. These thoughts or ideas can rapidly fade from view and disappear if they are not quickly written down. When introspection is allowed to occur in more depth, thoughts are examined more critically and in detail. Patterns or links between thoughts and ideas emerge, and you may recognize fallacies or weaknesses in your thinking. You may question what brought you to this point in your thinking and find yourself really enjoying the experience.

Imagine the following clinical situation in which you have just left John Brown's home. John has a colostomy and has been receiving home health care for several weeks. Although John is caring for his colostomy, he is still reluctant to leave home for any length of time. You experience feelings of irritation and frustration with this situation. You begin to review your nursing actions and to recall other patients who have reacted in similar ways. What were the patterns of their behavior?

You have an idea—perhaps the patient's behavior is linked to the level of family support. You feel unsure about your ability to help the patient and family deal with this situation effectively. You recall other nurses describing similar reactions of patients and wonder just how many patients with colostomies have this problem. Your thoughts jump to reviewing the charts of other patients with colostomies and reading relevant ideas discussed in the literature. Some research has been conducted on this topic recently, and you could critique the findings for use in practice. If the findings are inadequate, perhaps other nurses would be interested in studying this situation with you.

Intuition

Intuition is an insight or understanding of a situation or event as a whole that usually cannot be logically explained (Rew & Barrow, 1987). Since intuition is a type of knowing that seems to come unbidden, it may also be described as a gut feeling or a hunch. Because intuition cannot be scientifically explained with ease, many people are uncomfortable with it. Some even say that it does not exist. So, sometimes, the feeling or sense is pushed down, ignored, or dismissed as silly. However, intuition is not the lack of knowing; it is rather a result of deep knowledge—tacit knowing or personal knowledge (Benner, 1984; Polanyi, 1962, 1966). The knowledge is incorporated so deeply within that it is difficult to bring it consciously to the surface and express it in a logical manner (Beveridge, 1950; Kaplan, 1964).

Intuition is generally considered unscientific and unacceptable for use in research. In some instances, that concern is valid. For example, a hunch that there is a significant difference between one set of scores and another set of scores is not particularly useful as an analysis technique. But even though intuition is often unexplainable, it has some important scientific uses. Researchers do not always need to be able to explain something in order to use it. A burst of intuition may identify a problem for study, indicate important variables to measure, or link two ideas together in interpreting the findings. The trick is to recognize the feeling, value it, and hang onto the idea long enough to consider it.

Imagine the following situation. You have been working in an outpatient cardiac rehabilitation unit for the last three years. You and two other nurses working on the unit have been meeting with the clinical nurse specialist to plan a study to determine the factors important in promoting positive patient outcomes in the rehabilitation program. The group has met several times with a nursing professor at the university who is collaborating with the group to develop the study. At present, the group is concerned with identifying the factors that need to be measured and how to measure them.

You have had a busy morning. Mr. Green, a patient, stops by to chat on his way out of the clinic. He chats and you listen, but not attentively. Then you become more acutely aware of what he is saying. While listening, you begin to have a feeling about one variable that should be studied. You cannot really explain the origin of this feeling. You cannot identify any specific thing that Mr. Green said that triggered the idea, but somehow the flow of words stimulated a burst of intuition. The variable you have in mind has not been previously studied. You feel both excited and uncertain. What will the other nurses think? If it has not been studied, is it really significant? But somehow you feel that it is important to consider.

Reasoning

Reasoning is the processing and organizing of ideas in order to reach conclusions. Through reasoning, people are able to make sense of both their thoughts and experiences. This type of thinking is often evident in the verbal presentation of a logical argument in which each part is linked together to reach a logical conclusion. Patterns of reasoning are used to develop theories and to plan and implement research. Stevens (1984) identified four patterns of reasoning as being essential to nursing: (1) problematic, (2) operational, (3) dialectic, and (4) logistic. An individual uses all four types of reasoning, but frequently one type of reasoning is more dominant than the others. Reasoning is also classified by the discipline of logic into inductive and deductive modes (Bandman & Bandman, 1995; Chinn & Kramer, 1995).

Problematic Reasoning

Problematic reasoning involves identifying a problem and the factors influencing the problem, selecting solutions to the problem, and resolving the problem. For example, nurses use problematic reasoning in the nursing process to identify nursing diagnoses and to implement nursing interventions to resolve these problems. Problematic reasoning is also evident in the identification of a research problem.

Operational Reasoning

Operational reasoning involves the identification and discrimination between many alternatives and viewpoints. The focus is on the process (debating alternatives) rather than on resolution (Stevens, 1984). Nurses use operational reasoning in developing realistic, measurable goals with patients and families. Nurse practitioners use operational reasoning in debating which pharmacological and nonpharmacological treatments to use in treating patient illnesses. In research, operationalizing a treatment for implementation or debating which measurement methods or data analysis techniques to use in a study require operational thought.

Dialectic Reasoning

Dialectic reasoning involves looking at situations in a holistic way. A dialectic thinker believes that the whole is greater than the sum of the parts and that the whole organizes the parts (Stevens, 1984). For example, a nurse using dialectic reasoning would view a patient as a person with strengths and weaknesses who is experiencing an illness and not just the "gallbladder in room 219." Dialectic reasoning also includes examining factors that are opposites and making sense of them by merging them into a single unit or idea, which is greater than either alone. For example, analyzing studies with conflicting findings and summarizing these findings to determine the current knowledge base for a research problem requires dialectic reasoning.

Logistic Reasoning

Logic is a science that involves valid ways of relating ideas to promote understanding. The aim of logic is to determine "truth" or to explain and predict phenomena. The science of logic deals with thought processes, such as concrete and abstract thinking, and methods of reasoning, such as logistic, inductive, and deductive. *Logistic reasoning* is used to break the whole into parts that can be carefully examined, as can the relationships among the parts. In some ways, logistic reasoning is the opposite of dialectic reasoning. A logistic reasoner assumes that the whole is the sum of the parts and that the parts organize the whole. For

example, a patient states that she is cold, and the nurse logically examines the following parts and their relationships: (1) room temperature, (2) patient's temperature, (3) patient's clothing, and (4) patient's activity. The room temperature is 65°F; the patient's temperature is 98.6°F; and the patient is wearing lightweight pajamas and drinking ice water. The nurse concludes that the patient is cold because of external environmental factors (room temperature, lightweight pajamas, and drinking ice water). Logistic reasoning is used frequently in research to develop a study design, plan and implement data collection, and conduct statistical analyses.

INDUCTIVE AND DEDUCTIVE REASONING. The science of logic also includes inductive and deductive reasoning. These modes of reasoning are used constantly by individuals, although the choice of types of reasoning may not always be conscious (Kaplan, 1964). *Inductive reasoning* moves from the specific to the general where particular instances are observed and then combined into a larger whole or general statement (Bandman & Bandman, 1995; Chinn & Kramer, 1995). An example of inductive reasoning follows:

A headache is an altered level of health that is stressful.
A fractured bone is an altered level of health that is stressful.
A terminal illness is an altered level of health that is stressful.
Therefore, all altered levels of health are stressful.

In this example, inductive reasoning is used to move from the specific instances of altered levels of health that are stressful to the general belief that all altered levels of health are stressful. The testing of many different altered levels of health through research to determine whether they are stressful is necessary to confirm the general statement that all types of altered health are stressful.

Deductive reasoning moves from the general to the specific or from a general premise to a particular situation or conclusion (Bandman & Bandman, 1995; Chinn & Kramer, 1995). A premise or hypothesis is a statement of the proposed relationship between two or more variables. An example of deductive reasoning follows:

PREMISES

All human beings experience loss.
All adolescents are human beings.

CONCLUSION

All adolescents experience loss.

In this example, deductive reasoning is used to move from the two premises about human beings and adolescents experiencing loss to the conclusion that "All adolescents experience loss." However, the conclusions generated from deductive reasoning are valid only if they are based on valid premises.

PREMISES

All health professionals are caring.
All nurses are health professionals.

CONCLUSIONS

All nurses are caring.

The premise that all health professionals are caring is not valid or an accurate reflection of reality. Research is a means to test and confirm or refute a premise, so valid premises can be used as a basis for reasoning in nursing practice.

SCIENCE

Science is a coherent body of knowledge composed of research findings and tested theories for a specific discipline. Science is both a product (end point) and a process (mechanism to reach an end point) (Silva & Rothbart, 1984). An example in physics is Newton's law of gravity, which was developed through extensive research. The knowledge of gravity (product) is a part of the science of physics that evolved through formulating and testing theoretical ideas (process). The ultimate goal of science is to be able to explain the empirical world and, thus, to have increased control over it. In order to accomplish this goal, scientists must discover new knowledge, expand existing knowledge, and reaffirm previously held knowledge in a discipline (Andreoli & Thompson, 1977; Greene, 1979; Toulmin, 1960).

The science of a field determines the accepted process for obtaining knowledge within that field. Research is an accepted process for obtaining scientific knowledge in nursing. Some sciences will rigidly limit the types of research that can be used to obtain knowledge. The acceptable method for developing a science is the traditional research process or quantitative research. According to this process, the information gained from one study is not sufficient for its inclusion in the body of science. A study must be repeated (replicated) several times and must yield similar results each time before that information can be considered a *fact*. Consider the research on the relationship between smoking and lung cancer. Numerous studies of animals and humans have been done, and the findings all indicate a relationship between smoking and lung cancer, although certainly not everyone who smokes develops lung cancer. Enough research has been done so that it is now considered a fact that smoking is a major factor in the development of lung cancer.

Facts from studies are systematically related to each other in a way that seems to best explain the empirical world. Abstract thought processes are used to make these linkages. The linkages are called laws, principles, or axioms, depending on the certainty of the facts and relationships within the linkage. Laws are used to express the most certain relationships. The certainty is dependent on the amount of research conducted to test it and to some extent on skills in abstract thought processes. The truths or explanations of the empirical world reflected by these laws, principles, and axioms are never absolutely certain and may be disproved by further research.

Nursing science has been developed using predominantly quantitative research methods. However, in the last 20 years, there has been an increasing interest in developing a qualitative research tradition. Qualitative research is based on a different philosophical orientation toward reality than quantitative research. Within the qualitative research tradition, many of the long-held tenets about science and ways of obtaining knowledge are being questioned. The philosophical orientation of qualitative research is holistic, and the purpose of this research is to examine the whole rather than the parts. Qualitative researchers are more interested in understanding complex phenomena than in determining cause-and-effect relationships among specific variables. Both quantitative and qualitative research have proved valuable in the development of nursing knowledge (Clarke, 1995; Dzurec & Abraham, 1993; Ford-Gilboe, Campbell, & Berman, 1995). For this reason, this textbook provides a background for conducting different types of both quantitative and qualitative research.

Nursing is in the beginning stages of developing a science, since a limited number of original studies and replications have been conducted (Bednar, 1993; Gortner, 1990). Major studies with findings significant to nursing practice must be implemented and replicated. If researchers find the same results each time they replicate a study, they become increasingly certain that they are accurately describing the empirical world. The cluster of findings from replicated research then becomes a part of science (Beck, 1994).

might be developed, it is essential that there are a variety of them to provide nurses new insights into patient care and to stimulate the development of innovative interventions (Levine, 1995).

Research is conducted either to develop or to test theory. However, many nurse researchers do not recognize or value the link of theory and research. Thus, many nursing studies are not based on theory and the findings are not linked to theory (Moody, Wilson, Smyth, Schwartz, Tittle, & Van Cott, 1988). In order to be useful, information acquired through nursing research must be developed into nursing theories. Isolated facts from a study are not useful alone; they must be linked within nursing's knowledge base to form theories. These theories explain the meaning of research findings and must then be tested through further research and refined to enhance their usefulness in nursing practice. Of course, not all nursing theory will be originally developed from research findings. Sometimes a theory originates as an idea, and then research is conducted to test its accuracy. Either way, research has a role in furthering the development of nursing theories (Chinn & Kramer, 1995; Fawcett & Downs, 1986; Meleis, 1990).

THEORY

A *theory* is a way of explaining some segment of the empirical world and can be used to describe, explain, predict, and/or control that segment (Dubin, 1978). A theory consists of a set of concepts that are defined and interrelated to present a view of a phenomenon. For example, Selye developed a theory about stress; Freud, a theory of human personality; and Maslow, a theory about human needs. A theory is developed from a combination of personal experiences, research findings, and abstract thought processes. Findings from research may be used as a starting point, with the theory emerging as the theorist organizes the findings to best explain the empirical world. Or the theorist may use abstract thought processes, personal knowledge, and intuition to develop a theory of a phenomenon. However these theories

KNOWLEDGE

Knowledge is a complex, multifaceted concept. For example, you may say that you "know" your friend John, "know" that the earth rotates around the sun, "know" how to give an injection, and "know" pharmacology. These are examples of knowing—being familiar with a person, comprehending facts, acquiring a psychomotor skill, and mastering a subject. There are differences in types of knowing, yet there are also similarities. Knowing presupposes order or imposes order on thoughts and ideas (Engelhardt, 1980). People have a desire to know what to expect (Russell, 1948). There is a need for certainty in the world, and individuals seek it by trying to decrease uncertainty through knowledge (Ayer, 1966). Think of the questions you ask of a person related to some bit of knowledge. "Is it true?" "Are you sure?"

"How do you know?" Thus, knowledge is acquired in a variety of ways and is expected to be an accurate reflection of reality.

Ways of Acquiring Nursing Knowledge

An additional expectation of knowledge is that it be acquired through acceptable and accurate means (White, 1982). Nursing has historically acquired knowledge through traditions, authority, borrowing, trial and error, personal experience, role-modeling and mentorship, intuition, reasoning, and research. Intuition, reasoning, and research have been introduced earlier in this chapter and the other ways of acquiring knowledge are briefly described in this section.

Traditions

Traditions include "truths" or beliefs that are based on customs and past trends. Nursing traditions from the past have been transferred to the present by written and verbal communication and role-modeling and continue to influence the present practice of nursing. For example, many of the policy and procedure manuals in hospitals and other health care facilities contain traditional ideas. In addition, nursing interventions are commonly transmitted verbally from one nurse to another over the years. Traditions can positively influence nursing practice, because they were developed from effective past experiences. For example, the idea of providing a patient with a clean, safe, well-ventilated environment originated with Nightingale.

However, traditions can also narrow and limit the knowledge sought for nursing practice. For example, nursing units are frequently organized and run according to set rules or traditions. Tradition has established the time and pattern for giving baths, taking vital signs, giving medications, and selecting needle length for giving injections. The nurses on patient care units quickly inform new staff members about the accepted or traditional behaviors for the unit.

Traditions are difficult to change because they have existed for long periods of time and are fre-

quently supported by people with power and authority. Many traditions have not been evaluated or tested for accuracy or efficiency. However, even those traditions that have not been supported through research tend to persist. For example, many cardiac patients are required to take basin baths throughout their hospitalization despite the findings from nursing research. Research has shown "that the physiologic costs of the three types of baths (basin, tub, and shower) are similar; differences in responses to bathing seem more a function of subject variability than bath types; and many cardiac patients can take a tub bath or shower earlier in their hospitalization" (Winslow, Lane, & Gaffney, 1985, p. 164). Nursing's body of knowledge needs to have an empirical rather than a traditional base if nurses are to have a powerful impact on health care and patient outcomes.

Authority

An *authority* is a person with expertise and power who is able to influence opinion and behavior. A person is given authority because it is thought that she or he knows more in a given area than others do. Knowledge acquired from authority is illustrated when one person credits another person as the source of information. Nurses who publish articles and books or develop theories are frequently considered authorities. Students usually view their instructors as authorities, and clinical nursing experts are considered authorities within their clinical settings. However, persons viewed as authorities in one field are not authorities in other fields. An expert is only an authority when addressing his or her area of expertise (Bandman & Bandman, 1995). To be considered a source of knowledge, authorities in nursing must have both expertise and power. The use of only power and control does not make someone an authority.

Many customs or traditional ways of knowing are maintained by authorities, but the knowledge obtained from these authorities can be inaccurate. Like tradition, the knowledge acquired from authorities has frequently not been validated; and although it may be useful, it must be verified through research.

Borrowing

Some nursing leaders have described part of nursing's knowledge as information borrowed from disciplines such as medicine, psychology, physiology, and education (Andreoli & Thompson, 1977; McMurrey, 1982). *Borrowing* in nursing involves the appropriation and use of knowledge from other fields or disciplines to guide nursing practice. Nursing has borrowed in two ways. For years, some nurses have taken information from other disciplines and applied it directly to nursing practice. This information was not integrated within the unique focus of nursing. For example, some nurses have used the medical model to guide their nursing practice, thus focusing on the diagnosis and treatment of disease. This type of borrowing continues today as nurses use advances in technology to become highly specialized and focused on the detection and treatment of disease to the exclusion of health promotion and illness prevention.

Another way of borrowing, which is more functional in nursing, is the integration of information from other disciplines within the focus of nursing. Since disciplines share knowledge, it is sometimes difficult to know where the boundaries exist between nursing's knowledge base and that of other disciplines. There is a blurring of boundaries as the knowledge bases of disciplines evolve (McMurrey, 1982). For example, information about self-esteem as a characteristic of the human personality is associated with psychology; but this knowledge of self-esteem also directs the nurse in assessing the psychological needs of patients and families. However, borrowed knowledge has not been adequate for answering many questions generated in nursing practice.

Trial and Error

Trial and error is an approach with unknown outcomes used in a situation of uncertainty, when other sources of knowledge are unavailable. Since each patient responds uniquely to a situation, there is uncertainty in nursing practice. Because of this uncertainty, nurses must use trial and error in providing care. However, with trial and error, there is frequently no formal documentation of effective and ineffective nursing actions. Using this strategy, knowledge is gained from experience but is often not shared with others. The trial-and-error way of acquiring knowledge can also be time consuming, because multiple interventions might be implemented before one is found to be effective. There is also a risk of implementing nursing actions that are detrimental to a patient's health.

Personal Experience

Personal experience involves gaining knowledge by being personally involved in an event, situation, or circumstance. In nursing, personal experience enables one to gain skills and expertise by providing care to patients and families in clinical settings. Learning occurs during personal experience and enables the nurse to cluster ideas into a meaningful whole. For example, students may be told how to give an injection in a classroom setting, but they do not "know" how to give an injection until they observe other nurses giving injections to patients and actually give several injections themselves.

The amount of personal experience affects the complexity of a nurse's knowledge base. Benner (1984) described five levels of experience in the development of clinical knowledge and expertise: (1) novice, (2) advanced beginner, (3) competent, (4) proficient, and (5) expert. *Novice* nurses have no personal experience in the work that they are to perform, but they have preconceived notions and expectations about clinical practice that are challenged, refined, confirmed, or disconfirmed by personal experience in a clinical setting. The *advanced beginner* has just enough experience to recognize and intervene in recurrent situations. For example, the advanced beginner nurse is able to recognize and intervene to meet patients' mobility needs.

Competent nurses frequently have been on the job for two or three years, and their personal experiences enable them to generate and achieve long-range goals and plans. Through experience, the competent nurse is able to use personal knowledge to take conscious, deliberate actions that are efficient and organized. From a more complex knowledge base, the *proficient* nurse views the patient as a whole and as a member of a family and community. The proficient nurse recognizes that each patient and family responds differently to illness and health. The *expert* nurse has an extensive background of experience and is able to identify accurately and intervene skillfully in a situation. Personal experience increases an expert nurse's ability to grasp a situation intuitively with accuracy and speed. The dynamics of expert nursing practice need to be clarified through research. In addition, the methods that facilitate meaningful, personal experiences need to be identified for use in nursing education.

Role-Modeling and Mentorship

Role-modeling is learning by imitating the behaviors of an exemplar. An exemplar or role model is viewed as knowing the appropriate and rewarded roles for a profession, and these roles reflect the attitudes and include the standards and norms of behavior for that profession (Bidwell & Brasler, 1989). In nursing, role-modeling enables the novice nurse to learn through interaction with or examples set by highly competent nurses. Examples of role models are "admired teachers, practitioners, researchers, or illustrious individuals who inspire students through their examples" (Werley & Newcomb, 1983, p. 206).

An intense form of role-modeling is *mentorship*. In a mentorship, the expert nurse or *mentor* serves as a teacher, sponsor, guide, exemplar, and counselor for the novice nurse (Vance, 1982). There is an investment of time and active involvement that results in a close, personal mentor-mentee relationship (Bidwell & Brasler, 1989). This relationship promotes a mutual exchange of ideas and aspirations relative to the mentee's career plans. The mentee assumes the values, attitudes, and behaviors of the mentor while gaining intuitive knowledge and personal experience.

In nursing, a body of knowledge must be acquired (learned), incorporated, and assimilated by each member of the profession and collectively by the profession as a whole. This body of knowledge guides the thinking and behavior of the profession and individual practitioners. It will provide direction for further development and interpretation of science and theory in the discipline. Nursing's development of a body of knowledge will give nurses the confidence that they know what they are doing. This knowledge base is necessary for the recognition of nursing as a science by health professionals, consumers, and society.

PHILOSOPHY

Philosophy provides a broad, global explanation of the world. It is the most abstract and all-encompassing concept in the model (see Figure 1–1). Philosophy gives unity and meaning to nursing's world and provides a framework within which thinking, knowing, and doing occur. Nursing's philosophical position influences its knowledge. The way nurses use science and theories to explain the empirical world will depend on their philosophy. Ideas about truth and reality as well as beliefs, values, and attitudes are part of philosophy. Philosophy asks such questions as, "Is there an absolute truth or is truth relative?" "Is there one reality or is reality different for each individual?" "What are their purposes in life?"

Everyone's world is modified by her or his philosophy as a pair of glasses would modify vision. Perceptions are influenced first by philosophy and then by knowledge. For example, if what you see is not within your ideas of truth or reality, if it does not fit your belief system, you may not see it. Your mind may reject it altogether or modify it to fit within your philosophy (Scheffler, 1967; Tucker, 1979).

Philosophical positions commonly held by the nursing profession include the view of human beings as holistic, rational, and responsible. Nurses believe that people desire health and health is considered to be better than illness. Quality of life is as important as quantity of life. Good nursing care facilitates improved patterns of health and quality of life. In nursing, truth is seen as relative and reality tends to vary with perception (Silva, 1977).

For example, because nurses believe that reality varies with perception and that truth is relative, they would not try to impose their views of truth and reality on patients. Rather, they would accept patients' views of the world and help them seek health from within their world view.

Nursing's philosophical positions have a strong influence on the research conducted (Ford-Gilboe et al., 1995; Newman, 1992). These philosophical positions support the use of both quantitative and qualitative research in the development of a scientific knowledge base for nursing. The research problems selected for study, the methodologies implemented in research, and the interpretations of research findings are influenced by nursing's philosophy.

In conclusion, the most abstract concept (philosophy) links in a direct and meaningful way with the most concrete concept, the empirical world. Our philosophy directs how we view and interact with others in the world around us. Figure 1–1 demonstrates that research is not off to the side, disconnected from the rest of nursing. In order to utilize nursing's body of knowledge in practice, one must incorporate all the elements of the nursing world. If one element is missing, the rest of the elements lose meaning. One cannot be only concrete, only abstract, only theoretical, or only scientific. One cannot attend to only clinical practice and disregard the rest of the nursing world— not if one is a nurse in the whole sense of the word.

◾ SUMMARY

The purpose of this chapter is to introduce the reader to the world of research. Research is defined as diligent, systematic inquiry to validate and refine existing knowledge and generate new knowledge. Defining nursing research requires examining differing views about what is relevant knowledge for nursing. One view is that nursing research should be limited to only those studies that generate knowledge that is directly useful in clinical practice. Another view is that nursing research includes studies of nursing education, nursing administration, health services, and characteristics of nurses and the nursing role as well as clinical situations. Those who support this view argue that findings from these studies indirectly influence nursing practice. In this textbook, nursing research is defined as a scientific process that validates and refines existing knowledge and generates new knowledge that directly and indirectly influences nursing practice.

The primary goal of nursing research is to develop a scientific knowledge base for nursing practice. This knowledge base is derived from the focus or unique perspective of the discipline and provides an organizing framework for nursing practice. The knowledge generated through research is essential for description, explanation, prediction, and control of nursing phenomena.

This chapter presents a framework that links nursing research to the world of nursing (see Figure 1–1). This framework provides an organizing model for this textbook. The concepts in this framework range from concrete to abstract and include concrete and abstract thinking, empirical world (nursing practice), reality testing (research), abstract thought processes, science, theory, knowledge, and philosophy.

Nursing thought flows along a continuum of concrete and abstract thinking. Concrete thinking is oriented toward tangible things or events. Abstract thinking is oriented toward the development of an idea without application to, or association with, a particular instance. The empirical world is the concrete portion of human existence experienced through the

continued

continued

senses and is validated through reality testing. Research is a form of reality testing requiring skills in both concrete and abstract thinking. Abstract thought processes influence every element of the nursing world. Three major abstract thought processes, introspection, intuition, and reasoning, are important in nursing. These thought processes are used in practicing nursing, developing and evaluating theory, critiquing and using scientific findings, planning and implementing research, and building a body of knowledge.

Science and theory are two different but interdependent concepts that are linked by abstract thought processes. Science is a coherent body of knowledge composed of research findings and tested theories for a specific discipline. It is both a process (scientific methods) and a product (body of knowledge). Nursing science is slowly developing with the utilization of a variety of both quantitative and qualitative research methods. Theory is a way of explaining some segment of the empirical world. Theories are developed and tested through research, and when they are adequately tested, they become part of science.

Science and theory contribute to the development of a body of knowledge in a discipline. In nursing, a body of knowledge must be acquired (learned), incorporated, and assimilated by each member of the profession and collectively by the profession as a whole. Nursing has historically acquired knowledge through traditions, authority, borrowing, trial and error, personal experience, role-modeling and mentorship, intuition, reasoning, and research. The most abstract element of the framework is philosophy. Philosophy gives unity and meaning to the world of nursing and provides a structure within which thinking, knowing, and doing occur. Nursing's philosophical positions, such as the holistic perspective and importance of quality of life, have a strong influence on the research conducted and the knowledge developed in the discipline. The framework demonstrates that nursing research is not an entity disconnected from the rest of nursing but rather is influenced by and influences all other nursing activities.

References

Abbott, E. A. (1952). *Flatland.* New York: Dover Publications.

American Nurses Association. (1981). *Research priorities for the 1980s: Generating a scientific basis for nursing practice.* Kansas City, MO: Commission on Nursing Research, ANA.

Andreoli, K. G., & Thompson, C. E. (1977). The nature of science in nursing. *Image: Journal of Nursing Scholarship, 9*(2), 32–37.

Ayer, A. J. (1966). *The problem of knowledge.* Baltimore, MD: Penguin.

Bandman, E. L., & Bandman, B. (1995). *Critical thinking in nursing* (2nd ed.). Norwalk, CT: Appleton & Lange.

Beck, C. T. (1994). Replication strategies for nursing research. *Image: Journal of Nursing Scholarship, 26*(3), 191–194.

Bednar, B. (1993). Developing clinical practice guidelines: An interview with Ada Jacox. *ANNA Journal, 20*(2), 121–126.

Benner, P. (1984). *From novice to expert: Excellence and power in clinical nursing practice.* Menlo Park, CA: Addison-Wesley.

Beveridge, W. I. B. (1950). *The art of scientific investigation.* New York: Vintage Books.

Bidwell, A. S., & Brasler, M. L. (1989). Role modeling versus mentoring in nursing education. *Image: Journal of Nursing Scholarship, 21*(1), 23–25.

Carlson-Catalano, J., & Lunney, M. (1995). Quantitative methods for clinical validation of nursing diagnoses. *Clinical Nurse Specialist, 9*(6), 306–311.

Chinn, P. L., & Kramer, M. K. (1995). *Theory and nursing: A systematic approach* (4th ed.). St. Louis: Mosby.

Clarke, L. (1995). Nursing research: Science, visions, and telling stories. *Journal of Advanced Nursing, 21*(3), 584–593.

Dickoff, J., James, P., & Wiedenbach, E. (1968). Theory in a practice discipline: Practice oriented theory (Part I). *Nursing Research, 17*(5), 415–435.

Dubin, R. (1978). *Theory building* (rev. ed.). New York: Free Press.

Dzurec, L. C., & Abraham, I. L. (1993). The nature of inquiry: Linking quantitative and qualitative research. *Advances in Nursing Science, 16*(1), 73–79.

Engelhardt, H. T., Jr. (1980). Knowing and valuing: Looking for common roots. In H. T. Engelhardt & D. Callahan

(Eds.), *Knowing and valuing: The search for common roots* (Vol. 4, pp. 1–17). New York: Hastings Center.

Fawcett, J., & Downs, F. S. (1986). *The relationship of theory and research.* Norwalk, CT: Appleton-Century-Crofts.

Ford-Gilboe, M., Campbell, J., & Berman, H. (1995). Stories and numbers: Coexistence without compromise. *Advances in Nursing Science, 18*(1), 14–26.

Gortner, S. R. (1990). Nursing values and science: Toward a science philosophy. *Image: Journal of Nursing Scholarship, 22*(2), 101–105.

Greene, J. A. (1979). Science, nursing and nursing science: A conceptual analysis. *Advances in Nursing Science, 2*(1), 57–64.

Hegyvary, S. T. (1991). Issues in outcomes research. *Journal of Nursing Quality Assurance, 5*(2), 1–6.

Kaplan, A. (1964). *The conduct of inquiry.* New York: Harper & Row.

Kearney, M. H., Murphy, S., Irwin, K., & Rosenbaum, M. (1995). Salvaging self: A grounded theory of pregnancy on crack cocaine. *Nursing Research, 44*(4), 208–213.

Keller, M. J. (1981). Toward a definition of health. *Advances in Nursing Science, 4*(1), 43–64.

Levine, M. E. (1995). The rhetoric of nursing theory. *Image: Journal of Nursing Scholarship, 27*(1), 11–14.

McMurrey, P. H. (1982). Toward a unique knowledge base in nursing. *Image: Journal of Nursing Scholarship, 14*(1), 12–15.

Meleis, A. I. (1990). *Theoretical nursing: Development and progress* (2nd ed.). Philadelphia: Lippincott.

Moody, L. E., Wilson, M. E., Smyth, K., Schwartz, R., Tittle, M., & Van Cott, M. L. (1988). Analysis of a decade of nursing practice research: 1977–1986. *Nursing Research, 37*(6), 374–379.

Newman, M. A. (1992). Prevailing paradigms in nursing. *Nursing Outlook, 40*(1), 10–13, 32.

Polanyi, M. (1962). *Personal knowledge.* Chicago: University of Chicago Press.

Polanyi, M. (1966). *The tacit dimension.* New York: Doubleday.

Rew, L., & Barrow, E. M. (1987). Intuition: A neglected hallmark of nursing knowledge. *Advances in Nursing Science, 10*(1), 49–62.

Russell, B. (1948). *Human knowledge, its scope and limits.* Brooklyn: Simon and Schuster.

Scheffler, I. (1967). *Science and subjectivity.* Indianapolis: Bobbs-Merrill.

Silva, M. C. (1977). Philosophy, science, theory: Interrelationships and implications for nursing research. *Image: Journal of Nursing Scholarship, 9*(3), 59–63.

Silva, M. C., & Rothbart, D. (1984). An analysis of changing trends in philosophies of science on nursing theory development and testing. *Advances in Nursing Science, 6*(2), 1–13.

Stevens, B. J. (1984). *Nursing theory: Analysis, application, evaluation* (2nd ed.). Boston: Little, Brown.

Stevenson, J. S. (1988). Nursing knowledge development: Into era II. *Journal of Professional Nursing, 4*(3), 152–162.

Toulmin, S. (1960). *The philosophy of science.* New York: Harper & Row.

Tucker, R. W. (1979). The value decisions we know as science. *Advances in Nursing Science, 1*(2), 1–12.

U.S. Department of Health and Human Services (1994). *Health for the United States 1993.* Hyattsville, MD: DHHS Publication No. (PHS) 94–1232.

Vance, C. (1982). The mentor connection. *Journal of Nursing Administration, 12*(4), 7–13.

Werley, H. H., & Newcomb, B. J. (1983). The research mentor: A missing element in nursing? In N. L. Chaska (Ed.), *The nursing profession: A time to speak* (pp. 202–215). New York: McGraw-Hill.

White, A. R. (1982). *The nature of knowledge.* Totowa, NJ: Rowman and Littlefield.

Winslow, E. H., Lane, L. D., & Gaffney, F. A. (1984). Oxygen consumption and cardiovascular response in patients and normal adults during in-bed and out-of-bed toileting. *Journal of Cardiac Rehabilitation, 4*(8), 348–354.

Winslow, E. H., Lane, L. D., & Gaffney, F. A. (1985). Oxygen uptake and cardiovascular responses in control adults and acute myocardial infarction patients during bathing. *Nursing Research, 34*(3), 164–169.

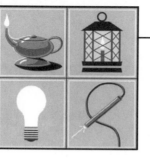

2

The Evolution
of Research in Nursing

Initially, research evolved slowly in nursing from the investigations of Nightingale in the nineteenth century to the studies of nursing education in the 1930s and 1940s and the research of nurses and nursing roles in the 1950s and 1960s. However, in the 1970s and 1980s, numerous studies were conducted that focused on clinical nursing practice. The conduct of clinical research continues to be a major focus of the 1990s, with the intent of developing a research-based practice. Reviewing the history of research in nursing increases our understanding of the current status and facilitates the projection of the future of nursing research. These historical events also provide a basis for the selection of the scientific methodologies that are used in developing the empirical or research knowledge base for nursing. Nurses have found that both quantitative and qualitative research methodologies are needed to develop nursing knowledge. In the 1990s, outcomes research has emerged as an important methodology for generating knowledge about the end-result of patient care. Outcomes research is conducted to examine both short-term and long-term results of health care, such as patient health status, quality of care, and cost-effectiveness of care. In this chapter, the historical events relevant to research are identified; the problem-solving process and nursing process are discussed as a basis for the research process; and the types of quantitative and qualitative research methods and outcomes research are introduced.

HISTORICAL DEVELOPMENT OF RESEARCH IN NURSING

Some people think that research is relatively new to nursing, but Florence Nightingale initiated nursing research more than 140 years ago (Nightingale, 1859). Following Nightingale's work (1850–1910), research received minimal attention until the 1950s. From 1960, the value of nursing research gradually increased; but few nurses had the educational background to conduct studies until the 1970s. However, in the 1980s and 1990s, research has become a major force in developing a scientific knowledge base for nursing practice. Table 2–1 identifies some of the key historical events that have influenced the development of nursing research and these events are discussed in the following sections.

FLORENCE NIGHTINGALE

Nightingale was described as a reformer, reactionary, and researcher. Her research has influenced health care in general, and nursing specifically. Nightingale's *Notes on Nursing* (1859) describe her initial research activities, which focused on the importance of a healthy environment in promoting the patient's physical and mental well-being. She identified the need to gather data on the environment, such as ventilation, cleanliness, temperature,

Table 2–1
Historical Events Influencing Nursing Research

Year	Historical Event
1850	Nightingale, first nurse researcher
1900	*American Journal of Nursing* (first published)
1923	Teacher's College at Columbia offers the first doctoral program for nurses
1929	First Master's in Nursing Degree is offered at Yale University
1932	The Association of Collegiate Schools of Nursing is organized
1950	American Nurses' Association study of nursing functions and activities
1952	*Nursing Research* (first published)
1953	Institute of Research and Service in Nursing Education
1963	*International Journal of Nursing Studies* (first published)
1965	ANA sponsored nursing research conferences
1967	*Image* (Sigma Theta Tau Publication) (first published)
1970	ANA Commission on Nursing Research
1972	ANA Council of Nurse Researchers
1973	First Nursing Diagnosis Conference was held
1978	*Research in Nursing & Health* (first published)
	Advances in Nursing Science (first published)
1979	*Western Journal of Nursing Research* (first published)
1982–83	Conduct and Utilization of Research in Nursing (CURN) Project (published)
1983	*Annual Review of Nursing Research* (first published)
1985	National Center for Nursing Research (NCNR) was established within the National Institutes of Health
1987	*Scholarly Inquiry for Nursing Practice* (first published)
1988	*Applied Nursing Research* (first published)
	Nursing Science Quarterly (first published)
1989	Agency for Health Care Policy and Research (AHCPR) was established
	Clinical practice guidelines were first published by the AHCPR
1992	*Healthy People 2000* was published by Department of Health and Human Services
1993	NCNR was renamed the National Institute of Nursing Research

purity of water, and diet to determine the influence on the patient's health (Herbert, 1981).

Nightingale is most noted for her data collection and statistical analyses during the Crimean War. She gathered data on soldier morbidity and mortality and the factors influencing these and presented her results in tables and pie diagrams, a sophisticated type of data presentation for this period (Palmer, 1977). Nightingale's research enabled her to instigate attitudinal, organizational, and social change. She changed the attitudes of the military and society toward the care of the sick. The military began to view the sick as having the right to adequate food, suitable quarters, and appropriate medical treatment. These interventions drastically reduced mortality from 43% to 2% in the Crimean War (Cook, 1913). She improved the organization of army administration, hospital management, and hospital construction. Because of

Nightingale's influence, society began to accept responsibility for testing public water, improving sanitation, preventing starvation, and decreasing morbidity and mortality (Palmer, 1977).

EARLY 1900s

From 1900 to 1950, research activities were limited, but a few studies advanced nursing education. These studies included the Nutting Report, 1912; Goldmark Report, 1923; and Burgess Report, 1926 (Abdellah, 1972; W. L. Johnson, 1977). Based on the recommendations of the Goldmark Report, more schools of nursing were established in university settings. The baccalaureate degree in nursing provided a basis for graduate nursing education, with the first Master of Nursing degree offered by Yale University in 1929. Teachers College at Columbia offered the first doctoral program for nurses in 1924 and granted a degree in education (Ed.D.). The first nursing doctoral degrees were in education to prepare teachers for the profession. The Association of Collegiate Schools of Nursing was organized in 1932 and promoted the conduct of research to improve education and practice. This organization later sponsored the publication of the first research journal in nursing, *Nursing Research* (Fitzpatrick, 1978).

In 1900, the *American Journal of Nursing* was first published, and late in the 1920s and 1930s, case studies began appearing in this journal. Case studies involve an in-depth analysis and systematic evaluation of one patient or a group of similar patients to promote understanding of nursing interventions. These case studies were the beginning of practice-related research.

A research trend that started in the 1940s and continued in the 1950s focused on the organization and delivery of nursing services. Studies were conducted on the numbers and kinds of nursing personnel, staffing patterns, patient classification systems, patient and personnel satisfaction, and unit arrangement. Types of care such as comprehensive care, home care, and progressive patient care were evaluated. These evaluations of care laid the foundation for the development of self-study manuals, which are similar to the quality assurance manuals of today (Gortner & Nahm, 1977).

NURSING RESEARCH IN THE 1950s AND 1960s

Major advances were made in nursing research during the 1950s for several reasons. Research became a higher priority with the support of such nursing leaders as Henderson and Abdellah. There were an increased number of master's-prepared nurses who had taken courses in research; some had completed theses, which provided them with a background for conducting research. In the 1950s and 1960s, schools of nursing began introducing research and the steps of the research process at the baccalaureate level. In addition, increased funding for research became available. In

1955, $500,000 was awarded for federal research grants in nursing (de Tornyay, 1977). The increase in research activities prompted the publication of the journal *Nursing Research* in 1952. This journal provided nurses an opportunity for communicating their findings.

In 1950, the American Nurses' Association (ANA) initiated a 5-year study on nursing functions and activities. The findings of this study were reported in *Twenty Thousand Nurses Tell Their Story*. As a result of this study, ANA developed statements on functions, standards, and qualifications for professional nurses in 1959. Also during this time, clinical research began expanding as specialty groups, such as community health, psychiatric, medical-surgical, pediatrics, and obstetrics, developed standards of care. The research conducted by ANA and the specialty groups provided the basis for the nursing practice standards that currently guide professional nursing practice (Gortner & Nahm, 1977).

Educational studies were conducted in the 1950s and 1960s to determine the most effective educational preparation for the registered nurse. Montag developed and evaluated the 2-year nursing preparation (associate degree) in the junior colleges. Student characteristics, such as admission and retention patterns, and the elements that promoted success in nursing education, were also studied (Downs & Fleming, 1979).

In 1953, an Institute for Research and Service in Nursing Education was established at Teacher's College, Columbia University, which provided research learning experiences for doctoral students (Werley, 1977). The American Nurse's Foundation was chartered in 1955. This foundation's functions included receiving and administering research funds, conducting research programs, consulting with nursing students, and engaging in research. In 1956, a Committee on Research and Studies was established to guide ANA research (See, 1977).

A Department of Nursing Research in the Walter Reed Army Institute of Research was established in 1957. This was the first nursing unit in a research institution that emphasized conducting clinical nursing research (Werley, 1977).

Also in 1957, the Southern Regional Educational Board (SREB), Western Interstate Commission on Higher Education (WICHE), and the New England Board of Higher Education (NEBHE) were developed. These organizations are actively involved in promoting research and disseminating the findings. ANA sponsored the first of a series of research conferences in 1965, and the conference sponsors required that the studies presented be relevant to nursing and be conducted by a nurse researcher (See, 1977). These ANA conferences continue to be an important means for disseminating research findings today.

In the 1960s, an increasing number of clinical studies focused on quality care and the development of criteria to measure patient outcomes. Intensive care units were being developed, which promoted the investigation of nursing interventions, staffing patterns, and cost-effectiveness of care (Gortner & Nahm, 1977).

NURSING RESEARCH IN THE 1970s

In the 1970s, the groundwork for clinical research was laid, and it remains a priority today. O'Connell and Duffey (1976) reviewed the studies published in *Nursing Research* from 1970 to 1974 and noted that of the 275 studies published, 71 (26%) involved nursing practice. Forty-six percent of these nursing practice studies focused on monitoring techniques, such as temperature, pulse, and blood pressure; 25% dealt with physical treatment procedures; and 29% with psychological treatment procedures. Subjects in these studies were mainly adults (65%) and inpatients (77%).

The nursing process became the focus of many nursing studies, such as investigations of assessment techniques and guidelines, goal-setting methods, and specific nursing interventions. In 1973, the first Nursing Diagnosis Conference was held, and these conferences continue to be held every two years. Studies are being conducted to identify appropriate diagnoses and to generate an effective diagnostic process (Carlson-Catalano & Lunney, 1995).

The educational studies of the 1970s were concerned with the evaluation of teaching methods and student learning experiences. For example, Newman and O'Brien (1978) developed a computer program to provide nursing students with an opportunity to experience the research process through computer simulation. A number of studies have been conducted to differentiate the practice of the baccalaureate-prepared nurse and the associate degree nurse. These studies, which primarily measured abilities to perform technical skills, were ineffective in differentiating the two levels of education.

In the service setting, primary patient care was the trend of the 1970s; studies were conducted related to its implementation and outcomes. In addition, researchers continued to study quality assurance methods related to clinical practice. The number of nurse practitioners and clinical nurse specialists (both master's-prepared clinicians) increased rapidly during the 1970s. Limited research has been conducted on the clinical nurse specialist role; however, the nurse practitioner role has been researched extensively to determine its impact on productivity, quality, and cost of health care (Downs & Fleming, 1979). In addition, these master's-prepared clinicians were provided the background to conduct research and to use research findings in practice.

In the late 1960s and 1970s, nursing scholars began developing models, conceptual frameworks, and theories to guide nursing practice. These nursing theorists' works provided direction for future nursing research. In 1978, Chinn began publishing the journal *Advances in Nursing Science,* which includes the works of the nursing theorists and the research conducted on theories relevant to nursing.

The number of doctoral programs in nursing and the number of nurses prepared at the doctoral level (approximately 2,500) increased in the 1970s (Jacox, 1980). This has increased the conduct of studies and has facilitated more sophisticated research. However, many doctorally prepared nurses did not become actively involved in research. Another event influencing research in the 1970s was the establishment of the ANA Commission on Nursing Research. In 1972, the commission established the Council of Nurse Researchers to advance research activities, provide an exchange of ideas, and recognize excellence in research. The commission also prepared position papers on subjects' rights in research and on federal guidelines concerning research and human subjects, and sponsored research programs nationally and internationally (See, 1977). Federal funds for nursing research increased significantly, with a total of just over $39 million awarded for research in nursing from 1955 to 1976. Even though federal funding increased for nursing studies, the funding was not comparable to the $493 million in federal research funds received by medicine in 1974 alone (de Tornyay, 1977).

The dissemination of research findings was a major issue in the 1970s (Barnard, 1980). Sigma Theta Tau, the International Honor Society for Nursing, sponsored national and international research conferences; and the chapters of this organization sponsored many local conferences to promote the dissemination of research. *Image*, initially published in 1967 by Sigma Theta Tau, includes many articles concerning the research process and relevant nursing studies. A major goal of Sigma Theta Tau is the advancement of scholarship in nursing by promoting the conduct, communication, and utilization of research in nursing. The communication of research findings was also facilitated by the addition of two new research journals in the 1970s, *Research in Nursing & Health* in 1978, and *Western Journal of Nursing Research* in 1979.

NURSING RESEARCH IN THE 1980s

The conduct of clinical nursing research was the focus of the 1980s. A variety of clinical journals (*Cancer Nursing, Cardiovascular Nursing, Dimensions of Critical Care Nursing, Heart & Lung, Journal of Obstetric, Gynecologic, and Neonate Nursing, Journal of Neurosurgical Nursing, Pediatric Nursing,* and *Rehabilitation Nursing*) published an increasing number of studies. One new research journal was published in 1987, *Scholarly Inquiry for Nursing Practice,* and two in 1988, *Applied Nursing Research* and *Nursing Science*

Quarterly. Even though the body of empirical knowledge generated through clinical research increased rapidly in the 1980s, little of this knowledge was used in practice. During 1982 and 1983, the materials from a federally funded project, Conduct and Utilization of Research in Nursing (CURN), were published to facilitate the use of research to improve nursing practice (Horsley, Crane, Crabtree, & Wood, 1983). In 1983, the first volume of the *Annual Review of Nursing Research* was published (Werley & Fitzpatrick, 1983). These volumes include experts' reviews of research in selected areas of nursing practice, nursing care delivery, nursing education, and the profession of nursing. These summaries of current research knowledge encourage the use of research in practice and provide direction for future research.

Another priority of the 1980s was to obtain increased funding for nursing research. Most of the federal funds in the 1980s were designated for studies involving the diagnosis and cure of diseases. Therefore, nursing received a very small percentage of the federal research and development (R&D) funds (approximately 2–3%) compared with medicine (approximately 90%), even though nursing personnel greatly outnumber medical personnel (Larson, 1984). However, ANA accomplished a major political victory for nursing research with the creation of the National Center for Nursing Research (NCNR) in 1985. This center was created after years of work and two presidential vetoes (Bauknecht, 1986). The purpose of NCNR was "the conduct, support, and dissemination of information regarding basic and clinical nursing research, training and other programs in patient care research" (Bauknecht, 1985, p. 2). The NCNR was established under the National Institutes of Health (NIH) and provides visibility for nursing research at the federal level. The first center director, Ada Sue Hinshaw, Ph.D., R.N., initiated the identification of the following nursing research priorities: (1) HIV-positive clients, partners, and families; (2) prevention and care of low birth weight infants; (3) long-term care; (4) symptom management; (5) information systems; (6) health promo-

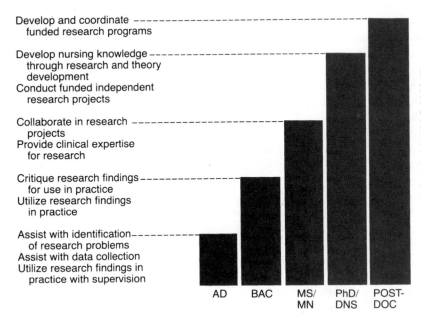

Develop and coordinate funded research programs

Develop nursing knowledge through research and theory development
Conduct funded independent research projects

Collaborate in research projects
Provide clinical expertise for research

Critique research findings for use in practice
Utilize research findings in practice

Assist with identification of research problems
Assist with data collection
Utilize research findings in practice with supervision

AD   BAC   MS/MN   PhD/DNS   POST-DOC

Figure 2–1
Research participation at various levels of education preparation. (Adapted from Maxine E. Loomis, Ph.D., R.N., C.S., F.A.A.N., unpublished work, 1989, by American Nurses Association [1989]. *Education for participation in nursing research.* Kansas City, MO: American Nurses Association, with permission.)

tion; and (7) technology dependency across the lifespan (Bloch, 1990).

In the 1980s, many nurses obtained master's and doctoral degrees, and postdoctoral education was encouraged for nurse researchers. The ANA Cabinet on Nursing Research identified the research participation for various levels of educational preparation. As indicated in Figure 2–1, nurses at all levels of education have a role in research (ANA, 1989). Through their educational preparation, the associate degree nurse is encouraged to assist with problem identification and data collection, the baccalaureate-prepared nurse to use research findings in practice, the master's-prepared nurse to collaborate in research projects, and the doctoral-prepared nurse to conduct independent, funded research projects (ANA, 1989; Davis & Burnard, 1992). The researcher's role expands with advanced education, and the maximal preparation of postdoctoral education provides a background for the development and coordination of funded research programs. Nursing research became a powerful force in the 1980s, and a strong base was developed to promote research productivity in the 1990s.

NURSING RESEARCH FOR THE 1990s

Under the direction of Dr. Hinshaw, the NCNR became the National Institute of Nursing Research (NINR) in 1993. This change in title increases the recognition of nursing as a research discipline and will hopefully increase the funding for nursing research. NINR has selected five research priorities that will guide funding for 1995 through 1999. These priorities include: community-based nursing models, effectiveness of nursing interventions in HIV/AIDS, cognitive impairment, living with chronic illness, and biobehavioral factors related to immunocompetence (NINR, 1993).

Research focused on health promotion and illness prevention is also expanding in the 1990s as people move toward improving the quality and quantity of their lives. *Healthy People 2000,* published by the Department of Health and Human Services, has identified priorities for health promotion research. Currently, little research exists to document the effectiveness of many of the health promotion and illness prevention interventions.

Outcomes research is emerging as an important methodology for documenting the effectiveness of health care service in the 1990s. This effectiveness research has evolved from the quality assessment and quality assurance functions that originated with the professional standards review organizations (the PSROs) in 1972 and more recently the peer review organizations (PROs). In the 1980s, outcomes research was promoted by William Roper, who was then the director of the Health Care Finance Administration (HCFA), to determine the quality and cost-effectiveness of patient care. Through the initiatives of Roper, Wennberg, and others, the need to expand health service research focused on outcomes has received extensive attention. In 1989, the Agency for Health Care Policy and Research (AHCPR) was established to facilitate the conduct of outcomes research (Rettig, 1991). AHCPR also has an active role in communicating research findings to health care practitioners and was responsible for publishing the first clinical practice guidelines in 1989. Several of these guidelines have been published in the 1990s and include the latest research findings with directives for practice. Predominantly, the focus of outcomes research in the 1980s was patient health status and cost related to medical care. Patient outcomes research related to nursing care has received limited attention in the early 1990s and needs to become a major focus for future nursing studies (Bowers, 1994; Hegyvary, 1991; Higgins, McCaughan, Griffiths, & Carr-Hill, 1992; Jennings, 1991; J. E. Johnson, 1993; Jones, 1993).

BACKGROUND FOR THE RESEARCH PROCESS

Research is a process and is similar in some ways to other processes. Therefore, the background acquired early in nursing education in problem solving and the nursing process is also useful in research. A process includes a purpose, a series of actions, and a goal. The purpose provides direction to the process, and the series of actions are organized into steps to achieve the identified goal. A process is continuous and can be revised and reimplemented in order to reach an end point or goal. The steps of the problem-solving process, nursing process, and research process are presented in Table 2–2. Relating the research process

Table 2–2
Comparison of the Problem-Solving Process, Nursing Process, and Research Process

Problem-Solving Process	Nursing Process	Research Process
Data collection	Assessment Data collection Data interpretation	Knowledge of the world of nursing Clinical experience Literature review
Problem definition	Nursing diagnosis	Problem and purpose identification
Plan Goal setting Identify solutions	Plan Goal setting Planned interventions	Methodology Design Sample Methods of measurement
Implementation	Implementation	Data collection and analysis
Evaluate and revise process	Evaluation and modification	Outcomes and dissemination of findings

to problem solving and the nursing process can be helpful in assisting the beginning researcher to use familiar ways of thinking to facilitate the incorporation of new skills and knowledge.

COMPARISON OF THE PROBLEM-SOLVING PROCESS AND THE NURSING PROCESS

The *problem-solving process* is the systematic identification of a problem, determination of goals related to the problem, identification of possible approaches to achieve those goals, implementation of selected approaches, and evaluation of goal achievement. Problem solving is frequently used in daily activities and in nursing practice. For example, problem solving is used when selecting clothing, deciding where to live, and turning a patient with a fractured hip.

The *nursing process* is a subset of the problem-solving process. The steps of the nursing process are assessment, diagnosis, plan, implementation, evaluation, and modification. Assessment involves the collection and interpretation of data for the development of nursing diagnoses. These diagnoses guide the remaining steps of the nursing process, just as the step of defining the problem directs the remaining steps of the problem-solving process. The planning step in the nursing process is the same as in the problem-solving process. Both processes involve implementation, or putting the plan into action, and evaluation or determination of the effectiveness of the process. The problem-solving process and the nursing process are cyclic. If the process is not effective, all steps are reviewed and revised (modified), and the process is reimplemented.

COMPARISON OF THE NURSING PROCESS AND THE RESEARCH PROCESS

The nursing process and research process have important similarities and differences. The two processes are similar because they both involve abstract, critical thinking and complex reasoning. Using these processes, one is able to identify new information, discover relationships, and make predictions about phenomena. In these two processes, information is gathered, observations are made, problems are identified, plans are developed (methodology), and actions are taken (data collection and analysis) (Blumer, 1969; Whitney, 1986). Both processes are reviewed for effectiveness and efficiency—the nursing process is evaluated, and outcomes are determined in the research process (see Table 2–2). These processes are also iterative and spiraling, which means that implementing them expand and refine the user's knowledge. With this growth in knowledge, the user is able to implement increasingly complex nursing processes and studies. The steps of the nursing process, assessment, planning, implementation, and evaluation, could also be used to coordinate a multidisciplinary, collaborative research project. For example, one might assess who will be involved in the research team and what problem will be investigated, plan the details of the research project, implement the project, and evaluate the collaborative research effort (Martin, 1994). Thus, the organizing steps of the nursing process can be used to facilitate the conduct of collaborative research.

The research process and nursing process also have definite differences. Knowledge of the nursing process will not enable one to conduct the research process. The research process is more complex than the nursing process, requires an understanding of a unique language, and involves the rigorous application of a variety of research methods (Burns, 1989). The research process also has a broader focus than the nursing process. In the nursing process, the nurse focuses on a specific patient and family. In the research process, the nurse must be aware of and knowledgeable about the world of nursing in order to identify a phenomenon requiring investigation. This knowledge of the world of nursing is obtained from clinical experience and a review of the empirical, theoretical, and clinical literature.

The nursing process and research process also differ in purposes. The nursing process organizes and directs the care for a particular patient and family. The purpose of research is to refine and generate knowledge that can improve care for a variety of patients and families. The theoretical underpinnings of the research process are much stronger than those of the nursing process. All steps of the research process are logically linked together and are also linked to the theoretical foundations of the study (Burns, 1989). The conduct of research requires greater precision, rigor, and control than the implementation of the nursing process. The outcomes from research are frequently shared with a large number of nurses through presentations and publications, and these outcomes have the potential to create a lasting impact on nursing practice.

NURSING RESEARCH METHODOLOGIES

Scientific method incorporates all procedures that scientists have used, currently use, or may use in the future to pursue knowledge (Kaplan, 1964). This definition eliminates the idea that there is "the" scientific method or that there is only one way to conduct research (Munhall, 1982, 1983; Silva, 1977; Tinkle & Beaton, 1983). This broad definition of scientific method includes quantitative and qualitative research and a relatively new methodology used to generate knowledge for clinical practice called outcomes research.

INTRODUCTION TO QUANTITATIVE AND QUALITATIVE RESEARCH

Since 1930, many researchers have narrowly defined scientific method to include only quantitative research. This research method is based in the philosophy of logical empiricism or positivism (Norbeck, 1987; Scheffler, 1967). Therefore, scientific knowledge is generated through an application of logical principles and reasoning, where the researcher adopts a distant and noninteractive posture with the research subject to prevent bias

(Newman, 1992; Silva & Rothbart, 1984). *Quantitative research* is a formal, objective, systematic process in which numerical data are utilized to obtain information about the world. This research method is used to describe variables, examine relationships among variables, and determine cause-and-effect interactions between variables. Currently, the predominantly used method of scientific investigation in nursing is quantitative research. Some researchers believe that quantitative research provides a sounder knowledge base to guide nursing practice than does qualitative research (Norbeck, 1987).

Qualitative research is a systematic, interactive, subjective approach used to describe life experiences and give them meaning (Ford-Gilboe, Campbell, & Berman, 1995; Leininger, 1985; Munhall, 1989). Qualitative research is not a new idea in the social or behavioral sciences (Baumrind, 1980; Glaser & Strauss, 1967). However, nurses' interest in qualitative research is more recent, having begun in the late 1970s. This type of research is conducted to describe and promote understanding of such human experiences as pain, caring, powerlessness, and comfort. Since human emotions are difficult to quantify (assign a numerical value), qualitative research seems to be a more effective method of investigating these emotional responses than is quantitative research. In addition, qualitative research focuses on understanding the whole, which is consistent with the holistic philosophy of nursing (Baer, 1979; Ford-Gilboe et al., 1995; Ludemann, 1979; Munhall & Oiler, 1986).

COMPARISON OF QUANTITATIVE AND QUALITATIVE RESEARCH

Quantitative and qualitative research complement each other because they generate different kinds of knowledge that are useful in nursing practice. The problem area to be studied determines the type of research to conduct, and the researcher's knowledge of both types of research will promote accurate selection of the research process for the problem identified. Quantitative

Table 2-3
Quantitative and Qualitative Research Characteristics

Quantitative Research	Qualitative Research
Hard science	Soft science
Focus: usually concise	Focus: usually broad
Reductionistic	Holistic
Objective	Subjective
Reasoning: logistic, deductive	Reasoning: dialectic, inductive
Basis of knowing: cause-and-effect relationships	Basis of knowing: meaning, discovery
Tests theory	Develops theory
Control	Shared interpretation
Instruments	Communication and observation
Basic element of analysis: numbers	Basic element of analysis: words
Statistical analysis	Individual interpretation
Generalization	Uniqueness

and qualitative research methodologies have some similarities, since both require researcher expertise, involve rigor in implementation, and result in the generation of scientific knowledge for nursing practice. Some of the differences between the two methodologies are presented in Table 2–3.

Quantitative research is thought to produce a "hard" science that is based on rigor, objectivity, and control. The quantitative approach toward scientific inquiry emerged from a branch of philosophy called logical positivism, which operates on strict rules of logic, truth, laws, axioms, and predictions (Watson, 1981). Quantitative researchers hold the position that "truth" is absolute and that there is a single reality that one could define by careful measurement. In order to find truth, one must be completely objective, which means that values, feelings, and personal perceptions cannot enter into the measurement of reality. Quantitative researchers believe that all human behavior is objective, purposeful, and measurable. The researcher needs only to find or develop the "right" instrument or tool to measure the behavior. However, today many nurse researchers base their quantitative studies on more of a postpositivist philosophy. This philosophy evolved from positivism but focuses on the discovery of reality that is characterized by patterns and trends that can be used to describe, explain, and predict phenomena. With postpositivist philosophy, "truth can be discovered only imperfectly and in a probabilistic sense, in contrast to the positivist ideal of establishing cause-and-effect explanations of immutable facts" (Ford-Gilboe et al., 1995, p. 16). The postpositivist approach also rejects the idea of complete objectivity between the researcher and what is to be discovered but continues to emphasize the need to control environmental influences (Newman, 1992).

Qualitative research is an artistic, philosophical approach that is thought to produce more of a "soft" science than quantitative research. The primary concern some researchers have with qualitative research is that it lacks the objectivity and control that are essential to "hard" scientific research. Qualitative research evolved from the behavioral and social sciences as a method of understanding the unique, dynamic, holistic nature of human beings. The philosophical base of qualitative research is interpretive, humanistic, or naturalistic and is concerned with understanding the meaning of social interactions by those involved. Qualitative researchers believe that "truth" is both complex and dynamic and can be found only by studying persons as they interact with and in their sociohistorical settings (Ford-Gilboe et al., 1995; Newman, 1992).

The focus or perspective for quantitative research is usually concise and reductionistic. Reductionism involves breaking the whole into parts so that the parts can be examined. Quantitative researchers remain detached from the study and try not to influence the study with their values (objectivity). Researcher involvement in the study is thought to bias or sway the study toward the perceptions and values of the researcher, and biasing a study is considered poor scientific technique.

The focus of qualitative research is usually broad, and the intent of the research is to give meaning to the whole (holistic). The qualitative researcher has an active part in the study, and the findings from the study are influenced by the researcher's values and perceptions. Thus, this research approach is subjective, but the approach assumes that subjectivity is essential for the understanding of human experiences.

Quantitative research is conducted to describe, examine relationships, and determine causality among variables. Thus, this method is useful in testing theory, by testing the validity of relationships that compose the theory. Quantitative research incorporates logistic, deductive reasoning as the researcher examines particulars in order to make generalizations about the universe.

Qualitative research is conducted to generate knowledge concerned with meaning and discovery. Inductive and dialectic reasoning are predominant in these studies. For example, the qualitative researcher studies the whole person's response to pain; this is accomplished by examining premises about human pain and by determining the meaning that pain has for a particular person. Since qualitative research is concerned with meaning, the findings from these studies can be used to identify the relationships among the variables, and these relational statements are used in theory development.

Quantitative research requires control (see Table 2–3). The investigator uses control to identify and limit the problem to be researched and attempts to limit the effects of extraneous or outside variables that are not being studied. For example, one might study the effects of nutritional education on serum lipid levels (total serum cholesterol, low-density lipoprotein (LDL), and high-density lipoprotein (HDL). The researcher would control the educational program by manipulating the type of education provided, the teaching methods, the length of the program, the setting for the program, and the instructor. Other extraneous variables, such as subjects' age, history of cardiovascular disease, and exercise level could be controlled because they might affect the serum lipid levels. The intent of this control is to provide a more precise examination of the effects of nutritional education on serum lipid levels.

Quantitative research also requires the use of instruments or tools that will generate numerical data. Statistical analyses are conducted to reduce and organize data, determine significant relationships, and identify differences among groups. Control, instruments, and statistical analyses are used to render the research findings an accurate reflection of reality, so the study findings can be generalized. Generalization involves the application of trends or general tendencies (that are identified by studying a sample) to the population from which the research sample was drawn. For example, a controlled, quasi-experimental study indicated that nutrition education was effective in lowering the total serum cholesterol and LDL levels and raising the HDL level in a selected sample of a population. Therefore, the researcher generalizes that nutrition education is an effective treatment for positively changing the serum lipid values of "similar" individuals. Researchers must be cautious in making generalizations, since a sound generalization requires the support of many studies.

Qualitative researchers use structured and unstructured observation and communication as means of gathering data. The data include the shared interpretations of the researcher and the subjects, and no attempts are made to control the interaction. For example, the researcher and subjects might share their experiences of powerlessness in the health care delivery system. The data are subjective and incorporate the perceptions and beliefs of the researcher and the subjects (Eisner, 1981).

Qualitative data are in the form of words and are analyzed in terms of individual responses, descriptive summaries, or both. The researcher identifies categories for sorting and organizing the data (Miles & Huberman, 1994; Munhall & Oiler, 1986). The intent of the analysis is to organize the data into a meaningful, individualized interpretation or framework that describes the phenomenon studied. The findings from a qualitative study are unique to that study, and it is not the intent of the researcher to generalize the findings to a larger population. However, understanding the meaning of a phenomenon in a particular situation is useful for understanding similar phenomena in similar situations.

USE OF TRIANGULATION TO COMBINE QUANTITATIVE AND QUALITATIVE RESEARCH METHODOLOGIES

In the last few years, some nurse researchers have advocated the use of triangulation to study the complex, dynamic human health phenomena relevant to nursing science (Duffy, 1987; Mitchell, 1986; Morse, 1991; Porter, 1989; Sohier, 1988). The idea of triangulation is not new to social scientists and was first used by Campbell and Fiske in 1959. *Triangulation* is the use of multiple methods, usually quantitative and qualitative research, in the study of the same research problem (Denzin, 1989). "When a single research method is inadequate, triangulation is used to ensure that the most comprehensive approach is taken to solve a research problem" (Morse, 1991, p. 120). The problem investigated is usually complex, like the human ability to cope with chronic illness, and requires in-depth study from a variety of perspectives to capture reality. Triangulation is a complex method that usually requires a research team of quantitative and qualitative researchers to maintain the integrity of both methodologies. The philosophic basis and assumptions for both quantitative and qualitative research must be maintained when these methodologies are combined, if the findings are to be meaningful (Dootson, 1995; Kimchi, Polivka, & Stevenson, 1991). The design of triangulation research is discussed in Chapter 10.

TYPES OF QUANTITATIVE AND QUALITATIVE RESEARCH

Research methods can be classified in many different ways. The classification system for this text-

Table 2–4
Classification System for Nursing Research Methodologies

I. Types of Quantitative Research
  Descriptive research
  Correlational research
  Quasi-experimental research
  Experimental research
II. Types of Qualitative Research
  Phenomenological research
  Grounded theory research
  Ethnographic research
  Historical research
  Philosophical inquiry
    1. Foundational inquiry
    2. Philosophical analyses
    3. Ethical analyses
  Critical social theory methodology
III. Outcomes Research

book is presented in Table 2–4 and includes both quantitative and qualitative research methodologies. The quantitative research methods are classified into four categories: descriptive, correlational, quasi-experimental, and experimental. These types of research are discussed briefly in this section and are described in more detail in Chapter 3. The qualitative research methods included in this textbook are phenomenological, grounded theory, ethnographic, historical, philosophical inquiry, and critical social theory. These approaches are introduced in this section and are described in depth in Chapter 4.

Quantitative Research Methods

Descriptive Research

Descriptive research provides an accurate portrayal or account of characteristics of a particular individual, situation, or group (Selltiz, Wrightsman, & Cook, 1976). Descriptive studies are a means of discovering new meaning, describing what exists, determining the frequency with which something occurs, and categorizing information (Marriner, 1981). Descriptive studies are usually

conducted when li[ttle] ... phenomenon. In ... ... rs
often use in...
structured obser...
checklist), and qu...
nomenon studied. ...
knowledge base and ...
the conduct of correl...
and experimental studie...

Correlational Research

Correlational research invol...
investigation of relationships be...
two or more variables. If the relat...
the researcher determines the type...
negative) and the degree or strength o...
tionships. The primary intent of correlatio...
ies is to explain the nature of relationships, ...
determine cause-and-effect. However, correlational studies are the means for generating hypotheses to guide quasi-experimental and experimental
studies that do focus on examining cause-and-
effect interactions.

Quasi-Experimental Research

The purpose of *quasi-experimental research* is
to explain relationships, clarify why certain events
happened, or both (Cook & Campbell, 1979).
These studies are also a means of examining
causal relationships; thus, they are a basis for
prediction of phenomena. Quasi-experimental studies are less powerful than experimental studies
because of the lower level of control. Quasi-
experimental studies have insufficient control
when compared with experimental studies in at
least one of three areas: (1) manipulation of the
treatment variable, (2) manipulation of the setting,
or (3) selection of subjects. When studying human
behavior, especially in clinical areas, researchers
are frequently unable to manipulate or control certain variables. In clinical nursing studies, subjects
are frequently not randomly selected but are samples of convenience. Thus, nurse researchers conduct more quasi-experimental than experimental
studies.

Experimental Research

Experimental research is an objective, system-
... controlled investigation for the purpose of
... ing and controlling phenomena. The pur-
... his type of research is to examine causal-
... ger, 1986; Lawson, 1981). Experimental
... onsidered the most powerful quantita-
... because of the rigorous control of
... rimental studies have three main
...) a controlled manipulation of at
... ment variable (independent vari-
... some of the subjects in the study receive
... reatment (experimental group) and some do
not (control group), and (3) random selection of
subjects so that each individual has a probability
greater than zero.

Qualitative Research Methods

Phenomenological Research

Phenomenological research is an inductive,
descriptive approach, developed from phenomenological philosophy. The focus of phenomenological philosophy is to understand the response of the
whole human being, not just understanding specific parts or behaviors (Omery, 1983, 1987). The
aim of phenomenological research is to describe
an experience as it is lived by the person, such as
describing a person's experience of pain as it is
lived by that person (Munhall, 1989; Munhall &
Oiler, 1986; Oiler, 1982).

Grounded Theory Research

Grounded theory research is an inductive research technique initially described by Glaser and
Strauss (1967). This research approach is useful
in discovering what problems exist in a social
scene and the process persons use to handle them.
Grounded theory methodology emphasizes obser-

vation and the development of practice-based intuitive relationships between variables. The research process involves formulation, testing, and redevelopment of propositions until a theory evolves. The theory developed is "grounded" or has its roots in the data from which it was derived (Simms, 1981).

Ethnographic Research

Ethnographic research was developed by the discipline of anthropology for investigating cultures through an in-depth study of the members of the culture. This type of research attempts to tell the story of people's daily lives while describing the culture they are a part of. The ethnographic research process is the systematic collection, description, and analysis of data to develop a theory of cultural behavior. The researcher (ethnographer) actually lives in or becomes a part of the cultural setting in order to gather the data. Using ethnographic research, different cultures are described, compared, and contrasted to add to the understanding of the impact of culture on human behavior and health (Aamodt, 1982; Leininger, 1985).

Historical Research

Historical research is a narrative description or analysis of events that occurred in the remote or recent past. Data are obtained from records, artifacts, or verbal reports (Krampitz, 1981). Through historical research, past mistakes are examined to facilitate an understanding of and an effective response to present situations. In addition, this type of research has the potential to provide a foundation for and direct the future movements of the profession. Only a minimal amount of historical research has been conducted in nursing, with the majority of the studies focusing on past and current nursing leaders (Newton, 1965).

Philosophical Inquiry

Philosophical inquiry involves using intellectual analyses to clarify meanings, make values

manifest, identify ethics, and study the nature of knowledge (Ellis, 1983). The philosophical researcher considers an idea or issue from all perspectives by extensively exploring the literature, examining conceptual meaning, raising questions, proposing answers, and suggesting the implications of those answers. The research is guided by philosophical questions that have been posed. There are three categories of philosophical inquiry covered in this textbook: foundational inquiry, philosophical analyses, and ethical inquiry. *Foundational inquiries* involve the analyses of the structure of a science and the process of thinking about and valuing certain phenomena held in common by members of a scientific discipline. The purposes of *philosophical analyses* are to examine meaning and develop theories of meaning that are accomplished through concept analysis or linguistic analysis (Rodgers, 1989). *Ethical inquiry,* another type of philosophical inquiry, involves intellectual analysis of problems of ethics related to obligation, rights, duty, right and wrong, conscience, justice, choice, intention, and responsibility. Ethical inquiry is a means of striving for rational ends when others are involved.

Critical Social Theory

Critical social theory provides the basis for research that focuses on understanding how people communicate and how they develop symbolic meanings in a society. Many of the meanings occur in a world where certain facts of the society are taken for granted, not discussed and not disputed. The established political, social, and/or cultural orders are perceived as closed to change and are not questioned. The researcher attempts to "uncover the distortions and constraints that impede free, equal, and uncoerced participation in society" (Stevens, 1989, p. 58). Through research, power imbalances are exposed and people are empowered to make changes (Newman, 1992). Empowerment involves recognizing the contradictions in a situation, reflecting on the reality of the situation, moving to a state of action, and making changes in the situation to correct the contradictions or imbalances. Critical social theory provides a philosophical basis for multiple research methods to generate knowledge that might promote empowerment and political change (Ford-Gilboe et al., 1995). Thus, critical social scientists might use both quantitative and qualitative research or a combination of the two, triangulation, because the knowledge generated can be the most persuasive to policymakers and the public. Critical nursing science provides a "framework from which one may ask how social, political, economic, gender, and cultural factors interact to influence health or illness experiences" (Ford-Gilboe et al., 1995). Nurses need to be aware of constraints and power imbalances in society that effect such areas as access to care, care of the chronically ill, and pain management of the terminally ill. The patients' and families' health needs and the health care system developed to meet these needs are continuously influenced by the social system that surrounds them.

OUTCOMES RESEARCH

The spiraling cost of health care has generated many questions about the quality and effectiveness of health care services and the patient outcomes related to these services. Consumers want to know what services they are buying and if these services will improve their health. Health care policymakers want to know if the care is cost-effective and high-quality. These concerns have promoted the development of outcomes research. An outcome is the end-result of care or a measure of the change in health status of the patient (Higgins et al., 1992; Jones, 1993; Rettig, 1991). In the past, outcome measures have been negative, such as mortality, morbidity (iatrogenic complications), length of stay, infection rate, unscheduled readmission, unscheduled repeat surgery, and unnecessary hospital procedures. These outcomes are only short-term and intermediate results of care and are primarily focused on hospital services (Hegyvary, 1991; J. E. Johnson, 1993; Jones, 1993). In the future, outcomes research must include determina-

tion of short-term and long-term end-results of care and examination of negative and positive results of care across a variety of settings, such as hospitals, rehabilitation centers, clinics, and homes. Some of the positive patient outcomes include quality of life, improved health status, increased functional status, improved mobility, patient satisfaction, and return to work or normal activities. Jones (1993, p. 146) identified four areas that require examination through outcomes research.

1. Clinical—patient response to medical and nursing interventions.
2. Functional—maintenance or improvement of physical functioning.
3. Financial—outcomes achieved with most efficient use of resources.
4. Perceptual—patient's satisfaction with outcomes, care received, and providers.

Currently, the Joint Commission on Accreditation of Healthcare Organizations (Joint Commission) and the AHCPR are major forces in promoting the examination of patient outcomes. The Joint Commission is concerned with hospital analysis of outcomes. The AHCPR is "developing clinical practice guidelines and emphasizing research in three areas: medical effectiveness and patient outcomes, database development, and dissemination methods" (Jennings, 1991). Nurses have made contributions to the AHCPR program but the current major focus of this agency is medical care. Nurses need to take an active role in the conduct of outcomes research and participate in the multidisciplinary teams that are examining the outcomes of health care services. The conduct of quality outcomes research can influence (1) patient health status, (2) the delivery of practitioners' services, (3) the use of limited resources, (4) the development of public policy, and (5) purchaser demand (Davies, Doyle, Lansky, Rutt, Stevic, & Doyle, 1994). Key ideas related to outcomes research are addressed throughout the text and Chapter 21 contains a detailed discussion of this methodology.

■ SUMMARY

The focus of this chapter is the evolution of research in nursing. Reviewing the history of research in nursing enables one to better understand the current status and project the future of nursing research. Historical events also provide a basis for the methods of scientific inquiry that are used in developing the empirical or research knowledge base for nursing. Some people think that research is relatively new to nursing, but Florence Nightingale initiated nursing research more than 140 years ago. Nightingale's research enabled her to instigate attitude, organizational, and social change. However, following her work, little research was conducted in nursing until the 1950s.

During the 1950s and 1960s, research became a high priority with the support of such nursing leaders as Henderson and Abdellah. The number of nurses with doctorates and masters' degrees increased and the research process was introduced at the baccalaureate level. The number of research conferences held at the local and national levels increased and the first research journal, *Nursing Research,* was published. The studies conducted during these two decades focused on such topics as nursing education, standards for nursing practice, nurses' characteristics, staffing patterns, and quality of care.

Research activities advanced extensively during the 1970s and 1980s. The major focus was on the conduct of clinical research to improve nursing practice. Several new research journals were initiated, numerous research conferences were held, and the educational level and research background of nurses drastically improved. The National Center for Nursing Research (NCNR) was created in 1985 to fund nursing research activities. Nursing research became a powerful force in the 1980s, developing a strong base for research productivity in the 1990s.

In 1993, the NCNR was renamed the National Institute for Nursing Research (NINR) to increase the visibility of nursing as a research discipline and to promote increased funding for nursing research. The NINR developed research priorities for funding to the year 2000. The conduct of health promotion and illness prevention research is a major focus of the 1990s with the publication of *Healthy People 2000.* Outcomes research is also emerging as an important methodology for documenting the effectiveness of health care services. Predominantly, the focus of outcomes research in the 1980s was patient health status and costs related to medical care. Patient outcome studies related to nursing care received limited attention by nurses in the early 1990s and need to become a major focus for future nursing research.

Research is a process and is similar in some ways to other processes. Therefore, the background acquired early in nursing education in problem solving and the nursing process is also useful in research. A comparison of the problem-solving process, nursing process, and research process shows the similarities and differences in these processes and provides a basis for understanding the research process.

Scientific method incorporates all procedures that scientists have used, currently use, or may use in the future to pursue knowledge. Nursing research incorporates both quantitative and qualitative research and a new methodology, outcomes research. Quantitative research is an objective, systematic process of using numerical data to obtain information about the world. This research method is used to describe, examine relationships, and determine cause-and-effect interactions. Qualitative research is a systematic, subjective approach used to describe life experiences and give them meaning. Knowledge generated from qualitative research will provide meaning and

continued

continued

understanding of the specific, not the general; of values; and of life experiences.

Quantitative and qualitative research complement each other, because they generate different kinds of knowledge that are useful in nursing practice. A comparison of quantitative and qualitative research methods is presented to clarify the similarities and differences of these two methods. Some researchers advocate combining quantitative and qualitative research methods in the study of the same research problem. Combining research methods is called triangulation and is used to ensure that the most comprehensive approach is taken to solve a research problem. If the findings from triangulation research are to be meaningful, the philosophical basis and assumptions for both quantitative and qualitative research must be maintained when these methodologies are combined.

Research methods can be classified in many different ways. In this textbook, three methodologies were identified: quantitative research, qualitative research, and outcomes research. Quantitative research is classified into four types: descriptive, correlational, quasi-experimental, and experimental. Six types of qualitative research are included in this text.

phenomenological, grounded theory, ethnographic, historical, philosophic inquiry, and critical social theory. The third methodology, outcomes research, is relatively new in nursing.

The spiraling cost of health care has generated many questions about the quality and effectiveness of health care services and the patient outcomes related to these services. These concerns have promoted the development of outcomes research. Outcomes are the end-results of care or a measure of the change in health status of the patient. Outcomes research must include determination of short-term and long-term end-results of care and examination of negative and positive results of care across a variety of settings, such as hospitals, rehabilitation centers, clinics, and homes. The conduct of quality outcomes research can influence (1) patient health status, (2) the delivery of practitioners' services, (3) the use of limited resources, (4) the development of public policy, and (5) purchaser demand. Nurses need to take an active role in the conduct of outcomes research and participate in the multidisciplinary teams to examine the outcomes of health care services.

References

Aamodt, A. M. (1982). Examining ethnography for nurse researchers. *Western Journal of Nursing Research, 4*(2), 209–221.

Abdellah, F. G. (1972). Evolution of nursing as a profession. *International Nursing Review, 19*(3), 219–235.

American Nurses Association (ANA). (1989). *Education for participation in nursing research.* Kansas City, MO: American Nurses Association.

Baer, E. D. (1979). Philosophy provides the rationale for nursing's multiple research directions. *Image: Journal of Nursing Scholarship, 11*(3), 72–74.

Barnard, K. E. (1980). Knowledge for practice: Directions for the future. *Nursing Research, 29*(4), 208–212.

Bauknecht, V. L. (1985). Capital commentary: NIH bill passes, includes nursing research center. *American Nurse, 17*(10), 2.

Bauknecht, V. L. (1986). Congress overrides veto, nursing gets center for research. *American Nurse, 18*(1), 24.

Baumrind, D. (1980). New directions in socialization research. *American Psychologist, 35*(7), 639–652.

Bloch, D. (1990). Strategies for setting and implementing the National Center for Nursing Research priorities. *Applied Nursing Research, 3*(2), 2–6.

Blumer, H. (1969). *Symbolic interactionism: Perspective and method.* Englewood Cliffs, NJ: Prentice-Hall, Inc.

Bowers, F. L. (1994). Research: Outcomes must be the focus. *Reflections, 20*(4), 4.

Burns, N. (1989). The research process and the nursing process: Distinctly different. *Nursing Science Quarterly, 2*(4), 157–158.

Carlson-Catalano, J., & Lunney, M. (1995). Quantitative methods for clinical validation of nursing diagnoses. *Clinical Nurse Specialist, 9*(6), 306–311.

Cook, Sir E. (1913). *The life of Florence Nightingale* (Vol. 1). London: Macmillan.

Cook, T. D., & Campbell, D. T. (1979). *Quasi-experimentation: Design and analysis issues for field settings.* Chicago: Rand McNally.

Davies, A. R., Doyle, M. A. T., Lansky, D., Rutt, W., Stevic, M. O., & Doyle, J. B. (1994). Outcomes assessment in clinical settings: A consensus statement on principles and best practices in project management. *The Joint Commission Journal of Quality Improvement, 20*(1), 6–16.

Davis, B. D., & Burnard, P. (1992). Academic levels in nursing. *Journal of Advanced Nursing, 17*(12), 1395–1400.

Denzin, N. K. (1989). *The research act* (3rd ed.). New York: McGraw-Hill.

de Tornyay, R. (1977). Nursing research—The road ahead. *Nursing Research, 26*(6), 404–407.

Downs, F. S., & Fleming, W. J. (1979). *Issues in nursing research.* New York: Appleton-Century-Crofts.

Dootson, S. (1995). An in-depth study of triangulation. *Journal of Advanced Nursing, 22*(1), 183–187.

Duffy, M. E. (1987). Methodological triangulation: A vehicle for merging quantitative and qualitative research methods. *Image: Journal of Nursing Scholarship, 19*(3), 130–133.

Eisner, E. W. (1981). On the differences between scientific and artistic approaches to qualitative research. *Educational Researcher, 10*(4), 5–9.

Ellis, R. (1983). Philosophic inquiry. In H. H. Werley & J. J. Fitzpatrick (Eds.). *Annual review of nursing research* (Vol. 1, pp. 211–228). New York: Springer.

Fitzpatrick, M. L. (1978). *Historical studies in nursing.* New York: Teachers College Press.

Ford-Gilboe, M., Campbell, J., & Berman, H. (1995). Stories and numbers: Coexistence without compromise. *Advances in Nursing Science, 18*(1), 14–26.

Glaser, B. G., & Strauss, A. L. (1967). *The discovery of grounded theory: Strategies for qualitative research.* Chicago: Aldine.

Gortner, S. R., & Nahm, H. (1977). An overview of nursing research in the United States. *Nursing Research, 26*(1), 10–33.

Herbert, R. G. (1981). *Florence Nightingale: Saint, reformer or rebel?* Malabar, FL: Robert E. Krieger.

Hegyvary, S. T. (1991). Issues in outcomes research. *Journal of Nursing Quality Assurance, 5*(2), 1–6.

Higgins, M., McCaughan, D., Griffiths, M., & Carr-Hill, R. (1992). Assessing the outcomes of nursing care. *Journal of Advanced Nursing, 17*(5), 561–568.

Horsley, J. A., Crane, J., Crabtree, M. K., & Wood, D. J. (1983). *Using research to improve nursing practice: A guide; CURN Project.* New York: Grune & Stratton.

Jacox, A. (1980). Strategies to promote nursing research. *Nursing Research, 29*(4), 213–218.

Jennings, B. M. (1991). Patient outcomes research: Seizing the opportunity. *Advances in Nursing Science, 14*(2), 59–72.

Johnson, J. E. (1993). Outcomes research and health care reform: Opportunities for nurses. *Nursing Connections, 6*(4), 1–3.

Johnson, W. L. (1977). Research programs of the National League for Nursing. *Nursing Research, 26*(3), 172–176.

Jones, K. R. (1993). Outcomes analysis: Methods and issues. *Nursing Economics, 11*(3), 145–152.

Kaplan, A. (1964). *The conduct of inquiry: Methodology for behavioral science.* New York: Chandler.

Kerlinger, F. N. (1986). *Foundations of behavioral research* (3rd ed.). New York: Holt, Rinehart, and Winston.

Kimchi, J., Polivka, B., & Stevenson, J. S. (1991). Triangulation: Operational definitions. *Nursing Research, 40*(6), 364–366.

Krampitz, S. D. (1981). Research design: Historical. In S. D. Krampitz & N. Pavlovich (Eds.), *Readings for nursing research* (pp. 54–58). St. Louis: Mosby.

Larson, E. (1984). Health policy and NIH: Implications for nursing research. *Nursing Research, 33*(6), 352–356.

Lawson, L. (1981). Research design: Experimental. In S. D. Krampitz & N. Pavlovich (Eds.), *Readings for nursing research* (pp. 67–74). St. Louis: Mosby.

Leininger, M. M. (1985). *Qualitative research methods in nursing.* Orlando, FL: Grune & Stratton.

Ludemann, R. (1979). The paradoxical nature of nursing research. *Image: Journal of Nursing Scholarship, 11*(1), 2–8.

Marriner, A. (1981). Research design: Survey/descriptive. In S. D. Krampitz & N. Pavlovich (Eds.), *Readings for nursing research* (pp. 59–66). St. Louis: Mosby.

Martin, K. M. (1994). Coordinating multidisciplinary, collaborative research: A formula for success. *Clinical Nurse Specialist, 8*(1), 18–22.

Miles, M. B., & Huberman, A. M. (1994). *Qualitative data analysis: A sourcebook of new methods* (2nd ed.). Beverly Hills, CA: Sage.

Mitchell, E. S. (1986). Multiple triangulation: A methodology for nursing science. *Advances in Nursing Science, 8*(3), 18–26.

Morse, J. M. (1991). Approaches to qualitative-quantitative methodological triangulation. *Nursing Research, 40*(1), 120–123.

Munhall, P. L. (1982). Nursing philosophy and nursing research: In apposition or opposition? *Nursing Research, 31*(3), 176–177, 181.

Munhall, P. L. (1983). Methodologic fallacies: A critical self-appraisal. *Advances in Nursing Science, 5*(4), 41–49.

Munhall, P. L. (1989). Philosophical ponderings on qualitative research methods in nursing. *Nursing Science Quarterly, 2*(1), 20–28.

Munhall, P. L., & Oiler, C. J. (1986). *Nursing research: A qualitative perspective.* Norwalk, CT: Appleton-Century-Crofts.

National Institute of Nursing Research (September 23, 1993). *National nursing research agenda: Setting nursing research priorities.* Bethesda, MD: National Institutes of Health.

Newman, M. A. (1992). Prevailing paradigms in nursing. *Nursing Outlook, 40*(1), 10–13, 32.

Newman, M. A., & O'Brien, R. A. (1978). Experiencing the research process via computer simulation. *Image: Journal of Nursing Scholarship, 10*(1), 5–9.

Newton, M. E. (1965). The case for historical research. *Nursing Research, 14*(1), 20–26.

Nightingale, F. (1859). *Notes on Nursing: What it is, and what it is not.* Philadelphia: Lippincott.

Norbeck, J. S. (1987). In defense of empiricism. *Image: Journal of Nursing Scholarship, 19*(1), 28–30.

O'Connell, K. A., & Duffey, M. (1976). Research in nursing practice: Its nature and direction. *Image: Journal of Nursing Scholarship, 8*(1), 6–12.

Oiler, C. (1982). The phenomenological approach in nursing research. *Nursing Research, 31*(3), 178–181.

Omery, A. (1983). Phenomenology: A method for nursing research. *Advances in Nursing Science, 5*(2), 49–63.

Omery, A. (1987). Qualitative research designs in the critical care setting: Review and application. *Heart & Lung, 16*(4), 432–436.

Palmer, I. S. (1977). Florence Nightingale: Reformer, reactionary, researcher. *Nursing Research, 26*(2), 84–89.

Porter, E. J. (1989). The qualitative-quantitative dualism. *Image: Journal of Nursing Scholarship, 21*(2), 98–102.

Rettig, R. (1991). History, development, and importance to nursing of outcomes research. *Journal of Nursing Quality Assurance, 5*(2), 13–17.

Rodgers, B. L. (1989). Concepts, analysis and the development of nursing knowledge: The evolutionary cycle. *Journal of Advanced Nursing, 14*(4), 330–335.

Scheffler, I. (1967). *Science and subjectivity.* Indianapolis: Bobbs-Merrill.

See, E. M. (1977). The ANA and research in nursing. *Nursing Research, 26*(3), 165–171.

Selltiz, C., Wrightsman, L. S., & Cook, S. W. (1976). *Research methods in social relations* (3rd ed.). New York: Holt, Rinehart, and Winston.

Silva, M. C. (1977). Philosophy, science, theory: Interrelationships and implications for nursing research. *Image: Journal of Nursing Scholarship, 9*(3), 59–63.

Silva, M. C., & Rothbart, D. (1984). An analysis of changing trends in philosophies of science on nursing theory development and testing. *Advances in Nursing Science, 6*(2), 1–13.

Simms, L. M. (1981). The grounded theory approach in nursing research. *Nursing Research, 30*(6), 356–359.

Sohier, R. (1988). Multiple triangulation and contemporary nursing research. *Western Journal of Nursing Research, 10*(6), 732–742.

Stevens, P. E. (1989). A critical social reconceptualization of environment in nursing: Implications for methodology. *Advances in Nursing Science, 11*(4), 56–68.

Tinkle, M. B., & Beaton, J. L. (1983). Toward a new view of science: Implications for nursing research. *Advances in Nursing Science, 5*(2), 27–36.

Watson, J. (1981). Nursing's scientific quest. *Nursing Outlook, 29*(7), 413–416.

Werley, H. H. (1977). Nursing research in perspective. *International Nursing Review, 24*(3), 75–83.

Werley, H. H., & Fitzpatrick, J. J. (1983). *Annual review of nursing research* (Vol. 1). New York: Springer.

Whitney, F. W. (1986). Turning clinical problems into research. *Heart & Lung, 15*(1), 57–59.

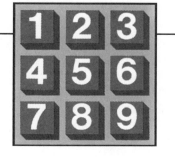

3

Introduction to Quantitative Research

What do you think of when you hear the word *research?* Frequently the word *experiment* comes to mind. One might equate experiments with randomizing subjects into groups, collecting data, and conducting statistical analyses. Frequently, one thinks that an experiment is conducted to "prove" something, such as proving that one pain medicine is more effective than another. These common notions are associated with the classic experimental design originated by Sir Ronald Fisher (1935). Fisher is noted for adding structure to the steps of the research process with such ideas as the null hypothesis, research design, and statistical analysis.

Fisher's experimentation provided the groundwork for what is now known as experimental research. Throughout the years, a number of other quantitative approaches have been developed. Campbell and Stanley (1963) developed quasi-experimental approaches. Karl Pearson developed statistical approaches for examining relationships between variables, which increased the conduct of correlational research. The fields of sociology, education, and psychology are noted for their development and expansion of strategies for conducting descriptive research. The steps of the research process used in these different types of quantitative studies are the same, but the philosophy and strategies for implementing these steps vary with the approaches.

A broad range of quantitative research approaches is needed to develop nursing's body of knowledge. Thus, quantitative research is a major focus throughout this textbook. This chapter pro-

vides an overview of quantitative research by (1) discussing concepts relevant to quantitative research, (2) identifying the steps of the quantitative research process, and (3) providing examples of different types of quantitative studies.

CONCEPTS RELEVANT TO QUANTITATIVE RESEARCH

Some concepts relevant to quantitative research include basic and applied research, rigor, and control. These concepts are defined and major points are reinforced with examples from quantitative studies.

BASIC RESEARCH

Basic, or pure, *research* is a scientific investigation that involves the pursuit of "knowledge for knowledge's sake" or for the pleasure of learning and finding truth (Nagel, 1961). The purpose of basic research is to generate and refine theory and build constructs; thus, the findings are frequently not directly useful in practice. However, since the findings are abstract (theoretical in nature), they can be generalized to various settings (Wysocki, 1983). Basic research is also conducted to examine the underlying mechanisms of actions of an intervention (Wallenstein, 1987). For example, what are the mechanisms of tumor-induced anorexia and what is its role in the nutritional decline of cancer patients? Are oral supplements with high calorie/high protein content effective in treating anorexia and promoting body weight gain in cancer patients? (Fridriksdottir & McCarthy, 1995). Bond and Heitkemper (1987) stressed the importance of basic nursing research on physiological variables that might involve investigations in laboratory settings on animals or humans. Studies might focus on "oxygenation, perfusion, fluid and electrolyte balance, acid-base status, eating and sleeping patterns, and comfort status, as well as pathophysiology" (p. 347).

Fridriksdottir and McCarthy (1995, p. 357) conducted basic research using "an animal model of tumor-induced anorexia to evaluate the effect of feeding a high caloric diet on food and caloric intake and body weight of tumor-bearing rats." The authors found that the tumor-bearing rats fed a 24% fat diet gradually reduced their food consumption until it was similar to the animals fed a 5% fat diet. These results indicate that the energy intake of tumor-bearing rats is similar to healthy animals. Thus, the high caloric diet intervention did not affect the tumor-bearing rats' body weight or tumor growth. "These data have implications for further study of the effects of nutritional supplements on food intake and nutritional status of cancer patients" (Fridriksdottir & McCarthy, 1995, p. 357). Basic research usually precedes or provides the basis for applied research. Thus, this basic research provides a basis for the conduct of applied studies to examine the effects of different nutritional interventions on the weight loss and anorexia of cancer patients. In this animal study, only increasing calories is an ineffective intervention to prevent weight loss in rats with cancer.

APPLIED RESEARCH

Applied, or practical, *research* is a scientific investigation conducted to generate knowledge that will directly influence or improve clinical practice. The purpose of applied research is to solve problems, make decisions, or predict or control outcomes in real-life practice situations (Abdellah & Levine, 1979). Since applied research focuses on specific problems, the findings are less generalizable than those from basic research. Applied research is also used to test theory and validate its usefulness in clinical practice. Often the new knowledge discovered through basic research is examined for usefulness in practice by applied research, making these approaches complementary (Wallenstein, 1987; Wysocki, 1983).

MacVicar, Winningham, and Nickel (1989) conducted an applied study to determine the "effect of a 10-week aerobic interval-training cycle ergometer protocol on the functional capacity (VO_2Lmax) of 45 women receiving chemotherapy for treatment of Stage II breast cancer" (p. 348). The experimental (EX) subjects "completed a 10-week, 3 times/week exercise training program"; placebo (PL) subjects "participated in 10 weeks of nonaerobic stretching and flexibility exercises"; and the control (CO) subjects "maintained normal activities" (p. 348). The EX group's functional capacity was significantly improved from pre- to post-test and was significantly better when compared with that of the PL and CO groups. The findings from this study have the potential, with replication, to impact nursing practice by validating the effectiveness of exercise in improving the functional capacity of Stage II breast cancer patients on chemotherapy. More research is needed before the information from this study can be generalized to other types of exercise programs and to "patients diagnosed with different cancers, at more advanced stages of disease, and with other treatment modalities such as radiation therapy, and combination radiation/chemotherapy protocols" (MacVicar et al., 1989, p. 351). Further research is also needed to determine the relationship between functional capacity and self-care and physical independence. Individuals with a serious illness like cancer, who have a strong functional capacity, could have an improved ability to care for themselves and a feeling of physical independence.

Many of the studies conducted in nursing are applied because researchers have chosen to focus on clinical problems such as developing and testing the effectiveness of nursing interventions. In addition, most federal funding has been granted for applied research (Wysocki, 1983). Since the future of any profession rests on its research base, both basic and applied research are needed to develop nursing knowledge.

RIGOR IN QUANTITATIVE RESEARCH

Rigor is the striving for excellence in research and involves discipline, scrupulous adherence to detail, and strict accuracy. A rigorous quantitative researcher constantly strives for more precise measurement methods, representative samples, and tightly controlled designs. Characteristics valued in these researchers include critical examination of reasoning and attention to precision.

Logistic and deductive reasoning are essential to the development of quantitative research. The research process includes specific steps that are developed with meticulous detail and logically linked together. These steps are critically examined and re-examined for errors and weaknesses in such areas as design, treatment implementation, measurement, sampling, statistical analysis, and generalization. Reducing these errors and weaknesses is essential to ensure that the research findings are an accurate reflection of reality.

Another aspect of rigor is precision, which encompasses accuracy, detail, and order. Precision is evident in the concise statement of the research purpose, detailed development of the study design, and the formulation of explicit treatment protocols. But the most explicit use of precision is evident in the measurement or quantification of the study variables. Measurement involves objectively experiencing the real world through the senses: sight, hearing, touch, taste, and smell. The researcher continually searches for new and more precise ways to measure elements and events of the world.

CONTROL IN QUANTITATIVE RESEARCH

Control involves the imposing of "rules" by the researcher to decrease the possibility of error and thus increase the probability that the study's findings are an accurate reflection of reality. The rules used to achieve control are referred to as *design.* Through control, the researcher can reduce the influence or confounding effect of extraneous variables on the research variables. For example, if a study focused on the effect of relaxation therapy on perception of incisional pain, the extraneous variables, such as type of surgical incision and time, amount, and type of pain medicine administered following surgery, would have to be controlled to prevent their influence on the patient's perception of pain. Controlling extraneous variables enables the researcher to accurately identify relationships among the study variables and examine the effect(s) of one variable on another. Extraneous variables can be controlled by randomly selecting a certain type of subject, such as individuals who have never been hospitalized before or those with a certain medical diagnosis. The selection of subjects is controlled with sample criteria and sampling method. The setting can be changed to control such extraneous variables as temperature, noise, and interactions with other people. The data collection process could be sequenced to control such extraneous variables as fatigue or discomfort.

Quantitative research requires varying degrees of control, ranging from uncontrolled to highly controlled depending on the type of study (see Table 3–1). Descriptive studies are usually conducted without researcher control, since subjects are examined as they exist in their natural setting, such as home, work, or school. Experimental studies are highly controlled and often conducted on animals in laboratory settings to determine the underlying mechanisms for and effectiveness of a treatment. Some common areas where control might be enhanced in quantitative research include (1) subject selection (sampling), (2) research setting selection, (3) development and implementation of a treatment, and (4) subject's knowledge of the study.

Sampling

Sampling is a process of selecting subjects who are representative of the population being studied.

Table 3–1
Control in Quantitative Research

Type of Quantitative Research	Researcher Control	Sampling	Research Setting
Descriptive	Uncontrolled	Nonrandom/random	Natural setting/ partially controlled
Correlational	Uncontrolled/ partially controlled	Nonrandom/random	Natural setting/ partially controlled
Quasi-experimental	Partially controlled/ highly controlled	Nonrandom/random	Partially controlled
Experimental	Highly controlled	Random	Highly controlled/ laboratory

Random sampling usually provides a sample that is representative of a population, because each member of the population has a probability greater than zero of being selected for a study. In quantitative research, both random and nonrandom samples are used (see Table 3–1). Descriptive and correlational studies are usually conducted with a nonrandom or nonprobability sample, in which the subjects are selected based on convenience. Quasi-experimental studies incorporate either nonrandom or random sampling methods, but experimental studies usually have a random sample. The research problem and purpose, the study design, and the number and type of subjects needed all affect the selection of a sampling method. The concepts of sampling theory, such as population, representative sample, and sampling methods, are presented in Chapter 12.

Research Settings

There are three common settings for conducting research: natural, partially controlled, and highly controlled (see Table 3–1). *Natural settings,* or field settings, are uncontrolled, real-life situations (Abdellah & Levine, 1979). Conducting a study in a natural setting means that the researcher does not manipulate or change the environment for the study. For example, Carrieri, Kieckhefer, Janson-Bjerklie, and Souza (1991) conducted a study "to describe the sensation of dyspnea in a sample of

39 school-age children with asthma and to identify strategies used to cope with the symptom" (p. 81). Data were gathered through interviews with the children that were conducted in natural settings, the children's homes and an ambulatory clinic.

A *partially controlled setting* is an environment that is manipulated or modified in some way by the researcher. An increasing number of nursing studies are being conducted in partially controlled settings. Younger, Marsh, and Grap (1995, p. 294) studied the "relationships among participation in outpatient rehabilitation, health locus of control, and mastery of stress with coronary artery disease." This was a two-phase study with Phase I taking place in the hospital and Phase II in the rehabilitation center. Within the hospital, Younger et al. (1995) controlled the assessment of patient and family needs, provided appropriate teaching, and enrolled the patients in the rehabilitation program. However, the researchers did not control other aspects of the hospital environment, such as family support and different types of nursing care on the hospital units, that might have influenced the research variables, patients' decision to participate in rehabilitation, health locus of control, and mastery of stress. In Phase II, the participants were enrolled in a rehabilitation program that involved attending a 60-minute session three days a week in a rehabilitation center. The content and activities of these sessions were controlled but no attempt was made to control the interactions of the participants as they exercised together, which could have influenced the research variables.

Highly controlled settings are artificially constructed environments that are developed for the sole purpose of conducting research. Laboratories, research or experimental centers, and test units are highly controlled settings for conducting research. This type of setting reduces the influence of extraneous and environmental variables, which enables the researcher to examine accurately the effect of the independent variable on the dependent variable. Only a limited number of nursing studies are conducted in highly controlled settings; most are conducted in natural settings. Fridriksdottir and McCarthy (1995) conducted an experimental study in a laboratory setting using animals. The purpose of their study was to determine the effect of feeding a high caloric diet on food and caloric intake and body weight of tumor-bearing rats. These researchers implemented precise control of the selection of animals, maintenance of their environment, implementation of the treatment, and measurement of the dependent variables.

"Thirty-two male Buffalo rats weighing between 100 to 120 grams were housed individually and maintained on 12-hour light-dark cycle commencing at 6:00 a.m. . . . The animals were conditioned to the housing for 5 days before the start of the experiment and were treated at all times in a manner consistent with Department of Health, Education, and Welfare Guidelines for the Care and Use of Laboratory Animals. (p. 358)

The tumor-selected animals were lightly anesthetized with ether fumes and 1 cm tumor fragment was implanted subcutaneously between the scapula with a sterile trochar needle . . . The experimental period lasted 28 days. For the first 15 days, all animals were maintained on standard rodent diet containing 5% fat . . . The dishes were weighed each morning on a portable electric digital scale which was zeroed each time before weighing. After day 15 of tumor growth, one half of the tumor-bearing and one half of the healthy controls were switched to a diet containing 24% fat. . . . " (p. 359) ■

Development and Implementation of Study Interventions

Quasi-experimental and experimental studies are conducted to examine the effect of an independent variable or intervention on a dependent variable(s) or outcome(s). More intervention studies are being conducted in nursing to establish a scientific basis for the interventions used in practice. Controlling the development and implementation of a study intervention increases the validity of the study design and the credibility of the findings. A study intervention needs to be described in detail and a protocol developed to ensure that the intervention is executed in the same manner in each treatment session (Egan, Snyder, & Burns, 1992). A detailed discussion of the development and implementation of interventions in research is provided in Chapter 11. Johnson and Frank (1995, p. 42) examined the "effectiveness of a telephone intervention in reducing anxiety of families of patients in an intensive care unit." They provided the following description of their intervention.

"Within the experimental group, a designated family member received a telephone call twice daily to inform them of the status of the patient. The primary care nurse for the patient was designated to call the family at a prearranged time in the morning and evening. The nurse used a protocol checklist to provide the status report that included information about any new treatments, stability of vital signs, level of pain, test reports, or other changes in the patient's condition since the previous call. This checklist was then placed on the patient's chart." (p. 42) ■

Subjects' Knowledge of a Study

Subjects' knowledge of a study could influence their behavior and possibly alter the outcome of a study. This creates a threat to the validity or accuracy of the study design. An example of this type of threat to design validity is the Hawthorne effect, which was identified during the classic experiments at the Hawthorne plant of the Western Electric Company during the late 1920s and early 1930s. The employees at this plant exhibited a particular psychological response when they became research subjects. They changed their behavior simply because they were subjects in a study, not because of the research treatment. In these studies, the researcher manipulated the working conditions (altered the lighting, decreased work hours, changed payment, and increased rest periods) to examine the effects on worker productivity (Homans, 1965). The subjects in both the treatment group (work conditions were changed) and control group (no change in work conditions) increased their productivity. Even those subjects in a group where lighting was decreased showed an increase in productivity. The subjects seemed to change their behaviors (increase their productivity) just because they were part of a study.

A study's design validity can also be threatened when the subjects guess the outcome of a study and change their behavior to achieve this outcome (Cook & Campbell, 1979). This problem is called hypothesis guessing, when the subjects change their behavior based on what they think a researcher wants them to do and not based on exposure to a treatment. An example of hypothesis guessing is demonstrated with the following hypothesis: Patients receiving preoperative instruction on coughing and deep breathing (treatment group) have better results on pulmonary function tests on the first, second, and third postoperative days than patients not receiving this planned instruction (control group). If the patients in both the treatment and control groups know the study hypothesis, they might alter their coughing and deep breathing patterns based on this information and not because of the preoperative instruction.

A researcher must take precautions not to influence or bias subjects' responses. Subjects could be given a simple or vague explanation of a study that does not include the outcome expected from the treatment. Another strategy is to not inform the subjects as to whether they are in the treatment or the control group, provided this can be done without infringing upon their rights (Cook &

Campbell, 1979). At the end of the study, subjects would receive a complete description of the study and the findings. Subjects in the treatment and control groups might be selected from two different hospital units, so they do not have an opportunity to discuss their involvement in the study. These strategies increase researcher control in an attempt to reduce the effects of subjects' knowledge of the study on the study outcomes.

STEPS OF THE QUANTITATIVE RESEARCH PROCESS

The quantitative research process involves conceptualizing a research project, planning and implementing that project, and communicating the findings. Figure 3–1 identifies the steps of the

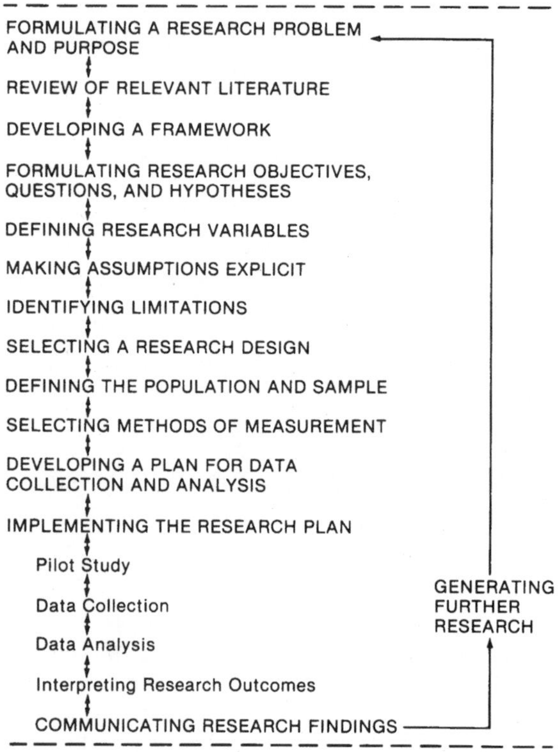

FORMULATING A RESEARCH PROBLEM AND PURPOSE

REVIEW OF RELEVANT LITERATURE

DEVELOPING A FRAMEWORK

FORMULATING RESEARCH OBJECTIVES, QUESTIONS, AND HYPOTHESES

DEFINING RESEARCH VARIABLES

MAKING ASSUMPTIONS EXPLICIT

IDENTIFYING LIMITATIONS

SELECTING A RESEARCH DESIGN

DEFINING THE POPULATION AND SAMPLE

SELECTING METHODS OF MEASUREMENT

DEVELOPING A PLAN FOR DATA COLLECTION AND ANALYSIS

IMPLEMENTING THE RESEARCH PLAN

  Pilot Study

  Data Collection

  Data Analysis

  Interpreting Research Outcomes

COMMUNICATING RESEARCH FINDINGS

GENERATING FURTHER RESEARCH

Figure 3–1

Steps of the quantitative research process.

quantitative research process and indicates the logical flow of this process as one step progressively builds upon another. This research process is also flexible and fluid, with a flow back and forth among the steps as the researcher strives to clarify the steps and strengthen the proposed study. This flow back and forth among the steps is indicated in the figure by the two-way arrows connecting the steps of the process. Figure 3–1 also contains a feedback arrow that indicates the research process is cyclic, for each study provides a basis for generating further research. The steps of the quantitative research process are briefly introduced in this chapter and presented in detail in Unit II, The Research Process (Chapters 5–23). The correlational study conducted by Hulme and Grove (1994) on the symptoms of female survivors of child sexual abuse is used as an example during the introduction of the steps of the research process.

FORMULATING A RESEARCH PROBLEM AND PURPOSE

A *research problem* is a "situation in need of a solution, improvement, or alteration" (Adebo, 1974, p. 53) or "a discrepancy between the way things are and the way they ought to be" (Diers, 1979, p. 12). The problem identifies an area of concern for a particular population and often indicates the concepts to be studied. The major sources for nursing research problems include nursing practice, researcher and peer interactions, literature review, theory, and research priorities. Using deductive reasoning, a research problem is generated from a research topic or a broad problem area of personal interest that is relevant to nursing.

The *research purpose* is generated from the problem and identifies the specific goal or aim of the study. The goal of a study might be to identify, describe, explain, or predict a solution to a situation. The purpose often indicates the type of study (descriptive, correlational, quasi-experimental, or experimental) to be conducted and includes the

variables, population, and setting for the study. As the research problem and purpose increase in clarity and conciseness, the researcher is able to determine the feasibility of conducting the study. Chapter 5 provides a background for formulating a research problem and purpose. Hulme and Grove (1994) identified the following problem and purpose for their study of female survivors of child sexual abuse.

Problem

"The actual prevalence of child sexual abuse is unknown but is thought to be high. Bagley and King (1990) were able to generalize from compiled research that at least 20% of all women in the samples surveyed had been victims of serious sexual abuse involving unwanted or coerced sexual contact up to the age of 17 years. Evidence indicates that the prevalence is greater for women born after 1960 than before (Bagley, 1990).

The impact of child sexual abuse on the lives of the girl victims and the women they become has only lately received the attention it deserves . . . the knowledge generated from research and theory has slowly forced the recognition of the long-term effects of child sexual abuse on both the survivors and society as a whole . . . Recently, Brown and Garrison (1990) developed the Adult Survivors of Incest (ASI) Questionnaire to identify the patterns of symptoms and the factors contributing to the severity of these symptoms in survivors of childhood sexual abuse. This tool requires additional testing to determine its usefulness in identifying symptoms and contributing factors of adult survivors of incest and other types of child sexual abuse." (pp. 519–520)

Purpose

"Thus, the purpose of this study was twofold: (a) to describe the patterns of physical and psychosocial symptoms in female sexual abuse survivors using the ASI Questionnaire, and (b) to examine relationships among the symptoms and identified contributing factors." (p. 520) ■

REVIEW OF RELEVANT LITERATURE

A *review of relevant literature* is conducted to generate a picture of what is known about a particular situation and the knowledge gaps that exist in the situation. Relevant literature refers to those sources that are pertinent or highly important in providing the in-depth knowledge needed to study a selected problem. This background enables the researcher to build upon the works of others. The concepts and interrelationships of the concepts in the problem guide the researcher in selecting relevant theories and studies for review. Theories are reviewed to clarify the definitions of concepts and to develop and refine the study framework. Reviewing relevant studies enables the researcher to clarify which problems have been investigated, which require further investigation or replication, and which have not been investigated. In addition, the literature review directs the researcher in designing the study and interpreting the outcomes. The process for reviewing relevant literature is described in Chapter 6. Hulme and Grove's (1994) review of the literature covered relevant theories and studies related to child sexual abuse and its contributing factors and long-term effects.

■

"Theorists indicated that . . . the act of child sexual abuse can be explained as an abuse of power by a trusted parent figure, usually male, on a dependent child, violating the child's body, mind, and spirit. The family, which normally functions to nurture and protect the child from harm, is viewed as not fulfilling this function, leaving the child to feel further betrayed and powerless. Acceptance of the immediate psychological trauma of child sexual abuse has given impetus for acknowledging the long-term effects.

Studies of both nonclinical and clinical populations have lent support to these theoretical developments. When compared with control groups consisting of women who had not been sexually abused as children, survivors of child sexual abuse consistently have higher incidence of depression and lower self-esteem. Other psycho-social long-term effects encountered include suicidal plans, anxiety, distorted body image, decreased sexual satisfaction, poor general social adjustment, lower positive affect, negative personality characteristics, and feeling different from significant others . . . The physical long-term effects suggested by research include gastrointestinal problems such as ulcers, spastic colitis, irritable bowel syndrome, and chronic abdominal pain; gynecological disorders; chronic headache; obesity; and increased lifetime surgeries." (p. 521)

"Studies of contributing factors that may affect the traumatic impact of child sexual abuse are less in number and less conclusive than those that identify long-term effects. However, poor family functioning, increased age difference between the victim and perpetrator, threat or use of force or violence, multiple abusers, parent or primary caretaker as perpetrator, prolonged or intrusive abuse, and strong emotional bond to the perpetrator with betrayal of trust may all contribute to the increased severity of the long-term effects." (pp. 521–522) ■

DEVELOPING A FRAMEWORK

A *framework* is the abstract, logical structure of meaning that guides the development of the study and enables the researcher to link the findings to nursing's body of knowledge. In quantitative research, the framework is a testable theory that has been developed in nursing or in another discipline, such as psychology, physiology, or sociology. The framework may also be developed inductively from clinical observations. The terms related to frameworks are concept, relational statement, theory, and framework map. A concept is a term to which abstract meaning is attached. A relational statement declares that a relationship of some kind exists between two or more concepts. A theory consists of an integrated set of defined concepts and relational statements that presents a view of a phenomenon and can be used to describe, explain, predict, or control the phenomenon. The statements of the theory, not the theory itself, are tested through research. A study framework can be expressed as a map or a diagram of the relationships

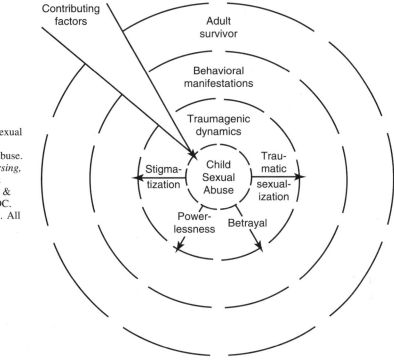

Figure 3–2
Long-term effects of child sexual abuse. (From Symptoms of female survivors of sexual abuse. *Issues in Mental Health Nursing*, *15*[5], 123. Hulme, P. A., & Grove, S. K. [1994]. Taylor & Francis, Inc., Washington, DC. Reproduced with permission. All rights reserved.)

that provide the basis for a study or can be presented in narrative format. The steps for developing a framework are described in Chapter 7. The framework for Hulme and Grove's (1994) study is based on Browne and Finkelhor's (1986) theory of traumagenic dynamics in the impact of child sexual abuse and is expressed in a map.

Framework

"As shown in Figure 3–2, child sexual abuse is at the center of the adult survivor's existence. Arising from the abuse are four trauma-causing dynamics: traumatic sexualization, betrayal, powerlessness, and stigmatization. These traumagenic dynamics lead to behavioral manifestations and collectively indicate a history of child sexual abuse. The behavioral manifestations were operationalized as physical and psychosocial symptoms for the purposes of this study. Piercing the adult survivor are the contributing factors, which are characteristics of the child sexual abuse or

other factors occurring later in the survivor's life, that affect the severity of behavioral manifestations (Follette, Alexander, & Follette, 1991). The contributing factors examined in this study were age when the abuse began, duration of the abuse, and other victimizations. Other victimizations included past or present physical and emotional abuse, rape, control by others, and prostitution." (pp. 522–523) ■

FORMULATING RESEARCH OBJECTIVES, QUESTIONS, AND HYPOTHESES

Research objectives, questions, or hypotheses are formulated to bridge the gap between the more abstractly stated research problem and purpose, and the study design and plan for data collection and analysis. Objectives, questions, and hypotheses are more narrow in focus than the purpose and often specify only one or two research variables, identify the relationship between the variables, and indicate the population to be studied. Some studies do not include objectives, questions, or hypotheses and the development of the study is directed by the research purpose. Many descriptive studies include only a research purpose, and other descriptive studies include a purpose and objectives or questions. Some correlational studies include a purpose and specific questions or hypotheses. Quasi-experimental and experimental studies often use hypotheses to direct the development and implementation of the studies and the interpretation of findings. The development of research objectives, questions, and hypotheses is discussed in Chapter 8. Hulme and Grove (1994) developed the following research questions to direct their study.

Research Questions

1. "What patterns of physical and psychosocial symptoms are present in women 18 to 40 years of age who have experienced child sexual abuse?
2. Are there relationships among the number of physical and psychosocial symptoms, the age when the abuse began, the duration of abuse, and number of other victimizations?" (p. 523) ■

DEFINING RESEARCH VARIABLES

The research purpose and the objectives, questions, or hypotheses identify the variables to be examined in a study. Research *variables* are concepts of various levels of abstraction that are measured, manipulated, or controlled in a study. The more concrete concepts like temperature, weight, or blood pressure are referred to as variables in a study. The more abstract concepts like creativity, empathy, or social support are sometimes referred to as research concepts.

The variables or concepts in a study are operationalized by identifying conceptual and operational definitions. A *conceptual definition* provides a variable or concept with theoretical meaning (Fawcett & Downs, 1986) and is derived from a

theorist's definition of the concept or is developed through concept analysis. An *operational definition* is developed so the variable can be measured or manipulated in a study. The knowledge gained from studying the variable will increase understanding of the theoretical concept the variable represents. A more extensive discussion of variables is provided in Chapter 8. Hulme and Grove (1994) provided conceptual and operational definitions of the study variables, physical and psychosocial symptoms, age abuse began, duration of abuse, and victimizations, identified in their purpose and research questions. Only the definitions for physical symptoms and victimizations are presented as examples.

Physical Symptoms

Conceptual Definition. "Behavioral manifestations that result directly from the traumagenic dynamics of child sexual abuse." (p. 522)
Operational Definition. ASI Questionnaire was used to measure physical symptoms.

Victimizations

Conceptual Definition. Adult survivor who has experienced multiple forms of abuse, including "past and present physical and emotional abuse, rape, control by others, and prostitution." (p. 523)
Operational Definition. ASI Questionnaire was used to measure victimizations. ■

MAKING ASSUMPTIONS EXPLICIT

Assumptions are statements that are taken for granted or are considered true, even though these statements have not been scientifically tested (Silva, 1981). Assumptions are often embedded (unrecognized) in thinking and behavior, and uncovering these assumptions requires introspection. Sources of assumptions are universally accepted truths (all humans are rational beings), theories, previous research, and nursing practice (Myers, 1982).

In studies, assumptions are embedded in the

philosophical base of the framework, study design, and interpretation of findings. Theories and instruments are developed based on assumptions that may or may not be recognized by the researcher. These assumptions influence the development and implementation of the research process. The recognition of assumptions by the researcher is a strength, not a weakness. Assumptions influence the logic of the study, and their recognition leads to more rigorous study development.

Williams (1980) reviewed published nursing studies and other health care literature to identify 13 commonly embedded assumptions:

1. People want to assume control of their own health problems.
2. Stress should be avoided.
3. People are aware of the experiences that most affect their life choices.
4. Health is a priority for most people.
5. People in underserved areas feel underserved.
6. Most measurable attitudes are held strongly enough to direct behavior.
7. Health professionals view health care in a different manner than do lay persons.
8. Human biological and chemical factors show less variation than do cultural and social factors.
9. The nursing process is the best way of conceptualizing nursing practice.
10. Statistically significant differences relate to the variable or variables under consideration.
11. People operate on the basis of cognitive information.
12. Increased knowledge about an event lowers anxiety about the event.
13. Receipt of health care at home is preferable to receipt of care in an institution. (p. 48)

Hulme and Grove (1994) did not identify assumptions for their study but the following assumptions seem to provide a basis for this study: (1) the child victim bears no responsibility for the sexual contact, (2) a relatively large portion of the survivors remember and are willing to report their past child sexual abuse, and (3) behavioral manifestations are not indicative of optimal health and functioning.

IDENTIFYING LIMITATIONS

Limitations are restrictions in a study that may decrease the generalizability of the findings. The two types of limitations are theoretical and methodological. *Theoretical limitations* restrict the abstract generalization of the findings and are reflected in the study framework and the conceptual and operational definitions. Theoretical limitations might include the following: (1) a concept might not be clearly defined in the theory used to develop the study framework; (2) the relationships among some concepts might not be identified or are unclear in the theorist's work; (3) a study variable might not be clearly linked to a concept in the framework; or (4) an objective, question, or hypothesis might not be clearly linked to the study framework.

Methodological limitations can limit the credibility of the findings and restrict the population to which the findings can be generalized. Methodological limitations result from such factors as unrepresentative samples, weak designs, single setting, limited control over treatment implementation, instruments with limited reliability and validity, limited control over data collection, and improper use of statistical analyses. Limitations regarding sampling (see Chapter 12), design (see Chapter 10), measurement (see Chapter 13), and data collection (see Chapter 15) are discussed later in the text. Hulme and Grove (1994) identified the following methodological limitation.

■───────────────────────────

Methodological Limitation

"This study has limited generalizability due to the relatively small nonprobability sample. . . ." (p. 528)

"Additional replications drawing from various social classes and age groups are needed to improve the generalizability of Brown and Garrison's (1990) findings and establish reliability and validity of their tool." (p. 529) ■

SELECTING A RESEARCH DESIGN

Research *design* is a blueprint for the conduct of a study that maximizes control over factors that

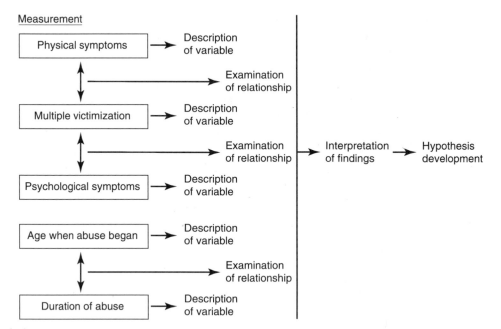

Figure 3–3
Proposed descriptive correlational design for Hulme and Grove (1994) study of symptoms of female survivors of child sexual abuse. (From Hulme, P. A., & Grove, S. K. [1994]. *Physical and Psychosocial Symptomatology of Female Survivors of Child Sexual Abuse,* 55. With permission.)

could interfere with the study's desired outcome. The type of design directs the selection of a population, sampling procedure, methods of measurement, and a plan for data collection and analysis. The choice of research design depends on the researcher's expertise, the problem and purpose for the study, and the desire to generalize the findings (Brophy, 1981).

Designs have been developed to meet unique research needs as they emerge; thus, a variety of descriptive, correlational, quasi-experimental, and experimental designs have been generated over time. In descriptive and correlational studies, no treatment is administered, so the focus of the study design is improving the precision of measurement. Quasi-experimental and experimental study designs usually involve treatment and control groups and focus on achieving high levels of control as well as precision in measurement. The purpose of a design and threats to design validity are covered in Chapter 10. Models and descriptions of several types of descriptive, correlational, quasi-experi-

mental, and experimental designs are presented in Chapter 11.

In the study by Hulme and Grove (1994), a descriptive correlational design was used to direct the conduct of the study. A diagram of the design is presented in Figure 3–3 and indicates the variables described and the relationships examined. The findings generated from correlational research provide a basis for generating hypotheses for testing in future research.

DEFINING THE POPULATION AND SAMPLE

The population is all elements (individuals, objects, or substances) that meet certain criteria for inclusion in a given universe (Kerlinger, 1986). A study might be conducted to describe patients' responses to their first hospitalization. The population could be defined in different ways and include all patients hospitalized for the first time in (1)

Hospital X on Unit Y, (2) all units in Hospital X, or (3) all hospitals in City Z. The definition of the population will depend on the sample criteria and the similarity of subjects in these various settings. The researcher must determine which population is accessible and can be best represented by the study sample.

A *sample* is a subset of the population that is selected for a particular study, and the members of a sample are the subjects. Sampling defines the process for selecting a group of people, events, behaviors, or other elements with which to conduct a study. A variety of probability and non-probability sampling methods are used in nursing studies. In probability sampling every member of the population has a probability greater than zero of being selected for the sample. With nonprobability sampling, not every member of the population has an opportunity for selection in the sample. Sampling theory and sampling methods are presented in Chapter 12. The following quote identifies the sampling method, setting, sample size, population, sample criteria, and sample characteristics for the study conducted by Hulme and Grove (1994).

■

Sample

"The convenience sample (sampling method) was obtained by advertising for subjects at three state universities in the southwest (setting). Despite the sensitive nature of the study, 22 (sample size) usable interviews were obtained. The sample included women between the ages of 18 and 39 years ($X = 28$ years, $SD = 6.5$ years) who were identified as survivors of child sexual abuse (population) (sample criteria). The majority of these women were white (91%) and students (82%). A little more than half (54%) were single, seven (32%) were divorced, and three (14%) were married. Most (64%) had no children. A small percentage (14%) were on some form of public assistance and only 14% had been arrested. Although 27% of the subjects had step family members, the parents of 14 subjects (64%) were still married. Half the fathers were work-

ing class or self-employed; the rest were professionals. Mothers were either working class or self-employed (50%), homemakers (27%), or professionals (11%). Most subjects (95%) had siblings, and 36% knew or suspected their siblings also had been abused (sample characteristics)." (pp. 523–524) ■

SELECTING METHODS OF MEASUREMENT

Measurement is the process of assigning "numbers to objects (or events or situations) in accord with some rule" (Kaplan, 1964, p. 177). A component of measurement is instrumentation, which is the application of specific rules to the development of a measurement device or instrument. An instrument is selected to examine a specific variable in a study. Data generated with an instrument are at the nominal, ordinal, interval, or ratio level of measurement. The level of measurement, with nominal being the lowest form of measurement and ratio being the highest, determines the type of statistical analyses that can be performed on the data.

Selection of an instrument requires extensive examination of its reliability and validity. Reliability is concerned with how consistently the measurement technique measures a concept. Validity of an instrument is the extent to which the instrument actually reflects the abstract concept being examined. Chapter 13 introduces the concepts of measurement and explains the different types of reliability and validity for instruments. Chapter 14 provides a background for selecting measurement methods for a study. Hulme and Grove (1994) used only the ASI Questionnaire to measure the study variables.

■

Measurement Method

"The ASI Questionnaire contains 10 sections: demographics; family origin; educational history, occupational history and public assistance; legal history; characteristics of the child sexual abuse (duration, perpetrator, pregnancy, type, and threats); past and present other victimizations; past and present physical symptoms; past and present psychosocial symptoms; and relationship with own children. Each section is followed by a response set that includes space for 'other.' Content validity was established by Brown and Garrison (1990) using an in-depth review of 132 clinical records . . . For this descriptive correlational study . . . content validity of the tool was examined by asking an open-ended question: Is there additional information you would like to share?" (p. 524) ■

DEVELOPING A PLAN FOR DATA COLLECTION AND ANALYSIS

Data collection is the precise, systematic gathering of information relevant to the research purpose or the specific objectives, questions, or hypotheses of a study. The data collected in quantitative studies are usually numerical. Planning data collection enables the researcher to anticipate problems that are likely to occur and to explore possible solutions. Usually detailed procedures for implementing a treatment and collecting data are developed, with a schedule that identifies the initiation and termination of the process. Planning and implementing data collection is the focus of Chapter 15.

Planning data analysis is the final step before the study is implemented. The analysis plan is based on the research objectives, questions, or hypotheses; data collected; research design; researcher expertise; and availability of computer resources. A variety of statistical analysis techniques are available to describe the sample, examine relationships, or determine significant differences. Most researchers consult a statistician for assistance in developing an analysis plan.

IMPLEMENTING THE RESEARCH PLAN

Implementing the research plan involves treatment implementation, data collection, data analysis, in-terpretation of research findings, and sometimes a pilot study.

Pilot Study

A *pilot study* is frequently defined as a smaller version of a proposed study conducted to refine the methodology (Van Ort, 1981). It is developed similarly to the proposed study, using similar subjects, the same setting, same treatment, and the same data collection and analysis techniques. Prescott and Soeken (1989), however, believe the pilot can have many other uses. A pilot study could be conducted to develop and refine the steps in the research process. For example, a pilot study could be conducted to develop and refine a research treatment, a data collection tool, or the data collection process. Thus, a pilot study could be used to develop a research plan rather than test an already-developed plan. Some of the reasons for conducting pilot studies include:

1. To determine whether the proposed study is feasible (e.g., are the subjects available, does the researcher have the time and money to do the study?).
2. To develop or refine a research treatment.
3. To develop a protocol for the implementation of a treatment.
4. To identify problems with the design.
5. To determine whether the sample is representative of the population or whether the sampling technique is effective.
6. To examine the reliability and validity of the research instruments.
7. To develop or refine data collection instruments.
8. To refine the data collection and analysis plan.
9. To give the researcher experience with the subjects, setting, methodology, and methods of measurement.
10. To try out data analysis techniques (Prescott & Soeken, 1989; Van Ort, 1981).

Prescott and Soeken (1989) reviewed 212 studies published in three research journals (*Nursing Research, Research in Nursing & Health,* and

Western Journal of Nursing Research) during 1985–1987. Only 18 (8.8%) of these studies reported a pilot. In 13 of the 18 studies, a pilot was conducted to assess instrument reliability. In the other five studies, the pilots were a smaller version of the published studies that were conducted to test the research plans. Pilot studies can be used to improve the quality of research conducted, and their findings need to be shared through presentations and publications. Wilkie, Williams, Grevstad, and Mekwa (1995, p. 8) conducted a "pilot study to develop and test a method of COACHING 18 patients with lung cancer to inform clinicians about their pain." COACHING is one method of improving clinicians' assessments of pain by encouraging patients to communicate their pain in ways that clinicians recognize. "Pilot study findings demonstrated feasibility of implementing the COACHING protocol and suggest a trend for COACHING to possibly be an effective method of reducing discrepancies between patients' self-reports and nurses' assessments of sensory pain" (Wilkie et al., 1995, p. 13). Thus, the focus of this pilot study was to test the completeness of the protocol for implementing the COACHING intervention and to determine the effectiveness of this intervention in increasing the recognition of cancer patients' pain.

Data Collection

In quantitative research, data collection involves the generation of numerical data to address the research objectives, questions, or hypotheses. In order to collect data, the researcher must obtain consent or permission from the setting or agency where the study is to be conducted. Getting approval to conduct a study is described in Chapter 26. Consent must also be obtained from the research subjects to indicate their willingness to participate in the study. Frequently, the subjects are asked to sign a consent form, which describes the study, promises the subjects confidentiality, and indicates that the subjects can stop participation at any time (see Chapter 9).

During data collection, the study variables are measured using a variety of techniques, such as observation, interview, questionnaires, or scales. In an increasing number of studies, nurses are measuring physiological variables with high technology equipment. The data are collected and recorded systematically on each subject and are organized in a way to facilitate computer entry. Hulme and Grove (1994) identified the following procedure for data collection.

"Although the tool can be self-reporting, it was administered by personal interview to allow for elaboration of 'other' responses. The interviews lasted about one hour and were conducted in a private room provided by The University of Texas at Arlington. Each interview started with a discussion of the study benefits and risks and included signing a consent form. Risks included possible painful memories and embarrassment during the interview as well as emotional and physical discomfort after the interview. Sources of public and private counseling were provided to assist subjects with any difficulties experienced related to the study." (pp. 524–525) ∎

Data Analysis

Data analysis is conducted to reduce, organize, and give meaning to the data. Analysis techniques conducted in quantitative research include descriptive and exploratory procedures (see Chapter 17); inferential analyses (see Chapter 18); and sophisticated, advanced analyses (see Chapter 19). Most analyses are performed by computer, so Chapter 15 provides a background for using computers in research. The analysis techniques implemented are determined primarily by the research objectives, questions, or hypotheses; the research design; and the level of measurement achieved by the research instruments. Hulme and Grove (1994) conducted frequencies, percents, means, standard deviations, and Pearson correlations to answer their research questions.

Results

"The first research question focused on patterns of physical and psychosocial symptoms. Six physical symptoms occurred in 50% or more of the subjects: insomnia, sexual dysfunction, overeating, drug abuse, severe headache, and two or more major surgeries . . . Eleven psychosocial symptoms occurred in 75% or more of the subjects: depression, guilt, low self-esteem, inability to trust others, mood swings, suicidal thoughts, difficulty in relationships, confusion, flashbacks of the abuse, extreme anger, and memory lapse . . . Self-injurious behavior was reported by eight subjects (33%)." (pp. 527–528)

"The second research question focused on the relationships among the number of physical and psychosocial symptoms and three contributing factors (age abuse began, duration of abuse, and other victimizations). There were five significant correlations among study variables: physical symptoms with other victimizations ($r = .59$, $p = .002$), physical symptoms with psychosocial symptoms ($r = .56$, $p = .003$), age abuse began with duration of abuse ($r = -.50$, $p = .009$), psychosocial symptoms with other victimizations ($r = .40$, $p = .033$), and duration of abuse with psychosocial symptoms ($r = .40$, $p = .034$)." (p. 528) ■

Interpreting Research Outcomes

The results obtained from data analysis require interpretation to be meaningful. *Interpretation of research outcomes* involves examining the results from data analysis, forming conclusions, considering the implications for nursing, exploring the significance of the findings, generalizing the findings, and suggesting further studies. The results obtained from data analyses are of five types: (1) significant as predicted by the researcher, (2) nonsignificant, (3) significant but not predicted by the researcher, (4) mixed, and (5) unexpected. The study results are then translated and interpreted to become findings, and conclusions are formed from the synthesis of findings. The conclusions provide a basis for identifying nursing implications, gen-

eralizing findings, and suggesting further studies. Interpreting research outcomes is the focus of Chapter 22. Hulme and Grove (1994) provided the following discussion of their findings, with implications for nursing and suggestions for further study.

Discussion

"While this study may have limited generalizability due to the relatively small nonprobability sample, the findings do support previous research . . . In addition, the findings support Browne and Finkelhor's (1986) framework that a wide range of behavioral manifestations (physical and psychosocial symptoms) comprise the long-term effects of child sexual abuse." (p. 528)

"Brown and Garrison's (1990) ASI Questionnaire was effective in identifying patterns of physical and psychosocial symptoms in women with a history of child sexual abuse . . . As data on the behavioral manifestations (physical and psychosocial symptoms) and the effect of each of the contributing factors accumulate, hypotheses need to be formulated to further test Browne and Finkelhor's (1986) framework explaining the long-term effects of child sexual abuse . . . With additional research, the ASI Questionnaire might be adapted for use in clinical situations. This questionnaire might facilitate identification and delivery of appropriate treatment to female survivors of child sexual abuse in clinical settings." (pp. 529–530) ■

COMMUNICATING RESEARCH FINDINGS

Research is not considered complete until the findings have been communicated. *Communicating research findings* involves the development and dissemination of a research report to appropriate audiences, including nurses, health professionals, health care consumers, and policymakers. The research report is disseminated through presentations and publication. The details for developing a research report and presenting and publishing the report are in Chapter 23.

TYPES OF QUANTITATIVE RESEARCH

Four types of quantitative research are included in this text: (1) descriptive, (2) correlational, (3) quasi-experimental, and (4) experimental. The type of research planned is influenced by the level of existing knowledge for the research problem. When little knowledge is available, often descriptive studies are conducted. As the knowledge level increases, correlational, quasi-experimental, and experimental studies are implemented. In this section, the purpose of each quantitative research approach is identified and an example of the steps of the research process from a published study are presented.

DESCRIPTIVE RESEARCH

The purpose of descriptive research is the exploration and description of phenomena in real life situations. This approach is used to generate new knowledge about concepts or topics that have limited or no research. Through descriptive research, concepts are described and relationships are identified that provide a basis for further quantitative research and theory testing. Carrieri et al. (1991, p. 81) conducted the following descriptive study on "the sensation of pulmonary dyspnea in school-age children."

Steps of the Research Process

1. **Research Problem.** "Dyspnea, the subjective perception of uncomfortable breathing, is a symptom that can have a significant impact on the daily routines and activities of a school-age child and is a common experience of children with asthma . . . The sensation of dyspnea has not been well described in children. Little is known about the intensity, quality, or range of responses to this experience in children . . . Little is known about the strategies children use to cope with the actual symptom of dyspnea." (p. 81)

2. **Research Purpose.** "The major purposes of this investigation were to describe the sensation of dyspnea in school-age children and to identify strategies children use to cope with shortness of breath. A secondary purpose was to test and compare three methods for the measurement of dyspnea intensity in children." (p. 81) The purpose includes three objectives that were used to develop and implement this study.

3. **Review of Literature.** The review of literature covers mainly empirical literature and is organized by two concepts, sensation of dyspnea and coping strategies.

4. **Framework.** A framework is not clearly presented in the study; however, the findings are discussed using Lazarus and Folkman's (1984) theory of stress, appraisal, and coping. Figure 3–4 presents a possible map for the study framework. When a child experiences a stressful situation (dyspnea), they appraise this situation (assess the sensation and intensity of dyspnea). The child then implements coping strategies (problem-focused and

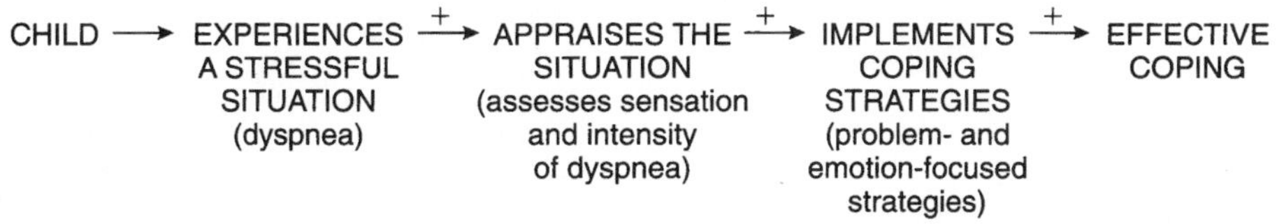

CHILD $\longrightarrow$ EXPERIENCES A STRESSFUL SITUATION (dyspnea) $\xrightarrow{+}$ APPRAISES THE SITUATION (assesses sensation and intensity of dyspnea) $\xrightarrow{+}$ IMPLEMENTS COPING STRATEGIES (problem- and emotion-focused strategies) $\xrightarrow{+}$ EFFECTIVE COPING

Figure 3–4
Proposed framework for the study by Carrieri and associates (1991) of the sensation of pulmonary dyspnea in school-age children.

emotion-focused) in an attempt to effectively respond to the stressful situation. The framework identifies the concepts and their interrelationships. To demonstrate the link between the concepts in the framework and the study variables, the variables are placed in parentheses below the concepts. The framework also guides the development of conceptual definitions of the variables and provides a basis for interpretations of research findings.

5. **Variables.** Research variables were examined in the study and included sensation of dyspnea, intensity of dyspnea, and coping strategies.

Sensation of Dyspnea

Conceptual Definition. Subjective perception of uncomfortable breathing, which is a stressful situation that requires appraisal.

Operational Definition. Interviews were conducted with open-ended questions and forced-choice items that focused on the subjects' descriptions (physical and emotional sensations) of dyspnea.

Intensity of Dyspnea

Conceptual Definition. Appraising the strength or degree of dyspnea experienced during a stressful situation.

Operational Definition. "Three methods were used to rate the intensity of recalled dyspnea: a word descriptor scale, a visual analogue scale, and a color shade scale." (p. 82)

Coping Strategies

Conceptual Definition. Problem-focused and emotion-focused strategies used to manage a stressful situation (dyspnea).

Operational Definition. An interview with open-ended questions and forced-choice items that addresses the problem-focused and emotion-focused coping strategies used with dyspnea.

6. **Design.** Typical descriptive design.
7. **Sample.** "A convenience sample of 23 males and 16 females aged 7 to 13 years with documented asthma and episodes of wheezing . . . The documentation of asthma was made by chart review or physician report. Almost all children ($N = 31$) used inhalers for bronchodi-

lator medications at least occasionally, while only six of the children required periodic oral steroids for symptom management . . . The duration of illness for the children ranged from two months to 13 years. Twenty-six of the children had an episode of shortness of breath within 24 hours of the interview and 13 within the previous month." (p. 82)

8. **Data Collection.** One interview was conducted with the child "either at home or in an ambulatory clinic. After a short interview with both parent and child to obtain information about medications and breathing problems, children were interviewed alone." (p. 82)

9. **Results.** Sensations of dyspnea were described using percentages, with wheezy (77%) being the most common physical sensation and worried (74%) being the most common emotional sensation. Means were calculated for the children's good, usual, and bad breathing days using the data from the three methods of dyspnea intensity measurement. The problem-focused, emotion-focused, and mixed coping strategies were described using frequencies and percentages. The most commonly used problem-focused coping strategy was self-adjustment of medications (90%) and the most commonly used emotion-focused coping strategy was conscious attempt to calm down (10%). The children used predominantly problem-focused coping strategies to manage their dyspnea.

10. **Discussion.** "School-age children with asthma are able to rate both the intensity of dyspnea and give qualitative descriptions of the sensations. There were striking similarities in the intensity and sensation of dyspnea between the children and an adult sample . . . All methods used in this study to measure dyspnea intensity were understandable to the children, demonstrated changes in the theoretically predicted direction, and distinguished among bad, usual, and good breathing days . . . The most common coping strategy used by all samples to cope with their dyspnea was medications . . . This preliminary investigation of dyspnea experienced by asthmatic children needs to be expanded with larger samples who have a

variety of illnesses to further understand the experience and impact of this persistent symptom." (pp. 84–85) ■

CORRELATIONAL RESEARCH

Correlational research is conducted to examine linear relationships between two or more variables and to determine the type (positive or negative) and degree (strength) of the relationship. The strength of a relationship varies from $a - 1$ (perfect negative correlation) to $a + 1$ (perfect positive correlation), with 0 indicating no relationship. The positive relationship indicates that the variables vary together, where both variables either increase or decrease together. The negative or inverse relationship indicates that the variables vary in opposite directions; thus, as one variable increases, the other will decrease. The correlational study conducted by Hulme and Grove (1994) was presented as an example when the steps of the research process were introduced.

QUASI-EXPERIMENTAL RESEARCH

The purpose of quasi-experimental research is to examine cause-and-effect relationships between selected independent and dependent variables. Quasi-experimental studies in nursing are conducted to determine the effects of nursing interventions (independent variables) on patient outcomes (dependent variables) (Cook & Campbell, 1979). Hastings-Tolsma, Yucha, Tompkins, Robson, and Szeverenyi (1993, p. 171) conducted a quasi-experimental study of the "effect of warm and cold applications on the resolution of IV infiltrations." Following is an outline of the steps of the study.

Steps of the Research Process

1. Research Problem. "It has been estimated that as many as 80% of hospitalized patients

receive intravenous (IV) therapy each day (Millam, 1988). IV infiltration, or extravasation, occurs in as many as 23% of all IV infusion failures (MacCara, 1983) and is second only to phlebitis as a cause of IV morbidity (Lewis & Hecker, 1991). The resulting tissue injury depends on the clinical condition of the patient, the nature of the infusate, and the volume infiltrated, and may range from little apparent injury to serious damage. In addition, considerable patient suffering, prolonged hospitalization, and significant costs may be incurred. Despite the frequency and potential severity of injury, little is known about how to treat IV infiltration effectively once it is identified." (p. 171)

2. Research Purpose. "The purpose of this research was to determine the effect of warm versus cold applications on the pain intensity and the speed of resolution of the extravasation of a variety of commonly used intravenous solutions." (p. 172)

3. Review of Literature. The literature review included relevant, current sources that ranged from 1976 to 1991. The journal article was received in April 1992 and accepted for publication in January 1993. The signs and symptoms of IV infiltration were identified and the tissue damage that occurs with an IV infiltration was described. The effects of the pH and osmolarity of different types of IV solutions on IV infiltration were also discussed. The literature review concluded with a description of the effects of a variety of treatments, including warm and cold applications, on the resolution of IV infiltrations. Hastings-Tolsma et al. (1993, p. 172) concluded that "examination of warm and cold application with less toxic infiltrates has not been studied carefully under controlled conditions."

4. Framework. Hastings-Tolsma and colleagues did not identify a framework for their study. They did identify relevant concepts (IV therapy, nature of infusate, vessel damage, extravasation, tissue damage, treatment, and resolution) and discuss the relationships among these concepts in their review of literature. A possible map for their study framework is presented in Figure 3–5. The map indicates that the more IV therapy patients receive, the more likely they are to experi-

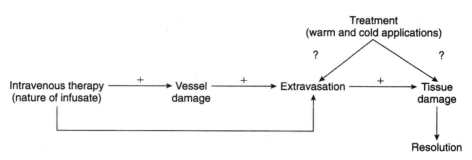

Figure 3–5
Proposed framework map in Hastings-Tolsma, Yucha, Tompkins, Robson, and Szeverenyi's (1993) study of the effect of warm and cold applications on the resolution of intravenous infiltrations.

ence vessel damage that leads to extravasation or IV infiltration. The nature of the IV infusate (IV solution) also effects the severity of the vessel damage and extravasation. The extravasation then leads to tissue damage and the greater the extravasation, the greater the tissue damage. The treatment with warm and cold applications has an unknown effect on the extravasation and tissue damage. If the extravasation and tissue damage are decreased by either the cold or warm treatment, then the patient experiences resolution of the extravasation.

5. **Research Questions.** "(a) What are the differences in tissue response as measured by pain, erythema and induration, and interstitial fluid volume between warm versus cold applications to infiltrated IV sites? (b) What is the effect of warm versus cold applications in the resolution of infiltrated solutions of varying osmolarity when pH is held constant?" (pp. 172–173)

6. **Variables.** The independent variables were temperature applications (warm and cold) and osmolarity of the IV solution. The dependent variables were pain, erythema, induration, and interstitial fluid volume.

Independent Variable—Temperature Applications

Conceptual Definition. Topical warm and cold applications to the sites of extravasation to promote the reabsorption of infusate and resolution of the infiltration.

Operational Definition. Warm (43°C) or cold (0°)

topical applications using a thermostated pad to the sites of IV infiltration.

Independent Variable—Osmolarity of the IV Solution

Conceptual Definition. The osmolar concentration expressed as osmoles per liter of solution.

Operational Definition. IV solutions of ½ saline (154 mOsm), normal saline (308 mOsm), or 3% saline (1027 mOsm).

Dependent Variable—Pain

Conceptual Definition. Sensation of discomfort caused by tissue damage and the inflammatory response.

Operational Definition. Pain was measured with the Analogue Chromatic Continuous Scale (ACCS), which is a self-report, unidimensional visual analogue scale for quantifying pain intensity.

Dependent Variable—Erythema

Conceptual Definition. Redness at the IV infiltration site due to inflammatory response.

Operational Definition. Indelible ink pen was used to mark the borders of erythema. Then a centimeter ruler was used to measure the widest perpendicular widths and the two widths were multiplied to estimate surface area of erythema.

Dependent Variable—Induration

Conceptual Definition. The swelling at the site of the IV infiltration created by the IV solution, tissue damage, and inflammatory response.

Operational Definition. Indelible ink pen was used to mark the borders of induration. Then a centimeter ruler was used to measure the widest perpendicular widths and the two widths were multiplied to estimate surface area of induration.

Dependent Variable—Interstitial Fluid Volume

Conceptual Definition. The amount of fluid that leaks outside of the damaged blood vessel into the surrounding tissues.

Operational Definition. Magnetic resonance imaging (MRI) was used to quantify the amount of infiltrate remaining at the IV site.

7. **Design.** The design most closely resembles an interrupted time series with each subject receiving both treatments of warm and cold applications.

8. **Sample.** "The sample was composed of 18 healthy adult volunteers. All participants were nonpregnant and taking no medications . . . Of the 18 participants studied, 78% were female ($n = 14$) and 22% were male ($n = 4$), and they ranged in age from 20 to 45 years with a mean age of 35 years ($SD = 7$). All subjects were Caucasian. The research was approved by the Health Science Center Institutional Review Board for the Protection of Human Subjects. After the study was explained to interested individuals, written informed consent was obtained from volunteers. All individuals were offered financial compensation for their participation." (p. 173)

9. **Procedures.** "All measurements were taken in the Health Science Center's Department of Radiology NMR Laboratory. After obtaining written informed consent, participants were taken to the MR imaging suite where infiltrations and subsequent measurements were made . . . Total data collection time was approximately 3½ hours. One of three solutions was infiltrated into the cephalic vein of the forearm: ½ saline (154 mOsm), normal saline (308 mOsm), or 3% saline (1027 mOsm). These solutions were selected because of the varying osmolarity range, as well as relatively common clinical use. Solutions were infil-

trated sequentially so that each participant was given a different solution in the order of recruitment into the study. Randomization was used to determine right or left arm, as well as which application, warm or cold, would be used." (p. 174)

10. **Results.** "Warm and cold treatments to the infiltrated IV sites using three solutions revealed significant differences in tissue response as measured by the interstitial fluid volume . . . For all three solutions, the volume remaining was always less with warm than with cold application, $F_{(1,15)} = 46.69$, $p < .001$.

There was no difference in pain with warm or cold applications . . . Surface area measurement failed to demonstrate the presence of erythema with any of the solutions . . . Surface induration reflected a significant decrease over time, $F_{(2,16)} = 14.38$, $p = .001$, although accurate measurement of the infiltrate was nearly impossible after the first or second imaging period as the borders were so poorly defined . . . There was no significant effect of warmth or cold on surface area." (p. 175)

11. **Discussion.** This section includes the study conclusions, recommendations for further research, and the implications of the findings for nursing practice. "These findings demonstrate that the application of warmth to sites of IV infiltration produces faster resolution of the extravasation than does cold, as monitored over one hour . . . It is interesting to note that cold appeared to have a more immediate dramatic effect on the increase in interstitial edema than warmth when applied to the hyperosmolar infiltrate. Presumably this is due to osmosis of fluid from the plasma and surrounding tissues into the area of infiltration . . .

Other factors that might influence accurate assessment and treatment of infiltrations need to be examined. These should include the use of larger amounts of extravasate and other more varied and caustic solutions, as well as other treatments such as elevation, differing IV site placement, differing gauge needles, and the study of patients of varying ages and clinical conditions . . . " (p. 176)

"The nurse generally has responsibility for IV therapy and criteria for accurate assessment and appropriate intervention clearly are needed. Findings from this research support the use of warm application to sites of infiltration of noncaustic solutions of varying osmolarity, but raise questions about the adequacy of currently used indicators of IV infiltrations. Continued scientific scrutiny should contribute to the development of standards useful in the assessment and treatment of IV extravasation." (p. 177) ∎

EXPERIMENTAL RESEARCH

The purpose of experimental research is to examine cause-and-effect relationships between independent and dependent variables under highly controlled conditions. The planning and implementation of experimental studies are highly controlled by the researcher, and often these studies are conducted in a laboratory setting on animals or objects. Few nursing studies are "purely" experimental. Metheny, Eisenberg, and McSweeney (1988, p. 165) conducted an experimental study to determine "the effect of feeding tube properties and three irrigants on clogging rates."

Steps of the Research Process

1. **Research Problem.** "Luminal obstruction of feeding tubes is one of the most common mechanical complications associated with enteral feedings . . . Inability to clear a clogged tube necessitates its removal and replacement with a new tube. Not only does this add to the patient's discomfort and risk of trauma, but it interrupts the administration of nutrients and results in increased cost." (p. 165)

2. **Research Purpose.** "The purpose of this laboratory study was to examine the effect of selected feeding tube properties (material and diameter) on the incidence of tube clogging and the efficacy of three irrigants (cranberry juice, water, and Coca-Cola) in preventing tube clogging." (p. 165)

3. **Review of Literature.** The literature review included mainly studies of the effects of feeding tube properties on flow rate and use of irrigants to maintain tube patency.

4. **Framework.** The authors did not identify a framework but the concepts of tube properties, irrigants, tube flow rate, and luminal obstruction were identified and the relationships among these concepts are presented in Figure 3–6. Certain tube properties and irrigants were proposed to affect the tube flow rate. An increase in flow rate would result in an increase in the delivery of a substance and a decrease in flow rate could result in luminal obstruction of the tube.

5. **Variables.** The independent variables were physical tube properties (material and diameter) and irrigants (cranberry juice, water, and cola beverage), and the dependent variable was tube clogging.

Independent Variable—Physical Tube Properties

Conceptual Definition. The physical elements or properties (material and diameter) of the tube that influence flow rate.

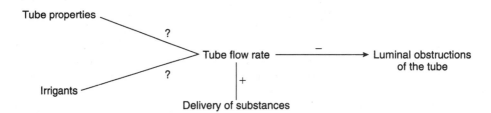

Figure 3–6

Map of the framework for the study by Metheny and associates (1988) of the effect of feeding tube properties and irrigants on clogging rates.

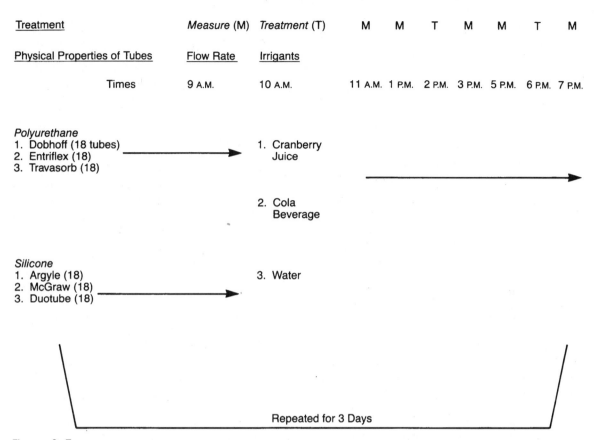

Treatment	Measure (M)	Treatment (T)	M	M	T	M	M	T	M
Physical Properties of Tubes	Flow Rate	Irrigants							
Times	9 A.M.	10 A.M.	11 A.M.	1 P.M.	2 P.M.	3 P.M.	5 P.M.	6 P.M.	7 P.M.

Polyurethane
1. Dobhoff (18 tubes)
2. Entriflex (18)
3. Travasorb (18)

1. Cranberry Juice

2. Cola Beverage

Silicone
1. Argyle (18)
2. McGraw (18)
3. Duotube (18)

3. Water

Repeated for 3 Days

Figure 3–7

Repeated measures design for Metheny and associates' (1988) study of the effect of feeding tube properties and irrigants on clogging rates.

Operational Definition. Polyurethane and silicone tubes of the following diameters were used: 12 Fr., 10 Fr., and 8 Fr.

Independent Variable—Irrigants

Conceptual Definition. The substance used to flush the internal surface of the tube.

Operational Definition. Three irrigants were used: cranberry juice, water, and cola beverage.

Dependent Variable—Tube Clogging

Conceptual Definition. Mechanical complication of the tube that results in decreased flow rate through the tube and ultimate obstruction of the lumen of the tube.

Operational Definition. Clogging was defined by flow rates. "Flow rates were considered free flowing if the volume was greater than

0.7 ml/minute, slowed if less than 0.7 ml/minute but greater than 0.4 ml/minute, almost stopped if less than 0.4 ml/minute but greater than zero, and completely stopped if zero ml/minute. When tubes became irreversibly clogged, they were removed from the study and not replaced." (pp. 166–167)

6. **Design.** An experimental design of repeated measures was used in this study (see Figure 3–7). The diagram indicates the manipulation of two treatments, physical tube properties (material and diameter), and irrigants (cranberry juice, water, and cola beverage). The treatment (T) of the irrigants was implemented three times a day for three days, and the flow rates through the different tubes were measured (M) every two hours for three days.

7. Sample. "One hundred and eight feeding tubes were studied over three consecutive 12-hour days. There were 54 polyurethane and 54 silicone tubes equally divided among external diameters of 8 Fr., 10 Fr., and 12 Fr." (p. 166)

8. Data Collection. "Each tube was connected to a gravity flow feeding bag containing 200 ml of isotonic enteral formula . . . To facilitate collection of data, six 'stations' were set up. At each station, there were three sets of tubes (a set was defined as one of each of the six types of tubes) . . . One set of tubes at each station was irrigated with cranberry juice, one with Coca-Cola, and one with tap water . . . Actual amounts of formula delivered per tube were monitored at 2-hour intervals (9:00 AM, 11:00 AM, 1:00 PM, 3:00 PM, 5:00 PM, and 7:00 PM) for three days" (see Figure 3–6). (p. 166)

9. Results. "On each of the three days, both the univariate and multivariate ANOVAs re-vealed significant, $p < .05$, effects of tube material, of cranberry juice contrasted with Coca-Cola and water as irrigants, and of time. Polyurethane was consistently superior to silicone as a tube material, and cranberry juice was consistently inferior to both Coca-Cola and water as an irrigant." (p. 167)

10. Discussion. "Among the tube properties examined the only significant finding was the superiority of polyurethane over silicone in promoting flow of enteral formula . . . Contrary to some reports in the literature, cranberry juice is not an effective irrigant to prevent tube clogging . . . Although it was hypothesized that Coca-Cola would be a more effective irrigant than water because of its carbonation and relatively low pH, this was not supported . . . Thus, considering all of the above factors, it is logical to use polyurethane tubes of 10 Fr. or 12 Fr. diameters" (p. 168) and to irrigate the tubes with water.

SUMMARY

Quantitative research is the traditional research approach in nursing. Nurses use a broad range of quantitative approaches, including descriptive, correlational, quasi-experimental, and experimental to develop nursing knowledge. Some of the concepts relevant to quantitative research include basic and applied research, rigor, and control. Basic or pure research is a scientific investigation that involves the pursuit of "knowledge for knowledge's sake" or for the pleasure of learning and finding truth. Applied or practical research is a scientific investigation conducted to generate knowledge that will directly influence or improve clinical practice. Many of the studies conducted in nursing are applied because researchers have chosen to focus on clinical problems, such as developing and testing the effectiveness of nursing interventions. Since the future of any profession rests on its research base, both basic and applied research are needed to develop nursing knowledge.

Conducting quantitative research involves rigor, which is the striving for excellence in research. Rigor involves discipline, scrupulous adherence to detail, and strict accuracy. A rigorous quantitative researcher constantly strives for more precise measurement tools, a representative sample, and tightly controlled study designs. Control involves the imposing of "rules" by the researcher to decrease the possibility of error and thus increase the probability that the study's findings are an accurate reflection of reality. Some of the mechanisms for enhancing control within quantitative research include (1) subject selection (sampling), (2) research setting selection, (3) development and implementation of study interventions, and (4) subject's knowledge of the study. Sampling is a process of selecting subjects who are

continued

continued

representative of the population being studied. The three settings for conducting research are natural, partially controlled, and highly controlled. Controlling the development and implementation of a study intervention increases the validity of the study design and the credibility of the findings. Subjects' knowledge of a study could influence their behavior and possibly alter the study outcome. This creates a threat to the validity and accuracy of the study design.

The quantitative research process involves conceptualizing a research project, planning and implementing that project, and communicating the findings. The steps of this research process are briefly introduced in this chapter and presented in detail in Unit II, The Research Process. The steps of the quantitative research process include:

1. **Formulating a research problem and purpose.** The research problem is a situation in need of a solution, improvement, or alteration or a discrepancy between the way things are and the way they ought to be. A problem stimulates interest and prompts investigation. The research purpose is generated from the problem and identifies the specific goal or aim of the study.

2. **Review of relevant literature.** The literature review is conducted to generate a picture of what is known about a particular situation and the knowledge gaps that exist in the situation.

3. **Developing a framework.** The framework is the abstract, logical structure of meaning that guides the development of the study and enables the researcher to link the findings to nursing's body of knowledge.

4. **Formulating research objectives, questions, and hypotheses.** Research objectives, questions, and hypotheses are formulated to bridge the gap between the more abstractly stated research problem and purpose and the study design and plan for data collection and analysis.

5. **Defining research variables.** Variables are concepts of various levels of abstraction that are measured, manipulated, or controlled in a study. Variables are operationalized by identifying conceptual and operational definitions.

6. **Making assumptions explicit.** Assumptions are statements that are taken for granted or are considered true, even though these statements have not been scientifically tested. Assumptions influence the logic of the study, and their recognition leads to more rigorous study development.

7. **Identifying limitations.** Limitations are restrictions in a study that may decrease the generalizability of the findings. The two types of limitations are theoretical and methodological.

8. **Selecting a research design.** Research design is a blueprint for the conduct of a study that maximizes control over factors that could interfere with the study's desired outcome. The type of design directs the selection of a population, sampling procedure, methods of measurement, and a plan for data collection and analysis.

9. **Defining the population and sample.** The population is all elements that meet certain criteria for inclusion in a given universe. A sample is a subset of the population that is selected for a particular study and the members of a sample are the subjects. Sampling defines the process for selecting a group of subjects with which to conduct a study.

10. **Selecting methods of measurement.** Measurement is the process of assigning numbers to objects, events, or situations in accord with some rule. A component of measurement is instrumentation, and an instrument is selected to examine a specific variable in a study.

continued

continued

11. **Developing a plan for data collection and analysis.** Data collection is the precise, systematic gathering of information relevant to the research purpose or the specific objectives, questions, or hypotheses of a study. The data collected in quantitative studies are usually numerical. Planning data analysis involves the selection of appropriate statistical techniques to analyze the study data.

12. **Implementing the research plan.** The research plan involves treatment implementation, data collection, data analysis, and interpretation of research outcomes. In some studies, implementing the research plan might include a pilot study. The reasons for conducting a pilot study might include refining a research treatment, refining a data collection sheet, examining an instrument's reliability or validity, and identifying problems in the design. Data collection involves the generation of numerical data to answer the research objectives, questions, or hypotheses. Data analysis is conducted to reduce, organize, and give meaning to the data. Interpretation of research outcomes involves examining the results from data analysis, forming conclusions, considering the implications for nursing, exploring the significance of the findings, generalizing the findings, and suggesting further studies.

13. **Communicating findings.** Research is communicated by developing and disseminating a research report to appropriate audiences, including nurses, other health professionals, health care consumers, and policy makers. The research report is disseminated through presentations and publication.

Four types of quantitative research are introduced in this chapter: descriptive, correlational, quasi-experimental, and experimental. The purpose of each quantitative approach is identified, followed by an example of the steps of the research process from a published study.

References

Abdellah, F. G., & Levine, E. (1979). *Better patient care through nursing research* (2nd ed.). New York: Macmillan.

Adebo, E. O. (1974). Identifying problems for nursing research. *International Nursing Review, 21*(2), 53–54, 59.

Bagley, C. (1990). Development of a measure of unwanted sexual contact in childhood, for use in community health surveys. *Psychology Reports, 66*(2), 401–402.

Bagley, C., & King, K. K. (1990). *Child sexual abuse: The search for healing.* New York: Travistock/Routledge.

Bond, E. F., & Heitkemper, M. M. (1987). Importance of basic physiologic research in nursing science. *Heart & Lung, 16*(4), 347–349.

Brophy, E. B. (1981). Research design: General introduction. In S. D. Krampitz & N. Pavlovich (Eds.), *Readings for nursing research* (pp. 40–48). St. Louis: Mosby.

Brown, B. E., & Garrison, C. J. (1990). Patterns of symptomatology of adult women incest survivors. *Western Journal of Nursing Research, 12*(5), 587–600.

Browne, A., & Finkelhor, D. (1986). Initial and long-term effects: A review of the research. In D. Finkelhor (Ed.), *A source book on child sexual abuse* (pp. 143–179). Beverly Hills: Sage.

Campbell, D. T., & Stanley, J. C. (1963). *Experimental and quasi-experimental designs for research.* Chicago: Rand McNally.

Carrieri, V. K., Kieckhefer, G., Janson-Bjerklie, S., & Souza, J. (1991). The sensation of pulmonary dyspnea in school-age children. *Nursing Research, 40*(2), 81–85.

Cook, T. D., & Campbell, D. T. (1979). *Quasi-experimentation: Design and analysis issues for field settings.* Chicago: Rand McNally.

Diers, D. (1979). *Research in nursing practice.* Philadelphia: Lippincott.

Egan, E. C., Snyder, M., & Burns, K. R. (1992). Intervention studies in nursing: Is the effect due to the independent variable? *Nursing Outlook, 40*(4), 187–190.

Fawcett, J., & Downs, F. S. (1986). *The relationship of theory and research.* Norwalk, CT: Appleton-Century-Crofts.

Fisher, Sir R. A. (1935). *The designs of experiments.* New York: Hafner.

Follette, N. M., Alexander, P. C., & Follette, W. C. (1991). Individual predictors of outcome in group treatment for incest survivors. *Journal of Consulting and Clinical Psychology, 59*(1), 150–155.

Fridriksdottir, N., & McCarthy, D. O. (1995). The effect of caloric density of food on energy intake and body weight in tumor-bearing rats. *Research in Nursing & Health, 18*(4), 357–363.

Hastings-Tolsma, M. T., Yucha, C. B., Tompkins, J., Robson, L., & Szeverenyi, N. (1993). Effect of warm and cold applications on the resolution of IV infiltrations. *Research in Nursing & Health, 16*(3), 171–178.

Homans, G. (1965). Group factors in worker productivity. In H. Proshansky & B. Seidenberg (Eds.), *Basic studies in social psychology* (pp. 592–604). New York: Holt, Rinehart and Winston.

Hulme, P. A., & Grove, S. K. (1994). Symptoms of female survivors of child sexual abuse. *Issues in Mental Health Nursing, 15*(5), 519–532.

Johnson, M. J., & Frank, D. I. (1995). Effectiveness of a telephone intervention in reducing anxiety of families of patients in an intensive care unit. *Applied Nursing Research, 8*(1), 42–43.

Kaplan, A. (1964). *The conduct of inquiry: Methodology for behavioral science.* New York: Chandler.

Kerlinger, F. N. (1986). *Foundations of behavioral research* (2nd ed.). New York: Holt, Rinehart and Winston.

Lazarus, R. S., & Folkman, S. (1984). *Stress, appraisal and coping.* New York: Springer.

Lewis, G. B. H., & Hecker, J. F. (1991). Radiological examination of failure of intravenous infusions. *British Journal of Surgery, 78*(4), 500–501.

MacCara, M. E. (1983). Extravasation: A hazard of intravenous therapy. *Drug Intelligence and Clinical Pharmacy, 17*(10), 713–717.

MacVicar, M. G., Winningham, M. L., & Nickel, J. L. (1989). Effects of aerobic interval training on cancer patients' functional capacity. *Nursing Research, 38*(6), 348–351.

Metheny, N., Eisenberg, P., & McSweeney, M. (1988). Effect of feeding tube properties and three irrigants on clogging rates. *Nursing Research, 37*(3), 165–169.

Millam, D. A. (1988). Managing complications of IV therapy. *Nursing 88, 18*(3), 34–42.

Myers, S. T. (1982). The search for assumptions. *Western Journal of Nursing Research, 4*(1), 91–98.

Nagel, E. (1961). *The structure of science: Problems in the logic of scientific explanation.* New York: Harcourt, Brace & World.

Prescott, P. A., & Soeken, K. L. (1989). Methodology corner: The potential uses of pilot work. *Nursing Research, 38*(1), 60–62.

Silva, M. C. (1981). Selection of a theoretical framework. In S. D. Krampitz & N. Pavlovich (Eds.), *Readings for nursing research* (pp. 17–28). St. Louis: Mosby.

Van Ort, S. (1981). Research design: Pilot study. In S. D. Krampitz & N. Pavlovich (Eds.), *Readings for nursing research* (pp. 49–53). St. Louis: Mosby.

Wallenstein, S. L. (1987). Research perspectives: A response. *Journal of Pain and Symptom Management, 2*(2), 103–106.

Wilkie, D. J., Williams, A. R., Grevstad, P., & Mekwa, J. (1995). Coaching persons with lung cancer to report sensory pain: Literature review and pilot study findings. *Cancer Nursing, 18*(1), 7–15.

Williams, M. A. (1980). Editorial: Assumptions in research. *Research in Nursing & Health, 3*(2), 47–48.

Wysocki, A. B. (1983). Basic versus applied research: Intrinsic and extrinsic considerations. *Western Journal of Nursing Research, 5*(3), 217–224.

Younger, J., Marsh, K. J., & Grap, M. J. (1995). The relationship of health locus of control and cardiac rehabilitation to mastery of illness-related stress. *Journal of Advanced Nursing, 22*(2), 294–299.

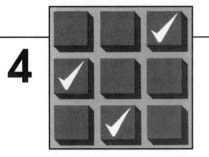

4

Introduction to Qualitative Research

Qualitative research is a way to gain insights through discovering meanings. However, these insights are obtained not through establishing causality but through improving our comprehension of the whole. Within a holistic framework, qualitative research is a means of exploring the depth, richness, and complexity inherent in phenomena. The insights from this process can guide nursing practice and aid in the important process of theory development for building nursing knowledge (Schwartz-Barcott & Kim, 1986).

Qualitative studies are beginning to appear more frequently in journals and books. Comprehension of these research methodologies is necessary in order to critique the studies in publications and utilize the findings in practice. The terminology used in qualitative research and the methods of reasoning are different from those of more traditional methods and are reflections of the philosophical orientations. The specific philosophical orientations differ with each approach and direct the methodology. Although each qualitative approach is unique, there are many commonalities. To facilitate comprehension of these methodologies, the logic underlying the qualitative approach is explored, using gestalt change as a model. A general overview of the following qualitative approaches is presented: phenomenology, grounded theory, ethnography, historical, philosophical inquiry, and critical social theory.

THE LOGIC OF QUALITATIVE RESEARCH

The qualitative approaches are based on a world view which is holistic and has the following be-

liefs: (1) There is not a single reality. Reality, based on perceptions, is different for each person and changes over time. (2) What we know has meaning only within a given situation or context. The reasoning process used in qualitative research involves perceptually putting pieces together to make wholes. From this process, meaning is produced. However, because perception varies with the individual, many different meanings are possible (Munhall & Oiler, 1986). This reasoning process can be understood by exploring the formation of gestalts.

GESTALTS

The concept of *gestalt* is closely related to holism and proposes that knowledge about a particular phenomenon is organized into a cluster of linked ideas, a gestalt. A theory is a form of gestalt. If we are trying to understand something new and are offered a theory that explains it, our reaction may be "Now that makes sense" or "Oh, I see." It has "come together" for us. One disadvantage of this process is that, once we understand a phenomenon through the interpretation of a particular theory, it is difficult for us to "see" the phenomenon outside of the meaning given it by that particular theory. Therefore, in addition to giving meaning, a theory can limit meaning. "Seeing" the phenomenon from the perspective of one point of view may limit our ability to see it from another point of view. For example, because Selye's theory of stress is so familiar to us, it would be difficult to examine the phenomenon of stress without using Selye's perception.

The purpose of qualitative research is to form new gestalts, and sometimes to generate new theories. To accomplish this, the researcher has to "get outside of" any existing theories or gestalts that explain the phenomenon of interest. The mind must be open to new gestalts emerging through the abstract thinking processes of the researcher during the personal experiences of the qualitative research process.

Experiencing Gestalt Change

One qualitative researcher, Ihde (1977), has explained the process of forming a gestalt, "getting outside of" that gestalt, and developing a new gestalt in such a way that you can experience the process. According to the qualitative point of view, experiencing the process is the best way to understand it.

Ihde's extensive research has been in the area of vision. He has studied how our eyes and brain perceive an image—for example, how our eyes sometimes see one line as shorter or longer than another when the lines are actually equal in length. Ihde has associated the vision of the eye with the way we "see" mentally. Consider the concrete thinking behind sayings such as "seeing makes it real," "seeing is believing," or "I saw it with my own eyes." It is easy to generalize from seeing to the other senses (hearing, touching, smelling, tasting), or empirical ways of knowing, and from there to perception. In fact, we often use phrases such as "I see" or "I hear" to mean "I understand."

Ihde proposes that we have an initial way of perceiving (or seeing) a phenomenon that is naive and inflexible, thought to be the one and only way of seeing it that is real. But "seeing" occurs within a specific context of beliefs, which Ihde calls a natural or *sedimented view*. In other words, we see things from the perspective of a specific frame of reference, world view, or theory. This is our reality, which gives us a sense of certainty, security, and control. Ihde uses line drawings to demonstrate this sedimented view. Examine the following line drawing.

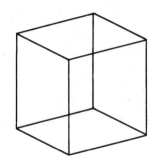

Most people who passively view this figure will see a cube. If you continue to gaze at it, you will find that the cube reverses itself. The figure actually seems to move. It jumps and then becomes fixed again in your view. With practice, you can see first one view and then the other, and then reverse it again. Ihde (1977) developed five alternative ways to view the drawing and suggests that there are more.

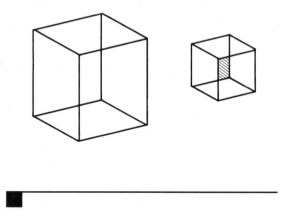

"Suppose, now, that the cube drawing is not a cube at all, but is an insect in a hexagonal opening . . . Suppose I tell you that the cube is not a cube at all, but is a very oddly cut gem. The central facet (the shaded area of the guide picture) is nearest you, and all the other facets are sloping downwards and away from it . . . Now, suppose I tell you that the gem is also reversible. Suppose you are now inside the gem, looking upwards, so that the central facet (the shaded area of the guide picture) is the one farthest away from you, and the oddly cut side facets are sloping down towards you." (pp. 96–98) ■

Ihde proposes that in order to see an alternate view of the drawing, you must first deconstruct your original sedimented view. Then you must reconstruct another view. This activity involves the use of intuition. He sees this as jumping from one gestalt to another. Try examining another line drawing. What is your sedimented view? Can you reconstruct another gestalt or view?

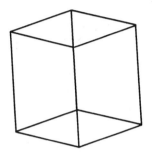

Ihde found that one of the important strategies in switching from one view of a drawing to another was to change your focus. Try focusing on a different point of the drawing or looking at it as two-dimensional rather than as three-dimensional. If you concentrate and gaze for a long enough period of time, you can experience the change in gestalt. Ihde cautions that a new reconstruction tends to be considered odd at first and unnatural, but attains stability and naturalness after a while.

Once you have accomplished this jump, you are no longer naive; you cannot go back to the idea that the phenomenon you have observed can be seen only in one way. You have become more open and receptive to experiencing the phenomenon; you can explore deeper layers of the phenomenon. Viewing these deeper layers requires a second-order deconstruction and an additional increase in openness. Ihde refers to this as *ascendance to the open context.* It allows you to see more depth and complexity within the phenomenon you examine; you have increased your capacity for insight. Ihde suggests that ascendance to the open context gives you multistability and greater control than the sedimented view.

Changing Gestalts in Nursing

Nursing has a strong traditional base. With this tradition comes a sedimented view of such phenomena as patients, illness situations, health, and nursing care and its effects. We are introduced to these sedimented views very early in our nursing experiences. Now, we are beginning to question many of these long-held ideas, and the insights gained are changing nursing practice. For example, for many years, nurses perceived the patient as being passive, dependent, and unable to take responsibility for his or her care. Now, patients are more often perceived as participating in their care and being responsible for their health. Ascendance to the open context requires more than just switching from one sedimented view to another. The nurse functioning within an open context would be able to view the patient from a variety of perspectives, passive and dependent in some ways, participating with health care givers in other ways, and directing his or her care in some cases.

Qualitative research provides a process through which we can examine a phenomenon outside of sedimented views. The earliest and perhaps most dramatic demonstration of the influence qualitative research can have on nursing practice was the 4-year study conducted by Glaser and Strauss (1965, 1968, 1971), who are credited with developing a qualitative approach referred to as grounded theory for health-related topics. This study was reported in three books, entitled *Awareness of Dying, Time for Dying,* and *Status Passage,* which described the social environment of dying patients in hospitals. At that time, the gestalt commonly held was that people could not cope with knowing that they were dying and must be protected from that knowledge. The environment of care was designed to protect the patient from that knowledge. Glaser and Strauss examined the meanings that social environment had to the patient. The study changed our gestalt. Instead of protecting, we saw the traditional care of the dying as creating loneliness and isolation. We began to "see" the patient in a new light, and our care began to change. Kubler-Ross (1969), perhaps influenced by the work of Glaser and Strauss, then began her studies of the dying, using an approach similar to that of phenomenology. From this new orientation of caring for the dying, hospice care began to develop, and now, 20 years later, the environment of care for the dying is different.

PHILOSOPHY AND QUALITATIVE RESEARCH

In qualitative research, frameworks are not used in the same sense as they are in quantitative studies since the goal is not theory testing. Nonetheless, each type of qualitative research is guided by a particular philosophical stance thought to be a paradigm. The philosophy directs the questions which are asked, the observations which are made, and the interpretation of data (Munhall, 1989). These philosophical bases and their methodologies, developed outside of nursing, will likely undergo evolutionary changes within nursing. The works of Parse (1981), Leininger (1985), Chenitz and Swanson (1984), and Artinian (1988), discussed later in the chapter, are illustrations of these changes.

RIGOR IN QUALITATIVE RESEARCH

Scientific rigor is valued because it is associated with the worth of research outcomes, and studies are critiqued as a means of judging rigor. Qualitative research methods have been criticized for lack of rigor. However, these criticisms have occurred because of attempts to judge the rigor of qualitative studies using rules developed to judge quantitative studies. Rigor needs to be defined differently for qualitative research since the desired outcome is different (Burns, 1989; Dzurec, 1989; Morse, 1989; Sandelowski, 1986). In quantitative research, rigor is reflected in narrowness, conciseness, and objectivity and leads to rigid adherence to research designs and precise statistical analyses. Rigor in qualitative research is associated with openness, scrupulous adherence to a philosophical

perspective, thoroughness in collecting data, and consideration of all of the data in the subjective theory development phase. Evaluation of the rigor of a qualitative study is based, in part, on the logic of the emerging theory and the clarity with which it sheds light on the studied phenomenon.

In order to be rigorous in conducting qualitative research, the researcher must ascend to an open context and be willing to continue to let go of sedimented views (*deconstructing*). Maintaining openness requires discipline. The researcher will be examining many dimensions of the area being studied and forming new ideas (*reconstructing*) while continuing to recognize that the present reconstructing is only one of many possible ways of organizing data. Lack of rigor in qualitative research is due to problems such as inconsistency in adhering to the philosophy of the approach being used, the failure to "get away from" older ideas, poorly developed methods, inadequate time spent collecting data, poor observations, failure to give careful consideration to all the data obtained, and inadequacy of theoretical development from the data.

APPROACHES TO QUALITATIVE RESEARCH

Six approaches to qualitative research being used in nursing are presented here: phenomenological, grounded theory, ethnographic, historical, philosophical inquiry, and critical social theory. In some ways, these approaches are very different. Ethnography and historical research are broad and are the accepted methodology for a discipline. Critical social theory is narrow in focus and controversial in its philosophical perspective. The world view of phenomenology is also controversial. However, in each method, the purpose is to examine meaning. The unit of analysis is words rather than numerical values.

Although the data are gathered using an open context, this does not mean that the interpretation is value-free. Each approach is based on a philosophical orientation that influences the interpretation of the data. Thus, it is critical to understand the philosophy on which the method is based. Each approach is discussed in relation to the philosophical orientation, nursing knowledge, and a brief overview of research methodology. Data collection strategies and the process of qualitative data analysis are described in more detail in Chapter 20. A list of published studies using each approach is provided in the student study guide.

PHENOMENOLOGICAL RESEARCH

Phenomenology is both a philosophy and a research method. The purpose of phenomenological research is to describe experiences as they are lived—in phenomenological terms, to capture the "lived experience" of study participants. The philosophers from which phenomenology emerged include Husserl, Kierkegaard, Heidegger, Marcel, Sartre, and Merleau-Ponty (Boyd, 1993a; Munhall, 1989). The philosophical positions taken by phenomenological researchers are very different from those common in nursing's culture and research traditions and thus are difficult to understand. However, discussions of this philosophical stance, appearing more frequently in the nursing literature, are introducing a broader audience to these ideas (Anderson, 1989; Beck, 1994; Boyd, 1993b; Leonard, 1989; Munhall, 1989; Salsberry, Smith, & Boyd, 1989; Walters, 1995).

Philosophical Orientation

Phenomenologists view the person as integral with the environment. The world is shaped by the self and also shapes the self. At this point, however, phenomenologists diverge in their beliefs. Heideggerian phenomenologists believe that the person is a self within a body. Thus, the person is referred to as *embodied*. "Our bodies provide the possibility for the concrete actions of self in the world" (Leonard, 1989, p. 48). The person has a world which is "the meaningful set of relationships, practices, and language that we have by virtue of being born into a culture" (Leonard, 1989, p. 43). The person is *situated* as a consequence of being

shaped by his or her world and thus is constrained in the ability to establish meanings by language, culture, history, purposes, and values. Thus the person has only *situated* freedom, not total freedom. A person's world is so pervasive that generally it is not noticed unless some disruption occurs. Not only is the world of each person different, but each person's concerns are qualitatively different. The body, the world, and the concerns, unique to each person, are the *context* within which that person can be understood. Husserlian phenomenologists believe that while self and world are mutually shaping, it is possible to bracket oneself from one's beliefs, to see the world firsthand in a naive way.

Heideggerians believe that the person experiences *being* within the framework of time. This is referred to as *being-in-time*. The past and the future influence the now, and thus are part of being-in-time (Leonard, 1989). All phenomenologists agree that there is not a single reality; each individual has his or her own reality. Reality is considered subjective; thus, an experience is considered unique to the individual. This is considered true even of the researcher's experiences in collecting data for a study and analyzing the data. "Truth is an interpretation of some phenomenon; the more shared that interpretation is, the more factual it seems to be, yet it remains temporal and cultural" (Munhall, 1989).

Methodology

The broad question that phenomenologists ask is "What is the meaning of one's lived experience?" Being a person is self-interpreting, therefore the only reliable source of information to answer this question is the person. Understanding human behavior or experience requires that the person interpret the action or experience for the researcher, and then the researcher must interpret the explanation provided by the person.

Developing Research Questions

The first step in conducting a phenomenological study is to identify the phenomenon to be explored. Next, the researcher will develop a research question. Two factors need to be considered in developing the research question: "(1) What are the necessary and sufficient constituents of this feeling or experience? (2) What does the existence of this feeling or experience indicate concerning the nature of the human being?" (Omery, 1983, p. 55).

Sampling

After developing the research question, the researcher identifies sources of the phenomenon being studied and from these sources seeks individuals who are willing to describe their experience(s) with the phenomenon in question. These individuals must understand and be willing to express inner feelings and describe the physiologic experiences that occur with the feelings.

Data Collection and Analysis

Data are collected through a variety of means: observation, interactive interviews, videotape, and written descriptions by subjects. Analysis begins when the first data are collected and will guide decisions related to further data collection. The meanings attached to the data are expressed within the phenomenological philosophy. The outcome of analysis is a theoretical statement responding to the research question. The statement is validated by examples of the data—often direct quotes from the subjects.

Nursing Knowledge and Phenomenology

Phenomenology is the philosophical base for three nursing theories: Parse's (1981) theory of man-living-health, Paterson and Zderad's (1976) theory of humanistic nursing, and Watson's (1985) theory of caring. By virtue of the assumptions of her theory, Parse states that the only acceptable method of testing her theory is through qualitative research (Parse, 1981, 1990). Parse (1990) states that any qualitative method—phenomenological, ethnographic, exploratory, or case method—can be used since all of these methods are consistent with phenomenological theory. She has also developed a man-living-health research methodology (Parse, 1987, 1995) which "includes the processes of dialogical engagement (researcher-person dialogues), extraction-synthesis (transforming the data across levels of abstraction to the level of science), and heuristic interpretation (specifying the findings in the light of the man-living-health theory and integrating them into the language of the theory)" (Parse, 1990, p. 140). A number of the published phenomenological nursing studies are based on her theory. Parse (1990) sees these studies as clarifying or substantiating her theory.

The meaning of grieving for families living with AIDS was the focus of a study by Cody (1995) using Parse's research method. Cody videotaped dialogue with ten diverse families living with AIDS. The researcher then constructed narratives of the grieving experiences of each family. One family consisted of Alice—age 43, Joe, who lived with Alice, a daughter Hannah—age 13, a son—age 8, who did not participate in the discussion, an adult son and a grandchild. Alice received a diagnosis of AIDS after a yearlong complicated illness. The following narrative was extracted from the family discussion.

"During her illness, Alice felt life leaving her; she had lost her self; she felt empty, unable to share, and hopeless. She was ready to die and 'death was warm and fuzzy.' Joe felt anger and helplessness that nothing could relieve her suffering. Hannah didn't want to leave her mother for fear she would die. Alice was angry when she got better; it was like 'being played with by God.' Now she misses the way the family used to be, but, with hope renewed, she is grateful for every moment she can share with her family; it is not always pleasant, but comfortable and good. Joe appreciates day-to-day things and special happenings more but worries whether he'll be there to guide his kids. Hannah is calmer now and thinks about her feelings more. She's not sure of anything, knowing that anybody could get sick and die but says, 'I'm mostly afraid for my Mom.' Alice felt like a burden and not a mother to her children, but with no energy there

was nothing she could do. Joe would never have walked away; 'in a situation like that you need help,' but this is something she has to do all alone. The others are not in the same mode, don't feel as strongly as she does. (Events) bring her to sudden tears and anger, and the others just back off. Joe doesn't deal much with pain. Alice says he feels nothing while she feels everything. Hannah tries to do everything right so her Mom will be happy, but she forgets. She only thinks about it a few minutes at a time unless she has to. They tease and joke even in talk of conflicts and dying. In the short time they have on earth, it's best to laugh; it doesn't hurt as much if you do. Alice was going to see her grandchild by autumn no matter what, but now she has to say, 'If there's any way possible.' She doesn't put her dreams into later but lives them now. Joe says they 'just take small bites of the future and nibble on them.' AIDS took away freedom of expression and action, and they are all cautious now, but that changes the focus from dying of AIDS to living with HIV. Alice cries at times because she can't be what she hopes to be. But with attention to what's most important, there is 'more freedom and unburdening' than she's ever experienced. Since Alice found out she had AIDS, she's thought a lot about her (deceased) Mama. She wants to know that Hannah has that same feeling when she's gone, so Alice strives to make memories that will last a long time." (Cody, 1995, p. 107)
(Used with permission of *Nursing Science Quarterly* 8[3], 1995, 107.) ∎

Through dwelling with the narrative, Cody extracted essences and synthesized a proposition. The essences and proposition for Alice, Joe, and Hannah are shown in Table 4–1 (on p. 74). Using the essences and propositions from each of the ten families, Cody integrated the findings to generate the structure of grieving for these families as shown in Table 4–2 (on p. 74).

This study provides insights useful to nursing practice that could not be obtained using quantitative methodologies. It leads us to ask questions we would not have asked within the more traditional research orientation. In a sense, knowledge generated using Parse's methodology redefines the potential of nursing's body of knowledge. References for published phenomenological studies can be found in the appendices of your student study guide.

GROUNDED THEORY RESEARCH

Grounded theory is an inductive research technique developed for health-related topics by Glaser and Strauss (1967). It emerged from the discipline of sociology. The term *grounded* means that the theory developed from the research is "grounded" or has its roots in the data from which it was derived.

Philosophical Orientation

Grounded theory is based on symbolic interaction theory, which holds many views in common with phenomenology. George Herbert Mead (1934), a social psychologist, was a leader in the development of symbolic interaction theory. Symbolic interaction theory explores how people define reality and how their beliefs are related to their actions. Reality is created by people through attaching meanings to situations. Meaning is expressed in terms of symbols such as words, religious objects, and clothing. These symbolic meanings are the basis for actions and interactions. Unfortunately, symbolic meanings are different for each individual. We cannot completely know the symbolic meanings of another individual. In social life, meanings are shared by groups. These shared meanings are communicated to new members through socialization processes. Group life is based on consensus and shared meanings. Interaction may lead to redefinition and new meanings and can result in the redefinition of self. Because of its theoretical importance, the interaction is the focus of observation in grounded theory research (Chenitz & Swanson, 1986).

Grounded theory has been used most frequently in studying areas in which little previous research has been conducted and in gaining a new viewpoint in familiar areas of research. However, because of the basic quality of theory generated through this methodology, further theory testing is not usually needed to enhance usefulness.

Methodology

The steps of grounded theory research occur simultaneously. The researcher will be observing,

Table 4-1
Alice, Joe, and Hannah

Essences—Participants' Language	Essences—Researcher's Language
1. Alice felt life leaving her empty and she welcomed death, while Joe felt helpless and got angry, and Hannah lived in fear. Alice misses the way things were but is grateful to share today with Joe, who worries about their future, and with Hannah as she explores her feelings.	1. Struggling together through harrowing personal agony confirms endearment.
2. Alice feels everything deeply while Joe and Hannah sometimes back off and keep quiet. Joe is committed to stay, and Hannah tries to make Alice happy as they tease and laugh so it doesn't hurt as much.	2. Bearing witness uncovers aloneness with togetherness in pulses of divulging-hiding and ease-unease.
3. Alice has to live her dreams now and plan on an if-possible basis. In living with HIV they lost some freedom but shifted the focus from dying of AIDS. Alice cries over unrealizable hopes, yet attention to what's important brings freedom and unburdening as she strives to make lasting memories with Hannah.	3. Opportunities and limitations emerging with ambiguity evolve new perspectives.

Proposition

For Alice, Joe, and Hannah, grieving is struggling together through harrowing personal agony confirming endearment as bearing witness uncovers aloneness with togetherness in pulses of divulging-hiding and ease-unease while opportunities and limitations emerging with ambiguity evolve new perspectives.

From "The Lived Experience of Grieving, for Families Living With AIDS," by W. K. Cody. In R. R. Parse (Ed.), *Illuminations: The human becoming theory in practice and research* (p. 213), 1995. New York: National League for Nursing. Table taken from *Nursing Science Quarterly, 8*(3), 1995, p. 107, with permission.

Table 4-2
Heuristic Interpretation

For the ten participant families living with AIDS, the structure of grieving is:		
Structure	*Structural Integration*	*Conceptual Interpretation*
easing-intensifying with the flux of change	pushing-resisting with diverse rhythms	powering
through bearing witness to aloneness with togetherness	of communion-solitude	the connecting-separating
as possibilities emerge with ambiguity	evolving with certainty-uncertainty	in originating
confirming realms of endearment.	through honoring the treasured.	valuing.

From "The Lived Experience of Grieving, for Families Living With AIDS," by W. K. Cody. In R. R. Parse (Ed.), *Illuminations: The human becoming theory in practice and research* (p. 220), 1995. New York: National League for Nursing. Table taken from *Nursing Science Quarterly, 8*(3), 1995, p. 110, with permission.

collecting data, organizing data, and forming theory from the data at the same time. An important methodological technique in grounded theory research is the constant comparative process in which every piece of data is compared with every other piece. The methodological techniques used in grounded theory research are explained in depth in a book by Glaser (1978) entitled *Theoretical Sensitivity.* More recently, Chenitz and Swanson (1986) published an excellent book, *From Practice to Grounded Theory: Qualitative Research in Nursing,* which can serve as a useful guide to the nurse researcher wishing to initiate a grounded theory study.

Data Collection and Analysis Techniques

Data may be collected by interview, observation, records, or a combination of these. Data collection usually results in large amounts of handwritten notes and/or typed interview transcripts that contain multiple pieces of data to be sorted and analyzed. This process is initiated by coding and categorizing the data.

Outcomes

The outcome is a theory explaining the phenomenon under study. The research report presents the theory supported by examples from the data. The literature review and numerical results are not used in the report. The report tends to be narrative discussions of the study process and findings.

Nursing Knowledge and Grounded Theory

Artinian (1988) has identified four qualitative modes of nursing inquiry within grounded theory, each used for different purposes: descriptive mode, discovery mode, emergent fit mode, and intervention mode. The descriptive mode provides rich detail and must precede all other modes. This mode, ideal for the beginning researcher, answers such questions as what is going on? How are activities

organized? What roles are evident? What are the steps in a process? What does a patient do in a particular setting? The discovery mode leads to the identification of patterns in life experiences of individuals and relates the patterns to each other. Through this mode, a theory of social process, referred to as substantive theory, is developed that explains a particular social world. The emergent fit mode is used when substantive theory has been developed in order to extend or refine this existing theory. This mode enables the researcher to focus on a selected portion of the theory, to build on previous work, or to establish a research program around a particular social process. The intervention mode is used to test the relationships in the substantive theory. The fundamental question for this mode is, How can I make something happen in such a way as to bring about new and desired states of affairs? This mode demands deep involvement on the part of the researcher/practitioner.

Pollack (1995), with funding from an American Nurses' Foundation grant, conducted a study that developed a grounded theory of strategies of information seeking and self-management by participants with bipolar disorder despite barriers they encountered throughout the process. Twenty women and thirteen men were interviewed. In-depth tape recorded interviews were conducted using an outline "constructed to elicit the participants' perceptions of their everyday life context as it related to informational search and need, and their self-management informational needs and activities" (p. 123). A sample question was "Can you help me to understand what actions, if any, you have taken to get information about the self-management of your bipolar disorder?" An excerpt from one of the interviews follows.

"Interviewer: So what you're saying is that denial is something that can crop up at various times throughout the whole cycle?

Participant: Not even meaning to deny you have the disorder, or that you have problems; you know you have problems, but you're thinking, 'well, these situations I've heard about and talked about, they don't fit.' 'Cause like me, I don't go out drinking and I talk to manic people who do go out drinking and heavily, and I'm thinking, 'well, I'm not manic depressive because I don't do things like that, but I know I am because the doctors tell me I am.' So you do fight with denial." (Pollack, 1995, p. 124) ■

The data obtained through the interviews were subjected to the constant comparative method of analysis, examining differences and similarities. The topologies that emerged where presented to the participants for verification. Then a theoretical model emerging from the topologies was presented to the participants for further verification. Participants' critiques and suggestions for revision were incorporated into the emerging theory until the participants were satisfied that the model (shown in Figure 4–1) was an accurate, ideal depiction of the phenomenon being studied.

As can be seen from the study described, grounded theory research examines a much broader scope of dimensions than is usually possi-

ble with quantitative research. The findings can be intuitively verified by the experiences of the reader. The clear, cohesive description of the phenomenon can allow greater understanding and, thus, more control of nursing practice. References for published grounded theory studies can be found in the appendices of your student study guide.

ETHNOGRAPHIC RESEARCH

Ethnographic research provides a mechanism for studying our own culture and that of others. The word ethnographic means "portrait of a people." Although ethnography originated as the research methodology for the discipline of anthropology, it is now a part of the cultural research conducted by a number of other disciplines including social psychology, sociology, political science, education, and nursing and is used in feminist research. Although all ethnography focuses on culture, not all cultural research is, or needs to be, ethnography. Ethnography describes and analyzes aspects

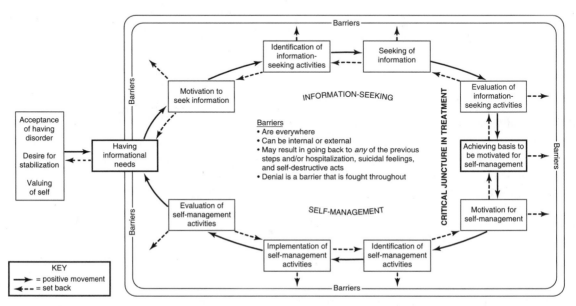

Figure 4–1
Conceptualization of striving for stability with bipolar disorder (From Pollack, L. E. [1995]. Striving for stability with bipolar disorder despite barriers. *Archives of Psychiatric Nursing, 9*[3], 125, with permission).

of the ways of life of particular cultures, subcultures, or subculture groups. Ethnographic studies result in theories of culture. Ethnography has been associated with studies of primitive, foreign, or remote cultures. This enabled the researcher to acquire new perspectives beyond his or her own ethnocentric perspective. Today, the emphasis has shifted to obtaining cultural knowledge within one's own society (Germain, 1993).

Philosophical Orientation

Anthropology, which began about the same time as the nursing discipline did, in the mid-nineteenth century, seeks to understand people: their ways of living, ways of believing, and ways of adapting to changing environmental circumstances. The philosophical base for anthropology has not been spelled out clearly, is in evolution, and needs considerable refinement (Sanday, 1983). Culture, the most central concept, is defined by Leininger (1970, pp. 48–49), a nurse anthropologist, as "a way of life belonging to a designated group of people . . . a blueprint for living which guides a particular group's thoughts, actions, and sentiments . . . all the accumulated ways a group of people solve problems, which are reflected in the people's language, dress, food, and a number of accumulated traditions and customs." The purpose of anthropological research is to describe a culture through examining these various cultural characteristics.

Anthropologists study the origin of people, their past ways of living, and their ways of surviving through time. These insights increase our ability to predict the future directions of cultures and the forces that guide their destiny, or they may provide opportunities to influence the direction of cultural development (Leininger, 1970). There are many cultural aspects of our own society that need to be understood in order to address issues related to health. Germain (1993, p. 238) points out that "cultures and subcultures in American society may be found in rural and urban ethnic and racial enclaves; nonethnic groups such as those located in prisons and bars; complex organizations; factories; the social institutions such as nursing homes, hospitals, or shelters for the homeless or the abused; community-based groups of various types such as street gangs, motorcycle gangs, and teenage groups such as jocks and skinheads; religious communities; and disciplines such as nursing and medicine. Thus, for example, nursing is a professional culture, a hospital is a sociocultural institution, and a unit of a hospital can be viewed as a subculture."

A number of dimensions of culture are of interest within anthropology. Material culture consists of all man-made objects associated with a given group. Ethnoscience ethnography focuses on the ideas, beliefs, and knowledge that a group holds that are expressed in language, and may address aspects such as symbolic referents, the network of social relations, and the beliefs reflected in social and political institutions. Cultures also have ideals which the people hold as desirable, even though they do not always live up to these standards. A relatively new approach, referred to as cognitive anthropology, holds the view that culture is an adaptive system that is in the minds of people, and is expressed in the language or semantic system of the group. Studies from this perspective will examine observable patterns of behavior, customs, and ways of life. Anthropologists seek to discover the many parts of a whole culture and how these parts are interrelated, so that a picture of the wholeness of the culture evolves. Ethnographic research is used in nursing not just to increase ethnic cultural awareness, but to enhance the provision of quality health care for all cultures (Germain, 1993; Leininger, 1970).

Methodology

There are two basic research approaches in anthropology, emic and etic. The *emic approach* to research involves studying behaviors from within the culture. The *etic approach* involves studying behaviors from outside the culture and examining similarities and differences across cultures. The steps of ethnographic research include the following: (1) identification of the culture to be studied, (2) identifying the significant variables within the culture, (3) literature review, (4) gaining entrance,

(5) cultural immersion, (6) acquiring informants, (7) gathering data (elicitation procedures), (8) analysis of data, (9) description of the culture, and (10) theory development.

Literature Review

The purpose of a literature review in ethnographic research is to provide background for the study. The researcher is seeking a broad general understanding of the variables to be considered in a specific culture or subculture.

Data Collection and Analysis

Data collection involves primarily observation and interview. The researcher may become a participant/observer in the culture through which he or she "becomes a part of the subculture being studied by physical association with the people in their setting during a period of fieldwork. . . . The researcher learns from informants the meanings they attach to their activities, events, behaviors, knowledge, rituals, and other aspects of their lifestyle" (Germain, 1993, p. 238). Analysis involves identifying the meanings attributed to objects and events by members of the culture. These meanings are often validated by members of the culture before finalizing the results.

Nursing Knowledge and Ethnography

A group of nurse scientists, lead by Madeleine Leininger, have developed a strategy of ethnonursing research, which emerged from Leininger's theory of transcultural nursing (Leininger, 1985, 1990, 1991). *Ethnonursing research* "focuses mainly on observing and documenting interactions with people of how these daily life conditions and patterns are influencing human care, health, and nursing care practices" (Leininger, 1985, p. 238). Munet-Vilero (1988) identifies three problems related to the use of ethnographic methodology by nurses. First, nurse researchers may not be sufficiently familiar with the cultural mores of the people being studied or their language. Second, studies sometimes use measures which are assumed, inaccurately, to be equivalent across cultures. Third, interpretation of findings may be inadequate due to the limited knowledge of the culture being studied. These concerns should be carefully considered by nurse researchers planning ethnographic studies.

Killion (1995) conducted an ethnographic study of homeless pregnant women in Southern California using participant observation over a 3-year period.

"The researcher 'buddied' with 15 homeless pregnant women from five different shelters. The time spent with each woman varied from several weeks to more than 1 year. The researcher spent time with the women in the shelters and accompanied them to the emergency department, the housing authority, the welfare office, and health clinics and while grocery shopping, apartment hunting, and job hunting. This intense social interaction with the women in their own milieu allowed the researcher to witness the homeless experience through the eyes of the women. . . . The researcher interacted with scores of other homeless pregnant women who served as informants through health education classes taught by the researcher at some of the shelters and through informal, unstructured interviews in various settings. In addition, shelter operators and directors, landlords, social workers, nurses, physicians, housing officials, and family members or significant others of the sample members were interviewed. Finally, general and focused observations were made of shelters, neighborhoods, and agencies frequented by the participants so that the intimacy of daily routine activities could be explored against the backdrop of the wider realm of community life." (Killion, 1995, p. 45)

"The women conceived because of victimization; dependent, abusive relationships; lack of access to contraceptives; the need for closeness and intimacy; cessation of menses resulting in uncertainty about fertility; and a sense that pregnancy was their only source of joy and gave them hope for the future. None had consistent prenatal care and were limited in means to relieve the discomforts of pregnancy. Common problems were difficulty finding places to void resulting in urinary tract infections, vaginal discharge resulting in difficulties staying dry and clean, morning sickness, and maintaining an adequate diet. During the last trimester, the women continued to look for a permanent living space and for other services even though they were exhausted. 'They did not want their infant born in a shelter, in unfamiliar surroundings among strangers' (Killion, 1995, p. 50). The mood swings of pregnancy were exacerbated by the struggle to survive day by day, complicated in some women by mental illness or substance abuse. Some women slipped deeper into substance abuse 'to escape their predicament and deal with their pain.'" (Killion, 1995, p. 50)

"The women went to great lengths to conceal their extreme poverty and homelessness. In health care settings they attempted to present an image of normalcy and avoided situations that would be stigmatizing, embarrassing, or cause them more shame. . . . The women were convinced that they risked having their children taken away. On health care entry or admissions forms, the women often gave erroneous addresses. Some nurses and physicians . . . who recognized seriously impoverished women and knew or suspected that they were homeless . . . 'turned their heads the other way.' They rationalized that the care they provided ended in the clinic or hospital, and they felt absolved of any responsibility once the woman left or was discharged. The combined effect of concealment on the part of the women and denial on the part of the health care provider led to a kind of collusion that promoted nonaction. The homeless pregnant woman unknowingly became a participant in her own neglect and consequently was not identified. Her living conditions were not acknowledged and her special health needs not adequately addressed. . . . However, in some instances, when the woman revealed her homeless status, the professional who managed her care shifted between being controlling and protective. Also, the health care professional's notions about why a woman was homeless (or simply the fact that she was homeless) seemingly guided the extent to which the woman was deemed worthy or unworthy of certain services and quality of care." (Killion, 1995, p. 52)

(Killion, C. M. [1995]. Special health care needs of homeless pregnant women. *Advances in Nursing Science, 18*[2], 44–56. Copyright © 1995 Aspen Publishers, Inc., with permission.) ■

The author concludes with extensive recommendations for addressing the care needs of pregnant homeless women.

Studies such as this provide insights that can be used in many clinical situations. Reading this type of study can lead the nurse to ask different questions about patients and their behavior. References for published ethnographic studies can be found in the appendices of your student study guide.

HISTORICAL RESEARCH

Historiography examines events of the past. Many historians believe that the greatest value of historical knowledge is an increased self-understanding, in addition to increasing nurses' understanding of their profession.

Philosophical Orientation

History is a very old science that dates back to the beginnings of humankind. The primary question of history is "Where have we come from, who are we, where are we going?" Although the questions do not change, the answers do. The most ancient form of history is the myth. The myth explains origins and gives justification to the order of existence. In the myth, past, present, and future are not distinguishable. Myths, a form of storytelling, provide an image of and legitimize the existing order. History then moved beyond the myth to the chronicling of events such as great deeds, victories, and stories about peoples and citizens. These descriptions blurred the distinction between the real and the ideal. Historians then moved to comparing histories, selecting histories based on values, and identifying patterns of regularity and change. More recently, there has been a move to interpretive history, an effort to make sense out of it, to search for meaning. This may be accomplished by concept development, by explaining causality through theory development, and by generalizing to other events and other times. Miller (1967, p. xxxi) suggests that "History is an estimate of the past from the standpoint of the present." Looking at history from the present, historians may see their role as that of patriots, as judges and censors of morals, or as detached observers. The values contained in each of these roles are reflected in the nature of the historical interpretation.

Philosophers found that understanding mankind as a historical phenomenon held out the promise of understanding the essence of mankind. To this extent, the development of a historical method was of interest to philosophy (Pflug, 1971). The initial philosophy of history and an associated research methodology were developed by Voltaire (Sakmann, 1971). His strategy was to look at general lines of development rather than an indiscriminate presentation of details, the common practice of historians of his period. Using this strategy, he moved history from chronicling to critical analysis. Voltaire recognized that in history there can be no certainty, but he searched for criteria by which historical truth could be ascertained.

One of the assumptions of historical philosophy is that "there is nothing new under the sun." Because of this assumption, the historian can search throughout history for generalizations. For example, the question can be asked: "What causes wars?" The historian could search throughout history for commonalities, and develop a theoretical explanation of the causes of wars. The questions asked, the factors that the historian selects to look for throughout history, and the nature of the explanation are all based on a world view (Heller, 1982).

Another assumption of historical philosophy is that one can learn from the past. The philosophy of history is a search for wisdom with the historian examining what has been, what is, and what ought to be. Historical philosophers have attempted to identify a developmental scheme for history, to explain all events and structures as elements of the same social process. Heller (1982) identifies three developmental schemes found in philosophies of history: (1) History reflects progression—the development from "lower" to "higher" stages; (2) history has a tendency to regress—development is from "higher" stages to "lower" stages; movement is toward a decrease in freedom and

the self-destruction of our species; and (3) history shows a repetition of developmental sequences in which patterns of progression and regression can be seen.

Fitzpatrick (1993, p. 361) suggests that "there is usually a tendency to justify historical research in professional fields like nursing from the standpoint of its helping to inform future decisions and to avoid repeating past mistakes. Such arguments have only slight merit because they serve a reductionist belief that historical facts can be distilled with a formula. History, although its goal is the establishment of fact that leads us to truth, cannot be reduced to statistical proof."

Nursing Knowledge and Historiography

Christy (1978, p. 9) asks "How can we in nursing today possibly plan where we are going when we don't know where we have been nor how we got here?" One criterion of a profession is that there is a knowledge of the history of the profession that is transmitted to those entering the profession. Until recently, historical nursing research has not been a valued activity and few nurse researchers had the skills or desire to conduct it. Therefore, our knowledge of our past is sketchy. However, there is now a growing interest in the field of historical nursing research. Sarnecky (1990) suggests that the increased interest in historiography is related to the move from a total focus on logical positivism to a broader perspective that is fully supportive of the type of knowledge provided by historical research.

Methodology

The methodology of historical research includes the following components: formulating an idea, developing research questions, developing an inventory of sources, clarifying validity and reliability of data, developing a research outline, and conducting data collection and analysis.

Formulating an Idea

The first step in historical research is selecting a topic. The following are some appropriate topics for historical research.

"Origins, epochs, events treated as units; movements, trends, patterns over stated periods; history of specific agencies or institutions; broad studies of the development of needs for specialized types of nursing; biographies and portrayals of the nurse in literature, art, or drama." (Newton, 1965, p. 20) ■

As with many types of research, the initial ideas for historical research tend to be broad. Initial ideas must be clearly defined and narrowed to a topic that is precisely defined so that the time required to search for related materials is realistic. In addition to narrowing the topic, it is often important to limit the historical period to be studied. Limiting this time period requires a knowledge of the broader social, political, and economic factors that would have an impact on the topic under study.

The researcher may spend much time extensively reading related literature before a final decision is made about the precise topic. Waring (1978) conducted her doctoral dissertation using historical research to examine the idea of the nurse experiencing a "calling" to practice nursing. She described the extensive process of developing a precise topic.

"Originally my idea was to pursue concepts in the area of Puritan social thought and to relate concepts such as altruism and self-sacrifice to nursing. Two years after the formulation of this first idea, I finally realized that the topic was too broad. Reaching that point was slow and arduous but quite essential to the development of my thinking and the prospectus that developed as an outcome.

When I first began the process, it seemed that I might have to abandon the topic 'calling.' Now, since the clarification and tightening up of my title and the clarification of my study thesis, I open volumes fearing that I will find yet another reference, once overlooked. It is only recently that I have become convinced that there was a

needle in the haystack and that I had indeed found it." (Waring, 1978, pp. 18–19) ■

In historical research, there frequently is no problem statement. Rather than define the research topic in a problem statement, it is usually expressed in the title of the study. For example, Waring's title was: "American Nursing and the Concept of the Calling."

Developing Research Questions

After the topic has been clearly defined, the researcher will identify the questions to be examined during the research process. These questions tend to be more general and analytical than those found in quantitative studies. Evans (1978), then a doctoral student, describes the research questions she developed for her historical study.

"I propose to study the nursing student. Who was this living person inside the uniform? Where did she come from? What were her experiences as a nursing student? I use the word 'experience' in terms of the dictionary definition of 'living through.' What did she live through? What happened to her and how did she respond, or react, as the case may be? What was her educational program like? We have a pretty good notion of what nurse educators and others thought about the educational program, but what about it from the students' point of view?

What were the functions of rituals and rites of passage such as bed check, morning inspection, and capping?

What kind of person did the nursing student tend to become in order to successfully negotiate studenthood? What are the implications of this in terms of her own personal and professional development and the development of the profession at large?" (Evans, 1978, p. 16) ■

Developing an Inventory of Sources

The next step is to determine whether sources of data for the study exist and are available. Many

Table 4-3
Sources of Archival Data for Historical Nursing Studies

The American Journal of Nursing Company
Bellevue Hospital
Boston University, Mugar Memorial Library
Columbia University
Hampton University
Johns Hopkins University
Massachusetts General Hospital, The Palmer-Davis Library
The Museum of Nursing History, Inc.
National Archives
National League for Nursing, National Library of Medicine
New York Hospital—Cornell Medical Center
New York Public Library, Manuscript Division
New York State Nurses' Association Library
Rockefeller Archive Center
Schlesinger Library at Radcliffe College
Simmons College
Sophia Smith Women's History Archive at Smith College in
   Massachusetts
Stanford University, Lane Medical Library
State University of New York at Buffalo
University of California at San Francisco
University of Illinois
University of Pennsylvania
University of Texas at Austin
University of Wisconsin—Milwaukee
Yale University

of the materials for historical research are contained within private archives in libraries or are privately owned. One must obtain written permission to gain access to library archives. Private materials are often difficult to ferret out, and, when discovered, access may again be a problem. However, Sorensen (1988) feels that the primary problem is the lack of experience of nurse researchers with the use of archival data. Sorensen (1988) and Fairman (1987) have identified the major sources of archival data for historical nursing studies (see Table 4–3).

Historical materials in nursing, such as letters, memos, handwritten materials, and mementos of significant leaders in nursing, are being discarded because no one recognizes their value. The same is true of materials related to the history of institutions and agencies within which nursing has been involved. Christy (1978, p. 9) states: "It seems obvious that interest in the preservation of historical materials will only be stimulated if there is a con-

comitant interest in the value of historical research." Sometimes when such material is found, it is in such poor condition that much of the data are unclear or completely lost. Christy describes one of her experiences in searching for historical data.

"M. Adelaide Nutting and Isabel M. Stewart are two of the greatest leaders we have ever had, and their friends, acquaintances, and former students were persons of tremendous importance to developments in nursing and nursing education throughout the world. Since both of these women were historians, they saved letters, clippings, manuscripts—primary source materials of inestimable value. Their friends were from many walks of life: physicians, lawyers, social workers, philanthropists—supporters and nonsupporters of nursing and nursing interests. Miss Nutting and Miss Stewart crammed these documents into boxes, files, and whatever other receptacles were available and—unfortunately—some of these materials are this very day in those same old boxes.

When I began my research into the Archives in 1966, the files were broken, rusty, and dilapidated. Many of the folders were so old and ill-tended that they fell apart in my hands, the ancient paper crumbled into dust before my eyes. My research was exhilaratingly stimulating, and appallingly depressing at the same time; stimulating due to the gold mine of data available, and depressing as I realized the lack of care provided for such priceless materials. In addition, there was little or no organization, and one had to go through each document, in each drawer, in each file, piece by piece . . . . The boxes and cartons were worse, for materials bearing absolutely no relationship to each other were simply piled, willy-nilly, one atop the other. Is it any wonder that it took me eighteen months of solid work to get through them?" (1978, pp. 8–9) ■

Currently, most historical nursing research has focused on nursing leaders. However, Noel (1988) suggests that "women in general are woefully underrepresented in the biographical form" (p. 107). She suggests that worthy nurses are those controversial figures who have influenced broad segments of their cultures, although any life well told can help the reader understand and value the individual and his or her contributions. She suggests two prerequisites for selecting a subject: "the biographers' interest, affinity, or fatal fascination for the subject (living or dead) . . . and the existence and availability of data" (p. 107). Life histories can provide insight into the lives of significant nursing figures. Gathering data for life histories involves collecting stories and interpretations told by the individual being studied. This method allows the individuals to present their views of their life in their own words. Life histories have been viewed with skepticism because findings are difficult to verify, results are vague, and generalization is very limited. In-depth repeated interviews longitudinally overcome some of these drawbacks but selective memory of the subject can be problematic. Triangulation of data collection methods and verification with other sources reduce this limitation (Admi, 1995).

Rosenberg (1987) has identified eight areas which are important to examine from a nursing history perspective: (1) history from below—the life of ordinary men and women in nursing, (2) gender and the professions, (3) knowledge and authority, (4) the role of technology, (5) the new institutional history, (6) the hospital as problematic, (7) the nurse as worker, and (8) history as meaning.

There seems to have been no examination of historical patterns of nursing practice. Since so much of nursing knowledge has been transmitted verbally or by role-modeling, we as nurses may lose much of the understanding of our roots unless studies are initiated to record them. We have no clear picture of how nursing practice has changed over the years (e.g., when, how, and for what reasons have nursing care patterns changed for individuals experiencing diabetes, cardiovascular disease, surgery, or stroke?). Changes in nursing procedures such as bed baths, enemas, and the feeding of patients could be examined. Procedure manuals, policy books, and nurses' notes in patient charts are useful sources for examining changes in nursing practice.

Some possible research questions might include:

1. Which nursing practice changes were due to medical actions and which were nursing innovations?
2. What factors in nursing influence changes in nursing practice?
3. What are the time patterns for changes in practice?
4. Have the time patterns for changes in practice remained fairly consistent, or have they changed over the history of nursing?
5. What has been the influence of levels of education (LVN, ADN, Diploma, BSN) on nursing practice?
6. What has been the influence of advanced nursing roles (Clinical Nurse Specialist, Nurse Practitioner, Administrator) on nursing practice?
7. How has the quality of nursing care changed over the decade? century?

This type of information might provide increased insight into future directions for nursing practice, research, and theory development. However, if quality historical research is to be conducted, those of us in the process of making history must accept responsibility for preserving the sources. References for published historical studies can be found in the appendices of your student study guide.

PHILOSOPHICAL INQUIRY

Philosophy is not generally thought of as a discipline within which one conducts research since philosophy is not a science. But philosophy does have strong links with science. Most importantly, philosophy guides the methods within any given science. It is the foundation of science. Furthermore, philosophy is used to develop theories about science and to debate issues related to science. The purpose of philosophical inquiry is to perform research using intellectual analyses to clarify meanings, make values manifest, identify ethics, and study the nature of knowledge (Ellis, 1983).

Philosophical Orientation

The philosophical researcher considers an idea or issue from all perspectives through an extensive exploration of the literature, examining conceptual meaning, raising questions, proposing answers, and suggesting the implications of those answers. The research is guided by philosophical questions that have been posed. As with other qualitative approaches, data collection occurs simultaneously with analysis, and focuses on words. However, because philosophy attends to ideas, meaning, and abstractions, the content the researcher seeks may be implied rather than clearly stated in the literature. It may be necessary for the researcher to come to some conclusions about what the author meant in a specific text. Ideas, questions, answers, and consequences are often explored and/or debated with colleagues during the analysis phase. The process is cyclical, with answers generating further questions, leading to further analysis. Therefore, the thoughtful posing of questions is considered more important than the answers.

To avoid bias in their analysis, philosophers cultivate detachment from any particular type of knowledge or method. Published reports of philosophical inquiries do not describe the methodology used but focus on discussing the conclusions of the analyses. There are three categories of philosophical inquiry: foundational inquiry, philosophical analyses, and ethical analyses.

Foundational Inquiry

The foundations of a science are its philosophical bases, concepts, and theories. A new science tends to borrow elements from the foundations of other sciences, although sometimes they are a poor fit. Even those developed within the science may have problems such as logical inconsistencies. Foundational inquiries examine the foundations for a science. The studies provide analyses of the structure of a science, and the process of thinking about and valuing certain phenomena held in common by the science. They are important to perform prior to theory development or developing programs of research. The debates related to qualitative and quantitative research methods and triangulation of methods emerge from foundational inquiries.

Nursing Knowledge and Foundational Inquiry

Philosophical analyses are expected to be carried out by scientists within a particular field, such as nursing, rather than by philosophers as such. What is recommended is that the nurse scientist desiring to perform a philosophical study seek consultation with a philosopher. An example of a foundational analysis is presented in Chapter 20.

Purposes

The purposes for a foundational study include:

1. Compare different philosophical bases, different theories, and different definitions of concepts.
2. Seek common meanings in radically different theories.
3. Critically examine operational definitions of concepts.
4. Explore the relationship between the concept and the science being examined.
5. Define the boundaries of a specific science by showing what phenomena belong to the field and what do not (boundary delineation).
6. Assist in the development of programs of research capable of shaping the empirical content of the field.
7. Draw attention to differences in ways of exploring, explaining, proving, and valuing.
8. Explain the rational or thoughtful consequences of choosing various ways to investigate phenomena.
9. Analyze the reasoning that underlies the science.
10. Describe productive reasoning activities from which the science may develop methods for conducting foundational inquiries as well as conceiving, planning, executing, and monitoring its programs of research.

Questions

Because philosophical questions are critical to the process of philosophical inquiry, the formation of questions of concern to the discipline is important. Ellis (1983) identified the following questions that need to be addressed in nursing from the perspective of philosophical inquiry: "What does it mean to be human? What is the meaning of dignity? What does it mean to be compassionate, humane, and caring? What is nursing? . . . What views of humans are appropriate, for what purpose, and for what questions?" (pp. 212, 224)

Philosophical Analysis

The primary purpose of philosophical analysis is to examine meaning and to develop theories of meaning. This is usually accomplished through concept analysis or linguistic analysis (Rodgers, 1989). In some cases, attempts are made to reconcile apparently different concepts. These analyses clarify the language of a science and use multiple concepts and their relationships to organize the phenomena of a science. Clarification of the process of theory development and the criteria for critiquing theories emerges from philosophical inquiry and is referred to as metatheory.

Critiques of these analyses are conducted to determine completeness, meaning, and an explanation of scientific significance. These analyses provide descriptions of the meaning of a word as it is used in theoretical models and in research programs using those models. Linguistic analysis requires an examination of the occasions, intentions, and practical consequences of using certain words relevant to the science. This includes their function when applied to various research problems in different sciences; their operational definitions; the kinds of research methods they dictate; their relationship to the theoretical goals and values of the science in which they function; and most important, their possible relationship to the idea of nursing science (Manchester, 1986).

Nursing Knowledge and Philosophical Analysis

Ellis (1983) suggests that many of the "nursing theories" are actually philosophies of nursing even though they were not developed using the method of philosophical analysis. These philosophies of nursing were developed to express the essence of nursing and the desired goals of nursing. They are statements of the way nursing ought to be. Concept analyses are strengthening our nursing theories and providing conceptual definitions for our research. An example of a concept analysis using the methods of philosophical analysis is presented in Chapter 20.

Ethical Inquiry

Ethics is the branch of philosophy that deals with morality. This discipline contains a set of propositions for the intellectual analysis of morality. The problems of ethics relate to obligation, rights, duty, right and wrong, conscience, justice, choice, intention, and responsibility. Ethics is a means of striving for rational ends when others are involved. The desirable rational ends are justice, generosity, trust, faithfulness, love, and friendship. All of these reflect respect for the other person. An ethical dilemma occurs when one must choose between conflicting values. In some cases, both choices are good and in other cases, neither choice is good but one must choose even so (Steele & Harmon, 1983).

Methodology

In ethical inquiry, the researcher identifies principles to guide conduct based on ethical theories. The research methodology is similar to other philosophical inquiries. The literature related to the problem is thoroughly examined. Using a selected ethical theory, an analysis is performed. The actions prescribed by the analysis may vary with the ethical theory used. The ideas are submitted to colleagues for critique and debate. Their conclusions reflect judgments of value which are prescriptive in nature. They are associated with rights and duties rather than preferences.

Nursing Knowledge and Ethics

Curtin (1979), a nurse ethicist, claims that the goals of nursing are not scientific, they are moral and seek good. To her, nursing is not a science;

it is an art. Scientific knowledge is used as a tool in the artful practice of nursing (Curtin, 1990). As such, ethical inquiry is a research method required to clarify the means and ends of nursing practice. Much of the ethical analyses in the nursing literature addresses three issues: combining the roles of nurse and scientist, the protection of human subjects, and peer and institutional review (Gortner, 1985). An example of a study using ethical inquiry is presented in Chapter 20. References for published philosophical studies can be found in the appendices of your student study guide.

CRITICAL SOCIAL THEORY

In recent years, another philosophy with a unique qualitative research methodology, critical social theory, has begun to appear in nursing journals. Feminist research, which is gaining increasing interest in nursing, uses critical social theory methods and could be considered a subset of critical social theory (Chinn & Wheeler, 1985; MacPherson, 1983). Allen (1985) suggests that critical social theory is important to nursing because nurses need to "be as conscious as possible about the constraints operating on both nurse and client" (p. 62). She also suggests that the way nurses define health, promote health, and define themselves as nurses is governed by factors explored within this philosophy (Allen, 1986).

Philosophical Orientation

Critical social theory contains the views of a number of philosophers, with its beginnings in Frankfurt, Germany, at the Institute for Social Research. In the 1920s and 1930s, critical social theory was influenced by the writings of Karl Marx. These philosophers, who contend that social phenomena must be examined within a historical context, believe that most societies function based on closed systems of thought that lead to patterns of domination and prevent personal growth of individuals within the society.

In the late 1960s, a second generation of German philosophers, the most prominent being

Habermas (1971), revised critical social theory, leading to a resurgence of interest in these ideas. Habermas sees the task of critical social theory as understanding how people communicate and how they develop symbolic meanings. Many of these meanings occur within a fact world (doxa) in which the "facts" of the society are taken for granted, not discussed, and not disputed. The established political order is perceived not as one possible order among others, but rather as self-evident, as going without saying, and as such, is unquestioned. The legitimacy and power of this fact world come from not recognizing that the established order is only one possible way of constructing reality. These tacit beliefs become visible and objectively real when someone challenges their legitimacy. Following this recognition comes the insight that the established order is maintained by power relations, or relations of domination that usually are not recognized or seen through (Thompson, 1987).

Using the defined research methodology to analyze these processes, the researcher can "uncover the distortions and constraints that impede free, equal, and uncoerced participation in society" (Stevens, 1989, p. 58). Habermas believes that researchers have a responsibility not only to study and identify constraining social, political, and economic circumstances in society, but also to be instrumental in the liberation from oppressive structures in order to facilitate the quest for human potential, completion, and authenticity (Stevens, 1989).

The structures of society that are of interest include kinds of work and wages; family; access to education; images of women, African Americans, Latinos, and gays; availability of health care; the profit motive; the distribution of wealth; and law enforcement. Within such structures, the researcher focuses on issues of privilege, exploitation, powerlessness, oppression, and liberation. To accomplish this, the researcher needs to construct a picture of society that exposes the prevailing system of domination, express the contradictions embedded in the domination, assess society's potential for emancipatory change, and criticize the system in order to promote that change (Stevens,

1989). An example of a study using critical social theory methods is presented in Chapter 20.

Friere's Theory of Cultural Action

Friere (1972), a Brazilian educator, used critical social theory methodology to develop a theory of cultural action through his experiences in attacking illiteracy in his country. Friere's theory is beginning to attract the interest of nurse researchers. Friere sees the world not as a static and closed order, but as a problem to be worked on and solved. He is convinced that every human being, no matter how "ignorant" or submerged in the "culture of silence," is capable of looking critically at the world in a dialogical encounter with others. "Provided with the proper tools for such an encounter, he can gradually perceive his personal and social reality as well as the contradictions in it, become conscious of his own perception of that reality, and deal critically with it" (Shaull, 1972, p. 12).

"Dialogue cannot exist, however, in the absence of a profound love for the world and for men" (Friere, 1972, p. 77). Redefining the world is an act of creation and is not possible if it is not infused with love.

"Love is an act of courage, not of fear, love is commitment to other men . . . If I do not love the world—if I do not love life—if I do not love men—I cannot enter into dialogue. On the other hand, dialogue cannot exist without humility . . . How can I dialogue if I always project ignorance onto others and never perceive my own? How can I dialogue if I regard myself as a case apart from other men? . . . Dialogue further requires an intense faith in man, faith in his power to make and remake, to create and re-create, faith in his vocation to be more fully human." (Friere, 1979, pp. 78–79) ■

A peasant can facilitate this process for his neighbor more effectively than a teacher brought in from outside (Shaull, 1972).

In his book *Pedagogy of the Oppressed,* Friere (1972) describes oppressed group behavior and the behavior of the oppressors. He describes an act of oppression as any act that prevents a person from being more fully human. He believes that both the oppressed and the oppressor must be liberated. If not, the liberated oppressed will simply become oppressors because both oppressors and oppressed fear freedom, autonomy, and responsibility. However, a person cannot be liberated by others, but must liberate himself or herself. Friere sees the fight against oppression as an act of love.

Friere points out that education can be a tool of conformity to present social situations or an instrument of liberation. He advocates working with groups, which leads to cultural synthesis, rather than trying to manipulate groups, which leads to cultural invasion. In a true educational experience, both teacher and student learn, and all grow as a consequence. This type of education is the practice of freedom. Friere's ideas are currently being applied to nursing situations.

Feminist research is considered by some to emerge from critical social theory. However, feminist researchers use a broad range of research methodologies—both qualitative and quantitative. A philosophical foundation and a defined methodology have not yet been broadly accepted by feminist researchers. Sigsworth (1995, p. 897), based on Harding (1987), suggests the following methodological conditions for feminist research:

1. Feminist research should be based on women's experiences, and the validity of women's perceptions as the "truth" for them should be recognized.
2. Artificial dichotomies and sharp boundaries are suspect in research involving women and other human beings. They should be carefully scrutinized as reflecting a logical positivist approach to research.
3. The context and relationship of phenomena, such as history and concurrent events, should always be considered in designing, conducting, and interpreting research.
4. Researchers should recognize that the questions asked are at least as important as the answers obtained.

5. Researchers should address questions that women want answered (i.e., the research should be for women).

6. The researcher's point of view (i.e., biases, background, and ethnic and social class) should be treated as part of the data. This involves ensuring that the researcher is on a plane with the person being researched.

References for published critical social theory studies can be found in the appendices of your student study guide.

SUMMARY

Although the writings of qualitative researchers began to appear in nursing journals occasionally in the 1970s, it was not until the mid to late 1980s that these works were published with any regularity. The concepts and methods of reasoning are very different from those of quantitative research. Some major concepts important to qualitative research include gestalt, sedimented view, and open context. A gestalt is a way of viewing the world that is closely related to holism. This view proposes that knowledge about a particular phenomenon is organized into a cluster of linked ideas. It is this clustering and interrelatedness that provides meaning. A gestalt is in some ways like a theory. A sedimented view is seeing things within a specific gestalt, frame of reference, or world view. This gives a sense of reality, certainty, and, seemingly, control. A sedimented view is a naive and inflexible way of perceiving a phenomenon. The opposite of a sedimented view is an open context. An open context requires deconstruction of the sedimented view, which allows you to see the depth and complexity within the phenomenon being examined. Ihde's work is used as a way of experiencing the jump from a sedimented view to an open context.

The conduct of qualitative research requires the rigorous implementation of qualitative research techniques such as openness, scrupulous adherence to a philosophical perspective, thoroughness in collecting data, and inclusion of all the data in the theory development phase.

Six approaches to qualitative research are described in this chapter: phenomenological, grounded theory, ethnographic, historical, philosophical inquiry, and critical social theory. The goal of phenomenological research is to describe experiences as they are lived. Grounded theory is an approach for discovering what problems exist in a social scene and how the persons involved handle them. The research process involves formulation, testing, and redevelopment of propositions until a theory is developed. Ethnographic research is the investigation of cultures through an in-depth study of the members of the culture. The ethnographic research process is the systematic collection, description, and analysis of data to develop a theory of cultural behavior. Historical research is a narrative description or analysis of events that occurred in the remote or recent past. The data of past events are obtained from records, artifacts, or verbal reports. Philosophical inquiry includes three types: foundational studies, philosophical analysis, and ethical analysis. Foundational inquiry provides analyses of the structures of a science, such as concepts and theories, and the process of thinking about and valuing certain phenomena held in common by the science. Philosophical analyses are used to examine conceptual meaning and develop theories of meaning. Ethical inquiry is intellectual analyses of morality. Critical social theory involves analysis of systems of thought which lead to patterns of domination and prevent personal growth of individuals within a society.

References

Admi, H. (1995). The life history: A viable approach to nursing research. *Nursing Research, 44*(3), 186–188.

Allen, D. G. (1985). Nursing research and social control: Alternative models of science that emphasize understanding and emancipation. *Image: The Journal of Nursing Scholarship, 17*(2), 58–64.

Allen, D. G. (1986). Using philosophical and historical methodologies to understand the concept of health. In P. L. Chinn (Ed.), *Nursing research methodology: Issues and implementation* (pp. 157–168). Rockville, MD: Aspen.

Anderson, J. M. (1989). The phenomenological perspective. In J. M. Morse (Ed.), *Qualitative nursing research: A contemporary dialogue* (pp. 15–26). Rockville, MD: Aspen.

Artinian, B. A. (1988). Qualitative modes of inquiry. *Western Journal of Nursing Research, 10*(2), 138–149.

Beck, C. T. (1994). Phenomenology: Its use in nursing research. *International Journal of Nursing Studies, 31*(6), 499–510.

Boyd, C. O. (1993a). Philosophical foundations of qualitative research. In P. Munhall and C. O. Boyd (Eds.), *Nursing research: A qualitative perspective,* 2nd ed., pp. 66–93. New York: National League for Nursing Press.

Boyd, C. O. (1993b). Phenomenology: The method. In P. Munhall and C. O. Boyd (Eds.), *Nursing research: A qualitative perspective,* 2nd ed., pp. 99–132. New York: National League for Nursing Press.

Burns, N. (1989). Standards for qualitative research. *Nursing Science Quarterly, 2*(1), 44–52.

Chenitz, W. C., & Swanson, J. M. (1984). Surfacing nursing process: A method for generating nursing theory from practice. *Journal of Advanced Nursing, 9*(7), 205–215.

Chenitz, W. C., & Swanson, J. M. (1986). *From practice to grounded theory: Qualitative research in nursing.* Menlo Park, CA: Addison-Wesley.

Chinn, P. L., & Wheeler, C. E. (1985). Feminism and nursing. *Nursing Outlook, 33*(2), 74–77.

Christy, T. E. (1978). The hope of history. In M. L. Fitzpatrick (Ed.), *Historical studies in nursing* (pp. 3–11). New York: Teachers College.

Cody, W. K. (1995). The meaning of grieving for families living with AIDS. *Nursing Science Quarterly, 8*(3), 104–114.

Curtin, L. L. (1979). The nurse as advocate: A philosophical foundation for nursing. *Advances in Nursing Science, 1*(3), 1–10.

Curtin, L. L. (1990). Integrating practice with philosophy, theory and methods of inquiry. *Proceedings: Symposium on knowledge development: I. Establishing the linkages between philosophy, theory, methods of inquiry and practice, September 6–9, 1990.* University of Rhode Island College of Nursing.

Dzurec, L. C. (1989). The necessity and evolution of multiple paradigms for nursing research. *Advances in Nursing Science, 11*(4), 69–77.

Ellis, R. (1983). Philosophic inquiry. In H. H. Werley & J. J. Fitzpatrick (Eds.), *Annual review of nursing research* (Vol. I, pp. 211–228). New York: Springer.

Evans, J. C. (1978). Formulating an idea. In M. L. Fitzpatrick (Ed.), *Historical studies in nursing* (pp. 15–17). New York: Teachers College.

Fairman, J. A. (1987). Sources and references for research in nursing history. *Nursing Research, 36*(1), 56–59.

Fitzpatrick, M. L. (1993). Historical research: The method. In P. Munhall & C. O. Boyd (Eds.), *Nursing research: A qualitative perspective,* 2nd ed., pp. 359–371. New York: National League for Nursing Press.

Friere, P. (1972). *Pedagogy of the oppressed* (trans. M. B. Ramos). New York: Herder and Herder.

Germain, C. P. (1993). Ethnography: The method. In P. Munhall & C. O. Boyd (Eds.), *Nursing research: A qualitative perspective,* 2nd ed., pp. 237–268. New York: National League for Nursing Press.

Glaser, B. G. (1978). *Theoretical sensitivity.* Mill Valley, CA: The Sociology Press.

Glaser, B. G., & Strauss, A. (1965). *Awareness of dying.* Chicago: Aldine.

Glaser, B. G., & Strauss, A. (1967). *The discovery of grounded theory: Strategies for qualitative research.* Chicago: Aldine.

Glaser, B. G., & Strauss, A. (1968). *Time for dying.* Chicago: Aldine.

Glaser, B. G., & Strauss, A. (1971). *Status passage.* London: Routledge & Kegan Paul.

Gortner, S. R. (1985). Ethical inquiry. In H. H. Werley & J. J. Fitzpatrick (Eds.), *Annual review of nursing research* (Vol. 3, pp. 193–214). New York: Springer.

Habermas, J. (1971). *Knowledge and human interests* (trans. J. J. Shapiro). Boston: Beacon.

Harding, S. (1987). *Feminism and methodology.* Indiana: Open University Press.

Heller, A. (1982). *A theory of history.* London: Routledge & Kegan Paul.

Ihde, D. (1977). *Experimental phenomenology: An introduction.* New York: Putnam.

Killion, C. M. (1995). Special health care needs of homeless pregnant women. *Advances in Nursing Science, 18*(2), 44–56.

Kubler-Ross, E. (1969). *On death and dying.* New York: Macmillan.

Leininger, M. M. (1970). *Nursing and anthropology: Two worlds to blend.* New York: Wiley.

Leininger, M. M. (1985). *Qualitative research methods in nursing.* Orlando, FL: Grune & Stratton.

Leininger, M. M. (1990). Ethnomethods: The philosophic and epistemic basis to explicate transcultural nursing knowledge. *Journal of Transcultural Nursing, 1*(2), 40–51.

Leininger, M. M. (1991). *Ethnonursing: A research method with enablers to study the theory of culture care.* NLN Publication (15–2402): 73–117.

Leonard, V. W. (1989). A Heideggerian phenomenologic perspective on the concept of the person. *Advances in Nursing Science, 11*(4), 40–55.

MacPherson, K. I. (1983). Feminist methods: A new paradigm for nursing research. *Advances in Nursing Science, 5*(2), 17–25.

Manchester, P. (1986). Analytic philosophy and foundational inquiry: The method. In P. L. Munhall & C. J. Oiler (Eds.), *Nursing research: A qualitative perspective* (pp. 229–249). Norwalk, CT: Appleton-Century-Crofts.

Mead, G. H. (1934). *Mind, self and society.* Chicago: University of Chicago.

Miller, P. S. (1967) Introduction. In M. A. Fitzsimons, A. G.

Pundt, & C. E. Nowell (Eds.), *The development of historiography* (pp. xxv–xxxii). Port Washington, NY: Kennikat.

Morse, J. M. (1989). Qualitative nursing research: A free-for-all? In J. M. Morse (Ed.), *Qualitative nursing research: A contemporary dialogue* (pp. 14–22). Rockville, MD: Aspen.

Munet-Vilaro, F. (1988). The challenge of cross-cultural nursing research. *Western Journal of Nursing Research, 10*(1), 112–116.

Munhall, P. L. (1989). Philosophical ponderings on qualitative research methods in nursing. *Nursing Science Quarterly, 2*(1), 20–28.

Munhall, P. L., & Oiler, C. J. (1986). *Nursing research: A qualitative perspective.* Norwalk, CT: Appleton-Century-Crofts.

Newton, M. E. (1965). The case for historical research. *Nursing Research, 14*(1), 20–26.

Noel, N. L. (1988). Historiography: Biography of "Women Worthies" in nursing history. *Western Journal of Nursing Research, 10*(1), 106–108.

Omery, A. (1983). Phenomenology: A method for nursing research. *Advances in Nursing Science, 5*(2), 49–63.

Parse, R. R. (1981). *Man-living-health: A theory of nursing.* New York: Wiley.

Parse, R. R. (1987). *Nursing science: Major paradigms, theories, and critiques.* Philadelphia: Saunders.

Parse, R. R. (1990). Health: A personal commitment. *Nursing Science Quarterly, 3*(3), 136–140.

Parse, R. R. (Ed.) (1995). *Illuminations: The human becoming theory in practice and research.* New York: National League for Nursing.

Paterson, J. G., & Zderad, L. T. (1976). *Humanistic nursing.* New York: Wiley.

Pflug, G. (1971). The development of historical method in the eighteenth century. In G. Pflug, P. Sakmann, & R. Unger (Eds.), *History and theory: Studies in the philosophy of history* (pp. 1–23). Middletown, CT: Wesleyan University Press.

Pollack, L. E. (1995). Striving for stability with bipolar disorder despite barriers. *Archives of Psychiatric Nursing, 9*(3), 122–129.

Rodgers, B. L. (1989). Concepts, analysis and the development of nursing knowledge: The evolutionary cycle. *Journal of Advanced Nursing, 14*(4), 330–335.

Rosenberg, C. (1987). Clio and caring: An agenda for American historians and nursing. *Nursing Research, 36*(1), 67–68.

Sakmann, P. (1971). The problems of historical method and of philosophy of history in Voltaire [1906]. In G. Pflug, P. Sakmann, & R. Unger (Eds.), *History and theory: Studies in the philosophy of history* (pp. 24–59). Middletown, CT: Wesleyan University Press.

Salsberry, P. J., Smith, M. C., & Boyd, C. O. (1989). Dialogue on a research issue: Phenomenological research in nursing—Commentary and responses. *Nursing Science Quarterly, 2*(1), 9–19.

Sanday, P. (1983). The ethnographic paradigm(s). In J. Van Maanen (Ed.), *Qualitative methodology* (pp. 19–36). Beverly Hills, CA: Sage. (Original work published 1979, in *Administrative Science Quarterly.*)

Sandelowski, M. (1986). The problem of rigor in qualitative research. *Advances in Nursing Science, 8*(3), 27–37.

Sarnecky, M. T. (1990). Historiography: A legitimate research methodology for nursing. *Advances in Nursing Science, 12*(4), 1–10.

Schwartz-Barcott, D., & Kim, H. S. (1986). A hybrid model for concept development. In P. L. Chinn (Ed.), *Nursing research methodology: Issues and implementation* (pp. 91–101). Rockville, MD: Aspen.

Shaull, R. (1972). Foreword. In P. Friere, *Pedagogy of the oppressed* (pp. 9–15). New York: Herder and Herder.

Sigsworth, J. (1995). Feminist research: Its relevance to nursing. *Journal of Advanced Nursing, 22*(5), 896–899.

Sorensen, E. S. (1988). Historiography: Archives as sources of treasure in historical research. *Western Journal of Nursing Research, 10*(5), 666–670.

Steele, S. M., & Harmon, V. M. (1983). *Values clarification in nursing* (2nd ed.). New York: Appleton-Century-Crofts.

Stevens, P. E. (1989). A critical social reconceptualization of environment in nursing: Implications for methodology. *Advances in Nursing Science, 11*(4), 56–68.

Thompson, J. L. (1987). Critical scholarship: The critique of domination in nursing. *Advances in Nursing Science, 10*(1), 27–38.

Walters, A. J. (1995). The phenomenological movement: Implications for nursing research. *Journal of Advanced Nursing, 22*(4), 791–799.

Waring, L. M. (1978). Developing the research prospectus. In M. L. Fitzpatrick (Ed.), *Historical studies in nursing* (pp. 18–20). New York: Teachers College.

Watson, J. (1985). *Nursing: Human science and human care: A theory of nursing.* Norwalk, CT: Appleton-Century-Crofts.

II

The
Research
Process

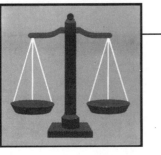

5

Research Problem and Purpose

We are constantly asking questions to gain a better understanding of ourselves and the world around us. This human ability to wonder and creatively ask questions about behaviors and situations in the world provides a basis for identifying research topics and problems. Identifying a problem is the initial, and one of the most significant, steps in conducting both quantitative and qualitative research. The research purpose evolves from the problem and provides direction for the subsequent steps of the research process.

Research topics are concepts or broad problem areas that contain numerous potential research problems. Nursing research topics focus on areas that are controlled by nursing and will influence nursing practice. Each problem provides the basis for developing many research purposes. Thus, the identification of a challenging, significant problem can direct a researcher in a lifetime of study. However, the abundance of research topics and potential problems are frequently not apparent to individuals struggling to identify their first research problem.

This chapter differentiates a research problem from a purpose, identifies sources for research problems, and provides a background for formulating a problem and purpose. The criteria for determining the feasibility of a study are also examined. The chapter concludes with examples of quantitative and qualitative research topics, problems, and purposes.

WHAT IS A RESEARCH PROBLEM AND PURPOSE?

A *research problem* is a "situation in need of a solution, improvement, or alteration" (Adebo,

1974, p. 53) or "a discrepancy between the way things are and the way they ought to be" (Diers, 1979, p. 12). Problematic situations and discrepancies in nursing practice stimulate interest and prompt the development of research problems. A research problem can be identified by asking questions such as: What is wrong or is of concern in this situation? Where are the discrepancies in this situation? What is known and not known about this situation? What information is needed to improve this situation? Will a particular intervention work in a clinical situation? Would another intervention be more effective? What changes need to be made to improve this intervention? Through questioning and a review of the literature, a research problem emerges that includes a specific area of concern and the knowledge gap that surrounds this concern. The knowledge gap related to a clinical problem determines the complexity and number of studies that need to be conducted to generate essential knowledge for clinical practice (Martin, 1994). Leske (1995) studied the effects of intraoperative progress reports on anxiety levels of surgical patients' family members and identified the following research problem.

"Surgery is an anxiety-producing situation for family members, especially during the time the patient is in the operating room (Kathol, 1984; Silva, Geary, Manning, & Zeccolo, 1984). Researchers suggest that families want to be involved in the care of their ill member (Raleigh, Lepczyk, & Rowley, 1990; Sigsbee & Geden, 1990), but a high level of anxiety can hamper such care. In addition, family members' anxiety may be transferred to the patient (Frederickson, 1989). Patients are being discharged "sooner and sicker" to the responsibility of their family members, and families require information about how to provide the needed postoperative care. If anxiety levels are too high, family members are not likely to make effective use of information provided by staff or to ask appropriate questions (Reider, 1994). Providing intraoperative progress reports appears to be a beneficial nursing intervention to reduce family members' anxiety (Leske, 1992). However, it remains unclear whether information provided by intraoperative progress reports or attention from a supportive person actually reduces family member anxiety." (p. 169) ■

In this example, the first six sentences identify the area of concern and provide background and significance for this concern. The last sentence indicates the knowledge gap or what is not known regarding this clinical problem. In this research problem, the area of concern is "interventions that decrease intraoperative anxiety levels" and the particular population of interest is surgical patients' family members. Problem statements include concepts such as anxiety-producing situation, anxiety, and nursing intervention identified in this example. The concept of interventions is abstract and a variety of nursing actions could be implemented to determine their effects on anxiety. Thus, each problem provides the basis for generating a variety of research purposes. The knowledge gap regarding the use of interventions, such as progress reports and attention from a supportive person to reduce family members' anxiety also directs the formulation of the purpose.

The *research purpose* is a concise, clear statement of the specific goal or aim of the study. The goal of a study might be to identify, describe, explain, or predict a solution to a clinical problem (Beckingham, 1974). The purpose usually indicates the type of study to be conducted and often includes the variables, population, and setting for the study. Every study has an explicit or implicit purpose statement. Leske (1995) explicitly stated the following purpose for her study.

"The purpose of this study was to examine the effects of current standards of care, intraoperative progress reports, and attention on family member ratings of anxiety during elective surgical procedures." (p. 169) ■

The goal of this study was to examine the effects of standard care, intraoperative progress reports, and attention from a supportive person on levels of anxiety as measured by state-anxiety scores, mean arterial pressure (MAP) level, and heart rate (HR). This is a quasi-experimental study to determine the effects of two independent variables or treatments (intraoperative progress reports and attention from a supportive person) on three dependent variables or outcomes (state-anxiety scores, MAP, and HR). The outcomes of the treatments were compared with the outcomes from the family members receiving standard care (comparison group). Other research purposes could have been formulated from the problem identified by Leske that focused on different interventions (independent variables) and/or different outcomes (dependent variables).

SOURCES OF RESEARCH PROBLEMS

Research problems are developed from many sources. However, one must be curious, astute, and imaginative to use these sources effectively. Moody, Vera, Blanks, and Visscher (1989) studied the source of research ideas and found that 87% came from clinical practice, 57% from the literature, 46% from interactions with colleagues, 28% from interactions with students, and 9% from funding priorities. These findings indicated that researchers often use more than one source in identifying a research problem. The sources for research problems included in this text are (1) nursing practice, (2) researcher and peer interactions, (3) literature review, (4) theory, and (5) research priorities identified by funding agencies and specialty groups.

NURSING PRACTICE

The practice of nursing needs to be based on knowledge generated through research. Thus, clinical practice is an extremely important source for research problems (Diers, 1979; Fuller, 1982; Jennings, 1991). Problems can evolve from clinical observations, such as observing the behaviors of a patient and family in crisis and wondering what interventions a nurse might use to improve their coping. A review of patient records, care plans, and procedure manuals might reveal concerns or raise questions about practice that could be the basis for research problems. For example, what procedures should be followed in providing mouth care to cancer patients or patients with endotracheal tubes? Is a particular procedure for changing an IV dressing effective? What nursing action will facilitate communication with a patient who has had a stroke? What is the impact of home visits on level of function, readjustment to the home environment, and rehospitalization pattern? What is the most effective treatment for hypertension?

Some students and nurses keep logs or journals of their practice that contain research ideas (Artinian & Anderson, 1980). They might record their experiences, thoughts, and observations of others. Analysis of these logs often reveals patterns and trends in a setting and facilitates the identification of patient care concerns. Some concerns might include: Why is emotional and spiritual care given less time and attention than physical care? Do the priority needs perceived by the patient direct the care received? What is the involvement of family members in patient care and how does this care delivery impact the family unit?

Questions about the effects of certain nursing interventions and the desire to improve these interventions and their outcomes have facilitated the development of many studies. For example, researchers have examined the effects of (1) a cognitive remediation intervention on the functional level of elderly with dementia of the Alzheimer's type (Quayhagen, Quayhagen, Corbeil, Roth, & Rodgers, 1995); (2) dynamic exercise on subcutaneous oxygen tension and temperature to promote wound healing (Whitney, Stotts, & Goodson, 1995);

(3) jaw relaxation and music on postoperative pain (Good, 1995); and (4) slow-stroke back massage on relaxation in hospice clients (Meek, 1993).

Nursing practice is constantly changing in response to consumer needs and trends in society. Some professional trends that have been researched include:

1. the impact of different types of nursing education (Cole, 1995; Thiele, Holloway, Murphy, Pendarvis, & Stucky, 1991);
2. the implementation of advanced nursing roles in practice, such as administrator (Ringerman, 1990; Schmieding, 1990), nurse practitioner (Lamb, 1991; Mahoney, 1994), and midwives (Brown & Grimes, 1995); and
3. the needs of chemically-dependent nurses (Trinkoff, Eaton, & Anthony, 1991).

Nurses have conducted many studies related to health trends in society, such as

1. the care of elderly patients (Glick & Swanson, 1995; Schrijnemaekers, & Haveman, 1995);
2. the care of persons with dementia (Boehm, Whall, Cosgrove, Locke, & Schlenk, 1995; McDougall, 1995);
3. the needs and care of HIV and AIDS patients (Lauver, Armstrong, Marks, & Schwarz, 1995; Rose, 1995);
4. the needs and care of chronically ill patients (Leidy & Traver, 1995; Packard, Haberman, Woods, & Yates, 1991);
5. promotion of a healthy lifestyle (Laffrey, 1990; Lusk, Kerr, & Ronis, 1995);
6. parenting and infant needs (Beck, 1995; Gross, Fogg, & Tucker, 1995; Hahn, 1995);
7. the needs and care of those experiencing sexual and physical abuse (Bradford, 1995; Brown & Garrison, 1990); and
8. health needs of different cultures (Phillips & Wilbur, 1995; Powe, 1995; Villarruel, 1995).

RESEARCHER AND PEER INTERACTIONS

Interactions with researchers and peers are valuable sources for generating research problems. Experienced researchers serve as mentors and share their knowledge with novice researchers in the identification of research topics and the formulation of problems. Nursing educators assist students in selecting research problems for theses and dissertations. When possible, students conduct studies in the same area of research as the faculty. The faculty can share their expertise regarding their research program, and the combined work of the faculty and students can build a knowledge base in a given area. This type of relationship could also be developed between an expert researcher and a nurse clinician. Some health care settings now employ nurse researchers to consult with nurses and other health professionals to identify research problems and priorities (Dennis, Howes, & Zelauskas, 1989).

Beveridge (1950) identified several reasons for discussing research ideas with others. Ideas are clarified and new ideas are generated when two or more people pool their thoughts. Interactions with others enable researchers to uncover errors in reasoning or information. These interactions are also a source of support in discouraging or difficult times. As well, another person can provide a refreshing or unique viewpoint, which prevents conditioned thinking or following an established habit of thought. A workplace that encourages interaction can stimulate nurses to identify research problems. Nursing conferences and professional organization meetings also provide excellent opportunities for nurses to discuss their ideas and brainstorm to identify potential research problems. Interactions with others are essential to broaden the perspective and knowledge base of researchers and to provide support in identifying significant research problems.

LITERATURE REVIEW

Reviewing research journals, such as *Advances in Nursing Science, Applied Nursing Research, Clinical Nursing Research, Image: Journal of Nursing Scholarship, Nursing Research, Research in Nursing & Health, Scholarly Inquiry for Nursing Practice: An International Journal*, and *Western Journal of Nursing Research*, and theses and dissertations will acquaint novice researchers with studies conducted in an area of interest. The nursing specialty journals, such as *Cancer Nursing, Dimensions of Critical Care, Heart & Lung, Journal of Obstetric, Gynecologic and Neonatal Nursing, Neurosurgical Nursing*, and *Oncology Nursing Forum* also place a high priority on publishing research findings. A literature review involves summarizing what is known and not known in an area of interest. What is not known or the gaps in the knowledge base provide direction for future research. The process of reviewing the literature is the focus of Chapter 6.

At the completion of a research project, an investigator often makes recommendations for further study. These recommendations provide opportunities for others to build upon a researcher's work and to strengthen the knowledge in a selected area. Leske (1995) examined the effects of intraoperative progress reports on anxiety levels of surgical patients' family members and made the following recommendations for further study.

"It appears that intraoperative progress reports are beneficial for family members during the waiting period, but the cost-effectiveness of such an intervention remains to be determined. Further studies that evaluate other methods of providing progress reports to family members, such as telephone calls, would be worthwhile. In addition, the beneficial effects of lowered family member anxiety on positive patient outcomes requires investigation." (pp. 172–173)

"The sample size is adequate and randomized. However, lack of pretest measures may require statistical control to examine causality about progress reports on anxiety levels, and replication is necessary. These results can be generalized only to family members of elective surgical patients. More research needs to be conducted to determine if similar results are obtained from family members of patients undergoing emergency, critical, or diagnostic surgery." (p. 173) ■

Leske (1995) provided direction for expanding her study findings using different populations and interventions and also encouraged validation of these findings through replication. In addition, this same study was a replication and extension of an earlier study (Leske, 1992).

Replication of Studies

Reviewing the literature is a way to identify a study to replicate. *Replication* involves reproducing or repeating a study to determine whether similar findings will be obtained (Taunton, 1989). Replication is essential for knowledge development since it (1) establishes the credibility of the findings, (2) extends the generalizability of the findings over a range of instances and contexts, (3) reduces the number of Type I and Type II errors, (4) provides support for theory development, and (5) decreases the acceptance of erroneous results (Beck, 1994). Some researchers replicate studies because they agree with the findings and wonder if the findings will hold up in different settings with different subjects over time. Others replicate studies because they want to challenge the findings or interpretations of prior investigators (Selltiz, Wrightsman, & Cook, 1981).

Four different types of replication are important in generating sound scientific knowledge for nursing: (1) exact, (2) approximate, (3) concurrent, and (4) systematic extension (Beck, 1994; Haller & Reynolds, 1986). An *exact,* or identical, *replication* involves duplicating the initial researcher's study to confirm the original findings. All conditions of the original study must be maintained; thus, "there must be the same observer, the same subjects, the same procedure, the same measures, the same locale, and the same time" (Haller & Reynolds, 1986, p. 250). Exact replications might be thought of as ideal to confirm original study findings but are frequently not attainable. In addition, one would not want to replicate the errors in an original study, such as small sample size, weak design, or poor quality measurement methods.

An *approximate,* or operational, *replication* involves repeating the original study under similar conditions, following the methods as closely as possible (Beck, 1994; Haller & Reynolds, 1986). The intent is to determine whether the findings from the original study hold up despite minor changes in the research conditions. If the findings generated through replication are consistent with the original study findings, these findings are more credible and have a greater probability of being an accurate reflection of the real world. If the replication fails to support the original findings, the designs and methods of both studies need to be examined for limitations and weaknesses, and further research needs to be conducted. Conflicting findings might also generate additional theoretical insights and provide new directions for research.

King and Tarsitano (1982) did an approximate replication of Lindeman and Van Aernam's (1971) study of the effects of structured and unstructured preoperative teaching. In the original study, Lindeman and Van Aernam developed the following research questions:

1. What are the effects of a structured and an unstructured preoperative teaching program upon the adult surgical patient's ability to deep breathe and cough 24 hours postoperatively?
2. What are the effects of a structured and an unstructured preoperative teaching program upon the adult surgical patient's length of hospital stay?
3. What are the effects of a structured and an unstructured preoperative teaching program upon the adult surgical patient's postoperative need for analgesia? (p. 321)

King and Tarsitano's (1982) research questions were:

1. What are the results of a structured and unstructured preoperative teaching program on the adult surgical patients' postoperative recovery as measured by pulmonary function tests?
2. What are the results of a structured and unstructured preoperative teaching program on the adult surgical patients' length of hospital stay? (p. 324)

King and Tarsitano elected to narrow the scope of the study to exclude the phenomenon of pain, as recommended by the original investigators. They also modified the measurement of respiratory function by including pulmonary function tests. They controlled the following factors that were not controlled in the original study.

"Restricting the sample to patients of three surgeons with similar techniques and to patients having lower or upper abdominal surgery. The structured preoperative teaching was conducted primarily by the principal investigator and associate and a checklist was used to indicate that the patients could perform the deep breathing, coughing and exercises." (p. 324) ■

Findings from both studies indicated that structured preoperative instruction significantly improved the ability of patients to cough and deep breathe postoperatively. Thus, the replication increased the credibility of this original finding. However, King and Tarsitano found that structured preoperative instruction did not significantly decrease the length of hospital stay, which is contradictory to the findings of Lindeman and Van Aernam. Additional research is needed to clarify the conflicting findings.

A *concurrent,* or internal, *replication* involves the collection of data for the original study and its replication simultaneously to provide a check of the reliability of the original study (Beck, 1994; Brink & Wood, 1979). The confirmation, through replication, of the original study findings is part of the original study's design. For example, a research team might collect data simultaneously at two different hospitals and compare and contrast the findings. Consistency in the findings increases the credibility and generalizability of the findings. Some expert researchers obtain funding to conduct multiple concurrent replications, in which a number of individuals are involved in the conduct of a single study but with different samples in different settings. As each study is completed, the findings are compiled in a report indicating the series of replications that were conducted to generate these findings (Brink & Wood, 1979).

A *systematic extension,* or constructive, *replication* is done under distinctly new conditions. The researchers conducting the replication do not follow the design or methods of the original researchers; rather, "the second investigative team begins with a similar problem statement but formulates new means to verify the first investigator's findings" (Haller & Reynolds, 1986, p. 250). The aim of this type of replication is to extend the findings of the original study and test the limits of generalizability.

Beck (1994) conducted a computerized and manual review of the nursing literature from 1983 through 1992 and found only 49 replication studies. Possibly, the number of replication studies is limited because replication is viewed by some as less scholarly or less important than original research. However, the lack of replication studies severely limits the use of research findings in practice and the development of a scientific knowledge base (Beck, 1994; Martin, 1995; Reynolds & Haller, 1986; Taunton, 1989). Thus, replicating a study should be respected as a legitimate scholarly activity for expert as well as novice researchers. Replication provides an excellent learning opportunity for the novice researcher to conduct a significant study, validate findings from a previous study, and generate new information from different populations and settings. Master's students could be encouraged to replicate studies for their theses, possibly to replicate faculty studies. Expert researchers could strengthen nursing knowledge with the conduct of concurrent and systematic replications.

The number of replication studies might be increased by supportive actions from journal editors, researchers, and funding agencies. Journal editors might increase the number of replications published in journals. When publishing a replication study, researchers need to indicate their study was a replication and designate the type of replication and how it was accomplished. Researchers might also identify the strengths and weaknesses of the original study and provide a rationale for the modifications made in the replication. Funding agencies might provide a higher priority for replication studies to encourage researchers to pursue this scientific activity (Beck, 1994; Martin, 1995).

Landmark studies are significant research projects that generate knowledge that influences a discipline and sometimes society. These studies are frequently replicated or are the basis for the generation of additional studies. For example, Williams (1972) studied factors that contribute to skin breakdown, and these findings provided the basis for numerous studies on the prevention and treatment of pressure ulcers. Many of these studies are summarized in the document *Pressure ulcers in adults: Prediction and prevention* published by the Agency for Health Care Policy and Research (Panel for the Prediction and Prevention of Pressure Ulcers in Adults, 1992).

THEORY

Theories are an important source for generating research problems because they set forth ideas about events and situations in the real world that require testing (Chinn & Kramer, 1991). In examining a theory, one notes that it includes a number of propositions and that each proposition is a statement of the relationship of two or more concepts. A research problem and purpose could be formulated to explore or describe a concept in a theory, such as a study to describe the concept of self-care in Orem's (1995) theory.

Propositions from a theory can also be the basis for generating research. For example, Jemmott and Jemmott (1991) applied the theory of reasoned action (Ajzen & Fishbein, 1980; Fishbein & Ajzen, 1975) in their study of condom use among black women. They identified the following proposition from the theory: "A behavioral intention is seen as determined by the attitude toward the specific behavior and the subjective norm regarding that behavior" (Jemmott & Jemmott, 1991, p. 228). The proposition was then linked to their study by stating: "Thus, a woman's intention to use condoms is a function of her attitude—positive or negative—toward using condoms and her perception of what significant others think she

should do" (Jemmott & Jemmott, 1991, p. 229). Based on this theoretical proposition, the following hypotheses were developed.

■

"First, women who express more favorable attitudes toward condoms will report stronger intentions to use condoms than will women who express less favorable attitudes. Second, women who perceive subjective norms more supportive of condom use will report stronger intentions to use condoms than will their counterparts who perceive subjective norms less supportive of condom use." (pp. 229–230) ■

Some researchers combine ideas from different theories to develop maps or models for testing through research. The map serves as the framework for the study and includes key concepts and relationships from the theories that the researcher wants to study (Chinn & Kramer, 1991). Phillips and Wilbur (1995) developed the breast cancer screening model (see Figure 5–1) to examine the breast cancer practice of African American women. Their model was based upon the health belief model (Becker, 1974), Ajzen and Fishbein's (1980) theory of reasoned action, and Cox's (1982) interaction model of client health behavior and provided a framework for their study. The purpose of the study was "to identify and compare the adherence to breast cancer screening guidelines (monthly breast self-examination [BSE], age-related mammography, and yearly professional breast exam [PBE] among African American women of different employment status" (Phillips & Wilbur, 1995, p. 261). The following questions addressed in this study show a clear relationship to the framework model:

1. To what extent do demographic characteristics (age, education, marital status), social influence (health-care provider recommendation), previous health-care experiences (personal risk factors, previous instruction in breast cancer screening) and environmental resources (income, insurance) influence adherence to breast

Element of Client Singularity

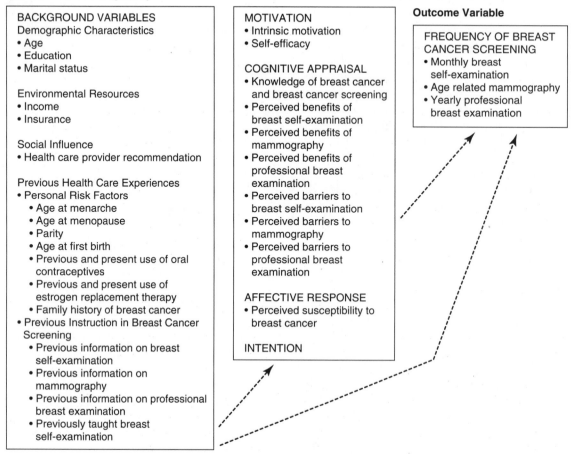

BACKGROUND VARIABLES
Demographic Characteristics
• Age
• Education
• Marital status

Environmental Resources
• Income
• Insurance

Social Influence
• Health care provider recommendation

Previous Health Care Experiences
• Personal Risk Factors
  • Age at menarche
  • Age at menopause
  • Parity
  • Age at first birth
  • Previous and present use of oral contraceptives
  • Previous and present use of estrogen replacement therapy
  • Family history of breast cancer
• Previous Instruction in Breast Cancer Screening
  • Previous information on breast self-examination
  • Previous information on mammography
  • Previous information on professional breast examination
  • Previously taught breast self-examination

MOTIVATION
• Intrinsic motivation
• Self-efficacy

COGNITIVE APPRAISAL
• Knowledge of breast cancer and breast cancer screening
• Perceived benefits of breast self-examination
• Perceived benefits of mammography
• Perceived benefits of professional breast examination
• Perceived barriers to breast self-examination
• Perceived barriers to mammography
• Perceived barriers to professional breast examination

AFFECTIVE RESPONSE
• Perceived susceptibility to breast cancer

INTENTION

Outcome Variable

FREQUENCY OF BREAST CANCER SCREENING
• Monthly breast self-examination
• Age related mammography
• Yearly professional breast examination

Figure 5–1

Phillips' (1993) breast cancer screening model, adapted with permission from Cox's (1982) Interaction model of client health behavior: Theoretical prescription for nursing. *Advances in Nursing Science 5*(1) 41–56. Copyright © 1982 Aspen Publishers, Inc. Phillips, J. M., & Wilbur, J. (1995). Adherence to breast cancer screening guidelines among African-American women of differing employment status. *Cancer Nursing, 18*(4), p. 260.

cancer screening guidelines (monthly BSE, age-related mammography, and yearly PBE)?

2. Do motivation (intrinsic motivation, BSE, self-efficacy), cognitive appraisal (knowledge of breast cancer, breast cancer screening, and benefits and barriers related to breast cancer screening), affective response (perceived susceptibility to breast cancer), and intention vary by employment status and age group?

3. How do motivation, cognitive appraisal, and intention influence adherence to breast cancer screening guidelines?

4. Which variables (demographic characteristics, social influence, previous health-care experiences, environmental resources, motivation, cognitive appraisal, and affective response) are most predictive of the adherence to breast cancer screening guidelines? (Phillips & Wilbur, 1995, p. 261)

The findings from a study either lend support to or do not support the relationships identified in the model. Phillips and Wilbur (1995, p. 268) found that "the Breast Cancer Screening Model was useful in explaining 74% of the variance in monthly BSE, 15% of the variance in age-related mammography, and 42% of the variance in yearly PBE." Thus, the relationships in this model were supported by this study.

RESEARCH PRIORITIES

Since 1975, expert researchers, specialty groups, and the National Institute for Nursing Research (NINR) have identified research priorities. Lindeman (1975, p. 434) developed an initial list of research priorities for clinical practice, which identified such priorities as "nursing interventions related to stress, care of the aged, pain, and patient education." The American Association of Critical-Care Nurses (AACN) determined initial research priorities in the early 1980s (Lewandowski & Kositsky, 1983) and revised these priorities for the 1990s (Lindquist et al., 1993). The process of identifying the research priorities for the 1990s involved three phases: (1) developing a comprehensive list of research topics, (2) surveying AACN members to determine priority topics, and (3) achieving a consensus on research priority rankings. The top clinical research priorities for critical-care nursing included:

1. Techniques to optimize pulmonary functioning and prevent pulmonary complications.
2. Weaning of mechanically ventilated patients.
3. Effect of nursing activities/interventions on hemodynamic parameters.
4. Techniques for real-time monitoring of tissue perfusion and oxygenation.
5. Nutritional support modalities and patient outcomes.
6. Interventions to prevent infection.
7. Pain assessment and pain management techniques. (Lindquist et al., 1993, p. 115)

The Council on Graduate Education for Administration in Nursing (CGEAN) conducted a 3-year study (1983–1986) to determine the research priorities for nursing administration (Henry et al., 1987). Twenty priority questions were identified and the top five questions follow.

1. What are the cost-effective components of clinical nursing care that yield high patient satisfaction, decrease number of complications, and shorten hospital stay for identified groups of patients?
2. How can nursing research in the practice setting be used to decrease cost, improve the quality of care, and increase patient and nurse satisfaction?
3. What is the relationship of patient acuity to cost of care, to nursing resource needs, and to nursing judgment of acuity?
4. How is nursing productivity measured in units of service or nursing care hours, and how does it compare with the quality of care patients receive?
5. What are the actual direct and indirect costs of providing nursing services for patients in selected intensity classifications? (Henry et al., 1987, p. 312)

The American Association of Occupational Health Nurses (AAOHN) identified research priorities for occupational health nursing. The top two priorities were "(1) the effectiveness of primary health care delivery at the worksite, and (2) effectiveness of health promotion nursing intervention strategies" (Rogers, 1989, p. 497).

In 1991, the Oncology Nursing Society (ONS) published the research priorities identified in a survey of 310 ONS members (Mooney, Ferrell, Nail, Benedict, & Haberman, 1991). The ONS members surveyed were involved in research or leadership. The top ten research topics identified were quality of life, symptom management, outcome measures, pain control and management, cancer survivorship, prevention and early detection, research utilization, cancer rehabilitation, cost containment, and economic influences.

As more health care is provided in the home, Albrecht (1992) recognized the importance of developing a list of the research priorities for home health nursing. These priorities were generated by surveying 50 experts in the field of home health and the top ten research priorities identified were (1) outcomes of care, (2) cost of home care, (3) policy analysis and reimbursement, (4) client classification systems, (5) uniform data set, (6) predictors of care/managed care, (7) coordination of care/managed care, (8) productivity, (9) documentation, and (10) use of health care services.

A major initiative of the National Institute for Nursing Research (NINR) is the development of a National Nursing Research Agenda that will involve identifying nursing research priorities, outlining a plan for implementing priority studies, and obtaining resources to support these priority projects (Hinshaw, 1988). Initially, seven broad priority areas (research topics) for nursing research were identified in 1989. The priority research topics were "(1) low birth weight: mothers and infants; (2) HIV infection: prevention and care; (3) long-term care for older adults; (4) symptom management; (5) information systems; (6) health promotion; and (7) technology dependency across the life span" (Bloch, 1990, p. 4). These topics were then refined by a Priority Expert Panel (PEP). The members of each PEP developed a report that included "(a) an assessment and critique of the state of the science; (b) the conclusions reached as a result of the review of the state of the science and the panel discussion; and (c) the panel's recommendations based on the identified scientific issues" (Bloch, 1990, p. 5).

Based on the work of the PEPs, five research priorities were selected to guide a portion of the NINR's funding from 1995 through 1999. The research priority for funding in 1995 was to develop and test community-based nursing models to promote access to, utilization of, and quality of health services by rural and other underserved populations. The funding priority for 1996 was research focused on the effectiveness of nursing interventions in HIV/AIDS, especially for individuals of different cultures and women. Cognitive impairment will be the research funding priority for 1997, with a focus on research to develop and test biobehavioral and environmental approaches to manage cognitive impairment. Living with chronic illness will be the funding priority for 1998, with a focus on research to test interventions that might increase individuals' resources in dealing with their chronic illness. In 1999, the research funding priorities will be biobehavioral factors related to immuno-competence, with research focused on identifying biobehavioral factors and testing interventions to promote immunocompetence (NINR, 1993).

Another federal agency that is having a major impact on setting research priorities for funding is the Agency for Health Care Policy and Research (AHCPR). This agency funds health services research that examines patient outcomes and the effectiveness of clinical practice (Rettig, 1990). The goals of outcomes research are to: (1) avoid adverse effects of care, (2) improve the patient's physiologic status, (3) reduce the patient's signs and symptoms, (4) improve the patient's functional status and well being, (5) achieve patient satisfaction, (6) minimize the cost of care, and (7) maximize revenues (Davies et al., 1994). Outcomes research is not a new methodology in nursing but has received limited attention over the last 25 years. Heater, Becker, and Olson (1988) conducted a meta-analysis of the studies from 1977 to 1984 that were focused on nursing interventions and patient outcomes. The researchers examined 84 studies and found that "patients who receive research-based nursing interventions can expect 28% better outcomes than 72% of the patients who receive standard care" (Heater et al., 1988, p. 303). Nurse researchers need to expand their conduct of outcomes research to increase the quality of care, improve the patient's health status, and decrease health care costs (Jennings, 1991).

FORMULATING A RESEARCH PROBLEM AND PURPOSE

Potential nursing research problems often emerge from observation of real-world situations, such as those in nursing practice (see Figure 5–2). A situation is a significant combination of circumstances that occur at a given time. Inexperienced researchers tend to want to study the entire situation, but it is far too complex for a single study. Multiple problems exist in a single situation, and each can be developed into a study. Each researcher's perceptions of what problems exist in a situation depends on that individual's clinical expertise,

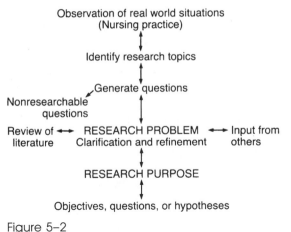

Figure 5–2
Formulating a research problem and purpose.

theoretical base, intuition, interests, and goals. Some researchers spend years developing different problem statements and new studies from the same clinical situation.

The exact thought processes used to extract problems from a situation have not been clearly identified because of the abstractness and complexity of the reasoning involved. However, the following steps appear to be used: the researcher examines the real-world situation, identifies research topics, generates questions, and ultimately clarifies and refines a research problem. From the problem, a specific goal or research purpose is developed for a study.

RESEARCH TOPICS

A nursing situation often includes a variety of research topics. Research topics are concepts or broad problem areas that provide the basis for generating questions. Some of the topics that have been investigated by nurses include coping patterns; developmental changes; teaching/learning process; health promotion; rehabilitation; emotional, psychological, and social support; and nursing interventions such as pain management, wound care, relaxation, biofeedback, oral hygiene, pulmonary hygiene, and bowel man-

agement (Lindsey, 1982, 1983). Gordon (1980) identified nursing diagnoses as research topics; example topics include self-care deficit, impaired skin integrity, ineffective family coping, and altered parenting. Outcomes research is focused on topics of health status, quality of life, cost-effectiveness, and quality of care that require examination in research. A specific outcome study might focus on a particular condition like terminal cancer and examine such outcomes as nutrition, hygiene, skin integrity, and pain control with a variety of treatments (Davies et al., 1994).

GENERATING QUESTIONS

Encountering situations in nursing stimulates the constant flow of questions. The questions fit into three categories: (1) questions answered by existing knowledge, (2) questions answered with problem solving, and (3) research-generating questions. The first two types of questions are nonresearchable and do not facilitate the formulation of research problems. Some of the questions raised have a satisfactory answer within nursing's existing body of knowledge, and these answers are available in the literature or from experts in nursing or other disciplines. For example, questions nurses have about performing some basic nursing skills, such as a protocol for taking a temperature or giving injections, are answered in the literature and procedure manuals. However, problems that focus on investigating new techniques to improve existing skills, patient responses to techniques, or ways to educate patients and families to perform techniques could add to nursing's knowledge base.

Some of the questions raised can be answered using problem solving or evaluation projects. Chapter 2 includes a comparison of the problem-solving process and the research process and indicates when and why to use each process. Many evaluation projects are conducted with minimal application of the rigor and control that are required in conducting research. These projects do not fit the criteria of research, and the findings are relevant for a particular situation. For example, quality assurance is an evaluation of client care implemented by a specific health care agency; the results of this evaluation project are usually relevant only to the agency conducting the review.

The type of question that can initiate the research process is one that requires further knowledge to answer. Some of the questions that come to mind about situations include: Is there a need to describe concepts, to know how they are related, or to be able to predict or control some event within the situation? What is known and what is not known about the concepts? What are the most urgent factors to know? Research experts have found that asking the right question is frequently more valuable than finding the solution to a problem. The solution identified in a single study might not withstand the test of time or might be useful only in a few situations. However, one well-formulated question can lead to the generation of numerous research problems, a lifetime of research activities, and possibly significant contributions to a discipline's body of knowledge.

CLARIFYING AND REFINING A RESEARCH PROBLEM

Fantasy and creativity are part of formulating a research problem, so imagine studies that could be done related to the situation. Imagine the difficulties likely to occur with each study, but avoid being too critical of potential research problems at this time. Which studies seem the most workable? Which ones appeal intuitively? Which problem is the most significant to nursing? Which study is of personal interest? Which problem has the greatest potential to provide a foundation for further research in the field? (Kahn, 1994)

The problems investigated need to have professional significance and potential or actual significance for society. A research problem is significant when it has the potential to generate or refine knowledge and/or influence nursing practice (Kahn, 1994; Rempusheski, 1990; Valiga & Mermel, 1985). Moody and colleagues (1989) surveyed nurse researchers and identified the following criteria for significant research problems: (1) focused on real world concerns (57%), (2) meth-

odologically sound (57%), (3) knowledge building (51%), (4) theory building (40%), and (5) focused on current or timely concerns (31%). The problems that are considered significant vary with time and the needs of society. The priorities identified earlier indicate some of the current, significant nursing research problems. Campbell, Daft, and Hulin (1982) indicated that the formation of a significant research problem results from extensive exposure to nursing practice and the literature; the convergence of several streams of thought and ideas; a creative, intuitive ability; and a concern with theoretical understanding and with real-world problems.

Personal interest in a problem influences the quality of the problem formulated and the study conducted. A problem of personal interest is one that an individual has pondered for a long time or one that is especially important in the individual's nursing practice or personal life. For example, a researcher who has had a mastectomy may be particularly interested in studying the emotional impact of a mastectomy or strategies for caring for mastectomy patients. This personal interest in the topic can become the driving force needed to conduct a quality study (Beveridge, 1950; Kahn, 1994).

Answering these questions regarding significance and personal interest often assists one in narrowing the number of problems. Without narrowing potential problems to only one idea, try some of the ideas out on colleagues. Let them play the devil's advocate, and explore the strengths and weaknesses of each idea. Then begin some preliminary reading in the area of interest. Examine literature related to the situation, the variables within the situation, measurement of the variables, and previous studies related to the situation. The literature review often enables one to refine the problem and clearly identify the gap in the knowledge base. As the problem statement is refined, the research purpose begins to emerge.

RESEARCH PURPOSE

The purpose is generated from the problem and clearly focuses the development of the study. In the research process, the purpose is usually stated after the problem, since the problem identifies the gap in knowledge in a selected area and the purpose clarifies the knowledge to be generated with a particular study. The research purpose needs to be stated objectively or in a way that does not reflect particular biases or values of the researcher. Researchers who do not recognize their values might include their biases in the research. This can lead them to generate the answers they want or believe to be true and might add inaccurate information to a discipline's body of knowledge (Kaplan, 1964). Based on the research purpose, specific research objectives, questions, or hypotheses are developed to direct the study (see Chapter 8).

The purpose of an outcomes research project is usually complex and requires a team of multidisciplinary health care providers to accomplish. The research team members are very cautious in the identification of a purpose that will make a significant contribution to the health care system and yet be feasible. Some possible purposes for outcomes research projects include:

1. comparing one treatment with another for effectiveness in the routine treatment of a particular condition;
2. describing in measurable terms the typical course of a chronic disease;
3. using variations in outcomes to identify opportunities for improving clinical process; and
4. developing decision support programs for use with individual patients when choosing among alternative treatment options. (Davies et al., 1994, p. 11)

EXAMPLE OF PROBLEM AND PURPOSE DEVELOPMENT

You might have observed the women receiving treatment at a psychiatric facility and noted that many were withdrawn and depressed and seemed to be unable to discuss certain events in their lives. Their progress in therapy was usually slow and they seemed to have similar physical and psychological symptoms. Often after a rapport was developed with a therapist, they would reveal that they were victims of incest as a child. This situation could lead you to identify research topics and generate searching questions. Research topics of interest include sexual abuse, childhood incest, physical and psychological symptoms of incest, history of incest, assessment of problems, and therapeutic interventions. Possible questions include: What are the physical and psychological symptoms demonstrated by someone who has experienced childhood incest? How would one assess the occurrence, frequency, and impact of rape or incest on a woman? What influences do age and duration of the abuse have on the woman's current behavior? How frequently is childhood sexual abuse a problem in the mentally disturbed adult female? What type of treatment is effective with an individual who has experienced child abuse? Questions such as these might have been raised by Brown and Garrison (1990) as they developed the following problem, purpose, and questions for their investigation.

Research Problem

"There is evidence that one in four girls and one in seven boys are sexually abused in some way prior to their 18th birthday . . . The long-term consequences of child sexual abuse makes it one of the most severe offenses against a child's dignity and sense of well-being . . . Unreported, untreated child sexual abuse results in long-term dysfunctional behavior requiring therapy (Browne & Finkelhor, 1986). Gold (1986) suggested that histories of incest are not often obtained by a systematic interviewing protocol or by specifically trained interviewers. Thus, the need for a systematic assessment tool to identify childhood incest in this high-risk population is imperative." (pp. 587–588)

Research Purpose

"The purpose of this study was to (a) identify physical and psychosocial patterns of symptomatology in adult women incest survivors, and (b) design a systematic assessment instrument to identify incest early in nonreporting adult women survivors." (p. 588)

Research Questions

1. "What patterns of physical symptoms are present in adult women incest survivors?
2. What patterns of psychosocial symptoms are present in adult women incest survivors?
3. Is there a correlation between the frequency of multiple victimization and the number of reported physical and psychosocial symptoms?
4. Is there a correlation between the age when the sexual abuse began and its duration?" (p. 588) ∎

FEASIBILITY OF A STUDY

As the research problem and purpose increase in clarity and conciseness, the researcher has greater direction in determining the feasibility of a study. The *feasibility of a study* is determined by examining the time and money commitment; the researcher's expertise; availability of subjects, facility, and equipment; cooperation of others; and the study's ethical considerations (Kahn, 1994; Rogers, 1987).

TIME COMMITMENT

Conducting research frequently takes more time than is anticipated, which makes it difficult for any researcher, especially the novice researcher, to estimate the time that will be involved. In estimating the time commitment, the researcher examines the purpose of the study; the more complex the purpose, the greater the time commitment. An approximation of the time needed to complete a study can be determined by assessing the following factors: (1) the type and number of subjects needed, (2) number and complexity of the variables to be studied, (3) methods for measuring the variables (are instruments available to measure the variables or must they be developed?), (4) methods for collecting data, and (5) the data analysis process. An often overlooked time commitment is

the writing of the research report for presentation and publication. The researcher must approximate the time needed to complete each step of the research process and must determine whether the study is feasible.

Most researchers propose a designated time period or set a specific deadline for their project. For example, an agency might set a 2-year deadline for studying the turnover rate of staff. The researcher needs to determine whether the identified purpose can be accomplished by the designated deadline; if not, the purpose could be narrowed or the deadline extended. Researchers are often cautious about extending deadlines, because a research project could continue for many years. The individual interested in conducting qualitative research frequently must make an extensive time commitment of years. Chapter 15 includes a discussion of the time commitment in research. Time is as important as money, and the cost of a study can be greatly affected by the time required to conduct it.

MONEY COMMITMENT

The problem and purpose selected are influenced by the amount of money available to the researcher. Potential sources for funding should be considered at the time the problem and purpose are identified. The cost of a research project can range from a few dollars for a student's small study (Holmstrom & Burgess, 1982) to hundreds of thousands of dollars for complex projects. In estimating the cost of a research project, the following questions need to be considered:

1. **Literature.** What will the review of the literature—including computer searches, copying articles, and purchasing books—cost?
2. **Subjects.** Will the subjects have to be paid for their participation in the study?
3. **Equipment.** What will the equipment cost for the study? Can the equipment be borrowed, rented, bought, or obtained through donation? Is the equipment available, or will it have to

be built? What type of maintenance will be required of the equipment during the study? What will the measurement instruments cost?

4. **Personnel.** Will assistants and/or consultants be hired to collect, computerize, and analyze the data and assist with the data interpretation? Will clerical help be needed to type and distribute the report and prepare a manuscript for publication?

5. **Computer time.** Will computer time be required to analyze the data? If so, what will be the cost?

6. **Transportation.** What will be the transportation costs for conducting the study and presenting the findings?

7. **Supplies.** Will any supplies, such as envelopes, postage, pens, paper, or photocopies, be needed? Will a beeper be needed to contact the researcher about potential subjects? Will long distance phone calls or overnight mailing be needed?

RESEARCHER EXPERTISE

A research problem and purpose needs to be selected based on the ability of the investigator. Initially one might work with another researcher (mentor) to learn the process and then investigate a familiar problem that fits one's knowledge base or experience. Selecting a difficult, complex problem and purpose can only frustrate and confuse the novice researcher. However, all researchers need to identify problems and purposes that are challenging and collaborate with other researchers as necessary to build their research background.

AVAILABILITY OF SUBJECTS

In selecting a research purpose, one must consider the type and number of subjects needed. Finding a sample might be difficult if the study involves investigating a unique or rare population, such as quadriplegic individuals who live alone. The more specific the population, the more difficult it is to obtain. The money and time available to the researcher will affect the subjects selected. With limited time and money, the researcher might want to investigate subjects who are accessible and do not require payment for participation. Even if a researcher identifies a population with a large number of potential subjects, those individuals may be unwilling to participate in the study because of the topic selected for study. For example, nurses could be asked to share their experiences with alcohol and drug use but many might fear that sharing this information would jeopardize their jobs and licenses. Researchers need to be prepared to pursue the attainment of subjects at whatever depth is necessary. Having a representative sample of reasonable size is critical to the generation of quality research findings (Kahn, 1994).

AVAILABILITY OF FACILITIES AND EQUIPMENT

Researchers need to determine whether their studies will require special facilities to implement. Will a special room be needed for an educational program, interview, or observations? If the study is conducted at a hospital, clinic, or school of nursing, will the agency provide the facilities that are needed? Setting up a highly specialized laboratory for the conduct of a study would be expensive and probably require external funding. Most nursing studies are done in natural settings like a hospital room or unit, a clinic, or a client's home.

Nursing studies frequently require a limited amount of equipment, such as a tape or video recorder for interviews or a physiological instrument such as a scale or thermometer. Equipment can often be borrowed from the facility where the study is conducted, or it can be rented. Some companies are willing to donate equipment if the study focuses on determining the effectiveness of the equipment and the findings are shared with the company. If specialized facilities or equipment are required for a study, the researcher needs to be aware what options are available before actively pursuing the study.

COOPERATION OF OTHERS

A study might appear feasible, but without the cooperation of others it is not. Some studies are conducted in laboratory settings and require minimal cooperation of others. However, most nursing studies involve human subjects and are conducted in hospitals, clinics, schools, offices, or homes. Having the cooperation of people in the research setting, the subjects, and the assistants involved in data collection is essential. People are frequently willing to cooperate with a study if they view the problem and purpose as significant or if they are personally interested. For example, nurses would probably be interested in cooperating in a study that examined the cost-effectiveness of nursing care in that institution. Gaining the cooperation of others in a research project is discussed in Chapter 15.

ETHICAL CONSIDERATIONS

The purpose selected for investigation must be ethical, which means that the subjects' rights and the rights of others in the setting are protected (Leino-Kilpi & Tuomaala, 1989). If the purpose appears to infringe upon the rights of the subjects, it should be reexamined and may have to be revised or abandoned. There are usually some risks in every study, but the value of the knowledge generated should outweigh the risks.

QUANTITATIVE, QUALITATIVE, AND OUTCOMES RESEARCH TOPICS, PROBLEMS, AND PURPOSES

Quantitative and qualitative research approaches enable nurses to investigate a variety of research problems and purposes. Examples of research topics, problems, and purposes for some of the different types of quantitative studies are presented in

Table 5–1. Not all published studies include a clearly expressed problem and purpose. The research purpose usually reflects the type of study that is to be conducted. The purpose of descriptive research is to describe concepts and identify relationships. The purpose of correlational research is to examine the type (positive or negative) and strength of relationships. Quasi-experimental and experimental studies are conducted to examine causal relationships or to determine the impact of a treatment on designated outcomes. If little is known about a topic, the researcher usually starts with a descriptive study and progresses to the other types of studies.

The problems formulated for qualitative research identify an area of concern that requires investigation. The purpose of a qualitative study indicates the focus of the study and whether it is a subjective concept, an event, a phenomenon, or a facet of a culture or society. Examples of research topics, problems, and purposes from some different types of qualitative studies are presented in Table 5–2 (on p. 110). Phenomenological research seeks an understanding of human experience from an individual researcher's perspective, like patients' lived experience of comfort (Morse, Bottorff, & Hutchinson, 1995). Some of the types of research problems investigated with phenomenological research include "(1) the interpretation of the single, unique event; (2) the interpretation of a single, unique individual; and (3) the interpretation of a general or repetitive psychological process (e.g., anger, learning, etc.)" (Knaack, 1984, p. 111).

In grounded theory research, the problem identifies the area of concern and the purpose indicates the focus of the theory to be developed from the research. In ethnographic research, the problem and purpose identify the culture and the specific attributes of the culture that are to be examined and described. The problem and purpose in historical research focus on a specific individual, a characteristic of society, an event, or a situation in the past and identify the time period in the past that will be examined in conducting the research. The problem and purpose in philosophical inquiry identify the focus of the analysis, whether it is

Table 5–1
Quantitative Research: Topics, Problems, and Purposes

Type of Research	Research Topic	Research Problem and Purpose
Descriptive	Coping strategies, dependency status, disabilities, illness	**Problem:** "Many physical, social, and emotional disabilities associated with multiple sclerosis (MS) result in social dependence on spouses and significant others during the long illness trajectory. Little is known about coping strategies used in responding to the dependency needs of persons with MS in the management of everyday activities. Knowledge about such coping strategies would be useful to health care providers in helping families deal with the changing and long-term demands required when living with MS" (Gulick, 1995, p. 220). **Purpose:** "The purposes of this study were twofold: to identify coping strategies used by spouses and significant others of persons with MS, and to determine if differences existed among the coping strategies with respect to frequency used, dependency status of the person with MS, presence or absence of illness in the spouse or significant other, and this person's gender and relationship to the person with MS" (Gulick, 1995, p. 221).
Correlational	Infant-mother attachment, maternal responsiveness, infant temperament, parenting	**Problem:** "The vast majority of attachment studies were focused on attachment of the mother or father to the infant, measuring parent rather than infant behaviors . . . Nurses are especially challenged to help parents gain insight into their own parenting behaviors and their influence on infant development. To guide practice in nursing, researchers need to expand the discipline's theoretical base to achieve a better understanding of the affectional ties between infants and parents" (Coffman, Levitt, & Guacci-Franco, 1995, p. 9). **Purpose:** "The purpose of this study was to explore the relationships between maternal responsiveness, infant temperament, and infant-mother attachment . . ." (Coffman et al., p. 9).
Quasi-experimental	Nonpharmacologic intervention, slow stroke back massage, relaxation, comfort	**Problem:** "Alleviation of symptoms and pain control to increase comfort are the primary goals of palliative nursing care . . . Therefore, it is essential to investigate nursing interventions such as relaxation techniques which may add to the comfort of terminally ill people" (Meek, 1993, p. 17). **Purpose:** "The purpose of this study was to examine the effects of a nonpharmacologic intervention, slow stroke back massage (SSBM), on systolic and diastolic blood pressure, heart rate, and skin temperature as indicators of relaxation in hospice clients" (Meek, 1993, p. 9).
Experimental	Caloric density of food, energy intake, body weight, anorexia	**Problem:** "Anorexia and weight loss are major problems for cancer patients and are associated with increased cancer morbidity and mortality . . . The effect of increasing the caloric density of food on energy intake of rats once tumor-induced anorexia has developed is not known" (Fridriksdottir & McCarthy, 1995, pp. 357–358). **Purpose:** "Therefore, the purpose of the present study was to examine the food and energy intake of tumor-bearing rats who are switched to a diet of higher caloric density after the onset of anorexia" (Fridriksdottir & McCarthy, 1995, p. 358).

Table 5-2
Qualitative Research: Topics, Problems, and Purposes

Type of Research	Research Topic	Research Problem and Purpose
Phenomenological	Comfort, illness, injury, lived experience	**Problem:** "What is comfort? In nursing, the term appears frequently in clinical texts, where 'making the patient comfortable' is a nursing goal . . . Interestingly, although relatively little attention has been paid to the concept of comfort, nurses are often judged by their ability to make their patients comfortable . . . comfort remains an illusive goal for nursing, and we know little about how it is experienced by patients" (Morse, Bottorff, & Hutchinson, 1995, p. 14).
		Purpose: "In this study, the phenomenological method as described by van Manen (1990) was used to explore and reflect on patients' experiences of illness or injury. The aim of this study was to uncover and gain a deeper understanding of the meaning of comfort as an everyday experience" (Morse et al., 1995, p. 15).
Grounded theory	Parenting experience, developmental delay, mental retardation, transformed parenting	**Problem:** "The birth of a child with a condition that will result in developmental delay including mental retardation (DD/MR) represents both an initial and an enduring crisis for parents . . . Findings from previous research have described specific components of parenting a child with DD/MR, such as stress, coping, chronic sorrow, and adaptation. Although these efforts have been helpful, a more comprehensive understanding is needed" (Seideman & Kleine, 1995, p. 38).
		Purpose: "Therefore, a grounded theory study was undertaken to enhance understanding of the total parenting experience. Within the grounded theory context, the basic social problem was identified as parenting a child with DD/MR at home. The basic social process that emerged was labeled Transformed Parenting" (Seideman & Kleine, 1995, p. 38).
Ethnography	Inner-city ghettos, survival, elders, drug activity	**Problem:** "In underserved, inner-city ghettos known for drug-related violence and crime, active participation in community life is dangerous and even life-threatening. This is especially true for elders burdened with the infirmities of aging and lacking the means to provide for alternatives to social isolation. Few researchers have ventured into inner-city communities known for troublesome and dangerous public spaces . . . Therefore, little is known about the social lives of people in these communities, in particular, vulnerable older people who are frequently victims of illegal drug activity" (Kauffman, 1995, p. 231).
		Purpose: "This urban ethnography was conducted over a period of three years in a predominantly African American inner-city ghetto. The main question to be answered was: How do elders survive in the midst of 'drug warfare' in an inner-city community known for its dangerous streets and public spaces?" (Kauffman, 1995, p. 231).

Table 5–2
Qualitative Research: Topics, Problems, and Purposes *Continued*

Type of Research	Research Topic	Research Problem and Purpose
Historical	Spirituality, beliefs, morals, religion	**Problem:** "Rigid morals characterize the nineteenth century in the minds of most twentieth-century people . . . While Nightingale's moral beliefs are well documented, less is known about why she held them. Moral and spiritual are not necessarily the same . . . To simply define Florence Nightingale's beliefs, however, does not describe her spirituality—the force that motivated her life" (Widerquist, 1992, p. 49).
		Purpose: "An examination of Nightingale's life—what influenced her beliefs, how she arrived at them, and what she did about them—offers a deeper understanding of her spirituality and a greater awareness of the spiritual issues surrounding nursing" (Widerquist, 1992, p. 49).
Philosophical analysis	Rights, human rights, patient rights, health care	**Problem:** "Nurses encounter the word right(s) in many aspects of their personal and professional lives. Patients' rights documents are displayed in healthcare institutions . . . Yet the idea of rights often is not understood clearly. For instance, controversy exists regarding whether access to healthcare is a human right. Furthermore, individual rights are not always honored. Sometimes rights are in conflict, as when one individual's right to confidentiality conflicts with another's right to information" (Reckling, 1994, p. 309).
		Purpose: "Philosophers have analyzed the ontology and epistemology of rights: Do rights exist? If so, what constitutes them? How do we recognize one when we see it? Where do rights originate? What does having a right imply?" (Reckling, 1994, p. 311).
Critical social theory	Oppressed group behaviors	**Problem:** "The study of the behavior of others sometimes reflects our own behaviors."
		Purpose: "A study was carried out in the Federal Republic of Germany (FRG) to analyze the social, economic, and political factors affecting the nursing education system . . . Theoretical constructs from the work of critical social theorist Jurgen Habermas and adult educator Paulo Freire were used to achieve a deeper understanding of the interrelations between the cultural context and the nursing education system as well as to provide direction for conceptualizing ways to transcend oppressive circumstances" (Hedin, 1986, p. 53).

Table 5–3
Outcomes Research: Topics, Problem, and Purpose

Type of Research	Research Topic	Research Problem and Purpose
Outcomes research	Patient outcomes, special care unit, intensive care unit, chronically critically ill	**Problem:** "The original purpose of intensive care units (ICUs) was to locate groups of patients together who had similar needs for specialized monitoring and care so that highly trained health care personnel would be available to meet these specialized needs. As the success of ICUs has grown and expanded, the assumption that a typical ICU patient will require only a short length of stay in the unit during the most acute phase of an illness has given way to the recognition that stays of more than one month are not uncommon . . . These long-stay ICU patients represent a challenge to the current system, not only because of costs, but also because of concern for patient outcomes . . . While ample evidence confirms that this subpopulation of ICU patients represents a drain on hospital resources, few studies have attempted to evaluate the effects of a care delivery system outside the ICU setting on patient outcomes, costs, and nurse outcomes" (Rudy, Daly, Douglas, Montenegro, Song, & Dyer, 1995, p. 324).
		Purpose: "The purpose of this study was to compare the effects of a low-technology environment of care and a nurse case management care delivery system (specific care unit, SCU) with the traditional high-technology environment (ICU) and primary nursing care delivery system on the patient outcomes of length of stay, mortality, readmission, complications, satisfaction, and cost" (Rudy et al., 1995, p. 324).

to clarify meaning, make values manifest, identify ethics, or examine the nature of knowledge. Of the three types of philosophical inquiry (foundational inquiry, philosophical analyses, and ethical analyses), only an example of philosophical analysis is provided with an analysis of the concept "rights" (Reckling, 1994). The problem and purpose in critical social theory identify a society and indicate the particular aspects of the society that will

be examined to determine their influence on an event, situation, or system in that society.

Outcomes research is conducted to examine the end-results of care. Table 5–3 includes the topics, problem, and purpose from an outcomes study. Rudy, et al. (1995) conducted a study to determine the patient outcomes for the chronically critically ill in the special care unit versus the intensive care unit.

SUMMARY

A research problem is a situation in need of a solution, improvement, or alteration, or a discrepancy between the way things are and the way they ought to be. The problem identifies an area of concern for a particular population and indicates the concepts to be studied. The major sources for nursing research problems include nursing practice; researcher and peer

interactions; literature review; theory; and research priorities identified by individuals, specialty groups, and funding agencies. Through the literature review, one might identify studies that require replication. Replication involves reproducing or repeating a study to determine whether similar findings will be obtained. Replication is essential to the develop

continued

continued

ment of a knowledge base and provides an excellent learning experience for novice researchers. Four types of replication are identified: exact, approximate, concurrent, and systematic.

The research purpose is a concise, clear statement of the specific goal or aim of the study. The goal of a study might be to identify, describe, explain, or predict a solution to a situation. The purpose indicates the type of study to be conducted and often includes the variables, population, and setting for the study. Several purposes can be generated from each research problem.

The exact thought processes used to formulate a research problem and purpose have not been clearly identified because of the abstractness and complexity of the reasoning involved. The researcher examines the real-world situation, identifies research topics, generates questions, and ultimately clarifies and refines a research problem. From the problem a specific goal or research purpose is developed for the study. The problem selected for investigation needs to have professional significance and be of personal interest to the researcher. The research priorities identified in nursing are useful in determining the significance of a problem.

The purpose is generated from the problem and clearly focuses the development of the study. Based on the research purpose, specific research objectives, questions, or hypotheses are developed to direct the study. As the research problem and purpose increase in clarity and conciseness, the researcher has greater direction in determining the feasibility of a study. The feasibility of conducting a study is determined by examining the time and money commitments; researchers' expertise; availability of subjects, facility, and equipment; cooperation of others; and the study's ethical considerations.

Quantitative, qualitative, and outcomes research enable nurses to investigate a variety of research problems and purposes. In quantitative research, the problem identifies an area of concern, and the purpose reflects the type of study (descriptive, correlational, quasi-experimental, or experimental) to be conducted. The problems formulated for qualitative research also identify an area of concern. The purpose of a qualitative study indicates the focus of the investigation, whether it is a subjective concept, an event, a phenomenon, or a facet of a culture or society. The purpose of outcomes research is to examine the end-results of patient care.

References

Adebo, E. O. (1974). Identifying problems for nursing research. *International Nursing Review, 21*(2), 53–54, 59.

Ajzen, I., & Fishbein, M. (1980). *Understanding attitudes and predicting social behavior.* Englewood Cliffs, NJ: Prentice-Hall.

Albrecht, M. (1992). Research priorities for home health nursing. *Nursing & Health Care, 13*(10), 538–541.

Artinian, B. M., & Anderson, N. (1980). Guidelines for the identification of researchable problems. *Journal of Nursing Education, 19*(4), 54–58.

Beck, C. T. (1994). Replication strategies for nursing research. *Image: Journal of Nursing Scholarship, 26*(3), 191–194.

Beck, C. T. (1995). The effects of postpartum depression on maternal-infant interaction: A meta-analysis. *Nursing Research, 44*(5), 298–304.

Becker, M. H. (1974). *The health belief model and personal health behaviors.* Thorofare, NJ: Charles B. Slack.

Beckingham, A. C. (1974). Identifying problems for nursing research. *International Nursing Review, 21*(2), 49–52.

Beveridge, W. I. B. (1950). *The art of scientific investigation.* New York: Vintage Books.

Bloch, D. (1990). Strategies for setting and implementing the National Center for Nursing Research priorities. *Applied Nursing Research, 3*(1), 2–6.

Boehm, S., Whall, A. L., Cosgrove, K. L., Locke, J. D., & Schlenk, E. A. (1995). Behavioral analysis and nursing interventions for reducing disruptive behaviors of patients with dementia. *Applied Nursing Research, 8*(3), 118–122.

Bradford, M. S. (1995). Health concerns and prevalence of

abuse and sexual activity in adolescents at a runaway shelter. *Applied Nursing Research, 8*(4), 187–190.

Brink, P. J., & Wood, M. J. (1979). Multiple concurrent replication. *Western Journal of Nursing Research, 1*(1), 117–118.

Brown, B. E., & Garrison, C. J. (1990). Patterns of symptomatology of adult women incest survivors. *Western Journal of Nursing Research, 12*(5), 587–600.

Brown, S. A., & Grimes, D. E. (1995). A meta-analysis of nurse practitioners and nurse midwives in primary care. *Nursing Research, 44*(5), 332–339.

Browne, A., & Finkelhor, D. (1986). Impact of child sexual abuse: A review of the research. *Psychological Bulletin, 99*(1), 66–77.

Campbell, J. P., Daft, R. L., & Hulin, C. L. (1982). *What to study: Generating and developing research questions.* Beverly Hills: Sage.

Chinn, P. L., & Kramer, M. K. (1991). *Theory and nursing: A systematic approach* (3rd ed.). St. Louis: Mosby.

Coffman, S., Levitt, M. J., & Guacci-Franco, N. (1995). Infant-mother attachment: Relationships to maternal responsiveness and infant temperament. *Journal of Pediatric Nursing, 10*(1), 9–18.

Cole, F. L. (1995). Implementation and evaluation of an undergraduate research practicum. *Journal of Professional Nursing, 11*(3), 154–160.

Cox, C. (1982). An interaction model of client health behavior: Theoretical prescription for nursing. *Advances in Nursing Science, 5*(1), 41–56.

Davies, A. R., Doyle, M. A. T., Lansky, D., Rutt, W., Stevic, M. O., & Doyle, J. B. (1994). Outcomes assessment in clinical settings: A consensus statement on principles and best practices in project management. *The Joint Commission Journal on Quality Improvement, 20*(1), 6–16.

Dennis, K. E., Howes, D. G., & Zelauskas, B. (1989). Identifying nursing research priorities: A first step in program development. *Applied Nursing Research, 2*(3), 108–113.

Diers, D. (1979). *Research in nursing practice.* Philadelphia: Lippincott.

Fishbein, M., & Ajzen, I. (1975). *Belief, attitude, intention, and behavior.* Boston: Addison-Wesley.

Frederickson, K. (1989). Anxiety transmission in the patient with myocardial infarction. *Heart & Lung, 18*(6), 617–622.

Fridriksdottir, N., & McCarthy, D. O. (1995). The effect of caloric density of food on energy intake and body weight in tumor-bearing rats. *Research in Nursing & Health, 18*(4), 357–363.

Fuller, E. O. (1982). Selecting a clinical nursing problem for research. *Image: Journal of Nursing Scholarship, 14*(2), 60–61.

Glick, O. J., & Swanson, E. A. (1995). Motor performance correlates of functional dependence in long-term care residents. *Nursing Research, 44*(1), 4–8.

Gold, E. (1986). Long-term effects of sexual victimization in childhood: An attributional approach. *Journal of Consulting and Clinical Psychology, 54*(4), 471–475.

Good, M. (1995). A comparison of the effects of jaw relaxation and music on postoperative pain. *Nursing Research, 44*(1), 52–57.

Gordon, M. (1980). Determining study topics. *Nursing Research, 29*(2), 83–87.

Gross, D., Fogg, L., & Tucker, S. (1995). The efficacy of parent training for promoting positive parent-toddler relationships. *Research in Nursing & Health, 18*(6), 489–499.

Gulick, E. E. (1995). Coping among spouses or significant others of persons with multiple sclerosis. *Nursing Research, 44*(4), 220–225.

Hahn, E. J. (1995). Predicting head start parent involvement in an alcohol and other drug prevention program. *Nursing Research, 44*(1), 45–51.

Haller, K. B., & Reynolds, M. A. (1986). Using research in practice: A case for replication in nursing: Part II. *Western Journal of Nursing Research, 8*(2), 249–252.

Heater, B. S., Becker, A. M., & Olson, R. K. (1988). Nursing interventions and patient outcomes: A meta-analysis of studies. *Nursing Research, 37*(5), 303–307.

Hedin, B. A. (1986). A case study of oppressed group behavior in nurses. *Image: Journal of Nursing Scholarship, 18*(2), 53–57.

Henry, B., Moody, L. E., Pendergast, J. F., O'Donnell, J., Hutchinson, S. A., & Scully, G. (1987). Delineation of nursing administration research priorities. *Nursing Research, 36*(5), 309–314.

Hinshaw, A. S. (1988). National Center for Nursing Research: Missions, programs and initiatives. *Nursing Connections, 1*(1), 42–45.

Holmstrom, L. L., & Burgess, A. W. (1982). Low-cost research: A project on a shoestring. *Nursing Research, 31*(2), 123–125.

Jemmott, L. S., & Jemmott J. B., III. (1991). Applying the theory of reasoned action to AIDS risk behavior: Condom use among black women. *Nursing Research, 40*(4), 228–234.

Jennings, B. M. (1991). Patient outcomes research: Seizing the opportunity. *Advances in Nursing Science, 14*(2), 59–72.

Kahn, C. R. (1994). Picking a research problem: The critical decision. *The New England Journal of Medicine, 330*(21), 1530–1533.

Kaplan, B. A. (1964). *The conduct of inquiry: Methodology for behavioral science.* New York: Harper & Row.

Kathol, D. (1984). Anxiety in surgical patient's families. *AORN Journal, 40*(1), 131–137.

Kauffman, K. S. (1995). Center as haven: Findings of an urban ethnography. *Nursing Research, 44*(4), 231–236.

King, I., & Tarsitano, B. (1982). The effect of structured and unstructured preoperative teaching: A replication. *Nursing Research, 31*(6), 324–329.

Knaack, P. (1984). Phenomenological research. *Western Journal of Nursing Research, 6*(1), 107–114.

Laffrey, S. C. (1990). An exploration of adult health behaviors. *Western Journal of Nursing Research, 12*(4), 434–447.

Lamb, G. S. (1991). Two explanations of nurse practitioner interactions and participatory decision-making with physicians. *Research in Nursing & Health, 14*(5), 379–386.

Lauver, D., Armstrong, K., Marks, S., & Schwarz, S. (1995). HIV risk status and preventive behaviors among 17,619 women. *JOGNN, 24*(1), 33–39.

Leidy, N. K., & Traver, G. A. (1995). Psychophysiologic factors contributing to functional performance in people with COPD: Are there gender differences? *Research in Nursing & Health, 18*(6), 535–546.

Leino-Kilpi, H., & Tuomaala, U. (1989). Research ethics and nursing science: An empirical example. *Journal of Advanced Nursing, 14*(6), 451–458.

Leske, J. S. (1992). Effects of intraoperative progress reports on anxiety levels of elective surgical patients' family members. *Clinical Nursing Research, 1*(3), 266–277.

Leske, J. S. (1995). Effects of intraoperative progress reports on anxiety levels of surgical patients' family members. *Applied Nursing Research, 8*(4), 169–173.

Lewandowski, A., & Kositsky, A. M. (1983). Research priorities for critical care nursing: A study by the American Association of Critical Care Nurses. *Heart & Lung, 12*(1), 35–44.

Lindeman, C. A. (1975). Delphi survey of priorities in clinical nursing research. *Nursing Research, 24*(6), 434–441.

Lindeman, C. A., & Van Aernam, B. (1971). Nursing intervention with the presurgical patient—The effects of structured and unstructured preoperative teaching. *Nursing Research, 20*(4), 319–332.

Lindquist, R., Banasik, J., Barnsteiner, J., Beecroft, P. C., Prevost, S., Riegel, B., Sechrist, K., Strzelecki, C., & Titler, M. (1993). Determining AACN's research priorities for the 90s. *American Journal of Critical Care, 2*(2), 110–117.

Lindsey, A. M. (1982). Phenomena and physiological variables of relevance to nursing, review of a decade of work: Part I. *Western Journal of Nursing Research, 4*(4), 343–364.

Lindsey, A. M. (1983). Phenomena and physiological variables of relevance to nursing, review of a decade of work: Part II. *Western Journal of Nursing Research, 5*(1), 41–63.

Lusk, S. L., Kerr, M. J., & Ronis, D. L. (1995). Health-promoting lifestyles of blue-collar, skilled trade, and white-collar workers. *Nursing Research, 44*(1), 20–24.

McDougall, G. J. (1995). Metamemory and depression in cognitively impaired elders. *Nursing Research, 44*(5), 306–311.

Mahoney, D. F. (1994). Appropriateness of geriatric prescribing decisions made by nurse practitioners and physicians. *Image: Journal of Nursing Scholarship, 26*(1), 41–46.

Martin, P. A. (1994). The utility of the research problem statement. *Applied Nursing Research, 7*(1), 47–49.

Martin, P. A. (1995). More replication studies needed. *Applied Nursing Research, 8*(2), 102–103.

Meek, S. S. (1993). Effects of slow stroke back massage on relaxation in hospice clients. *Image: Journal of Nursing Scholarship, 25*(1), 17–21.

Moody, L., Vera, H., Blanks, C., & Visscher, M. (1989). Developing questions of substance for nursing science. *Western Journal of Nursing Research, 11*(4), 393–404.

Mooney, K. H., Ferrell, B. R., Nail, L. M., Benedict, S. C., & Haberman, M. R. (1991). 1991 Oncology Nursing Society research priorities survey. *Oncology Nursing Forum, 18*(8), 1381–1388.

Morse, J. M., Bottorff, J. L., & Hutchinson, S. (1995). The paradox of comfort. *Nursing Research, 44*(1), 14–19.

National Institute of Nursing Research (NINR) (September 23, 1993). *National nursing research agenda: Setting nursing research priorities.* Bethesda, MD: National Institutes of Health.

Orem, D. E. (1995). *Nursing concepts of practice* (5th ed.). St. Louis: Mosby.

Packard, N. J., Haberman, M. R., Woods, N. F., & Yates, B. C. (1991). Demands of illness among chronically ill women. *Western Journal of Nursing Research, 13*(4), 434–457.

Panel for the Prediction and Prevention of Pressure Ulcers in Adults. (1992, May). *Pressure ulcers in adults: Prediction and preventions. Clinical practice guideline.* AHCPR Pub. No. 92-0047. Rockville, MD: Agency for Health Care Policy and Research, Public Health Service, U.S. Department of Health and Human Services.

Phillips, J. M., & Wilbur, J. (1995). Adherence to breast cancer screening guidelines among African-American women of differing employment status. *Cancer Nursing, 18*(4), 258–269.

Powe, B., (1995). Fatalism among elderly African Americans: Effects on colorectal cancer screening. *Cancer Nursing, 18*(5), 385–392.

Quayhagen, M. P., Quayhagen, M., Corbeil, R. R., Roth, P. A., & Rodgers, J. A. (1995). A dyadic remediation program for care recipients with dementia. *Nursing Research, 44*(3), 153–159.

Raleigh, E. H., Lepczyk, M., & Rowley, C., (1990). Significant others benefit from preoperative information. *Journal of Advanced Nursing, 15*(8), 941–945.

Reckling, J. B (1994). Conceptual analysis of rights using a philosophic inquiry approach. *Image: Journal of Nursing Scholarship, 26*(4), 309–314.

Reider, J. A. (1994). Anxiety during critical illness of a family member. *Dimensions of Critical Care Nursing, 13*(5), 272–279.

Rempusheski, V. F. (1990). Ask an expert. *Applied Nursing Research, 3*(1), 44–46.

Rettig, R. (1990). History, development, and importance to nursing of outcomes research. *Journal of Nursing Quality Assurance, 5*(2), 13–17.

Reynolds, M. A., & Haller, K. B. (1986). Using research in practice: A case for replication in nursing: Part I. *Western Journal of Nursing Research, 8*(1), 113–116.

Ringerman, E. S. (1990). Characteristics associated with decentralization experienced by nurse managers. *Western Journal of Nursing Research, 12*(3), 336–346.

Rogers, B. (1987). Research corner: Is the research project feasible? *AAOHN Journal, 35*(7), 327–328.

Rogers, B. (1989). Establishing research priorities in occupational health nursing. *AAOHN Journal, 37*(12), 493–500.

Rose, M. A. (1995). Knowledge of human immunodeficiency virus and acquired immunodeficiency syndrome, perception of risk, and behaviors among older adults. *Holistic Nursing Practice, 10*(1), 10–17.

Rudy, E. B., Daly, B. J., Douglas, S., Montenegro, H. D., Song, R., & Dyer, M. A. (1995). Patient outcomes for the chronically critically ill: Special care unit versus intensive care unit. *Nursing Research, 44*(6), 324–330.

Schmieding, N. J. (1990). A model for assessing nurse administrators' actions. *Western Journal of Nursing Research, 12*(3), 293–306.

Schrijnemaekers, V. J. J., & Haveman, M. J. (1995). Effects of preventive outpatient geriatric assessment: Short-term results of a randomized controlled study. *Home Health Care Services Quarterly, 15*(2), 81–97.

Selltiz, C., Wrightsman, L. S., & Cook, S. W. (1981). *Research methods in social relations* (4th ed.). New York: Holt, Rinehart and Winston.

Seideman, R. Y., & Kleine, P. F. (1995). A theory of transformed parenting: Parenting a child with developmental delay/mental retardation. *Nursing Research, 44*(1), 38–44.

Sigsbee, M., & Geden, E. A. (1990). Effects of anxiety on family members of patients with cardiac disease learning cardiopulmonary resuscitation. *Heart & Lung, 19*(6), 662–665.

Silva, M. C., Geary, M. L., Manning, C. B., & Zeccolo, P. G. (1984). Caring for those who wait. *Today's OR Nurse, 6*(6), 26–30.

Taunton, R. L. (1989). Replication: Key to research application. *Dimensions of Critical Care Nursing, 8*(3), 156–158.

Thiele, J. E., Holloway, J., Murphy, D., Pendarvis, J., & Stucky, M. (1991). Perceived and actual decision making by novice baccalaureate students. *Western Journal of Nursing Research, 13*(5), 616–626.

Trinkoff, A. M., Eaton, W. W., & Anthony, J. C. (1991). The prevalence of substance abuse among registered nurses. *Nursing Research, 40*(3), 172–175.

Valiga, T. M., & Mermel, V. M. (1985). Formulating the researchable question. *Topics in Clinical Nursing, 7*(2), 1–14.

van Manen, M. (1990). *Researching lived experience: Human science for an action sensitive pedagogy.* London, Ontario: Althouse Press.

Villarruel, A. M. (1995). Mexican-American cultural meanings, expressions, self-care and dependent-care actions associated with experiences of pain. *Research in Nursing & Health, 18*(5), 427–436.

Whitney, J. D., Stotts, N. A., & Goodson, W. H. (1995). Effects of dynamic exercise on subcutaneous oxygen tension and temperature. *Research in Nursing & Health, 18*(2), 97–104.

Williams, A. (1972). A study of factors contributing to skin breakdown. *Nursing Research, 21*(3), 238–243.

Widerquist, J. G. (1992). The spirituality of Florence Nightingale. *Nursing Research, 41*(1), 49–55.

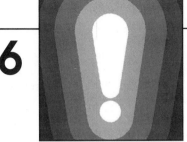

6

Review of Relevant Literature

A *review of relevant literature* is conducted to generate a picture of what is known and not known about a particular situation. *Relevant literature* refers to those sources that are important in providing the in-depth knowledge needed to make changes in practice or to study a selected problem. Thus, a literature review is conducted to ascertain whether research findings are ready for use in practice or whether additional study is needed. In conducting research, the literature review facilitates selecting a problem and purpose, developing a framework, and formulating a research plan. The literature is reviewed before, during, and after the conduct of a study, so the study builds on and is compared with previous research.

Since the number of nursing journals has increased by more than 565% from 1961, the literature review process has become more challenging but also more enlightening (Kilby, Fishel, & Gupta, 1989). To assist you in conducting a literature review, this chapter focuses on the purpose, scope, process, and end product of the review of relevant literature. The end product of a literature review is the generation of a written report that summarizes what is known and not known about a phenomenon.

PURPOSE FOR REVIEWING RELEVANT LITERATURE

The primary purpose for reviewing relevant literature is to gain a broad background or understanding of the information that is available related to a problem. This background enables a researcher

to build upon the works of others, since major breakthroughs or discoveries of new information in a field are based on previous works (Kaplan, 1964). The researcher's knowledge of the literature should include familiarity with what work (theoretical and empirical) has been done concerning a specific problem, what is considered to be the current knowledge regarding the problem, and what further research is needed. The type of quantitative or qualitative study planned determines the purpose and timing for the literature review.

PURPOSE OF THE LITERATURE REVIEW IN QUANTITATIVE RESEARCH

The review of literature in quantitative research influences the development of several steps in the research process (see Table 6–1). The purpose of the literature review is similar for the different types of quantitative research (descriptive, correlational, quasi-experimental, and experimental). The review is instigated at the beginning of the research process and continues throughout the development of the research proposal, collection and analysis of data, and interpretation of findings.

The initial identification of a research topic frequently evolves from a clinical experience; however, a topic may be identified and clarified through the literature review. The research problem, which emerges from the topic, is initially broad and general. The problem is refined and clarified many times throughout the literature review. With a solid background of the relevant

Table 6–1
Purpose of the Literature Review in Quantitative Research

Clarify the research topic
Clarify the research problem
Verify the significance of the research problem
Specify the purpose of the study
Describe relevant studies
Describe relevant theories
Summarize current knowledge
Facilitate development of the framework
Specify research objectives, questions, or hypotheses
Develop definitions of major variables
Identify limitations and assumptions
Select a research design
Identify methods of measurement
Direct data collection and analysis
Interpret findings

objectives, questions, or hypotheses are formulated and study variables are operationally defined based on information from the literature. The limitations and assumptions for a study are identified by reviewing other researchers' and theorists' works.

The design selected for a study reflects a thorough understanding of the designs used in similar studies. The strengths and weaknesses of previous study designs are examined in developing a stronger, more effective design. Reviewing relevant studies can also suggest effective methods of measurement and data collection and analysis techniques. Lastly, the findings from previous research form the basis for comparison when interpreting the findings from a recent study.

literature, the researcher is ultimately able to formulate a research purpose, which is clearly focused, significant for nursing, and feasible to study.

The researcher gains essential information from existing studies and theories through a literature review. This information is logically organized and presented in the review of literature section of the research proposal and the final research report. Theories are also reviewed to clarify the definitions and relationships of concepts and to develop a framework for the study. Specific research

PURPOSE OF THE LITERATURE REVIEW IN QUALITATIVE RESEARCH

In qualitative research, the purpose and timing of the literature review vary, based on the type of study to be conducted (see Table 6–2). Phenomenologists believe the literature should be reviewed after data collection and analyses so the information in the literature will not influence the researcher's objectivity (Oiler, 1982, 1986). The researcher's description of a real-world phenome-

Table 6–2
Purpose of the Literature Review in Qualitative Research

Phenomenological research	Compare and combine findings from the study with the literature to determine current knowledge of a phenomenon
Grounded theory research	Use the literature to explain, support, and extend the theory generated in the study
Ethnographic research	Review the literature to provide a background for conducting the study as in quantitative research
Historical research	Literature is reviewed to develop research questions and is a source of data in the study
Philosophical inquiry	Literature is reviewed to raise philosophical questions, and answers are sought in analyzing a variety of sources
Critical social theory	Study findings are compared and combined with existing literature to determine current knowledge of a social situation

non should include only what is seen in the situation and not what is read in the literature. For example, if a researcher decided to describe the phenomenon of dying, the review of literature would include Kubler-Ross's (1969) five stages of grieving. Knowing the details of these stages could influence the way the researcher views the phenomenon during data collection and analysis. After data analyses, the information from the literature is compared with findings from the present study to determine similarities and differences. Then the findings are combined to reflect the current knowledge of the phenomenon (Oiler, 1986).

Grounded theory research includes the following steps: (1) collection of empirical data, (2) concept formation, (3) concept development, (4) concept modification and integration, and (5) production of the research report (Stern, 1980). In grounded theory research, a minimal review of relevant studies is done at the beginning of the research process. This review is only a means of making the researcher aware of what studies have been conducted, but the information from these studies is not used to direct data collection or theory development from that data. A more extensive literature review is conducted in steps three (concept development) and four (concept modification and integration). The literature is used to define selected concepts and to verify the relationships in the theory developed from the empirical data. Using the literature, researchers are able to explain, support, and extend their emerging theories (Hutchinson, 1986; Stern, 1980).

The review of literature in ethnographic research is similar to that of quantitative research. The literature is reviewed early in the research process to provide a general understanding of the variables to be examined in a selected culture. The literature is usually theoretical because few studies have typically been conducted in the area of interest. From these sources, a framework is developed for examining complex human situations in the selected culture (Germain, 1986). The literature review also provides a background for conducting the study and interpreting the findings. The intent of the research is to generate new insights regarding the culture that would expand and refine the current knowledge of that culture (Aamodt, 1982).

In historical research, an initial literature review is conducted to select a research topic and to develop research questions (Christy, 1975). Then the investigator develops an inventory of sources, locates these sources, and examines them. Thus, the literature is a major source of data in historical research. The information gained from the literature is analyzed and organized into a report to explain how an identified phenomenon has evolved over a particular time period (Matejski, 1986). Historical research requires an extensive review of relevant literature, with the researcher spending months and even years locating and examining sources. To facilitate the work of historical researchers, Fairman (1987) developed a selective list of archival collections and nursing history research centers (see Chapter 4).

Philosophical inquiry involves intellectual analyses to clarify meanings, make values manifest, identify ethics, and study the nature of knowledge (Ellis, 1983). An extensive exploration of the literature is guided by the philosophical questions raised by the researcher. The researcher locates, analyzes, and abstracts meaning from a variety of sources, which generates more questions. Additional sources are sought and analyzed until the researcher is able to formulate descriptions and conclusions regarding the area of study (Ellis, 1983; Manchester, 1986).

Critical social theory involves the critique of a social situation to raise consciousness and identify actions to take against oppressive forces. Some of the techniques used are similar to those in phenomenology. The researcher interacts with persons in the society and constantly collects and analyzes data to describe the situation under study in a historical, cultural, and political context. The intent is to promote self-knowledge and self-reflection in those interviewed so they might experience increased autonomy and responsibility in their social setting (Holter, 1988). The findings from these interactions are compared and combined with the literature to determine the current knowledge of the social situation (Hedin, 1986).

SCOPE OF A LITERATURE REVIEW

The scope of a literature review should be broad enough for the investigator to become knowledgeable about the research problem and narrow enough to include predominantly relevant sources. To determine the scope of a literature review, the following areas are evaluated: (1) the types of information and sources available, (2) the approximate depth and breadth of the review needed, and (3) the time frame for conducting the review.

TYPES OF INFORMATION AND SOURCES AVAILABLE

Predominately two types of information are cited in the review of literature for research, theoretical and empirical. Other types of published information such as descriptions of clinical situations, educational literature, and position papers are reviewed but are rarely cited because of their subjectivity (Marchette, 1985; Pinch, 1995). *Theoretical literature* includes concept analyses, models, theories, and conceptual frameworks that support a selected research problem and purpose. Theoretical and conceptual sources are described and summarized to reflect the current understanding of the research problem and to facilitate developing the study framework.

Empirical literature includes relevant studies in journals and books as well as unpublished studies, such as master's theses and doctoral dissertations. The empirical literature reviewed depends on the problem, purpose, and type of study selected. Research problems that were frequently investigated in the past or are currently being investigated have more extensive empirical literature than new or unique problems. Some problems have been the focus of theorists more than researchers, such as the problem of "What is health to a human being?"; therefore, the literature review for this problem is predominately theoretical.

The published literature includes primary and secondary sources. A *primary source* is written by the person who originated or is responsible for generating the ideas published. In research publications, a primary source is written by the person(s) who conducted the research. A primary theoretical source is written by the theorist who developed the theory or conceptual content. A *secondary source* summarizes or quotes content from primary sources. Thus, authors of secondary sources paraphrase the works of researchers and theorists. The problem with secondary sources is that the author has interpreted the works of someone else, and this interpretation is influenced by that author's perception and bias. Sometimes errors and misinterpretations have been promulgated by authors using secondary sources rather than primary sources. Predominately primary sources need to be used in developing research proposals and reports. Secondary sources are used only if primary sources cannot be located or if the secondary source provides creative ideas or a unique organization of information not found in a primary source.

DEPTH AND BREADTH OF THE REVIEW

The *depth of a literature review* refers to the number and quality of the sources that are examined on a topic. The *breadth* is determined by the number of different topics examined. If the literature review is too broad, the researcher will be examining many irrelevant sources. When the review lacks sufficient depth and breadth, important sources may be overlooked. The depth and breadth of the literature review depend on the background of the researcher, the complexity of the research project, and the amount of literature available on a selected research problem.

Researcher's Background

When a research topic is new to an investigator, an extensive review of the literature is needed to gain the in-depth understanding needed to conduct the study. Some researchers spend their lives studying a specific problem, and they are aware of the relevant information available. However, these researchers continue to review the literature to update their knowledge base. An experienced researcher with a broad background of a research problem can help novice researchers find relevant sources.

Complexity of the Research Project

Major research projects that involve numerous variables and complex methodologies require more extensive literature reviews than do studies that focus on one or two variables and include simple methodology. Funded research projects are usually complex and require extensive coverage of the literature. Master's theses are usually narrow in focus and doctoral dissertations are frequently more complex. For both a thesis and dissertation, the depth of the review is extensive but the breadth of the review is frequently greater for a dissertation. An extensive literature review is conducted to provide the student with a background for planning and implementing the study.

Availability of Sources

The amount of information available continues to escalate with the production of approximately 6,000 new scientific articles a day. At this rate, scientific knowledge will double about every five years (Naisbitt, 1982). The number of new book titles and editions is rapidly escalating, rising from 41,000 in 1977 to 55,483 in 1988 (Naisbitt & Aburdene, 1990). If researchers attempted to read every source that is somewhat related to a selected problem, they would be well read but would probably never begin conducting their study. Some researchers believe they do not know enough about their area of study, so they continue to read; however, ultimately this becomes an excuse for not progressing with their research. The opposite of this is the researcher who wants to move rapidly through the review of literature to get on with the important part of conducting the study. In both situations, the researcher has not been able to set realistic goals for conducting the literature review.

The literature available is influenced by the problem selected for study. In quantitative research, a descriptive study is considered the initial investigation of a research problem, so there are few, if any, studies available on the problem. The review of literature would include primarily theoretical information and a few related studies. If a problem is investigated using a correlational study, the literature review usually includes theoretical information and a few relevant studies. In quasi-experimental and experimental studies, the information reviewed is both theoretical and empirical and usually many studies are available on the selected problem.

The sources available on problems investigated with qualitative research are predominantly theoretical, with some empirical information that is usually generated from related studies. Qualitative research is relatively new in nursing; therefore, the empirical information is frequently obtained from literature in related fields. However, even in other fields, prior studies on many qualitative research problems relevant to nursing are limited. Qualitative research is often a methodology of choice in areas of limited or no previous research (Munhall & Oiler, 1986). In examining sources, the concern should be with quality rather than quantity. Many sources are reviewed but only relevant, quality sources are included in the research proposal and study report.

TIME FRAME FOR A LITERATURE REVIEW

The time required to review the literature is influenced by the problem studied, sources available, and goals of the researcher. There is no set length of time for reviewing the literature, but there are guidelines for directing the review process. The narrower the focus of the study, the less time that will be required for reviewing the literature. The difficulty in identifying and locating sources and the number of sources to be located will also influence the time involved. If a researcher's goal is to conduct a study within a set time frame, the review of literature might have to be limited in order to meet the deadline. If a study is to be conducted within one year, the review of literature will probably take a minimum of a month but should not exceed three months. The intensity of the effort will determine the time required to complete the review. Only through experience do researchers become knowledgeable about the time frame for a literature review. Novice researchers frequently underestimate the time needed for the review and ought to plan at least twice the amount of time originally projected.

PROCESS OF REVIEWING THE LITERATURE

The quality (accuracy and completeness) of the literature review depends on the researcher's knowledge of and organization in conducting this review process. The process of reviewing the literature in quantitative and qualitative research involves: (1) using the library, (2) identifying sources, (3) locating sources, (4) reading sources, and (5) critiquing sources.

USING THE LIBRARY

Using library facilities requires current knowledge of the available libraries and their resources. The three major categories of libraries are (1) public, (2) academic, and (3) special (Strauch & Brundage, 1980). *Public libraries* serve the needs of the communities where they are located and frequently do not contain the sources required for nursing research. *Academic libraries* are located within institutions of higher learning and contain numerous resources for researchers. For example, there is a network of seven Regional Medical Libraries that contain relevant sources for health care providers. These libraries can be contacted directly or through a local librarian.

The *special library* contains a collection of materials on a selected topic or for a specialty area, such as nursing or medicine. Large hospitals, health care centers, health research centers, and certain organizations have special libraries that contain sources that are relevant to health care providers and researchers. For example, the most comprehensive collection of national and international nursing materials is available in the Center for Nursing Scholarship located in Indianapolis, Indiana. This center was dedicated on November 15, 1989 and was funded by gifts from Sigma Theta Tau International members and chapters, corporations, foundations, and friends of nursing.

When using a library for the first time, a formal orientation is helpful to identify and locate the resources and sources available in the library. Essential library resources include: the library personnel, interlibrary loan department, circulation department, reference department, audiovisual department, computer search department, and photocopy services. The circulation department provides information on the library's borrowing policies, and some libraries provide interlibrary loan cards that make it possible to check out books and materials from other libraries. The library personnel in the reference department are familiar with the library's collections and operations and can provide assistance in using the catalog, indexes, abstracts, and other reference materials in the facility. The common sources of interest to nurse researchers in the library include dictionaries, encyclopedias, books, journals, monographs, conference proceedings, bibliographies, directories, government documents, audiovisuals, master's theses, doctoral dissertations, research in progress, and professional publications of the American Nurses Association (ANA), National League for Nursing (NLN), and National Institute for Nursing Research (NINR).

IDENTIFYING SOURCES

To identify relevant sources, you must first clarify your research topic, conduct a brief manual literature search, and then conduct a computer search. A *manual search* involves examining the catalog, indexes, and abstracts for relevant sources. Many of the citations found in these documents are now entered in a variety of databases. Through the advancement of technology, *computer searches* can

Table 6–3
Clarifying a Research Topic

Research Topic	Synonymous Terms	Subheadings
Postoperative experience	Postoperative care	Postoperative ambulation
	Postoperative recovery	Postoperative attitude
	Postsurgical experience	Postoperative complications
	Surgical care	Postoperative hospitalization
	Surgical recovery	Postoperative pain
		Postoperative teaching

be conducted to scan the citations in different databases and identify sources relevant to a research problem. A brief manual search often helps to clarify a research topic and provide direction for a computer search.

Clarifying a Research Topic

A researcher selects a topic for study and then proceeds to clarify and narrow that topic by identifying synonymous terms and appropriate subheadings. Synonymous terms can be found in thesauruses, such as the *International Nursing Index's Nursing Thesaurus*. Subheadings can be located in the *Cumulative Index to Nursing & Allied Health Literature's (CINAHL) Nursing Subject Headings* and the *National Library of Medicine's Medical Subject Headings*. These documents sometimes organize sources under different subheadings. Frequently, word processing programs, dictionaries, and encyclopedias are helpful in identifying synonymous terms and subheadings. Some of the synonymous terms and subheadings for the research topic of postoperative experience are outlined in Table 6–3.

Using the Catalog, Indexes, and Abstracts

An orientation to the library provides a background for using its resources. The research topic, synonymous terms, and subheadings identified are used to guide a brief search of the catalog listings, indexes, and abstracts for relevant sources.

Catalog

The *catalog* identifies what is available in the library. These listings are usually available on an on-line computer. The catalog listings include books, monographs, conference proceedings, audiovisuals, professional organizations' publications, theses, and dissertations. Some individuals overlook the value of books, because they believe the content is too old. However, books can be excellent sources of theoretical information and frequently contain in-depth information on a specific topic. Many qualitative studies are published in books. Most books also include extensive bibliographies that might direct the researcher to additional sources.

Monographs and conference proceedings usually contain current empirical and theoretical information, but the content included is frequently limited to an abstract or a brief paper. The researcher or theorist can be contacted for more information. Theses and dissertations frequently provide a complete review of the literature for a specific research problem and an extensive bibliography.

Indexes

An *index* provides assistance in identifying journal articles and other publications relevant to a topic of interest. Indexes are organized into two major sections, subject and author. The research topic, synonymous terms, and subheadings identified by the researcher are used to guide the search through the subject section of the index. The subject section includes headings and subheadings; and under these headings, several publications (predominantly articles) are listed. Many of these publications are listed under more than one subject heading and subheading for easy access by the searcher. For example, a nursing study of the measurement of chronic pain in the elderly might be listed under the subject headings of *pain measurement, elderly,* and *nursing research* and under the subheadings of *old age* and *chronic pain.* An example of an index listing from the *Cumulative Index to Nursing & Allied Health Literature* follows:

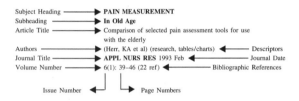

If you are familiar with the names of key researchers for a specific topic, you can search the author section of the index to identify recent publications by these individuals. The author section is organized alphabetically by the first author's name; no more than three authors are listed. The second and third authors' names appear as cross-references to the full citation under the first author's name. The author's name is followed by the same bibliographic content that is included in the subject section.

Some of the key indexes used by nursing researchers are *Cumulative Index to Nursing & Allied Health Literature, Index Medicus, International Nursing Index,* and *Hospital Literature Index.* These indexes are presented in order of importance for nurse researchers; the content, availability, and use of these indexes are briefly discussed.

CUMULATIVE INDEX TO NURSING & ALLIED HEALTH LITERATURE (CINAHL) (formerly, *Cumulative Index to Nursing Literature*).

This index is usually consulted first by nurse researchers, because it is published frequently, references a large number of relevant nursing sources, and is the original index for nursing literature. *CINAHL* was first published in 1956 and is currently published in five bimonthly issues and a cumulative annual bound volume. The index references more than 300 nursing journals, along with publications of the American Nurses' Association (ANA) and the National League for Nursing (NLN). The index also provides access to allied health and health-related journals and includes more than 3,200 pertinent citations from the biomedical journals listed in *Index Medicus.* The index includes an explanation on how to use it, criteria for selection of materials, *CINAHL* services, regional medical libraries, new journals indexed, U.S. government publications, subject section, author section, and appendices (audiovisual materials, book reviews, and pamphlets).

INDEX MEDICUS (IM).
IM is the oldest health-related index and was first published in 1879. This index cites articles from approximately 3,500 domestic and foreign journals. *IM* is published monthly and issues a bound annual volume of cumulated listings. This index covers all aspects of biomedicine and includes allied health fields, such as nursing, the biological and physical sciences, veterinary medicine, and the humanities. *IM* also includes listings of books related to biomedicine and publications from selected proceedings.

INTERNATIONAL NURSING INDEX (INI).
This index was first published in 1966 by the American Journal of Nursing Company in cooperation with the National Library of Medicine. *INI* is published quarterly, and the fourth issue is an annual cumulation of listings. This index includes more than 200 nursing journals in all languages, as well as all nursing articles in non-nursing journals currently indexed for *Index Medicus.* In addition, *INI* includes a nursing thesaurus and listings of publications of nursing organizations and agencies, nursing books, and dissertations.

HOSPITAL LITERATURE INDEX (HLI).
This index is published quarterly, and the fourth issue is the annual cumulation of listings. *HLI* was first published in 1945 by the American Hospital Asso-

ciation in cooperation with the National Library of Medicine. This index includes citations from more than 700 English language journals and relevant listings from *Index Medicus.* The listings in *HLI* focus on the administration and delivery of health care in hospitals.

Abstracts

Abstracts include the same bibliographical data as indexes, with an additional brief, objective summary (abstract) of the content covered in the publication. Abstracts are helpful in determining whether sources are relevant to the research problem identified. Some of the most commonly used abstracts in nursing research include *Nursing Abstracts, Psychological Abstracts, Dissertation Abstracts,* and *Master's Abstracts.*

NURSING ABSTRACTS. This resource was first published in 1979 and is currently published bimonthly, with an annual cumulative bound volume. The abstracts are generated from the articles in 53 nursing journals. *Nursing Abstracts* is indexed by subject, author, and journal. An example of a listing from this resource follows:

Subject Heading → **NURSING RESEARCH**
Article Title ⟶ **Effectiveness of the Auscultatory Method in Predicting Feeding Tube Location**
Authors ⟶ Metheny, Norma, et al
Publication ⟶
Nurs Res. 39:5, Sept/Oct 90, pp 262–67
Abstract ⟶ The auscultatory method is used to ensure patients' correct placement of nasogastric or nasointestinal feeding tubes. However, conflicting reports exist as to its utility. One area of this study was to determine to what extent sounds generated by air insufflations through feeding

tubes can be used to predict where the tubes' ports end in the gastrointestinal tract, and if these sounds can be used to differentiate between gastric and respiratory placement.

PSYCHOLOGICAL ABSTRACTS (PA). This resource was first published in 1927 by the American Psychological Association and is currently published monthly, with semiannual cumulative bound volumes. *PA* covers over 1,300 journals and publications in psychology and related disciplines such as psychiatry, sociology, anthropology, education, linguistics, and pharmacology. *PA* is organized into two sections (author and subject), and the citations included are journal articles, technical reports, monographic series, and dissertations. The citations and abstracts included in *PA* are available through the computer search PSYCINFO (formerly *Psychological Abstracts*). This resource was initiated in 1967 and the listings are updated monthly.

DISSERTATION ABSTRACTS INTERNATIONAL (DAI). This resource includes citations and abstracts of virtually every doctoral dissertation accepted at North American universities since 1861. *DAI* was first published in 1938 and is currently published monthly, with an annual cumulative author index. The authors determine under which heading(s) and subheading(s) their dissertations will be listed. Some nurses indexed their dissertations under "Nursing" in the health sciences section; however, many nurse-written dissertations are indexed under other headings. Consequently, it is important to search a variety of headings to locate relevant dissertations. Dissertation citations can also be identified with the *Dissertation Abstracts Online (DISS)* computer search. In 1980, abstracts were included for the dissertations; master's theses citations and abstracts were added after 1988. The database covers 1861 to present and is updated monthly.

MASTER'S ABSTRACTS (MA). This resource includes abstracts of master's theses from a variety of fields, including science, social sciences, and humanities. This index was first published in 1962/1963 and is currently a quarterly publication with a cumulative subject and author index published annually. Few abstracts of nursing master's theses were included in *MA* before 1985. Therefore, many of these studies completed before 1985 are relatively unavailable to researchers and have essentially been lost to nursing's body of knowledge. Since 1988, citations and abstracts of master's theses can be accessed using the *Dissertation Abstracts Online* computer search.

Conducting a Computer Search

After a brief manual search of the literature, you have clear direction for conducting a computer search. Computer searches are comprehensive, readily available, and affordable. The rapid expansion of published materials has made computer searchers invaluable. A computer search will generate a list of references with complete bibliographic information; for many of the references, abstracts are also available on request. (Nicoll, 1993; Saba, Oatway, & Rieder, 1989; Sinclair, 1987).

You can search the literature on your own or request a search be conducted by library personnel. Most academic libraries have the facilities for you to conduct your own on-line computer search. The computer system provides you access to catalog listings of library materials and to databases with lists of journal articles. Some libraries have on-line access to the catalogs of other libraries in the local area or within the state. Thus, when you are searching the literature for a topic, you have access to all the materials in your library and the surrounding libraries. In many libraries, you can direct the computer to print a copy of the sources selected for review.

Microcomputers can now be used to access and search *databases* (computerized lists of references). If you have a microcomputer, you can conduct literature searches from your home or worksite. You need to contact your university library to determine what you will need to conduct on-line searchers with your microcomputer. In addition to your microcomputer, you will probably need a modem and telephone line and a communication software package. The library personnel will provide you with information on how to access the university on-line system, how to search the library collections, and how to sign off of the system. You also need a number to call if you have any problems or questions while using the system. Most universities now provide students accounts that make it possible to access the World Wide Web (WWW), which has a wealth of information.

When you are searching databases, you need to organize your search. You can search by subject, journal, or author. You will probably want to start with a search of relevant topics or subjects. For example if you want information on prevention of pressure ulcers in the elderly, you might search under the topics of *pressure ulcer, pressure sore,* or *decubitus ulcer.* You also might want to search selective journals, such as *Applied Nursing Research, Decubitus, Journal of Gerontological Nursing, Nursing Research,* or *Research in Nursing & Health* for relevant sources. If you know authors that publish regularly on the topic of pressure ulcers, you might search under their name for current research articles. Some of the authors who have published on prevention of pressure ulcers include Braden and Bergstrom (1987) and Norton (1989).

Available Databases

Several databases are pertinent to nursing. Conducting a computer search involves identifying which databases to search to generate the references for a selected research problem. The most common databases used by nurse researchers are briefly introduced below.

NURSING & ALLIED HEALTH (NAHL). This database is the on-line version of the *Cumulative Index to Nursing and Allied Health Literature (CINAHL).* NAHL includes over 300 English-language nursing journals, publications of ANA and NLN, and primary journals from over a dozen allied health disciplines. The database also includes citations from approximately 3,200 biomedical journals from *Index Medicus*. The materials are indexed using *CINAHL*'s annually updated thesaurus, which is adapted from the U.S. National Library of Medicine's *Medical Subject Headings (MeSH)*. No abstracts are included. The database was initiated in 1983 and is updated every two months.

MEDLINE (MEDICAL LITERATURE ANALYSIS AND RETRIEVAL SYSTEM ONLINE). This database is supplied by the National Library of Medicine and is the most comprehensive on-line resource for national and international medical literature. MEDLINE includes about six million articles from approximately 3,500 biomedical journals. This database also contains a separate file called "Special List Nursing" that includes citations from approximately 260 nursing journals that are in the *International Nursing Index*. A MEDLINE search generates the following information: author, title, abstract (since 1975 for some citations), language, and indexing terms. This database covers the time period from 1966 to the present and is updated semimonthly.

COMBINED HEALTH INFORMATION DATABASE (CHID). This database contains over 44,000 citations and abstracts of information for health professionals, patients, and the general public. Just a few of the topics covered are Alzheimer's disease, AIDS information and education, cholesterol education, and high blood pressure. CHID was initiated in 1973 and is updated four times a year.

HEALTH PLANNING AND ADMINISTRATION (HLTH). This database contains more than 460,000 citations and is produced by the National Library of Medicine. The subjects covered include management, health care planning, organization, financing, manpower, patient education, accreditation, and other related subjects. The database includes citations from 1975 to the present and is updated every month. The information obtained by searching this database includes author, title, abstract, language, and indexing terms.

CATLINE (CATALOG ONLINE). This database contains about 500,000 references for books and serials cataloged at the National Library of Medicine. The information obtained includes author, title, source, language, indexing terms, and other data such as edition, series, title, and notes. CATLINE was originated in 1965 and is currently updated weekly.

HEALTH AND PSYCHOLOGICAL INSTRUMENTS ONLINE (HAPI). This database includes national and international instruments published in English for researchers, administrators, educators, and practitioners in the health fields and the behavioral and psychosocial sciences. Questionnaires, interview schedules, index measures, observation checklists/manuals, rating scales, coding schemes, projective techniques, tests, and scenarios/vignettes are included in the database. HAPI is produced by Behavioral Measurement Database Services (BMDS) and is organized using key terms from *Medical Subject Headings (MeSH)* and the *Thesaurus of Psychological Index Terms*. The database was initiated in 1985 and is updated quarterly.

AVLINE (AUDIOVISUAL CATALOG ONLINE). This database includes more than 11,000 audiovisual packages covering a broad range of health-related subjects, such as nurse-patient relationships, nursing care, nursing audit, and legal aspects of nursing. The supplier of AVLINE is the National Library of Medicine and it is updated every month. An AVLINE search produces the following information: title, media type, authorship, physical description, indexing terms, run time, audience level, review rating and date, reviewer, learning method, abstract, continuing education credit note, price, and source for purchase or loan.

BIOETHICSLINE. This database covers citations that deal with ethical questions arising in health care or biomedical research, such as human experimentation, patients' rights, death and dying, and resources allocation. The supplier of BIOETHICSLINE is the National Library of Medicine and the Kennedy Institute of Ethics. This database includes citations from 1973 to the present and is updated three times a year. The information obtained from this database includes author, title, source, indexing terms, language, and type of publication.

CANCERLIT (CANR). This database contains more than 685,000 citations from over 3,000 journals, books, conference proceedings, theses, and reports. The supplier of CANCERLIT is the National Library of Medicine and the Cancer Institute. This database covers all aspects of cancer from 1963 to the present and is updated monthly. The information obtained from this database includes author, author's affiliation, title, abstract, language, type of publication, and indexing terms.

LOCATING SOURCES

You are now ready to locate the sources identified by the manual and computer searches. Locating sources involves the following steps: (1) organizing the list of identified sources, (2) searching the library for those sources, (3) determining additional ways to locate sources, and (4) systematically recording references.

Organizing the List of Sources

The list of identified sources can be organized in several ways to facilitate locating them within the library. Journal sources might be organized by journal name and year, which can greatly reduce the time spent wandering from journal to journal. You can then methodically locate all sources within a specific journal and then proceed to the next one. Sources included in the library catalog (such as books, monographs, organizational publications, and conference proceedings) can be organized by author or subject. This organization will not only make it easier to find these sources in the library but will also assist you in eliminating any duplicated references.

Searching the Library for Sources

Your search for sources in the library can be facilitated by talking with library personnel to determine the classification system; the availability of resources and publications; and the location of journals, books, dictionaries, indexes, and abstracts. When locating books, the library call number should be recorded in case you need to find the source a second time. Persistence is required to find library sources, so do not mark a source off the list simply because it was not located on the first search.

Determining Additional Ways to Locate Sources

You need to identify the sources that were located in the available library(ies), the sources that are available in the library but were not found, and those sources that are unavailable. If certain sources cannot be located in the local library facilities, you should attempt to locate them through the *interlibrary loan department.* Locating a source might also require contacting the author when a journal article is incomplete or when requesting reprints of a study, instruments, or other relevant information. Reviewing the literature is an additive process, in which identifying and locating sources leads to further identification and location of sources until the relevant sources related to a research problem are exhausted.

Journal articles can also be obtained by computer. For example, Sigma Theta Tau International has just instigated *The Online Journal of Knowledge Synthesis for Nursing.* With a computer and a modem, access is possible through a network such as the Internet or CompuServe, or by a modem dial access through the Online Computer Library Center (OCLC) (Barnsteiner, 1994). Using this system, journal articles can be delivered across commercial telecommunications to a personal computer. Subscriptions for the online journal can be initiated through Sigma Theta Tau International. The OCLC will then provide the software, user documentation, user password, and technical support for the system. Many universities and colleges have purchased this system for use by faculty and students. Obtaining journal articles electronically is still quite expensive, and many students prefer to locate sources in their university libraries.

Systematically Recording References

The bibliographical information on a source should be recorded in a systematic manner, according to the format that will be used in developing the review of literature section and the reference list. Many journals and academic institutions use the American Psychological Association (APA) (1994) format. The reference lists in this textbook are presented in a modified APA format. A complete bibliographic citation (according to APA) should be recorded on all articles at the time they are copied. If the article is obtained from interlibrary loan, the complete citation is stapled to the article and should be kept or copied onto the article. Computerized lists of sources usually contain complete citations for references and should be filed for future use. With the use of your personal computer, you can also easily search a computerized database and obtain complete reference citations.

A systematic recording process increases the accuracy of the references in your research proposal and report. Anyone reviewing the literature has at some time been frustrated by inaccurate references in publications. Foreman and Kirchhoff (1987) studied the accuracy of references in 17 nursing journals. Sixty-five of the references were from clinical journals and 47 were from nonclinical journals. The errors were classified as major (preventing retrieval of the source) or minor (not preventing retrieval). Errors occurred more frequently in clinical journals (38.4%) than in nonclinical journals (21.3%). Clinical references also had a 4.5% incidence of major errors, while the nonclinical references had no major errors. The incidence of errors in these references reinforces the importance of recording complete, accurate citations for each source.

READING AND CRITIQUING SOURCES

Reading and critiquing sources promotes understanding of the current knowledge of a research problem and involves skimming, comprehending, analyzing, and synthesizing content from sources. An expertise in reading and critiquing sources is essential in developing a quality literature review. Many projects require a review of the literature and a summary of current knowledge, such as a project to use research findings in practice, a research proposal, and a research report. This section focuses mainly on reading skills with a brief introduction to the critique process.

Skimming Sources

Skimming is a quick review of a source to gain a broad overview of the content. You would probably read the title, author's name, and an abstract or introduction for the source. Then you would read the major headings and sometimes one or two sentences under each heading. Lastly, the conclusion or summary is reviewed. Skimming enables you to make a preliminary judgment about the value of a source and to determine whether it is a primary or secondary source. Secondary sources are reviewed and used to locate primary sources but frequently are not cited in a research proposal or report.

Comprehending Sources

Comprehending a source requires that the entire source be read carefully. You focus on understanding major concepts and the logical flow of ideas within the source. The content that is considered significant is highlighted and sometimes ideas are recorded in the margins. Notes might be recorded on photocopies of articles, indicating where the information will be used in developing a research proposal. The information highlighted on theoretical sources might include relevant concepts, definitions of those concepts, and relationships among the concepts. The notes recorded on empirical literature might include relevant information about the researcher, such as whether this is a critical or major researcher of a selected problem and other studies this individual has conducted. The research problem, purpose, framework, major variables, study design, sample size, data collection and analysis techniques, and findings are usually highlighted in a research article. You may wish to record quotes (including page numbers) that might be used in a review of literature section. The decision to paraphrase these quotes can be made later. You might also record creative ideas about content that develop while reading a source. At this point, relevant categories are identified for sorting and organizing sources. These categories will ultimately serve as a guide for writing the review of literature section, and some may even be major headings in this section.

Analyzing Sources

Through *analysis,* you can determine the value of a source for a particular study. The content of the source is divided into parts; and the parts are examined in-depth for accuracy, completeness, uniqueness of information, organization, and relevance of each part of the source for the study to be conducted. At this point, relevant content in sources is clearly identified and sources are sorted into a sophisticated system of categories. Conducting an analysis of sources to be used in a research proposal requires some knowledge of the subject to be critiqued, some knowledge of the research process, and the ability to exercise judgment in evaluation (Fleming & Hayter, 1974; Pinch, 1995). The critique process, including the steps of comprehension, comparison, analysis, evaluation, and conceptual clustering, is detailed in Chapter 24.

Synthesis of Source Content

Through *synthesis,* one can cluster and interrelate ideas from several sources to form a gestalt. Synthesis involves clarifying the meaning obtained from the source as a whole. This meaning should then be paraphrased. *Paraphrasing* involves ex-

pressing clearly and concisely the ideas of an author in your own words. The meanings of these sources are then connected to the proposed study. Lastly, the meanings obtained from all sources are combined, or clustered, to determine the current knowledge of the research problem (Pinch, 1995). Synthesis is the basis for developing the review of literature section for a research proposal, report, or utilization project. A comprehensive, scholarly synthesis of the literature is evident in published integrative reviews of research and meta-analyses. This type of synthesis is called *cognitive clustering* and requires knowledge of the literature and expertise in conducting and critiquing research. Integrative research reviews are introduced in this chapter, and Chapter 25 describes the use of integrative reviews and meta-analysis to summarize research findings for use in practice.

Integrative Reviews of Nursing Research

Integrative reviews are conducted to identify, analyze, and synthesize the results from independent studies to determine the current knowledge (what is known and not known) in a particular area (Ganong, 1987; Smith & Stullenbarger, 1991). These reviews include a comprehensive list of references and summarize empirical literature for selected topics (Cooper, 1984). In 1983, the first volume of the *Annual Review of Nursing Research* was published by Werley and Fitzpatrick. These volumes include integrative reviews of research in the areas of nursing practice, nursing care delivery, nursing education, and the profession of nursing. Integrative reviews have also been published in a variety of clinical and nonclinical journals. A list of integrative reviews of nursing research, organized by clinical topics, is included in the student study guide that accompanies this text.

WRITING THE REVIEW OF LITERATURE

A thorough, organized literature review will facilitate developing a research proposal. Writing the review of literature involves the selection of relevant sources, organization of those sources, and the mechanics of writing the review.

SELECTION OF RELEVANT SOURCES

Sources are selected for inclusion in the literature review based on their quality and relationship to the problem and purpose of the proposed study. Analysis of each source determines its quality and usefulness in developing the research proposal or report. The review of literature needs to build a case and provide direction for the proposed study.

ORGANIZATION OF SOURCES

Relevant sources (theoretical and empirical) are organized for inclusion in the different chapters of the research proposal. The sources to be included in the review of literature chapter are organized to reflect the current knowledge of the research problem. Those sources that provide background and significance for the study are included in the introduction chapter. Certain theoretical sources will provide the framework for the study. Other relevant sources become the basis for defining research variables and identifying assumptions and limitations. Methodologically strong studies will direct the development of the research design, guide the selection of instruments, influence data collection and analysis, and provide a basis for interpretation of findings. At this point, many researchers are beginning to get a complete picture of their study and are excited about its potential. They frequently feel confident about their knowledge of the research problem and their ability to make the study a reality.

The literature review for theses and dissertations is often organized into two major sections: empirical and theoretical. Within these two sections, the literature is then organized by concepts that are relevant to the research problem. The literature review for a research proposal often includes the following headings and essential content.

1. Introduction indicates the focus or purpose of the study; identifies the purpose of the literature review; describes the organization of sources (by concepts or theoretical or empirical sections); and indicates the basis for ordering the sources; for example, from least to most important or from least to most current. This section should be brief and catch the interest of the reader.

2. Theoretical literature includes concept analyses, models, theories, and conceptual frameworks that support the research purpose. Concepts, definitions of concepts, relationships among concepts, and assumptions are presented and analyzed to build a theoretical knowledge base for the study. This section is often organized by concepts appropriate to the study. These concepts are usually identified when searching for relevant theoretical and empirical sources and critiquing studies.

3. Empirical literature includes quality studies that support the research purpose. For each study, the purpose, sample size, design, and specific findings should be presented with a scholarly but brief critique of the study's strengths and weaknesses. Work for conciseness and clarity, with only the most relevant studies being included. This section is often organized by concepts or variables that are the focus of the study.

4. Summary includes a concise presentation of the current knowledge base for the research problem. The gaps in the knowledge base are identified, with a discussion of how the proposed study will generate essential information.

MECHANICS OF WRITING THE REVIEW OF LITERATURE

Writing the review of literature requires the development of a detailed outline that will be used as a guide. Often the introduction is written and rewritten based on the development of other sections in the literature review. In writing the main section of the literature review, the empirical and theoretical sources must be presented in a concise, accurate manner. The content from these sources is best paraphrased or summarized in the researcher's own words. If a direct quote is used, it should be kept short to promote the flow of ideas. Long quotes are often unnecessary and interfere with the reader's train of thought.

The researcher should discuss in depth those studies that are most relevant in guiding the investigation. Studies with similar methodologies or findings need to be discussed in relation to each other to show similarities and differences and to prevent repetition. Some novice researchers tend to randomly list sources, with a paragraph about each. This strategy indicates no analysis and synthesis of the meaning obtained from various sources (Pinch, 1995). The findings from the studies should logically build on each other so that the reader can see how the body of knowledge in the research area evolved.

Ethical issues must be considered in presenting sources (Gunter, 1981). The content from sources should be presented honestly, not distorted to support the selected problem. Researchers will frequently read studies and wish that the authors had studied slightly different problems or that the studies had been designed or conducted differently. However, they must recognize their own opinions and be objective in presenting information. The defects of a study need to be addressed, but it is not necessary to be highly critical of another researcher's work. The criticisms need to focus on the content that is in some way relevant to the proposed study and be stated as possible or plausible explanations, so that they are more neutral and scholarly than negative and blaming. Authors' works must be accurately documented so they receive credit for their publications. The reference list includes only those sources that have been cited in the development of the proposal or report.

EXAMPLE OF A LITERATURE REVIEW

The literature review from a published study is presented to reinforce the points that were ad-

dressed in this chapter. The study focuses on "behavioral analysis and nursing interventions for reducing disruptive behaviors of patients with dementia" (Boehm, Whall, Cosgrove, Locke, & Schlenk, 1995). Only selected content from this literature review is presented to demonstrate (1) the introduction; (2) organization of empirical and theoretical information by the concepts of behavioral therapy, behavioral gerontology, and disruptive behaviors; and (3) the summary. The complete literature review can be found on pages 118–119 and the references on page 122 (Boehm et al., 1995).

Introduction

Behavioral gerontological research has successfully developed a number of effective behavioral interventions that have implications for nursing practice. (McCormick, Scheve, & Leahy, 1988)

Behavioral Therapy and Behavioral Gerontology

The majority of the literature in behavioral gerontology is built on the conceptual underpinnings that "behavior therapy includes interventions that attempt to change the frequency, intensity, duration, or location of a specific behavior or set of behaviors through systematic varying antecedent stimuli or consequential events." (Hussian & Davis, 1985, p. 15)

Behavioral analysis provides the basis for identification and development of behavioral interventions and is the process by which behavior is observed, documented, and analyzed from three perspectives. The three perspectives include (1) antecedent events that precede and serve as stimuli for the behavior, (2) small steps of behavior that comprise the whole behavior, and (3) consequences that follow the behavior. (Brigham, 1982)

Behavior interventions have been used successfully to treat a variety of problems in elderly, institutionalized individuals (Vaccaro, 1990). The challenge in addressing behavioral problems of individuals with dementia, however, is that many of the successful behavioral interventions rely on memory and thus are not suitable for the patient with dementia (Carstensen & Erickson, 1986). Techniques must be developed to teach nurses to provide cues and consequences that may elicit desirable patient behavior instead of abusive behavior (Lewin & Lundervold, 1990). . . . One such technique is behavioral modeling, which is the acquisition of behavior by observing other persons' behaviors and the consequences of their behaviors . . .

Disruptive Behaviors

According to the 1989 National Nursing Home Survey (National Center for Health Statistics, 1989), 80% of nursing home patients required extra nursing care because of disruptive behaviors associated with dementia, such as Alzheimer's disease. Behavioral gerontology has directed considerable attention to such areas as depression, paranoia, pain, insomnia, incontinence, memory and cognition, alcohol abuse, anxiety, and social behavior, such as dependence . . .

Summary

However, few behavioral researchers have used behavioral analysis techniques as a means of changing patients' disruptive behaviors (Fisher & Carstensen, 1990). Indeed, research evaluating behavioral analysis approaches for reducing such disquieting behaviors as wandering, inappropriate sexual behavior, and verbal and physical aggressive outbursts is needed by nurses and other caregivers for individuals with dementia (Carstensen & Erickson, 1986). (Boehm et al., 1995, pp. 118–119) ■

▌ SUMMARY

A review of literature is conducted to generate a picture of what is known and not known about a particular situation. Relevant literature refers to those sources that are important in providing the in-depth knowledge needed to make changes in practice or to study a selected problem. The primary purpose for reviewing the literature is to gain a broad background or understanding of the information that is available related to a problem. This background enables the researcher to build upon the works of others. The purpose and timing of the literature review vary with quantitative and qualitative research. In quantitative research, the review is instigated at the beginning of the research process and continues throughout the development of the research proposal, collection and analysis of data, and interpretation of findings. In qualitative research, the purpose and timing of the literature review vary based on the type of study (phenomenology, grounded theory, ethnographic, historical, philosophical inquiry, or critical social theory) to be conducted.

The scope of the literature review should be broad enough for the investigator to be knowledgeable about the research problem and narrow enough to include predominantly relevant sources. To determine the scope of a literature review, the following areas are evaluated: (1) the types of information and sources available, (2) the approximate depth and breadth of the review needed, and (3) the time frame for conducting the review. Predominately two types of information are cited in the review of literature for research: theoretical and empirical. The published literature includes two types of sources, primary and secondary sources. A primary source is written by the person who originated and is responsible for generating the ideas published. A secondary source summarizes or quotes content from primary sources. Predominately primary sources should be used in developing research proposals and reports. The depth and breadth of the literature review depend on the background of the researcher, the complexity of the research project, and the amount of literature available on a selected problem. The time

continued

continued

required to review the literature is influenced by the problem studied, sources available, and goals of the researcher.

The process of reviewing the literature involves (1) using the library, (2) identifying sources, (3) locating sources, (4) reading sources, and (5) critiquing sources. Academic and special libraries are used in research. To identify relevant sources, one must first clarify the research topic and then search the literature manually and with the computer. Manual searches involve examining the catalog, indexes, and abstracts for relevant sources. Through the advancement of technology, computer searches can be conducted to scan the citations in different databases and identify sources relevant to a research problem. The process of locating sources involves organizing a list of identified sources, searching the library for those sources, systematically recording references, and determining additional

ways to locate sources. Reading and critiquing sources promotes understanding of the current knowledge of a research problem and involves skimming, comprehending, analyzing, and synthesizing content from sources. Integrative reviews of nursing research are being conducted to identify, analyze, and synthesize the results from independent studies to determine the current knowledge of a phenomenon.

Writing the review of literature involves the selection of relevant sources, the organization of those sources, and the mechanics of writing a review. Sources are selected for inclusion in the literature review based on their quality and relationship to the problem and purpose of the proposed study. The review of literature chapter usually begins with an introduction, includes empirical and theoretical sources, and provides a summary of current knowledge. An example of a literature review from a published study is provided.

References

Aamodt, A. M. (1982). Examining ethnography for nurse researchers. *Western Journal of Nursing Research, 4*(2), 209–221.

American Psychological Association (APA). (1994). *Publication manual of the American Psychological Association* (4th ed.). Washington, DC: American Psychological Association.

Barnsteiner, J. H. (1994). The Online Journal of Knowledge Synthesis for Nursing. *Reflections, 20*(2), 10–11.

Boehm, S., Whall, A. L., Cosgrove, K. L., Locke, J. D., & Schlenk, E. A. (1995). Behavioral analysis and nursing interventions for reducing disruptive behaviors of patients with dementia. *Applied Nursing Research, 8*(3), 118–122.

Braden, B., & Bergstrom, N. (1987). A conceptual schema for the study of the etiology of pressure sores. *Rehabilitation Nursing, 12*(1), 8–12.

Brigham, T. (1982). Self-management: A radical behavioral perspective. In P. Karoly & F. H. Kanfer (Eds.), *Self-management and behavior change: From theory to practice* (pp. 32–59). New York: Pergamon.

Carstensen, L. L., & Erickson, R. J. (1986). Enhancing the social environments of elderly nursing home residents: Are high rates of interaction enough? *Journal of Applied Behavior Analysis, 19*(4), 349–355.

Christy, T. E. (1975). The methodology of historical research: A brief introduction. *Nursing Research, 24*(3), 189–192.

Cooper, H. M. (1984). *The integrative research review: A systematic approach.* Beverly Hills: Sage.

Ellis, R. (1983). Philosophic inquiry. In H. H. Werley & J. J. Fitzpatrick (Eds.), *Annual review of nursing research: Vol. 1* (pp. 211–228). New York: Springer.

Fairman, J. A. (1987). Sources and references for research in nursing history. *Nursing Research, 36*(1), 56–59.

Fisher, J. E., & Carstensen, L. L. (1990). Behavior management of the dementias. *Clinical Psychology Review, 10*(6), 611–629.

Fleming, J. W., & Hayter, J. (1974). Reading research reports critically. *Nursing Outlook, 22*(3), 172–175.

Foreman, M. D., & Kirchhoff, K. T. (1987). Accuracy of references in nursing journals. *Research in Nursing & Health, 10*(3), 177–183.

Ganong, L. H. (1987). Integrative reviews of nursing research. *Research in Nursing & Health, 10*(1), 1–11.

Germain, C. (1986). Ethnography: The method. In P. L. Munhall & C. J. Oiler (Eds.), *Nursing research: A qualitative perspective* (pp. 147–162). Norwalk, CT: Appleton-Century-Crofts.

Gunter, L. (1981). Literature review. In S. D. Krampitz & N. Pavlovich (Eds.), *Readings for nursing research* (pp. 11–16). St. Louis: Mosby.

Hedin, B. A. (1986). Nursing, education, and emancipation:

Applying the critical theoretical approach to nursing research. In P. L. Chinn (Ed.), *Nursing research methodology: Issues and implementation* (pp. 133–146). Rockville, MD: Aspen.

Holter, I. M. (1988). Critical theory: A foundation for the development of nursing theories. *Scholarly Inquiry for Nursing Practice: An International Journal, 2*(3), 223–232.

Hussian, R. A., & Davis, R. L. (1985). *Responsive care: Behavioral interventions with elderly persons.* Champaign, IL: Research.

Hutchinson, S. (1986). Grounded theory: The method. In P. L. Munhall & C. J. Oiler (Eds.), *Nursing research: A qualitative perspective* (pp. 111–130). Norwalk, CT: Appleton-Century-Crofts.

Kaplan, A. (1964). *The conduct of inquiry: Methodology for behavioral science.* New York: Chandler.

Kilby, S. A., Fishel, C. C., & Gupta, A. D. (1989). Access to nursing information resources. *Image: Journal of Nursing Scholarship, 21*(1), 26–30.

Kubler-Ross, E. (1969). *On death and dying.* New York: Macmillan.

Lewin, L. M., & Lundervold, D. A. (1990). Behavioral analysis of separation-individuation conflict in the spouse of an Alzheimer's disease patient. *The Gerontologist, 30*(5), 703–705.

Manchester, P. (1986). Analytic philosophy and foundational inquiry: The method. In P. L. Munhall & C. J. Oiler (Eds.), *Nursing research: A qualitative perspective* (pp. 229–249). Norwalk, CT: Appleton-Century-Crofts.

Marchette, L. (1985). Research: The literature review process. *Perioperative Nursing Quarterly, 1*(4), 69–76.

Matejski, M. (1986). Historical research: The method. In P. L. Munhall & C. J. Oiler (Eds.), *Nursing research: A qualitative perspective* (pp. 175–193). Norwalk, CT: Appleton-Century-Crofts.

McCormick, K. A., Scheve, A. A., & Leahy, E. (1988). Nursing management of urinary incontinence in geriatric inpatients. *Nursing Clinics of North America, 23*(1), 231–264.

Munhall, P. L., & Oiler, C. J. (1986). *Nursing research: A qualitative perspective.* Norwalk, CT: Appleton-Century-Crofts.

Naisbitt, J. (1982). *Megatrends: Ten new directions transforming our lives.* New York: Warner Books.

Naisbitt, J., & Aburdene, P. (1990). *Megatrends 2000: Ten new directions for the 1990's.* New York: William Morrow.

National Center for Health Statistics. (1989). *The national nursing home survey* (DHHS Publication No. PHS 8901758, Series 13, No. 97). Hyattsville, MD: Public Health Service.

Nicoll, L. H. (1993). Keeping abreast of the literature electronically. *Nursing Research, 42*(5), 315–317.

Norton, D. (1989). Calculating the risk: Reflections on the Norton Scale. *Decubitus, 2*(3), 24–31.

Oiler, C. (1982). The phenomenological approach in nursing research. *Nursing Research, 31*(3), 178–181.

Oiler, C. J. (1986). Phenomenology: The method. In P. L. Munhall & C. J. Oiler (Eds.), *Nursing research: A qualitative perspective* (pp. 69–84). Norwalk, CT: Appleton-Century-Crofts.

Pinch, W. J. (1995). Synthesis: Implementing a complex process. *Nurse Educator, 20*(1), 34–40.

Saba, V. K., Oatway, D. M., & Rieder, K. A. (1989). How to use nursing information sources. *Nursing Outlook, 37*(4), 189–195.

Sinclair, V. G. (1987). Literature searches by computer. *Image: Journal of Nursing Scholarship, 19*(1), 35–37.

Smith, M. C., & Stullenbarger, E. (1991). A prototype for integrative review and meta-analysis for nursing research. *Journal of Advanced Nursing, 16*(11), 1272–1283.

Stern, P. N. (1980). Grounded theory methodology: Its uses and processes. *Image: Journal of Nursing Scholarship, 12*(1), 20–23.

Strauch, K. P., & Brundage, D. J. (1980). *Guide to library resources for nursing.* Norwalk, CT: Appleton-Century-Crofts.

Vaccaro, F. J. (1990). Application of social skills training in a group of institutionalized aggressive elderly subjects. *Psychology and Aging, 5*(3), 369–378.

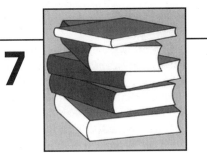

7 Frameworks

A *framework* is the abstract, logical structure of meaning that guides the development of the study and enables the researcher to link the findings to nursing's body of knowledge. Frameworks are used in both quantitative and qualitative research. In quantitative studies, the framework is a testable theory that may emerge from a conceptual model or be developed inductively from clinical observations. In qualitative research, the initial framework is a philosophy or world view; a theory consistent with the philosophy is developed as an outcome of the study.

Every study has a framework. The framework should be well integrated with the methodology, carefully structured, and clearly presented. This is true whether the study is physiological or psychosocial. In order to critique studies for application in clinical practice or for use in further research, the reader needs to be able to identify and evaluate the framework. Each person's understanding of the meaning of study findings, which is based on the framework, determines how that individual will use those findings. Thus, utilization is enhanced when the reader understands the framework and can relate it to the findings for their use in nursing practice.

Unfortunately, in some studies, the ideas that compose the framework remain nebulous and vaguely expressed. The researcher holds in his or her mind the notion that the variables being studied are related in some fashion. In fact, the variables are selected because the researcher thinks there may be one or more important links among them. Otherwise, why would the study be conducted? These ideas are the rudiments of a framework. In some rudimentary frameworks, the ideas may be expressed in the literature review; but then the researcher stops without fully developing the ideas as a framework. Many studies have these implicit frameworks. Forty-nine percent of nursing practice studies published between 1977 and 1986 had no identifiable theoretical perspective (Moody et al., 1988). According to Sarter (1988, p. 2) "nursing research shows an alarming absence of theoretical relevance."

There is, however, an increasing expectation that frameworks be an integral part of nursing research and be introduced when the research process, critique, and utilization are taught to undergraduate nursing students. This knowledge can then later be expanded as the learner participates in the process of developing a framework while being taught to plan and implement studies. To facilitate development of the knowledge and skills needed to critique and/or develop a framework, this chapter explains relevant terms, describes framework development, and discusses the critique of frameworks.

DEFINITION OF TERMS

The first step in understanding theories and frameworks is to become familiar with the terms related to theoretical ideas and their application. These terms and the ways they are used come from the philosophy of science, the main concern of which is the nature of scientific knowledge (Feyerabend, 1975; Foucault, 1970; Frank, 1961; Gibbs, 1972; Hemple, 1966; Kaplan, 1964; Kerlinger, 1986; Kuhn, 1970; Laudan, 1977, 1981; Merton, 1968; Popper, 1968; Reynolds, 1971; Scheffler, 1967; Suppe, 1972; Suppe & Jacox, 1985). As nurses have studied philosophies of science, philosophies of nursing science are beginning to emerge. This is an exciting development in nursing. But, because of differences of opinion in the philosophies of nursing science, some confusion exists in the nursing literature regarding the use of terms related to theory and research. However, a growing consensus is emerging in nursing regarding the terms that should be used and their meanings. These terms include *concept, relational statement, conceptual model, theory,* and *conceptual map.* The greatest confusion has involved differences in the uses of the terms *theory* and *conceptual model.* Within philosophies of science, the term theory is used in a variety of ways that could include both specific theories and conceptual models (Suppe & Jacox, 1985). However, in philosophies of nursing science, theory tends to be defined narrowly and be differentiated from conceptual model. The definitions used in this text reflect the predominant use of these terms in nursing.

CONCEPT

A *concept* is a term that abstractly describes and names an object or phenomenon, thus providing it with a separate identity or meaning. An example of a concept is the term anxiety. At high levels of abstraction, concepts have very general meanings and are sometimes referred to as *constructs.* For example, a construct associated with the concept of anxiety might be "emotional responses." At a more concrete level, terms are referred to as variables and are narrow in their definitions. A variable is more specific than a concept and implies that the term is defined so that it is measurable. The word *variable* means that numerical values of the term *vary* from one instance to another. A variable related to anxiety might be "palmar sweating" if a method could be found to assign numerical values to varying amounts of palmar sweat. The linkages among constructs, concepts, and variables is illustrated here:

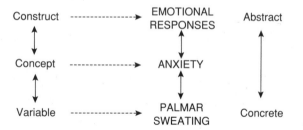

Defining concepts allows consistency in the way the term is used. A *conceptual definition* differs from the denotative (or dictionary) definition of a word. A conceptual definition (connotative meaning) is more comprehensive than a denotative definition and includes associated meanings the word may have. For example, a fireplace may connote hospitality and warm comfort. A conceptual definition can be established through concept synthesis, concept derivation, or concept analysis.

Concept Synthesis

In nursing, many phenomena have not yet been identified as discrete entities. The recognition and description of these phenomena are often critical to understanding the process and outcomes of nursing practice. The process of describing and naming a previously unrecognized concept is *concept synthesis.* In the discipline of medicine, Selye performed concept synthesis to identify and define the concept of stress. Prior to his work, stress as a phenomenon was unknown. Nursing studies often involve previously unrecognized and unnamed phenomena that need to be named and carefully defined. Concept synthesis is also important in nursing theory development (Walker & Avant, 1995).

Concept Derivation

In some cases, the conceptual definition may be derived from theories in other disciplines. These definitions—or *concept derivations*—are extracted from theories developed to explain a phenomenon important to that discipline. However, these conceptual definitions need to be carefully evaluated in terms of their fit with nursing knowledge. They often need to be modified so that they are meaningful within nursing and consistent with nursing thought (Walker & Avant, 1995).

Concept Analysis

Concept analysis is a strategy through which a set of characteristics essential to the connotative meaning of a concept is identified. The procedure requires the reader to explore the various ways the term is used and to identify a set of characteristics that can be used to clarify the range of objects or ideas to which that concept may be applied. These characteristics are also used to distinguish the concept from similar concepts (Chinn & Kramer, 1995; Walker & Avant, 1995). A number of concept analyses have been published in the nursing literature. Concept analysis is a form of philosophical inquiry and is described in Chapter 20 where an example of a concept analysis is given.

Importance of a Conceptual Definition— An Example

The importance of a conceptual definition is illustrated in a study by Morse, Solberg, Neander, Bottorff, and Johnson (1990), who performed an analysis of published definitions of the concept of "caring," a project funded by the National Center for Nursing Research. Although the concept caring is central to the essence of nursing, efforts to define it have led to confusion rather than consensus. For example, it is difficult to separate meanings for caring, care, and nursing care. Caring may be an action such as "taking care of" or a concern such as "caring about." Caring may be viewed from the perspective of the nurse or of the patient. Research examining caring in nursing practice is limited by the inadequacies in the conceptual definition of caring.

Morse and colleagues (1990) used content analysis to examine 35 authors' definitions of caring. The analysis included definitions of caring from three nursing theorists: Orem, Watson, and Leininger. Five categories of caring were identified: (1) caring as a human trait, (2) caring as a moral imperative, (3) caring as an affect, (4) caring as an interpersonal relationship, and (5) caring as a therapeutic intervention. In addition, two outcomes of caring were identified: (1) the subjective experience of the patient and (2) the physical response of the patient.

Morse and colleagues developed a model illustrating the interrelationships between the categories discussed in the literature and identifying the authors who had explored each category and each relationship (see Figure 7–1 on p. 140). The model

looks really complex but it is not. Each letter in the model refers to one of the authors listed at the bottom of the figure. These authors are identified in the reference list at the end of the chapter. If the letter is within a circle, the author identified that element as essential to the conceptual meaning of caring. If the letter is on an arrow, the author suggested that the two elements linked by the arrow were related. Arrows with solid lines show that the author directly stated the relationship. Arrows with dotted lines indicate that the author implied the relationship without directly discussing it.

After examining this model, the researchers concluded that there was little consistency in the way caring was being defined by these authors. Questions that emerged from the analysis and need to be considered in developing a conceptual definition include: (1) "Is caring a constant and uniform characteristic, or may caring be present in various degrees within individuals?" (p. 9), (2) Is caring an emotional state that can be depleted?, (3) "Can caring be nontherapeutic? Can a nurse care too much?" (p. 10), (4) Can cure occur without caring? Can a nurse provide safe practice without caring?, (5) "What difference does caring make to the patient?" (p. 11).

The authors concluded that a clear conceptual definition of caring did not exist. Until caring can be more satisfactorily defined conceptually, measuring it will be difficult since measurement is dependent upon the conceptual definition. The inadequacy of the conceptual definition of caring impedes the development of studies examining caring in nursing practice.

RELATIONAL STATEMENTS

A *relational statement* declares that a relationship of some kind exists between two or more concepts (Walker & Avant, 1995). Relational statements, sometimes referred to as propositions, are the core of the framework. Without statements, the framework is not complete. A framework must have clearly expressed relational statements in order to be well integrated into the methodology of the study since it is the statements that are tested through research. The type of statement expressed

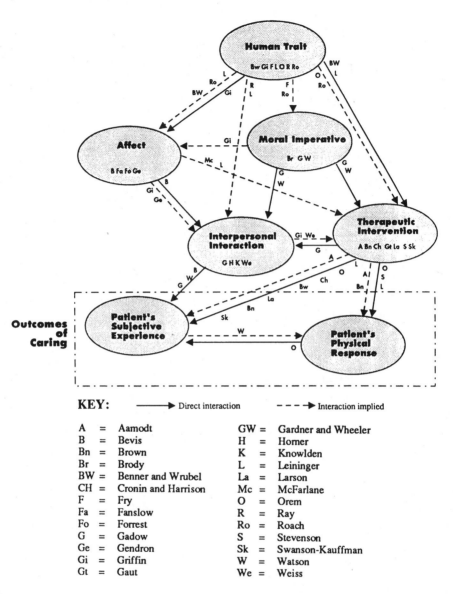

Figure 7-1
The interrelationship of five perspectives of caring. (Reprinted from *Advances in Nursing Science, 13*[1], 3, with permission of Aspen Publishers, Inc., © 1990.)

in a framework determines the objective, question, or hypothesis formulated; the design of the study; the statistical analyses that will be performed; and the type of findings that can be expected.

Understanding the various types of relational statements is essential to the critique of frameworks. Evaluation of the link between the hypothesis, the design, and the framework is a critical part of critiquing a study. Judging whether the study was successful is dependent, in part, on identifying the statements in the framework and tracking their examination by the study.

Skills in selecting or developing statements are essential for constructing an integrated framework that will, in turn, lead to a well-designed study. The adequacy of the study design is therefore dependent on the precision of statements in the framework. Frameworks developed with inadequate knowledge and skills in statement development serve only to provide a broad orientation for the study and do not guide the research process.

Characteristics of Relational Statements

Relational statements describe the direction, shape, strength, symmetry, sequencing, probability of occurrence, necessity, and sufficiency of a relationship (Fawcett & Downs, 1986; Stember, 1986; Walker & Avant, 1995). One statement may have several of the characteristics described earlier. Thus, each characteristic is not exclusive of the others. Statements may be expressed in literary form (such as a sentence), in diagrammatic form (such as a map), or in mathematical form (such as an equation). Statements in nursing tend to be expressed primarily in literary and diagrammatic form.

Direction

The direction of a relationship may be positive, negative, or unknown. A *positive linear relationship* implies that as one concept changes (the value or amount of the concept increases or decreases), the second concept will also change in the same direction. For example, the literary statement that "the risk of illness (A) increases as

stress (B) increases" expresses a positive relationship. This positive relational statement could also be expressed as "the risk of illness decreases as stress decreases." Diagrammatically this could be depicted as:

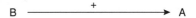

A *negative relationship* implies that as one concept changes, the other concept changes in the opposite direction. For example, the literary statement that "as relaxation (A) increases, blood pressure (B) decreases" expresses a negative relationship. Diagrammatically, this could be depicted as:

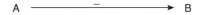

If a relationship is believed to exist, but the nature of that relationship is *unclear,* that could be depicted as:

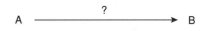

This type of statement might be appropriate for discussing the relationship between coping and social support. We might say that there is evidence that a relationship exists between these two concepts, but studies examining that relationship have conflicting findings. Some researchers find coping to be positively related to social support, whereas others find that as social support increases, coping decreases. Thus the nature of the relationship between coping and social support is uncertain. It is possible that the conflicting findings may be due to differences in the ways coping and social support have been defined and measured in various studies.

Shape

Most relationships are assumed to be linear, and statistical tests are conducted looking for linear relationships. In a *linear relationship,* the relationship between the two concepts will remain

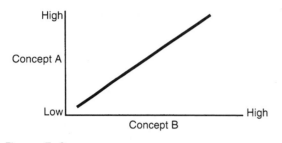

Figure 7–2
Example of a linear relationship.

consistent regardless of the values of each of the concepts. For example, if the value of A increases by 1 point each time the value of B increases by 1 point, the values will continue to increase at the same rate whether the value is 2 or 200. The relationship can be illustrated by a straight line as in Figure 7–2.

Relationships can be curvilinear or some other shape. In a *curvilinear relationship,* the relationship between two concepts varies depending on the relative values of the concepts. The relationship between anxiety and learning is a good example of a curvilinear relationship. Very high or very low levels of anxiety are associated with low levels of learning, whereas moderate levels of anxiety are associated with high levels of learning (Fawcett & Downs, 1986). This type of relationship is illustrated by a curved line as in Figure 7–3.

Strength

The *strength of a relationship* is the amount of variation explained by the relationship. Some

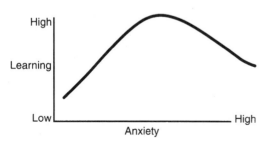

Figure 7–3
Example of a curvilinear relationship.

of the variation in a concept, but not all, is associated with variation in another concept. The strength of a relationship is sometimes discussed using the term *effect size.* The effect size explains how much "effect" variation in one concept has on variation in the second concept. In some cases a large portion and in others only a moderate or a small portion of the variation can be explained by the relationship. For example, one might examine the strength of the relationship between coping and compliance. Although a portion of the variance in a measure of compliance is associated with the measure of a person's coping ability, there is another portion of variation in the measure of compliance that cannot be explained by measuring how well a person copes. Conversely, only a portion of variation in a measure of a person's ability to cope can be explained by variation in a measure of their compliance. The portions of the two concepts that are associated are explained by the strength of the relationship. Strength is usually determined by correlational analysis and is expressed mathematically by a correlation coefficient such as:

$$r = .35$$

The statistic r is the coefficient obtained by performing the statistical procedure Pearson's product moment correlation. A value of 0 would indicate no strength, whereas $a +1$ or $a -1$ would indicate the greatest strength, as indicated in the diagram below.

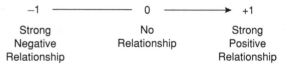

The + or − does not have an impact on strength. For example, $r = -.35$ is as strong as $r = +.35$. A weak relationship is usually considered one with an r value of .1 to .3; a moderate relationship one of .3 to .5; and a strong relationship one greater than .5. The greater the strength, the easier it is to detect differences in groups being studied.

This idea will be explored further in the chapters on sampling, measurement, and data analysis.

Symmetry

Relationships may be symmetrical or asymmetrical. In an *asymmetrical relationship,* if A occurs (or changes), then B will occur (or change), but there may be no indication that if B occurs (or changes), A will occur (or change) (Fawcett & Downs, 1986). A previous example was given showing that when changes in relaxation level (A) occurred, changes in blood pressure (B) occurred. However, can one say that when changes in blood pressure occur, changes in relaxation levels occur? The relationship, then, is asymmetric. An asymmetric relationship may be diagramed as:

A ———————————➤ B

A *symmetrical relationship* is complex and actually contains two statements. If A occurs (or changes), B will occur (or change); if B occurs (or changes), A will occur (or change) (Fawcett & Downs, 1986). An example of this is the symmetrical relationship between the occurrence of cancer and impaired immunity. As cancer increases, impaired immunity increases; as impaired immunity increases, cancer increases. A symmetrical relationship may be diagramed as:

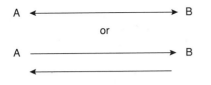

Sequencing

Time is the important factor in explaining the sequential nature of a relationship. If both concepts occur simultaneously, the relationship is *concurrent* (Fawcett & Downs, 1986). The relationship between relaxation (A) and blood pressure (B) may seem to be concurrent. If so, it would be expressed as follows.

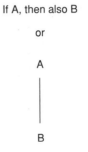

If A, then also B

or

A

|

B

If one concept occurs later than the other, the relationship is *sequential.* If relaxation (A) was thought to occur first, and then blood pressure (B) decreased, the relationship is sequential. This is expressed as follows.

If A, then later B

or

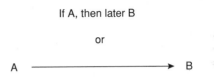

A ———————————➤ B

Probability of Occurrence

A relationship can be deterministic or probabilistic based on the degree of certainty that it will occur. *Deterministic* (or *causal*) *relationships* are statements of what always occurs in a particular situation. A scientific law is one example of a deterministic relationship (Fawcett & Downs, 1986). This is expressed as:

If A, then always B

Another deterministic relationship describes what always happens if there are no interfering conditions. This is referred to as a *tendency statement.* A tendency statement might propose that an immobilized patient lying in a typical hospital bed (A) will always develop pressure sores (B) after 6 weeks if there are no interfering conditions. A tendency statement would be expressed in the following form:

If A, then always B
if there are no interfering conditions

A *probability statement* expresses the probability that something will happen in a given situation. (Fawcett & Downs, 1986). This is expressed as:

If A, then probably B

Probability statements are tested statistically to determine the extent of probability of B occurring in the event of A. For example, one could state that there is greater than a 50% probability that a patient who has an indwelling catheter for one week will develop a urinary bladder infection. This probability could be expressed mathematically as:

$$p > .50$$

The p is a symbol for probability. The $>$ is a symbol for "greater than." This mathematical statement asserts that there is more than a 50% probability that the relationship will occur.

Necessity

In a *necessary relationship,* one concept must occur for the second concept to occur. For example, one could propose that if sufficient fluids are administered (A), and only if sufficient fluids are administered, then the unconscious patient will remain hydrated (B). This is expressed as:

If A, and only if A, then B

In a *substitutable relationship,* a similar concept can be substituted for the first concept and the second concept will still occur. A substitutable relationship might propose that if tube feedings are administered (A_1), but also if hyperalimentation is administered (A_2), the unconscious patient can remain nourished (B). This is expressed as:

If A_1, but also if A_2, then B

Sufficiency

A *sufficient relationship* states that when the first concept occurs, the second concept will oc-

cur, regardless of the presence or absence of other factors (Fawcett & Downs, 1986). A statement could propose that if a patient is immobilized in bed longer than a week, bone calcium will be lost, regardless of anything else. This is expressed as:

If A, then B, regardless of anything else

A *contingent relationship* will occur only if a third concept is present. For example, a statement might claim that if a person experiences a stressor (A), stress management (B) occurs, but only if effective coping strategies (C) are used. The third concept, in this case effective coping strategies, is referred to as an intervening variable. Intervening variables can affect the occurrence, strength, or direction of a relationship. A contingent relationship can be expressed as:

If A, then B, but only if C

or

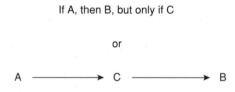

Statement Hierarchy

Statements about the same two conceptual ideas can be made at various levels of abstractness. The statements found in conceptual models (general propositions) are at high levels of abstraction. Statements found in theories (specific propositions) are at a moderate level of abstraction. Hypotheses, which are a form of statement, are at a low level of abstraction and are specific. As statements are expressed in a less abstract way, they become narrower in scope (Fawcett & Downs, 1986).

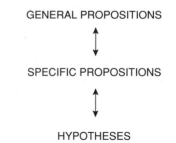

Statements at varying levels of abstraction that express relationships between or among the same conceptual ideas can be arranged in hierarchical form, from general to specific. This will allow the reader to see the logical links among the various levels of abstraction. Statement sets link the relationships expressed in the framework with the hypotheses, research questions, or objectives that guide the methodology of the study.

Roy and Roberts (1981, p. 90) developed statement sets related to Roy's nursing model that could be used in frameworks for research. An example follows.

General Proposition

The magnitude of the internal and external stimuli will positively influence the magnitude of the physiological response of an intact system.

Specific Proposition

The amount of mobility in the form of exercising positively influences the level of muscle integrity.

Hypothesis

If the nurse helps the patient maintain muscle tone through proper exercising, the patient will experience fewer problems associated with immobility. ■

CONCEPTUAL MODELS

A *conceptual model* is a set of highly abstract, related constructs that broadly explains phenomena of interest, expresses assumptions, and reflects a philosophical stance. A number of conceptual models have been developed in nursing. For example, Roy's (1984, 1988, 1990) model describes adaptation as the primary phenomenon of interest to nursing. Her model identifies the constructs she considers essential to adaptation and how these constructs interact to produce adaptation. Orem (1995) considers self-care to be the phenomenon central to nursing. Her model explains how nurses facilitate the self-care of clients. Rogers (1970, 1980, 1983, 1986, 1988) sees human beings as the central phenomenon of interest to nursing and her model is designed to explain the nature of human beings. A conceptual model may use the same or similar constructs as other models but define them in different ways. Thus, Roy, Orem, and Rogers may all use the construct "health" but define it in different ways.

Most disciplines have several conceptual models, each with a distinctive vocabulary. Fawcett and Downs (1986) identify seven conceptual models in nursing: Johnson's behavioral system model (1980), King's open systems model (1981), Levine's conservation model (1973), Neuman's systems model (1989), Orem's self-care model (1995), Rogers's science of unitary human beings model (1970, 1980, 1983, 1986, 1988), and Roy's adaptation model (1984, 1988, 1990). Walker and Avant (1995) identify nineteen conceptual models, which they refer to as grand nursing theories (see Table 7–1). These conceptual models vary in their level of abstraction and the breadth of phenomena they explain. However, all of them provide a broad, overall picture, a gestalt of the phenomena they explain. It is not their purpose to provide detail or to be specific. These models are not directly testable through research and thus cannot be used alone as the framework for a study (Fawcett & Downs, 1986; Walker & Avant, 1995). However, a framework could include a combination of a conceptual model and a theory.

Relatively few nursing studies have frameworks that include a conceptual nursing model. Moody and colleagues (1988), who examined nursing practice research from 1977 to 1986, found an increase in studies using a nursing model as a framework from 8% in the first half of the decade under study to 13% in the second half. The most frequently used models were Orem, Rogers, and Roy. Silva (1986), who studied the extent to which five nursing models (Johnson, Roy, Orem, Rogers, and Newman) had been used as frameworks for nursing research, found 62 studies between 1952 and 1985 that had used these models. However, only nine of these met her specified criteria as actually testing nursing theory. Only in

Table 7–1
Representative Grand Nursing Theories

Author	Date	Publication
Peplau	1952	Interpersonal Relations in Nursing
Orlando	1961	The Dynamic Nurse–Patient Relationship
Wiedenbach	1964	Clinical Nursing: A Helping Art
Henderson	1966	The Nature of Nursing
Levine	1967	The Four Conservation Principles of Nursing
Ujhely	1968	Determinants of the Nurse–Patient Relationship
Rogers	1970	An Introduction to the Theoretical Basis of Nursing
King	1971	Toward a Theory of Nursing
Orem	1971	Nursing: Concepts of Practice
Travelbee	1971	Interpersonal Aspects of Nursing
Neuman	1974	The Betty Neuman Health-Care Systems Model
Roy	1976	Introduction to Nursing: An Adaptation Model
Newman	1979	Toward a Theory of Health
Johnson	1980	The Behavioral System Model for Nursing
Parse	1981	Man-Living-Health
Erickson et al	1983	Modeling & Role-Modeling
Leininger	1985	Transcultural Care Diversity and Universality
Watson	1985	Nursing: Human Science and Human Care
Newman	1986	Health as Expanding Consciousness

(From Walker, L. O., & Avant, K. C. [1995]. *Strategies for theory construction in nursing.* Norwalk, CT: Appleton & Lange, p. 9, with permission.)

these nine studies were statements extracted and tested by the study design.

An organized program of research is important for building a body of knowledge related to the phenomena explained by a particular conceptual model. This program of research is referred to as a *research tradition*. Development of a research tradition for a particular model requires the commitment of a group of scholars who are willing to dedicate their time and energy to this endeavor. Theories compatible with the model need to be developed. The research tradition for the conceptual model will need to be defined, including identifying acceptable strategies for developing and testing theory based on the model, defining the phenomena to be studied, selecting the research questions, developing research methods and measurement techniques, describing data collection strategies, and selecting acceptable approaches to data analyses. Researchers conducting studies con-

sistent with this tradition may be scattered across the country (or the world) but often maintain a network of communication regarding their work. In some cases, annual conferences focused on the model are held to share research findings, explore theoretical ideas, and maintain network contacts. Conceptual models of nursing do not have well-established research traditions (Fawcett, 1995). However, research traditions are developing for some nursing models.

One example of a nursing model with an emerging research tradition is Orem's model of self-care. Orem's (1995) model focuses on the domain of nursing practice and on what nurses actually do when they practice nursing. She proposes that individuals generally know how to take care of themselves (self-care). If they are dependent in some way, such as a child, aged, or handicapped, family members take on this responsibility (dependent care). If individuals are ill or have some defect (such as diabetes or a colostomy), these individuals or their family members acquire special skills to provide that care (therapeutic self-care). An individual's capacity to provide self-care is referred to as self-care agency. A self-care deficit occurs when self-care demand exceeds self-care agency.

Nursing care is provided only when there is a deficit in the self-care or dependent care that the individual and his or her family can provide (self-care deficit). In this case, the nurse or nurses develop a nursing system to provide the needed care. This system involves prescribing, designing, and providing the needed care. The goal of nursing care is to facilitate resumption of self-care by the person and/or family. There are three types of nursing systems: wholly compensatory, partly compensatory, and supportive-educative. The selection of one of these systems is based on the capacity of the person to perform self-care.

The notion of self-care as an important construct for nursing has drawn nurse researchers to Orem's work. Multiple studies have been performed examining self-care in a variety of nursing situations (Bakker, Kastermans, & Dassen, 1995; Brugge, 1981; Davies, 1993; Frey & Denyes, 1989; Laskey & Eichelberger, 1985; McCaleb & Edgil, 1994; McDermitt, 1993; Moore, 1987a, 1987b, 1993; Rew, 1987; Saucier & Clark, 1993). The following instruments, consistent with Orem's model, have been developed:

1. Self-Care Agency Questionnaire (Bottorff, 1988)
2. Self-Care Agency in Adolescents (Deynes, 1982)
3. Self-Care Behavior Questionnaire (Dodd, 1984a)
4. Self-Care Behavior Log (Dodd, 1984b, 1987)
5. ADL Self-Care Scale (Gulick, 1987, 1988, 1989)
6. Perception of Self-Care Agency (Hanson & Bickel, 1985; Weaver, 1987)
7. Exercise of Self-Care Agency Scale (Kearney & Fleischer, 1979; McBride, 1987; Riesch & Hauch, 1988)

8. Nurse Performance Evaluation Tool (Kostopoulos, 1988)
9. Nursing Care Role Orientation (Stemple, 1988)
10. Children's Self-Care Performance Questionnaire (Moore, 1993)
11. Mother's performance of self-care activities for children (Moore & Gaffney, 1989)

Orem (1995) has developed three theories related to her model: the theory of self-care deficits, the theory of self-care, and the theory of nursing systems (also referred to as the general theory of nursing). Studies testing statements emerging from Orem's theories are appearing in the literature. Research methodologies acceptable for testing Orem's theories have not been specified. Orem did suggest that research be designed to examine the qualitative characteristics of self-care as well as its presence or absence. She also recommends studying the investigative and decision-making phase of self-care and the capability to engage in the production phase of self-care. Considerable work remains to be done in establishing a research tradition for Orem's model.

THEORY

A theory is more narrow and specific than a conceptual model and is directly testable. A theory consists of an integrated set of defined concepts, existence statements, and relational statements that present a view of a phenomenon and can be used to describe, explain, predict, and/or control that phenomenon. Existence statements declare that a given concept exists or that a given relationship occurs. For example, an existence statement might claim that a condition referred to as "stress" exists and that there is a relationship between stress and health. Relational statements clarify the type of relationship that exists between or among concepts. For example, a relational statement might propose that high levels of stress are related to declining levels of health. It is the statements of a theory that are tested through research, not the theory itself. Thus, identification of statements within theory is critical to the research endeavor and forms the basis for the framework of the study. Types of theory include scientific, substantive, and tentative.

Scientific Theory

The term *scientific theory* is restricted to those theories with valid and reliable methods of measuring each concept and whose relational statements have been repeatedly tested through research and demonstrated to be valid. Scientific theories have *empirical generalizations.* These are statements that have been repeatedly tested and have not been disproved. There are no scientific theories within nursing. Scientific theories from other disciplines are commonly used within nursing practice. For example, most physiological theories are scientific in nature.

Substantive Theory

Substantive theory is recognized within the discipline as useful for explaining important phenomena. Although there are few substantive theories within nursing, substantive theories developed within other disciplines are commonly used within nursing. The knowledge provided by a substantive theory may be in use in practice settings. An example of a substantive theory is the theory of reasoned action (Ajzen & Fishbein, 1980; Fishbein & Ajzen, 1975) which proposes that a person's expectation that a particular behavior will lead to a given outcome increases their intention to perform the behavior. Intention has been found to be predictive of behavior. Studies examining the capacity of this theory to predict engagement in exercise programs have been reviewed by Blue (1995). Substantive theories do not have the validity of a scientific theory. Some of the statements may have been tested and verified while others have not. In some cases, the statements in the theory may not have been clearly identified by the theorist or by those using the theory. Most theory testing has been performed by researchers in other disciplines. Few nursing studies actually test statements from substantive theory. The substantive theory has been used rather shallowly to provide an overall orientation for the study. Concepts are defined for use in the framework and may be linked with the methods of measurement, but because statements are not extracted from the theory and used to develop research questions or hypotheses, the framework does not guide the research process.

Most substantive theories (or conceptual models) used in nursing research frameworks are from outside of nursing (Walker & Avant, 1995). Moody and colleagues (1988) found that in 1986, 49% of nursing research frameworks were based on theoretical works from psychology. This was followed by frameworks based on theoretical works from physiology and sociology. Theoretical works from other disciplines are an important source of nursing knowledge but they need to be tested in nursing studies before incorporating them in nursing practice. Sources of some substantive theories and conceptual models from other disciplines that have been included in nursing frameworks are in Appendicies in the student study guide. Sources of theoretical works from nursing that have been cited in nursing frameworks are also provided in Appendices of the student study guide.

Tentative Theory

Tentative theory is newly proposed, has had minimal exposure to critique by the discipline, and has had little testing. Tentative theories are developed to propose an integrated set of relationships among concepts that have not been satisfactorily addressed in a substantive theory. Because these are newly emerging and untested theories, they tend to be less well developed than substantive theory. Many tentative theories have short lives but others may eventually be more extensively developed and validated through multiple studies. Tentative theories may be developed from clinical insights, from elements of existing theories not previously related, or from conceptual models.

Tentative theories developed in nursing often contain concepts and relational statements derived

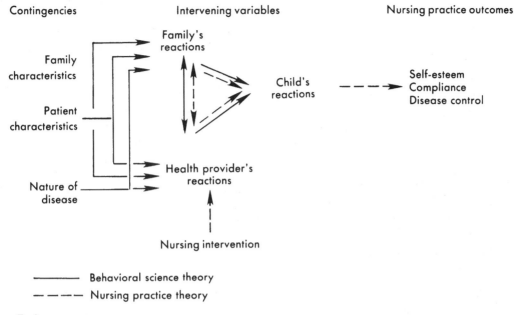

Figure 7–4

Illustration of the merger of concepts using theory from other sciences with concepts from nursing science theories. (From Wooldridge, P. J., Schmitt, M. J., Skipper, J. K., Jr., & Leonard, R. C. [1983]. *Behavioral science and nursing theory.* St. Louis: C. V. Mosby Company, 283.)

from sociological, psychosocial, psychological, and physiological theories. In some cases, the framework may require that the nurse researcher merge concepts using theory from other sciences with concepts from nursing science theories. Figure 7–4 illustrates the merger of behavioral science variables and nursing science variables used in Benoliel's research (Wooldridge, Schmitt, Skipper, & Leonard, 1983, p. 283). The solid lines indicate concepts and relationships taken from behavioral science theory. However, this theory was not sufficient to explain the phenomenon from a nursing practice perspective. Therefore, concepts and relationships from nursing practice theory were added to the behavioral science theory. These are indicated by dotted lines. Theory explaining reactions of family, health provider, and child were found in both nursing practice theory and behavioral science theory, as is indicated by combining solid lines and dotted lines to illustrate these relationships.

Tentative theories in nursing often emerge

from questions related to identified nursing problems or from the clinical insight that a relationship exists between or among elements important to desired outcomes. These situations tend to be concrete and require that the researcher express these concrete ideas in more abstract language. This is particularly difficult for the beginning researcher. The neophyte researcher's awareness of theoretical ideas related to the situation may be limited or the situation may be perceived in such concrete terms that even though the theories are known, the novice fails to make the link between the situation and available theory.

For example, one nurse, a novice researcher who worked in a newborn intensive care unit, was convinced from her clinical experiences that the frequency of visits by the mother was related to the infant's weight gain. Her ideas could be diagramed as:

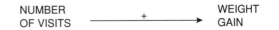

She wanted to study this relationship but was having difficulty expressing her ideas as a framework. Number of visits and weight gain are very concrete ideas. From the perspective of research, these ideas are variables. However, to develop a framework, the variables must be expressed in a more abstract and general way as concepts. This novice researcher lacked the knowledge and skills needed to accomplish this task. She was stuck at a concrete level of viewing her problem.

Many students recognize that they are concrete thinkers and feel that they are incapable of moving beyond that very limited way of thinking. However, the capacity for abstract thinking is not an innate ability; it is a learned skill. Acquiring it simply requires that one invest the energy to obtain the knowledge and practice the skills.

Converting a concretely expressed term to a higher level of abstractness—from variable to concept—is a form of translation. Since the translation in this case is from a lower level of abstractness to a higher level, inductive reasoning is used.

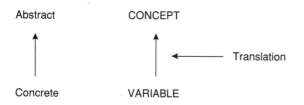

However, knowledge of equivalent terms at both the concrete and abstract level is required to perform the translation. Conducting a literature search can be useful in identifying equivalent abstract terms. The search may be difficult if the novice researcher is blind to theoretical ideas presented in the literature and picks up only the concrete ideas. Sometimes, probing questions facilitate the process of moving from concrete to more abstract thinking. For example, one could ask: Why is it important that the mother visit? What happens when the mother visits? Answering these questions may help in labeling what happens when the mother visits. Existing theories have named this bonding or attachment. There might be other names for it also.

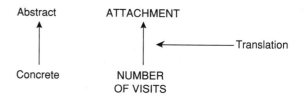

Then one can ask: What happens when the baby gains weight? Why is this important? How is it different from the baby who gains weight more slowly or fails to gain weight? One name for this phenomenon is growth; another is thriving. There might be other ways the phenomenon could be described.

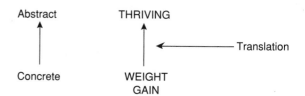

At this point, the novice nurse researcher is ready to search the literature more thoroughly. Theories related to bonding, attachment, growth, and thriving can be examined. The novice researcher may find literature that proposes a positive relationship between attachment and thriving. This relationship could be expressed as follows:

Abstract   ATTACHMENT ——— + ——→ THRIVING

When the aforementioned ideas are linked, we have the beginning of a tentative theory. The illustration—the beginning of a conceptual map—will have this appearance:

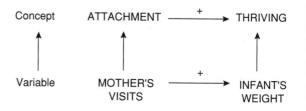

However, the ideas for a framework and a tentative theory are still incomplete. One needs to ask: What other factors are important in influencing the relationship between mother's visits and infant's weight gain, between attachment and thriving? Again, the literature can be consulted. Researchers in this field have examined elements relevant to this question. What concepts did they include? What relationships did they find? Are their findings consistent with the emerging framework? Clinically, what other elements seem to be associated with this phenomenon? Do the newly found concepts need to be included in the framework? While the researcher is pondering these questions, conceptual definitions for attachment and thriving and statements expressing the relationship between the two concepts can be obtained from the existing theories.

As the framework expressing a tentative theory takes shape, it is time to consider moving to an even higher level of abstraction, that of conceptual models. Is there a possible fit between a conceptual model and the tentative theory expressed in the developing framework? Can the study concepts be translated to the even more abstract constructs of a conceptual model? Are the study statements linked in any way with the broad statements of a conceptual model? If a conceptual model is included in the framework, the links between the conceptual model and the tentative theory need to be made clear.

CONCEPTUAL MAPS

One strategy for expressing a framework is a *conceptual map* that diagrams the interrelationships of the concepts and statements (Artinian, 1982; Fawcett & Downs, 1986; Moody, 1989; Newman, 1979; Silva, 1981). Figures 7–4 through 7–10 in this chapter are examples of conceptual maps. A conceptual map summarizes and integrates what is known about a phenomenon more succinctly and clearly than a literary explanation and allows one to grasp the gestalt of a phenomenon. A conceptual map should be supported by references from the literature (Artinian, 1982).

A conceptual map is developed to explain which concepts contribute to or partially cause an outcome. Conditions, direct and indirect, that may produce the outcome are specified. The process in which factors must cumulatively interact across time in some sequence to have a causal effect is illustrated by a conceptual map. Conceptual maps vary in complexity and accuracy, depending on the available body of knowledge related to the phenomenon. Mapping is also useful in identifying gaps in the logic of the theory being used as a framework and reveals inconsistencies, incompleteness, and errors (Artinian, 1982).

Conceptual maps are useful beyond the study for which they were developed. Hypotheses may be suggested that can be tested in future studies. In addition, through map development, insight may occur about different situations in which the same process may be occurring. Publication of the map may stimulate interest of other researchers who may then use it in their own studies. Thus, a well-developed conceptual map may facilitate building a body of knowledge related to a particular theory. In addition to conceptual maps included as the framework for a study, more maps are being published that are outcomes of extensive reviews of the literature that are expressed as tentative theories. For example, Leidy (1994) has developed a framework proposing a functional status trajectory pattern in chronic illness. The conceptual map for this framework is illustrated in Figure 7–5 (on p. 152). O'Connor (1994) has proposed a framework for symptom regulation in schizophrenia. The conceptual map for this framework is illustrated in Figure 7–6 (on p. 152). Brown and Hedges (1994) have extended this idea to develop a conceptual map predicting metabolic control in diabetes using the results of a meta-analysis. In addition to showing the concepts and relationships, they provide the effect size (ES) of the concepts. Effect size is discussed in Chapter 12. The conceptual map for this framework is illustrated in Figure 7–7 (on p. 153).

THE STEPS OF CONSTRUCTING A STUDY FRAMEWORK

Developing a framework is one of the most important steps in the research process but perhaps also

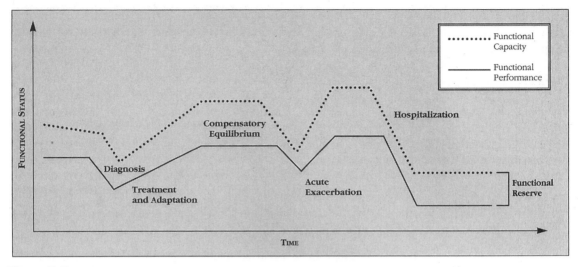

Figure 7–5
Possible functional status trajectory pattern in chronic illness. (From Leidy, N. K. [1994]. Functional status and the forward progress of merry-go-rounds: Toward a coherent analytical framework. *Nursing Research, 43*[4], 200. Used with permission of Lippincott–Raven Publishers, Philadelphia, PA.)

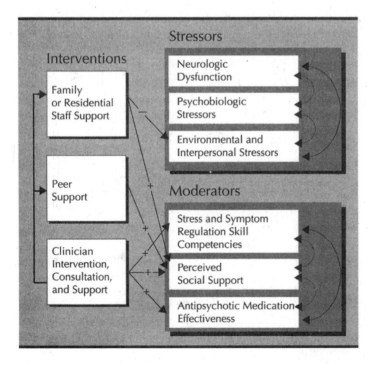

Figure 7–6
Effects of interventions on stressors and moderators. Straight lines denote causal relationships; curved lines denote correlations without a specified causal direction. (From O'Connor, F. W. [1994]. A vulnerability-stress framework for evaluating clinical interventions in schizophrenia. *Image: Journal of Nursing Scholarship, 26*[3], 234, with permission.)

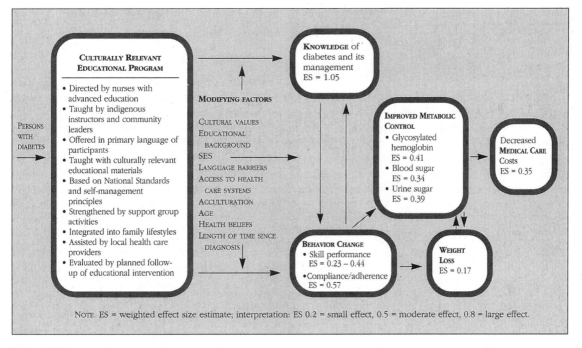

Figure 7–7
Model of diabetes patient education intervention and outcomes. (From Brown, S. A., & Hedges, L. V. [1994]. Predicting metabolic control in disease: A pilot study using meta-analysis to estimate a linear model. *Nursing Research, 43*[6], 363.)

one of the most difficult. Examples of frameworks from the literature are helpful but not sufficient as a guide to framework development. The brief but impressive presentation of a framework in a published study often belies the careful, thoughtful work required to arrive at that point. Yet, the neophyte researcher needs to learn how to perform that thoughtful work.

As the body of knowledge related to a phenomenon increases, the development of a framework to express the knowledge becomes easier. Therefore, frameworks for quasi-experimental and experimental studies, which should have a background of descriptive and correlational studies and perhaps some substantive theory, should be more easily and fully developed than those for descriptive studies. Descriptive studies often examine multiple factors to understand a phenomenon not previously well studied. Previous theoretical work related to the phenomenon may be tentative or

nonexistent. Therefore, the framework may be less comprehensive. In qualitative studies, in which the framework development is an outcome of the study, even identification of concepts may not be clear at the beginning of the study and statements will be synthesized from the data. The basis for the development of qualitative studies is more philosophical than theoretical.

A study by Fink (1995) examining the influence of family resources and family demands on the strains and well-being of caregiving families will be used to illustrate the development of a framework. However, keep in mind that the nicely turned phrases in Fink's framework required much time, effort, thought, and reflection. They did not easily and miraculously appear in their present form. You will be examining the finished framework, and will not be able to see the process of thinking or the work involved as Fink developed her ideas.

To explain the process of framework development, a series of steps are identified and described. The steps are a way of introducing the reasoning used in developing a framework. The steps of the process include selecting and defining concepts, developing statements relating the concepts, expressing the statements in hierarchical fashion, and developing a conceptual map expressing the framework. The steps presented are not usually performed in order. In reality, there is a movement of the flow of thought from one step to another, back and forth, as ideas are developed and refined.

SELECTING AND DEFINING CONCEPTS

Concepts are selected for a framework based on their relevance to the phenomenon of concern. Thus, the problem statement, which describes the phenomenon of concern, will be a rich source of concepts for the framework. If the researcher begins from a concrete clinical perspective, the concepts may first be identified as variables and then be translated to concepts. Every major variable included in the study should be a reflection of a concept included in the framework. The framework may be modified as the rest of the study is developed. As the researcher gains additional insight into the phenomenon through a thorough search of theoretical, research, and clinical publications, additional relevant concepts may be identified or new relationships proposed. As these are incorporated into the framework, their implications in terms of the study design also need to be considered.

Fink (1995) stated the purpose of her study was to "examine the influence of family resources and demands on the well-being of families providing care to an elderly parent and on the strains experienced by the family unit" (p. 139). The concepts she selected were family systems resources, family demands, family strains, and family well-being. Two types of family system resources were included: social support resources and internal system resources.

Each concept included in a framework needs to be conceptually defined. When available and appropriate, conceptual definitions from existing theoretical works need to be used, quoting definitions and citing the source. If theories that define the concept are not available, the researcher needs to develop the definition. Conceptual definitions may be available in the literature in the absence of theories that use the concept. For an illustration of extracting conceptual definitions from the literature, see Chapter 5 in *Understanding Nursing Research* (Burns & Grove, 1995). One source of conceptual definitions is published concept analyses. Previous studies using the concept may also provide a conceptual definition. Another source of a conceptual definition is literature associated with instrument development related to the concept. Although the instrument itself is an operational definition of the concept, the author will often provide a conceptual definition on which the instrument development was based. The general literature can sometimes provide a conceptual definition. These definitions may not have been as carefully thought out as those in a theory or a concept analysis, but may reflect the only definition available in the discipline.

When acceptable conceptual definitions are not available, concept synthesis or concept analysis needs to be performed in order to develop the definition. Various definitions of the concept from the literature need to be presented to validate the conceptual definition selected for the study.

Fink (1995) provided these conceptual definitions with discussion following, offering rationale and further clarification for the definitions.

Family Social Support. "Perceived support from friends, relatives, and community resources. Supportive interactions with social networks provide resources families draw upon in meeting the needs of their members. Antonovsky (1974) suggested that ties to a place or community may be a significant resource over and above those of interpersonal ties. . . . Although social support has usually been conceptualized at the individual level, support is also available to the family unit through a network of friends, relatives, and community resources (Kane, 1988; McCubbin & Thompson, 1987)." (p. 139)

Internal Family System Resources. "Strengths and assets of the family system that can be drawn upon to meet the needs of the family unit and its individual . . . The internal system resources of interest in this study were problem solving, sense of mastery, and perception that changes can be managed. In previous family studies, the constructs of family sense of coherence and family hardiness have been operationally defined as the ability to work together on solving problems, confidence that the family can master problems, and ability to view problems or changes as challenges rather than as threats." (p. 140)

Family Demands. "Stimuli or stressors that require a response from the family unit. Developmental and situational changes require altered roles, rules, and task allocations. The needs of the older adult for care and assistance combine with other developmental and situational changes the family already faces and add to their demands." (p. 140)

Family Strains. "A condition of felt tension or difficulty were indicators of stress within the family system." (p. 140)

Family Well-Being. "The members' satisfaction with the functioning of the family unit, their perception of their own health and emotional well-being, and their perception of the family's health. In this definition, the focus is on the outcomes of family functioning rather than on the process or structure. Family well-being has been described as an index of the fit between supplies or resources and demands that affect both the family unit and its members (Meister, 1991). The family with a high degree of well-being is able to meet its own self-maintenance needs and has the capacity to contribute to the health and well-being of its members." (p. 140) ∎

DEVELOPING RELATIONAL STATEMENTS

The next step in framework development is to link all of the concepts through relational statements.

Whenever possible, relational statements need to be obtained from theoretical works and the sources cited. If such statements are unavailable, relationships need to be proposed by the researcher. Evidence for the validity of each relational statement needs to be provided whenever available. This support needs to include a discussion of previous studies that have examined the proposed relationship and published observations from the clinical practice perspective.

The researcher developing a framework may need to extract statements that are embedded in the literary text of an existing theory. When one first begins extracting statements, the task seems overwhelming since it may seem that every sentence in the text is a relational statement. A little practice will make the task easier. These are the steps of extracting statements: (1) Select a portion of a theory discussing the relationships between or among two or three concepts. (2) Write down a single sentence from the theory that seems to be a relational statement. (3) Express it diagrammatically using the statement diagrams presented earlier in the chapter. (4) Move to the next statement and express it diagrammatically. (5) Continue until all of the statements related to the selected concepts have been diagrammatically expressed. (6) Examine the linkages among the diagrammatic statements you have developed. The logic of what the theorist is saying will gradually become clearer. This process is illustrated in greater detail in *Understanding Nursing Research,* Chapter 5 (Burns & Grove, 1995).

If statements relating the concepts of interest are not available in the literature, *statement synthesis* will be necessary. This means that the researcher will have to develop statements proposing specific relationships among the concepts being studied. Knowledge for use in statement synthesis may be obtained through clinical observation and integrative literature review (Walker & Avant, 1995).

In descriptive studies, theoretical statements related to the phenomenon may be sparse. In this case, developing a framework requires more synthesis and will have a higher level of uncertainty. The statement set may include a statement that a relationship between A and B is proposed but the type of relationship is unknown. This may be followed by a research question related to this relationship rather than a hypothesis. For example, one might ask, "What is the nature of the relationship between A and B?" An objective might be to examine the nature of the relationship between A and B.

Fink (1995) offered the following relational statements:

1. In this study, the resources of family social supports and internal family system resources were expected to increase family well-being both directly and indirectly by decreasing strains. (Fink, 1995, p. 140)

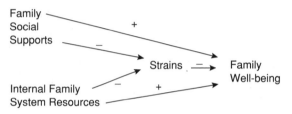

2. Family system resources and social supports were expected to decrease strains and to increase well-being. (Fink, 1995, pp. 140–141).

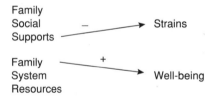

3. Family demand (family life changes, care provided to the elder, and appraisal of caregiving) were expected to increase strains directly and to affect well-being indirectly through their impact on strains. (Fink, 1995, p. 141)

Family demand
Family life changes $\xrightarrow{+}$ Strains $\longrightarrow$ Well-being
Care provided to elderly
Appraisal of caregiving

4. Family strains were expected to have a direct negative impact on well-being. (Fink, 1995, p. 141)

Strains $\xrightarrow{\quad - \quad}$ Well-being

DEVELOPING HIERARCHICAL STATEMENT SETS

A hierarchical statement set is composed of a specific proposition and a hypothesis or research question. If a conceptual model is included in the framework, the set may also include a general proposition. The proposition is listed first, with the hypothesis or research question immediately following. In some cases, there may be more than one hypothesis related to a particular proposition. However, there must be a proposition for each hypothesis stated. This statement set indicates the link between the framework and the methodology.

CONSTRUCTING A CONCEPTUAL MAP

Conceptual maps are initiated early in the development of the framework but refinement of the map will probably be one of the last steps accomplished. Before the map can be completed, the following information needs to be available:

1. A clear problem and purpose statement.
2. The concepts of interest, including conceptual definitions.
3. Results of an integrative review of the theoretical and empirical literature.
4. Relational statements linking the concepts, expressed literally and diagrammatically.
5. Identification and analysis of existing theories that address the relationships of interest.
6. Identification of existing conceptual models congruent with the developing framework.
7. Linking of proposed relationships with hypotheses, questions, or objectives (hierarchical statement sets).

Some believe that the map should be limited to those concepts included in the study (Fawcett & Downs, 1986). However, Artinian (1982) suggests including in the map all of the concepts necessary to explain the phenomenon, plainly delineating that portion of the map to be studied. This strategy is illustrated by Artinian's map of the conceptualization of the effects of role supplementation pre-

Conceptualization of the Effects of Role Supplementation

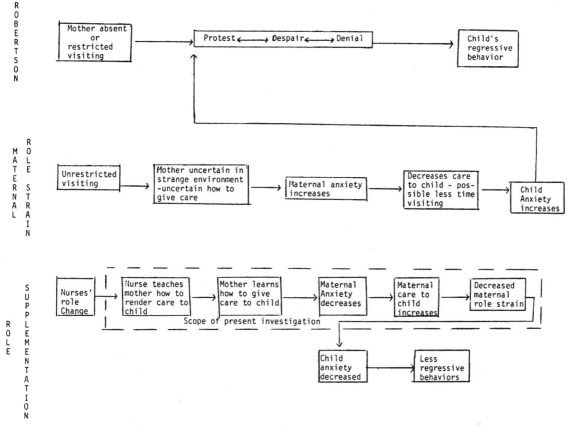

Figure 7–8

Conceptual map outlining scope of present study: conceptualization of the effects of role supplementation. (From Artinian, B. M. [1982]. Conceptual mapping: Development of the strategy. *Western Journal of Nursing Research, 4*[4], 385. © 1982. Reprinted by permission of Sage Publications, Inc.)

sented in Figure 7–8. The scope of the study is enclosed by dashed lines.

To develop a map, arrange the concepts on the page in sequence of occurrence (or causal linkage) from left to right, with the concept(s) reflecting the outcome(s) located on the far right. Concepts that are elements of a more abstract construct can be placed in a frame or box. Sets of closely interrelated concepts can be linked by enclosing them in a frame or circle. Using arrows, link the concepts in a way consistent with the diagrammatic statements you have previously developed. In some cases, at some point on the map, the path of relationships may diverge, so that there are then

two or more paths of concepts. The paths may again converge at a later point. Every concept should be linked to at least one other concept. Examine the map for completeness. Are all the concepts that are included in the study on the map? Are all the concepts on the map defined? Does it clearly portray the phenomenon? Does it accurately reflect all the statements? Is there a statement for each of the linkages portrayed by the map? Is the sequence accurate?

Developing a well-constructed conceptual map requires repeated tries. But persistence pays off. You may need to go back and re-examine the statements identified. Are there some missing

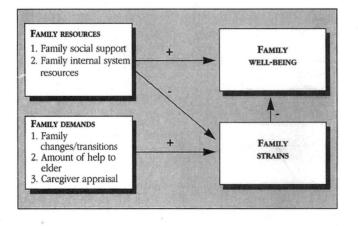

Figure 7–9

Theoretical model developed to explain strains and well-being in families providing care to an elderly parent. (From Fink, S. V. [1995]. The influence of family resources and family demands on the strains and well-being of caregiving families. *Nursing Research, 44*[3], 140.)

links? Are some of the links inaccurately expressed? As the map takes shape and begins to seem right, show it to trusted colleagues. Can they follow your logic? Do they agree with your linkages? Can they identify missing elements? Can you explain the map to them? Seek out individuals who have experienced the phenomenon you are mapping. Does the process depicted seem valid to them? Seek out someone more experienced than you in conceptual mapping who will closely and critically examine your map. Continue to revise it until you achieve some degree of consensus and you feel a sense of rightness about the map. Examine Fink's conceptual map in Figure 7–9. Is it consistent with her concepts and statements? Does the process described seem valid to you?

CONSTRUCTING A STUDY FRAMEWORK FROM SUBSTANTIVE THEORY

Developing a framework designed to test a substantive theory requires that all concepts in the framework be obtained from the substantive theory. These concepts must be defined as they are defined by the theorist. Operational definitions must be consistent with the conceptual definition and should be an accepted method of measurement used for testing the selected theory. Statements (propositions) must be extracted from the theory for testing. Hypotheses must emerge from these statements. Previous studies designed to test these relational statements need to be discussed in the literature review. The following study by O'Connell, Gerkovich, and Cook (1995) illustrates a framework developed to test components of reversal theory. In the following explanation of the theory, concepts are in bold print, while statements are underlined.

O'Connell and colleagues (1995) used reversal theory (Apter, 1982a, 1989; O'Connell, 1991) to examine success in smoking cessation. According to the researchers, reversal theory "holds that human beings are inherently inconsistent and that they reverse back and forth between opposing **metamotivational states.** The states are called 'metamotivational' because they are not about motivation themselves but pertain to how certain motivational variables are interpreted. Four pairs of metamotivational states have been identified: **telic** (serious minded) versus **paratelic** (playful), **negativistic** versus **conformist, mastery** versus **sympathy,** and **autic** (self-centered) versus **alloic** (other-centered). The theory holds that the states of each pair are mutually exclusive. Thus, one cannot be telic and paratelic at the same time. However, the same individual is in one state of each pair during all of waking life. Therefore, a person can be in the combination of telic, conformist, mastery, and autic states. Moreover, reversal theory holds that normal individuals **reverse** several times a day between the states of each of the pairs of states and that these reversals are largely involuntary." (pp. 311–312)

"Reversal Theory is not a theory about relapse to smoking. Instead, reversal theory is a general theory that has been applied to a variety of areas including psychopathology (Thomas-Peter & McDonagh, 1988), sports psychology (Kerr, 1987), muscle tension (Svebak, 1984), psychophysiology (Svebak, 1985; Svebak, 1986), and humor (Apter, 1982b, Svebak & Apter, 1987). Previous studies have shown that hypotheses derived from reversal theory explain behavior during highly tempting situations. In particular, ex-smokers who were abstinent 3 months after cessation attempt were more likely to lapse during highly tempting situations when they were paratelic or negativistic than when they were telic and conformist (O'Connell et al., 1990; Potocky et al., 1991). In another study, ex-smokers who had been abstinent for 2 weeks were more likely to lapse in paratelic than in telic states, but no relationship was found between negativistic/conformist states and the tendency to lapse during an episode (Cook, Gerkovich, O'Connell, & Potocky, 1995). One study (O'Connell et al., 1990) showed that the amount of effort required to get a cigarette interacted with the telic/paratelic pair to predict resisting or lapsing." (p. 312)

"The mastery/sympathy pair has received less attention in the reversal theory literature than the telic/paratelic and negativistic/conformist pairs. Reversal theory holds that people reverse from the mastery state, in which individual is oriented to control and competition, to the sympathy state, in which individual is oriented toward caring and cooperation (Apter & Smith, 1985; Apter, 1988; O'Connell & Apter, 1993; O'Connell, 1993). Although these orientations usually involve controlling or caring for individuals, objects, or situations external to the self, sometimes it is oneself that one wants to control or care for. One's preference for feeling tough versus tender reverses when one switches between the mastery and the sympathy state. In the mastery state one prefers to be tough (rugged, disciplined, hardy); tenderness is construed as being soft (meek, wimpish, overly indulgent). Positive feelings associated with the mastery state include feeling proud, strong, and competent. Negative feelings

associated with the mastery state include feeling humiliated and weak. In the sympathy state, on the other hand, one prefers to be tender (sensitive, caring, gentle), while being tough is construed as being insensitive (harsh, unfeeling, unsympathetic). Positive feelings associated with the sympathy state include feeling grateful, appreciated, nurtured, or kind to oneself. Negative feelings associated with the sympathy state include feeling neglected and deprived. 'Thus, one can experience both the mastery and sympathy states in positive and negative ways. . . . Reversal theorists propose that one's feelings and motivations about the same activity may be opposite when one switches from the mastery to the sympathy state.' Figure 7–10 illustrates the decision tree which serves as a conceptual map for a study examining changes in the metamotivational state of mastery/sympathy in individuals in highly tempting situations who are attempting to quit smoking. As the figure suggests, the state a subject is in affects perceived consequences of smoking. When a subject who is trying to quit smoking encounters a highly tempting situation while in the mastery state, the subject regards control and toughness as important. In the mastery state, the usual perceived consequences of having a cigarette are negative feelings, while the usual perceived consequence of resisting the urge are positive feelings. In the mastery state, the likely outcome is that the subject abstains from smoking. On the other hand, when a highly tempting situation is encountered while in the sympathy state, caring and tenderness are important. In the sympathy state, subjects often see smoking a cigarette as a way of being kind to themselves and this leads to positive feelings, while the usual perceived consequences of resisting a cigarette are negative feelings. The likely outcome in this case is that the subject lapses."

"Two hypotheses are posed to test these ideas. (1) 'temptations occurring when subjects are in the sympathy state are more likely to result in lapses to smoking than temptations occurring when subjects are in the mastery state' (p. 312); and (2) 'lapses will be more likely when cigarettes are available without effort than when effort is required to get cigarettes' (p. 312). 'Two additional research questions were addressed: (a) does the effort to get cigarettes interact with mastery/sympathy states to explain whether the

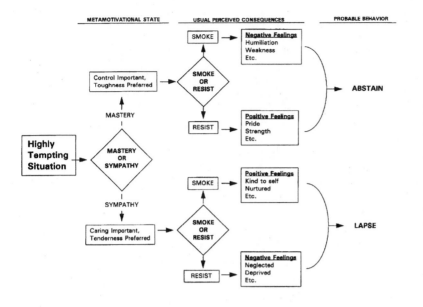

Figure 7–10

Hypothesized effects of mastery and sympathy states on smoking outcome of typical highly tempting situations. (From O'Connell, K. A., Gerkovich, M. M., & Cook, M. R. [1995]. Reversal theory's mastery and sympathy states in smoking cessation. *Image: Journal of Nursing Scholarship, 27*[4], 315, with permission.)

subject lapses or abstains during highly tempting episodes? And (b) is gender related to experiencing mastery and sympathy states during highly tempting situations?'" (p. 312)
(Reprinted with permission from O'Connell, K. A., Gerkovich, M. M., & Cook, M. R. [1995]. Reversal theory's mastery and sympathy states in smoking cessation. *Image: Journal of Nursing Scholarship, 27*[4], 311–316.) ■

CONSTRUCTING A STUDY FRAMEWORK BASED ON A CONCEPTUAL MODEL

The inclusion of a conceptual model as well as a theory in a framework is a relatively new idea in nursing. Few published studies have frameworks that include a conceptual model, a theory, and a conceptual map illustrating the linkage between the model and the theory. The map for such a framework needs to include both the conceptual model and a testable theory.

A framework that includes a conceptual model has the following elements:

1. Constructs from the conceptual model.
2. Definitions of constructs from the conceptual model.
3. Statements linking the constructs.
4. Concepts that represent portions of the selected constructs.
5. Conceptual definitions compatible with construct definitions.
6. Statements linking the concepts that express a tentative or substantive theory.
7. Selection of variables that represent portions of the concepts.
8. Operational definitions of the variables compatible with conceptual definitions.
9. Statement sets.
10. A conceptual map linking the constructs, concepts, and variables. In some cases, methods of measurement are also included in the map.

When a conceptual model is included, the portion of the model relevant to the phenomenon to be studied needs to be identified. If theory emerging from that portion of the model is available and relevant to the research problem, the framework is developed from that theory. Otherwise, a tentative theory needs to be developed using statements and constructs from the model as a guide. Methods of measurement selected to operationalize the concepts would need to be philosophically and logically compatible with the model and with the research tradition associated with the conceptual model.

In some cases, rather than beginning with the choice of a model, the development of the framework begins with identification of concepts relevant to a particular nursing problem. A theory related to the phenomenon of interest is identified or developed; and simultaneously or perhaps later, all or a portion of a conceptual model compatible with the researcher's interests is selected. The important issue is not where the development of the framework begins, but rather how well the various elements of the framework are logically linked together and the completeness of the end product.

Calvillo and Flaskerud (1993) conducted a cross-cultural study of pain using Roy's adaptation model and the gate control theory of pain as a framework. Their framework (as published) is presented in its entirety to show the careful connections made by these scholars between Roy's model and Melzack and Wall's gate control theory of pain. Figure 7–11 identifies the adaptation model constructs, gate control concepts, and empirical indicators for the framework. The researchers provide conceptual definitions and statements related to the concepts which are presented below. Can you underline the statements in their framework? Can you map the statements? A map illustrating the concepts and relationships was not provided in their publication. Can you develop a conceptual map from the description they provide? An example of a

Major Concepts of the Adaptation Model							
Environmental Stimuli Independent Variables				Adaptive Modes: Limits of Adaptation Dependent Variables			
Adaptation Model Concepts	Focal	Contextual	Residual	Physiological	Self-Concept	Role Function	Interdependence
Gate Control Theory Concepts	Noxious Stimulus	Psychologic/ Emotional Factors	Sociocultural Factors	Regulation of Senses: Pain	Self-Consistency and Self-Esteem	Sick Role	Support System
Empirical Indicators	Elective Cholecystectomy	1. State-Trait Anxiety Scale	1. Sample Selection Criteria	1. McGill Pain Questionnaire	1. Self-Esteem Inventory	1. Activities of Daily Living Scale	1. Zich's Social Support Scale
		2. Anxiety Analog Scale	2. Socio-demo-graphic Items	2. Total Number of Pain Medications	2. Sense of Coherence Scale	2. Length of Hospital Stay	2. Number of Visitors
			3. Accultur-ation Scale	3. Blood Pressure, Pulse, and Respirations			3. Identity of Visitors
				4. Pain Evaluation by Nurse (PPI)			
				5. Total Amount of Pain Medication Taken			

Figure 7–11

Conceptual-theoretical-empirical structure for study of the pain response. (From Calvillo, E. R., & Flaskerud, J. H. [1993]. The adequacy and scope of Roy's adaptation model to guide cross-cultural pain research. *Nursing Science Quarterly, 6*[3], 119, with permission.)

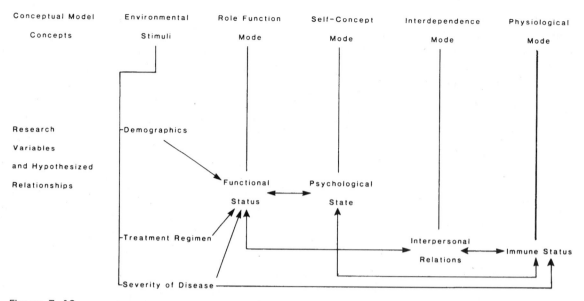

Figure 7–12

Conceptual map including conceptual nursing model (Roy) and tentative theory: Framework for studying functional status after diagnosis of breast cancer. (From Tulman, L., & Fawcett, J. [1990]. A framework for studying functional status after diagnosis of breast cancer. *Cancer Nursing, 13*[2], 98, with permission.)

conceptual map including both a conceptual model and a theory is illustrated in Figure 7–12.

"According to the adaptation model of nursing, persons are biopsychosocial beings in constant interaction with a changing environment (Andrews & Roy, 1991). Persons cope with the changing environment by a positive response known as adaptation. Internal or external stimuli (focal, contextual, and residual) affect the behavior of a person. The person adapts to these stimuli through four adaptive modes: physiologic, self-concept, interdependence, and role function." (Andrews & Roy, 1991, qtd. in Calavillo & Flaskerud, 1993, p. 119)

"The gate control theory of pain developed by Melzack and Wall (1975, 1983) and research literature related to pain and culture, anxiety, social support, self-esteem, and sick role provided operational definitions of the concepts and propositions to be tested. This theory proposes that pain is not just a physiologic response to tissue damage but that sociocultural and psychologic variables influence the perception of pain as well. The gate control theory suggests that many pre-existing factors, such as expectations of a culture, influence pain impulses in the

brain and how the person responds overtly during the pain experience." (Calavillo & Flaskerud, 1993, p. 119)

Independent Variables

Environmental Stimuli. According to Roy (Andrews & Roy, 1991), "an internal or an external change or stimulus affects the behavior of a person. There are three classifications of stimuli which affect adaptation: focal, contextual, and residual. These environmental stimuli affect the person's ability to adapt physiologically, psychologically, socially, and interpersonally.

Focal Stimulus. A focal stimulus is the internal or external stimulus immediately confronting the person. In this study elective cholecystectomy was the focal stimulus. Previous studies of pain have demonstrated that a person's culture may affect the discomfort experienced after surgery (Zborowski, 1952, 1969). Cross-cultural studies have focused on obstetrical pain, chronic facial pain, and electric shock (Lipton & Marbach, 1980; Sternbach & Tursky, 1965; Winsberg & Greenlick, 1967). However, each of these pain stimuli was considered to have an emotional component that might confound the measurement of pain. Elective cholecystectomy was considered to be relatively free of emotional content and to offer a similar stimulus to all participants. For a person experiencing pain following an elective cholecystectomy, the focal stimulus is the surgery itself. Pain, a behavioral response to surgery, primarily affects physiologic adaptation. According to the gate control theory (Melzack & Wall, 1983), noxious stimuli activate small diameter afferent nerves that transmit pain signals to the spinal cord. If nothing blocks the conduction of the signals at the level of the spinal cord, the messages cross over the spinal cord and ascend to the brain and the physiologic adaptation process begins. However, because of the complexity of the pain response, disruption can occur in psychologic adaptation (self-concept), in social adaptation (the ability to perform usual roles), and in interpersonal adaptation (relationships with others) (Andrews & Roy, 1991)." (p. 120)

Contextual Stimulus. "The contextual stimuli are all the other stimuli confronting the person in the immediate environment such as sounds, smells, sights, and compounding characteristics of the focal stimulus. The contextual stimuli contribute to the behavior caused by the focal stimulus. For example, in the patient having a cholecystectomy, the pain response to the surgery may be aggravated by a coughing episode in which the person does not support the incision. Other contextual stimuli that may contribute to the pain behavior caused by the focal stimulus are complications commonly seen with a cholecystectomy such as incisional infection, obstruction of the T-tube, respiratory complications, and circulatory complications. Emotional factors or stimuli may influence the behavioral response to pain and operate as contextual stimuli. Melzack and Wall (1983) established that pain is not just a physiologic response to tissue damage, but that psychologic variables may influence the transmission and perception of pain. Anxiety may influence the response to pain (Seyle, 1976). It has been determined that acute pain is closely associated with anxiety (Meinhart & McCaffery, 1983). Because anxiety can cause the same adaptive physiologic response as pain, it is important that identification of the type of stimulus be distinguished. Anxiety may be a focal or contextual stimulus; however, in this case, it was considered contextual." (p. 120)

Residual Stimulus. "Residual stimuli are those personal and ideological factors that may affect the person. Neither the person nor the observer may be aware of the influence these factors are having on the behavioral response to the focal stimulus unless specific measures are taken to observe them. The person's age, sex, socioeconomic status, family structure, and culture may operate as residual stimuli and contribute to the pain response. It is difficult to validate the effect that residual stimuli have unless they are carefully defined and measured. In this study, culture was considered a major residual stimulus. Culture is an important variable in determining an individual's behavioral response to pain. Leininger (1979) stated that a person's reaction to illness, health maintenance, body discomforts, and caring and curing practices are linked with cultural beliefs, values, and experiences. A person learns what is expected and accepted by his or her culture regarding painful experiences. According to Meinhart and McCaffery (1983), cultural expectations may specify: (a) different reactions according to age, sex, and occupation; (b) what treatment to seek; (c) the intensity and duration of pain that should be tolerated; (d) what responses should be made; (e) to whom to report when pain occurs; and (f) what types of pain require attention. It is possible that a patient's cultural background influences not only attitude toward pain but the overt response to it as well." (p. 120)

Dependent Variables: Adaptive Modes

"According to Roy (Andrews & Roy, 1991) adaptation to internal and external environmental stimuli may be observed in behaviors indicating four adaptive modes: physiologic needs, self-concept, role and interdependence functions. Underlying each mode are basic needs of the individual which stimulate a response to facilitate integrity or wholeness." (p. 120)

Physiologic Mode. The underlying need of the physiologic mode is physiologic integrity. In this mode the person responds physiologically to stimuli from the environment, that is, an excessive physiologic demand on the regulation of the senses, or in this study, pain (Andrews & Roy, 1991). Regulation of the senses is an important process for achieving physiologic integrity. Stimuli activate adaptive mechanisms manifested as physiologic behaviors in response to the excess.

According to the gate control theory (Melzack & Wall, 1983), noxious stimuli activate adaptive mechanisms manifested as physiologic behaviors. Surgery, the focal stimulus, causes the pain response, which initiates endocrine and central nervous system activity to produce physiologic adaptive responses. Roy's model proposes that these responses are primarily activated by the regulator subsystem which is an automatic neural, chemical, and endocrine response process (Andrews & Roy, 1991). This process, in response to the stressor (surgery) is manifested by activation of the sympathetic nervous system (Seyle, 1976). The activation of the sympathetic nervous system increases the pulse and respiratory rates, produces a rise in blood pressure, causes pallor, dilates the pupils, and produces cold perspiration among other physiologic responses.

Self-Concept Mode. Self-concept is the composite beliefs and feelings a person holds about himself/herself at any given time. The basic need of this mode is psychologic integrity. The self-concept consists of two areas: (a) physical self and (b) personal self. The personal self, which was of concern in this study, has the components of self-consistency and self-esteem, among others. Integrity of the personal self is thought to lead to a positive psychologic adaptation, in this case blocking pain impulses from reaching the level of awareness.

Self-consistency is continuity of self over time and avoidance of disequilibrium in the self-concept (Andrews & Roy, 1991). Self-esteem is a feeling of personal worth. Anything that threatens self-consistency or self-esteem may result in anxiety, a painful uneasiness of mind due to an impending or anticipated threat. As previously stated, anxiety and pain are closely related. A person who has surgery may experience pain and in turn may experience anxiety which may exacerbate pain. The brain does not distinguish between a physiologic threat or psychologic threat, and in fact, anxiety can initiate or increase the pain experience. In response to a threat to self-consistency or self-esteem, the autonomic nervous system may be activated, resulting in adaptive responses, similar to those in the physiologic adaptive mode. Behavior in the self-concept mode is manifested through the person's appearance, facial expression, and through statements the person makes about himself or herself (Andrews & Roy, 1991).

Role Function Mode. A person sometimes has to alter his or her usual social roles because of a change in health status and may take on temporary roles such as the sick role. The sick role may be a tertiary or a temporary role as used in Roy's conceptual model (Andrews & Roy, 1991). The person electing to have a cholecystectomy is temporarily in the sick role. The basic need in this mode is social integrity or the need to know who one is in relation to others. Adaptation to the sick role can assist the individual in accepting help to perform activities of daily living and thereby return to former (pre-surgical) social roles as expeditiously as possible.

In this mode, culture may be influencing role performance (Melzack & Wall, 1983). A person's reaction to illness is linked to cultural beliefs, values, and expectations. These cultural values and expectations may conflict with the sick role expectations of health care providers, which in turn may result in the inability of the patient to meet his or her social integrity needs.

Interdependence Mode. "The interdependence mode focuses on interactions related to giving and receiving love, respect, and value (Andrews & Roy, 1991). The basic need of this mode is affectional adequacy or the feeling of security in nurturing, interpersonal relationships. It is through the social interactions of the interdependence mode that a person's need for affectional adequacy is met. Two specific relationships are the focus of this mode: (a) significant others and (b) social support system. A significant other is a person who is most important to the individual such as a spouse; a support system may be family members and friends. Support systems provide the love, respect, and value that significant others bring to a relationship but that are different in intensity and meaning. It is believed that the presence or absence of a trusting, supporting person or significant other may increase or decrease the pain threshold (Andrews & Roy, 1991). Separation from a significant other or a support person may lead to anxiety, which could increase pain intensity."

The following specific propositions were tested.

1. Culture is related to the response to cholecystectomy pain.
2. Anxiety might act as a confounding variable and be related to the response to pain.
3. Physiologic adaptation is related to the pain response.
4. Self-concept adaptation is related to the pain response.
5. Sick role adaptation is related to the pain response.
6. Social support is related to the pain response. (From Calvillo, E. R., & Flaskerud, J. H. [1993]. The adequacy and scope of Roy's Adaptation Model to guide cross-cultural pain research. *Nursing Science Quarterly*, 6[3], 118–129, with permission.) ■

THE CRITIQUE OF FRAMEWORKS: THEORETICAL SUBSTRUCTION

In the past, the common approach to critiquing a framework was to search for a statement by the author that the study was based on a particular theory. Strategies had not been developed for evaluating the extent to which the study was actually guided by the theory. This information was often not included in the published version of the study. In 1979, Hinshaw proposed using theoretical substruction as a strategy for evaluating study frameworks. However, the method proposed needed further development. The process has been further refined by Dulock and Holzemer (1991) and now offers a viable approach to critiquing frameworks.

The term substruction is the opposite of construction and means "to take apart." With *theoretical substruction,* a framework of a published study is separated into component parts to evaluate the logical consistency of the theoretical system and interaction of the framework with the study methodology. It essentially reverses the process described in this chapter. If components of the framework are inferred rather than clearly stated, the evaluator extracts those components and states them as clearly as possible. If a conceptual map is not presented, the evaluator may construct one.

Theoretical substruction needs to answer two questions: (1) Is the framework logically adequate? and (2) Did the framework guide the methodology of the study? Gaps and inconsistencies are identified. The conclusions of the study are evaluated in terms of whether they are logical, defensible, and congruent with the framework.

To perform theoretical substruction, the following elements need to be extracted from the published description of the framework:

1. Concepts (and constructs if included).
2. Conceptual definitions (and construct definitions if used).
3. Operational definitions.
4. Sets linking constructs, concepts, and variables.
5. General propositions linking the constructs.
6. Specific propositions linking the concepts.
7. Hypotheses, research questions, or objectives.
8. Statement sets linking general propositions; specific propositions; and hypotheses, questions, or objectives.
9. A conceptual map.
10. Sampling method and size.
11. Design.
12. Data analysis performed in relation to each hypothesis, question, or objective.
13. Findings related to each hypothesis, question, or objective.
14. Author's interpretation of findings in relation to the framework.

This information will be used to analyze the logical structure of the framework and its link with the methodology. The following questions can be used to guide that analysis:

1. Is the framework based on a substantive theory or a tentative theory?
2. Was a conceptual model included in the framework?
3. Is the definition of constructs consistent with the theorist's definition?
4. Do the concepts reflect the constructs identified in the framework?
5. Do the variables reflect the concepts identified in the framework?
6. Are the conceptual definitions validated by references to the literature?
7. Are the operational definitions reflective of the conceptual definitions?
8. Are the reliability and validity of the operational definitions adequate?
9. Are the propositions logical and defensible?
10. Is evidence from the literature used to validate the propositions?
11. Are the hypotheses, questions, or objectives logically linked to the propositions?
12. Can diagrams of the propositions be linked to the conceptual map?
13. Is the conceptual map adequate to explain the phenomenon of concern?
14. Is the design appropriate to test the propositions?
15. Is the sample size adequate to avoid a Type II error? (Type II errors are discussed in Chapter 16.)
16. Are the data analyses appropriate for the hypotheses, questions, or objectives?
17. Are the findings for each hypothesis, question, or objective consistent with that proposed by the framework? If not, was the methodology adequate to test the hypothesis, question, or objective?
18. Were the findings interpreted by the author in terms of the framework?
19. Do the findings validate the framework?
20. Are the findings consistent with those of other studies using the same framework (or testing the same propositions)?

Critical reviews are now being published that examine studies related to selected areas of research. Theoretical substruction is being used to evaluate these studies. One example of this is Silva's (1986) examination of studies asserting to test nursing models. The use of substruction should strengthen frameworks appearing in published studies. In addition, it will assist in building a body of knowledge related to a specific theory that can then be applied to clinical practice situations with greater confidence. For further information on critiquing frameworks, see Chapter 24.

SUMMARY

A framework is the abstract, logical structure of meaning that guides the development of the study and enables the researcher to link the findings to nursing's body of knowledge. Every study has a framework. The framework should be well integrated with the methodology, carefully structured, and clearly presented. This is true whether the study is physiological or psychosocial. If a well-established theory is being tested, the framework is derived deductively from the theory. However, many theoretical ideas in nursing have not been formally expressed as theories yet. Nursing studies often emerge from questions related to identified nursing problems or from the clinical insight that a relationship exists between or among elements important to desired outcomes.

The first step in understanding theories and frameworks is to become familiar with the

continued

continued

terms related to theoretical ideas and their application. A concept is a term that abstractly describes and names an object or phenomenon, thus providing it with a separate identity or meaning. A relational statement declares that a relationship of some kind exists between two or more concepts. Relational statements are the core of the framework; it is these statements that are tested through research. The type of statement expressed in a framework determines the design of the study, the statistical analysis that will be performed, and the type of findings that can be expected. Relational statements describe the direction, shape, strength, symmetry, sequencing, probability of occurrence, necessity, and sufficiency of a relationship.

Statements about the same two conceptual ideas can be made at various levels of abstractness. The statements found in conceptual models (general propositions) are at high levels of abstraction. Statements found in theories (specific propositions) are at a moderate level of abstraction. Hypotheses, which are a form of statement, are concrete and specific. As statements become more concrete, they become narrower in scope.

A conceptual model is a set of highly abstract, related constructs that broadly explains phenomena of interest, expresses assumptions, and reflects a philosophical stance. A theory is narrower and more specific than a conceptual model and is directly testable. A theory consists of an integrated set of defined concepts, existence statements, and relational statements that present a view of a phenomenon and can be used to describe, explain, predict, and/or control that phenomenon. A scientific theory has valid and reliable methods of measuring each concept and relational statements that have been repeatedly tested through research and demonstrated to be valid. A substantive theory has some recognition of its worth or meaning in the discipline and has been validated to some extent through research. A tentative theory is newly proposed, has minimal exposure to critique by the discipline, and has had little testing.

One strategy for expressing a framework is a conceptual map that diagrams the interrelationships of the concepts and statements. A conceptual map succinctly summarizes and integrates what is known about a phenomenon and allows one to grasp the gestalt of a phenomenon.

Developing a framework is one of the most important steps in the research process. The steps of the process include selecting and defining concepts, developing statements relating the concepts, expressing the statements in hierarchical fashion, and developing a conceptual map. Developing a framework designed to test a substantive theory requires that all concepts and statements in the framework be obtained from the substantive theory. When conceptual models are used in a framework, the framework must also include a testable theory. The map for such a framework must also include both.

Frameworks are evaluated using theoretical substruction. The term substruction is the opposite of construction and means "to take apart." A framework of a published study is separated into its component parts to evaluate the logical consistency of the theoretical system and its interaction with the study methodology. This provides a means of critiquing frameworks in published studies. The critique of frameworks strengthens their development and ultimate usefulness to practice.

References

Aamodt, A. M. (1984). Themes and issues in conceptualizing care. In M. M. Leininger (Ed.), *Care: The essence of nursing and health* (pp. 75–79). Thorofare, NJ: Slack.

Ajzen, I., & Fishbein, M. (1980). *Understanding attitudes and predicting social behavior.* Englewood Cliffs, NJ: Prentice-Hall.

Andrews, H. A., & Roy, C. (1991). *The Roy adaptation model: The definitive statement.* Norwalk, CT: Appleton & Lange.

Antonovsky, A. (1974). Conceptual and methodological problems in the study of resistance resources and stressful life events. In B. S. Dohrenwend & B. P. Dohrenwend (Eds.), *Stressful life events: Their nature and effects* (pp. 245–255), New York: Wiley.

Apter, M. J. (1982a). *The experience of motivation: The theory of psychological reversals.* London: Academic Press.

Apter, M. J. (1982b). Fawlty towers: A reversal theory analysis of a popular television comedy series. *Journal of Popular Culture, 16*(3), 128–138.

Apter, M. J. (1988). Reversal theory as a theory of emotions. In M. J. Apter, J. H. Kerr, & M. P. Cowles (Eds.), *Progress in reversal theory* (pp. 43–62). Amsterdam: Elsevier.

Apter, M. J. (1989). *Reversal theory: Motivation, emotion, and personality.* London: Routledge.

Apter, M. J., & Smith, K. C. P. (1985). Experiencing personal relationships. In M. J. Apter, D. Fontana, & S. Murgatroyd (Eds.), *Reversal theory: Applications and developments* (pp. 161–178). Cardiff, Wales: University College Cardiff Press.

Artinian, B. (1982). Conceptual mapping: Development of the strategy. *Western Journal of Nursing Research, 4*(4), 379–393.

Bakker, R. H., Kastermans, M. C., & Dassen, T. W. N. (1995). An analysis of the nursing diagnosis ineffective management of therapeutic regimen compared to noncompliance and Orem's self-care deficit theory of nursing. *Nursing Diagnosis, 6*(4), 161–166.

Benner, P., & Wrubel, J. (1989). *The primacy of caring: Stress and coping in health and illness.* Menlo Park, CA: Addison Wesley.

Bevis, E. O. (1981). Caring: A life force. In M. M. Leininger (Ed.), *Caring: An essential human need. Proceedings of Three National Caring Conferences* (pp. 49–60). Thorofare, NJ: Slack.

Blue, C. L. (1995). The predictive capacity of the theory of reasoned action and the theory of planned behavior in exercise research: An integrated literature review. *Research in Nursing & Health, 18*(2), 105–121.

Bottorff, J. L. (1988). Assessing an instrument in a pilot project: The self-care agency questionnaire. *The Canadian Journal of Nursing Research, 20*(1), 7–16.

Brody, J. K. (1988). Virtue ethics, caring, and nursing. *Scholarly Inquiry in Nursing Practice, 2*(2), 31–42.

Brown, L. (1986). The experience of care: Patient perspectives. *Topics in Clinical Nursing, 8*(2), 56–62.

Brown, S. A., & Hedges, L. V. (1994). Predicting metabolic control in diabetes: A pilot study using meta-analysis to estimate a linear model. *Nursing Research, 43*(6), 362–368.

Brugge, P. (1981). The relationship between family as a social support system, health status, and exercise of self-care agency in the adult with a chronic illness. *Dissertation Abstracts International, 42,* 1704B. (University Microfilms No. 82–09, 277)

Calvillo, E. R., & Flaskerud, J. H. (1993). The adequacy and scope of Roy's adaptation model to guide cross-cultural pain research. *Nursing Science Quarterly, 6*(3), 118–129.

Chinn, P. L., & Kramer, M. K. (1995). *Theory and nursing: A systematic approach* (4th ed.). St. Louis: Mosby.

Cook, M. R., Gerkovich, M. M., O'Connell, K. A., & Potocky, M. (1995). Reversal theory constructs predict lapse early in smoking cessation. *Research in Nursing & Health, 18*(3), 217–224.

Cronin, S. N., & Harrison, B. (1988). Importance of nurse caring behaviors as perceived by patients after myocardial infarction. *Heart & Lung, 17*(4), 374–380.

Davies, L. K. (1993). Comparison of dependent-care activities for well siblings of children with cystic fibrosis and well siblings in families without children with chronic illness. *Issues in Comprehensive Pediatric Nursing, 16*(2), 91–98.

Deynes, M. J. (1982). Measurement of self-care agency in adolescents (abstract). *Nursing Research, 31*(1), 63.

Dodd, M. J. (1984a). Measuring informational intervention for chemotherapy knowledge and self-care behavior. *Research in Nursing & Health, 7*(1), 43–50.

Dodd, M. J. (1984b). Patterns of self-care in cancer patients receiving radiation therapy. *Oncology Nursing Forum, 10*(3), 23–27.

Dodd, M. J. (1987). Efficacy of proactive information on self-care in radiation therapy patients. *Heart & Lung, 16*(5), 538–544.

Dulock, H. L., & Holzemer, W. L. (1991). Substruction: Improving the linkage from theory to method. *Nursing Science Quarterly, 4*(2), 83–87.

Fanslow, J. (1987). Compassionate nursing care: Is it a lost art? *Journal of Practical Nursing, 37*(2), 40–43.

Fawcett, J. (1995). *Analysis and evaluation of conceptual models of nursing* (3rd ed.). Philadelphia: Davis.

Fawcett, J., & Downs, F. (1986). *The relationship of theory and research.* Norwalk, CT: Appleton-Century-Crofts.

Feyerabend, P. (1975). *Against method.* London: Verso.

Fink, S. V. (1995). The influence of family resources and family demands on the strains and well-being of caregiving families. *Nursing Research, 44*(3), 139–146.

Fishbein, M., & Ajzen, I. (1975). *Belief, attitude, intention and behavior.* Boston: Addison-Wesley.

Forrest, D. (1989). The experience of caring. *Journal of Advanced Nursing, 14*(10), 815–823.

Foucault, M. (1970). *The order of things: An archaeology of the human sciences.* New York: Vintage.

Frank, P. (1961). The variety of reasons for the acceptance of scientific theories. In P. Frank (Ed.), *The validation of scientific theories* (pp. 13–25). New York: Collier.

Frey, M. A., & Denyes, M. J. (1989). Health and illness self-care in adolescents with IDDM: A test of Orem's theory. *Advances in Nursing Science, 12*(1), 67–75.

Fry, S. T. (1988). The ethic of caring: Can it survive in nursing? *Nursing Outlook, 36*(1), 48.

Gadow, S. A. (1985). Nurse and patient: The caring relationship. In A. N. Bishop & J. R. Scudder (Eds.), *Caring, curing, coping* (pp. 31–43). Birmingham, AL: University of Alabama.

Gardner, K. G., & Wheeler, E. C. (1981). The meaning of

caring in the context of nursing. In M. M. Leininger (Ed.), *Caring: An essential human need. Proceedings of three national caring conferences* (pp. 69–82). Thorofare, NJ: Slack.

Gaut, D. A. (1983). Development of a theoretically adequate description of caring. *Western Journal of Nursing Research, 5*(4), 313–324.

Gendron, D. (1988). *The expressive form of caring.* Toronto, Canada: University of Toronto.

Gibbs, J. (1972). *Sociological theory construction.* Hinsdale, IL: Dryden.

Griffin, A. P. (1983). A philosophical analysis of caring in nursing. *Journal of Advanced Nursing, 8*(4), 289–295.

Gulick, E. E. (1987). Parsimony and model confirmation of the ADL self-care scale for multiple sclerosis persons. *Nursing Research, 36*(5), 278–283.

Gulick, E. E. (1988). The self-administered ADL scale for persons with multiple sclerosis. In C. Waltz & O. Strickland (Eds.), *The measurement of nursing outcomes* (Vol. 1, pp. 128–159). New York: Springer.

Gulick, E. E. (1989). Model confirmation of the MS-related symptom checklist. *Nursing Research, 38*(3), 147–153.

Hanson, B. R., & Bickel, L. (1985). Development and testing of the questionnaire on perception of self-care agency. In J. Riehl-Sisca, *The science and art of self-care* (pp. 271–278). Norwalk, CT: Appleton-Century-Crofts.

Hemple, C. G. (1966). *Philosophy of natural science.* Englewood Cliffs, NJ: Prentice-Hall.

Hinshaw, A. S. (1979). Theoretical substruction: An assessment process. *Western Journal of Nursing Research, 1*(4), 319–324.

Horner, S. (1988). Intersubjective co-presence in a caring model. In *Caring and nursing explorations in the feminist perspectives.* Denver, Colorado: School of Nursing, University of Colorado Health Sciences Center.

Johnson, D. E. (1980). The behavioral system model for nursing. In J. P. Riehl & C. Roy (Eds.), *Conceptual models for nursing practice* (2nd ed., pp. 206–216). New York: Appleton-Century-Crofts.

Kane, C. (1988). Family social support: Toward a conceptual model. *Advances in Nursing Science, 10*(2), 13–25.

Kaplan, A. (1964). *The conduct of inquiry.* San Francisco: Chandler.

Kearney, B., & Fleischer, B. (1979). Development of an instrument to measure exercise of self-care agency. *Research in Nursing & Health, 2*(1), 25–34.

Kerlinger, F. N. (1986). *Foundations of behavioral research* (3rd ed.). New York: Holt, Rinehart and Winston.

Kerr, J. H. (1987). Cognitive intervention with elite performers: Reversal theory. *British Journal of Sports Medicine, 21*(2), 29–33.

King, I. M. (1981). *A theory for nursing: Systems, concepts, process.* New York: Wiley.

Knowlden, V. (1988). Nurse caring as constructed knowledge. In *Caring and nursing explorations in the feminist perspectives.* Denver, Colorado: School of Nursing, University of Colorado Health Sciences Center.

Kostopoulos, M. R. (1988). The reliability and validity of a nurse performance evaluation tool. In O. L. Strickland & C. F. Waltz (Eds.), *Measurement of nursing outcomes* (Vol. 2, pp. 77–95). New York: Springer.

Kuhn, T. (1970). *The structure of scientific revolutions* (2nd ed.). New York: Holt, Rinehart & Winston.

Larson, P. (1987). Comparison of cancer patients' and professional nurses' perceptions of important caring behaviors. *Heart & Lung, 16*(2), 187–193.

Lasky, P. A., & Eichelberger, K. M. (1985). Health-related views and self-care behaviors of young children. *Family Relations, 34*(1), 13–18.

Laudan, L. (1977). *Progress and its problems: Toward a theory of scientific growth.* Berkeley: University of California.

Laudan, L. (1981). A problem-solving approach to scientific progress. In I. Hacking (Ed.), *Scientific revolutions* (pp. 144–155). Fair Lawn, NJ: Oxford University.

Leidy, N. K. (1994). Functional status and the forward progress of merry-go-rounds: Toward a coherent analytical framework. *Nursing Research, 43*(4), 196–202.

Leininger, M. (1979). *Transcultural nursing.* New York: Masson.

Leininger, M. M. (1981). *Caring: An essential human need. Proceedings of three national caring conferences.* Thorofare, NJ: Slack.

Leininger, M. M. (1984). *Care: The essence of nursing and health.* Thorofare, NJ: Slack.

Leininger, M. M. (1988). *Care: Discovery and uses in clinical and community nursing.* Thorofare, NJ: Slack.

Levine, M. E. (1973). *Introduction to clinical nursing* (2nd ed.). Philadelphia: Davis.

Lipton, J. A., & Marbach, J. J. (September 20, 1980). Pain differences, similarities found. *Science News, 118,* 182–183.

McBride, S. (1987). Validation of an instrument to measure exercise of self-care agency. *Research in Nursing & Health, 10*(5), 311–316.

McCaleb, A., & Edgil, A. (1994). Self-concept and self-care practices of healthy adolescents. *Journal of Pediatric Nursing, 9*(4), 233–238.

McCubbin, H., & Thompson, A. (1987). *Family assessment inventories for research and practice.* Madison, WI: University of Wisconsin-Madison.

McDermitt, M. A. N. (1993). Learned helplessness as an interacting variable with self-care agency: Testing a theoretical model. *Nursing Science Quarterly, 6*(1), 28–38.

McFarlane, J. (1976). A charter for caring. *Journal of Advanced Nursing, 1,* 187–196.

Meinhart, N. T., & McCaffrey, M. (1983). *Pain: A nursing approach to assessment and analysis.* Norwalk, CT: Appleton-Century-Crofts.

Meister, S. (1991). Family well-being. In A. Whall & J. Fawcett (Eds.), *Family theory development in nursing: State of the science and art* (pp. 209–231). Philadelphia: Davis.

Melzack, R. (1975). McGill pain questionnaire: Major properties and scoring methods. *Pain, 1*(3), 277–299.

Melzack, R. & Wall, P. (1983). *Pain measurement and assessment.* New York: Raven.

Merton, R. K. (1968). *Social theory and social structure.* New York: Free Press.

Moody, L. E. (1989). Building a conceptual map to guide research. *Florida Nursing Review, 4*(1), 1–5.

Moody, L. E., Wilson, M. E., Smyth, K., Schwartz, R., Tittle, M., & Van Cott, M. L. (1988). Analysis of a decade of nursing practice research: 1977–1986. *Nursing Research, 37*(6), 374–379.

Moore, J. B. (1987a). Determining the relationship of autonomy to self-care agency or locus of control in school-age children. *Maternal-Child Nursing Journal, 16*(1), 47–60.

Moore, J. B. (1987b). Effects of assertion training and first aid instruction on children's autonomy and self-care agency. *Research in Nursing & Health, 10*(2), 101–109.

Moore, J. B. (1993). Predictors of children's self-care performance: Testing the theory of self-care deficit. *Scholarly Inquiry for Nursing Practice: An International Journal, 7*(3), 199–217.

Moore, J. B., & Gaffney, K. F. (1989). Development of an instrument to measure mother's performance of self-care activities for children. *Advances in Nursing Science, 12*(1), 76–84.

Morse, J. M., Solberg, S. M., Neander, W. L., Bottorff, J. L., & Johnson, J. L. (1990). Concepts of caring and caring as a concept. *Advances in Nursing Science, 13*(1), 1–14.

Neuman, B. (1989). *The Neuman systems model.* Norwalk, CT: Appleton & Lange.

Newman, M. A. (1979). *Theory development in nursing.* Philadelphia: Davis.

O'Connell, K. A. (1991). Why rational people do irrational things: The theory of psychological reversals. *Journal of Psychosocial Nursing, 29*(1), 11–14.

O'Connell, K. A. (1993). A lexicon for the mastery/sympathy and autic/alloic states. In J. H. Kerr, S. J. Murgatroyd, & M. J. Apter (Eds.). *Advances in reversal theory* (pp. 53–65). Amsterdam: Swets & Zeitlinger.

O'Connell, K. A., & Apter, M. J. (1993). Mastery and sympathy: Conceptual elaboration of transactional states. In J. H. Kerr, S. J. Murgatroyd, & M. J. Apter (Eds.). *Advances in reversal theory* (pp. 41–51). Amsterdam: Swets & Zietlinger.

O'Connell, K. A., Cook, M. R., Gerkovich, M. M., Potocky, M., & Swan, G. E. (1990). Reversal theory and smoking: A state-based approach to ex-smokers' highly tempting situations. *Journal of Consulting and Clinical Psychology, 58*(4), 498–494.

O'Connell, K. A., Gerkovich, M. M., & Cook, M. R. (1995). Reversal theory's mastery and sympathy states in smoking cessation. *Image: Journal of Nursing Scholarship, 27*(4), 311–316.

O'Connor, F. W. (1994). A vulnerability-stress framework for evaluating clinical interventions in schizophrenia. *Image: Journal of Nursing Scholarship, 26*(3), 231–237.

Orem, D. E. (1995). *Nursing: Concepts of practice* (5th ed.). New York: McGraw-Hill.

Popper, K. (1968). *The logic of scientific discovery.* New York: Harper & Row.

Potocky, M., Gerkovich, M. M., O'Connell, K. A., & Cook, M. R. (1991). State-outcome consistency in smoking relapse crises: A reversal theory approach. *Journal of Consulting and Clinical Psychology, 59*(2), 351–353.

Ray, M. A. (1984). The development of a classification system of institutional caring. In M. M. Leininger (Ed.), *Care: The essence of nursing and health* (pp. 95–112). Thorofare, NJ: Slack.

Ray, M. A. (1987a). Health care economics and human caring in nursing: Why the moral conflict must be resolved. *Family and Community Health, 10*(1), 35–43.

Ray, M. A. (1987b). Technological caring: A new model in critical care. *Dimensions of Critical Care Nursing, 6*(3), 166–173.

Rew, L. (1987). The relationship between self-care behaviors and selected psychosocial variables in children with asthma. *Journal of Pediatric Nursing, 2*(5), 333–341.

Reynolds, P. D. (1971). *A primer in theory construction.* Indianapolis: Bobbs-Merrill.

Riesch, S. K., & Hauch, M. R. (1988). The exercise of self-care agency: An analysis of construct and discriminant validity. *Research in Nursing & Health, 11*(4), 245–255.

Roach, M. S. (1987). *The human act of caring: A blueprint for health professions.* Toronto, Canada: Canadian Hospital Association.

Rogers, M. E. (1970). *An introduction to the theoretical basis of nursing.* Philadelphia: Davis.

Rogers, M. E. (1980). Nursing: A science of unitary man. In J. P. Riehl & C. Roy (Eds.), *Conceptual models for nursing practice* (2nd ed., pp. 329–337). Norwalk, CT: Appleton-Century-Crofts.

Rogers, M. E. (1983). A paradigm for nursing. In I. W. Clements & F. B. Roberts (Eds.), *Family Health: A theoretical approach to nursing care* (pp. 219–227). New York: Wiley.

Rogers, M. (1986). Science of unitary human beings. In V. M. Malinski (Ed.), *Explorations on Martha Rogers' science of unitary human beings* (pp. 3–8). Norwalk, CT: Appleton-Century-Crofts.

Rogers, M. E. (1988). Nursing science and art: A prospective. *Nursing Science Quarterly, 1*(3), 99–102.

Roy, C. (1984). *Introduction to nursing: An adaptation model* (2nd ed.). Englewood Cliffs, NJ: Prentice-Hall.

Roy, C. (1988). An explication of the philosophical assumptions of the Roy adaptation model. *Nursing Science Quarterly, 1*(1), 26–34.

Roy, C. (1990). Response to dialogue on a theoretical issue: Strengthening the Roy adaptation model through conceptual clarification. *Nursing Science Quarterly, 3*(2), 64–66.

Roy, C., & Roberts, S. L. (1981). *Theory construction in nursing: An adaptation model.* Englewood Cliffs, NJ: Prentice-Hall.

Sarter, B. (1988). *The stream of becoming: A study of Martha Rogers's theory.* New York: National League for Nursing.

Saucier, C. P., & Clark, L. M. (1993). The relationship between self-care and metabolic control in children with insulin-dependent diabetes mellitus. *Diabetes Education, 19*(2), 133–135.

Scheffler, I. (1967). *Science and subjectivity.* Indianapolis: Bobbs-Merrill.

Seyle, H. (1976). *The stress of life.* New York: McGraw-Hill.

Silva, M. C. (1981). Selection of a theoretical framework. In S. D. Krampitz & N. Pavlovich (Eds.), *Readings for nursing research* (pp. 17–28). St. Louis: Mosby.

Silva, M. C. (1986). Research testing nursing theory: State of the art. *Advances in Nursing Science, 9*(1), 1–11.

Stember, M. L. (1986). Model building as a strategy for theory development. In P. L. Chinn (Ed.), *Nursing research methodology: Issues and implementation* (pp. 103–119). Rockville, MD: Aspen.

Stemple, J. (1988). Measuring nursing care role orientation. In O. L. Strickland & C. F. Waltz (Eds.), *Measurement of nursing outcomes* (Vol. 2, pp. 19–31). New York: Springer.

Sternbach, R. A., & Tursky, B. (1965). Ethnic differences among housewives in psychophysical and skin potential responses to electric shock. *Psychophysiology, 1*(3), 241–246.

Stevenson, J. (1990). Quantitative care research: Review of content, process and product. In J. Stevenson & T. Tripp-Reimer (Eds.), *Knowledge about care and caring: State of the art and future development* (pp. 97–118). Kansas City, KS: American Academy of Nursing.

Suppe, F. (1972). What's wrong with the received view on the structure of scientific theories? *Philosophy of Science, 39*(1), 1–19.

Suppe, F., & Jacox, A. K. (1985). Philosophy of science and the development of nursing theory. In H. H. Werley & J. J. Fitzpatrick (Eds.), *Annual review of nursing research* (Vol. 3, pp. 241–267). New York: Springer.

Svebak, S. (1984). Active and passive forearm flexor tension patterns in the continuous perceptual-motor task paradigm: The significance of motivation. *International Journal of Psychophysiology, 2*(3), 167–176.

Svebak, S. (1985). Serious-mindedness and the effect of self-induced respiratory changes upon parietal EEG. *Biofeedback and Self-Regulation, 10*(1), 49–62.

Svebak, S. (1986). Cardiac and somatic activation in the continuous perceptual-motor task: The significance of threat and serious-mindedness. *International Journal of Psychophysiology, 3*(3), 155–162.

Svebak, S., & Apter, M. J. (1987). Laughter: An empirical test of some reversal theory hypotheses. *Scandinavian Journal of Psychology, 28*(3), 189–198.

Swanson-Kauffman, K. M. (1986). Caring in the instance of unexpected early pregnancy loss. *Topics in Clinical Nursing, 8*(2), 37–46.

Swanson-Kauffman, K. M. (1988). Caring needs of women who miscarried. In M. M. Leininger (Ed.), *Care: Discovery and uses in clinical and community nursing* (pp. 55–70). Detroit, MI: Wayne State University.

Thomas-Peter, B. A., & McDonagh, J. D. (1988). Motivational dominance in psychopaths. *British Journal of Clinical Psychology, 27*(Pt. 2), 153–158.

Tulman, L., & Fawcett, J. (1990). A framework for studying functional status after diagnosis of breast cancer. *Cancer Nursing, 13*(2), 98.

Walker, L. O., & Avant, K. C. (1995). *Strategies for theory construction in nursing* (3rd ed.). Norwalk, CT: Appleton-Lange.

Watson, J. (1988). *Nursing: Human science and human care. A theory of nursing.* New York: National League for Nursing.

Weaver, M. T. (1987). Perceived self-care agency: A LISREL factor analysis of Bickel and Hanson's questionnaire. *Nursing Research, 36*(6), 381–387.

Weiss, C. J. (1988). Model to discover, validate, and use care in nursing. In M. M. Leininger (Ed.), *Care, discovery and uses in clinical and community nursing* (pp. 139–150). Detroit, MI: Wayne State University.

Winsberg, B., & Greenlick, M. (1967). Pain response in Negro and white obstetrical patients. *Journal of Health and Social Behavior, 8*(3), 222–227.

Wooldridge, P. J., Schmitt, M. J., Skipper, J. K., Jr., & Leonard, R. C. (1983). *Behavioral science and nursing theory.* St. Louis: Mosby.

Zborowski, M. (1952). Cultural components in responses to pain. *Journal of Social Issues, 8*(4), 16–30.

Zborowski, M. (1969). *People in pain.* San Francisco: Jossey-Bass.

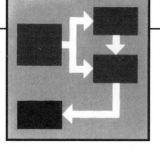

8

Objectives, Questions, and Hypotheses

Research objectives, questions, or hypotheses are formulated to bridge the gap between the more abstractly stated research problem and purpose, and the detailed design and plan for data collection and analysis. Objectives, questions, and hypotheses delineate the research variables, the relationships among the variables, and often the population to be studied. Research *variables* are concepts at various levels of abstraction that are measured, manipulated, or controlled in a study. Concrete concepts such as temperature, weight, or blood pressure are referred to as variables in a study; abstract concepts such as creativity, empathy, or social support are sometimes referred to as research concepts. Variables and concepts are conceptually defined, based on the study framework and either measured or manipulated in research.

This chapter focuses on formulating research objectives, questions, and hypotheses, with an emphasis on testing different types of hypotheses. The process of selecting objectives, questions, or hypotheses to direct studies is described. This selection process is influenced by a variety of factors, such as the number and quality of relevant studies conducted on a selected problem, the type of study to be conducted (quantitative or qualitative), and the expertise and preference of the researcher. Different types of variables are introduced and a background is provided for developing conceptual and operational definitions for research variables and concepts.

FORMULATING RESEARCH OBJECTIVES

Research objectives are clear, concise, declarative statements that are expressed in the present tense. For clarity, an objective usually focuses on one or two variables (or concepts) and indicates whether the variables are to be identified or described. Sometimes, their focus is to identify relationships or associations among variables or to determine differences between two groups regarding selected variables. Possible formats for developing objectives include:

1. to identify the elements or characteristics of variable X in a specified population. (Identification)
2. to describe the existence of variable X in a specified population. (Description)
3. to determine the difference between group one and group two regarding variable X in a specified population. (Difference)
4. to determine or identify the relationship between variable X and variable Y in a specified population. (Relational)
5. to determine if certain independent variables are predictive of a dependent variable. (Prediction)

Objectives are developed from the research problem and purpose, and clarify the variables (or concepts) and population to be studied. A descriptive study by Savedra, Tesler, Holzemer, and Brokaw (1995) demonstrates the logical flow from research problem and purpose to research objectives.

Research Problem

"Pain is a complex, multifaceted phenomenon with four major dimensions: location, intensity, quality, and temporal patterning (McCaffery & Beebe, 1989). Variability in pain responses to a given stimulus can be attributed to physiologic as well as psychologic factors. It is the individual variability and the subjective nature of the pain experience that demands that approaches be found to enable children and adolescents to communicate the nature of their pain." (p. 272)

Research Purpose

"The purpose of this study was to develop a strategy to assist school-aged children and adolescents to describe the changing temporal nature of their pain." (p. 272)

Research Objectives

"More specifically, the aims (objectives) of the study were: (a) to identify words or phrases used by school-aged children and adolescents to communicate how pain starts and how pain changes over time, and (b) to test the ability of school-aged children and adolescents to use a dot matrix format to draw how pain changes." (p. 272) ∎

The first objective focused on *identification* of words or phrases to communicate pain over time (variable) in school-aged children and adolescents (population). The second objective focused on *description* of the use of dot matrix format (variable) to draw how pain changes. "Analyses of the dot matrix markings revealed six patterns of pain: steady decrease, steady increase, ongoing sharp increases and decreases, stair-step increase and decrease, steady increase and decrease, and constant. The 12 words and phrases described how pain be-

gan as well as how the pattern of pain changed over time" (Savedra et al., 1995, p. 272).

The objectives in some studies are complex and include several variables. Kemp, Keithley, Smith, and Morreale (1990, p. 293) conducted a prospective study to examine "factors that contribute to pressure sores in surgical patients." The objectives for this study were:

1. To determine whether there was a relationship between (a) time on the operating table, (b) proportion of diastolic hypotensive episodes during surgery (diastolic blood pressure < 60 mm Hg), (c) age, (d) preoperative albumin levels, (e) preoperative total protein levels, and (f) preoperative Braden scores, and the development of pressure sores.
2. To determine how time on the operating table, proportion of diastolic hypotensive episodes during surgery, age, preoperative albumin and total protein levels, and preoperative Braden scores could be combined to best predict the development of pressure sores. (p. 295)

The first objective focuses on the *relationships* of six variables to pressure sore development. The second objective is concerned with *prediction* of the development of pressure sores (dependent variable) using the independent variables time on the operating table, proportion of diastolic hypotensive episodes during surgery, age, preoperative albumin and total protein levels, and preoperative Braden scores. Kemp et al. (1990) found that age, time on the operating table, and extracorporeal circulation were the most useful in predicting patients who are at risk for developing pressure sores during elective surgery. The relationships identified in this study could be developed into hypotheses for testing through further research.

FORMULATING RESEARCH QUESTIONS

A *research question* is a concise, interrogative statement that is worded in the present tense and includes one or more variables (or concepts). The foci of research questions are description of variable(s), determination of differences between two or more groups regarding selected variable(s), examination of relationships among variables, and use of independent variables to predict a dependent variable. The format for research questions is as follows:

1. How is variable *X* described in a specified population? (Description)
2. What is the perception of variable *X* in a specified population? (Description)
3. Is there a difference between groups one and two regarding variable *X?* (Difference)
4. Is variable *X* related to variables *Y* and *Z* in a specified population? (Relational)
5. What is the relationship between variables *X* and *Y* in a specified population? (Relational)
6. Are independent variables *W, X,* and *Y* useful in predicting dependent variable *Z?*

Zauszniewski (1995) developed research questions to direct her descriptive correlational study. The flow from research problem and purpose to research questions is demonstrated in the following example.

▌▬▬▬▬▬▬▬▬▬▬▬▬▬

Research Problem

"Depression remains the most commonly diagnosed mental disorder in the United States, with approximately 15% to 30% of the population affected each year. . . . Recent changes in the delivery of mental health services have shifted from traditional inpatient psychiatric care for clinical depression to community-based treatment. . . . Nursing interventions that enhance such health-seeking resources as social interest and learned resourcefulness may be useful in promoting adaptive functioning among depressed outpatients. Relationships among these concepts have been examined within the context of Schlotfeldt's (1975) health-seeking model for depressed inpatients, but not for outpatients (Zauszniewski, 1994). . . . Therefore, health-

seeking resources and adaptive functioning of depressed persons treated outside the hospital environment may differ from resources of inpatients." (p. 179)

Research Purpose

"This study, therefore, examined relationships among social interest, learned resourcefulness, depressive symptoms, and adaptive functioning in two groups of depressed persons being treated in community settings." (p. 180)

Research Questions

"The following research questions were addressed: 1. What are the differences between depressed outpatients recently discharged from the hospital and those never hospitalized in health-seeking resources, depressive symptoms, and adaptive functioning? 2. What are the relationships among health-seeking resources (social interest, learned resourcefulness), depressive symptoms, and adaptive functioning? 3. Of social interest, learned resourcefulness, and depressive symptoms, which best predicts adaptive functioning?" (p. 1995) ■

The first question focuses on examining *differences* between two groups (depressed outpatients recently discharged from the hospital and those never hospitalized) for the variables of health-seeking resources, depressive symptoms, and adaptive functioning. The second question focuses on examining *relationships* among the variables health-seeking resources, depressive symptoms, and adaptive functioning. The third question examines the use of social interest, learned resourcefulness, and depressive symptoms (independent variables) to *predict* adaptive functioning (dependent variable).

The research questions formulated for quantitative and qualitative studies have many similarities. However, the questions directing qualitative studies are frequently broader in focus and include concepts that are more complex and abstract than in quantitative studies. The ethnographic study by Allan (1989, p. 657) that focused on "women who successfully manage their weight" is presented as an example.

Research Problem

"Approximately 30% of Americans are overweight (Abraham, 1983). Moreover, overweight and obesity are more prevalent among women, particularly women of lower socioeconomic class. Despite widespread concern among health professionals, most view overweight and obesity as difficult conditions to treat. . . . Most weight research and treatment programs tend to focus on a self-selected population (Weiss, 1977). Because most individuals desiring to lose weight do not attend such programs (Schachter, 1982), little is known about the self-care experiences of women with regard to weight management." (p. 657)

Research Purpose

"To explore the characteristics of those women who successfully manage their weight." (p. 659)

Research Questions

1. "What methods for weight management are used by women who successfully manage their weight?
2. What factors influence the selection of particular methods?" (p. 659) ■

The first question focuses on the *description* of the complex concept of weight management methods. The second question is concerned with *identification* and *description* of factors influencing weight management methods.

FORMULATING HYPOTHESES

A *hypothesis* is the formal statement of the expected relationship(s) between two or more variables in a specified population. The hypothesis translates the research problem and purpose into a clear explanation or prediction of the expected results or outcomes of the study. This section includes the purpose, sources, and types of hypotheses and the process for developing and testing hypotheses.

PURPOSE OF HYPOTHESES

The purpose of a hypothesis is similar to that of research objectives and questions. A hypothesis includes the variables to be manipulated or measured, identifies the population to be examined, indicates the type of research, and directs the conduct of the study. Hypotheses also influence the study design, sampling technique, data collection and analysis methods, and the interpretation of findings. Hypotheses differ from objectives and questions by predicting the outcomes of a study, and the researcher indicates rejection, nonrejection, support, or nonsupport of each hypothesis. Hypothesis testing is a means of generating knowledge through the testing of theoretical statements or relationships that have been identified in previous research, proposed by theorists, or observed in practice. In addition, hypotheses are developed to direct the testing of new treatments and are often viewed as tools for uncovering ideas rather than ends in themselves (Beveridge, 1950).

SOURCES OF HYPOTHESES

Hypotheses are generated by observing phenomena or problems in the real world, analyzing theory, and reviewing the literature. Many hypotheses originate from real-life experiences. Clinicians and researchers observe events in the world and identify relationships among these events (theorizing), which is the basis for formulating hypotheses. For example, clinicians might have noticed that the hospitalized patient who complains the most receives the most pain medicine. The relationship identified is a prediction about events in the world that has potential for empirical testing. Theory to support this relationship could be identified through a literature review. Fagerhaugh and Strauss (1977) developed a theory of pain management identifying the following relationship: "As

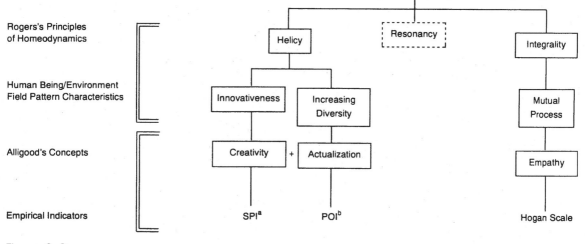

Rogers's Conceptual System and Theory of Accelerating Change

Rogers's Principles of Homeodynamics	Helicy Resonancy	Integrality
Human Being/Environment Field Pattern Characteristics	Innovativeness Increasing Diversity	Mutual Process
Alligood's Concepts	Creativity + Actualization	Empathy
Empirical Indicators	SPI[a] POI[b]	Hogan Scale

Figure 8–1

Illustration of derivation of Alligood's concepts from Rogers's principles. (From Alligood, M. R. [1991]. Testing Rogers's theory of accelerating change: The relationships among creativity, actualization, and empathy in persons 18 to 92 years of age. *Western Journal of Nursing Research, 13*[1], 85. © 1991. Reprinted by permission of Sage Publications, Inc.)

expressions of pain increase, pain management increases." This theory was developed using grounded theory research but requires additional testing to determine its usefulness in describing pain expression and management in a variety of situations. Based on theory and clinical observation, the following hypothesis might be formulated: "The more frequent a hospitalized patient complains of pain, the more often doses of analgesic medications are administered."

The nursing diagnoses formulated in caring for patients can be the basis for developing hypotheses. The development of hypotheses from a nursing diagnosis requires that the theoretical formulations from which the diagnosis was derived be identified. For example, the theoretical relationships identified in Orem's (1995) theory of self-care and the nursing diagnosis "self-care deficit of hygiene and dressing related to joint pain and restricted mobility" could serve as the basis for developing hypotheses. One could examine the effectiveness of interventions in reducing joint pain and improving mobility and their impact on individuals' self-care abilities. An example hypothesis might include: "Individuals with arthritis who use

relaxation therapy have less perceived joint pain and require less time to dress and bathe themselves than those not using the therapy."

Some hypotheses are initially generated from theory, when the intent of the researcher is to test statements of a theory that will ultimately have an impact on nursing practice (Chinn & Kramer, 1995). The relationships expressed in theory can be used to generate hypotheses. Alligood used two principles, *helicy* and *integrality,* from Martha Rogers's theory as a basis for her study. "Helicy is the continuous, innovative, probabilistic increasing diversity of human and environmental field pattern. Integrality is the continuous mutual human and environmental field process" (1991, p. 84). Alligood chose to study the interrelationship of the concepts creativity, actualization, and empathy (see Figure 8–1). The link between Rogers's principles and the study variables is as follows: "Helicy (Rogers, 1986) sets forth the innovative (creativity) and increasingly diverse (actualizing) nature of human and environmental field pattern in development. Integrality describes the mutual (empathic) character of the human and environmental energy field process" (Alligood,

1991, p. 89). Figure 8–1 demonstrates the link of Rogers's principles, the constructs in the principles, Alligood's study concepts, and the empirical indicators or instruments used to measure the concepts. The hypotheses formulated by Alligood (1991) were:

1. There is a positive correlation between creativity and empathy.
2. There is a positive correlation between actualization and empathy.
3. Creativity and actualization, combined, account for more of the variance in empathy than either one does separately. (p. 89)

Hypotheses can be generated by reviewing the literature. A researcher might restate a hypothesis that was tested previously by another researcher and focus on a different variable. For example, the hypothesis stated by Leske (1995, p. 169), that "family members of surgical patients who received intraoperative progress reports would report less anxiety than families who did not receive such an intervention or attention" might be restated as, "family members of surgical patients who received intraoperative progress reports express greater *satisfaction with care* than families who did not receive such an intervention or attention." A researcher could also choose to replicate Leske's study and test the original hypothesis.

In reviewing the literature, researchers analyze and synthesize the findings from different studies. The relationships identified from synthesis of study findings are valuable in generating hypotheses. Bull (1990) studied the factors influencing family caregivers' burdens and health. The hypotheses she formulated were based on a synthesis of previous findings.

"The findings of previous cross-sectional studies indicate that caregiver's health, recipient's health, and social support are important predictors of caregiver burden. The extent to which these factors are applicable to situations of caregiver burden two weeks and two months following hospital discharge and identification of the best predictors form the basis of this study. The following hypotheses were tested:

H1. Poor physical health, poor functional ability, and poor mental health of family caregivers and recipients prior to hospital discharge and limited social support following hospitalization are associated with greater caregiver burden at two weeks and two months postdischarge.

H2. Greater subjective burden and greater objective burden at two weeks postdischarge are associated with poor physical health, functional ability, and mental health for family caregivers at two weeks and two months postdischarge." (pp. 758–759) ∎

TYPES OF HYPOTHESES

Different types of relationships and numbers of variables are identified in hypotheses. Studies might have one, three, five, or more hypotheses, depending on the complexity of the study. The type of hypothesis developed is based on the purpose of the study. Hypotheses can be described using four categories: (1) associative versus causal, (2) simple versus complex, (3) directional versus nondirectional, and (4) null versus research.

Associative Versus Causal Hypotheses

The relationships identified in hypotheses are associative or causal. An associative relationship identifies variables that occur or exist together in the real world (Reynolds, 1971). In an associative relationship, when one variable changes, the other variable changes. A format for expressing an associative hypothesis follows:

1. Variable X is related to variable Y in a specified population. (Predicts a relationship.)
2. Variable X increases as variable Y increases in a specified population. (Predicts a positive relationship.)
3. Variable X decreases as variable Y decreases in a specified population. (Predicts a positive relationship.)

4. Variable *X* increases as variable *Y* decreases in a specified population. (Predicts a negative or inverse relationship.)

5. Variable *X* decreases as variable *Y* increases in a specified population. (Predicts a negative or inverse relationship.)

Georges and Heitkemper (1994) examined the relationship between "dietary fiber and distressing gastrointestinal (GI) symptoms in midlife women" and formulated the following associative hypotheses to direct their study.

II. "An inverse relationship exists between fiber intake and symptom reports in this group.

III. A positive relationship exists between caffeine/alcohol intake and symptom reports in this group." (p. 357) ∎

Hypothesis II presents a negative or inverse relationship, indicating that a decrease in fiber intake (*X*) is associated with an increase in GI symptom reports (*Y*). A diagram of this relationship follows:

↓ *X* ——————— − ↑ *Y*

Hypothesis III presents a positive relationship, indicating that an increase in caffeine/alcohol intake (*X*) is associated with an increase in GI symptom reports (*Y*) or a decrease in caffeine/alcohol intake (*X*) is associated with a decrease in GI symptom reports (*Y*). A diagram of these two relationships follows:

↑ *X* —— + —— ↑ *Y*   ↓ *X* —— + —— ↓ *Y*

Causal relationships identify a cause-and-effect interaction between two or more variables, which are referred to as independent and dependent variables. The *independent variable* (treatment or experimental variable) is manipulated by the researcher to cause an effect on the dependent variable. The *dependent variable* (outcome or criterion variable) is measured to examine the effect

created by the independent variable. A format for stating a causal hypothesis is: The subjects exposed to the independent variable demonstrate greater change as measured by the dependent variable than the subjects not exposed to the independent variable.

Poroch (1995) studied the "effect of preparatory patient education (PPE) on the anxiety and satisfaction of cancer patients receiving radiation therapy" and formulated the following causal hypothesis: patients receiving the "PPE intervention experience lower levels of anxiety than those who receive routine information" (p. 208). In this hypothesis, cancer patients receiving radiation are the population; PPE intervention is the independent variable (*X*); and anxiety level is the dependent variable (*Y*). The arrow in the following diagram indicates that the independent variable (*X*) causes an effect on the dependent variable (*Y*).

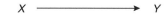

X ⟶ *Y*

Simple Versus Complex Hypotheses

A *simple hypothesis* states the relationship (associative or causal) between two variables. One format for stating a simple associative hypothesis is: Variable *X* is related to variable *Y*. A simple causal hypothesis identifies the relationship between one independent variable and one dependent variable.

A *complex hypothesis* predicts the relationship (associative or causal) among three or more variables. A complex associative hypothesis would indicate the relationships among variables *X, Y,* and *Z*. In complex causal hypotheses, relationships are predicted between two (or more) independent variables and/or two (or more) dependent variables. For example, Gross, Fogg, and Tucker (1995) examined the effect of "parent training for promoting positive parent-toddler relationships" and hypothesized that "following a 10-week parent training program, parents would report greater self-efficacy, less stress and depression, and reductions in difficult child behaviors than parents in the control group" (p. 490). This complex hypothesis has one independent variable, parent training program (*X*), and four dependent variables, self-

Table 8–1
Simple and Complex Hypotheses

	Independent Variables	Dependent Variables
Simple Hypotheses		
"Motor activity over all states as well as within a given state will be (is) reduced during the on-waterbed period.	Waterbed flotation	Motor activity
Heart rate will be (is) reduced during the on-waterbed period.	Waterbed flotation	Heart rate
There will be (is) a greater percentage of time spent in sleep states versus awake states during the on-waterbed period.	Waterbed flotation	Sleep versus awake states
There will be (are) fewer sleep-to-wake transitions during the on-waterbed period" (Deiriggi, 1990, p. 141).	Waterbed flotation	Sleep-to-wake transitions
Complex Hypothesis		
"The duration of sleep state epochs will be (are) greater during the on-waterbed period. The duration of waking activity and fuss state epochs will be (are) greater during the off-waterbed period. (Expressed as one hypothesis)" (Deiriggi, 1990, p. 141).	Waterbed flotation	Sleep state epochs Waking activity Fuss state epochs

efficacy (Y_1), stress (Y_2), depression (Y_3), and difficult child behaviors (Y_4). A diagram of this hypothesis follows:

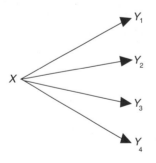

In real-life situations, often multiple variables cause an event or a treatment results in multiple outcomes. Therefore, complex rather than simple causal hypotheses are often more representative of real-life events.

Some studies include both simple and complex hypotheses. Deiriggi (1990) conducted a quasi-experimental study "to test the effects of nonoscillating waterbed flotation on indicators of energy expenditure in preterm infants: motor activity, heart rate, and behavioral state" (p. 140). Table 8–1 includes the study's hypotheses, which are labeled as simple or complex based on the number of independent and dependent variables in each hypothesis. These hypotheses might have been more reflective of the population studied rather than the sample if they had been expressed in the present tense (is or are) rather than the future tense (will be). This idea is expanded in the section on developing hypotheses.

Nondirectional Versus Directional Hypotheses

A *nondirectional hypothesis* states that a relationship exists but does not predict the nature of the relationship. If the direction of the relationship being studied is not clear in clinical practice or the theoretical or empirical literature, the researcher has no clear indication of the nature of the relationship. Under these circumstances, nondirectional hypotheses are developed, such as those developed by Jirovec and Kasno (1990) to direct their study.

1. Elderly nursing home residents' self-appraisals of their self-care abilities are related to the basic conditioning factors of sex, sociocultural orientation, health, and family influences.
2. Elderly nursing home residents' self-appraisals of their self-care abilities are related to their perceptions of the nursing home environment. (p. 304)

The first hypothesis is complex (five variables), associative, and nondirectional. The second hypothesis is simple (two variables), associative, and nondirectional. Both hypotheses state that a relationship exists but do not indicate the direction of the relationship.

A *directional hypothesis* states the nature of the relationship between two or more variables. These hypotheses are developed from theoretical statements, findings of previous studies, and clinical experience. As the knowledge on which a study is based increases, the researcher is able to make a prediction about the direction of a relationship between the variables being studied. The use of such terms as *less, more, increase, decrease,* and *greater* indicate the directions of relationships in hypotheses. Directional hypotheses can be associative or causal and simple or complex. For example, Gross, Conrad, Fogg, Willis, and Garvey (1995, p. 96) examined the "relationship between maternal depression and preschool children's mental health in a community sample" and hypothesized that preschool children's lower social competence and increased behavior problems are related to higher maternal depression scores (associative, directional, complex hypothesis).

A *causal hypothesis* predicts the effect of an independent variable on a dependent variable, specifying the direction of the relationship. Thus, all causal hypotheses are directional. An example

of a complex, causal hypothesis is: "Patients with transcutaneous electrical nerve stimulation (TENS) have less postoperative pain arising from clinical wound care procedures than patients with the placebo-TENS or no-treatment" (Hargreaves & Lander, 1989, p. 159). This hypothesis predicts that the independent variables TENS, placebo-TENS, and no-treatment affect the dependent variable postoperative pain. Gross et al. (1995, p. 490) formulated the following simple causal hypothesis: families experiencing a parent training program "demonstrate more positive parent-toddler interactions than control group families."

Null Versus Research Hypotheses

The *null hypothesis (Ho)*, also referred to as a statistical hypothesis, is used for statistical testing and interpreting statistical outcomes. Even if the null hypothesis is not stated, it is implied, since it is the converse of the research hypothesis (Kerlinger, 1986). A null hypothesis can be simple or complex, associative or causal. An associative null hypothesis states: There is no relationship between the variables. An example of a simple associative null hypothesis is: "There is no relationship between the number of experiences performing a developmental assessment skill and learning of the skill, as measured by clinical performance test scores" (Koniak, 1985, p. 85).

A causal null hypothesis might be stated in the following format:

1. There is no effect of one variable on another.
2. There is no difference in the experimental group exposed to the independent variable and the control group as measured by the dependent variable.

Fahs and Kinney (1991, p. 204) developed the following complex null hypothesis to direct their study: "There is no difference in the occurrence of a bruise at injection site with low-dose heparin therapy when administered in three different subcutaneous sites" (abdomen, thigh, and arm). There was no statistically significant difference in bruising at 60 and 72 hours postinjection for the three sites. Thus, this null hypothesis was supported.

A *research hypothesis* is the alternative hypothesis (H_1 or H_A) to the null. The research hypothesis states that there is a relationship between two or more variables and can be simple or complex, nondirectional or directional, and associative or causal. Researchers have different beliefs about when to state a research hypothesis or a null hypothesis. Some researchers state the null because it is more easily interpreted based on the results of statistical analyses. The null is also used when the researcher believes there is no relationship between two variables and when there is inadequate theoretical or empirical information to state a research hypothesis (Kerlinger, 1986). A research hypothesis is used to make a prediction about the existence or direction of a relationship between variables. The prediction in a research hypothesis needs to be based on theoretical statements, previous research findings, or clinical experience. Jadack, Hyde, and Keller (1995, p. 313) formulated both research and null hypotheses to "examine gender differences in knowledge about HIV, the reported incidence of risky sexual behavior, and comfort with safer sexual practices among young adults."

"(a) There will be no difference between men and women in knowledge about HIV transmission routes (sexual, needle sharing, casual); (b) there will be no difference between men and women in knowledge about the effectiveness of measures to prevent sexual transmission of HIV; (c) men and women will differ with respect to reported frequency and type of behaviors that could lead to the transmission of HIV; and (d) men and women will differ with respect to reported level of comfort and safer sexual practices." (p. 315) ∎

DEVELOPING HYPOTHESES

Developing hypotheses requires inductive and deductive thinking. Most people have a predominant way of thinking and will use that thinking pattern in developing hypotheses. Inductive thinkers have a tendency to focus on relationships that are observed in clinical practice and will synthesize these observations to formulate a general statement about the relationships observed (Chinn & Kramer, 1995). For example, inductive thinkers might note that elderly patients who are not instructed about the reasons for early postoperative ambulation make no effort to get out of bed. Deductive thinkers examine more abstract statements from theories or previous research and then formulate a hypothesis for study. Deductive thinkers might translate a statement such as "people who receive instruction in self-care are more responsible in caring for themselves" into a hypothesis.

Neither the inductive nor the deductive thinker has completed the process of formulating a hypothesis. The inductive thinker must link the relational statement that was developed from clinical observations with a theoretical framework to increase the usefulness of the study findings. This requires deductive thinking. The deductive thinker must use inductive thinking to determine whether the relationship of events in clinical practice is accurately predicted based on the theoretical statement. Without this real-world experience, the selection of subjects and the identification of ways to measure the variables would be unclear. Thus, hypothesis development requires both inductive and deductive thinking. An example hypothesis for potential study is: "Elderly patients who receive self-care instruction on early ambulation get out of bed earlier and are discharged sooner after surgery than elderly patients who receive no self-care instruction on early ambulation."

In formulating a hypothesis, a researcher has several decisions to make. These decisions will be directed by the problem studied and the expertise and preference of the researcher. The researcher must decide whether the problem to be studied is best investigated using simple or complex hypotheses. Complex hypotheses frequently require complex methodology and the outcomes may be difficult to interpret. Some researchers prefer the clarity of simple hypotheses. The research problem and purpose determine whether an associative or causal relationship is to be studied. Testing a hypothesis that states a causal relationship requires expertise in implementing a treatment and controlling extraneous variables. Another decision involves the formulation of a research or a null hypothesis. This decision must be made based on what the researcher believes is the most accurate prediction of the relationship between the variables.

A hypothesis that is clearly and concisely stated provides the greatest direction in conducting a study. For clarity, hypotheses are expressed as declarative statements written in the present tense. Thus, hypotheses need to be written without the phrase "There *will be* no relationship . . ." because the future tense refers to the sample being studied. Hypotheses are statements of relationships about populations, not about study samples. According to mathematical theory related to generalization, one cannot generalize to the future (Kerlinger, 1973).

Hypotheses are clearer without the phrase "There is no *significant* difference . . ." because the level of significance is only a statistical technique applied to sample data (Armstrong, 1981). In addition, hypotheses should not identify methodological points such as techniques of sampling, measurement, and data analysis (Kerlinger, 1973, 1986). Therefore, statements such as *"measured by,"* "in a *random sample* of," or *"using ANOVA* (analysis of variance)" are not appropriate. Thus, hypotheses are not limited to the variables, methodology, and sample identified for one study. Hypotheses need to reflect the variables (or concepts) and population outlined in the research purpose.

A well-formulated hypothesis clearly identifies the relationship between the variables to be studied. For clarity, novice researchers often state a simple, concise hypothesis that identifies a relationship between two variables. A study might contain as few as one or as many as five to ten hypotheses. There is no set number of hypotheses that are needed to direct the study of a problem. The number of hypotheses developed is usually reflective of the researcher's expertise and the complexity of the problem studied. However, most studies include one to five hypotheses, and the relationships identified in these hypotheses set the limits for the study.

TESTING HYPOTHESES

A hypothesis's value is ultimately derived from whether or not it is testable in the real world. A *testable hypothesis* is one that contains variables that are measurable or manipulatable in the world, such as the one developed by Corff, Seideman, Venkataraman, Lutes, and Yates (1995).

Research Purpose

The purpose was to determine the "effectiveness of facilitated tucking, a nonpharmacologic nursing intervention, as a comfort measure in modulating preterm neonates' physiologic and behavioral responses to minor pain." (p. 143)

Hypothesis

The hypothesis for this prospective study was that "preterm neonates would have less variation in heart rate, oxygen saturation, and sleep state (shorter crying and sleep disruption time and less fluctuation in sleep states) in response to the painful stimulus of a heelstick with facilitated tucking than without." (p. 144)

Independent Variable—Facilitate Tucking

Conceptual Definition. A nonpharmacologic comfort measure that involves the motoric containment of an infant's arms and legs.

Operational Definition. The infant's arms and legs are contained in "a flexed, midline position close to the infant's trunk with the infant in a side-lying or supine position." (p. 144) (See Figure 8–2.)

Dependent Variables—Heart Rate and Oxygen Saturation

Conceptual Definition. Physiologic responses that are influenced by painful stimuli.

Operational Definition. Heart rate and oxygen saturation per pulse oximetry "were recorded

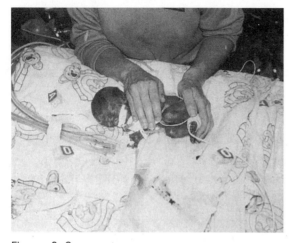

Figure 8–2
Facilitated tucking of a premature infant. (From Corff, K. E., Seideman, R., Venkataraman, P. S., Lutes, L., & Yates, B. [1995]. Facilitated tucking: A nonpharmacologic comfort measure for pain in preterm neonates. *JOGNN*, *24*[2], 144, with permission.)

visually and were graphed using a System VI Air Shields Infant Monitor With Data Logger." (p. 145)

Dependent Variable—Sleep State

Conceptual Definition. Behavioral responses of crying, sleep disruption time, and fluctuation in sleep state that are influenced by painful stimuli.

Operational Definition. "Sleep states were recorded by one of two observers who reached 90% reliability in reading sleep states, as defined in the Neonatal Individualized Developmental Care and Assessment Program. Sleep states are defined as state 1 = deep sleep; state 2 = light sleep; state 3 = drowsiness; state 4 = awake, alert; state 5 = aroused, fussy; and state 6 = crying . . . Sleep states were recorded during a 12-minute baseline period, the heelstick period, and a 15-minute post-stick period for both control and experimental trials." (p. 145) ∎

Hypotheses are evaluated with statistical analyses. If the hypothesis states an associative relationship, correlational analyses, such as Spearman rank order correlation or Pearson's correlation, are conducted to determine the existence, type, and degree of the relationship between the variables studied. The hypothesis that states a causal relationship is analyzed using statistics that examine differences, such as Mann-Whitney U, *t*-test, and analysis of variance (ANOVA). These statistical tests are explained in Chapter 18. It is the null hypothesis (stated or implied) that is tested. The intent is to determine whether the independent variable caused a significant effect on the dependent variable. The level of significance, alpha (α) = .05, .01, .001, is set following the generation of causal hypotheses. Further discussion on selecting a level of significance for testing a hypothesis is included in Chapter 16.

The results obtained from testing a hypothesis are described using certain terminology. Hypotheses are not proved true or false by the findings from research. Hypotheses are statements of relationships or differences in populations; the findings from one study do not prove a hypothesis. Even after a series of studies, the word "proved" is not used in scientific language because of the tentative nature of science. Research hypotheses are described as being supported or not supported in a study. When testing a null hypothesis, the hypothesis is either rejected or not rejected. Not rejecting the null hypothesis indicates that there was no relationship or effect found among the variables. Rejecting the null hypothesis indicates the possibility that a relationship or difference exists.

In the Corff et al. (1995, p. 145) study, the hypothesis identified a causal relationship between facilitated tucking and heart rate, oxygen saturation, and sleep state. The results "suggest that facilitated tucking is an effective comfort measure in attenuating preterm neonates' physiologic and behavioral responses to minor painful stimuli. Significantly improved homeostasis and stability were demonstrated within the parameters of heart rate, sleep state changes, crying time, and sleep disruption" but not with oxygen saturation. Thus, the causal relationships between facilitated tucking, heart rate, and sleep state were supported but the causal relationship between facilitated tucking and oxygen saturation was not supported.

SELECTING OBJECTIVES, QUESTIONS, OR HYPOTHESES FOR QUANTITATIVE OR QUALITATIVE RESEARCH

Selecting objectives, questions, or hypotheses for a study is often based on (1) the number and quality of relevant studies conducted on a selected problem (existing knowledge base), (2) the framework of the study, (3) the expertise and preference of the researcher, and (4) the type of study to be conducted (quantitative or qualitative). If minimal or no research has been conducted on a problem, frequently investigators will state objectives or questions because inadequate knowledge is available to formulate hypotheses. The framework for a study indicates whether the intent is to develop or test theory. Objectives and questions are usually stated to guide theory development, and the focus of a hypothesis is to test theory.

Researcher expertise and preference can also influence the selection of objectives, questions, or hypotheses to direct a study. Moody, Wilson, Smyth, Schwartz, Tittle, and Van Cott (1988) analyzed the focus of nursing practice research from 1977–1986 and found that 16% of the studies had research questions and 31% included hypotheses. The number of nursing studies containing hypotheses seems to be increasing, and there appears to be a "trend away from descriptive and fact-finding studies toward efforts to establish relationships between variables and to test hypotheses" (Brown, Tanner, & Padrick, 1984, p. 31). The increased use of hypotheses to direct research could indicate the growth of knowledge in selected problem areas and the increasing sophistication of nurse researchers. However, Brown et al. (1984) noted in the studies they reviewed that only 51% of these studies included explicitly stated hypotheses, and the others had implicit or implied hypotheses. The explicit statement of hypotheses is important to provide clear direction for the conduct of a study and the use of the findings in practice.

The objectives, questions, or hypotheses designated for study frequently indicate a pattern that

Table 8–2
Selecting Objectives, Questions, or Hypotheses for Different Types of Research

Types of Research	Use of Objectives, Questions or Hypotheses
Qualitative research	Objectives, questions, or none
Quantitative research	
Descriptive studies	Objectives, questions, or none
Correlational studies	Objectives, questions, hypotheses, or none
Quasi-experimental studies	Questions or hypotheses
Experimental studies	Hypotheses

the researcher uses in conducting investigations. Problems can be investigated in a variety of ways; some researchers start at the core of a problem and work their way outward. Other investigators study a problem from the outside edge and work to the core (Kaplan, 1964). Each study needs to logically build on the other, as the researcher establishes a pattern for studying a problem area that will affect the quality and quantity of the knowledge generated in that area.

Researchers select objectives, questions, or hypotheses based on the type of study to be conducted. Objectives and questions are typically stated when the intent of the study is to identify or describe characteristics of variables and/or examine relationships among variables. Thus, objectives or questions are sometimes formulated to direct qualitative and selected quantitative (descriptive and correlational) studies (see Table 8–2). However, some experienced researchers can clearly focus and develop their study without objectives or questions. In these studies, a research purpose directs the research process.

In some qualitative research, only a problem and purpose are used to direct the study. The specification of objectives or questions might limit the scope of the study and the methods of data collection and analysis. Discovery is important in qualitative research, and sometimes the "research questions may be unclear, the objectives ambiguous and the final outcome uncertain. . . . Hypotheses and detailed accounts of precise research strategies are not necessary nor desirable in a well constructed qualitative design" (Aamodt, 1983, p. 399).

Researchers often develop hypotheses when the relationships or results of a study can be anticipated or predicted. Hypotheses are typically used in quantitative research to direct correlational, quasi-experimental, and experimental studies.

DEFINING RESEARCH VARIABLES

The research purpose and objectives, questions, and hypotheses identify the variables or concepts to be examined in a study. Variables are qualities, properties, or characteristics of persons, things, or situations that change or vary. In research, variables are characterized by degrees, amounts, and differences. Variables are also concepts of various levels of abstraction that are concisely defined to facilitate their measurement or manipulation within a study (Kaplan, 1964; Moody, 1990).

The concepts examined in research can be concrete and directly measurable in the real world, such as heart rate, hemoglobin, and lung tidal volume. These concrete concepts are usually referred to as variables in a study. Other concepts, such as anxiety, psychosocial needs, and pain are more abstract and are indirectly observable in the real world (Fawcett & Downs, 1986). Thus, the properties of these concepts are inferred from a combination of measurements. For example, the properties of anxiety are inferred by combining information obtained from observing signs and symptoms of anxiety (frequent movement and verbalization of anxiety), examining completed questionnaires or scales (A-state and trait anxiety scales), and measuring physiological responses (galvanic skin response). The concept of anxiety might be represented by the variables "reported anxiety" or "perceived level of anxiety."

In many qualitative studies and in some quantitative studies (descriptive and correlational), the focus of the study is abstract concepts, such as grieving, caring, and health promotion. Researchers identify the elements of the study as concepts, not variables. For example, Alligood (1991) identified the concepts of her study as creativity, actualization, and empathy. Thus, the elements examined in a study can range from concrete to abstract and can be identified as variables or concepts.

TYPES OF VARIABLES

Variables have been classified into a variety of types to explain their use in research. Some variables are manipulated; others are controlled. Some variables are identified but not measured; others are measured with refined measurement devices. The types of variables presented in this section include independent, dependent, research, extraneous, and demographic.

Independent and Dependent Variables

The relationship between independent and dependent variables is the basis for formulating hypotheses for correlational, quasi-experimental, and experimental studies. An *independent variable* is a stimulus or activity that is manipulated or varied by the researcher to create an effect on the dependent variable. The independent variable is also called a treatment or experimental variable. A *dependent variable* is the response, behavior, or outcome that the researcher wants to predict or explain. Changes in the dependent variable are presumed to be caused by the independent variable. The dependent variable can also be called an effect variable or a criterion measure (Kerlinger, 1986).

Leske (1995) hypothesized that those family members of surgical patients who received intraoperative progress reports have less anxiety than families who did not receive such an intervention or attention from a supportive person. The independent variable was intraoperative progress reports that were provided to the experimental group; the comparison group received standard care; and a third group received attention from a supportive person. The dependent variable was anxiety that was measured by state-anxiety scores, mean arterial pressure (MAP) levels, and heart rate.

Research Variables or Concepts

Qualitative studies and some quantitative (descriptive and correlational) studies involve the investigation of research variables or concepts. Research variables or concepts are the qualities, properties, or characteristics identified in the research purpose and objectives or questions that are observed or measured in a study. Research variables (or concepts) are used when the intent of the study is to observe or measure variables as they exist in a natural setting without the implementation of a treatment. Thus, no independent variables are manipulated and no cause-and-effect relationships are examined.

Allan (1989, p. 659) conducted an ethnographic study of women who successfully managed their weight. The study included the following questions: "(1) What methods for weight management are used by women who successfully manage their weight? and (2) What factors influence the selection of particular methods?" The research concepts studied were "methods for weight management" and "factors influencing the selection of particular methods."

Olson (1995) investigated the relationships between a nurse's empathy and selected patient outcomes. This study provided an increased understanding of the concepts of nurse empathy and patient outcomes by examining the research variables: nurse-expressed empathy, patient-perceived empathy, and patient distress. These variables are conceptually and operationally defined later in this chapter.

Extraneous Variables

Extraneous variables exist in all studies and can affect the measurement of study variables and the relationships among these variables. Extraneous variables are of primary concern in quantitative

studies, since they can interfere with obtaining a clear understanding of the relational or causal dynamics within these studies. Extraneous variables are classified as recognized or unrecognized and controlled or uncontrolled. Some extraneous variables are not recognized until the study is in progress or is completed but their presence influences the study outcome. Researchers attempt to recognize and control as many extraneous variables as possible in quasi-experimental and experimental studies and specific designs have been developed to control the influence of these variables (see Chapter 11). Corff et al. (1995) controlled some of the extraneous variables in their study by the use of inclusion and exclusion criteria for sample selection.

"Inclusion criteria included neonates of 25–35 weeks gestational age at birth, appropriate for gestational age, 36 weeks or less postconceptual age, and less than 22 days postnatal age at time of testing. Exclusion criteria included neonates with chromosomal or genetic anomalies; significant central nervous system abnormalities (congenital or acquired, including grade II or greater intraventricular hemorrhage); Apgar scores of less than 5 at 5 minutes; congenital heart disease; dysmorphic syndrome; and infants receiving paralytic, analgesic, or sedating medications." (p. 144) ∎

The authors also disqualified six infants to control extraneous variables that might have influenced the implementation of the treatment or measurement of the dependent variables. The infants were disqualified "because of changes in their physiologic or respiratory status ($n = 3$), infiltrated intravenous site as a source of additional pain ($n = 1$), or transfer out of NICU ($n = 2$) between the first and second observations" (Corff et al., 1995, p. 144).

The extraneous variables that are not recognized until the study is in process or are recognized before the study is initiated but cannot be controlled are referred to as *confounding vari-*

ables. Sometimes these variables can be measured during the study and controlled statistically during analysis. However, in other cases, measurement of the confounding variable is not possible and thus hinders the interpretation of findings. As control decreases in quasi-experimental and experimental studies, the potential influence of confounding variables increases. In a study of the impact of social support on adherence to a treatment protocol, variables such as stage of illness, knowledge of treatment, attitudes of health care professionals, home environment, and the value placed on health by the patient could be confounding variables.

Environmental variables are a type of extraneous variable that make up the setting where the study is conducted. Examples of these variables include climate, family, health care system, and governmental organizations. If a researcher is studying humans in an uncontrolled or natural setting, it is impossible and undesirable to control all the extraneous variables. In qualitative and some quantitative (descriptive and correlational) studies, little or no attempt is made to control environmental variables. The intent is to study subjects in their natural environment without controlling or altering that setting. The environmental variables in quasi-experimental and experimental research can be controlled by using a laboratory setting or a specially constructed research unit in a hospital.

Demographic Variables

Demographic variables are characteristics or attributes of the subject that are collected to describe the sample. Some common demographic variables are age, educational level, gender, income, job classification, length of hospital stay, medical diagnosis, and race. Demographic variables are selected by the researcher based on experience and previous research and subjects are asked to provide this information on a demographic or information sheet. When a study is completed, the demographic information is analyzed to provide a picture of the sample or the *sample characteristics.* Nokes, Wheeler, and Kendrew (1994) administered a tool to assess the perception of the severity of human immunodeficiency virus (HIV) related symptoms and general well-being in a sam-

ple of 156 volunteer subjects. The subjects included three groups: 53 healthy college students, 60 patients who are HIV positive, and 43 patients who have AIDS. The characteristics of these three groups in this study are presented in Table 8–3.

Sample characteristics are also presented in narrative form in the research report. For example, Allan (1989), who studied women who successfully manage their weight, described her sample as follows.

"The typical demographic characteristics reflected in the study group were: well-educated, young, white collar, married, and Protestant. The mean age was 30 years with a range of 19–52. Forty-eight percent were married, 43% were single, and 10% were divorced. Only 5 (24%) women had a full-term pregnancy. All informants were high school graduates and 57% had earned a college degree. All but 2 of the 21 women worked. They were employed primarily in the private sector in clerical and sales jobs and had individual annual incomes ranging from $10,500 to $60,000. The two subgroups, working class (9 women) and middle class (12 women), were not significantly different on any non-class-related characteristics except marital status; more middle-class women were married." (p. 660) ■

OPERATIONALIZING VARIABLES OR CONCEPTS

Operationalizing a variable or concept involves developing conceptual and operational definitions. A *conceptual definition* provides the theoretical meaning of a concept or variable (Fawcett & Downs, 1986) and is derived from a theorist's definition of that concept or is developed through concept analysis. The study framework, which includes concepts and their definitions, provides a basis for conceptually defining the variables. Hargreaves and Lander (1989) studied the "effects of transcutaneous electrical nerve simulation (TENS) on incisional pain" (p. 159). The analgesic effects

Table 8–3
Frequencies of Selected Demographic Variables

	Healthy (n = 53)	HIV+ (n = 60)	AIDS (n = 43)
AGE			
19–29	29	1	2
30–39	16	19	15
40–49	5	27	20
50–59	2	4	2
60+	1	9	4
	(range 19–60)	(range 28–67)	(range 27–68)
SEX			
Male	7	59	43
Female	46	1	
ETHNICITY			
Black	12(23%)	27(45%)	12(30%)
White	25(47%)	13(22%)	14(33%)
Hispanic	7(13%)	20(33%)	17(40%)
Other	4(8%)	0	0
INCOME			
On assistance	0	1(2%)	25(58%)
$10,–20,000	18(34%)	14(23%)	8(19%)
$21,–30,000	5(9%)	20(33%)	4(9%)
$31,–50,000	16(30%)	11(18%)	3(7%)
Over $50,000	4(8%)	6(10%)	1(2%)
No answer	10(19%)	8(13%)	2(5%)
EMPLOYMENT STATUS			
Not working	16(30%)	37(62%)	29(67%)
Work 10–20[hrs/wk]	14(26%)	3(5%)	4(9%)
Work 20–30[hrs/wk]	7(13%)	3(5%)	2(4%)
Work 40[hrs/wk]	11(21%)	11(18%)	7(16%)
Over 40[hrs/wk]	4(8%)	4(7%)	1(2%)
No answer	1(2%)	2(3%)	0
RISK BEHAVIORS ASSOCIATED WITH HIV INFECTION			
Male/male sex	3(6%)	26(43%)	20(47%)
Injection drugs	0	22(37%)	16(37%)
Male/male sex + IDU	0	2(3%)	1(2%)
Sex partner (IDU)	1(2%)	3(5%)	1(2%)
Blood product	0	2(3%)	1(2%)
Other, missing	49(92%)	5(8%)	4(9%)

(From Nokes, K. M., Wheeler, K., & Kendrew, J. [1994]. Development of an HIV assessment tool. *Image: Journal of Nursing Scholarship, 26*[2], p. 135, with permission.)

of the TENS (independent variable) was conceptually defined using gate-control theory.

Conceptual Definition of TENS

"TENS is thought to activate the large diameter, myelinated A-beta fibers which have a low threshold for electrical stimulation. The increased activity in these fibers would serve to decrease the transmission of painful stimuli through the small diameter A-delta and C fibers." (Melzack & Wall, 1984, p. 159) ∎

This conceptual definition links the TENS variable to the concepts and relationships in the gate-control theory developed by Melzack and Wall (1984). This conceptual definition provides a basis for formulating an operational definition.

An *operational definition* is derived from a set of procedures or progressive acts that a researcher performs to receive sensory impressions (such as sounds or visual or tactile impressions) that indicate the existence or degree of existence of a variable (Reynolds, 1971). Operational definitions need to be independent of time and setting, so that variables can be investigated at different times and in different settings using the same operational definitions. An operational definition is developed so that a variable can be measured or manipulated in a concrete situation, and the knowledge gained from studying the variable will increase the understanding of the theoretical concept that variable represents. Hargreaves and Lander (1989) operationalized the TENS as follows.

Operational Definition of TENS

"Piece of equipment with a portable GRASS SD9 stimulator (Grass Instrument Co., Quincy, MA) and two pre-jelled, sterile surface electrodes 3 cm in diameter (Myo-Trode II, No. 410)." (p. 160) ∎

The variables in quasi-experimental and experimental research are narrow and specific in focus and are capable of being quantified (converted to numbers) or manipulated using specified steps. In addition, the variables are objectively defined to decrease researcher bias. The concepts or variables in descriptive and correlational studies are usually more abstract and broadly defined than the variables in quasi-experimental studies.

Olson (1995) conducted a correlational study to examine the relationships among three research variables, nurse-expressed empathy, patient-perceived empathy, and patient distress. The author developed three hypotheses that indicated there is: (a) . . . negative relationships between nurse-expressed empathy and measures of patient distress, (b) . . . negative relationships between patient-perceived empathy and measures of patient distress, and (c) . . . positive relationships between measures of nurse-expressed empathy and patient-perceived empathy" (Olson, 1995, p. 318). These three variables were conceptually and operationally defined as indicated.

Variable—Nurse-expressed Empathy

Conceptual Definition. "Understanding what a patient is saying and feeling, then communicating this understanding verbally to the patient." (p. 318)

Operational Definition. Nurse-expressed empathy was measured using two instruments, Behavioral Test of Interpersonal Skills (BTIS) and Staff-Patient Interaction Response Scale (SPIRS).

Variable—Patient-perceived Empathy

Conceptual Definition. "The patient's feeling of being understood and accepted by the nurse." (p. 318)

Operational Definition. Patient-perceived empathy was measured with one instrument, Barrett-Lennard Relationship Inventory (BLRI).

Variable—Patient Distress

Conceptual Definition. "A negative emotional state." (p. 318)

Operational Definition. Patient distress was measured with two instruments, Profile of Mood States Inventory (POMS) and Multiple Affect Adjective Check List (MAACL). ∎

Some researchers believe that the concepts in qualitative studies do not require operational definitions because sensitizing or experiencing the real situation rather than operationalizing the concepts is most important (Benoliel, 1984). Operational definitions are thought to limit the focus of the investigation so that a phenomenon such as pain or a characteristic of a culture such as the health practices is not completely experienced or understood from the investigation. In other qualitative studies, the phenomena being examined are not named until the data analysis step. Thus, some concepts may not be identified or defined until late in the study.

However, some qualitative researchers develop broad definitions of their concepts to direct their investigations. Norman (1989) conducted a qualitative study of the factors that influenced the wartime experiences of military nurses in the Vietnam war, 1965–1973. Norman (1989) "defined *factors that influenced the wartime experience* as the clinical jobs and off-duty experiences that were prevalent for the nurses in Vietnam and the potential for these shared occurrences to sway the nurses' wartime experience" (p. 219) (conceptual definition). "In this study, 35 open- and closed-ended questions in an interview schedule measured the wartime experience" (Norman, 1989, pp. 219–220) (operational definition).

◼ SUMMARY

Research objectives, questions, or hypotheses are formulated to bridge the gap between the more abstractly stated research problem and purpose, and the detailed design and plan for data collection and analysis. Research objectives are clear, concise, declarative statements that are expressed in the present tense. For clarity, an objective usually focuses on one or two variables (or concepts) and indicates whether the variables are to be identified or described. Sometimes, the foci of objectives include identifying relationships among variables and determining differences between two groups regarding selected variables.

A research question is a concise, interrogative statement that is worded in the present tense and includes one or more variables (or concepts). The foci of questions are description of variables, examination of relationships among variables, and determination of differences between two or more groups regarding selected variables.

A hypothesis is the formal statement of the expected relationship(s) between two or more variables in a specified population. The hypothesis translates the research problem and purpose into a clear explanation or prediction of the expected results or outcomes of the study. Hypotheses are generated by observing phenomena or problems in the real world, analyzing theory, and reviewing the literature. Hypotheses can be described using four categories: (1) associative versus causal, (2) simple versus complex, (3) nondirectional versus directional, and (4) null versus research. A hy-

pothesis is developed using inductive and deductive thinking and is expressed as a declarative statement in the present tense. Testable hypotheses contain variables that are measurable or manipulatable and these hypotheses are evaluated using statistical analyses.

Selecting objectives, questions, or hypotheses for a study is based on (1) the number and quality of relevant studies conducted on a selected problem (existing knowledge base), (2) the framework of the study, (3) the expertise and preference of the researcher, and (4) the type of study to be conducted (quantitative or qualitative). The research purpose and objectives, questions, and hypotheses identify the variables to be examined in a study. Variables are concepts of various levels of abstraction that are measured, manipulated, or controlled in a study. The concepts examined in research can be concrete and directly measurable in the real world, such as heart rate, hemoglobin, and lung tidal volume. These concrete concepts are usually referred to as variables in a study. Other concepts, such as anxiety, psychosocial needs, and pain, are more abstract and are indirectly observable in the world.

Variables are qualities, properties, and/or characteristics of persons, things, or situations that change or vary. The types of variables discussed in this chapter include independent, dependent, research, extraneous, and demographic. An independent variable is a stimulus or activity that is manipulated or varied by the researcher to create an effect on the dependent variable. A dependent variable is the response,

continued

◼

continued

behavior, or outcome that the researcher wants to predict or explain. Research variables or concepts are the qualities, properties, or characteristics that are observed or measured in a study. Extraneous variables exist in all studies and can affect the measurement of study variables and the relationships among these variables. These variables are of primary concern in quantitative studies, since they can interfere with obtaining a clear understanding of the relational or causal dynamics within these studies. Environmental variables are a type of extraneous variable that makes up the setting where the study is conducted. Demographic variables are characteristics or attributes of the subjects that are collected to describe the sample. These variables are collected using a demographic or information sheet and the data are analyzed to provide a picture of the sample or sample characteristics.

The variables or concepts in a study require conceptual and operational definitions. A conceptual definition provides the theoretical meaning of a concept or variable and is derived from a theorist's definition of the concept or is developed through concept analysis. The study framework, which includes concepts and their definitions, provides a basis for conceptually defining the variables. The conceptual definition provides a basis for formulating an operational definition. An operational definition is derived from a set of procedures or progressive acts that a researcher performs to receive sensory impressions that indicate the existence or degree of existence of a variable. Operational definitions need to be independent of time and setting, so that variables can be investigated at different times and in different settings using the same definitions. Operational definitions in quasi-experimental and experimental studies are specific and precisely developed. In qualitative studies, the definitions of concepts are fairly abstract and broad, so the scope of the investigation is not limited.

References

Aamodt, A. M. (1983). Problems in doing nursing research: Developing a criteria for evaluating qualitative research. *Western Journal of Nursing Research, 5*(4), 398–402.

Abraham, S. (1983). Obese and overweight adults in the United States. *Vital Health Statistics* (DHHS Pub. No. 83-1980). Hyattsville, MD: U.S. Public Health Service, National Center for Health Statistics.

Allan, J. D. (1989). Women who successfully manage their weight. *Western Journal of Nursing Research, 11*(6), 657–675.

Alligood, M. R. (1991). Testing Rogers's theory of accelerating change: The relationships among creativity, actualization, and empathy in persons 18 to 92 years of age. *Western Journal of Nursing Research, 13*(1), 84–96.

Armstrong, R. L. (1981). Hypothesis formulation. In S. D. Krampitz & N. Pavlovich (Eds.), *Readings for nursing research* (pp. 29–39). St. Louis: Mosby.

Benoliel, Q. (1984). Advancing nursing science: Qualitative approaches. *Western Journal of Nursing Research, 6*(3), 1–8.

Beveridge, W. B. (1950). *The art of scientific investigation.* New York: Vintage Books.

Brown, J. S., Tanner, C. A., & Padrick, K. P. (1984). Nursing's search for scientific knowledge. *Nursing Research, 33*(1), 26–32.

Bull, M. J. (1990). Factors influencing family caregiver burden and health. *Western Journal of Nursing Research, 12*(6), 758–776.

Chinn, P. L., & Kramer, M. K. (1995). *Theory and nursing: A systematic approach* (4th ed.). St. Louis: Mosby.

Corff, K. E., Seideman, R., Venkataraman, P. S., Lutes, L., & Yates, B. (1995). Facilitated tucking: A nonpharmacologic comfort measure for pain in preterm neonates. *Journal of Obstetric Gynecologic & Neonatal Nursing, 24*(2), 143–147.

Deiriggi, P. M. (1990). Effects of waterbed flotation on indicators of energy expenditure in preterm infants. *Nursing Research, 39*(3), 140–146.

Fagerhaugh, S. Y., & Strauss, A. (1977). *Politics of pain management.* Menlo Park, CA: Addison-Wesley.

Fahs, P. S. S., & Kinney, M. R. (1991). The abdomen, thigh, and arm as sites for subcutaneous sodium heparin injections. *Nursing Research, 40*(4), 204–207.

Fawcett, J., & Downs, F. S. (1986). *The relationship of theory and research.* Norwalk, CT: Appleton-Century-Crofts.

Georges, J. M., & Heitkemper, M. M. (1994). Dietary fiber and distressing gastrointestinal symptoms in midlife women. *Nursing Research, 43*(6), 357–361.

Gross, D., Conrad, B., Fogg, L., Willis, L., & Garvey, C. (1995). A longitudinal study of maternal depression and preschool children's mental health. *Nursing Research, 44*(2), 96–101.

Gross, D., Fogg, L., & Tucker, S. (1995). The efficacy of parent training for promoting positive parent-toddler relationships. *Research in Nursing & Health, 18*(6), 489–499.

Hargreaves, A., & Lander, J. (1989). Use of transcutaneous electrical nerve stimulation for postoperative pain. *Nursing Research, 38*(3), 159–161.

Jadack, R. A., Hyde, J. S., & Keller, M. L. (1995). Gender and knowledge about HIV, risky sexual behavior, and safer sex practices. *Research in Nursing & Health, 18*(4), 313–324.

Jirovec, M. M., & Kasno, J. (1990). Self-care agency as a function of patient-environmental factors among nursing home residents. *Research in Nursing & Health, 13*(5), 303–309.

Kaplan, A. (1964). *The conduct of inquiry: Methodology for behavioral science.* New York: Harper & Row.

Kemp, M. G., Keithley, J. K., Smith, D. W., & Morreale, B. (1990). Factors that contribute to pressure sores in surgical patients. *Research in Nursing & Health, 13*(5), 293–301.

Kerlinger, F. N. (1973). *Foundations of behavioral research* (2nd ed.). New York: Holt, Rinehart and Winston.

Kerlinger, F. N. (1986). *Foundations of behavioral research* (3rd ed.). New York: Holt, Rinehart and Winston.

Koniak, D. (1985). Autotutorial and lecture-demonstration instruction: A comparative analysis of the effects upon students' learning of a developmental assessment skill. *Western Journal of Nursing Research, 7*(1), 80–100.

Leske, J. S. (1995). Effects of intraoperative progress reports on anxiety levels of surgical patients' family members. *Applied Nursing Research, 8*(4), 169–173.

McCaffery, M., & Beebe, A. (1989). *Pain: Clinical manual for nursing practice.* St. Louis: Mosby.

Melzack, R., & Wall, P. D. (1984). *The challenge of pain.* Suffolk, Great Britain: Chaucer Press.

Moody, L. E. (1990). *Advancing nursing science through research:* Vol. 1. Newbury Park, CA: Sage.

Moody, L. E., Wilson, M. E., Smyth, K., Schwartz, R., Tittle, M., & Van Cott, M. L. (1988). Analysis of a decade of nursing practice research: 1977–1986. *Nursing Research, 37*(6), 374–379.

Nokes, K. M., Wheeler, K., & Kendrew, J. (1994). Development of an HIV assessment tool. *Image: Journal of Nursing Scholarship, 26*(2), 133–138.

Norman, E. M. (1989). The wartime experience of military nurses in Vietnam, 1965–1973. *Western Journal of Nursing Research, 11*(2), 219–233.

Orem, D. E. (1995). *Nursing: Concepts of practice* (5th ed.). New York: McGraw-Hill.

Olson, J. K. (1995). Relationships between nurse-expressed empathy, patient-perceived empathy and patient distress. *Image: Journal of Nursing Scholarship, 27*(4), 317–322.

Poroch, D. (1995). The effect of preparatory patient education on the anxiety and satisfaction of cancer patients receiving radiation therapy. *Cancer Nursing, 18*(3), 206–214.

Reynolds, P. D. (1971). *A primer in theory construction.* Indianapolis: Bobbs-Merrill.

Rogers, M. E. (1986). Science of unitary human beings. In V. Malinski (Ed.), *Exploration on Martha Rogers' science of unitary human-beings* (pp. 3–8). Norwalk, CT: Appleton-Century-Crofts.

Savedra, M. C., Tesler, M. D., Holzemer, W. L., & Brokaw, P. (1995). A strategy to assess the temporal dimension of pain in children and adolescents. *Nursing Research, 44*(5), 272–276.

Schachter, S. (1982). Recidivism and self-cure of smoking and obesity. *American Psychologist, 37*(4), 436–444.

Schlotfeldt, R. M. (1975). The need for a conceptual framework. In P. Verhonick (Ed.), *Nursing research* (pp. 3–23). Boston: Little Brown.

Weiss, A. (1977). Characteristics of successful weight reducers: A brief review of predictor variables. *Addictive Behaviors, 2*(2), 193–201.

Zauszniewski, J. A. (1994). Health-seeking resources and adaptive functioning in depressed and nondepressed adults. *Archives of Psychiatric Nursing, 8*(3), 159–168.

Zauszniewski, J. A. (1995). Health-seeking resources in depressed outpatients. *Archives of Psychiatric Nursing, 9*(4), 179–187.

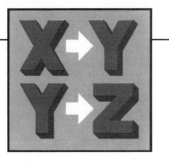

9

Ethics and Research

The conduct of nursing research requires not only expertise and diligence but also honesty and integrity. Conducting research ethically starts with the identification of the study topic and continues through the publication of the study. Ethical codes and regulations provide guidelines for (1) the selection of the study purpose, design, methods of measurement, and subjects; (2) the collection and analysis of data; (3) the interpretation of results; and (4) the publication of the study. One would like to believe that unethical research, such as the Nazi experiments of World War II, is a thing of the past. However, this is not the case since published studies continue to include evidence that subjects' rights were violated (Beecher, 1966).

An ethical problem that escalated in the 1980s and continues today is scientific fraud or misconduct (Garfield & Welljams-Dorof, 1990; Hawley & Jeffers, 1992; Henderson, 1990). Scientific misconduct involves such practices as fabrication, falsification, or forging of data; dishonest manipulation of the design or methods; and plagiarism (Larson, 1989). Scientific misconduct has occurred during the conduct, reporting, and publication of research, with "one half of the top 50 research institutions in the United States having had fraud investigations" (Chop & Silva, 1991, p. 166). Medicine is struggling with this problem (Friedman, 1990); but many disciplines, including nursing, are concerned about the quality of their research-generated knowledge base (Wocial, 1995).

Ethical research is essential to generate knowledge, but what does conducting research ethically involve? This is a question that has been debated without resolution for many years by researchers, politicians, philosophers, lawyers, and even research subjects. The debate about ethics and re-

search continues, probably because of the complexity of human rights issues, the abstractness of the ethical codes and regulations governing research, and the variety of interpretations of these codes and regulations.

Even though the phenomenon of conducting research ethically defies precise delineation, there are certain historical events, ethical codes, and regulations that are presented in this chapter to provide guidance for nurse researchers. This chapter also includes the following ethical actions essential in research: (1) protecting the rights of human subjects, (2) balancing benefits and risks in a study, (3) obtaining informed consent, and (4) submitting a research proposal for institutional review. This chapter concludes with a discussion of two timely ethical issues in research, scientific misconduct and the use of animals as research subjects.

HISTORICAL EVENTS AFFECTING THE DEVELOPMENT OF ETHICAL CODES AND REGULATIONS

Since the 1940s, the ethical conduct of researchers has received increasing attention because of the mistreatment of human subjects. Four experimental projects have been highly publicized for their unethical treatment of human subjects: (1) the Nazi medical experiments, (2) the Tuskegee syphilis study, (3) the Willowbrook study, and (4) the Jewish Chronic Disease Hospital study. Although these were biomedical studies and the primary investigators were physicians, there is evidence that nurses were aware of the research, identified potential research subjects, delivered treatments to the subjects, and/or served as data collectors in these studies. These unethical studies demonstrate the importance of ethical conduct when reviewing, participating in, and conducting nursing or biomedical research. These studies also influenced the formulation of ethical codes and regulations to direct the conduct of research.

NAZI MEDICAL EXPERIMENTS

From 1933 to 1945, atrocious, unethical activities were implemented by the Third Reich in Europe (Steinfels & Levine, 1976). The programs of the Nazi regime included sterilization, euthanasia, and numerous medical experiments to produce a population of racially pure Germans or Aryans who were destined to rule the world. The Nazis encouraged population growth in the Aryans ("good Nazis") and sterilized those regarded as racial enemies, such as the Jews. They also practiced what they called euthanasia, which involved killing various groups of people who they considered racially impure, such as the insane, deformed, or senile. In addition, numerous medical experiments were conducted on prisoners of war and racially "valueless" persons, who had been confined to the concentration camps.

The medical experiments involved exposing subjects to high altitudes, freezing temperatures, malaria, poisons, spotted fever (typhus), and untested drugs and operations, usually without any form of anesthesia (Steinfels & Levine, 1976). For example, in the hypothermia studies, subjects were immersed in bath temperatures ranging from 2 to 12°C. The researchers noted that "immersion in water 5°C is tolerated by clothed men for 40 to 60 minutes, whereas raising the water temperature to 15°C increases the period of tolerance to four to five hours" (Berger, 1990, p. 1436). These medical experiments were conducted not only to generate knowledge about human beings but also to destroy certain groups of people. Extensive examination of the records from some of these studies indicated they were poorly conceived and conducted. Thus, little if any useful scientific knowledge was generated by these studies.

The Nazi experiments violated numerous rights of human research subjects. The selection of subjects for these studies was racially based, demonstrating an unfair selection process. The subjects also had no opportunity to refuse participation; they were prisoners who were coerced or forced to participate. As a result of these experiments, subjects were frequently killed or sustained permanent physical, mental, and social damage (Levine, 1986; Steinfels & Levine, 1976). These studies were not conducted by a few isolated scientists and doctors; they were "the product of coordinated policy-making and planning at high governmental, military, and Nazi Party levels, conducted as an integral part of the total war effort" (Nuremberg Code, 1986, p. 425).

NUREMBERG CODE

Those involved in the Nazi experiments were brought to trial before the Nuremberg Tribunals, who publicized these unethical activities. The mistreatment of human subjects in these studies led to the development of the *Nuremberg Code* in 1949. This ethical code of conduct contains rules, some general, others specific, that were developed to guide investigators in conducting research ethically. The code includes guidelines for voluntary consent; withdrawal of subjects from studies; protection of subjects from physical and mental suffering, injury, disability, and death; and the balance of benefits and risks in a study (see Table 9–1). This code was formulated mainly to direct the conduct of biomedical research; however, the rules in this code are essential to the conduct of research in other sciences, such as nursing, psychology, and sociology.

DECLARATION OF HELSINKI

The Nuremberg Code provided the basis for the development of the Declaration of Helsinki, which

Table 9–1
The Nuremberg Code

1. The voluntary consent of the human subject is absolutely essential.
2. The experiment should be such as to yield fruitful results for the good of society, unprocurable by other methods or means of study, and not random and unnecessary in nature.
3. The experiment should be so designed and based on the results of animal experimentation and a knowledge of the natural history of the disease or other problem under study that the anticipated results will justify the performance of the experiment.
4. The experiment should be so conducted as to avoid all unnecessary physical and mental suffering and injury.
5. No experiment should be conducted where there is an a priori reason to believe that death or disabling injury will occur, except, perhaps, in those experiments where the experimental physicians also serve as subjects.
6. The degree of risk to be taken should never exceed that determined by the humanitarian importance of the problem to be solved by the experiment.
7. Proper preparations should be made and adequate facilities provided to protect the experimental subject against even remote possibilities of injury, disability, or death.
8. The experiment should be conducted only by scientifically qualified persons. The highest degree of skill and care should be required through all stages of the experiment of those who conduct or engage in the experiment.
9. During the course of the experiment the human subject should be at liberty to bring the experiment to an end if he has reached the physical or mental state where continuation of the experiment seems to him to be impossible.
10. During the course of the experiment the scientist in charge must be prepared to terminate the experiment at any stage, if he has probable cause to believe, in the exercise of the good faith, superior skill, and careful judgment required of him that a continuation of the experiment is likely to result in injury, disability, or death to the experimental subject.

(From The Nuremberg Code, 1949, pp. 285–286.)

was adopted in 1964 and revised in 1975 by the World Medical Assembly (Declaration of Helsinki, 1986). The Declaration of Helsinki differentiated therapeutic research from nontherapeutic research. *Therapeutic research* provides the patient an opportunity to receive an experimental treatment that might have beneficial results. *Nontherapeutic research* is conducted to generate knowledge for a discipline, and the results from the study might benefit future patients but will probably not benefit those acting as research subjects (Purtilo & Cassel, 1981). The Declaration of Helsinki provided that (1) greater care should be exercised to protect subjects from harm in nontherapeutic research; (2) strong, independent justification is required for exposing a healthy volunteer to substantial risk of harm just to gain new scientific information; and (3) the investigator must protect the life and health of the research subject (Oddi & Cassidy, 1990). The Declaration of Helsinki was adopted by most institutions in which clinical research is conducted. However, neither this document nor the Nuremberg Code have prevented some investigators from conducting unethical research (Beecher, 1966).

TUSKEGEE SYPHILIS STUDY

In 1932, the United States Public Health Service (USPHS) initiated a study of syphilis in black men in the small, rural town of Tuskegee, Alabama (Brandt, 1978; Rothman, 1982). The study, which continued for 40 years, was conducted to determine the natural course of syphilis in the adult black man. The research subjects were black men who were organized into two groups: one group included 400 men who had untreated syphilis; and the second group included 200 men without syphilis, who served as a control group. Many of the subjects who consented to participate in the study were not informed about the purpose and procedures of the research. Some individuals were unaware that they were subjects in a study. By 1936, it was apparent that the men with syphilis developed more complications than the control group. Ten years later the death rate of those with syphilis was twice as high as it was for the control group. The subjects were examined periodically but did not receive treatment for syphilis, even when penicillin was determined to be an effective treatment for the disease in the 1940s (Levine, 1986). Information about an effective treatment for syphilis was withheld from the subjects, and deliberate steps were taken to keep the subjects from receiving treatment (Brandt, 1978).

Published reports of the Tuskegee syphilis

study first started appearing in 1936, and additional papers were published every four to six years. No effort was made to stop the study; in fact, in 1969, the Center for Disease Control decided that the study should continue. Numerous individuals were involved in conducting this study, including "three generations of doctors serving in the venereal disease division of the USPHS, numerous officials at the Tuskegee Institute and its affiliated hospital, hundreds of doctors in the Macon County and Alabama medical societies, and numerous foundation officials at the Rosenwald Fund and the Milbank Memorial Fund" (Rothman, 1982, p. 5). In 1972, an account of the study in the *Washington Star* sparked public outrage. Only then did the Department of Health, Education, and Welfare stop the study. The study was investigated and found to be ethically unjustified, but the racial implications of the study were never addressed (Brandt, 1978). There are still many unanswered questions related to this study, such as: Where were the checks and balances in the government and health care systems that should have stopped this unethical study from continuing for 40 years? Why was an effective treatment withheld from the subjects for several years? Why was public outrage the only effective means for halting the study?

WILLOWBROOK STUDY

From the mid-1950s to the early 1970s, research on hepatitis was conducted by Dr. Saul Krugman at Willowbrook, an institution for the mentally retarded (Rothman, 1982). The subjects were all children who were "deliberately infected with the hepatitis virus; early subjects were fed extracts of stool from infected individuals and later subjects received injections of more purified virus preparations" (Levine, 1986, p. 70). During the 20-year study, Willowbrook closed its doors to new inmates because of overcrowded conditions. However, the research ward continued to admit new inmates. Parents were forced to give permission for their child to be in the study in

order to gain their child's admission to the institution.

From the late 1950s to early 1970s, Krugman's research team published several articles describing the study protocol and findings. In 1966, the Willowbrook study was cited by Beecher as an example of unethical research in the *New England Journal of Medicine*. The investigators defended injecting the children with the virus because they believed most of them would acquire the infection upon admission to the institution. They also stressed the benefits the subjects received, which were a cleaner environment, better supervision, and a higher nurse/patient ratio on the research ward (Rothman, 1982). Despite the controversy, this unethical study continued until the early 1970s.

JEWISH CHRONIC DISEASE HOSPITAL STUDY

Another highly publicized example of unethical research was a study conducted at the Jewish Chronic Disease Hospital in the 1960s. The purpose of this study was to determine the patients' rejection responses to live cancer cells. Twenty-two patients were injected with a suspension containing live cancer cells that had been generated from human cancer tissue (Hershey & Miller, 1976; Levine, 1986).

The rights of these patients were not protected, because they were not informed that they were taking part in research and that the injections they received were live cancer cells. In addition, the study was never presented to the research committee of the Jewish Chronic Disease Hospital for review; and the physicians caring for the patients were unaware that the study was being conducted. The physician directing the research was an employee of the Sloan-Kettering Institute for Cancer Research, and there was no indication that this institution had conducted a review of the research project (Hershey & Miller, 1976). The research project was conducted without the informed consent of the subjects and without institutional review and had the potential to cause the human subjects injury, disability, or even death.

OTHER UNETHICAL STUDIES

In 1966, Henry Beecher published a classic article that included 22 of 50 examples of unethical or questionably ethical studies that he had identified in the published literature. The examples, which included the Willowbrook and Jewish Chronic Disease Hospital studies, indicated a variety of ethical problems that were relatively widespread. Consent was mentioned in only two of the 50 studies and many of the investigators had unnecessarily risked the health and lives of their subjects. Beecher (1966, p. 1356) believed that many of the abuses in the research were due to "thoughtlessness and carelessness, not a willful disregard of patients' rights." These studies reinforce the importance of conscientious institutional review and ethical conduct by researchers.

DEPARTMENT OF HEALTH, EDUCATION, AND WELFARE (DHEW) REGULATIONS

The continued conduct of harmful, unethical research made additional controls necessary. In 1973, the DHEW published its first set of regulations on the protection of human subjects. By May 1974, clinical researchers were presented with very stiff regulations for research involving humans. The DHEW also published additional regulations to protect persons having limited capacities to consent, such as the ill, mentally impaired, and dying (Levine, 1986).

In the 1970s, researchers went from a few vague regulations to almost overwhelming guidelines that controlled the research they conducted. All research involving human subjects had to undergo full institutional review. Nursing studies, which frequently involved minimal risks to human subjects, required complete review. Institutional review increased the protection of human subjects; but reviewing all studies, without regard for the

degree of risk involved, overwhelmed the review process and greatly increased the time required for a study to be approved.

NATIONAL COMMISSION FOR THE PROTECTION OF HUMAN SUBJECTS OF BIOMEDICAL AND BEHAVIORAL RESEARCH

Since the issue of protecting human subjects in research was far from resolved by the DHEW regulations, the National Commission for the Protection of Human Subjects of Biomedical and Behavioral Research (1978) was formed. This commission was established by the National Research Act (Public Law 93–348) passed in 1974. The goals of the commission were to identify the basic ethical principles that should underlie the conduct of biomedical and behavioral research involving human subjects and to develop guidelines based on these principles.

The commission identified three ethical principles as relevant to the conduct of research involving human subjects: the principles of respect for persons, beneficence, and justice. The *principle of respect for persons* indicates that persons have the right to self-determination and the freedom to participate or not participate in research. The *principle of beneficence* encourages the researcher to do good and "above all, do no harm." The *principle of justice* states that human subjects should be treated fairly. The commission developed ethical research guidelines based on these three principles and made recommendations to the Department of Health and Human Services (DHHS). The commission summarized its findings in the Belmont Report and was dissolved in 1978 (National Commission for the Protection of Human Subjects of Biomedical and Behavioral Research, 1978).

In 1980, the DHHS developed a set of regulations in response to the commission's recommendations; these regulations were much more reasonable than those proposed in 1973 and 1974. The DHHS regulations were published in 1981 and revised in 1983 and 1991. These regulations include (1) general requirements for informed consent,

(2) documentation of informed consent, (3) Institutional Review Board (IRB) membership, (4) exempt and expedited review procedures for certain kinds of research, and (5) criteria for IRB approval of research (DHHS, 1983, 1991). These regulations are discussed in depth in this chapter.

PROTECTION OF HUMAN RIGHTS

Human rights are claims and demands that have been justified in the eyes of an individual or by the consensus of a group of individuals. Having rights is necessary for the self-respect, dignity, and health of an individual (Sasson & Nelson, 1971). Researchers and reviewers of research have an ethical responsibility to recognize and protect the rights of human research subjects. The human rights that require protection in research include the rights to (1) self-determination, (2) privacy, (3) anonymity and confidentiality, (4) fair treatment, and (5) protection from discomfort and harm (American Nurses' Association [ANA], 1985a, 1985b; American Psychological Association [APA], 1982).

RIGHT TO SELF-DETERMINATION

The right to *self-determination* is based on the ethical principle of respect for persons, which states that humans are capable of self-determination or controlling their own destiny. Thus, humans should be treated as autonomous agents, who have the freedom to conduct their lives as they choose without external controls. Prospective subjects are treated as autonomous agents by informing them about a proposed study and allowing them to voluntarily choose to participate or not participate. In addition, subjects have the right to withdraw from a study at any time without a penalty (Levine, 1986).

Violation of the Right to Self-Determination

A subject's right to self-determination can be violated through the use of coercion, covert data collection, and deception. *Coercion* occurs when an overt threat of harm or excessive reward is intentionally presented by one person to another in order to obtain compliance (National Commission for the Protection of Human Subjects of Biomedical and Behavioral Research, 1978). Some subjects are coerced to participate in research because they fear harm or discomfort if they do not participate. For example, some patients feel that their medical or nursing care will be negatively affected if they do not agree to be research subjects. Sometimes students feel forced to participate in research to protect their grades or prevent negative relationships with the faculty conducting the research. Other subjects are coerced to participate in studies because they believe that they cannot refuse the excessive rewards offered, such as large sums of money, special privileges, and jobs.

An individual's right to self-determination is violated when he or she becomes a research subject without realizing it. Some researchers have exposed persons to experimental treatments without their knowledge, which is exemplified by the Jewish Chronic Disease Hospital study. Most of the patients and their physicians were unaware of the study. The subjects were informed that they were receiving an injection of cells but the word cancer was omitted (Beecher, 1966). With *covert data collection,* subjects are unaware that research data are being collected because the investigator develops "descriptions of natural phenomena using information that is provided as a matter of normal activity" (Reynolds, 1979, p. 76). This type of data collection was more commonly used by psychologists to describe human behavior in a variety of situations but it has also been used by nursing and other disciplines (APA, 1982). Covert data collection is considered acceptable in some situations but not when research deals with sensitive aspects of a subject's behavior, such as illegal conduct, sexual behavior, or drug and alcohol use (DHHS, 1991). When covert data collection is used, subjects must be informed of the research activities and the findings at the end of the study.

The use of deception in research can also violate a subject's right to self-determination. *Deception* is the actual misinforming of subjects for research purposes (Kelman, 1967). A classic example of deception is the Milgram (1963) study, in which the subjects were to administer electric shocks to another person. During the study, the subjects thought that they were giving the shocks to another person, but the person was really a professional actor who pretended to feel the shocks. Some subjects experienced severe mental tension, almost to the point of collapse, by participating in this study. The use of deception is not uncommon in social and psychological research, but it is a controversial research activity (Kelman, 1967). Nurse researchers considering the use of deception in their studies should examine the ethical and methodological implications of this activity as well as the implications that deception has for the future of nursing research.

Persons with Diminished Autonomy

Some persons have diminished autonomy or are vulnerable and less advantaged because of legal or mental incompetence, terminal illness, or confinement to an institution (Levine, 1986; Watson, 1982). These persons require additional protection of their right to self-determination because they have a decreased ability, or inability, to give informed consent. In addition, these persons are vulnerable to coercion and deception. Researchers must provide justification for the use of subjects with diminished autonomy, and the need for justification increases as the subject's risk and vulnerability increases (DHHS, 1991; Levine, 1986). However, in many situations, the knowledge needed to improve nursing care to vulnerable populations can be gained only by studying them.

Legally and Mentally Incompetent Subjects

Children (minors), the mentally impaired, and unconscious patients are legally or mentally incompetent to give informed consent. These individuals lack the ability to comprehend information about a study and to make decisions regarding participation in or withdrawal from the study. These persons have a range of vulnerability from minimal to absolute. The use of persons with diminished autonomy as research subjects is more acceptable (1) if the research is therapeutic, when the subjects have the potential to benefit from the experimental process (Watson, 1982); (2) if the researcher is willing to use both vulnerable and nonvulnerable individuals as subjects; and (3) if the risk is minimized and the consent process is strictly followed to secure the rights of the prospective subjects (DHHS, 1991; Levine, 1986).

CHILDREN. The laws defining the minor status of a child are statutory and vary from state to state. Often a child's competency to consent is governed by age, with incompetence being nonrefutable up to age seven years (Broome & Stieglitz, 1992; Thompson, 1987). Thus, a child is not believed to be mature enough to give assent or consent to research under the age of seven. However, by age seven, "children are capable of concrete operations of thought and are capable of providing meaningful assent to participation as research subjects" (Thompson, 1987, pp. 394–395). With advancing age and maturity, the child should have a stronger role in the consent process.

The DHHS (1991, Section 46.404) regulations require "soliciting the assent of the children (when capable) and the permission of their parents or guardians . . . Assent means a child's affirmative agreement to participate in research. Permission means the agreement of parent(s) or guardian to the participation of their child or ward in research" (DHHS, 1991, Section 46.402). Using children as research subjects is also influenced by the therapeutic nature of the research and the risks versus benefits. Thompson (1987) developed a guide for obtaining informed consent based on the child's level of competence, the therapeutic nature of the research, and the risks versus benefits (see Table 9–2). Children who are experiencing a developmental delay, cognitive deficit, emotional disorder, or physical illness must be considered individually (Broome & Stieglitz, 1992).

Unless otherwise specified, nurses conducting research with children must obtain permission from the child's parent or guardian for the child's participation. In studies of minimal risk, permission from one parent is usually sufficient for the

Table 9–2
Guide to Obtaining Informed Consent, Based on the Relationship Between a Child's Level of Competence, the Therapeutic Nature of the Research, and Risk Versus Benefit

	Nontherapeutic		Therapeutic	
	MMR-LB	*MR-LB*	*MR-HB*	*MMR-HB*
Child, incompetent (generally 0–7 yr)				
Parents' consent	Necessary	Necessary	Sufficient*	Sufficient
Child's assent	Optional†	Optional†	Optional	Optional
Child, relatively competent (7 yr and older)				
Parents' consent	Necessary	Necessary	Sufficient‡	Recommended
Child's assent	Necessary	Necessary	Sufficient§	Sufficient

Key: MMR, more than minimal risk; MR, minimal risk; LB, low benefit; HB, high benefit.
* A parent's refusal can be superseded by the principle that a parent has no power to forbid the saving of a child's life.
† Children making "deliberate objection" would be precluded from participation by most researchers.
‡ In cases not involving the privacy rights of a "mature minor."
§ In cases involving the privacy rights of a "mature minor."
(From Thompson, P. J. [1987]. Protection of the rights of children as subjects for research. *Journal of Pediatric Nursing, 2*[6], 397, with permission.)

research to be conducted. However, for research that involves more than minimal risk and has no prospect of direct benefit to the individual subject, the "permission is to be obtained from the parents, both parents must give their permission unless one parent is deceased, unknown, incompetent, or not reasonably available, or when only one parent has legal responsibility for the care and custody of the child" (DHHS, 1991, Section 46.408b).

ADULTS. Certain adults, due to mental illness, cognitive impairment, or a comatose state, are incompetent and incapable of giving informed consent. Persons are "said to be incompetent if in the judgment of a qualified clinician they have those attributes that ordinarily provide the grounds for adjudicating incompetence" (Levine, 1986, p. 261). Incompetence can be temporary (e.g., inebriation), permanent (e.g., advanced senile dementia), or subjective or transitory (e.g., behavior or symptoms of psychosis). If an individual is judged incompetent and incapable of consent, the researcher must seek approval from the prospective subject and his or her legally authorized representative. A "legally authorized representative means an individual or judicial or other body authorized under applicable law to consent on behalf of a prospective subject to the subject's participation in the procedure(s) involved in the research" (DHHS,

1991, Section 46.102). However, individuals can be judged incompetent and can still assent to participate in certain minimal risk research if they have the ability to understand what they are being asked to do, to make reasonably free choices, and to communicate their choices clearly and unambiguously (Levine, 1986).

An increasing number of individuals have become permanently incompetent from the advanced stages of senile dementia of the Alzheimer type (SDAT). A minimum of 60% of nursing home residents have this condition (Floyd, 1988). Most long-term care (LTC) settings have no institutional review board (IRB) for research and many of the LTC patients' families or guardians are reluctant to give consent for research. Nursing research is needed to establish methods of comforting and caring for individuals with SDAT. Floyd (1988) recommended the development of IRBs in LTC settings and the use of client advocates to assist in the consent process. Levine (1986) identified two approaches that families, guardians, researchers, or IRBs might use when making decisions on behalf of these incompetent individuals: (1) best interest standard and (2) substituted judgment standard. The former involves doing what is best for the individual based on a balancing of risks and benefits. The latter is concerned with determining the course of action incompetent individuals would have taken if they were capable of making a choice.

Terminally Ill Subjects

In conducting research on terminally ill subjects, the investigator should determine (1) who will benefit from the research and (2) if it is ethical to conduct research on individuals who might not benefit from the study. Participating in research could have increased risks and minimal or no benefits for these subjects. In addition, the dying subject's condition could affect the study results and lead the researcher to misinterpret the results (Watson, 1982). For example, cancer patients have become an overstudied population, in whom "it is not unusual for the majority of bloods, bone marrows, lumbar punctures, and biopsies to be conducted for purposes of research, to fulfill protocol requirements" (Strauman & Cotanch, 1988, p. 666). Many ethical issues have been raised regarding the conduct of research on children with HIV (Twomey, 1994). These biomedical research projects can easily compromise the care of these individuals, which poses ethical dilemmas for clinical nurses. More and more nurses will be responsible for assuring ethical standards in research as they participate in institutional review of research and serve as patient advocates in the clinical setting (Carico & Harrison, 1990; Davis, 1989; McGrath, 1995).

Some terminally ill individuals are willing subjects because they believe that participating in research is a way to contribute to society before they die. Others want to take part in research because they believe that the experimental process will benefit them. In AIDS research, many individuals want to participate in research to gain access to experimental drugs and hospitalized care. However, researchers are concerned because these individuals are often noncompliant with the research protocol (Arras, 1990). This is a serious dilemma for researchers studying subjects with any type of terminal illness, since they must consider the rights of the subjects and be responsible for conducting quality research.

Subjects Confined to Institutions

Hospitalized patients have diminished autonomy because they are ill and are confined in settings that are controlled by health care personnel (Besch, 1979; Levine, 1986). Some hospitalized patients feel obligated to be research subjects, because they want to assist a particular practitioner (nurse or physician) with his or her research. Others feel coerced to participate, because they fear that their care will be adversely affected if they refuse. Nurses conducting research with hospitalized patients must make every effort to protect these subjects from feelings of coercion.

In the past, prisoners have experienced diminished autonomy in research projects because of their confinement. They might feel coerced to participate in research because they fear harm or desire the benefits of early release, special treatment, or monetary gain. Prisoners were frequently used for drug studies in which there were no health-related benefits and possible harm for them (Levine, 1986). Federal regulations regarding research involving prisoners require that "the risks involved in the research are commensurate with risks that would be accepted by nonprisoner volunteers and procedures for the selection of subjects within the prison are fair to all prisoners and immune from arbitrary intervention by prison authorities or prisoners" (DHHS, 1991, Section 46.305). Researchers must evaluate each prospective subject's capacity for self-determination and protect subjects with diminished autonomy.

RIGHT TO PRIVACY

Privacy is the right an individual has to determine the time, extent, and general circumstances under which private information will be shared with or withheld from others. Private information includes one's attitudes, beliefs, behaviors, opinions, and records. The research subject's privacy is protected if the subject is informed and consents to participate in a study and voluntarily shares private information with a researcher (Hayter, 1979; Levine, 1986).

Invasion of Privacy

An *invasion of privacy* occurs when private information is shared without an individual's knowledge or against his or her will. Invading an individual's privacy might cause loss of dignity, friendships, or employment, or create feelings of anxiety, guilt, embarrassment, or shame. Research subjects experience an invasion of privacy most frequently during the data collection process. For example, invasive questions might be asked during an interview, such as (1) Are you an illegitimate child? (2) Were you an abused child? (3) What are your sexual activities? or (4) Do you use drugs? Some researchers have gathered data from subjects without their knowledge by taping conversations, observing through one-way mirrors, and using hidden cameras and microphones. In these situations, subjects have no knowledge that their words and actions are being shared with a researcher, which is an invasion of privacy (Kelman, 1977).

The invasion of subjects' right to privacy brought about the Privacy Act of 1974. As a result of this act, data collection methods are to be scrutinized to protect subjects' privacy, and data cannot be gathered from subjects without their knowledge. Individuals also have the right to access and to prevent access of others to their records (Hayter, 1979). One of the reasons for the Privacy Act was the increased technology that made it possible to collect and rapidly disseminate data without the knowledge or control of the subject.

RIGHT TO ANONYMITY AND CONFIDENTIALITY

Based on the right to privacy, the research subject has the right to anonymity and the right to assume that the data collected will be kept confidential. Complete *anonymity* exists if the subject's identity cannot be linked, even by the researcher, with his or her individual responses (ANA, 1985b; Sasson & Nelson, 1971). In most studies, researchers know the identity of their subjects and they promise them their identity will be kept anonymous from others. *Confidentiality* is the researcher's management of private information shared by a

subject. The researcher must refrain from sharing that information without the authorization of the subject. Confidentiality is grounded in the following premises: (1) individuals can share personal information to the extent they wish and are entitled to have secrets; (2) one can choose with whom to share personal information; (3) those accepting information in confidence have an obligation to maintain confidentiality; and (4) professionals, such as researchers, have a "duty to maintain confidentiality that goes beyond ordinary loyalty" (Levine, 1986, p. 164).

Breach of Confidentiality

A *breach of confidentiality* can occur when a researcher by accident or direct action allows an unauthorized person to gain access to raw data of a study. Confidentiality can also be breached in reporting or publishing a study when a subject's identity is accidentally revealed, violating the subject's right to anonymity (Ramos, 1989). Breaches of confidentiality can harm subjects psychologically and socially as well as destroy the trust they had in the researcher. Breaches of confidentiality regarding religious preferences; sexual practices; income; racial prejudices; drug use; child abuse; and personal attributes such as intelligence, honesty, and courage can be especially harmful to subjects.

Some nurse researchers have encountered health care professionals who believe that they should have access to information about the patients in the hospital and will request to see the data collected. Sometimes family members or close friends would like to see the data collected on specific subjects. Sharing research data in these circumstances is a breach of confidentiality. When requesting permission to conduct a study, health care professionals, family members, and others in the setting should be told that the raw data will not be shared.

Maintaining Confidentiality

Researchers have a responsibility to protect the anonymity of subjects and to maintain the confidentiality of data collected during a study. The anonymity of subjects can be protected by giving each subject a code number. The researcher keeps a master list of the subjects' names and their code number in a locked place. For example, a subject Mary Jones might be assigned the code number 001. All instruments and forms completed by Mary and data collected by the researcher on her during the study will be identified with the 001 code number, not her name. The master list of subjects' names and code numbers is best kept separate from the data collected to protect subjects' anonymity. Signed consent forms should not be stapled to instruments or other data collection tools. This would make it easy for unauthorized persons to readily identify the subjects and their responses. Consent forms are often stored with the master list of subjects' names and code numbers. The data collected should be entered in the computer using code numbers for identification. The original data collection tools should then be locked in a secure place.

The anonymity of subjects could also be protected by the generation of their own identification codes (Damrosch, 1986). Each subject could generate an individual code from personal information, such as the first letter of a mother's name, the first letter of a father's name, the number of brothers, the number of sisters, and middle initial. Thus, the code would be composed of three letters and two numbers, such as BD21M. This code would be identified on each form that the subject completes. The subject's identity would be anonymous even from the researcher who would know only the subject's code. If the data collected are highly sensitive, researchers might want to use this type of coding system.

The data collected should be group-analyzed so that an individual cannot be identified by his or her responses. If the subjects are divided into groups for data analysis and there is only one subject in a group, that subject's data should be combined with another group or the data should be deleted. In writing the research report, the investigator should report the findings so that an individual or group of individuals cannot be identified by their responses.

Maintaining confidentiality in qualitative re-

search is often more difficult than in quantitative research. The nature of qualitative research requires that the "investigator must be close enough to understand the depth of the question under study, and must present enough direct quotes and detailed description to answer the question" (Ramos, 1989, p. 60). The small number of subjects used and the depth of detail gathered on each subject make it difficult to disguise the subject's identity. To maintain confidentiality, Ford and Reutter (1990) recommend using pseudonyms instead of the participants' names and distorting certain details in the subjects' stories while leaving the contents unchanged. Researchers must respect subjects' privacy as they decide the amount of detail and editing of private information that is necessary to publish a study (Robley, 1995).

Researchers should also take precautions during data collection to maintain confidentiality. The interviews conducted with subjects are frequently taped and later transcribed so the subject's name should not be mentioned on tape. The subject has the right to know if anyone other than the researcher will be transcribing information from the interview. In addition, subjects should be informed on an ongoing basis that they have the right to withhold information (Ford & Reutter, 1990; Robley, 1995).

RIGHT TO FAIR TREATMENT

The right to fair treatment is based on the ethical principle of justice. This principle states that each person should be treated fairly and should receive what he or she is due or owed. In research, the selection of subjects and their treatment during the course of a study should be fair.

Fair Selection of Subjects

In the past, injustice in subject selection has resulted from social, cultural, racial, and sexual biases in society. For many years, research was conducted on categories of individuals who were thought to be especially suitable as research subjects: the poor, charity patients, prisoners, slaves, peasants, dying persons, and others who were considered undesirable (Reynolds, 1972, 1979). Researchers often treated these subjects carelessly and had little regard for the harm and discomfort they experienced. The Nazi medical experiments, Tuskegee syphilis study, and Willowbrook study all exemplify unfair subject selection.

The selection of a population to study and the specific subjects to study should be fair; and the risks and benefits of a study should be fairly distributed based on the subject's efforts, needs, and rights. Subjects should be selected for reasons directly related to the problem being studied and not for "their easy availability, their compromised position, or their manipulability" (National Commission for the Protection of Human Subjects of Biomedical and Behavioral Research, 1978, p. 10). Another concern with subject selection is that some researchers select subjects because they like them and want them to receive the specific benefits of a study. Other researchers have been swayed by power or money to make certain individuals subjects so that they can receive potentially beneficial treatments. Random selection of subjects can eliminate some of the researcher's biases that might influence subject selection.

A current concern in conducting research is finding an adequate number of appropriate subjects to take part in certain studies. As a solution to this problem, some biomedical researchers have offered physicians finder's fees for identifying research subjects. For example, an investigator might be studying patients with lung cancer and the physician would receive a fee for every patient with lung cancer who was referred to the researcher. The ethics of this practice are questionable since the physician is receiving money for the referral. Are the rights of the patient being protected? Researchers using finders' fees should indicate this in their proposal and the human rights review committees must make a decision regarding this practice. Some agencies like Massachusetts General Hospital have reviewed the pros and cons of using finders' fees to obtain research subjects and decided against it (Lind, 1990).

Fair Treatment of Subjects

Researchers and subjects should have a specific agreement about what the subject's participation involves and what the role of the researcher will be (APA, 1982). While conducting a study, the researcher should treat the subjects fairly and respect that agreement. If the data collection requires appointments with the subjects, the researcher should be on time and should terminate the data collection process at an agreed-upon time. The activities or procedures that the subject is to perform should not be changed without the subject's consent. The benefits promised the subjects should be provided. For example, if subjects are promised a copy of the study findings, they should receive those findings when the study is completed. In addition, subjects who participate in studies should receive equal benefits, regardless of age, race, and socioeconomic level. Treating subjects fairly often facilitates the data collection process and decreases subjects' withdrawal from a study.

RIGHT TO PROTECTION FROM DISCOMFORT AND HARM

The right to protection from discomfort and harm is based on the ethical principle of beneficence that states one should do good and above all, do no harm. This principle indicates that members of society should take an active role in preventing discomfort and harm and promoting good in the world around them (Frankena, 1973). Therefore, researchers should conduct their studies to protect subjects from discomfort and harm and try to bring about the greatest possible balance of benefits over harm. Discomfort and harm can be physiological, emotional, social, and economical in nature. Reynolds (1972) identified five categories of studies based on levels of discomfort and harm: (1) no anticipated effects, (2) temporary discomfort, (3) unusual levels of temporary discomfort, (4) risk of permanent damage, and (5) certainty of permanent damage.

No Anticipated Effects

In some studies, there are no positive or negative effects that are expected for the subjects. For example, studies that involve reviewing patients' records, students' files, pathology reports, or other documents have no anticipated effects on the subjects. In these types of studies, the researcher does not interact directly with the research subjects. However, even in these situations, there is a potential risk of invading a subject's privacy.

Temporary Discomfort

Studies that cause temporary discomfort are described as minimal risk studies, in which the discomfort encountered is similar to what the subject would experience in his or her daily life and ceases with the termination of the experiment (DHHS, 1991). Many nursing studies require the completion of questionnaires or participation in interviews, which usually involve minimal risk for the subjects. The physical discomforts might include fatigue, headache, or muscle tension. The emotional and social risks might include anxiety or embarrassment associated with responding to certain questions. The economic risks might include the time of being involved in the study or travel costs to the study site. Participation in many nursing studies is considered a mere inconvenience for the subject with no foreseeable risks or harm.

Most clinical nursing studies examining the impact of a treatment involve minimal risk. For example, a study might involve examining the effects of exercise on the blood glucose levels of diabetics. During the study, the subjects would be asked to test their blood glucose level one extra time per day. There is discomfort when the blood is drawn, and a potential risk of physical changes that might occur with exercise. The subjects might also experience anxiety and fear associated with the additional blood testing, and the testing could be an added expense. The diabetic subjects in this study would experience similar discomforts in their daily lives, and the discomforts would cease with the termination of the study.

Unusual Levels of Temporary Discomfort

In studies that have unusual levels of temporary discomfort, the subjects frequently experience discomfort during the study and after the study has been terminated. For example, subjects might experience prolonged muscle weakness, joint pain, and dizziness after participating in a study that required them to be confined to bed for 10 days to determine the effects of immobility. Studies that require subjects to experience failure, extreme fear, or threats to their identity, or to act in unnatural ways involve unusual levels of temporary discomfort. In some qualitative studies, subjects are asked questions that open old wounds or involve reliving traumatic events (Ford & Reutter, 1990). For example, asking subjects to describe their rape experience could precipitate feelings of extreme fear, guilt, and shame. In these types of studies, investigators should be vigilant in assessing the subjects' discomfort and should refer them for appropriate professional intervention as necessary.

Risk of Permanent Damage

Subjects participating in some studies have the potential to suffer permanent damage, but this is more common in biomedical research than in nursing. For example, medical studies of new drugs and surgical procedures have the potential to cause subjects permanent physical damage. Some topics investigated by nurses have the potential to damage subjects permanently, both emotionally and socially. Studies examining sensitive information, such as sexual behavior, child abuse, or drug use, can be very risky for subjects. These types of studies have the potential to cause permanent damage to a subject's personality or reputation. There are also potential economic risks, such as less efficient job performance or loss of employment.

Certainty of Permanent Damage

In some research, such as the Nazi medical experiments and the Tuskegee syphilis study, the subjects experienced permanent damage. Conducting research that will permanently damage subjects is highly questionable, regardless of the benefits that will be gained. Frequently the benefits gained are for other individuals but not for the subjects. Studies causing permanent damage to subjects violate the fifth principle of the Nuremberg Code (1986, p. 426) that states: "No experiment should be conducted where there is an a priori reason to believe that death or disabling injury will occur except, perhaps, in those experiments where the experimental physicians (or other health professionals) also serve as subjects."

BALANCING BENEFITS AND RISKS FOR A STUDY

Researchers and reviewers of research must examine the balance of benefits and risks in a study. To determine this balance or benefit-risk ratio, the researcher must predict the outcome of a study, assess the actual and potential benefits and risks based on this outcome, and then maximize the benefits and minimize the risks (see Figure 9–1). The outcome of a study is predicted based on previous research, clinical experience, and theory.

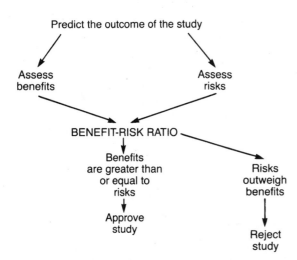

Figure 9–1
Balancing benefits and risks for a study.

ASSESS THE BENEFITS

The probability and magnitude of a study's potential benefits need to be assessed. In most proposals, these benefits are described for the individual subjects, the subjects' families, and society. Frequently, optimistic researchers will have a tendency to overestimate these benefits (Levine, 1986). Reviewers of research need to be cautious in examining study benefits and balancing those benefits with risks. An important benefit of research is the development and refinement of knowledge that can affect the individual subject; but, more important, this knowledge can have a forceful influence on a discipline and members of society.

The type of research conducted, therapeutic or nontherapeutic, affects the potential benefits for the subjects. In therapeutic research, the individual subject has the potential to benefit from the procedures, such as skin care, range of motion, touch, and other nursing interventions that are implemented in the study. The benefits might include improvement in the subject's physical condition, which could facilitate emotional and social benefits. In addition, the knowledge generated from the research might expand the subjects' and their families' understanding of health. The conduct of nontherapeutic nursing research does not benefit the subject directly but is important to generate and refine nursing knowledge. By participating in research, subjects have the potential to increase their understanding of the research process and an opportunity to know the findings from a particular study.

ASSESS THE RISKS

Researchers must assess the type, degree, and number of risks the subjects experience or might experience by participating in a study. The risks involved depend on the purpose of the study and the procedures used to conduct the study. Risks can be physical, emotional, social, and economical in nature and can range from no risk or mere inconvenience to the risk of permanent damage

(Levine, 1986; Reynolds, 1972). Studies can have actual (known) risks and potential risks for subjects. In a study of the effects of bed rest, an actual risk would be muscle weakness and a potential risk might be severe muscle cramps. Some studies have actual or potential risks for the subjects' families and society. The researcher must try to determine the likelihood of the risks and take precautions to protect the rights of subjects when implementing the research.

BENEFIT-RISK RATIO

The *benefit-risk ratio* is determined based on the maximized benefits and the minimized risks. The researcher attempts to maximize the benefits and minimize the risks by making changes in the purpose and/or procedures of the study. If the risks cannot be eliminated or further minimized, the researcher should be able to justify their existence (Levine, 1986). If the risks outweigh the benefits, the study should be revised or a new study developed. If the benefits equal or outweigh the risks, the researcher can justify conducting the study and it will probably be approved by an institutional review board (IRB) (see Figure 9–1).

For example, you wanted to balance the benefits and risks in a study that would examine the effect of an exercise and diet program on the participants' serum lipid values (serum cholesterol, low density lipoprotein [LDL], and high density lipoprotein [HDL]) and cardiovascular (CV) risk level. The benefits to the participants are exercise and diet instruction and information on their serum lipid values and CV risk level at the start of the program and one year later. Potential benefits include improved serum lipid values, lowered CV risk level, and improved exercise and diet habits. The risks include the discomfort of having the serum lipid levels drawn twice and the time spent participating in the study (Bruce & Grove, 1994). These discomforts are temporary and are no more than what the subject would experience in his or her daily life and cease with the termination of the study. The subjects' time participating in the study can be minimized through organization and

precise scheduling of research activities. In examining the ratio of benefits to risks, the benefits are greater in number and importance than the risks; and the risks are temporary and can be minimized. Thus, you could justify conducting this study and it would receive approval from the IRB.

The obligation to balance the benefits and risks of studies is the responsibility of the researcher, professionals, and society. The researcher needs to balance the benefits and risks of a particular study and protect the subjects from harm during the study. Professionals need to participate on IRBs to ensure the conduct of ethical research. Society needs to be concerned with the benefits and risks of the entire enterprise of research and with the protection of all human research subjects from harm.

OBTAINING INFORMED CONSENT

Obtaining *informed consent* from human subjects is essential for the conduct of ethical research (Brent, 1990; Cassidy & Oddi, 1986; Nusbaum & Chenitz, 1990). *Informing* is the transmission of essential ideas and content from the investigator to the prospective subject. *Consent* is the prospective subject's agreement to participate in a study as a subject, which is reached after assimilation of essential information. Prospective subjects, to the degree that they are capable, should have the opportunity to choose whether or not to participate in research. The phenomenon of informed consent was formally defined in the first principle of the Nuremberg Code.

■

"The voluntary consent of the human subject is absolutely essential. . . . This means that the person involved should have *legal capacity* to give consent; should be so situated as to be able to exercise *free power of choice*, without the intervention of any element of force, fraud, deceit, duress, over-reaching or other ulterior form of constraint or coercion; and should have *suffi-*

cient knowledge and *comprehension* of the elements of the subject matter involved as to enable him to make an understanding and enlightened decision." (Nuremberg Code, 1986, p. 425) ∎

This definition of informed consent provided a basis for the discussion of consent in all subsequent codes and regulations and has general acceptance in the research community (Levine, 1986). As indicated in the definition, informed consent includes four elements: (1) disclosure of essential information, (2) comprehension, (3) competency, and (4) voluntarism. This section describes the elements of informed consent and the methods of documenting consent.

ESSENTIAL INFORMATION FOR CONSENT

Informed consent requires the researcher to disclose specific information to each prospective subject. The following information is identified by the Code of Federal Regulations for the Protection of Human Subjects to be essential for informed consent in research (DHHS, 1991).

1. **Introduction of Research Activities.** Each prospective subject is provided "a statement that the study involves research" and the individual is being asked to participate as a subject (DHHS, 1991, Section 46.116a). In clinical nursing research, the patient, serving as a subject, needs to know which nursing activities are research activities and which are routine nursing interventions.

2. **Statement of the Research Purpose.** The researcher must provide "an explanation of the purposes of the research and the expected duration of the subject's participation" (DHHS, 1991, 46.116a). The purposes of some qualitative studies are broad, so additional information regarding the study goals might be supplied during the study (Ford & Reutter, 1990; Ramos, 1989). If at any point the prospective subjects disagree with the researcher's goals or the intent of the study, they can decline participation.

3. **Explanation of Procedures.** Prospective subjects receive a complete "description of the procedures to be followed and identification of any procedures which are experimental in the study" (DHHS, 1991, Section 46.116a). Thus, the investigator describes the research variables and the procedures or mechanisms that will be used to observe, examine, manipulate, and/or measure these variables. In addition, the prospective subjects are informed about when the study procedures will be implemented, how many times, and in what setting.

4. **Description of Risks and Discomforts.** Prospective subjects are informed of any "reasonably foreseeable risks or discomforts" (physical, emotional, social, or economical) that might result from the study (DHHS, 1991, Section 46.116a). The investigator then indicates how the risks of the study have been or will be minimized.

If the study involves greater than minimal risk, the researcher usually encourages the prospective subjects to consult another person regarding their participation. A trusted advisor, such as a friend, family member, or another nurse could serve as a consultant (Levine, 1986).

5. **Description of Benefits.** The investigator also describes "any benefits to the subject or to others which may reasonably be expected from the research" (DHHS, 1991, Section 46.116a). Any financial advantages or other rewards for participating in the study are described.

6. **Disclosure of Alternatives.** The investigator needs to disclose the "appropriate, alternative procedures or courses of treatment, if any, that might be advantageous to the subject" (DHHS, 1991, Section 46.116a). For example, the researchers of the Tuskegee syphilis study should have informed the subjects with syphilis that penicillin was an effective treatment for the disease.

7. **Assurance of Anonymity and Confidentiality.** Prospective subjects must be provided a "statement describing the extent, if any, to which confidentiality of records identifying the subject will be maintained" (DHHS, 1991, 46.116a). Thus, subjects need to know that their responses

and the information obtained from their records during a study will be kept confidential. They also need to be assured that their identity will remain anonymous in reports and publications of the study.

8. **Compensation for Participation in Research.** For research involving more than minimal risks, the prospective subjects must be given an explanation as to whether any compensation and/or medical treatments are available if injury occurs (DHHS, 1991, Section 46.116a). If medical treatments are available, the type and extent of the treatments are described. When appropriate, the prospective subject is informed as to whether "the particular treatment or procedure may involve risks to the subject (or to the embryo or fetus, if the subject is or may become pregnant) which are currently unforeseeable" (DHHS, 1991, Section 46.116b).

9. **Offer to Answer Questions.** The researcher offers to answer any questions that are raised by the prospective subjects. Prospective subjects are provided an "explanation of whom to contact for answers to pertinent questions about the research and research subjects' rights, and whom to contact in the event of a research-related injury" (DHHS, 1991, Section 46.116a) and a mechanism for contacting that person.

10. **Noncoercive Disclaimer.** A noncoercive disclaimer is "a statement that participation is voluntary, refusal to participate will involve no penalty or loss of benefits to which the subject is otherwise entitled" (DHHS, 1991, Section 46.116a). This statement can facilitate a relationship between prospective subjects and the investigator, especially if the relationship has a potential for coercion.

11. **Option to Withdraw.** Subjects "may discontinue participation (withdraw from a study) at any time without penalty or loss of benefits" (DHHS, 1991, Section 46.116a). However, researchers do have the right to ask subjects if they think that they will be able to complete the study, in order to decrease the number of subjects withdrawing early.

There may be circumstances "under which the subject's participation may be terminated by the investigator without regard to the subject's consent" (DHHS, 1991, Section 46.116b). For example, if a particular treatment becomes potentially dangerous to a subject, the researcher has an obligation to discontinue the subject's participation in the study. Thus, prospective subjects are told under what circumstances they might be withdrawn from a study. The researcher also makes a general statement about the circumstances that could lead to the termination of the entire project (Levine, 1986).

12. **Consent to Incomplete Disclosure.** In some studies, subjects are not completely informed of the study purpose, because that knowledge will alter the subjects' actions. However, prospective subjects need to know when certain information is being withheld deliberately. The researcher ensures that there are no undisclosed risks to the subjects that are more than minimal, and the subjects' questions regarding the study are answered truthfully.

Subjects who are exposed to nondisclosure of information need to know when and how they will be debriefed about the study. The researcher *debriefs* the subjects by informing them of the actual purpose of the study and the results that were obtained. If the subjects experience adverse effects related to the study, the researcher ought to make every attempt to reconcile them (Jacobson, 1973).

COMPREHENSION OF CONSENT INFORMATION

Informed consent implies not only the imparting of information by the researcher but also the comprehension of that information by the subjects. Studies have been done to determine subjects' levels of comprehension after receiving the essential information for consent, and their comprehension was frequently low (Levine, 1986). The researcher needs to take the time to teach prospective subjects about the study. The amount of information to be taught depends on the subjects' knowledge of research and the specific research topic. The benefits and risks of a study need to be discussed in detail, using examples that are relevant to the prospective subject. The specific procedures to be used in the study and the subjects' rights are best outlined and described in terms the subjects can understand.

The DHHS Regulations (1991, Section 46.116) designate that the information given to the "subject or the representative shall be in language understandable to the subject or representative." Thus, the consent information needs to be written and verbalized in lay terminology, not professional jargon, and presented without loaded or biased terms that might coerce a subject into participating in a study. The wording of the consent form will depend on the educational level of the subjects, with the general public on average having an eighth grade level of education.

Assessing Subjects' Comprehension

The researcher can take steps to determine the prospective subject's level of comprehension. Silva (1985) studied the comprehension of information for informed consent by spouses of surgical patients and found that 72 of the 75 spouses had adequate comprehension of the consent information. The subjects' comprehension of consent information was assessed using the following questions: "(1) What is the purpose of this study? (2) What risks are involved in the study procedures? (3) What does your participation in this study involve? (4) Approximately how long will your participation in this study take? (5) When can you withdraw from this study? (6) How will your name be associated with the study data? (7) With whom will the study information be shared? and (8) What direct personal benefit will come to you as a result of participating in this study?" (Silva, 1985, p. 121). Comprehension of consent information becomes more difficult in complex, high-risk studies. In some high-risk studies, the prospective subjects are tested on consent information, and they do not become subjects unless they pass the tests (Hershey & Miller, 1976).

COMPETENCY TO GIVE CONSENT

Autonomous individuals, who are capable of understanding and weighing the benefits and risks of a proposed study, are competent to give consent. The competence of the subject is often determined by the researcher (Douglas & Larson, 1986). Persons with diminished autonomy because of legal or mental incompetence, terminal illness, or confinement to an institution might not be legally competent to consent to participate in research (see the section on right to self-determination) (Cassidy & Oddi, 1986). However, the researcher makes every effort to present the consent information at a level these potential subjects can understand, so they can assent to the research. In addition, the researcher presents the essential information for consent to the legally authorized representative, such as the parents or guardian, of the prospective subject (DHHS, 1991; Levine, 1986).

VOLUNTARY CONSENT

Voluntary consent means the prospective subject has decided to take part in a study of his or her own volition without coercion or any undue influence (Douglas & Larson, 1986). Voluntary consent is obtained after the prospective subject has been given essential information about the study and has shown comprehension of this information. Some researchers, because of their authority, expertise, or power, have the potential to coerce subjects into participating in research. Researchers need to be cautious that their persuasion of prospective subjects does not become coercion. Thus, the rewards offered in a study ought to be congruent with the risks the subjects must take.

DOCUMENTATION OF INFORMED CONSENT

The documentation of informed consent depends on the degree of risk involved in the study and the discretion of the researcher and those reviewing the study. Most studies require a written consent form; but in some studies, the consent form is waived.

Written Consent Waived

The requirements for written consent may be waived in research that "presents no more than minimal risk of harm to subjects and involves no procedures for which written consent is normally required outside of the research context" (DHHS, 1991, Section 46.117c). For example, researchers collecting relatively harmless data using questionnaires would not need to obtain a signed consent form from the subjects. The subject's completion of the questionnaire may serve as consent. The top of the questionnaire might contain a statement: "Your completion of this questionnaire indicates your consent to participate in this study."

Written consent is also waived in a situation when "the only record linking the subject and the research would be the consent document and the principal risk would be potential harm resulting from a breach of confidentiality. Each subject will be asked whether the subject wants documentation linking the subject with the research, and the subject's wishes will govern" (DHHS, 1983, Section 46.117c). Thus, in this situation, subjects are given the option to sign or not sign a consent form that links them to the research. The four elements of consent (disclosure, comprehension, competency, and voluntariness) are essential in all studies whether written consent is waived or required.

Written Consent Documents

"Short Form" Written Consent Document

The "short form" consent document includes the following statement: "The elements of informed consent required by Section 46.116 [see the section on essential information for consent] have been presented orally to the subject or the subject's legally authorized representative" (DHHS, 1991, Section 46.117a). The researcher must develop a written summary of what is to be said to the subject in the oral presentation and the summary must be approved by an institutional review board (IRB). When the oral presentation is made to the subject or his or her representative, a witness is required. The subject or representative must sign the short form consent document. "The witness shall sign both the short form and a copy of the summary, and the person actually obtaining consent shall sign a copy of the summary" (DHHS, 1991, Section 46.117a). Copies of the summary and short form are given to the subject and the witness; the original documents are retained by the researcher. These documents need to be kept by the researcher for three years. The short form written consent documents might be used in studies that present minimal or moderate risk to the subjects.

The Formal Written Consent Document

The written consent document includes the elements of informed consent required by the DHHS Regulation Section 46.116 (see the section on essential information for consent). In addition, a consent form might include other information required by the institution where the study is to be conducted or by the agency funding the study. A sample *consent form* is presented in Figure 9–2 with descriptors of the essential consent information. The consent form can be read by the subject or read to the subject by the researcher; however, it is wise also to explain the study to the subject. The form is signed by the subject and is witnessed by the investigator or research assistant collecting the data. This type of consent can be used for any type of study from minimal to high-risk. All persons signing the consent form need to receive a copy of it, which includes the subject, researcher, and any other witnesses. The original consent form is kept by the researcher for three years.

Studies that involve subjects with diminished autonomy require a written consent form. If these prospective subjects have some comprehension of the study and agree to participate as subjects, they need to sign the consent form. However, the form also needs to be signed by the subject's legally authorized representative. The representative indi-

Study Title: The Needs of Family Members of Critically Ill Adults

Investigator: Linda L. Norris, R.N.

Ms. Norris is a registered nurse studying the emotional and social needs of family members of patients in the Intensive Care Units (**research purpose**). Although the study will not benefit you directly, it will provide information that might enable nurses to identify family members' needs and to assist family members with those needs (**potential benefits**).

The study and its procedures have been approved by the appropriate people and review boards at The University of Texas at Arlington and X hospital (**IRB approval**). The study procedures involve no foreseeable risks or harm to you or your family (**potential risks**). The procedures include: (1) responding to a questionnaire about the needs of family members of critically ill patients and (2) completing a demographic data sheet (**explanation of procedures**). Participation in this study will take approximately 20 minutes (**time commitment**). You are free to ask any questions about the study or about being a subject and you may call Ms. Norris at (999) 999-9999 (work) or (111) 111-1111 (home) if you have further questions (**offer to answer questions**).

Your participation in this study is voluntary; you are under no obligation to participate (**voluntary consent**). You have the right to withdraw at any time and the care of your family member and your relationship with the health care team will not be affected (**option to withdraw**).

The study data will be coded so they will not be linked to your name. Your identity will not be revealed while the study is being conducted or when the study is reported or published. All study data will be collected by Ms. Norris, stored in a secure place, and not shared with any other person without your permission (**assurance of anonymity and confidentiality**).

I have read this consent form and voluntarily consent to participate in this study.

(If Appropriate)

_____   _____   _____   _____
Subject's Signature   Date   Legal Representative   Date

                                          _____
                                          Relationship to Subject

I have explained this study to the above subject and have sought his/her understanding for informed consent.

_____   _____
Investigator's Signature   Date

Figure 9–2
Sample consent form.

cates his or her relationship to the subject under the representative's signature (see Figure 9–2).

The written consent form used in a high-risk study often includes the signatures of two witnesses: (1) the researcher, and (2) an additional person. The additional person signing as a witness needs to observe the informed consent process and must not be otherwise connected with the study (Hershey & Miller, 1976). The best witnesses are research subject advocates or patient advocates who are employed in the institution. Sometimes nurses are asked to sign a consent form as a witness for a biomedical study. They need to know the study purpose and procedures and the subject's comprehension of the study before signing the form (Carico & Harrison, 1990; Chamorro & Appelbaum, 1988). The role of the witness is more important in the consent process if the prospective subject is in awe of the investigator and does not feel free to question the procedures of the study.

Tape Recording or Videotaping the Consent Process

A researcher might elect to tape record or videotape the consent process. These methods document what was said to the prospective subject and record the subject's questions and the investigator's answers. However, tape recording and video-taping are time consuming and costly and are not appropriate for studies of minimal or moderate risk. If a study is considered high-risk, complete documentation of the consent process with a tape might be wise to protect the subjects and the re-searcher. Both the researcher and the subject would retain a copy of the tape recording or video-tape.

Documenting Consent Rates

Informed consent can be documented in a variety of ways as previously discussed. Researchers need to report the way informed consent was obtained and to document the consent rates. *Consent rate* is the percentage of people that indicated a will-ingness to participate in a study based on the total number of people approached. If the consent rate is low, this indicates several people refused to par-ticipate in the study, which limits the generaliz-ability of the results. Low consent rates can also indicate biased results because only certain people are willing to participate in a study. A recent sur-vey of research articles indicated that only 41% of the studies reported their consent rate. Of those reporting a consent rate, the mean consent rate was 72%, with the consent rate higher for clinical than nonclinical studies (Douglas, Briones, & Chronis-ter, 1994). Schaefer and Moos (1996) studied the effects of work stressors and work climate on long-term care staff's job morale and functioning and provided the following information on the consent rate and informed consent process.

"Of the 695 staff who met the study criteria, 84% (585) agreed to participate, and 74% (435) com-pleted the inventories." (p. 65)

"Staff were screened and recruited both by per-sonal contact at work and by telephone at home. A cover letter, the inventories, and a con-sent form were mailed to staff members who agreed to participate. To ensure confidentiality, staff returned the inventories and signed consent forms in separate postage-paid envelopes." (p. 66) ■

In this study, the consent rate was 84% and the documentation of informed consent was done with a formal consent form. However, even though 84% consented to participate, only 74% of the po-tential subjects actually participated.

INSTITUTIONAL REVIEW

In *institutional review,* a study is examined for ethical concerns by a committee of peers. The first federal policy statement on protection of human subjects by institutional review was issued by the United States Public Health Service (USPHS) in 1966. The USPHS indicated that research involv-ing human subjects must be reviewed by a com-mittee of peers or associates to determine: "(1) the rights and welfare of the individual or individuals involved, (2) the appropriateness of the methods used to secure informed consent, and (3) the risks and potential medical benefits of the investigation" (Levine, 1986, p. 323).

In 1974, DHEW passed the National Research Act, which required that all research involving hu-man subjects undergo institutional review. The DHHS reviewed and revised these guidelines in 1981, 1983, and 1991. These regulations describe the membership, functions, and operations of an institutional review board (IRB). An IRB is a committee that reviews research to ensure that the investigator is conducting the research ethically. Universities, hospital corporations, and many managed care centers have IRBs to promote the conduct of ethical research and protect the rights of prospective subjects.

Each IRB has at least five members of varying background (cultural, economic, educational, gen-der, racial) to promote complete and adequate re-view of research that is commonly conducted in an institution. The members need to have sufficient experience and expertise to review research and not have conflicting interest related to the research conducted in the institution. The IRB also needs to include other members whose primary concern is nonscientific, such as an ethicist, lawyer, or minister. At least one of the members ought to be someone who is not affiliated with the institution

Table 9–3
Research Qualifying for Exemption from IRB Review

Unless otherwise required by department or agency heads, research activities in which the only involvement of human subjects will be in one or more of the following categories are exempt from review.

(1) Research conducted in established or commonly accepted educational settings, involving normal educational practices, such as (i) research on regular and special education instructional strategies, or (ii) research on the effectiveness of or the comparison among instructional techniques, curricula, or classroom management methods.

(2) Research involving the use of educational tests (cognitive, diagnostic, aptitude, achievement), survey procedures, interview procedures or observation of public behavior, unless:

(i) information obtained is recorded in such a manner that human subjects can be identified, directly or through identifiers linked to the subjects; and (ii) any disclosure of the human subjects' responses outside the research could reasonably place the subjects at risk of criminal or civil liability or be damaging to the subjects' financial standing, employability, or reputation.

(3) Research involving the use of educational tests (cognitive, diagnostic, aptitude, achievement), survey procedures, interview procedures, or observation of public behavior that is not exempt under paragraph (b)(2) of this section, if:

(i) the human subjects are elected or appointed public officials or candidates for public office; or (ii) Federal statute(s) require(s) without exception that the confidentiality of the personally identifiable information will be maintained throughout the research and thereafter.

(4) Research involving the collection or study of existing data, documents, records, pathological specimens, or diagnostic specimens, if these sources are publicly available or if the information is recorded by the investigator in such a manner that subjects cannot be identified, directly or through identifiers linked to the subjects.

(5) Research and demonstration projects which are conducted by or subject to the approval of Department or Agency heads, and which are designed to study, evaluate, or otherwise examine:

(i) Public benefit or service programs; (ii) procedures for obtaining benefits or services under those programs; (iii) possible changes in or alternatives to those programs or procedures; or (iv) possible changes in methods or levels of payment for benefits or services under those programs.

(6) Taste and food quality evaluation and consumer acceptance studies, (i) if wholesome foods without additives are consumed or (ii) if a good is consumed that contains a food ingredient at or below the level and for a use found to be safe, or agricultural chemical or environmental contaminant at or below the level found to be safe, by the Food and Drug Administration or approved by the Environmental Protection Agency or the Food Safety and Inspection Service of the U.S. Department of Agriculture.

(Excerpted from *Federal Register* of June 18, 1991 [DHHS, 1991, Section 46.101b].)

(DHHS, 1991, Section 46. 107a-f). The IRBs in hospitals are often composed of physicians, lawyers, scientists, clergy, community lay persons, and, more recently, nurses (Chamorro & Appelbaum, 1988).

The functions and operations of an IRB involve the review of research. The DHHS regulations (1991) identify three levels of review: (1) exempt from review, (2) expedited review, and (3) complete review. The level of the review required for each study is decided by the IRB chairperson and/or committee and not by the researcher. Studies are usually *exempt* from review if they have no apparent risks for the research subjects. The studies that are exempted from review by the DHHS (1991, Section 46.101b) are identified in Table 9–3. Nursing studies that have no foreseeable risks or are a mere inconvenience for subjects are usually identified as exempt from review by the chairperson of the IRB committee.

Studies that have some risks, but the risks are viewed as minimal, are expedited in the review

Table 9–4
Research Qualifying for Expedited IRB Review

Expedited review (by committee chairpersons or designated members) for the following research involving no more than minimal risk is authorized:

1. Collection of: hair and nail clippings, in a nondisfiguring manner; deciduous teeth and permanent teeth if patient care indicates a need for extraction.
2. Collection of excreta and external secretions including sweat, uncannulated saliva, placenta removed at delivery, and amniotic fluid at the time of rupture of the membrane prior to or during labor.
3. Recording of data from subjects 18 years of age or older using noninvasive procedures routinely employed in clinical practice. This includes the use of physical sensors that are applied either to the surface of the body or at a distance and do not involve input of matter or significant amounts of energy into the subject or an invasion of the subject's privacy. It also includes such procedures as weighing, testing sensory acuity, electrocardiography, electroencephalography, thermography, detection of naturally occurring radioactivity, diagnostic echography, and electroretinography. It does not include exposure to electromagnetic radiation outside the visible range (for example, x-rays, microwaves).
4. Collection of blood samples by venipuncture, in amounts not exceeding 450 milliliters in an eight-week period and no more than two times per week, from subjects 18 years of age or older and who are in good health and not pregnant.
5. Collection of both supra- and subgingival dental plaque and calculus, provided the procedure is not more invasive than routine prophylactic scaling of the teeth and the process is accomplished in accordance with accepted prophylactic techniques.
6. Voice recordings made for research purposes such as investigations of speech defects.
7. Moderate exercise by health volunteers.
8. The study of existing data, documents, records, pathological specimens, or diagnostic specimens.
9. Research on individual or group behavior or characteristics of individual, such as studies of perception, cognition, game theory, or test development, where the investigator does not manipulate subjects' behavior and research will not involve stress to subjects.
10. Research on drugs or devices for which an investigational new drug exemption or an investigational device exemption is not required.

(Excerpted from the *Federal Register* of June 18, 1991 [DHHS, 1991, Section 46.110]. Additional regulations that apply to research involving fetuses, pregnant women, human in vitro fertilization, and prisoners are available in the *Federal Register*, 1991, part 46.)

process. *Minimal risk* means "that the risks of harm anticipated in the proposed research are not greater, considering probability and magnitude, than those ordinarily encountered in daily life or during the performance of routine physical or psychological examinations or tests" (DHHS, 1991, Section 46.102i). Expedited review procedures can also be used to review minor changes in previously approved research (DHHS, 1991, Section 46.110b). Under *expedited review* procedures, "the review may be carried out by the IRB chairperson or by one or more experienced reviewers designated by the chairperson from among members of the IRB. In reviewing the research, the reviewers may exercise all of the authorities of the IRB except disapproval of the research. A research activity may be disapproved only after review in accor-

dance with the nonexpedited procedure" (DHHS, 1991, Section 46.110b). Table 9–4 identifies research that qualifies for expedited review.

Studies that have greater than minimal risks must receive a complete review by an IRB. To obtain IRB approval, researchers need to ensure that (1) risks to subjects are minimized, (2) risks to subjects are reasonable in relation to anticipated benefits, (3) selection of subjects is equitable, (4) informed consent will be sought from each prospective subject or the subject's legally authorized representative, (5) informed consent will be appropriately documented, (6) the research plan makes adequate provision for monitoring data collection for subjects' safety, and (7) adequate provisions are made to protect the privacy of subjects and to maintain the confidentiality of data (DHHS,

1991, Section 46.111a). The process of seeking approval from a research review committee to conduct a study is described in Chapter 26.

Published studies often indicate that the research project was approved by an IRB. Jarrett, Cain, Heitkemper, and Levy (1996) studied the relationship between gastrointestinal and dysmenorrheic symptoms at menses and identified the IRB approval and consent process for their study.

"Following approval by the university's institutional human subjects review board, women were recruited by posted advertisements throughout a large northwestern university . . . Women who called in response to the advertisement were screened over the telephone to determine whether they met the inclusion criteria. Those who met the criteria were then scheduled for an initial interview, during which informed consent was obtained. . . ." (p. 47) ∎

SCIENTIFIC MISCONDUCT

The goal of research is to generate scientific knowledge, which is possible only through the honest conduct, reporting, and publication of research. However, during the last 15 years, an increasing number of fraudulent studies have been published in prestigious scientific journals. In the late 1980s, scientific misconduct was deemed a serious problem that was investigated by the DHHS. In a final ruling in 1989, the DHHS defined scientific fraud (misconduct) as "fabrication, falsification, plagiarism, or other practices that seriously deviate from those that are commonly accepted within the scientific community for proposing, conducting, or reporting research. It does not include honest error or honest differences in interpretation or judgments of data" (DHHS, 1989, p. 32449). Thus, scientific fraud includes intentional, not unintentional, misconduct.

In 1989, two new federal agencies were organized for the reporting and investigating of scientific misconduct. The Office of Scientific Integrity

Table 9–5 **Dishonesty in Research**	
Type	**Description**
Fabrication, falsification, or forging	Deliberate invention of nonexistent information
Manipulation of design or methods	Intentional planning of the study design or data collection methods so that the results will be biased toward the research hypothesis
Selective retaining or manipulation of data	Choosing only data that are consistent with the research hypothesis and discarding the rest
Plagiarism	Intentional representation of the work or ideas of others as one's own, or rewording one's own work to produce a new paper based on the same data; abuse of confidentiality of information from others
Irresponsible collaboration	Failure to participate appropriately in an investigative team or fulfill responsibilities as a coauthor

(From Larson, E. [1989]. Maintaining quality in clinical research and evaluation: When corrective action is necessary. Reprinted from the *Journal of Nursing Care Quality, 3*[4], 30, with permission of Aspen Publishers, Inc., © 1989.)

Review (OSIR) was established to manage scientific misconduct by grant recipients. The Office of Scientific Integrity (OSI) supervises the implementation of the rules and regulations related to scientific misconduct and manages any investigations (DHHS, 1989; Hawley & Jeffers, 1992). The investigations by these federal agencies revealed a variety of fraudulent behaviors. In some situations, the fraudulent studies were never conducted and the data and results were fabricated by the researchers. In other cases, the findings were consciously distorted. Some of the common types of dishonest or fraudulent research are identified and described in Table 9–5.

An example of scientific misconduct was evident in the publications of Dr. Robert Slutsky, a heart specialist at the University of California, San Diego, School of Medicine. He resigned in 1986 when confronted with inconsistencies in his research publications. His publications contained "statistical anomalies that raised the question of data fabrication" (Friedman, 1990, p. 1416). In six years, Slutsky published 161 articles, and at one time he was completing an article every 10 days. Eighteen of the articles were found to be fraudulent and have retraction notations, and 60 articles were questionable (Friedman, 1990; Henderson, 1990).

Stephen Breuning, a psychologist at the University of Pittsburgh, engaged in deceptive and misleading practices in reporting his research on retarded children. He used his fraudulent research to obtain more than $300,000 in federal grants. In 1988, he was criminally charged with research fraud, pleaded guilty, was fined $20,000, and was sentenced to up to 10 years in prison (Chop & Silva, 1991; Garfield & Welljams-Dorof, 1990; Leino-Kilpi & Tuomaala, 1989).

More recently, Dr. Roger Poisson, principle investigator at St. Luc Hospital in Montreal, was found guilty of scientific misconduct by the ORI due to his actions during the breast cancer trials. The first evidence of misconduct was noted in 1990 and was not confirmed until 1993. The data from Dr. Poisson's setting were removed and the remaining data were reanalyzed with similar results that a lumpectomy was as effective as a mastectomy in the treatment of early breast cancer. There was a significant delay in the identification of the scientific misconduct and the publication of the reanalyzed results in 1994 (Angell & Kassirer, 1994).

Friedman identified criteria for classifying a publication as fraudulent, questionable, or valid. Research articles were classified as *fraudulent* if there was documentation or testimony from coauthors that the publication did not reflect what had actually been done" (Friedman, 1990, p. 1416). Articles were considered *questionable* if no coauthor could produce the original data or if no coauthor had personally observed or performed each phase of the research or participated in the research publication. A research article was considered valid "if some coauthor had personally performed or participated in each aspect of the research and publication" (Friedman, 1990, p. 1416).

Preventing the publication of fraudulent research will require the efforts of authors, coauthors, reviewers, and editors (Hansen & Hansen, 1995; Hawley & Jeffers, 1992; Relman, 1990). Authors who are primary investigators for research projects must be responsible in their conduct, reporting, and publication of research. Coauthors and coworkers should question and if necessary challenge the integrity of a researcher's claims. Sometimes well-known scientists have been added as coauthors to give credibility to a research publication. Individuals should not be listed as coauthors unless they were actively involved in the conduct and publication of the research. Peer reviewers have a key role in determining the quality and publishability of a manuscript. They are considered experts in the field and their role is to examine research for inconsistencies and inaccuracies. Editors need to monitor the peer review process and be cautious in their publication of manuscripts if they are at all questionable. Editors also need procedures to respond to allegations of research misconduct (Friedman, 1990). They must decide what actions to take if the journal contains an article that has proved to be fraudulent. Usually fraudulent publications require retraction notations and are not to be cited by authors in future publications. Pfeifer and Snodgrass (1990) studied the continued citation of retracted, invalid scientific literature and noted that authors frequently continued to cite retracted articles in the United States and even more so in foreign countries.

The publication of fraudulent research is a major concern in medicine and a growing concern in nursing. The decreased funds available for research and the increased emphasis on research publications could lead to an increased incidence in fraudulent publications. The following issues are relevant in addressing the problem of scientific misconduct: (1) definition of scientific fraud, (2) development of a policy, (3) identification of mechanisms to distribute the policy to scientists, (4) determination of the membership of investigating committees, (5) development of a process for notifying funding agencies and journals, (6) public disclosure of the alleged incidents, (7) identification of legal ramifications, and (8) prevention and the role of peer review (Chop & Silva, 1991). Each researcher is responsible for monitoring the integrity of his or her research protocols, results, and publications. In addition, nursing professionals need to foster a spirit of intellectual inquiry; mentor prospective scientists regarding the norms for good science; and stress quality, not quantity, in publications (Wocial, 1995).

ANIMALS AS RESEARCH SUBJECTS

The use of animals as research subjects is a controversial issue of growing concern to nurse researchers. A small but increasing number of nurse scientists are conducting physiological studies that require the use of animals. Many scientists, especially physicians, believe the current animal rights movement could threaten the future of health research. These groups are active in antiresearch campaigns and are backed by massive resources, with a treasury that was estimated at $50 million in 1988 (Pardes, West, & Pincus, 1991). Some of the animal rights groups are trying to raise the consciousness of researchers and society to ensure that animals are used wisely in the conduct of research and treated humanely.

Other animal rights groups have tried to frighten the public with sometimes distorted stories of inhumane treatment of animals in research. Some of the activist leaders have made broad comparisons between human life and animal life. For example, a major animal rights group called People for the Ethical Treatment of Animals (PETA) stated, "There is no rational basis for separating out the human animal. A rat is a pig is a dog is a boy. They're all mammals" (Pardes et al., 1991, p. 1641). Some of these activists have now progressed to violence with "physical attacks, including real bombs, arson, and vandalism" (Pardes et al., 1991, p. 1642). Even more damage is being done to research through lawsuits that have blocked the conduct of research and the development of new research centers. "Medical schools are now spending over $15 million annually for

security, public education, and other efforts to defend research" (Pardes et al., 1991, p. 1642).

Two important questions need to be addressed: (1) Should animals be used as subjects in research? (2) If animals are used in research, what mechanisms ensure that they are treated humanely? The type of research project developed influences the selection of subjects. Animals are just one of a variety of subjects used in research; others include human beings, plants, and computer data sets. If possible, most researchers will use nonanimal subjects because they are generally less expensive. If the studies are low-risk, which most nursing studies are, human beings are frequently used as subjects. However, some studies require the use of animals to answer the research question. "In practice, the selection of an animal subject means that the scientific, political, and legal arguments for using a particular animal species outweigh the scientific, cultural, and ethical arguments against its uses" (Thomas, Hamm, Perkins, Raffin, & the Stanford University Medical Center Committee on Ethics, 1988, p. 1630). Approximately 17 to 22 million animals are used in research each year and 90% of them are rodents, with the combined percentage of dogs and cats being only 1 to 2% (Pardes et al., 1991).

Since animals are deemed valuable subjects for selected research projects, what mechanisms ensure that animals are treated humanely? At least five separate types of regulations exist to protect research animals from mistreatment. "The federal government, some state governments, an independent accreditation organization, professional societies, and individual institutions are involved in ensuring that research animals are used only when necessary and only under humane conditions" (Thomas et al., 1988, p. 1632). In addition, over 700 institutions conducting health-related research have sought accreditation by the American Association for Accreditation of Laboratory Animal Care (AAALAC), which was developed to ensure the humane treatment of animals in research (Pardes et al., 1991). In conducting research, the type of subject needs to be carefully selected; and if animals are used as subjects, they require humane treatment.

■ SUMMARY

The conduct of nursing research requires not only expertise and diligence but also honesty and integrity. Conducting research ethically starts with the identification of the study topic and continues through the publication of the study. The ethical issues of conducting research have been debated for many years. This debate will probably continue because of the complexity of human rights issues, the abstractness of the codes and regulations governing research, and the variety of interpretations of these codes and regulations. Even though the phenomenon of conducting research ethically defies precise delineation, certain historical events, ethical codes, and regulations provide guidelines for nurse researchers. Two historical documents that have had a strong impact on the conduct of research are the Nuremberg Code and the Declaration of Helsinki. More recently, the Department of Health and Human Services (DHHS) (1981, 1983, 1991) has promulgated regulations that direct the ethical conduct of research. These regulations include (1) general requirements for informed consent, (2) documentation of informed consent, (3) Institutional Review Board (IRB) review of research, (4) exempt and expedited review procedures for certain kinds of research, and (5) criteria for IRB approval of research.

Conducting research ethically requires protection of the human rights of subjects. Human rights are claims and demands that have been justified in the eyes of an individual or by the consensus of a group of individuals. The human rights that require protection in research include (1) self-determination, (2) privacy, (3) anonymity and confidentiality, (4) fair treatment, and (5) protection from discomfort and harm.

The rights of the research subjects can be protected by balancing benefits and risks of a study, securing informed consent, and submitting the research for institutional review. To balance the benefits and risks of a study, the type, degree, and number of risks are examined, and the potential benefits are identified. If possible, the risks need to be minimized and the benefits maximized to achieve the best possible benefit-risk ratio. Informed consent involves the transmission of essential information, comprehension of that information, competency to give consent, and voluntary consent of the prospective subject. The guidelines for seeking consent from subjects and for institutional review are described. In institutional review, a study is examined for ethical concerns by a committee of peers called an institutional review board (IRB). The IRB conducts three levels of review—exempt, expedited, and complete.

A serious ethical problem of the 1980s and 1990s is the conduct, reporting, and publication of fraudulent research. Researchers have fabricated data and research results for publication, distorted or incorrectly reported research findings, or mismanaged the implementation of study protocols. Authors, coauthors, reviewers of research, and editors of journals must take an active role to decrease the incidence of fraudulent publications. All disciplines have a responsibility to protect the integrity of scientific knowledge.

Another current ethical concern in research is the use of animals as subjects. Some of the animal right groups with their antiresearch campaigns are threatening the future of health research. Two important questions are addressed: (1) Should animals be used as research subjects? (2) If animals are used in research, what mechanisms ensure that they are treated humanely?

References

American Nurses Association (ANA). (1985a). *Code for nurses with interpretive statements.* Kansas City, MO: American Nurses Association.

American Nurses Association (ANA). (1985b). *Human rights guidelines for nurses in clinical and other research.* (Document No. D-46 5M). Kansas City, MO: American Nurses Association.

American Psychological Association (APA). (1982). *Ethical principles in the conduct of research with human participants.* Washington, DC: American Psychological Association.

Angell, M., & Kassirer, J. P. (1994). Setting the record straight in the breast-cancer trials. *The New England Journal of Medicine, 330*(20), 1448–1449.

Arras, J. D. (1990). Noncompliance in AIDS research. *Hastings Center Report, 20*(5), 24–32.

Beecher, H. K. (1966). Ethics and clinical research. *New England Journal of Medicine, 274*(24), 1354–1360.

Berger, R. L. (1990). Nazi science: The Dachau hypothermia experiments. *New England Journal of Medicine, 322*(20), 1435–1440.

Besch, L. (1979). Informed consent: A patient's right. *Nursing Outlook, 27*(1), 32–35.

Brandt, A. M. (1978). Racism and research: The case of the Tuskegee syphilis study. *Hastings Center Report, 8*(6), 21–29.

Brent, N. J. (1990). Legal issues in research: Informed consent. *Journal of Neuroscience Nursing, 22*(3), 189–191.

Broome, M. E., & Stieglitz, K. A. (1992). The consent process and children. *Research in Nursing & Health, 15*(2), 147–152.

Bruce, S. L, & Grove, S. K. (1994). The effect of a coronary artery risk evaluation program on serum lipid values and cardiovascular risk levels. *Applied Nursing Research, 7*(2), 67–74.

Carico, J. M., & Harrison, E. R. (1990). Ethical considerations for nurses in biomedical research. *Journal of Neuroscience Nursing, 22*(3), 160–163.

Cassidy, V. R., & Oddi, L. F. (1986). Legal and ethical aspects of informed consent: A nursing research perspective. *Journal of Professional Nursing, 2*(6), 343–349.

Chamorro, T., & Appelbaum, J. (1988). Informed consent: Nursing issues and ethical dilemmas. *Oncology Nursing Forum, 15*(6), 803–808.

Chop, R. M., & Silva, M. C. (1991). Scientific fraud: Definitions, policies, and implications for nursing research. *Journal of Professional Nursing, 7*(3), 166–171.

Damrosch, S. P. (1986). Ensuring anonymity by use of subject-generated identification codes. *Research in Nursing & Health, 9*(1), 61–63.

Davis, A. J. (1989). Informed consent process in research protocols: Dilemmas for clinical nurses. *Western Journal of Nursing Research, 11*(4), 448–457.

Declaration of Helsinki. (1986). In R. J. Levine (Ed.), *Ethics and regulations of clinical research* (2nd ed., pp. 427–429). Baltimore-Munich: Urban & Schwarzenberg.

Department of Health and Human Services (DHHS). (January 26, 1981). Final regulations amending basic HHS policy for the protection of human research subjects. *Code of Federal Regulations,* Title 45 Public Welfare, Part 46.

Department of Health and Human Services (DHHS). (March 8, 1983). Protection of human subjects. *Code of Federal Regulations,* Title 45 Public Welfare, Part 46.

Department of Health and Human Services (DHHS). (1989). Final rule: Responsibilities of awardee and applicant institutions for dealing with and reporting possible misconduct in science. *Federal Register, 54,* 32446–32451.

Department of Health and Human Services (DHHS). (June 18, 1991). Protection of human subjects. *Code of Federal Regulations,* Title 45 Public Welfare, Part 46.

Douglas, S., Briones, J., & Chronister, C. (1994). The incidence of reporting consent rates in nursing research articles. *Image: Journal of Nursing Scholarship, 26*(1), 35–40.

Douglas, S., & Larson, E. (1986). There's more to informed consent than information. *Focus on Critical Care, 13*(2), 43–47.

Floyd, J. (1988). Research and informed consent: The dilemma of the cognitively impaired client. *Journal of Psychosocial Nursing and Mental Health Services, 26*(3), 13–21.

Ford, J. S., & Reutter, L. I. (1990). Ethical dilemmas associated with small samples. *Journal of Advanced Nursing, 15*(2), 187–191.

Frankena, W. K. (1973). *Ethics* (2nd ed.). Englewood Cliffs, NJ: Prentice-Hall.

Friedman, P. J. (1990). Correcting the literature following fraudulent publication. *Journal of the American Medical Association, 263*(10), 1416–1419.

Garfield, E., & Welljams-Dorof, A. (1990). The impact of fraudulent research on the scientific literature: The Stephen E. Breuning case. *Journal of the American Medical Association, 263*(10), 1424–1426.

Hansen, B. C., & Hansen, K. D. (1995). Academic and scientific misconduct: Issues for nursing educators. *Journal of Professional Nursing, 11*(1), 31–39.

Hawley, D. J., & Jeffers, J. M. (1992). Scientific misconduct as a dilemma for nursing. *Image: Journal of Nursing Scholarship, 24*(1), 51–55.

Hayter, J. (1979). Issues related to human subjects. In F. S. Downs & J. W. Fleming (Eds.), *Issues in nursing research* (pp. 107–147). Norwalk, CT: Appleton-Century-Crofts.

Henderson, J. (1990, March). When scientists fake it. *American Way,* pp. 56–101.

Hershey, N., & Miller, R. D. (1976). *Human experimentation and the law.* Germantown, MD: Aspen.

Jacobson, S. F. (1973). Ethical issues in experimentation with human subjects. *Nursing Forum, 12*(1), 58–71.

Jarrett, M., Cain, K. C., Heitkemper, M., & Levy, R. L. (1996). Relationship between gastrointestinal and dysmenorrheic symptoms at menses. *Research in Nursing & Health, 19*(1), 45–51.

Kelman, H. C. (1967). Human use of human subjects: The problem of deception in social psychological experiments. *Psychological Bulletin, 67*(1), 1–11.

Kelman, H. C. (1977). Privacy and research with human beings. *Journal of Social Issues, 33*(3), 169–195.

Larson, E. (1989). Maintaining quality in clinical research and evaluation: When corrective action is necessary. *Journal of Nursing Quality Assurance, 3*(4), 28–35.

Leino-Kilpi, H., & Tuomaala, U. (1989). Research ethics and nursing science: An empirical example. *Journal of Advanced Nursing, 14*(6), 451–458.

Levine, R. J. (1986). *Ethics and regulation of clinical research* (2nd ed.). Baltimore-Munich: Urban & Schwarzenberg.

Lind, S. E. (1990). Sounding board: Finder's fees for research subjects. *New England Journal of Medicine, 323*(3), 192–195.

McGrath, P. (1995). It's ok to say no! A discussion of ethical issues arising from informed consent to chemotherapy. *Cancer Nursing, 18*(2), 97–103.

Milgram, S. (1963). Behavioral study of obedience. *Journal of Abnormal and Social Psychology, 67*(4), 371–378.

National Commission for the Protection of Human Subjects of Biomedical and Behavioral Research. (1978). *Belmont report: Ethical principles and guidelines for research involving human subjects.* Washington, DC: U. S. Government Printing Office, DHEW Publication No. (05) 78-0012.

Nuremberg Code. (1986). In R. J. Levine (Ed.), *Ethics and regulation of clinical research* (2nd ed., pp. 425–426). Baltimore-Munich: Urban & Schwarzenberg.

Nusbaum, J. G., & Chenitz, W. C. (1990). A grounded theory study of the informed consent process for pharmacologic research. *Western Journal of Nursing Research, 12*(2), 215–228.

Oddi, L. F., & Cassidy, V. R. (1990). Nursing research in the United States: The protection of human subjects. *International Journal of Nursing Studies, 27*(1), 21–34.

Pardes, H., West, A., & Pincus, H. A. (1991). Physicians and the animal-rights movement. *New England Journal of Medicine, 324*(23), 1640–1643.

Pfeifer, M. P., & Snodgrass, G. L. (1990). The continued use of retracted, invalid scientific literature. *Journal of the American Medical Association, 263*(10), 1420–1423.

Purtilo, R. B., & Cassel, C. K. (1981). *Ethical dimensions in the health professions.* Philadelphia: Saunders.

Ramos, M. C. (1989). Some ethical implications of qualitative research. *Research in Nursing & Health, 12*(1), 57–63.

Relman, A. S. (1990). Publishing biomedical research: Roles and responsibilities. *Hastings Center Report, 20*(5), 23–27.

Reynolds, P. D. (1972). On the protection of human subjects and social science. *International Social Science Journal, 24*(4), 693–719.

Reynolds, P. D. (1979). *Ethical dilemmas and social science research.* San Francisco, CA: Josey-Bass.

Robley, L. R. (1995). The ethics of qualitative nursing research. *Journal of Professional Nursing, 11*(1), 45–48.

Rothman, D. J. (1982). Were Tuskegee and Willowbrook studies in nature? *Hastings Center Report, 12*(2), 5–7.

Sasson, R., & Nelson, T. M. (1971). The human experimental subject in context. In J. Jung (Ed.), *The experimenter's dilemma* (pp. 265–296). New York: Harper & Row.

Schaefer, J. A., & Moos, R. H. (1996). Effects of work stressors and work climate on long-term care staff's job morale and functioning. *Research in Nursing & Health, 19*(1), 63–73.

Silva, M. C. (1985). Comprehension of information for informed consent by spouses of surgical patients. *Research in Nursing & Health, 8*(2), 117–124.

Steinfels, P., & Levine, C. (1976). Biomedical ethics and the shadow of Naziism. *Hastings Center Report, 6*(4), 1–20.

Strauman, J. J., & Cotanch, P. H. (1988). Oncology nurse research issues: Overstudied populations. *Oncology Nursing Forum, 15*(5), 665–667.

Thomas, J. A., Hamm, T. E., Perkins, P. L., Raffin, T. A., & Stanford University Medical Center Committee on Ethics. (1988). Animal research at Stanford University: Principles, policies and practices. *New England Journal of Medicine, 318*(24), 1630–1632.

Thompson, P. J. (1987). Protection of the rights of children as subjects for research. *Journal of Pediatric Nursing, 2*(6), 392–399.

Twomey, J. G. (1994). Investigating pediatric HIV research ethics in the field. *Western Journal of Nursing Research, 16*(4), 404–413.

Watson, A. B. (1982). Informed consent of special subjects. *Nursing Research, 31*(1), 43–47.

Wocial, L. D. (1995). The role of mentors in promoting integrity and preventing scientific misconduct in nursing research. *Journal of Professional Nursing, 11*(5), 276–280.

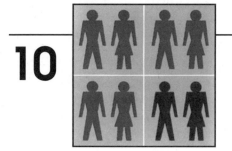

10

Understanding Research Design

A *research design* is a blueprint for conducting the study that maximizes control over factors that could interfere with the validity of the findings. The research design guides the researcher in planning and implementing the study in a way that is most likely to achieve the intended goal. The control provided by the design increases the probability that the study results are accurate reflections of reality. Skill in selecting and implementing research design is important to improving the quality of the study and thus the usefulness of the findings. Skill in identifying the study design and evaluating the threats to validity of findings due to design flaws are important parts of critiquing studies.

The term *research design* is used in two ways. Some consider research design to be the entire strategy for the study, from identifying the problem to final plans for data collection. Others limit design to clearly defined structures within which the study is implemented. In this text, the first definition refers to the research methodology and the second is a definition of the research design.

The design of a study is the end-result of a series of decisions made by the researcher concerning how the study will be implemented. The design is closely associated with the framework of the study and guides planning for implementing the study. As a blueprint, the design is not specific to a particular study. The design is a broad pattern or guide that can be applied to many studies. Just as the blueprint for a house must be individualized to the specific house being built, so must the design be made specific to a study. Using the problem statement, framework, research questions, and clearly defined variables, the design can be mapped out to provide a detailed research plan for data collection and analysis. This research plan specifically directs the implementation of the study. Developing a research plan is discussed in Chapter 15.

Elements central to the study design include the presence or absence of a treatment, number of groups in the sample, number and timing of measurements to be performed, sampling method, the time frame for data collection, planned comparisons, and control of extraneous variables. Decisions regarding the following questions lead to development of the design.

1. Is the primary purpose of the study to describe variables and groups within the study situation, to examine relationships, or to examine causality within the study situation?
2. Will a treatment be used?
3. If so, will the treatment be controlled by the researcher?
4. Will the sample be pretested before the treatment?
5. Will the sample be randomly selected?
6. Will the sample be studied as a single group or divided into groups?
7. How many groups will there be?
8. What will be the size of each group?
9. Will there be a control group?
10. Will groups be randomly assigned?
11. Will there be repeated measures of variables?
12. Will the data be collected cross-sectionally or across time?
13. Have extraneous variables been identified?
14. Are data being collected on extraneous variables?

15. What strategies are being used to control for extraneous variables?
16. What strategies are being used for comparison of variables or groups?
17. Will data be collected at a single site or at multiple sites?

Developing a design for a study requires consideration of multiple details such as the foregoing. The more carefully thought out these details are, the stronger the design. These questions are important because of their link to the logic on which research design is based. To provide you with the information necessary to understand and answer the foregoing questions, this chapter will discuss the concepts important to design, the elements of a good design, and triangulation, a relatively recent approach to research design.

CONCEPTS IMPORTANT TO DESIGN

There are many terms used in discussing research design that have special meanings within this context. An understanding of the meaning of these concepts is critical to understanding the purpose of a specific design. Some of the major concepts used in relation to design are causality, bias, manipulation, control, and validity.

CAUSALITY

The first assumption one must make in examining *causality* is that things have causes and that causes lead to effects. Some of the ideas related to causation emerged from the logical positivist philosophical tradition. Hume, a positivist, proposed that three conditions must be met in order to establish causality: (1) There must be a strong correlation between the proposed cause and the effect, (2) the proposed cause must precede the effect in time, and (3) the cause has to be present whenever the effect occurs. Cause, according to Hume, is not directly observable but must be inferred (Cook & Campbell, 1979).

Another philosophical group, essentialists, proposed that two concepts must be considered in determining causality: necessary and sufficient. The proposed cause must be necessary for the effect to occur. (The effect cannot occur unless the cause first occurs.) The proposed cause must also be sufficient (requiring no other factors) for the effect to occur. This leaves no room for a variable that may sometimes, but not always, serve as the cause of an effect.

John Stuart Mill, another philosopher, added another idea related to causation. He suggested that in addition to the above criteria for causation, there could be no alternative explanations for why a change in one variable seemed to lead to a change in a second variable (Cook & Campbell, 1979).

Causes are frequently expressed within the propositions of a theory. Testing the accuracy of these theoretical statements indicates the usefulness of the theory. A theoretical understanding of causation is considered important because it improves the ability to predict and, in some cases, to control events in the real world. The purpose of an experimental design is to examine cause and effect. The independent variable in a study is expected to be the cause, and the dependent variable is expected to reflect the effect of the independent variable.

MULTICAUSALITY

Multicausality, the recognition that a number of interrelating variables can be involved in causing a particular effect, is a more recent idea related to causality. Because of the complexity of causal relationships, a theory is unlikely to identify every variable involved in causing a particular phenomenon. A study is unlikely to include every component influencing a particular change or effect. Cook and Campbell (1979) have suggested three levels of causal assertions that must be considered in establishing causality. Molar causal laws relate to large and complex objects. Intermediate mediation considers causal factors operating between molar and micro levels. Micromediation examines causal connections at the level of small particles such as atoms. Cook and Campbell (1979) use the example of turning on a light switch causing the light to come on (molar). An electrician would tend to explain the cause of the light coming on in terms of wires and electrical current (intermediate mediation). However, the physicist would explain the cause of the light coming on in terms of ions, atoms, and subparticles (micromediation).

The essentialists' ideas of necessary and sufficient do not hold up well when one views a phenomenon from the perspective of multiple causation. The light switch may not be necessary to turn on the light if the insulation has worn off the electrical wires. Additionally, the light will not come on even though the switch is turned on if the light bulb is burned out. Although this is a rather concrete example, it is easy to relate to common situations in nursing.

Very few phenomena in nursing can be clearly pinned down to a single cause and a single effect. However, the greater the proportion of causal factors that can be identified and explored, the clearer the understanding of the phenomenon. This greater understanding will increase the ability to predict and control. For example, currently nurses have only a limited understanding of patients' preoperative attitudes, knowledge, and behaviors and their effects on postoperative attitudes and behaviors. Nurses assume that high preoperative anxiety leads to less healthy postoperative responses and that providing information before surgery will improve healthy responses in the postoperative period. Many nursing studies have examined this particular phenomenon. However, the causal factors involved are complex and have not been clearly delineated. This lack of knowledge limits the effectiveness of nursing actions in facilitating the healthiest response to the surgical experience.

PROBABILITY

The original criteria for causation required that a variable should cause an identified effect each time the cause occurred. Although this may occur in the basic sciences, such as chemistry or phys-

ics, it is unlikely to occur in the health sciences or social sciences. Because of the complexity of nursing's field, nurses deal in probabilities. *Probability* addresses relative, rather than absolute, causality. From the perspective of probability, a cause will not produce a specific effect each time that particular cause occurs.

Reasoning changes when one thinks in terms of probabilities. The researcher investigates the probability of an effect occurring under specific circumstances. Rather than seeking to prove that A causes B, a researcher would state that if A occurred, there was a 50% probability that B would occur. The reasoning behind probability is more in keeping with the complexity of multicausality. Using the surgical example, nurses could seek to predict the probability of unhealthy patient outcomes postoperatively when anxiety levels are high preoperatively.

CAUSALITY AND NURSING PHILOSOPHY

Traditional theories of prediction and control are built on theories of causality. The first research designs were also based on causality theory. Nursing science needs to be built within a philosophical framework of multicausality and probability. The strict sense of single causality and of "necessary and sufficient" are not in keeping with the progressively complex, holistic philosophy of nursing. Acquiring an understanding of multicausality and increasing the probability of being able to predict and control the occurrence of an effect will require an understanding of both wholes and parts.

Nursing knowledge for practice will require understanding of molar, intermediate mediational, and micromediational aspects of a particular phenomenon. A variety of differing approaches, reflecting both qualitative and quantitative, descriptive, and experimental research are necessary to develop a knowledge base for nursing. Explanation and causality have been seen by some as different and perhaps opposing forms of knowledge, yet these forms of knowledge need to be joined, sometimes within the design of a single study, to acquire the knowledge needed for nursing practice.

BIAS

The term *bias* means to slant away from the true or expected. A biased opinion has failed to include both sides of the question. Cutting fabric on the bias means to cut across the grain of the woven fabric. A biased witness is one who is strongly for or against one side of the situation. A biased scale is one that does not provide a valid measure.

Bias is of great concern in research because of the potential effect on the meaning of the study findings. Any component of the study that deviates or causes a deviation from true measure leads to distorted findings. Many factors related to research can be biased: the researcher, the measurement tools, the individual subjects, the sample, the data, and the statistics. Thus, an important concern in designing a study is to identify possible sources of bias and eliminate or avoid them. If they cannot be avoided, the study needs to be designed to control these sources of bias. Designs, in fact, are developed to reduce the possibilities of bias.

MANIPULATION

In nursing, manipulation tends to have a negative connotation and is associated with one person underhandedly causing another person to behave in a desired way. To *manipulate* means to move around or to control the movement of, such as manipulating a syringe. In research, manipulation is used in experimental or quasi-experimental research and is sometimes called the *treatment.* Thus, in a study on preoperative care, preoperative teaching might be manipulated so that one group received the treatment and another did not. In a study on oral care, the frequency of care might be manipulated.

In nursing research, when experimental designs are used to explore causal relationships, the nurse must be free to manipulate the variables under

study. If the freedom to manipulate a variable (e.g., pain control measures) is under the control of someone else, a bias is introduced into the study. In qualitative, descriptive, and correlational studies, no attempt is made to manipulate variables. Instead, the purpose is to describe a situation as it exists.

CONTROL

Control means having the power to direct or manipulate factors to achieve a desired outcome. The idea of control is very important in research, particularly in experimental and quasi-experimental studies. The greater the amount of control of the researcher over the study situation, the more credible the study findings. The purpose of research designs is to maximize control factors in the study situation.

STUDY VALIDITY

Study validity is a measure of the truth or accuracy of a claim and is an important concern throughout the research process. Questions of validity refer back to the propositions from which the study was developed. Thus, validity is an examination of the approximate truth or falsity of the propositions (Cook & Campbell, 1979). Is the theoretical proposition an accurate reflection of reality? Was the study designed well enough to provide a valid test of the proposition? Validity is a very complex idea that is important to the researcher and to those who read and consider using the findings in their practice. Critical analysis of research involves being able to think through threats to validity that have occurred and make judgments about how seriously these threats affect the integrity of the findings. Validity provides a major basis for making decisions about which findings are useful for patient care.

Cook and Campbell (1979) have described four types of validity: statistical conclusion validity, internal validity, construct validity, and external validity. When conducting a study, the researcher is confronted with major decisions regarding the four types of validity. In order to make decisions about validity, a variety of questions need to be addressed.

1. Is there a relationship between the two variables? (statistical conclusion validity)
2. Given that there is a relationship, is it plausibly causal from one operational variable to the other, or would the same relationship have been obtained in the absence of any treatment of any kind? (internal validity)
3. Given that the relationship is plausibly causal and is reasonably known to be from one variable to another, what are the particular cause-and-effect constructs involved in the relationship? (construct validity)
4. Given that there is probably a causal relationship from construct A to construct B, how generalizable is this relationship across persons, settings, and times? (external validity) (p. 39)

Statistical Conclusion Validity

The first step in inferring cause is to determine whether the independent and dependent variables are related. The determination of a relationship (covariation) is made through statistical analysis. *Statistical conclusion validity* is concerned with whether the conclusions about relationships or differences drawn from statistical analysis are an accurate reflection of the real world. The second step is to identify differences between groups. However, there are reasons why false conclusions can be drawn about the presence or absence of a relationship or difference. The reasons for the false conclusions are called threats to statistical conclusion validity. These threats include the following:

1. **Low Statistical Power.** Low statistical power increases the probability of concluding that there is no significant difference between samples when actually there is a difference (Type II error). A Type II error is most likely to occur when the sample size is small or when the power of the statistical test to determine differences is low. The concept of statistical power

and strategies to improve it are discussed in Chapters 12 and 16.
2. **Violated Assumptions of Statistical Tests.** Most statistical tests have assumptions about the data being used, such as assuming that the data are interval data, that the sample was randomly obtained, or that there is a normal distribution of scores to be analyzed. If these assumptions are violated, the statistical analysis may provide inaccurate results. The assumptions of each statistical procedure are provided in Chapters 17, 18, and 19.
3. **Fishing and the Error Rate Problem.** A serious concern in research is incorrectly concluding that a relationship or difference exists when it does not (Type I error). The risk of Type I error increases when the researcher conducts multiple statistical analyses of relationships or differences. This is referred to as fishing. When fishing is used, a given portion of the analyses will show significant relationships or differences simply by chance. For example, commonly, the *t*-test is used to make multiple statistical comparisons of mean differences in a single sample. This procedure increases the risk of a Type I error because some of the differences found in the sample occurred by chance and are not actually present in the population. Multivariate statistical techniques have been developed to deal with this error rate problem (Goodwin, 1984). Fishing and error rate problems are discussed in Chapter 16.
4. **The Reliability of Measures.** The technique of measuring variables must be reliable if true differences are to be found. A measure is reliable if it gives the same result each time the same situation or factor is measured. For example, a thermometer would be reliable if it showed the same reading when tested repeatedly on the same patient. If a scale is used to measure anxiety, it should give the same score if repeatedly given to the same person in a short period of time (unless, of course, repeatedly taking the same test caused anxiety to increase or decrease).
5. **The Reliability of Treatment Implementation.** If the method of administering a research

treatment varies from one person to another, the chance of detecting a true difference decreases. The lack of standardization in administering the treatment must be controlled during the planning phase by ensuring that the treatment will be provided in exactly the same way each time it is administered.

6. **Random Irrelevancies in the Experimental Setting.** Environmental (extraneous) variables in complex field settings can influence scores on the dependent variable. These variables will increase the difficulty of detecting differences. Consider the activities occurring on a nursing unit. The numbers and variety of staff, patients, crises, and work patterns merge into a complex arena for the implementation of a study. Any of the dynamics of the unit can influence manipulation of the independent variable or measurement of the dependent variable.

7. **Random Heterogeneity of Respondents.** Subjects in a treatment group can differ in ways that are correlated with the dependent variable. This difference can have an influence on the outcome of the treatment and prevent detection of a true relationship between the treatment and the dependent variable. For example, subjects may vary in response to preoperative attempts to lower anxiety because of unique characteristics associated with differing levels of anxiety.

Internal Validity

Internal validity is the extent to which the effects detected in the study are a true reflection of reality, rather than being the result of the effects of extraneous variables. Although internal validity should be a concern in all studies, it is addressed more frequently in relation to studies examining causality than in other studies. In studies examining causality, the researcher needs to determine whether the independent and dependent variables may have been caused by a third, often unmeasured, variable (an extraneous variable). The possibility of an alternative explanation of cause is sometimes referred to as a rival hypothesis. Any study can contain threats to internal validity, and these

validity threats can lead to a false-positive or false-negative conclusion. The following question needs to be considered: Is there another reasonable (valid) explanation (rival hypothesis) for the finding other than that proposed by the researcher? Threats to internal validity include the following:

1. **History.** This is an event that is not related to the planned study but occurs during the time of the study. History could influence the responses of subjects to the treatment.

2. **Maturation.** In research, maturation is defined as growing older, wiser, stronger, hungrier, more tired, or more experienced during the study. These unplanned and unrecognized changes can influence the findings of the study.

3. **Testing.** Sometimes, the effect being measured can be due to the number of times the subject's responses have been tested. The subject may remember earlier, inaccurate responses that can be modified, thus altering the outcome of the study. The test itself may influence the subject to change attitudes or increase the subject's knowledge.

4. **Instrumentation.** Effects can be due to changes in measurement instruments between the pretest and the post-test rather than an effect of the treatment. For example, a scale, accurate when the study began, could weigh subjects 2 lb. less than they actually weigh on the post-test. Instrumentation is also involved when people serving as observers or data collectors become more experienced between the pretest and the post-test, thus altering in some way the data they collect.

5. **Statistical Regression.** Statistical regression is the movement or regression of extreme scores toward the mean in studies using a pretest–post-test design. The process involved in statistical regression is difficult to understand. When a test or scale is used to measure a variable, some subjects will achieve very high or very low scores. In some studies, subjects are selected to be included in a particular group because their scores on a pretest are high or low. A treatment is then performed, and a post-test is administered. However, with no

treatment, subjects who initially achieve very high or very low scores will tend to have more moderate scores when retested. Their scores will regress toward the mean. The treatment did not necessarily cause the change. If the pretest scores were low, the post-test may show statistically significant differences (higher scores) from the pretest, leading to the conclusion that the treatment caused the change (Type I error). If the pretest scores were high, the post-test scores would tend to be lower (because of a tendency to regress toward the mean) even with no treatment. In this situation, the researcher may mistakenly conclude that there is no difference caused by the treatment (Type II error).

6. **Selection.** Selection addresses the process by which subjects are chosen to take part in a study and how subjects are grouped within a study. A selection threat is more likely to occur in studies in which randomization is not possible. In some studies, people selected for the study may differ in some important way from people not selected for the study. In other studies, the threat is due to differences in subjects selected for study groups. For example, people included in the control group could be different in some important way from people included in the experimental group. This difference in selection could lead to the two groups reacting differently to the treatment, rather than the treatment causing the differences in group responses.

7. **Mortality.** This threat is due to subjects who drop out of a study before completion. Mortality becomes a threat when those who drop out of a study are a different type of person from those who remain in the study, or when there is a difference in the kinds of people who drop out of the experimental group and the control group.

8. **Interactions with Selection.** The aforementioned threats can interact with selection to further complicate the validity of the study. The threats most likely to interact with selection include history, maturation, and instrumentation. For example, if a control group selected for the study has a different history than the experimental group has, responses to the treatment may be due to this interaction rather than to the treatment.

9. **Ambiguity About the Direction of Causal Influence.** This threat occurs most frequently in correlational studies that address causality. In a study in which variables are measured simultaneously and only once, it may be impossible to determine whether A caused B, B caused A, or the two variables interact in a noncausal way.

10. **Diffusion or Imitation of Treatments.** This threat occurs when the control group gains access to the treatment intended for the experimental group or a similar treatment available from another source. For example, suppose a study examined the effect of teaching specific information to hypertensive patients as a treatment and then measured the effect of the teaching on blood pressure readings and adherence to treatment protocols. Suppose the control group patients communicated with the experimental patients and the teaching information was shared. The control group patients' responses to the outcome measures may show no differences from those of the experimental group when the teaching actually did make a difference (Type II error).

11. **Compensatory Equalization of Treatments.** When the experimental group receives a treatment that is seen as desirable, such as a new treatment for AIDS, administrative people and other health professionals may not tolerate the difference and insist that the control group receive the treatment. If this occurs, the researcher no longer has a control group and cannot document the effectiveness of the treatment through the study. In health care, this has ethical implications on both sides.

12. **Compensatory Rivalry by Respondents Receiving Less Desirable Treatments.** In some studies, the design and plan of the study are publicly known. The control group subjects then know the expected difference between their group and the experimental group and may attempt to reduce or reverse the differ-

ence. This phenomenon may have occurred in the national hospice study funded by the Health Care Financing Administration and conducted by Brown University (Greer, Mor, Sherwood, Morris, & Birnbaum, 1983). In this study, 26 hospices were temporarily reimbursed through Medicare while a comparison of the care between hospices and hospitals was examined. The study made national headlines and was widely discussed in Congress. Health policy decisions related to reimbursement of hospice care hinged on the findings of the study. The study found no significant differences in care between the two groups although there were cost differentials. In addition to a selection threat (hospitals providing poor care to dying cancer patients were unlikely to agree to participate in the study), health care professionals in the hospitals selected may have been determined to counter the criticism that the care they provided was poor in quality. The rivalry in this situation could have influenced the outcomes of the study and thus threatened validity.

13. **Resentful Demoralization of Respondents Receiving Less Desirable Treatments.** If control group subjects believe that they are receiving less desirable treatment, they may react by withdrawing, giving up, or becoming angry. Changes in behavior resulting from this reaction rather than from the treatment can lead to differences that cannot be attributed to the treatment.

Construct Validity

Construct validity examines the fit between the conceptual definitions and operational definitions of variables. Theoretical constructs or concepts are defined within the framework (conceptual definitions). These conceptual definitions provide the basis for the development of operational definitions of the variables. Operational definitions (methods of measurement) need to reflect validly the theoretical constructs. (Theoretical constructs are discussed in Chapter 7. Conceptual and opera-

tional definitions of concepts and variables are discussed in Chapter 8.)

Is use of the measure a valid inference about the construct? Examination of construct validity determines whether the instrument actually measures the theoretical construct it purports to measure. The process of developing construct validity for an instrument often requires years of scientific work. When selecting methods of measurement, the researcher needs to determine previous development of instrument construct validity. (Instrument construct validity is discussed in Chapter 13.) The threats to construct validity are related both to previous instrument development and to the development of measurement techniques as part of the methodology of a particular study.

Threats to construct validity include the following:

1. **Inadequate Preoperational Explication of Constructs.** Measurement of a construct stems logically from a concept analysis of the construct, either by the theorist who developed the construct or by the researcher. The conceptual definition should emerge from the concept analysis, and the method of measurement (operational definition) should clearly reflect both. A deficiency in the conceptual or operational definitions leads to low construct validity.

2. **Mono-Operation Bias.** Mono-operation bias occurs when only one method of measurement is used to measure a construct. When only one method of measurement is used, fewer dimensions of the construct are measured. Construct validity is greatly improved if the researcher uses more than one instrument. For example, if anxiety were a dependent variable, more than one measure of anxiety could be used. More than one measurement of the dependent variable can often be accomplished with little increase in time, effort, or cost.

3. **Mono-Method Bias.** In mono-method bias, the researcher uses more than one measure of a variable, but all measures use the same method of recording. Attitude measures, for example, may all be paper and pencil scales. Attitudes that are personal and private may not

be detected using paper and pencil tools. Paper and pencil tools may be influenced by feelings of nonaccountability for responses, acquiescence, or social desirability. For example, construct validity would be improved if anxiety were measured by a paper and pencil test, verbal messages of anxiety, the galvanic skin response, and observer recording of incidence and frequency of behaviors that have been validly linked with anxiety.

4. **Hypothesis-Guessing Within Experimental Conditions.** Many subjects within a study can guess the hypotheses of the researcher. The validity concern is related to behavioral changes that may occur in the subjects as a consequence of knowing the hypothesis. The extent to which this modifies study findings is not presently known.

5. **Evaluation Apprehension.** Subjects wish to be seen in a favorable light by researchers. They want to be seen as competent and psychologically healthy. Their responses in the experiment may be due to this desire rather than being an effect of the independent variable.

6. **Experimenter Expectancies (Rosenthal Effect).** The expectancies of the researcher can bias the data. For example, if the researcher expected a particular intervention to be effective in pain relief, the data may reflect this expectation. If another researcher who did not believe the intervention would be effective had collected the data, results could be different. The extent to which this actually influences studies is not known. Because of this concern, some researchers are not involved in the data collection process. In other studies, data collectors do not know which subjects are assigned to treatment and control groups.

Another way to control this threat is to design the study so that data collectors differ in expectations. If the sample size is large enough, comparisons could be made in data collected by the different data collectors. Failing to determine a difference in the data collected by the two groups would give evidence of construct validity.

7. **Confounding Constructs and Levels of Constructs.** When developing the methodology of a study, the researcher makes decisions about the intensity of a variable that will be measured or provided as a treatment. The intensity of the variable measured influences the level of the construct that will be reflected in the study. These decisions can affect validity, since the method of measuring the variable influences the outcome of the study and the understanding of the constructs in the study framework.

For example, the researcher might find that variable A does not affect variable B when, in fact, it does, but not at the level of A that was manipulated, or perhaps not at the level of B that was measured. This is particularly a problem when A is not linearly related to B or when the effect being studied is weak. Control of this threat involves including several levels of A in the design and measuring many levels of B. For example, if A is preoperative teaching and B is anxiety, the instrument being used to measure anxiety may measure only high levels of anxiety. The preoperative teaching may be provided for 15 minutes when 30 minutes or an hour is required to cause significant changes in anxiety.

In some cases, there is confounding of variables, which leads to mistaken conclusions. Few measures of a construct are pure measures. Rather, a selected method of measuring a construct can measure a portion of the construct and also other related constructs. Thus, the measure can lead to confusing results, since the variable measured does not provide an accurate reflection of the construct.

8. **Interaction of Different Treatments.** The interaction of different treatments is a threat if subjects receive more than one treatment in a study. For example, a study might examine the effectiveness of pain relief measures, and subjects might receive medication, massage, distraction, and relaxation strategies. In this case, each one of the treatments will interact with the others, and the effect of any single treatment on pain relief would be impossible to ex-

tract. The findings cannot be generalized to any situation in which patients did not receive all four pain treatments.

9. **Interaction of Testing and Treatment.** In some studies, pretesting the subject is thought to modify the effect of the treatment. In this case, the findings can be generalized only to subjects who have been pretested. Although there is some evidence that pretest sensitivity does not have the extent of impact that was once feared, it needs to be considered in examining the validity of the study. One design, the Solomon Four-Group Design (discussed in Chapter 11) tests this threat to validity. Repeated post-tests can also lead to an interaction of testing and treatment.

10. **Restricted Generalizability Across Constructs.** When designing studies, the researcher needs to consider the impact of the findings on constructs other than those originally conceived in the problem statement. Often, by including another measure or two, the generalization of the findings to clinical settings and the translation back to theoretical dimensions can be much broader.

External Validity

External validity is concerned with the extent to which study findings can be generalized beyond the sample used in the study. The most serious threat would lead to the findings being meaningful only for the group being studied. To some extent, the significance of the study is dependent on the number of types of people and situations to which the findings can be applied. Sometimes, the factors influencing external validity are subtle and may not be reported in research papers; however, the researcher needs to be responsible for these factors. Generalization is usually more narrow for a single study than for multiple replications of a study using different samples, perhaps from different populations in different settings. The threats to the ability to generalize the findings (external validity) in terms of study design include the following.

1. **Interaction of Selection and Treatment.** Seeking subjects who are willing to participate in a study can be difficult, particularly if the study requires extensive amounts of time or other types of investment by subjects. If a large number of the persons approached to participate in a study decline to participate, the sample actually selected tends to be limited in ways that might not be evident at first glance. Only the researcher knows the subjects well. Subjects might tend to be volunteers, "do-gooders," or those with nothing better to do. In this case, generalizing the findings to all members of a population such as all nurses, all hospitalized patients, or all persons experiencing diabetes is not easy to justify.

The study needs to be planned to limit the investment demands on subjects in order to increase participation. The number of persons who were approached and refused to participate in the study needs to be reported so that threats to external validity can be judged. As the percentage of those who decline to participate increases, external validity decreases. Sufficient data need to be collected on the subjects so that the researcher can be familiar with the characteristics of subjects and, to the extent possible, the characteristics of those who decline to participate. Handwritten notes of verbal remarks made by those who decline and observations of behavior, dress, or other significant factors can be useful in determining selection differences.

2. **Interaction of Setting and Treatment.** Bias exists in types of settings and organizations that agree to participate in studies. This bias has been particularly evident in nursing studies. For example, some hospitals welcome nursing studies and encourage employed nurses to conduct studies. Others are resistant to the conduct of research. These two types of hospitals may be different in important ways; thus, there might be an interaction of setting and treatment that limits the generalizability of the findings. This factor needs to be considered in making statements about the population to which the findings can be generalized.

3. **Interaction of History and Treatment.** The circumstances during which a study was conducted (history) influence the treatment and thus the ability to generalize findings. Logically, one can never generalize to the future; however, replication of the study during various time periods gives further strength to the usefulness of findings across time. In critiquing studies, one needs always to consider the period of history during which the study was conducted and the impact of nursing practice and societal events during that time period on the reported findings.

ELEMENTS OF A GOOD DESIGN

The purpose of design is to set up a situation that maximizes the possibilities of obtaining accurate answers to objectives, questions, or hypotheses. The design selected needs to be appropriate to the purpose of the study, feasible given realistic constraints, and effective in reducing threats to validity. In most studies, comparisons are the basis of obtaining valid answers. A good design provides the subjects, the setting, and the protocol within which those comparisons can be clearly examined. The comparisons may focus on differences, relationships, or both. The study may require that comparisons be made between or among individuals, groups, or variables. A comparison may also be made of measures taken before a treatment (pretest) and measures taken after a treatment (post-test). Following these comparisons, the sample values are compared with statistical tables reflecting population values. In some cases, the study may involve comparing group values with population values.

Designs were developed to reduce threats to the validity of the comparisons. However, some designs are more effective in reducing threats than others. In some cases, it may be necessary to modify the design to reduce a particular threat. Before selecting a design, the researcher needs to identify the threats to validity most likely to occur in a particular study.

Strategies for reducing threats to validity are sometimes addressed in terms of control. Selecting a design involves decisions related to control of the environment, sample, treatment, and measurement. Increasing control (in order to reduce threats to validity) requires that the researcher carefully think through every facet of the design.

CONTROLLING THE ENVIRONMENT

The study environment has a major impact on research outcomes. An uncontrolled environment introduces many extraneous variables into the study situation. Therefore, the study design may include strategies for controlling that environment. In many studies, it is important that the environment be consistent for all subjects. Elements in the environment that may influence the application of a treatment or the measurement of variables need to be identified and, when possible, controlled.

CONTROLLING EQUIVALENCE OF SUBJECTS AND GROUPS

When comparisons are made, the assumption is that the individual units of the comparison are relatively equivalent except for the variables being measured. The researcher does not want to be comparing apples and oranges. To establish equivalence, sampling criteria are defined. Deviation from this equivalence is a threat to validity. Deviation occurs when sampling criteria have not been adequately defined or when unidentified extraneous variables increase variation in the group. The most effective strategy for achieving equivalence is random sampling followed by random assignment to groups. However, this strategy does not guarantee equivalence. Even when randomization has been used, the extent of equivalence needs to be examined by measuring and comparing characteristics on which the groups need to be equivalent. This comparison is usually reported in the description of the sample.

Contrary to the aforementioned need for equivalence, groups need to be as different as possible in relation to the research variables. Small differences or relationships are more difficult to distinguish than large differences. These differences are often addressed in terms of effect size. Although sample size plays an important role, effect size will be maximized by a good design. Effect size is greatest when variance within groups is small.

Control Groups

If the study includes a treatment, the design usually calls for a comparison of outcome measures of individuals who receive the treatment with those who do not receive the treatment. This comparison requires a *control group,* subjects who do not receive the treatment. One threat to validity is the lack of equivalence between the experimental and the control groups. This threat is best controlled by random assignment to groups. Another strategy used in some designs is for the subjects to serve as their own controls. Using this design strategy, pre- and post-test measures are taken of the subjects in the absence of a treatment as well as before and after the treatment. In this case, the timing of measures needs to be comparable between control and treatment conditions.

CONTROLLING THE TREATMENT

In a well-designed experimental study, the researcher has complete control of any treatment provided. The first step in achieving control is a detailed description of the treatment. The next step is to use strategies to ensure consistency in implementing the treatment. Consistency may involve such elements of the treatment as equipment, time, intensity, sequencing, and staff skill.

Variations in the treatment reduce the effect size. It is likely that subjects who receive less optimal applications of the treatment will have a re-duced response, resulting in more variance in post-test measures of the experimental group. To avoid this problem, the treatment is administered to each subject exactly the same way. This means that the researcher needs to carefully think through every element of the treatment in order to reduce variation wherever possible.

For example, if information is being provided as part of the treatment, some researchers will videotape the information, present it to each subject in the same environment, and attempt to decrease variation in the experience of the subject before and during the viewing of the videotape. This variation could include such elements as time of day, mood, anxiety, experience of pain, interactions with others, and period of time waiting.

There are many nursing studies in which the researcher does not have complete control of the treatment. It may be costly to carefully control the treatment, it may be difficult to persuade staff to be consistent in the treatment, or the time required to implement a carefully controlled treatment may seem prohibitive. The researcher may feel it is more important to examine a treatment as it is typically provided in the clinical setting. In some cases, the researcher may be studying causal outcomes of an event occurring naturally in the environment.

Regardless of the reason for the researcher's decision, internal validity is reduced when the treatment is inconsistently applied. There is an increased risk of a Type II error because of increased variance and a smaller effect size. Thus, studies with uncontrolled treatments need larger samples to reduce the risk of a Type II error. External validity may be increased if the treatment is studied as it typically occurs clinically. If a statistically significant difference is not found, it may be the case that, as the treatment is typically applied clinically, it does not have an important effect on patient outcomes. The question would still arise as to whether a difference might have been found if the treatment had been consistently applied. Another question might be whether current clinical practice in relation to the treatment is acceptable.

The researcher needs to decide whether the study is addressing outcomes when the treatment is consistently well performed or results from typical nursing practice. In other words, is the study examining nursing practice as it could be or nursing practice as it currently is?

Counterbalancing

In some studies, each subject will receive several different treatments (e.g., relaxation, distraction, or visual imagery) or various levels of the same treatment (e.g., different doses of a drug or varying lengths of relaxation time). Sometimes the application of one treatment can influence the response to following treatments, which is referred to as a *carryover effect*. If a carryover effect is known to occur, it is not advisable to use this design strategy. However, even when no carryover effect is known, the researcher may choose to take precautions against the possibility of this effect influencing outcomes. When counterbalancing is used, the various treatments are administered in random order rather than being provided consistently in the same sequence.

CONTROLLING MEASUREMENT

Measurements play a key role in the validity of a study. Measures need to have documented validity and reliability. When measurement is crude or inconsistent, variance within groups is high and it is more difficult to detect differences or relationships among groups. Thus, the study does not provide a valid test of the hypotheses. Validity is enhanced by consistent implementation of measurements. For example, each subject needs to receive the same instructions regarding completing scales. Data collectors need to be trained and observed for consistency. Designs define the timing of measures (e.g., pretest, post-test). Sometimes, the design calls for multiple measures across time. The researcher needs to specify the points in time during which measures will be taken. The research report needs to include a rationale for the timing of measures.

CONTROLLING EXTRANEOUS VARIABLES

In designing the study, it is important to identify variables not included in the design (extraneous variables) that could explain some of the variance in measurement of the study variables. In a good design, the effect of these variables on variance is controlled. Extraneous variables that are commonly encountered in nursing studies include age, education, gender, social class, severity of illness, level of health, functional status, and attitudes. For a specific study, the researcher needs to think carefully through the variables that could have an impact on that study. Design strategies used to control extraneous variables include random sampling, random assignment to groups, selecting subjects that are homogeneous in terms of a particular extraneous variable, selecting a heterogeneous sample, blocking, stratification, matching subjects between groups in relation to a particular variable, and statistical control. Table 10–1 (on pp. 238–239) identifies some recent nursing studies that have used various strategies to control extraneous variables.

Random Sampling

Random sampling increases the probability that subjects with various levels of an extraneous variable are included and are randomly dispersed throughout the groups within the study. This strategy is particularly important for controlling unidentified extraneous variables. However, whenever possible, extraneous variables need to be identified, measured, and reported in the description of the sample.

Random Assignment

Random assignment increases the probability that subjects with various levels of extraneous

Table 10–1
Studies Using Control Strategies for Extraneous Variables

Aim	Design Strategies	Extraneous Variable	Control Method

To examine the effects of standardized rest periods on the sleep–wake states of preterm infants who were convalescing (Holditch-Davis, Barham, O'Hale, & Tucker, 1995)	Random assignment
	Controlled treatment
	  Feeding schedule
	  Nap schedule
	  Bed darkened for nap
	  Nap disturbed only for urgent care
	  Checked every 15 min.
	  Awakened gently
	Trained observers
		Gestational age
		Race
		Sex
		Body size
		Multiple birth
		Chronological age on admission
		> 40 weeks gest. age
		Major congenital anomalies
		Terminal condition
			Matching
			Matching
			Matching
			Matching
			Matching
			Matching
			
			Exclusion
			Exclusion
			Exclusion

To compare the effects of a low-technology environment of care based on a nurse-managed care delivery system (special care unit [SCU] environment) with the traditional high-technology ICU environment based on a primary nursing care delivery system (Rudy, Daly, Douglas, Montenegro, Song, & Dyer, 1995)	Random assignment using biased-coin format Controlled treatment	Acuity of illness	Homogeneity
To determine the effect of exercise on subcutaneous tissue oxygen tension (Whitney, Stotts, & Goodson, 1995)	Convenience sample Repeated measures	Gender Smoking behavior Ambient temperature Humidity Fitness	Homogeneity Homogeneity Homogeneity Homogeneity Heterogeneity
Evaluate the effect of feeding a high caloric diet on food and caloric intake and body weight of tumor-bearing rats (Fredriksdottir & McCarthy, 1995)	Random assignment Experimental and control groups Controlled treatment Repeated measures	Type of rat Tumor type Gender Initial weight Light-dark cycle	Homogeneity Homogeneity Homogeneity Matching Homogeneity
To compare the individual and combined effects of jaw relaxation and music on the sensory and affective components of pain after the first postoperative ambulation (Good, 1995)	Random assignment four treatment groups, including control Tape used to explain each treatment, practice by patient, coaching, and mastery Assessment of mastery	Protocol for pain medication Preoperative anxiety Preambulatory sensation & distress	Homogeneity Statistical control Statistical control
To determine the impact over time on the cognitive and behavioral functioning of the care recipient with dementia from a home-based intervention program of active cognitive stimulation implemented by the family caregiver (Quayhagen, Quayhagen, Corbeil, Roth, & Rodgers, 1995)	Random assignment Treatment group, placebo group, control group Repeated measures Caregiver training for 12 weekly in-home sessions for treatment group Return demonstrations by caregivers Caregiver recorded weekly log of successes or problems Data collectors blinded to treatment group assignment	Stage of Alzheimer's Cognitive impairment Gender	Homogeneity Stratification Statistical control

Table 10–1
Studies Using Control Strategies for Extraneous Variables *Continued*

Aim	Design Strategies	Extraneous Variable	Control Method
Comparing the effectiveness of (a) a combination of mutual goal setting and the operant behavioral management techniques of prompting, shaping, and positive reinforcement, (b) mutual goal setting alone, and (c) usual nursing care in fostering morning self-care behaviors in dependent nursing home residents (Blair, 1995)	Random assignment of nursing homes Staff training Reacquisition-of-skills phase of 6 weeks during which staff helped subjects overcome self-care deficits 16-week phase during which staff helped subjects maintain gains in self-care	Reliance on staff to perform morning self-care Judgment by staff of capability to do tasks without assistance Cognitive intactness	Homogeneity Homogeneity Homogeneity
To examine nongenetic influences of obesity on the lipid profile and systolic and diastolic blood pressure (cross-sectionally) during two phases of development—the school-age years and adolescence—and (longitudinally) in the transition between these two developmental phases (Hayman, Meininger, Coates, & Gallagher, 1995)	Longitudinal design with cross-sectional elements random assignment for risk factor assessment Assignment of school-age twin to heavy/light group based on measure of obesity Assignment of adolescent twin to heavy/light group based on change in obesity	Genetic influences on Obesity Gender Age	Matching (twins) Heterogeneity Stratification

variables are equally dispersed in treatment and control groups. However, this dispersion needs to be evaluated whenever possible, rather than assumed.

Homogeneity

Homogeneity is a more extreme form of equivalence in which the researcher limits the subjects to only one level of an extraneous variable to reduce its impact on the study findings. In order to use this strategy, the researcher needs to have previously identified the extraneous variables. Using this strategy, the researcher might choose to include subjects with only one level of an extraneous variable in the study. For example, only subjects between the ages of 20 and 30 years may be included, or only male subjects. The study may include only breast cancer patients who have been

diagnosed within one month, are at a particular stage of their disease, and are receiving a specific treatment for cancer. The difficulty with this strategy is that it limits generalization to only those types of subjects included in the study. Findings could not justifiably be generalized to those excluded from the study.

Heterogeneity

In studies in which random sampling is not used, the researcher may attempt to obtain subjects with a wide variety of characteristics (or who are *heterogeneous*) to reduce the risk of biases. Using this strategy, subjects may be sought from multiple diverse sources. The strategy is designed to increase generalizability. Characteristics of the sample need to be described in the research report.

Table 10-2				
Example of Blocking Using Age and Ethnic Background				
Age	Ethnic Group		Experimental	Control
Under 18 years $n = 160$	African American	$n = 40$	$n = 20$	$n = 20$
	Hispanic	$n = 40$	$n = 20$	$n = 20$
	Caucasian	$n = 40$	$n = 20$	$n = 20$
	Asian	$n = 40$	$n = 20$	$n = 20$
19 to 60 years $n = 160$	African American	$n = 40$	$n = 20$	$n = 20$
	Hispanic	$n = 40$	$n = 20$	$n = 20$
	Caucasian	$n = 40$	$n = 20$	$n = 20$
	Asian	$n = 40$	$n = 20$	$n = 20$
Over 60 yrs $n = 160$	African American	$n = 40$	$n = 20$	$n = 20$
	Hispanic	$n = 40$	$n = 20$	$n = 20$
	Caucasian	$n = 40$	$n = 20$	$n = 20$
	Asian	$n = 40$	$n = 20$	$n = 20$

Blocking

In *blocking,* the researcher includes subjects with various levels of an extraneous variable in the sample but controls the numbers of subjects at each level of the variable and their random assignment to groups within the study. This is referred to as a randomized block design. The extraneous variable is then used as an independent variable in the data analysis. Therefore, the extraneous variable needs to be included in the framework and the study hypotheses. Using this strategy, the researcher might randomly assign equal numbers of subjects by three age categories (under 18 years, 18 to 60 years, and over 60 years) to each group in the study. The researcher could use blocking for several extraneous variables. For example, the study might be blocked in relation to both age and ethnic background (African American, Hispanic, Caucasian, and Asian). This could be illustrated as shown in Table 10-2.

During data analysis for the randomized block design, each cell in the analysis is treated as a group. Therefore, the cell size for each group and the effect size need to be evaluated to ensure adequate power to detect differences. A minimum of 20 subjects per group is recommended. The foregoing example would require a minimum sample of 480 subjects.

Stratification

Using *stratification,* subjects are distributed throughout the sample, using sampling techniques similar to those used in blocking, but the purpose of the procedure is even distribution throughout the sample. The extraneous variable is not included in analysis of the data. Distribution of the extraneous variable is included in the description of the sample.

Matching

Because of the importance of subjects in the control group being equivalent to subjects in the experimental group, some studies are designed to match subjects in these two groups. *Matching* is used when an experimental subject is randomly selected and a subject similar in relation to important extraneous variables is randomly selected for inclusion in the control group. Clearly, the pool of available subjects would need to be large to accomplish this. In quasi-experimental studies, matching may be performed without randomization.

Statistical Control

In some studies, it is not considered feasible to control extraneous variables through the design.

However, the researcher recognizes the possible impact of extraneous variables on variance and effect size. Therefore, measures are obtained on the identified extraneous variables. Data analysis strategies are planned that have the capacity to remove (partial out) the variance explained by the extraneous variable before performing analysis of differences or relationships between or among the variables of interest in the study. One statistical procedure commonly used for this purpose is analysis of covariance, described in Chapter 19. Although this seems to be a quick and easy solution to the problem of extraneous variables, the results are not as satisfactory as the various methods of design control.

TRIANGULATION

There has been much controversy among researchers in recent years regarding the relative validity of various approaches to research. Designing quantitative experimental studies with rigorous controls may provide strong internal validity but questionable or limited external validity. Qualitative studies may have strong external validity but questionable internal validity. A single approach to measuring a concept may be inadequate to justify a claim that it is a valid measure of a theoretical concept. Testing a single theory may leave the results open to the challenge of rival hypotheses from other theories.

Researchers have been exploring alternative design strategies that might increase the overall validity of studies. The strategy generating the most interest recently is referred to as triangulation. *Triangulation*, first used by Campbell and Fiske in 1959, is the combined use of two or more theories, methods, data sources, investigators, or analysis methods in the study of the same phenomenon. Denzin (1989) identified four types of triangulation: (1) data triangulation, (2) investigator triangulation, (3) theoretical triangulation, and (4) methodological triangulation. Kimchi, Polivka, and Stevenson (1991) have suggested a fifth type: analysis triangulation. *Multiple triangulation* is the combination of more than one of these types.

DATA TRIANGULATION

Data triangulation involves the collection of data from multiple sources for the same study. To be considered triangulation, the data must all have the same foci. The intent is to obtain diverse views of the phenomenon under study for purposes of validation (Kimchi et al., 1991). These data sources provide an opportunity to examine how an event is experienced by different individuals, groups of people, or communities; at different times; or in different settings (Mitchell, 1986). Longitudinal studies are not a form of triangulation since their purpose is to identify change. When time is triangulated, the purpose is validation of the congruence of the phenomenon across time. In order for a multiple site study to be triangulated, data from the settings must be cross-validated for multisite consistency. When person triangulation is used, data from individuals might be compared for consistency with data obtained from groups. The intent is to use data from one source to validate data from another source (Kimchi et al., 1991).

Kirkevold (1993) used data triangulation in a study of caring for patients with chronic skin disease. Data were obtained through semistructured group interviews, collection of critical incidents, and participant observation. The intent of the triangulation was to increase validity.

INVESTIGATOR TRIANGULATION

In *investigator triangulation,* two or more investigators with diverse research training backgrounds examine the same phenomenon (Mitchell, 1986). For example, a qualitative researcher and a quantitative researcher might cooperatively design and conduct a study of interest to both. Kimchi and colleagues (1991) indicate that investigator triangulation has occurred when "(a) each investigator has a prominent role in the study, (b) the expertise of each investigator is different, and (c) the expertise (disciplinary bias) of each investigator is evident in the study" (p. 365). The use of investigator triangulation removes the potential for bias that may occur in a single-investigator study (Denzin, 1989; Duffy, 1987).

Kimchi and colleagues (1991) suggest that investigator triangulation is difficult to discern from published reports. They advise that, in the future, authors claim it and describe how it was achieved in their study. They identified investigator triangulation in a study of the relationships between stress, job satisfaction, and job performance of hospital nurses (Packard & Motowidlo, 1987).

THEORETICAL TRIANGULATION

Theoretical triangulation is the use of all the theoretical interpretations "that could conceivably be applied to a given area" (Denzin, 1989, p. 241) as the framework for a study. Using this strategy, the various theoretical points of view are critically examined for utility and power. Competing hypotheses are developed based on the different theoretical perspectives and are tested using the same data set. Increased confidence is then placed in the accepted hypotheses because they have been pitted against rival hypotheses (Denzin, 1989; Mitchell, 1986). This is a tougher test of existing theory in a field of study when alternative theories are examined rather than a single test of a proposition(s) from one theory. Theoretical triangulation can lead to the development of more powerful substantive theories that have some scientific validation. Denzin recommends the following steps to achieve theoretical triangulation:

1. A comprehensive list of all possible interpretations in a given area is constructed. This will involve bringing a variety of theoretical perspectives to bear upon the phenomena at hand (including interactionism, phenomenology, Marxism, feminist theory, semiotics, cultural studies, and so on).
2. The actual research is conducted, and empirical materials are collected.
3. The multiple theoretical frameworks enumerated in Step 1 are focused on the empirical materials.

4. Those interpretations that do not bear on the materials are discarded or set aside.
5. Those interpretations that map and make sense of the phenomena are assembled into an interpretive framework that addresses all of the empirical materials.
6. A reformulated interpretive system is stated based at all points on the empirical materials just examined and interpreted. (1989, p. 241)

Currently, few nursing studies meet Denzin's criteria for theoretical triangulation, although some frameworks for nursing studies are developed to compare propositions from more than one theory. Braden (1986, 1990b) performed a competitive test of four theories: Seligman's (1975) learned helplessness theory, Baltes's (1982) instrumental passivity theory, Rosenbaum's (1983) learned resourcefulness theory, and Miller and Mangan's (1983) theory of information-seeking behavior. An outcome of this analysis was the development of the self-help model (Braden, 1990a).

METHODOLOGICAL TRIANGULATION

Methodological triangulation is the use of two or more research methods in a single study (Mitchell, 1986). The difference can be at the level of design or data collection. Methodological triangulation, the most common type of triangulation, is frequently used in the examination of complex concepts. Complex concepts of interest in nursing might include caring, hope in terminal illness, coping with chronic illness, and promotion of health.

There are two different types of methodological triangulation: (1) within-method triangulation and (2) across-method triangulation (Denzin, 1989). *Within-method triangulation* is the simplest form and is used when the phenomenon being studied is multidimensional. For example, two or three different quantitative instruments might be used to measure the same phenomenon. Conversely, two or more qualitative methods might be used. Examples of different data collection methods are questionnaires, physiological instruments, scales, interviews, and observation techniques. *Across-method* or *between-method triangulation* involves combining research strategies from two or more research traditions in the same study. For example, methods from qualitative and quantitative research might be used in the same study (Duffy, 1987; Mitchell, 1986; Morse, 1991; Porter, 1989). From these research traditions, different types of designs, methods of measurement, data collection processes, or data analysis techniques might be used to examine a phenomenon to try to achieve convergent validity.

Mitchell (1986, pp. 22–23) identified four principles to apply with methodological triangulation: "(1) the research question must be clearly focused; (2) the strengths and weaknesses of each chosen method need to complement each other; (3) the methods need to be selected according to their relevance to the phenomenon being studied; and (4) the methodological approach needs to be monitored throughout the study to make sure the first three principles are followed."

Wiener and Dodd (1993) used methodological triangulation in a prospective longitudinal study following 100 cancer patients and their families at three time periods to describe family coping and self-care during chemotherapy. The triangulation is described as follows.

"In addition to the quantitative component of this study (Dodd, Thomas, & Dibble, 1991; Dodd, Dibble, & Thomas, 1992) a 14-item structured interview, the Problem Centered Family Coping Inventory (PCFCI) (Lewis, Wood, & Ellison, 1989) was used at each data collection point, with all participating family members present. These family members remained consistent over time. All family PCFCI interviews were conducted in the family's home and by the same nurse-interviewer. Respondents were asked to 'brainstorm' problems or concerns that had occurred for the family in the last month. Using a 6-point Likert scale, respondents were then asked to select the most important problem or challenges they as a family had to deal with; how much it

distressed the family; and how satisfied they were with the way the problem/challenge was managed. Interviews were audiotaped and transcribed verbatim onto Ethnograph software. In addition, a nurse-recorder was present at each interview to write down key phrases as a backup to the audiotape system. A 5-item questionnaire was completed independently by each interviewer and recorder, who reported his/her overall impression of the interview, as well as his/her assessment of the family's willingness to be open, how well the family was managing, and any environmental factors which may have influenced the family's responses. Although the rationale of interviewing at three time periods was to determine shifts in the problems, challenges and activities that occurred over time, major shifts were not discernable. The patients' physical cancer status and the social/psychological consequences of the illness and of treatment . . . remained central at all three times.

This paper stems from the discovery by the principal investigator and coauthor (MJD) that significant findings existed in the qualitative data gleaned from the PCFCI. She enlisted the assistance of the primary author (CLW) to plumb the data for meanings and interpretations of respondents that would enrich the quantitative findings. The verbatim transcriptions of 100 family interviews (at three time periods) were scrutinized to that end. This provided a unique opportunity to partially adapt an established qualitative methodology, Grounded Theory . . . to secondary data.

Among the tenets of the Grounded Theory method is that data collection and analysis are interrelated processes. Sampling proceeds on theoretical grounds, in terms of concepts, their dimensions, and variations. Thus, pure Grounded Theory cannot proceed without analytical memos through which concepts are developed, related and tested as part of the research process, guiding the direction of continuing data collection. These requirements cannot be utilized when analyzing secondary data–especially data which have been restricted by structured interview schedules designed with a different goal in mind. Nevertheless, the coding paradigm of Grounded Theory proved to be adaptable to retrospective data and led to the emergence of the core social/psychological process of living with cancer reported by respondents in this study: tolerating the uncertainty that permeates the disease. The method also enhanced the discovery of the dimensions of that uncertainty and of the management processes people employ as they deal with the disease and its consequences. In that regard, this research collaboration is an experiment in re-examining existing data from a perspective that departs from the original intent of the research project and examining the internal consistency of a developed theoretical perspective, that of illness trajectory." (pp. 18–19)

(From Weiner, C. L., & Dodd, M. J. [1993]. Coping amid uncertainty: An illness trajectory perspective. *Scholarly Inquiry for Nursing Practice: An International Journal* 7[1], 17–35, with permission.) ■

ANALYSIS TRIANGULATION

In *analysis triangulation,* the same data set is analyzed using two or more differing analyses techniques. The purpose is to evaluate the similarity of findings. The intent is to provide a means of cross-validation of the findings (Kimchi et al., 1991).

PROS AND CONS OF TRIANGULATION

It is possible that triangulation will be the research trend of the future. However, before jumping on this bandwagon, it would be prudent to consider the implications of using these strategies. There is concern that triangulation will be used in studies for which it is not appropriate. There is additional concern that the popularization of the method will generate a number of triangulated studies that have been poorly conducted. Sohier (1988) points out that "multiple methods will not compensate for poor design or sloppy research. Ill-conceived measures will compound error rather than reduce it. Unclear questions will not become clearer" (p. 740).

The suggestion that qualitative and quantitative methods be included in the same study has generated considerable controversy in the nursing research community (Clarke & Yaros, 1988; Mitchell, 1986; Morse, 1991; Phillips, 1988a, 1988b). Myers and Haase (1989) believe the inte-

gration of these two research approaches is inevitable and essential. Clarke and Yaros (1988) suggest that combining methods is the first step in the development of new methodologies, which are greatly needed to investigate nursing phenomena. Hogan and DeSantis (1991) believe that triangulation of qualitative and quantitative methods will lead to the development of substantive theory. Phillips (1988a, 1988b) holds the position that the two methods are incompatible because they are based on different world views. If a single investigator attempted to use both methods in one study, it would be necessary to interpret the meaning of the data from two different philosophical perspectives. Because researchers tend to acquire their research training within a particular research tradition, attempts to incorporate another research tradition may be poorly achieved. Sandelowski (1995) states that "a misplaced ecumenicism, definitional drift, and conceptual misappropriation are evident in discussions of triangulation, which has become a technique for everything" (p. 569).

Mitchell (1986) identifies a number of problems that may be encountered by investigators using this method. These strategies require many observations and result in large volumes of data for analysis. The investigator needs to have the ability and desire to deal with complex design, measurement, and analysis issues with limited resources. Mitchell identifies the following concerns regarding data analysis:

- how to combine numerical (quantitative) data and linguistic or textual (qualitative) data;
- how to interpret divergent results between numerical data and linguistic data;
- what to do with overlapping concepts that emerge from the data and are not clearly differentiated from each other;
- whether and how to weight data sources; and
- whether each different method used should be considered equally sensitive and weighted equally.

Myers and Haase (1989) provide guidelines that they believe are necessary if qualitative and quantitative methods are merged. Their guidelines are based on the assumption that at least two investigators (one qualitative and one quantitative) will be involved in any study combining these two methods.

1. The world is viewed as a whole, an interactive system with patterns of information exchange between subsystems or levels of reality.
2. Both subjective and objective data are recognized as legitimate avenues for gaining understanding.
3. Both atomistic and holistic thinking are used in design and analysis.
4. The concept of research "participant" includes not only those who are the subjects of the methodology but also those who administer or operate the methodology.
5. Maximally conflicting points of view are sought with provision for systematic and controlled confrontation. Respectful, honest, open confrontation on points of view between investigators is essential. Here, conflict is seen as a positive value because it offers potential for expanding questioning and consequent understanding. Confrontation occurs between co-investigators with differing expertise who recognize that both approaches are equally valid and vulnerable. Ability to consider participants' views which may differ from the investigator's perspective is equally important. (p. 300)

Morse (1991) suggests that qualitative and quantitative methods cannot be equally weighted in a research project. The project can either be theoretically driven by qualitative methods and incorporate a complementary quantitative component, or theoretically driven by the quantitative method and incorporate a complementary qualitative component. However, each method used must be complete in itself and must meet appropriate criteria for rigor. For example, if qualitative interviews are conducted, "the interviews should be continued until saturation is reached, and the content analysis conducted inductively, rather than forcing the data into some preconceived categories to fit the quantitative study or to prove a point" (p. 121).

Morse (1991) also suggests that the greatest threat to validity of methodological triangulation is not philosophical incompatibility but the use of inadequate or inappropriate samples. The quantitative requirement for large, randomly selected samples is inconsistent with the qualitative requirement that subjects be selected based on how well they represent the phenomena of interest, and sample selection ceases when saturation of data is reached. However, she does not consider it necessary for the two approaches to use the same samples for the study. In all aspects of a methodologically triangulated study, Morse believes that strategies need to be implemented to maintain the validity for each method. Overall, Morse (1991) supports the use of methodological triangulation, believing it "will strengthen research results and contribute to theory and knowledge development" (p. 122).

Duffy (1987) suggests that triangulation, "when used appropriately, combines different methods in a variety of ways to produce richer and more insightful analyses of complex phenomena than can be achieved by either method separately" (p. 133). Coward (1990) suggests that the combining of qualitative and quantitative methods will increase support for validity. "Construct validity is enhanced when results are stable across multiple measures of a concept. Statistical conclusion validity is enhanced when results are stable across many data sets and methods of analysis. Internal validity is enhanced when results are stable across many potential threats to causal inference. External validity is supported when results are stable across multiple settings, populations and times" (p. 166).

Sandelowski (1995) recommends that "the concept of triangulation ought to be reserved for designating a technique for conformation employed within paradigms in which convergent and consensual validity are valued and in which it is deemed appropriate to use information from one source to corroborate another. Whether triangulation or not, the purpose, method of execution, and assumptions informing any research combinations should be clearly delineated" (p. 573).

SUMMARY

Research design is a blueprint for the conduct of a study that maximizes control over factors that could interfere with the desired outcomes from studies. The design of a study is the end-result of a series of decisions made by the researcher concerning how the study will be implemented. Elements central to the study design include the presence or absence of a treatment, number of groups in the sample, number and timing of measurements to be performed, sampling method, the time frame for data collection, planned comparisons, and control of extraneous variables.

Selecting a design requires an understanding of certain concepts: causality, bias, manipulation, control, and validity. In causality, there is an assumption that things have causes and that causes lead to effects. Nursing science needs to be built within a philosophical framework of multicausality and probability. Multicausality is the recognition that a number of interrelating variables can be involved in causing a particular effect. Probability deals with the likelihood that a specific effect will occur following a particular cause. Bias is of great concern in research because of the potential effect on the meaning of the study findings. Any component of the study that deviates or causes a deviation from true measure leads to distorted findings. Manipulation means to move around or to control the movement, such as the manipulation of the independent variable. If the freedom to manipulate a variable is under the control of someone else, a bias is introduced into the study. Control means having the power to direct or manipulate factors to achieve a desired outcome. The greater the amount of control of the researcher over the study situation, the more credible the study findings.

Validity is a measure of the truth or accuracy of a claim. When conducting a study, the researcher is confronted with major decisions regarding four types of validity: statistical conclusion validity, internal validity, construct validity, and external validity. Statistical conclusion validity is concerned with whether the conclusions about relationships drawn from statistical analysis are an accurate reflection of the real world. However, there are reasons why false conclusions can be drawn about the presence or absence of a relationship; these are called threats to statistical conclusion validity. Internal validity is the extent to which the effects detected in the study are a true reflection of reality, rather than being a result of the effects of extraneous variables. Any study can have threats to internal validity, and these validity threats can lead to a false-positive or false-negative conclusion. Construct validity examines the fit between the conceptual definitions and operational definitions of variables. The threats to construct validity are related to both previous instrument development and the development of measurement techniques as part of the methodology of a particular study. External validity is concerned with the extent to which study findings can be generalized beyond the sample used in the study. The most serious threat would lead to the findings being meaningful only for the group being studied.

The purpose of design is to set up a situation that maximizes the possibilities of obtaining valid answers to research questions or hypotheses. The design selected needs to be appropriate to the purpose of the study, feasible given realistic constraints, and effective in reducing threats to validity. In most studies, comparisons are the basis of obtaining valid answers. A good design provides the subjects, the setting, and the protocol within which these comparisons can be clearly examined. Designs were developed to reduce threats to the validity of the comparisons. However,

continued

continued

some designs are more effective in reducing threats than others. Selecting a design involves decisions related to control of the environment, the sample, the treatment, and measurement.

An uncontrolled environment introduces many extraneous variables into the study situation. The study design may include strategies for controlling that environment. When comparisons are made, the assumption is that the individual units of the comparison are relatively equivalent except for the variables being measured. To establish equivalence, sampling criteria are defined. Deviation occurs when sampling criteria have not been adequately defined or when unidentified extraneous variables result in deviation in parts of the sample. The most effective strategy for achieving equivalence is random sampling followed by random assignment to groups. If the study includes a treatment, the design usually calls for a comparison of outcome measures of individuals who receive the treatment with those who do not receive the treatment. This comparison requires a control group, subjects who do not receive the treatment. One threat to validity is the lack of equivalence between the experimental and the control groups.

In a well-designed experimental study, the researcher has complete control of any treatment provided. The first step in achieving control is a detailed description of the treatment. The next step is to use strategies to ensure consistency in implementing the treatment. When the subject will receive several different treatments or various levels of the same treatment, counterbalancing is used. The various treatments are administered in random order. Designs define the timing of measures (e.g., pretest, post-test). Sometimes, the design calls for multiple measures across time.

In designing the study, it is important to identify variables not included in the design (extraneous variables) that could explain some of the variance in measurement of the study variables. In a good design, the effect of these variables on variance is controlled. Design strategies used to control extraneous variables include random sampling, random assignment to groups, selecting subjects that are homogeneous in terms of a particular extraneous variable, selecting a heterogeneous sample, blocking, stratification, matching subjects between groups in relation to a particular variable, and statistical control.

Researchers have been exploring alternative design strategies that might increase the overall validity of studies. The strategy generating the most interest recently is referred to as triangulation. Triangulation is the combined use of two or more theories, methods, data sources, investigators, or analysis methods in the study of the same phenomenon. Five types of triangulation have been identified: data triangulation, investigator triangulation, theoretical triangulation, methodological triangulation, and analysis triangulation.

There is concern that triangulation will be used in studies for which it is not appropriate. There is additional concern that the popularization of the method will generate a number of triangulated studies that have been poorly conducted. The suggestion that qualitative and quantitative methods be included in the same study has generated considerable controversy in the nursing research community. Some hold that the two methods are incompatible because they are based on different world views. Because researchers tend to acquire their research training within a particular research tradition, attempts to incorporate another research tradition may be poorly achieved. A number of problems may be encountered by investigators using this method. Other researchers believe that combining the two methods has great promise for strengthening research results and contributing to theory and knowledge development.

References

Baltes, M. M. (1982). Environmental factors in dependency among nursing home residents: A social ecology analysis. In T. A. Wills (Ed.), *Basic processes in helping relationships* (pp. 405–425). New York: Academic Press.

Blair, C. E. (1995). Combining behavior management and mutual goal setting to reduce physical dependency in nursing home residents. *Nursing Research, 44*(3), 160–165.

Braden, C. J. (1986). Self-help as a learned response to chronic illness experience: A test of four alternative theories. (Doctoral dissertation, University of Arizona, Tucson). *Dissertation Abstracts International, 47*(9-B), 3704, March 1987.

Braden, C. J. (1990a). A test of the self-help model: Learned response to chronic illness experience. *Nursing Research, 39*(1), 42–47.

Braden, C. J. (1990b). Learned self-help response to chronic illness experience: A test of three alternative learning theories. *Scholarly Inquiry for Nursing Practice, 4*(1), 23–42.

Campbell, D. T., & Fiske, D. W. (1959). Convergent and discriminant validation by the multitrait-multimethod matrix. *Psychological Bulletin, 56*(2), 81–105.

Clarke, P. N., & Yaros, P. S. (1988). Research blenders: Commentary and response. *Nursing Science Quarterly, 1*(4), 147–149.

Cook, T. D., & Campbell, D. T. (1979). *Quasi-experimentation: Design and analysis issues for field settings.* Chicago: Rand McNally.

Coward, D. D. (1990). Critical multiplism: A research strategy for nursing science. *Image: Journal of Nursing Scholarship, 22*(3), 163–167.

Denzin, N. K. (1989). *The research act: A theoretical introduction to sociological methods* (3rd ed.). New York: McGraw-Hill.

Dodd, M., Dibble, S., & Thomas, M. (1992). Outpatient chemotherapy: Patients' and family members' concerns and coping strategies. *Public Health Nursing, 9*(1), 37–44.

Dodd, M., Thomas, M., & Dibble, S. (1991). Self care for patients experiencing cancer chemotherapy side effects: A concern for home care nurses. *Home Healthcare, 9*(6), 21–26.

Duffy, M. E. (1987). Methodological triangulation: A vehicle for merging quantitative and qualitative research methods. *Image: Journal of Nursing Scholarship, 19*(3), 130–133.

Fredriksdottir, N., & McCarthy, D. O. (1995). The effect of caloric density of food on energy intake and body weight in tumor-bearing rats. *Research in Nursing & Health, 18*(4), 357–363.

Good, M. (1995). A comparison of the effects of jaw relaxation and music on postoperative pain. *Nursing Research, 44*(1), 52–57.

Goodwin, L. D. (1984). Increasing efficiency and precision of data analysis: Multivariate vs. univariate statistical techniques. *Nursing Research, 33*(4), 247–249.

Greer, D. S., Mor, V., Sherwood, S., Morris, J. M., & Birnbaum, H. (1983). National hospice study analysis plan. *Journal of Chronic Disease, 36*(11), 737–780.

Hayman, L. L., Meininger, J. C., Coates, P. M., & Gallagher, P. R. (1995). Nongenetic influences of obesity on risk factors for cardiovascular disease during two phases of development. *Nursing Research, 44*(5), 277–283.

Hogan, N., & DeSantis, L. (1991). Development of substantive theory in nursing. *Nursing Education Today, 11*(3), 167–171.

Holditch-Davis, D., Barham, L. N., O'Hale, A., & Tucker, B. (1995). Effect of standard rest periods on convalescent preterm infants. *Journal of Gynecologic and Neonatal Nursing, 24*(5), 424–432.

Kimchi, J., Polivka, B., & Stevenson, J. S. (1991). Triangulation: Operational definitions. *Nursing Research, 40*(6), 364–366.

Kirkevold, M. (1993). Toward a practice theory of caring for patients with chronic skin disease. *Scholarly Inquiry for Nursing Practice, 7*(1), 37–57.

Lewis, F., Wood, H., & Ellison, E. (1989). [Family impact study: The impact of cancer on the family.] Unpublished preliminary analysis report.

Miller, S. M., & Mangan, C. (1983). Interacting effects of information and coping style in adapting to gynecologic stress: Should the doctor tell all? *Journal of Personality and Social Psychology, 45*(1), 223–236.

Mitchell, E. S. (1986). Multiple triangulation: A methodology for nursing science. *Advances in Nursing Science, 8*(3), 18–26.

Morse, J. M. (1991). Approaches to qualitative-quantitative methodological triangulation. *Nursing Research, 40*(1), 120–123.

Myers, S. T., & Haase, J. E. (1989). Guidelines for integration of quantitative and qualitative approaches. *Nursing Research, 38*(5), 299–301.

Packard, J. S., & Motowidlo, S. J. (1987). Subjective stress, job satisfaction, and job performance of hospital nurses. *Research in Nursing & Health, 10*(4), 253–261.

Phillips, J. R. (1988a). Research issues: Research blenders. *Nursing Science Quarterly, 1*(1), 4–5.

Phillips, J. R. (1988b). Dialogue on research issues: Diggers of deeper holes. *Nursing Science Quarterly, 1*(4), 149–151.

Porter, E. J. (1989). The qualitative-quantitative dualism. *Image: Journal of Nursing Scholarship, 21*(2), 98–102.

Quayhagen, M. P., Quayhagen, M., Corbeil, R. R., Roth, P. A., & Rodgers, J. A. (1995). A dyadic remediation program for care recipients with dementia. *Nursing Research, 44*(3), 153–159.

Rosenbaum, M. (1983). Learned resourcefulness as a behavioral repertoire for the self-regulation of internal events: Issues and speculations. In M. Rosenbaum, C. Franks, & Y. Jaffe (Eds.), *Perspectives on behavior therapy in the eighties* (pp. 54–73). New York: Springer.

Rudy, E. B., Daly, B. J., Douglas, S., Montenegro, H. D., Song, R., & Dyer, M. A. (1995). Patient outcomes for the chronically critically ill: Special care unit versus intensive care unit. *Nursing Research, 44*(6), 324–331.

Sandelowski, M. (1995). Triangles and crystals: On the geometry of qualitative research. *Research in Nursing & Health, 18*(6), 569–574.

Seligman, M. E. P. (1975). *Helplessness: On depression, development, and death.* San Francisco: Freeman.

Sohier, R. (1988). Multiple triangulation and contemporary nursing research. *Western Journal of Nursing Research, 10*(6), 732–742.

Whitney, J. D., Stotts, N. A., & Goodson, W. H. III. (1995). Effects of dynamic exercise on subcutaneous oxygen tension and temperature. *Research in Nursing & Health, 18*(2), 97–104.

Wiener, C. L., & Dodd, M. J. (1993). Coping amid uncertainty: An illness trajectory perspective. *Scholarly Inquiry for Nursing Practice: An International Journal, 7*(1), 17–35.

11

Selecting a Research Design

The purpose of a design is to achieve greater control and thus improve the validity of the study in examining the research problem. Determining the appropriate research design for a study requires integrating many elements of the study. The individual critiquing a nursing study is confronted with a similar dilemma. Many published studies do not identify the design used in the study. Identifying the design may require putting together bits of information from various parts of the research report. The questions at the beginning of Chapter 10 will be helpful in selecting a design or identifying the design of a study for a critique. This chapter describes the designs most commonly used in nursing research using the categorization of studies described in Chapter 3 of descriptive, correlational, quasi-experimental, and experimental. Descriptive and correlational designs examine variables in natural environments and do not include researcher-designed treatments. Quasi-experimental and experimental designs examine the effects of an intervention by comparing differences between groups who have received the intervention and those who have not received the intervention. As you review the designs, note the threats to validity controlled by the design, keeping in mind that uncontrolled threats in the design you choose may weaken the validity of your study. Table 11–1 (on p. 250) lists the designs discussed in this chapter. After describing the designs, a series of decision trees are provided to assist in the selection of the appropriate design, or the identification of the design used in published studies for purposes of critique.

Designs have been developed by researchers to meet unique research needs as they emerged.

The first experimental designs were developed in the 1930s by Sir Ronald A. Fisher (1935) and published in a book entitled *The Design of Experiments*. However, most work on design has been conducted in the last 30 years (Abdellah & Levine, 1979; Anderson & McLean, 1974; Cook & Campbell, 1979; Cox, 1958). During this time, designs have become much more sophisticated and varied. There is no universal standard for categorizing designs. Names of designs change as they are discussed by various authors. Researchers sometimes merge elements of several designs to meet the research needs of a particular study. From these, new designs sometimes emerge.

Originally, only experimental designs were considered of value. In addition, many believe the only setting in which an experiment can be conducted is a laboratory, which allows much stricter controls to be maintained than does a field or natural setting. This is appropriate for the natural sciences but not for the social sciences. From the social sciences have emerged additional quantitative designs (descriptive, correlational, and quasi-experimental) and qualitative designs.

At present, nurse researchers are using designs developed in other disciplines that meet the needs of that discipline. Will these designs be effective in adding to nursing's knowledge base? These designs are a useful starting point, but nurse scientists need to go beyond these designs to develop designs that will more appropriately meet the needs of nursing's knowledge base. To go beyond the present designs, nurse scientists need to have a working knowledge of available designs and the logic on which they are based. Designs created to

Table 11–1 Research Designs

Descriptive Designs
   Typical Descriptive Study Design
   Comparative Descriptive Design
   Time Dimensional Designs
      Longitudinal Designs
      Cross-Sectional Designs
      Trend Designs
      Event-Partitioning Designs
   Case Study Design
Correlational Designs
   Descriptive Correlational Design
   Predictive Design
   Model Testing Designs
Quasi-Experimental Designs
   Nonequivalent Control Group Designs
      The One-Group Post-test–Only Design
      The Post-test–Only Design with Nonequivalent Groups
      The One-Group Pretest–Post-test Design
      The Untreated Control Group Design with Pretest and Post-test
      The Removed-Treatment Design with Pretest and Post-test
      The Reversed-Treatment Nonequivalent Control Group Design with Pretest and Post-test
   Interrupted Time-Series Designs
      Simple Interrupted Time Series
      Interrupted Time Series with a Nonequivalent No-Treatment Control Group Time Series
      Interrupted Time Series with Multiple Replications
Experimental Study Designs
   Pretest–Post-test Control Group Design
   Post-test–Only Control Group Design
   Randomized Block Design
   Factorial Designs
   Nested Designs
   Crossover or Counterbalanced Designs
   Randomized Clinical Trials

meet nursing needs need to be congruent with nursing philosophy. They need to provide means to examine dimensions of nursing within a holistic framework and allow examination of nursing dimensions across time. Designs need to be developed that can seek answers to important nursing questions rather than answering only questions that can be examined by existing designs.

Innovative design strategies are beginning to appear within nursing research. The use of time series analysis strategies (described later in the chapter) holds great promise for examining important dimensions of nursing. Developing designs to study the outcomes of prevention interventions is also important for nursing. However, nurse researchers need to see themselves as credible scientists in order to dare to develop new design strate-

gies that facilitate examination of little understood aspects of nursing. Developing a new design requires careful consideration of possible threats to validity and ways to diminish them. Design development also requires a willingness to risk the temporary failures that are always inherent in developing something new.

DESCRIPTIVE STUDY DESIGNS

Descriptive studies (see Table 11–1) are designed to gain more information about characteristics within a particular field of study. Their purpose is to provide a picture of situations as they naturally happen. A descriptive design may be used for the purpose of developing theory, identifying prob-

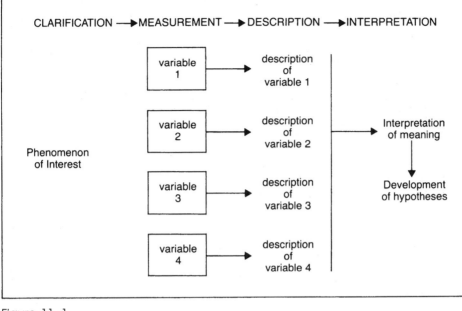

CLARIFICATION ➝ MEASUREMENT ➝ DESCRIPTION ➝ INTERPRETATION

Figure 11-1
Descriptive study design.

lems with current practice, justifying current practice, making judgments, or determining what others in similar situations are doing (Waltz & Bausell, 1981). No manipulation of variables is involved. Dependent and independent variables should not be used within a descriptive design because there is no attempt to establish causality. In many aspects of nursing there is a need for a clearer delineation of the phenomenon before causality can be examined.

Descriptive designs vary in levels of complexity. Some contain only two variables, whereas others may include multiple variables. The relationships among variables are identified to obtain an overall picture of the phenomenon being examined, but examination of types and degree of relationships is not the primary purpose of a descriptive study. Protection against bias is achieved through (1) linkages between conceptual and operational definitions of variables, (2) sample selection and size, (3) valid and reliable instruments, and (4) data collection procedures that achieve some environmental control.

TYPICAL DESCRIPTIVE STUDY DESIGN

The most commonly used design within the category of descriptive studies is presented in Figure 11-1. The design is used to examine characteristics of a single sample. The design includes identifying a phenomenon of interest, identifying the variables within the phenomenon, developing conceptual and operational definitions of the variables, and describing the variables. The description of the variables leads to an interpretation of the theoretical meaning of the findings and provides knowledge of the variables and the population that can be used for future research in the area.

Very few studies use a typical descriptive design; however, many contain descriptive components. An example of a descriptive design is Zahr and Balian's (1995) study of responses of premature infants to routine nursing interventions and noise in the NICU. The following describes the design of the study.

■

"This study documents the effects of routine nursing procedures and loud noise events on the behavioral and physiological responses of premature infants in the neonatal intensive care unit (NICU). The subjects were 55 premature infants ranging in weight from 480 to 1930 g and in age from 23 to 37 weeks gestation. Nineteen nursing activities common in the NICU as well as loud noises such as alarms, telephones, loud speech, or infant crying were recorded every 5 minutes. The infants' physiological and behavioral responses were recorded at 5-minute intervals for 2 hours in the morning and 2 hours in the evening. Nursing interventions and noise results in significant changes in both the behavioral and physiological responses of infants. The presence of noise alone and nursing interventions alone resulted in similar physiological responses; however, the combination of these events was not cumulative. Infants changed their behavioral states an average of six times each hour during the 12 observation periods, and the number of enduring states (10 minutes or longer) averaged 10 times in the 48 observation periods of 4 hours." (p. 179) ■

COMPARATIVE DESCRIPTIVE DESIGN

The comparative descriptive design (see Figure 11–2) examines and describes differences in variables in two or more groups that occur naturally in the setting. Descriptive statistics and inferential statistical analyses may be used to examine differences between or among groups. The results obtained from these analyses are frequently not generalized to a population. An example of this design is the Prescott, Soeken, and Griggs (1995) study "Identification and referral of hospitalized patients in need of home care." The following describes the study.

■

"The purpose of this exploratory study was to determine the degree to which patients with identifiable levels of need for services were referred for home health care and if selected clinical and functional status measures are useful in distinguishing need for service. Using a convenience sample of 145 patients ready for hospital discharge, data were collected on physical function, dependency at discharge, perceived helpfulness of others, social support, readiness for self-care, and planned adherence to treatment as well as demographic and medical variables. Using a combination of study variables, 93% of patients not in need of services could be correctly classified. In addition, patients in need of service but not referred by their physicians were found to differ significantly from patients not in need of care on all dimensions." (p. 85) ■

TIME DIMENSIONAL DESIGNS

Time dimensional designs were developed within the discipline of epidemiology, in which the oc-

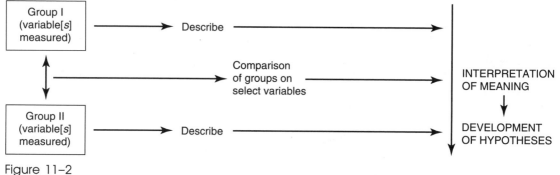

Figure 11–2
Comparative descriptive design.

currence and distribution of disease among populations are studied. These designs examine sequences and patterns of change, growth, or trends across time. The dimension of time, then, becomes an important factor. Within the field of epidemiology, the samples in time dimensional studies are called *cohorts*. Cohorts were originally age categories; however, the idea has been expanded to include many other variables. Other means of classifying populations that have relevance in relation to time include time of diagnosis, point of entry into a treatment protocol, point of entry into a new lifestyle, or age at which the subject started smoking. An understanding of temporal sequencing is an important prerequisite to examining causality between variables. Thus, the results of these designs lead to the development of hypotheses and are often forerunners of experimental designs.

Epidemiological studies that use time dimensional designs are developed to determine the risk factors or causal factors of illness states. Cause determined in this manner is called *inferred causality*. The best-known studies in this area are those on smoking and cancer. Because of the strength of multiply repeated studies, the causal link is strong. The strategy is not as powerful as experimental designs in supporting causality; however, in this situation, as in many others, one can never ethically conduct a true experiment.

Epidemiologists use two strategies to examine a situation across time: retrospective studies and prospective studies. The norm in epidemiological studies is to use the term cohort in reference to groups of subjects in prospective studies; but it is generally not used in retrospective studies. In retrospective studies, both the proposed cause and the proposed effect have already occurred. For example, the subjects could have a specific type of cancer and the researcher could be searching for commonalities among subjects that may have led to the development of that type of cancer. In a prospective study, causes may have occurred, but the proposed effect has not.

The Framingham study is the best-known example of a prospective study (USDHHS, 1968). In this study, members of a community were followed for 20 years by researchers who examined such variables as dietary patterns, exercise, weight, and blood lipid levels. As the subjects developed illnesses, such as heart disease, hypertension, or lung disease, their illnesses could be related to previously identified variables.

Prospective studies are considered more powerful than retrospective studies in inferring causality, because it can be demonstrated that the risk factors occurred prior to the illness and are positively related to the illness. These are important designs for use in nursing studies because a person's responses to health situations are patterns that developed long before the health situation occurred (Newman, 1986). These patterns then influence responses to nursing interventions.

Several designs are used to conduct time dimensional studies: longitudinal, cross-sectional, trend, and treatment partitioning.

Longitudinal Designs

Longitudinal designs examine changes in the same subjects over an extended period of time. This design is sometimes called a *panel design* (Figure 11–3). Longitudinal designs are expensive and require researcher and subject commitment over a long period of time. The area to be studied, the variables, and their measurement need to be clearly identified before data collection begins.

	Time 1	Time 2	Time 3	Time 4	Time . . *n*
	measure variables	measure variables	measure variables	measure variables	measure variables
	Sample 1	Sample 1	Sample 1	Sample 1	Sample 1

Figure 11–3
Longitudinal design.

Measurement needs to be carefully planned and implemented since repeated measures will be used across time. If children are being studied, the measures need to be valid across all the ages being studied. The researcher needs to be familiar with how the construct being measured is patterned across time, and clear rationale is given for the points of time selected for measurement. There is often a bias in selection of subjects because of the requirement for a long-term commitment. In addition, loss of subjects (mortality) can be high and can lead to decreased validity of findings.

Power analysis needs to be calculated based on the number of subjects expected to complete the study, not the number recruited initially. The researcher needs to invest considerable energy in developing effective strategies for maintaining the sample; some strategies for this purpose are discussed in Chapter 10. The period of time over which subjects will be recruited into the study needs to be carefully planned and a time line needs to be developed depicting data collection points for each subject in order to plan the numbers and availability of data collectors. If this is not carefully thought out, data collectors may be confronted with the need to continue to recruit new subjects while they are simultaneously attempting to collect data scheduled for subjects recruited earlier. Decisions also need to be made about whether all data from a particular subject will be collected by a single data collector or a different data collector will be used at each point to insure that data are collected blind.

Because of the large volumes of data acquired in a longitudinal study, careful attention needs to be placed on strategies for managing the data. Because of the repeated measures, data analysis is carefully thought through. Analyses commonly used are repeated-measures analyses of variance, multivariate analyses of variance (MANOVA), regression analysis, cluster analysis, and time series analysis (Barnard, Magyary, Booth, & Eyres, 1987).

An example of a longitudinal design is Bloom's (1995) study "The development of attachment behaviors in pregnant adolescents." The following is an abstract of that study.

"The development of attachment behaviors over time in a group of pregnant adolescents, ages 12–19, was investigated with Rubin's theoretical framework. Seventy-nine low-income pregnant adolescents enrolled in the study in their first trimester. Follow-up data were collected in the second and third trimesters . . . and after delivery. . . . Multivariate analysis, using profile analysis, indicated that maternal attachment in adolescents begins in pregnancy and increases over time, especially after quickening. Age-related differences were noted in the development of maternal-fetal attachment behaviors related to giving of self. Results showed a positive relationship between attachment in the third trimester and demonstration of affectionate behaviors toward the infant after birth. These findings are consistent with the theoretical framework." (p. 284) ∎

Cross-Sectional Designs

Cross-sectional designs are used to examine groups of subjects in various stages of development simultaneously (Figure 11–4). The assumption is that the stages are part of a process that will progress across time. Selecting subjects at various points in the process will provide important information about the totality of the process, even though the same subjects are not followed through the entire process. The processes of development selected for the study might be related to age, position in an educational system, growth pattern, or stages of maturation or personal growth (if these could be clearly enough defined to develop criteria for inclusion within differentiated groups). Subjects are then categorized by group, and data on the selected variables are collected at a single point in time.

For example, one might wish to study grief reactions at various periods after the death of a spouse. Using a cross-sectional design, a group of individuals whose spouse had died 1 week ago could be tested, another whose loss was 6 months ago, another 1 year, another 2 years, and another 5 years. All these groups could be studied at one time period, but a pattern of grief reactions over

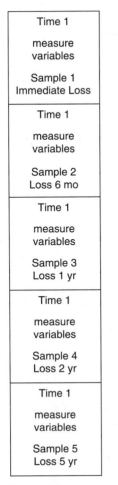

Figure 11–4
Cross-sectional study design.

Gottlieb and Baillies (1995) conducted a cross-sectional study of firstborns' behaviors during a mother's second pregnancy. The following is an abstract of their study.

"Distress and autonomy behaviors were examined in 80 preschool children of pregnant mothers and nonexpectant mothers. Four groups of only children participated: three groups of 20 children of expectant mothers who were in their early, middle, or late stages of pregnancy and a comparison group of 20 children of nonexpectant mothers. The groups were balanced for age (young: 18–36 months; old: 37–60 months) and sex. At 12 weeks, young firstborn girls were more dependent than either young boys or older girls and boys. Firstborns in the middle pregnancy group were more dependent at 20 weeks than at 24 and 28 weeks; however, boys reacted more to separation and expressed more anger than did girls. During the late phase of pregnancy, boys reacted to separation more negatively than girls did only at 28 weeks. Old firstborns were generally more autonomous than young firstborns; however, by the 32 week of pregnancy, the groups did not differ. Compared with children in the comparison group, those in the early pregnancy group showed fewer reactions to separation, and those in the middle pregnancy group were less dependent at 24 and 28 weeks. At 38 weeks of pregnancy, late pregnancy boys reacted less to separation and expressed less anger than did comparison group boys. Late pregnancy girls were angrier than boys in both the comparison and pregnancy groups." (p. 356) ■

a 5-year period could be described. The design is not as strong as the longitudinal design but allows some understanding of the phenomenon over time when time allowed for the study is limited.

Aaronson and Kingry (1988) describe a strategy for mixing cross-sectional data and longitudinal data to maximize the strengths of both designs. In their study of health behavior and beliefs during pregnancy, data were collected cross-sectionally on subjects, subjects were asked to recall previous attitudes, and a small portion of the sample were followed longitudinally in order to validate the cross-sectional findings.

Trend Designs

Trend designs examine changes in the general population in relation to a particular phenomenon (Figure 11–5). Different samples of subjects are selected from the same population at preset intervals of time, and, at each selected time, data are collected from that particular sample. The researcher needs to be able to justify generalizing from the samples to the population under study.

Time 1	Time 2	Time 3	Time 4	Time .. n
measure variables	measure variables	measure variables	measure variables	measure variables
Sample 1	Sample 2	Sample 3	Sample 4	Sample .... n

$\longrightarrow$ PREDICTION

Figure 11–5
Trend study design.

Analysis will involve strategies to predict future trends from examination of past trends. An example of this design is Wilbur, Zoeller, Talashek, and Sullivan's (1990) study, "Career trends of master's-prepared family nurse practitioners." They described their design as follows.

"The study consisted of FNPs (family nurse practitioners) who had completed graduate studies between 1974 and 1984 . . . A structured survey questionnaire was used to obtain information on employment, NP practice, professional, and demographic variables . . . A second questionnaire was used to structure the past employment and demographic variables . . . The subjects were asked to recall employment information for a maximum of four jobs held since graduation . . . To identify and compare career trends, the decision was made to group graduating classes into three cohorts representing the early, intermediate, and recent graduates. To identify career trends, the role characteristics of both the first job held following graduation and the present job were examined." (pp. 71–72) ■

Event-Partitioning Designs

A merger of the cross-sectional or longitudinal and trend designs is used in some cases to increase sample size and to avoid the effects of history on the validity of findings. Cook and Campbell (1979) refer to these as cohort designs with *treatment partitioning* (see Figures 11–6 and 11–7). The term *treatment* is used loosely here to mean a key event that is thought to lead to change. In a descriptive study, the researcher would not cause or manipulate the key event, but rather clearly define it so that when it occurred naturally it would be recognized.

For example, the event-partitioning design could be used to study subjects who have completed programs to stop smoking. Smoking behaviors and incidence of smoking-related diseases might be measured at intervals of 1 year for a 5-year period. However, the number of subjects available at one time period might be insufficient for adequate analysis of findings. Therefore, subjects from several programs offered at different times could be used. Data would be examined in terms of the relative length of time since the subjects' completion of the stop-smoking program, not the absolute length of time. Data are assumed to be comparable, and a larger sample size is available for analysis of changes across time. An example of this design is Lepczyk, Raleigh, and Rowley's (1990) study, "Timing of preoperative patient teaching."

"The convenience sample was selected from a population of patients who presented themselves for preoperative classes before coronary artery bypass surgery at two large metropolitan hospitals. Group 1 (from one hospital, $n = 32$) received teaching 2–7 days prior to hospital admission. Group 2 (from the other hospital, $n = 42$) received teaching on the afternoon of hospital admission. Seventy-four patients consented to participate. Data were collected over 8 months." (p. 302) ■

CASE STUDY DESIGN

The *case study design* involves an intensive exploration of a single unit of study: a person, family, group, community, or institution or a very small

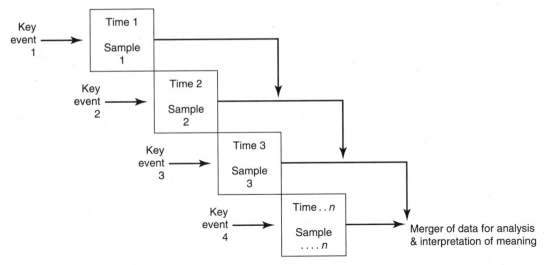

Figure 11-6
Cross-sectional study with treatment partitioning.

number of subjects who are examined intensively. Although the number of subjects tends to be small, the number of variables involved is usually large. In fact, it is important to examine all variables that might have an impact on the situation being studied.

Case studies were a commonly used design in nursing 30 years ago but appear in the literature less frequently today. Well-designed case studies are a good source of descriptive information and can be used as evidence for or against theories. A variety of sources of information can be collected on each concept of interest using different data collection methods. This strategy can greatly ex-

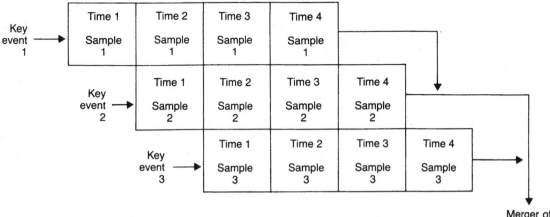

Figure 11-7
Longitudinal design with treatment partitioning.

pand the understanding of the phenomenon under study. Case studies are also useful in demonstrating the effectiveness of specific therapeutic techniques. In fact, the reporting of a case study can be the vehicle by which the technique is introduced to other practitioners. The case study design also has potential for revealing important findings that can generate new hypotheses for testing. Thus, the case study can lead to the design of large sample studies to examine factors identified by the case study.

The design of a case study is dependent on the circumstances of the case but usually includes an element of time. History and previous behavior patterns are usually explored in detail. As the case study proceeds, the researcher may become aware of components important to the phenomenon being examined that were not originally built into the study. A case study is likely to have both quantitative and qualitative elements, and these components need to be incorporated into the study design. Organizing the findings of a case study into a coherent whole is a difficult but critical component of the study. Generalization of study findings in the statistical sense is not appropriate; however, generalizing the findings to theory is appropriate and important (Barnard, Magyary, Booth, & Eyres, 1987; Yin, 1984).

An example of a case study design is Lewis's (1995) study, "One year in the life of a woman with premenstrual syndrome: A case study." The following is an abstract of that study.

◼️▬▬▬▬▬▬▬▬▬▬▬▬▬▬▬▬▬▬▬

"Over the course of 1 year (13 menstrual cycles), data were collected on a daily basis using Likert-scale ratings of symptom presence and severity, as well as narrative journal entries. The participant was a 37-year-old healthy woman (mean cycle length = 26.7 days, *SD* ± 1.8) with prospectively screened well-defined premenstrual syndrome (PMS), not on hormones or other drugs, and without a psychiatric history. Using the autocorrelation function (ACF), there was evidence for a statistically significant predictive cycle-to-cycle symptom pattern (ACF *r* = .49, *p* < .05; Bartlett Band range of significance = ± .13).

Cycle-phase–dependent coexistence of symptoms was noted, along with particular narrative themes, most dramatically exemplified by the theme of death. For this subject, the findings provided evidence for predictive symptom patterns and an effect of symptom presence on her interpretation of her environment and herself." (p. 111) ◼️

SURVEYS

There are two ways in which the term *survey* is used within scientific thought. It is used in a broad sense to mean any descriptive or correlational study. In this sense, survey tends to mean nonexperimental. In a narrower sense, survey is used to describe a technique of data collection in which questionnaires (collected by mail or in person) or personal interviews are used to gather data about an identified population. Surveys are used to gather data that can be acquired through self-report. Because of this limitation in data, some researchers view surveys as rather shallow and as contributing in a limited way to scientific knowledge. This belief has led to a bias in the scientific community against survey research. Used this way, the term survey is used in a derisive way. However, surveys can be an extremely important source of data. In this text, the term survey is used to designate a data collection technique, not a design. Surveys can be used within many designs, including descriptive, correlational, or quasi-experimental studies.

CORRELATIONAL STUDIES

Correlational studies examine relationships between variables. This examination can occur at several levels. The researcher can seek to describe a relationship, predict relationships among variables, or test the relationships proposed by a theoretical proposition. In any correlational study, a representative sample needs to be selected for the study, a sample reflecting the full range of scores possible on the variables being measured. In correlational designs, a large variance in the variable scores is necessary to determine the existence of a relationship. Therefore, correlational designs are unlike experimental designs, in which variance in variable scores is controlled (limited).

In correlational designs, if the range of scores is truncated, the obtained correlation will be artificially depressed. Truncated means that the lowest scores and the highest scores are not measured or are condensed and merged with less extreme scores. For example, if an attitude scale were scored from a low score of 1 to a high score of 50, truncated scores might indicate only scores in the range from 10 to 40. More extreme scores would be combined with scores within the designated range. If this occurs, the researcher may not find a correlation when the variables are actually correlated.

Neophyte researchers tend to make two serious errors with correlational studies. First, they often attempt to establish causality by correlation, reasoning that if two variables are related, one must cause the other. Second, they confuse studies in which differences are examined with studies in which relationships are examined. Although the existence of a difference assumes the existence of a relationship, the design and statistical analysis of studies examining differences are different from those examining relationships. When one is examining two or more groups in terms of one or more

variables, one is examining differences between groups as reflected in scores on the identified variables. When one is examining a single group in terms of two or more variables, one is examining relationships between variables. In a correlational study, the relationship examined is that between two or more research variables within an identified situation.

DESCRIPTIVE CORRELATIONAL DESIGN

The purpose of a descriptive correlational design is to examine the relationships that exist in a situation. Using this design will facilitate the identification of many interrelationships in a situation in a short period of time. These studies are also used to develop hypotheses for later studies (see Figure 11–8). The study may examine variables in a situation that has already occurred or a currently occurring situation. No attempt is made to control or manipulate the situation. As with descriptive studies, variables need to be clearly identified and defined. An example of a descriptive correlational design is Robinson and Kaye's (1994) study examining the relationships among spiritual perspective, social support, and depression in caregiving and noncaregiving wives. The following is an abstract of their study.

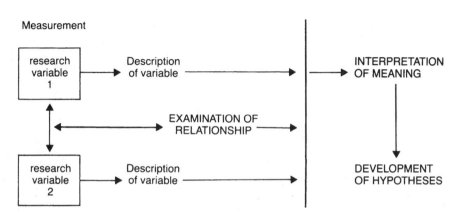

Figure 11–8
Descriptive correlational design.

"The purpose of this study was to compare the relationships between spiritual perspective, social support, and depression in two groups of adults: caregiving wives of dementia victims and noncaregiving wives of healthy adults. Hypotheses predicted that increased spiritual perspective would be associated with increased social support and decreased depression in caregiving wives. Hypotheses also predicted that spiritual perspective would be more strongly associated with these variables in caregiving wives. Spiritual perspective was not significantly related to social support or depression in the caregivers. The relationships between these variables, however, were noted to be stronger in caregiving wives than in noncaregivers. Employment and increased availability of support were associated with decreased depression in caregivers." (p. 375) ■

PREDICTIVE DESIGN

Predictive designs are developed to predict the value of one variable based on values obtained from another variable(s). Prediction is one approach to examining causal relationships between variables. Since causal phenomena are being examined, the terms *dependent* and *independent* are used to describe the variables. One variable is classified as the dependent variable and all other variables as independent variables. The aim of a predictive design (see Figure 11–9) is to predict the level of the dependent variable from the independent variables. Independent variables most effective in prediction are highly correlated with the dependent variable but not highly correlated with other independent variables used in the study. Predictive designs require the development of a theory-based mathematical hypothesis proposing variables expected to predict the dependent variable effectively. The hypothesis is then tested using regression analysis.

Johnson (1995) conducted a predictive correlational study to examine healing determinants in older people with leg ulcers. The ankle brachial pressure index (ABPI) was measured using the Medasonics ultrasound stethoscope. The Edema Index was a 4-point index ranging from 0 (no evidence of swelling) to 3 (severe swelling of the limb). The Wound Status Index consisted of four levels of characteristics—black (necrosis) = 1, yellow (exudate/yellow necrosis) = 2, red (revascularization granulation tissue present) = 3, and pink (new tissue, reepithelialization) = 4. The Pain in Mobility Index from the Functional Status Index (FSI) was used to determine pain when mobilizing. Bandage compression measurement was achieved with a medical stocking tester Kompritest II. The Time Use Pilot Survey was used to determine the number of hours per day the affected limb was in various positions (elevated, horizontal, dependent, and walking). Healing or monthly changes in surface area were measured by stereophotogrammetry. The Self-Efficacy scale and the Medical Outcomes Study Social Support scale were administered. Cognitive function was assessed using the Short Portable Mental Status questionnaire. Hierarchical multiple regression procedures were used to examine the amount of variance in healing rate explained by each set of variables—physiologic, therapeutic, and psychosocial. Their findings were abstracted as follows.

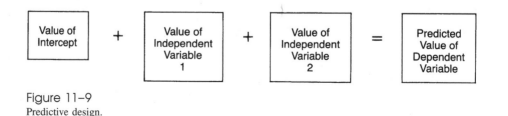

Figure 11–9
Predictive design.

"A regression model with healing rate as the dependent variable explained 49% of the variance. Increased pain when mobilizing, increased hours with limbs horizontal to the torso, and moderate and severe liposclerosis (hardening and induration of the skin) were associated with poorer healing rates. Higher wound status scores were associated with more rapid healing rates. Self-efficacy beliefs and social support were not significant factors. The findings suggest the need for early detection and management of limb pain that interferes with normal mobility. Limb position and edema assessment prior to the application of compression bandages is recommended, with bandages that provide clients with high compression when ambulant and low compression when resting being potentially beneficial." (p. 395) ■

MODEL TESTING DESIGNS

Some studies are designed specifically to test the accuracy of a hypothesized causal model. The design requires that all variables relevant to the model be measured. A large, heterogeneous sample is required. All the paths expressing relationships between concepts are identified and a conceptual map is developed (see Figure 11–10). The analysis determines whether or not the data are consistent with the model. In some studies, data from some subjects are set aside and not included in the initial path analysis. These data are used to test the fit of the paths defined by the initial analysis in another data set.

Variables are classified into three categories: exogenous variables, endogenous variables, and residual variables. Exogenous variables are within the theoretical model but are caused by factors outside of this model. Endogenous variables are those whose variation is explained within the theoretical model. Exogenous variables influence the variation of endogenous variables. Residual variables indicate the effect of unmeasured variables not included in the model. These variables explain some of the variance found in the data but not the variance within the model (Mason-Hawkes & Holm, 1989).

In Figure 11–10, paths are drawn demonstrating directions of cause and effect. The arrows (paths) from the exogenous variables 1, 2, and 3 lead to the endogenous variable 4, indicating that

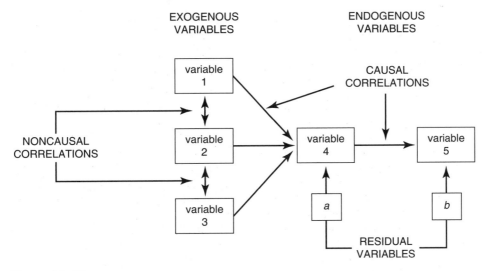

Figure 11–10
Model testing design.

variable 4 is theoretically proposed to be caused by variables 1, 2, and 3. The arrow (path) from endogenous variable 4 to endogenous variable 5 indicates that variable 4 causes variable 5.

Exogenous and endogenous variables are measured by collecting data from the experimental subjects, and the accuracy of the proposed paths is analyzed. Initially, these analysis procedures were performed using a series of regression analyses. Now, statistical procedures have been developed specifically for path analysis using LISREL and EQS. These computer programs are described in Chapter 19. Path coefficients are calculated that indicate the effect one variable has on another. The amount of variance explained by the model as well as the fit between the path coefficients and the theoretical model indicates the accuracy of the theory. Variance not accounted for in the statistical analysis is attributed to residual variables (variables *a* and *b*) not included in the analyses (Mason-Hawkes & Holm, 1989).

An example of this design is Pohl, Boyd, Liang, and Given's (1995) study, "Analysis of the impact of mother-daughter relationships on the commitment to caregiving." Exogeneous variables were mother's level of disability and mother-daughter relationships (attachment and conflict). Endogeneous variables were (step 1) employment and living arrangements and (step 2) instrumental commitment (direct care and supervising care) and affective commitment (positive and negative beliefs). Step 1 variables were proposed to explain step 2 variables. The following is the abstract from that study.

"Path analysis was used to test a model to examine the impact of mother-daughter relationships on the commitment to caregiving by 98 adult daughters during the first three months. Findings generally supported the model. Although significant, magnitude of mothers' limitations did not solely explain commitment, either instrumental or affective. Mother-daughter relationships were powerful predictors of commitment, especially affective commitment. Although predicted, employment status did not function as a mediator in this model, while living arrangements did." (p. 68) ■

DEFINING THERAPEUTIC NURSING INTERVENTIONS

In quasi-experimental and experimental studies, an intervention (or protocol) is developed that is expected to result in differences in post-test measures of the treatment and control or comparison groups. This intervention may be physiologic, psychosocial, educational, or a combination of these and should be designed to maximize the differences between the groups. Thus, it should be the best intervention that could be provided in the circumstances of the study, an intervention that is expected to improve the outcomes of the experimental group.

The methodology for designing interventions for nursing studies has not been adequately addressed in the nursing literature. In addition, descriptions of nursing interventions in published studies lack the specificity and clarity given to describing measurement instruments (Egan, Snyder, & Burns, 1992). To some extent, this may reflect nursing's state of knowledge regarding the provision of nursing interventions in clinical practice. Clinical nursing interventions are not well defined; thus, different terminology may be used by each nurse to describe a particular intervention. In addition, an intervention tends to be applied differently in each case by a single nurse and even less consistently by different nurses.

NURSING INTERVENTIONS CLASSIFICATION (NIC)

The Iowa Intervention Project is currently addressing this inconsistency by developing a Nursing Interventions Classification (NIC) in which a standardized language is used to describe treatments performed by nurses (Bulechek & McCloskey, 1994; Caldwell, 1994; Daly, McCloskey, &

Bulechek 1994; Iowa Intervention Project, 1992a, 1992b, 1993, 1995; McCloskey & Bulechek, 1993, 1994a, 1994b; Moorhead, McCloskey, & Bulechek, 1993; Tripp-Reimer, Woodworth, McCloskey, & Bulechek, 1996). The taxonomy has a three-tiered hierarchical structure with the top level including six domains, the second level 27 classes, and the third level more than 400 interventions. The domains include physiological: basic; physiological: complex, behavioral, family, health system, and safety. Each intervention consists of a label, a definition, and a set of activities performed by nurses carrying out the intervention. The intervention labels were derived from nursing education and nursing practice. The research methods used to develop the classification included content analysis, surveys, focus groups, similarity analysis, and hierarchical clustering. Field testing of the interventions is ongoing at five clinical sites.

Tripp-Reimer and colleagues (1996), in their analysis of the structure of the NIC interventions, identified three dimensions: focus of care, intensity, and complexity. High intensity of care would be associated with the physiological illness level of the patient and the emergent nature of the illness. The dimension of intensity of care includes indicators of (1) intensity (or acuity) and (2) whether the care is typical or novel. The dimension of focus of care addresses (1) the target of the intervention—ranging from the individual to the system, (2) whether the care action is direct or on behalf of the patient, and (3) the continuum of practice from independent to collaborative actions. The dimension of complexity of care includes continua of degree of knowledge, skill, and urgency of the interventions.

The interventions in the NIC need to be subjected to multiple studies examining the effects on different populations and the effects of varying degrees of intensity. Links need to be established between the intervention and outcomes at varying points in time after the intervention has been implemented. Researchers could develop a program of research examining these issues in relation to a selected intervention. Studies are also needed to determine the outcomes of each intervention. Outcomes that occur immediately following the intervention are easiest to determine. However, the most important outcomes may be those that occur after discharge from care, or several weeks or months after the intervention. This information is critical to justifying nursing actions in a cost-conscious market (Stewart & Archbold, 1992, 1993). For a more extensive discussion of the importance of linking interventions with outcomes measures, see Chapter 21.

DESIGNING AN INTERVENTION FOR A NURSING STUDY

The therapeutic nursing intervention provided in a nursing study needs to be carefully designed, clearly described, and well linked to the outcome measures (dependent variables) to be used in the study. Each of these dimensions needs to be considered to develop consistency of the intervention. The intervention needs to be provided consistently to all subjects. In some studies, controlling consistency may involve developing a step-by-step protocol. Educational treatments, or educational components of treatments, might be audio or videotaped for consistency.

The first step in designing an intervention should be a thorough review of the clinical and research literature related to the intervention. Because of the sparsity of information in the literature on nursing interventions, the researcher(s) may need to place considerable reliance on a personal knowledge base emerging from expertise in clinical practice. The nursing actions which are included in the intervention need to be spelled out sequentially to the extent needed for other nurses to be able to follow the description and provide the intervention in a consistent manner. The intervention needs to be consistent in such areas as content, intensity, and length of time. If a number of caregivers are involved in providing the intervention, care must be taken to protect the integrity of the intervention. A pilot study may be needed to refine the intervention so that it can be applied consistently.

Kirchhoff and Dille (1994) described their efforts to maintain the integrity of their nursing intervention as follows.

"In 1983 a study was conducted on the Rehabilitation Nursing Unit at University of Utah Hospital to test the effectiveness of a decontamination procedure on vinyl urinary leg and bed bags. Rehabilitation patients with bladder dysfunction use two urine bags, a daytime leg bag (for concealment under clothing) and a nighttime larger-volume bed bag. Because the usually closed urinary drainage system is disrupted at least twice daily, a procedure for decontamination was necessary if the bags were to be reused safely rather than discarded daily.

The solution instilled into bags daily was a 1:3 solution of bleach to water with a contact time of at least 30 minutes (Hashisaki, 1984). Based on that study's results of effective decontamination, the bag replacement schedule was changed from daily to weekly at a considerable savings.

Four years later cost-conscious nurses proposed a 4-week in-hospital reuse for the bags. Because the bags are marketed as single-use disposable items, this time frame needed to be carefully tested." (p. 32)

"In the decontamination study, the frequency, regularity, and daily nature of the intervention called for several individuals participating solely from a scheduling perspective. Because of the long-term nature of this study (3-year funding period), vacation time and other leave time had to be considered.

Discussion occurred about using a select group of nurses to administer the intervention. Those chosen would be highly motivated, trained in the protocol, and monitored in their performance. This decision would have enhanced the internal validity of the study. However, the trade-off would be a decrease in the external validity of the study. Another approach would have been to involve the entire nursing staff of the unit. This would be an advantage because 24-hour staffing and 7-day-a-week coverage would be ensured. . . . The disadvantage of involvement of the entire staff is reflected in the consistency of the implementation. The disad-vantage is compounded by the possibility of variable unit staffing and the use of per diem staff who may be unfamiliar with the intervention. The focal point of implementation of the study then becomes an issue of managing the staff." (pp. 33–34)

"In this study, communication occurred with the obvious: the Rehabilitation Unit nursing staff, the attending physicians, nursing and hospital administration, and the epidemiology nurses. Inadvertently, the not so obvious did not receive or recall study information: the per diem nurses who floated to the unit, the rehabilitation residents who rotated in and out of the unit every 3 months, and the housekeepers. These three groups of people had the potential to influence results, affect subject accrual, and contribute to missing or altered data if they were not informed about the study requirements. Per diem staff either had not been taught about the protocol or performed the former standard for the procedure. Residents who were not informed believed that the study would limit a patient's progression in bladder management and were reluctant to have their patients entered into the study. At times the housekeepers inadvertently discarded the drainage equipment as it was air drying, which resulted in the loss of data and affected costs of the grant.

For the per diem staff, regular staff performed the procedure when the charge nurse assigned a study patient to per diem nurses. Per diem staff who regularly came to the Rehabilitation Unit were in-serviced and were approved to do the procedure after successful return demonstrations. In addition, investigators attended a staff meeting of per diem nurses to inform them about requirements of the study. The residents and the housekeepers were in-serviced, and residents were given weekly reports on patients' progress." (p. 34)

"Using the procedure as a performance checklist, observations of the staff's performance of the procedure were completed before and during the study at least every 6 months. At the same time, the study progress was reviewed and the staff was questioned about activities they were required to perform for the study. These included how to label and use the bags, what to do when problems arise, the criteria for inclusion in the study, and the differences between the experimental and control groups. On subsequent observations, this time period also was used to discuss reported or discovered concerns about the individual's performance.

Despite the intensive planning and compliance checks, problems arose. Housekeeping personnel discarded bags that were air-drying. Per diem staff discarded the bags, performed the procedure incorrectly, or neglected to do it at all. Discoveries were made by the nursing staff or study staff that bags had been mislabeled, applied to the wrong patient, or had incomplete information on the bag label. When a few staff devised a method of hanging the leg bag to dry by knotting its tubing, the effect of air-drying was reduced. In all these instances, individual staff members were contacted and the situation was corrected.

Although it appears that a number of problems were uncovered, close monitoring showed these problems before there was major impact on the integrity of the study. When close monitoring does not occur, a lack of problems may really be a lack of discovery. A false sense of security can result." (pp. 35–36)
(From Kirchhoff, K. T., & Dille, C. A. (1994). Issues in intervention research: Maintaining integrity. *Applied Nursing Research*, 7(1) 32–46, with permission.) ∎

Difficulties in implementing the protocol as designed may also occur because of situational problems or environmental effects. Egan and colleagues (1992) describe problems they encountered in implementing their intervention and means of assessing the problem.

∎

"When conducting a pilot intervention study with persons in a care unit for patients with Alzheimer's disease, we became acutely aware of the need to attend to the execution of protocols. We developed very precise protocols for hand massage, therapeutic touch, and presence to examine their effectiveness in decreasing agitation behavior in persons in advanced stages of dementia. Initially, after each treatment session the researcher recorded comments about the implementation of the protocol. After reading the comments made during the first week of the study, the researchers became aware that the protocol had not always been implemented as it had been designed. Subjects' interactions differed from day to day; these changes prevented the researcher from performing the intervention in the same manner each day. Differentiation in the degree of implementation of the protocol was needed for analyses. Otherwise, the findings would not reflect the effect of the specific intervention. We developed a rating system that would allow the intervener to rate, on a 5-point scale, the degree to which the protocol was carried out during that session. Although these subjects posed unique problems because of their severe cognitive impairment, researchers using other populations may encounter similar problems in trying to implement precise protocols. Did some subjects fall asleep during the intervention? Was it necessary to shorten the time for the intervention because a subject had fatigue or pain? Was a teaching plan changed to adapt to a subject's specific needs? Few reports provide information regarding protocol adaptations made during the studies.

A second area that has an impact on the effectiveness of the independent variable is the environment in which the intervention is performed. Because most nursing intervention studies are conducted in clinical settings, control over many environmental variables is not always possible. When conducting the study with persons in advanced stages of dementia, we realized that variations in the environment affected the desired outcomes. Although we sought a quiet place for conducting the intervention, distractions were not uncommon. For example, another resident would enter the subject's room to see what was happening or some resident would pull on the subject's sleeve or arm. It also was difficult to control for noise. Therefore, we developed a 3-point scale for rating the environment." (p. 189) ∎

QUASI-EXPERIMENTAL STUDY DESIGNS

The purpose of quasi-experimental and experimental designs is to examine causality. The power of the design to accomplish this purpose is dependent on the degree to which the actual effects of the experimental treatment (the independent variable) can be detected by measurement of the dependent variable. Obtaining an understanding of the true effects of an experimental treatment requires action to control threats to the validity of the findings. Threats to validity are controlled through selection of subjects, control of the environment, manipulation of the treatment, and reliable and valid measurement of the dependent variables.

Experimental designs with their strict control of variance are the most powerful method of examining causality. However, in social science research, for many reasons—ethical and practical—experimental designs cannot always be used. Quasi-experimental designs were developed to provide alternate means for examining causality in situations not conducive to experimental controls. *Quasi-experimental designs* were first described as a group by Campbell and Stanley in 1963 at a time when only experimental designs were considered of any worth. Cook and Campbell expanded this description in 1979. The quasi-experimental designs facilitated the search for knowledge and examination of causality in situations in which complete control is not possible. These designs have been developed to control as many threats to validity as possible in a situation in which at least one of the three components of true experimental design (random sampling, control groups, and manipulation of the treatment) is lacking.

There are differences of opinion in nursing regarding the classification of a particular study as quasi-experimental or experimental. The experimental designs emerged from a logical positivist perspective with the purpose of determining cause and effect. The focus is on determining differences between groups using statistical analyses based on decision theory (see Chapter 16 for an explanation of decision theory). The true experimental design (from a logical positivist view) requires the use of random sampling to obtain control and experimental groups, rigorous control of the treatment, and designs that controlled threats to validity. A less rigorous type of experimental design, referred to

as comparative experimental designs, are being used by some researchers in nursing and medicine, in clinical situations in which the expectation of random sampling is difficult if not impossible to achieve. These studies use convenience samples with random assignment to groups. For example, clinical trials do not use randomly obtained samples but tend to be considered experimental in nature. The rationale for classifying these studies as experimental is that these studies have internal validity if the two groups are comparable on variables important to the study even though there are biases in the original sample. However, threats to statistical conclusion validity and threats to external validity by the nonrandom sample are not addressed by these designs. Threats to external validity have not, in the past, been considered to be a serious concern since these threats do not effect the claim that the treatment caused a difference, but rather effect the ability to generalize the findings. The importance of external validity, although discounted in the past, is taking on greater importance in the current political and health policy climate. See Chapter 21 on outcomes research for a discussion of concerns related to the validity of clinical trials. In this text, we focus on the ideal on which the experimental designs were based. Studies without random samples will continue to be classified as quasi-experimental. However, because of the difficulty in finding examples of experimental studies in nursing using random samples, some of our examples of particular experimental designs will not have random samples. Please keep in mind that nursing scholars have differing opinions on this issue. We recommend more dialogue related to this issue in the nursing literature.

Each of the quasi-experimental designs described below has threats to validity owing to constraints in controlling variance. Some achieve greater amounts of control than others. When choosing designs, one selects the design that offers the greatest amount of control possible within the study situation. Even the first designs described in this section, which have very low power in terms of establishing causality, can provide useful information on which to design later studies.

NONEQUIVALENT CONTROL GROUP DESIGNS

Random selection is the only acceptable way of maximizing the probability of equivalence between groups. A nonequivalent control group is one in which the control group is not selected by random means. Some groups are more nonequivalent than others, and some quasi-experimental designs involve using groups (control and treatment) that evolved naturally rather than being developed randomly. These groups cannot be considered equivalent because the individuals in the control group may be different from individuals in the treatment group. Individuals have selected the group in which they are included rather than being selected by the researcher. Thus, selection becomes a threat to validity.

The approach to statistical analysis is problematic in quasi-experimental designs. Although many researchers use the same approaches to analysis as are used for experimental studies, the selection bias inherent in nonequivalent control groups makes this a questionable practice. Reichardt (1979) recommends using multiple statistical analyses to examine the data from various perspectives and to compare levels of significance obtained from each analysis. The researcher needs to carefully assess the potential threats to validity in interpreting statistical results since statistical analysis cannot control for threats to validity. The following are examples of nonequivalent control group designs.

The One-Group Post-test–Only Design

This design is referred to as pre-experimental rather than quasi-experimental because of its weaknesses and the numerous threats to validity. It is inadequate for making causal inferences (see Figure 11–11). In this design, no attempt is usually made to control the selection of those who receive the treatment (the experimental group). Generalization of findings beyond those tested is

Manipulation of independent variable	Measurement of dependent variable(s)
TREATMENT ————————————————➤	**POST-TEST**

Treatment—often ex post facto

Experimental group—those who receive the treatment and the post-test

Pretest—inferred—norms of measures of dependent variables(s) of population from which pretreatment experimental group taken

Control group—implied—norms of measures of dependent variables(s) of population from which experimental group taken

Approach to Analysis: • comparison of post-test scores with inferred norms
• confident inferences about change

Example: Lamb (1979). Effect of positioning of postoperative fractured-hip patients as related to comfort.

Uncontrolled threats to validity: • no link between treatment and change
• no control group
• maturation
• undetected confounding variables
• inabilty to assess threats to validity

Figure 11–11
One-group post-test–only design.

difficult to justify. The group is not pretested; therefore, there is no direct way to measure change. The researcher cannot claim that the post-test score was a consequence (effect) of the treatment when scores before the treatment are unknown. Because there is no control group, one does not know whether groups not receiving the treatment would have similar scores on the dependent variable. This one-group post-test–only design is commonly used by the inexperienced researcher to evaluate a treatment program or a nursing intervention.

Cook and Campbell (1979) suggest situations in which the one-group post-test–only design can be appropriate and adequate for inferring causality. For example, this design could be used to determine that a single factory's use of vinyl chloride is causing an increase in neighborhood and employee cancers. The incidence of cancer in the community at large is known. The fact that vinyl chloride causes cancer and the types of cancer caused by it are also known. These norms would then take the place of the pretest and the control group. Thus, in order to use this design intelligently, one needs to know a great deal about causal factors interacting within the situation.

The Post-test–Only Design with Nonequivalent Groups

Although this design offers an improvement on the previous design, with the addition of a nonequivalent control group, it is still referred to as pre-experimental (see Figure 11–12). The addition of a nonequivalent control group can lead to a false confidence in the validity of the findings. Selection threats are a problem with both groups. The lack of a pretest remains a serious impediment to defining change. Differences in post-test scores

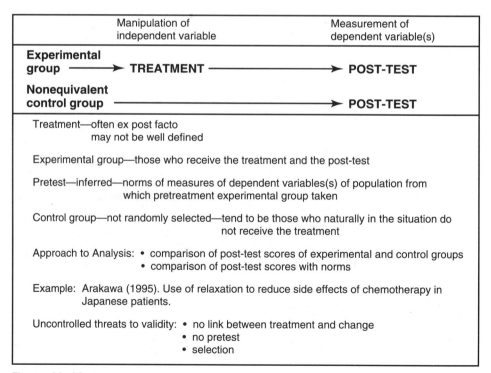

Figure 11–12
Post-test–only design with nonequivalent groups.

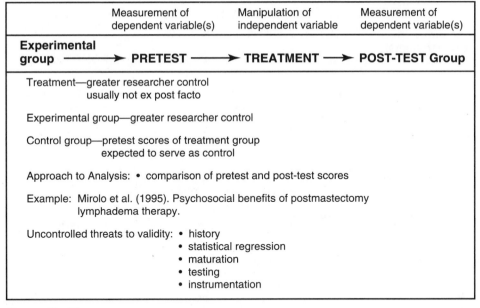

	Measurement of dependent variable(s)	Manipulation of independent variable	Measurement of dependent variable(s)
Experimental group ⟶	**PRETEST** ⟶	**TREATMENT** ⟶	**POST-TEST Group**

Treatment—greater researcher control
      usually not ex post facto

Experimental group—greater researcher control

Control group—pretest scores of treatment group
      expected to serve as control

Approach to Analysis: • comparison of pretest and post-test scores

Example: Mirolo et al. (1995). Psychosocial benefits of postmastectomy
      lymphadema therapy.

Uncontrolled threats to validity: • history
                              • statistical regression
                              • maturation
                              • testing
                              • instrumentation

Figure 11–13
One-group pretest–post-test design.

between groups may be caused by the treatment or by differential selection processes.

The One-Group Pretest–Post-test Design

This pre-experimental design is one of the more frequently used designs but has such serious weaknesses that findings are often uninterpretable (see Figure 11–13). Pretest scores cannot adequately serve the same function as a control group. Events can occur between the pretest and post-test that alter responses to the post-test. These events then serve as alternate hypotheses to the proposal that the change in post-test scores is due to the treatment. Post-test scores might be altered by (1) maturation processes, (2) administration of the pretest, and (3) changes in instrumentation. Additionally, subjects in many studies using this design are selected based on high or low scores on the pretest. Thus, there is an additional threat that changes in the post-test may be due to regression toward the

mean. The addition of a nonequivalent control group, as described in the next design, can greatly strengthen the validity of the findings.

The Untreated Control Group Design with Pretest and Post-test

This design is the one that is most frequently used in social science research (see Figure 11–14). This quasi-experimental design is the first design discussed that is generally interpretable. The uncontrolled threats to validity are primarily due to the nonequivalent control group. For the researcher planning to use this design, the effects of these threats on interpreting study findings are discussed in detail by Cook and Campbell (1979). Variations in this design include using proxy pretest measures (a different pretest that correlates with the post-test), separate pretest and post-test samples, and pretest measures at more than one time interval. The first two variations weaken the design, but the latter variation greatly strengthens it.

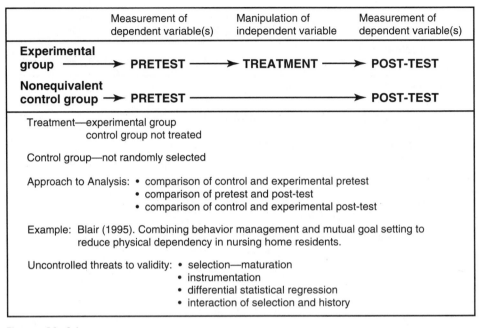

Figure 11–14
Untreated control group design with pretest and post-test.

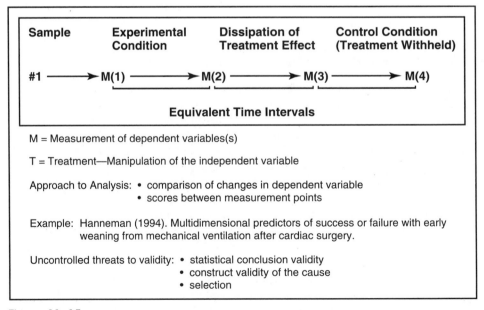

Figure 11–15
Removed-treatment design with pretest and post-test.

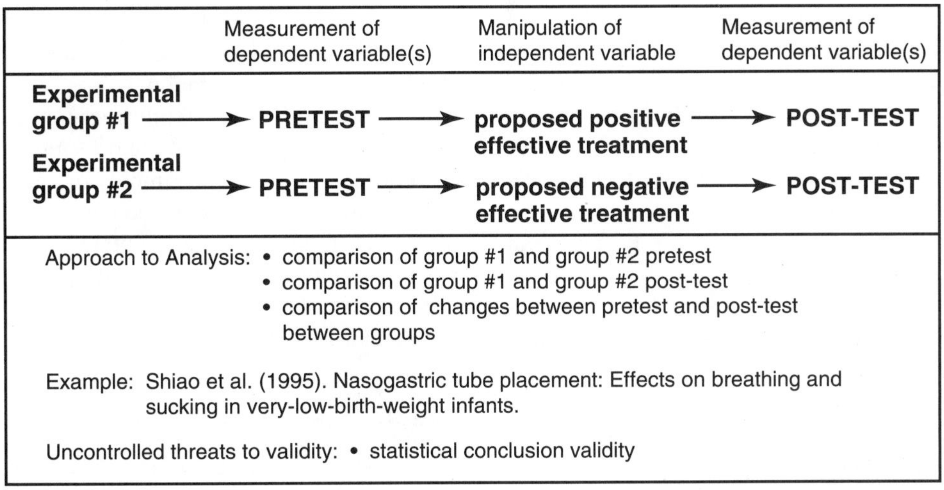

	Measurement of dependent variable(s)	Manipulation of independent variable	Measurement of dependent variable(s)
Experimental group #1 ⟶	PRETEST ⟶	proposed positive ⟶ effective treatment	POST-TEST
Experimental group #2 ⟶	PRETEST ⟶	proposed negative ⟶ effective treatment	POST-TEST

Approach to Analysis: • comparison of group #1 and group #2 pretest
 • comparison of group #1 and group #2 post-test
 • comparison of changes between pretest and post-test between groups

Example: Shiao et al. (1995). Nasogastric tube placement: Effects on breathing and sucking in very-low-birth-weight infants.

Uncontrolled threats to validity: • statistical conclusion validity

Figure 11–16
The reversed-treatment nonequivalent control group design with pretest and post-test.

The Removed-Treatment Design with Pretest and Post-test

In some cases, gaining access to even a nonequivalent control group is not possible. The removed-treatment design with pretest and post-test creates conditions that approximate the conceptual requirements of a control group receiving no treatment. The design is basically a one-group pretest–post-test design. However, after a delay of time, a third measure of the dependent variable is taken, followed by an interval of time in which the treatment is removed, followed by a fourth measure of the dependent variable (see Figure 11–15). The period of time between each measure needs to be equivalent. In nursing situations, the ethics of removing an effective treatment needs to be considered. Even if it is ethically acceptable, the response of subjects to the removal may make interpreting changes difficult.

The Reversed-Treatment Nonequivalent Control Group Design with Pretest and Post-test

This design introduces two independent variables: one expected to produce a positive effect, and one expected to produce a negative effect (see Figure 11–16). There are two experimental groups, each

exposed to one of the treatments. The design tests differences in response to the two treatments. This design is more useful for theory testing than the no-treatment control group design because of its high construct validity of the cause. The theoretical causal variable needs to be rigorously defined to allow differential predictions of directions of effect. In order to be maximally interpretable, two additional groups need to be added: (1) a placebo control group in which the treatment is not expected to affect the dependent variable, and (2) a no-treatment control group to provide a baseline.

INTERRUPTED TIME-SERIES DESIGNS

The interrupted time-series designs are similar to descriptive time designs except that a treatment is applied at some point in the observations. Time-series analyses have some advantages over other quasi-experimental designs. Repeated pretest observations can assess trends in maturation before the treatment. The repeated pretest observations also allow measures of trends in scores before the treatment, which decreases the risk of statistical regression, leading to misinterpretation of findings. If records are kept of events that could influence subjects in the study, the researcher can determine whether historical factors that could modify responses to the treatment were in operation between the last pretest and the first post-test.

There are, however, threats that are particularly problematic in time-series designs. Record-keeping procedures and definitions of constructs used for data collection tend to change over time. Thus, maintaining consistency can be a problem. The treatment can result in attrition so that the sample before treatment may be different in important ways from the post-treatment group. Seasonal variation or other cyclical influences can be interpreted as treatment effects. Therefore, identifying cyclical patterns that may be occurring and controlling for them is critical to the analysis of study findings.

McCain and McCleary (1979) suggest the use of the ARIMA statistical model (see Chapter 19)

to analyze time-series data. ARIMA is a relatively new model but has some distinct advantages over regression analysis techniques. For adequate statistical analysis, at least 50 measurement points are needed; however, Cook and Campbell (1979) believe that even small numbers of measurement points can provide information greater than that obtained in cross-sectional studies. Numbers of measures shown in the illustrated designs are limited by space and are not meant to suggest limiting measures to the numbers shown.

Simple Interrupted Time Series

This design is similar to the descriptive study, with the addition of a treatment that occurs or is applied at a given point in time (see Figure 11–17). The treatment, which in some cases is not

Measurement of dependent variable(s)	Manipulation of independent variable	Measurement of dependent variable(s)
PRETESTS ———————➤	**TREATMENT** ———————➤	**POST-TESTS**
Experimental group M(1) M(2) M(3) M(4)	T	M(5) M(6) M(7) M(8)

Subjects: may remain the same across the study or different individuals may be selected at each measurement period (as in the descriptive time-dimensional designs)

Pretest dependent variable measures: In addition to researcher-initiated tools, measures may be obtained from archival data sources such as patient records, scores available in student records, or employee records.

Treatment: may be a key event occurring at one specific point in time that is expected to modify subject responses to the dependent variable; that is, curriculum change, administrative change, change in nursing care of particular type of patient. The treatment tends to continue after implementation rather than occurring and then being withdrawn.

Approach to Analysis: • changes in trends of scores before and after treatment

Example: Whitney, Stotts, & Goodson (1995). Effects of dynamic exercise on subcutaneous oxygen tension and temperature.

Uncontrolled threats to validity: • history
　　　　　　　　　　　　　　　• seasonal trends
　　　　　　　　　　　　　　　• instrumentation
　　　　　　　　　　　　　　　• selection
　　　　　　　　　　　　　　　• mono-operation bias
　　　　　　　　　　　　　　　• cyclic influences interpreted as treatment effects

Figure 11–17
Simple interrupted time series.

completely under the control of the researcher, needs to be clearly defined. The use of multiple methods to measure the dependent variable greatly strengthens the design. Threats that are well controlled by this design include maturation and statistical regression.

Interrupted Time Series with a Nonequivalent No-Treatment Control Group Time Series

The addition of a control group to this design greatly strengthens the validity of the findings. The control group allows examination of differences in trends between groups after the treatment and the persistence of treatment effects over time (see Figure 11–18). Although the treatment may continue (e.g., a change in nursing management practices or patient teaching strategies), the initial response to the change may differ from later responses.

Interrupted Time Series with Multiple Replications

This is a powerful design for inferring causality (see Figure 11–19). It requires greater researcher control than is usually possible in social science research outside closed institutional settings such as laboratories or research units. The studies that led to the adoption of behavior modification techniques used this design. In order for significant differences to be interpretable, the pretest and

Measurement of dependent variable(s)	Manipulation of independent variable		Measurement of dependent variable(s)
PRETESTS ⟶	**TREATMENT ⟶**		**POST-TESTS**
Experimental group M(1) M(2) M(3) M(4)	T		M(5) M(6) M(7) M(8)
Control group M(1) M(2) M(3) M(4)			M(5) M(6) M(7) M(8)

Subjects: may remain the same across the study or may be part of a group in which some individuals may change (e.g., class, work group, patient teaching, or patient care group)

Pretest dependent variable measures: In addition to researcher-initiated tools, measures may be obtained from archival data sources.

Treatment: may be a key event occurring at one specific point in time that is expected to modify experimental subjects' responses to dependent variable measures. Treatment tends to continue after implementation rather than occurring and then being withdrawn.

Approach to Analysis: • changes in trends of scores before and after treatment
• comparison of trends in experimental and control groups
• temporal persistence of treatment effects

Example: Quayhagen et al. (1995). A dyadic remediation program for care recipients with dementia.

Uncontrolled threats to validity: • selection and history interaction
• as experimental and control groups increase in noncomparability, threats to validity increase
• interaction of populations and treatment
• cyclic influences interpreted as treatment effects

Figure 11–18
Interrupted time series with a nonequivalent no-treatment control group time series.

PRETEST → T → POST-TEST → PRETEST → T → POST-TEST etc.
Single sample
M(1) M(2) T M(3) M(4) T M(5) M(6) T M(7) M(8) T M(9) M(10)

Treatment: • provided repeatedly
• effects must dissipate rapidly
• should be scheduled randomly

Approach to Analysis: • powerful for inferring causal effects
• differences in pretest and post-test scores must be in opposite directions to be interpretable

Example: Fridriksdottir & McCarthy (1995). The effect of caloric density of food on energy intake and body weight in tumor-bearing rats.

Figure 11–19

Interrupted time series with multiple replications.

post-test scores must be in different directions. Within this design, treatments can be modified, substituting one treatment for another or combining two treatments and examining interaction effects.

EXPERIMENTAL STUDY DESIGNS

Experimental designs are set up to provide the greatest amount of control possible in order to examine causality more closely. To examine cause, one must eliminate all factors influencing the dependent variable other than the cause (independent variable) being studied. Other factors are eliminated by controlling them. The study is designed to prevent any other element from intruding into observation of the specific cause and effect that the researcher wishes to examine.

The three essential elements of experimental research are (1) random sampling; (2) researcher-controlled manipulation of the independent variable; and (3) researcher control of the experimental situation, including a control or comparison group. Experimental designs exert much effort to control variance. Sample criteria are explicit, the independent variable is provided in a precisely defined way, the dependent variables are carefully

operationalized, and the situation in which the study is conducted is rigidly controlled to prevent the interference of unstudied factors from modifying the dynamics of the process being studied.

PRETEST–POST-TEST CONTROL GROUP DESIGN

This design is the most commonly used experimental design (see Figure 11–20). The experimental and control groups are both randomly assigned from a sample that was randomly selected. Comparison of pretest scores allows evaluation of the effectiveness of randomization in providing equivalent groups. The treatment is under control of the researcher. The dependent variable is measured twice, before and after the manipulation of the independent variable. As with all well-designed studies, the dependent and independent variables will be conceptually linked, conceptually defined, and operationalized. Instruments used to measure the dependent variable will clearly reflect the conceptual meaning of the variable. Often, more than one means to measure the dependent variable is advisable to avoid mono-operation and mono-method bias.

Multiple groups (both experimental and control) can be used to great advantage in the pretest–

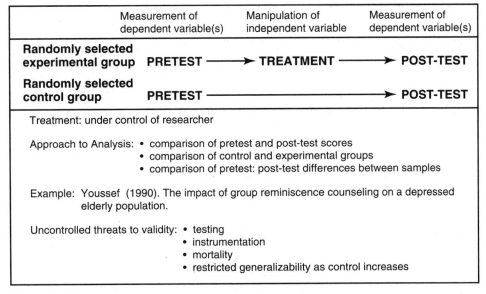

Figure 11-20
Pretest–post-test control group design.

post-test design and the post-test–only design. For example, one control group could receive no treatment while another control group could receive a placebo treatment. Multiple experimental groups could receive varying levels of the treatments, such as differing frequency, intensity, or length of nursing care measures. These additions greatly increase the generalizability of the study findings.

POST-TEST–ONLY CONTROL GROUP DESIGN

In some studies, the dependent variable cannot be measured before the treatment. For example, it is not possible meaningfully to measure responses to interventions designed to control nausea from chemotherapy or postoperative pain prior to the beginning of treatment. Additionally, in some cases, subjects' responses to the post-test can be due, in part, to learning from or subjective reaction to the pretest (pretest sensitization). If this is a concern in a specific study, the pretest may be eliminated and a post-test–only control group design can be

used (see Figure 11–21). However, this elimination prevents the use of many powerful statistical analysis techniques within the study. Additionally, the effectiveness of randomization in obtaining equivalent experimental and control groups cannot be evaluated in terms of the study variables. However, the groups can be evaluated in terms of sample characteristics and other relevant variables.

RANDOMIZED BLOCK DESIGN

The randomized block design uses the two-group pretest–post-test pattern or the two-group post-test pattern with one addition, a blocking variable. The blocking variable, if uncontrolled, is expected to confound the findings of the study. To prevent confounding the findings, the subjects are rank-ordered in relation to the blocking variable. For example, if effectiveness of a nursing intervention to relieve postchemotherapy nausea was the independent variable, severity of nausea could confound the findings. Subjects would be ranked according to severity of nausea. The two subjects

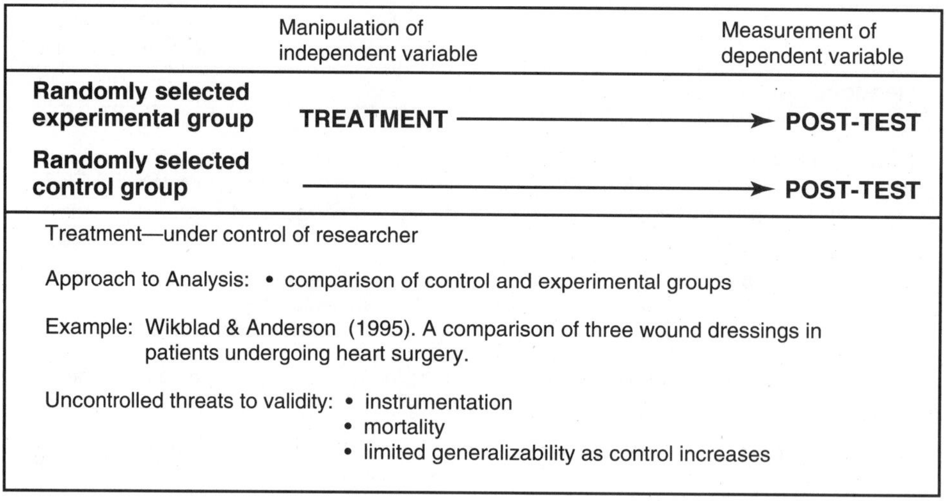

	Manipulation of independent variable	Measurement of dependent variable
Randomly selected experimental group	TREATMENT ——————————→	POST-TEST
Randomly selected control group	——————————————————→	POST-TEST

Treatment—under control of researcher

Approach to Analysis: • comparison of control and experimental groups

Example: Wikblad & Anderson (1995). A comparison of three wound dressings in patients undergoing heart surgery.

Uncontrolled threats to validity: • instrumentation
• mortality
• limited generalizability as control increases

Figure 11–21
Post-test–only control group design.

with the most severely classified nausea would be identified and randomly assigned, one to the experimental group and one to the control group. The two subjects next in rank would then be identified and randomly assigned. This pattern would be followed until the entire sample was randomly assigned as matched pairs. This procedure ensures that the experimental group and the control group are equal in relation to the potentially confounding variable.

The effect of blocking can also be accomplished statistically (using analysis of covariance) without categorizing the confounding variable into discrete components. However, for this analysis to be accurate, one must be careful not to violate the assumptions of the statistical procedure (Spector, 1981). An example of this design is Lauver's (1989) study "Instructional information and breast self-examination practice." The following excerpt describes the study design.

■————————————————

"A randomized experimental design was used. The four interventions were: (a) basic information on the steps of BSE, (b) tactile sensory information in addition to basic steps of BSE, (c) coping techniques instruction in addition to basic steps of BSE, and (d) tactile sensory information and coping techniques in addition to basic steps of BSE. Women were randomly assigned to interventions, stratified by level of BSE performance in the preceding 3 months. This approach was used to control for preintervention differences in BSE performance and to test for interactions between prior performance and the interventions. The outcome variables were frequency and thoroughness of BSE." (p. 13) ■

FACTORIAL DESIGNS

In a factorial design, two or more different characteristics, treatments, or events are independently varied within a single study. This design is a logical approach to examining multiple causality. The simplest arrangement is one in which two treatments or factors are involved, and, within each factor, two levels are manipulated (for example, the presence or absence of the treatment). This is referred to as a 2×2 factorial design. This design is illustrated in Figure 11–22, using the two inde-

Level of Relaxation	Level of Distraction	
	Distraction	No Distraction
Relaxation	A	B
No Relaxation	C	D

Figure 11–22
Example of factorial design.

pendent variables of relaxation and distraction as means of pain relief.

A 2 × 2 factorial design produces a study with four cells. Each cell must contain an equivalent number of subjects. Cells B and C allow examination of each separate intervention. Cell D subjects receive no treatment and serve as a control group. Cell A allows examination of interaction between the two independent variables. The design can be used, as in the randomized blocks design, to control for confounding variables. The confounding variable is included as an independent variable, and interactions between it and the other independent variable are examined (Spector, 1981).

Extensions of the factorial design to more than two levels of variables are referred to as $M \times N$ factorial designs. Within this design, independent variables can have any number of levels within practical limits. Note that a 3 × 3 design involves 9 cells and requires a much larger sample size. A 4 × 4 design would require 16 cells. A 4 × 4 design would allow relaxation to be provided at four levels of intensity, such as no relaxation, relaxation 10 minutes twice a day, 15 minutes three times a day, and 20 minutes four times a day. Distraction would be provided in similar levels. Factorial designs are not limited to two independent variables; however, interpretation of larger numbers becomes more complex, and increased knowledge of statistical analysis is required. Factorial designs do allow the examination of theoretically proposed interrelationships between multiple independent variables. However, very large samples are required.

An example of this design is Henker, Bernardo, O'Connor, and Sereika's (1995) study evaluating four methods of warming intravenous fluids. An excerpt from that study follows.

"The methods of warming IVF (intravenous fluids) and the control were evaluated with a 5 × 5 factorial experimental design. Each method of warming and the control were evaluated at each flow rate and replicated two times, yielding three measurements for each warming method at each rate." (p. 386) ∎

NESTED DESIGNS

In some experimental situations, the researcher wishes to consider the effect of variables that are found only at some levels of the independent variables being studied. Variables found only at certain levels of the independent variable are called *nested variables*. Possible nested variables include gender, race, socioeconomic status, and education, or may be such factors as patients who are cared for on specific nursing units or at different hospitals. The statistical analysis is then conducted as though the unit or hospital were the subject, rather than the individual patient. Figure 11–23 illustrates the nesting design. In actual practice, nursing units used in this manner would have to be much larger in number than those illustrated, since each unit would be considered a subject and would be randomly assigned to a treatment.

The following excerpt from Harris and Hyman's (1984) study, "Clean vs. sterile tracheotomy care and level of pulmonary infection" is an example of this design.

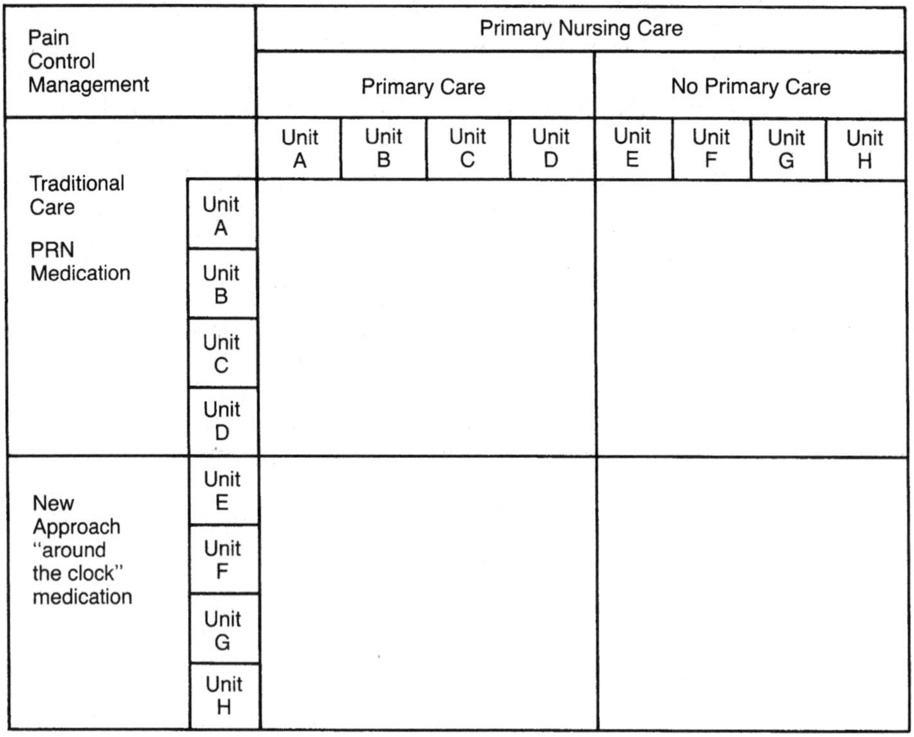

Pain Control Management		Primary Nursing Care							
		Primary Care				No Primary Care			
		Unit A	Unit B	Unit C	Unit D	Unit E	Unit F	Unit G	Unit H
Traditional Care PRN Medication	Unit A								
	Unit B								
	Unit C								
	Unit D								
New Approach "around the clock" medication	Unit E								
	Unit F								
	Unit G								
	Unit H								

Figure 11–23
Design using nesting.

"The purpose of this research was to determine if clean tracheotomy care was more effective than sterile as measured by levels of postoperative pulmonary infection. Ten hospitals with large Head and Neck/ENT services were selected as data collection sites . . . To increase external validity, possible unique effects associated with hospitals were controlled by use of a nested design-hospital nested within treatment procedure. . . . At these centers a minimum of 15 tracheostomy patient charts were reviewed pre- and postoperatively for clinical and laboratory data related to infection. Patient level of infection was defined using the Weighted Level of Pulmonary Infection Tool, which was constructed for this study." (pp. 80–83) ■

CROSSOVER OR COUNTERBALANCED DESIGNS

In some studies, more than one treatment is administered to each subject. The treatments are provided sequentially, rather than concurrently. Comparisons are then made on the effects of the different treatments on the same subject. For example, two different methods known to achieve relaxation might be used as the two treatments. One difficulty encountered in this type of study is that exposure to one treatment may result in effects (called *carryover effects*) that persist and influence responses of the subject to later treatments. Subjects can improve as they become more familiar with the experimental protocol, which is called a *practice effect*. They may become tired or bored with the study, which is called a *fatigue effect.* The direct interaction of one treatment with another, such as the use of two drugs, can confound differences in the two treatments.

Crossover, or *counterbalancing,* is a design strategy to guard against possible erroneous conclusions resulting from carryover effects. Using counterbalancing, subjects are randomly assigned to a specific sequencing of treatment conditions. This distributes the carryover effects equally across all the conditions of the study, thus canceling them out. To prevent an effect related to time, the same amount of time needs to be allotted to each treatment, and the crossover point needs to be related to time, not to the condition of the subject. In addition, the design must allow for an adequate interval between treatments to dissipate the effects of the first treatment. This is referred to as a washout period. For example, the design would specify that each treatment would last 6 days and on the 8th day, each subject would cross over to the alternate treatment after a 2-day washout period.

The researcher also needs to be alert to the possibility that changes may be due to such factors as disease progression, the healing process, or effects of treatment of the disease rather than the study treatment. The process of counterbalancing can become quite complicated when more than two treatments are involved. Counterbalancing is effective only if the carryover effect is essentially the same from treatment A to treatment B as it is from treatment B to treatment A. If one is more fatiguing than the other or more likely to modify response to the second treatment, counterbalancing will not be effective. The crossover design controls the variance in the study and thus allows the sample size to be smaller. The sample size required to detect a significant effect is considerably less since the subjects serve as their own controls. However, because the data collection period is longer, subject dropouts may increase (Beck, 1989).

An example of this design is Legault and Goulet's (1995) study, "Comparison of kangaroo and traditional methods of removing preterm infants from incubators."

"The intervention was use of the kangaroo or traditional method of maintaining body temperature of preterm infants. The dependent variables were physiologic parameters (skin temperature, heart rate, respiratory rate, and oxygen saturation) measured five times with each method. Mother's satisfaction was measured at the end of each testing period and mother's preference at the end of the experiment. The kangaroo method produced less variation in oxygen saturation and longer duration of testing, and it was preferred by most of the mothers." (p. 501) ∎

RANDOMIZED CLINICAL TRIALS

Randomized clinical trials have been used in medicine since 1945. However, until recently, they have not been used in nursing. Clinical trials can be used to examine areas of nursing practice or to test theory-based nursing practice (Tyzenhouse, 1981; Woods, 1990). Because of the involvement of large numbers of people, time, and costs, a carefully designed treatment with demonstrated effectiveness needs to be used in a clinical trial. Before the large study is initiated, several pilot studies need to be performed testing instruments, the methodology, and the treatment. Efforts need to be made to identify and resolve as many problems as possible prior to implementing the clinical trial. These activities need to be clearly documented in proposals seeking funding for a clinical trial.

The clinical trial uses large numbers of subjects to test the effects of a treatment and compare the results with those of a control group who have not received the treatment (or who have received a more traditional treatment). Subjects are drawn from a reference population, using clearly defined criteria, and then randomly assigned to treatment or control groups. Baseline states must be comparable in all groups included in the study. The treatment must be equal and consistently applied, and outcomes need to be measured consistently. Care also needs to be taken to ensure that randomization procedures are rigidly adhered to.

Because of the need for large samples and to be able to generalize to a variety of types of clinical settings and types of patients, the study is carried out simultaneously in multiple geographic locations and coordinated by the primary researcher. Several problems need to be confronted by the researcher using this technique. Coordination of a project of this type requires much time and effort. Keeping up with subjects is critical but may be difficult. Communication with and cooperation of nurses assisting with the study in the various geographic locations are essential but sometimes difficult. Costs of conducting studies such as these can be higher than those of most nursing studies, and such studies usually require obtaining grant funding from outside sources. Nurses are often so convinced that current nursing practice is effective that they may resist following a protocol for care that does not coincide with their beliefs. Thus, the

researcher may encounter attempts to ignore the protocol and provide traditional care. However, utilization of this design has the potential to improve greatly the scientific base for nursing practice (Fetter et al., 1989; Tyzenhouse, 1981).

Only a few clinical trials have been conducted in nursing. These include Brooten and colleagues' (1986) trial of early hospital discharge and home follow-up of very low birth weight infants and Burgess and colleagues' (1987) trial of cardiac rehabilitation. Recently, Gilliss and Kulkin (1991) described the administrative management of a clinical trial designed to examine nursing strategies for improving recovery from cardiac surgery. The study was funded by the National Center for Nursing Research. Baseline data were collected on individual health, psychological status, self-

150 pairs
Random Assignment

71 pairs
(Experimental Protocol)

79 pairs
(Usual Care/Intervention 1)

Schedule of Intervention and Evaluation

Pre-op/ Baseline	Prior to discharge (in hospital)	Postdischarge (weeks 1–8 in home)	3 months/12 weeks	6 months/24 weeks
Consent POMS (P & S) APGAR (P & S) Family profile/ Expected benefits Medical abstract Self-efficacy + Activity (P)	F-COPES (P & S)[a] FACES III (P & S) Self-efficacy (P)	Telephone call Self-efficacy + Activity (P) Self-report/ Recovery index (P) (weeks 4 and 8)	Telephone call Self-efficacy + Activity (P) Self-report/ Recovery index (P)	Telephone call Self-efficacy + Activity (P) Self-report/ Recovery index (P)
		Mail follow-up POMS (P & S) (week 4) ZCI/SSS (S) (week 4) SSS (P) (week 4)	Mail follow-up POMS (P & S) APGAR (P & S) F-COPES (P & S) FACES III (P & S) Caregiving index (S) Social support (P & S)	Mail follow-up POMS (P & S) APGAR (P & S) F-COPES (P & S) FACES III (P & S)
Experimental group	Interventions 1 and 2	Intervention 3 (calls at weeks 1, 2, 3, 4, 6, and 8)		
Control group	Intervention 1			

[a] P = patient; S = spouse/family caregiver

Figure 11–24
Design model for clinical trial by Gilliss and Kulkin (1991).

efficacy, family functioning, and coping. These variables were also used as outcome measures. A model of the design is illustrated in Figure 11–24. Gilliss and Kulkin's (1991) description of their study follows.

■

"Improving Recovery from Cardiac Surgery, or the Family Heart Study, was a randomized clinical trial of in-hospital and postdischarge nursing interventions designed to improve individual and family recovery from cardiac surgery. Eligible patients were between 25 and 75 years of age, spoke English, were scheduled for CABG (coronary artery bypass graft) or valve repair, were available for telephone contact for 6 months, and had a consenting partner who would care for them in early recovery. Subjects who experienced postsurgical complications of significance were excluded after surgery. All pairs inducted into the study were assigned to experimental or control status using a block randomization scheme. Patients received 'standard care' (Intervention 1) at the two study hospitals. This involved viewing a slide-tape presentation ('Move into Action') on cardiac risk reduction prepared by the Santa Clara (California) Heart Association. Experimental patient/caregiver pairs received additional education and counseling (Intervention 2) prior to discharge. This included an original slide-tape presentation ('Working Together for Recovery') that was patterned after the American Heart Association tapes and educated the pairs about common psychological and relationship responses to recovery from surgery. Following the viewing, each pair met with a study nurse to discuss the applicability of the slide-tape content to their particular situation.

Finally, experimental patients and caregivers were contacted at 1, 2, 3, 4, 6, and 8 weeks after discharge by graduate nurse researcher assistants for outcall telephone monitoring and recovery coaching (Intervention 3). These calls followed a semistructured guide and were intended to reinforce hospital-based education programs, detect early complications and drug effects, answer questions, and offer support for recovery; however, an overriding aim was to offer personalized nursing care" (pp. 416–417) ■

STUDIES THAT DO NOT USE TRADITIONAL RESEARCH DESIGNS

In some approaches to research, the research designs described in this chapter cannot be used. These studies tend to be in highly specialized areas that require unique design strategies to accomplish their purposes. Designs for primary prevention and health promotion, secondary analysis, meta-analysis, and methodological studies are described.

PRIMARY PREVENTION AND HEALTH PROMOTION STUDIES

Studying primary prevention and health promotion involves applying a treatment of primary prevention (the cause) and then attempting to measure the effect (an event that does not occur if the treatment was effective). Primary prevention studies, then, attempt to measure things that do not happen. One cannot select a sample to study, apply a treatment, and then measure an effect. The sample must be the community. The design involves examining changes in the community, and the variables are called indicators. A change in an identified indicator is inferred to be a consequence of the effectiveness of the prevention program (treatment). Specific indicators would depend on the focus of prevention. For example, the indicators identified by the National Institution on Drug Abuse include changes in drug-related perceptions, attitudes, knowledge, and action; changes in prevalence and incidence of drug use, drug-related mortality/morbidity; institutional policy/programs; youth/parent involvement in the community; and accident rates (French & Kaufman, 1981). Since one indicator alone would be insufficient to infer effect, multiple indicators and statistical analyses appropriate for these indicators must be used.

Van Rossum and colleagues (1991) describe the design of a study to determine the effect of preventive home visits to the elderly by public health nurses. The goals of the visits were to increase independence of the elderly and prevent or postpone institutional care. Outcome measures, or indicators, used in the study included perceived state of health, well-being, functional state, mental state, use of health care services, institutionalization, and mortality. A parallel group randomized trial was used. Subjects were limited to those 75 to 84 years of age. A questionnaire and letter were sent to all individuals of this age group living in Weert, a town in The Netherlands with a population of 60,000. The response rate was 85% with 92% of those responding agreeing to participate. Those already receiving home nursing care were excluded. A sample of 600 subjects was randomly selected using a computer from the possible pool of 1,285 questionnaire respondents. Before randomly assigning the subjects to groups, the participants were stratified by four variables: (1) gender; (2) composition of household; (3) perceived state of health; and (4) social class, to control for extraneous variables. Subjects were then randomly assigned to treatment and control groups within each stratum, using a computer. Those receiving the treatment were randomly assigned to a public health nurse. Subjects were followed for 3 years. Those receiving public health nursing visits were visited every 3 months by the same public health nurse. The nurse could be contacted daily, and additional visits were made when needed. Control group subjects received no visits but had access to all traditional health care services.

SECONDARY ANALYSIS

Secondary analysis design involves studying data previously collected in another study. Data are re-examined using different organizations of the data and different statistical analyses than those previously used. The design involves analyzing data to validate the reported findings, examining dimensions previously unexamined, or redirecting the focus of the data to allow comparison with data from other studies (Gleit & Graham, 1989). As data sets accumulate from research programs of groups of faculty, secondary analyses can be expected to increase. This approach allows the inves-

tigators to examine questions related to the data that were not originally posed. These data sets may provide opportunities for junior faculty members or graduate students to become involved in a research program. Of concern in secondary analyses of data is the tendency of some researchers to write as many papers as possible from the planned analyses of a study in order to increase their number of publications—a strategy referred to as "salami slicing." Researchers performing secondary analyses should always identify the original source of data and previous publications emerging from the analysis of that data set. Aaronson (1994) points out the problem.

"Fundamentally, each paper written from the same study or the same dataset must make a distinct and significant scientific contribution. Presumably this is not only the major overriding criterion used by reviewers, but also the author's intent when writing the paper. When a particular paper is one of several from the same study, project, or dataset, the author's responsibility to identify the source of the data is that much greater. To lead readers to think a report is from a new study or a different dataset than that used in the authors' previous work is dishonest, particularly if the second paper purports to substantiate findings of the first one. . . . Apart from the overriding concern about 'milking the data,' the most common objection to multiple articles from a single study is concern about the age of the data . . . Concerns in nursing about the number of papers generated from a single study may reflect the emerging status of secondary analysis as a legitimate approach to nursing research . . . All of the reasons offered for using secondary analysis—answering new questions with existing data, applying new methods to answer old questions, the real exigencies of cost and feasibility—serve equally to justify the continued use of data collected years ago, by the original investigator of a large project, as well as by others . . . The issue remains one of sound science. The question that needs to be asked is: Does this particular paper make a meaningful and distinct contribution to the scientific literature?" (pp. 61–62) ■

An example of secondary analysis is Lauver and Tak's (1995) study, "Optimism and coping with a breast cancer symptom."

"This cross-sectional study was a part of a larger investigation to explain care seeking for breast cancer symptoms. Complementary findings have been described elsewhere (Lauver, 1992, 1994). Data were collected in a breast surgery clinic of an urban hospital that provided care for the medically indigent. Participants were seeking evaluation for self-identified breast cancer symptoms, such as a lump or discharge. Eligible participants were older than 18 years of age, had no personal history of cancer, and could communicate in English." (p. 203) ■

META-ANALYSIS DESIGNS

Meta-analysis design involves merging findings from many studies that have examined the same phenomenon. The design uses specific statistical analyses to determine the overall findings from combined examination of reports of statistical findings of each study. The statistical values used include the means and standard deviations for each group in the study. One of the outcomes of a meta-analysis is the estimation of a population effect size for the topic under study. Since studies seldom have exactly the same focus, conclusions are never absolute but do give some sense of unity to knowledge within that area (O'Flynn, 1982).

One problem consistently encountered in meta-analyses is that the studies being examined are inconsistent in design quality. However, those conducting meta-analyses have not been successful in identifying a generally acceptable means to measure the research quality of studies. Brown (1991) proposed a research quality scoring method to accomplish this important task. Another problem encountered by researchers performing meta-analyses is that basic research information is often missing from research reports. Calculating effect sizes requires means and standard deviations in each study for both experimental and control groups. In addition, the beginning sample size needs to be reported as well as the sample size at the time of the post-test. Often the treatment has

been poorly described, making it difficult to determine the most effective treatments (Brown, 1991).

An example of a meta-analysis is Brown and Grimes (1995) meta-analysis of nurse practitioners and nurse midwives in primary care. The following is an abstract of that study.

"This meta-analysis was an evaluation of patient outcomes of nurse practitioners (NPs) and nurse midwives (NMs), compared with those of physicians, in primary care. The sample included 38 NP and 15 NM studies. Thirty-three outcomes were analyzed. In studies that employed randomization to provider, greater patient compliance with treatment recommendations was shown with NPs than with physicians. In studies that controlled for patient risk in ways other than randomization, patient satisfaction and resolution of pathological conditions were greater for NP patients. NPs were equivalent to MDs on most other variables in controlled studies. In studies that controlled for patient risk, NMs used less technology and analgesia than did physicians in intrapartum care of obstetric patients. NMs achieved neonatal outcomes equivalent to those of physicians. Limitations in data from primary studies precluded answering questions of why and under what conditions these outcomes apply and whether these services are cost-effective." (p. 332) ■

METHODOLOGICAL DESIGNS

Methodological designs are used to develop the validity and reliability of instruments to measure constructs used as variables in research. The process is lengthy and complex. The average length of researcher time required to develop a research tool to the point appropriate to use in a study is 5 years. An example of this design is Ludington-Hoe and Kasper's (1995) study, "A physiologic method for monitoring premature infants." The abstract from that study follows.

"Instrumentation capable of handling 12 continuous hours of nine-channel real-time physiologic data sampled at 10Hz was needed to test within and between subject variability and preterm infant responses to skin-to-skin contact with the mother. A review of basic electrical components, electrical principles related to physiologic monitoring, and electrophysiology concepts generic to physiologic monitoring is presented. The development, specification and applications of a new instrument to monitor premature infant cardiorespiratory adaptations are discussed." (p. 13) ■

Decision Trees for Selecting Research Designs

Selecting a research design involves following paths of logical reasoning. A calculating mind is needed to explore all the possible consequences of using a particular design in a study. In some ways, selecting a design is like thinking through the moves in a chess game. One needs to carefully think through the consequences of each option. The research design organizes all the components of the study in a way that is most likely to lead to valid answers to the questions that have been posed.

To assist in selecting the most appropriate design, a series of decision trees have been provided. The first decision tree, Figure 11–25, assists in identifying the type of study being conducted. The next four figures (see Figures 11–26, 11–27, 11–28, and 11–29) assist in the selection of spe-

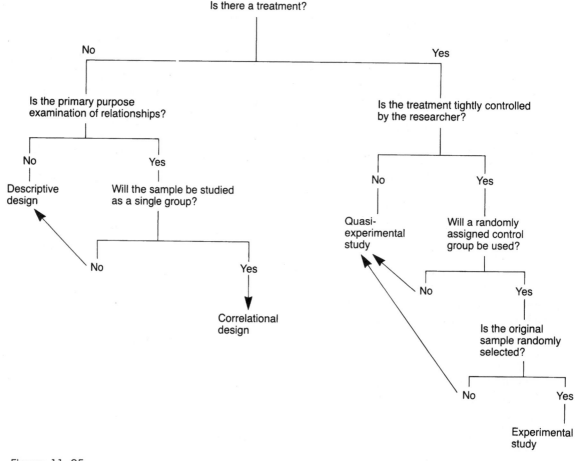

Figure 11–25
Type of study.

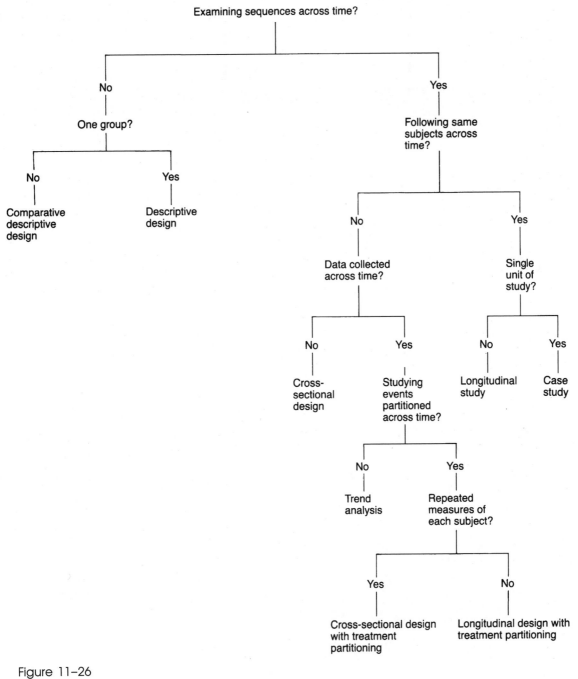

Figure 11–26
Descriptive studies.

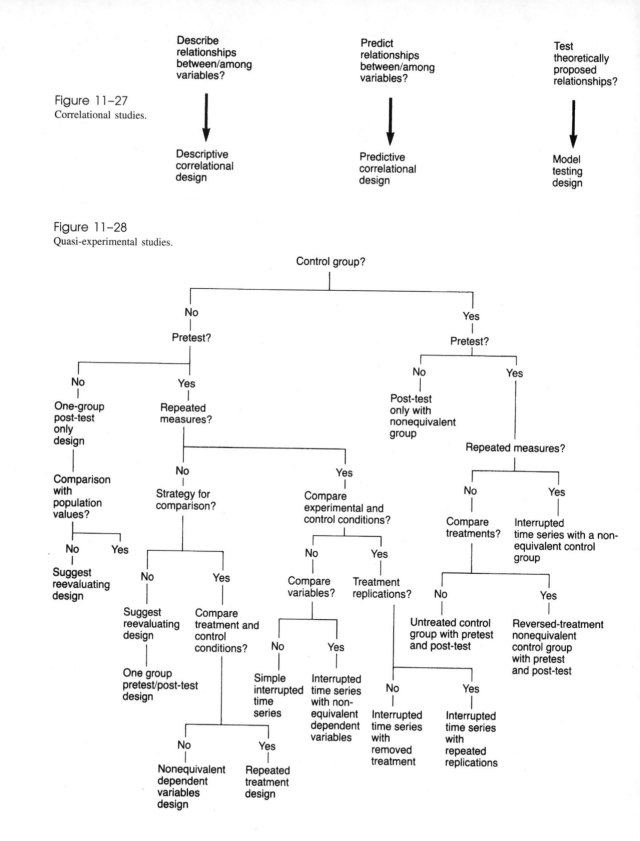

Figure 11-27
Correlational studies.

Figure 11-28
Quasi-experimental studies.

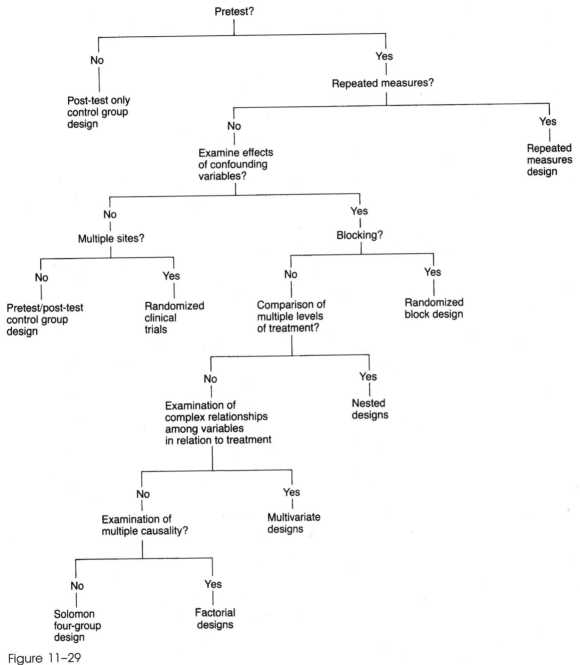

Figure 11–29
Experimental studies.

cific designs for each of the types of studies. The selection of a design is not a rigid, rule-guided task. The researcher has considerable flexibility in choosing a design. The pathways within the decision trees are not absolute and are to be used as guides. Note that we have included random sampling as a criterion for determining that the study is experimental rather than quasi-experimental. You, or the faculty members with whom you are working, may choose to disregard this criterion.

SUMMARY

Designs have been developed by researchers to meet unique research needs as they emerge. At present, nursing research is using designs developed by other disciplines. These designs are a useful starting point but nurse scientists need to go beyond these to develop designs that will more appropriately meet the needs of nursing's knowledge base. Descriptive studies are designed to gain more information about variables within a particular field of study. Their purpose is to provide a picture of situations as they naturally happen. No manipulation of variables is involved. Descriptive designs vary in levels of complexity. Some contain only two variables, whereas others may include multiple variables. The relationships between variables are identified to obtain an overall picture of the phenomenon being examined. Protection against bias is achieved through conceptual and operational definitions of variables, sample selection and size, valid and reliable instruments, and data collection procedures that achieve some environmental control.

Correlational studies examine relationships between variables. This examination can occur at several levels. The researcher can seek to describe a relationship, predict relationships among variables, or test the relationships proposed by a theoretical proposition. In correlational designs, a large variance in the variable scores is necessary to determine the existence of a relationship. Researchers tend to make two serious errors with correlational studies. First, they often attempt to establish causality by correlation, reasoning that if two variables are related, one must cause the other. Second, they confuse studies in which differences are examined with studies in which relationships are examined.

The purpose of quasi-experimental and experimental designs is to examine causality. The power of the design to accomplish this purpose is dependent on the degree to which the actual effects of the experimental treatment (the independent variable) can be detected by measurement of the dependent variable. Obtaining an understanding of the true effects of an experimental treatment requires action to control threats to the validity of the findings. Threats to validity are controlled through selection of subjects, manipulation of the treatment, and reliable measurement of variables. Experimental designs with their strict control of variance are the most powerful method of examining causality. Quasi-experimental designs were developed to provide alternate means for examining causality in situations not conducive to experimental controls. Experimental designs are set up to provide the greatest amount of control possible in order to more closely examine causality. To examine cause, one needs to eliminate all factors influencing the dependent variable other than the cause (independent variable) being studied. Other factors are eliminated by controlling them. The three essential elements of experimental research are (1) randomization; (2) researcher-controlled manipulation of the independent variable; and (3) researcher control of the ex-

continued

continued

perimental situation, including a control or comparison group.

There are studies in highly specialized areas that require unique design strategies to accomplish their purposes. Studying primary prevention and health promotion involves applying a treatment of primary prevention (the cause) and then attempting to measure the effect (an event that does not occur if the treatment was effective). The design involves examining changes in the community, and the variables are called indicators. Secondary analysis involves studying data previously collected in another study. Data are re-examined using different organizations of the data and different statistical analyses than those previously used. Meta-analysis involves merging findings from many studies that have examined the same phenomenon. Specific statistical analyses are used to determine the overall findings from joint examination of reported statistical findings. Methodological studies are designed to develop the validity and reliability of instruments to measure constructs used as variables in research. The average length of researcher time required to develop a research tool to the point appropriate to use in a study is 5 years.

References

Aaronson, L. S. (1984). Health behavior in pregnancy: Testing a general model. *Dissertation Abstracts International, 44–*11A, 3498.

Aaronson, L. S. (1994). Milking data or meeting commitments: How many papers from one study? *Nursing Research, 43*(1), 60–62.

Aaronson, L. S., & Kingry, M. J. (1988). A mixed method approach for using cross-sectional data for longitudinal inferences. *Nursing Research, 37*(3), 187–198.

Abdellah, F. G., & Levine, E. (1979). *Better patient care through nursing research.* New York: Macmillan.

Anderson, V. L., & McLean, R. A. (1974). *Design of experiments: A realistic approach.* New York: Marcel Dekker.

Arakawa, S. (1995). Use of relaxation to reduce side effects of chemotherapy in Japanese patients. *Cancer Nursing, 18*(1), 60–66.

Barnard, K. E., Magyary, D. L., Booth, C. L., & Eyres, S. J. (1987). Longitudinal designs: Considerations and applications to nursing research. *Recent Advances in Nursing, 17,* 37–64.

Beck, S. L. (1989). The crossover design in clinical nursing research. *Nursing Research, 38*(5), 291–293.

Blair, C. E. (1995). Combining behavior management and mutual goal setting to reduce physical dependency in nursing home residents. *Nursing Research, 44*(3), 160–165.

Bloom, K. C. (1995). The development of attachment behaviors in pregnant adolescents. *Nursing Research, 44*(5), 284–289.

Brooten, D., Kuman, S., Brown, L. P., Butts, P., Finkler, S. A., Bakewell-Sachs, S., Gibbons, A., & Delivoria-Papadopoulos, M. (1986). A randomized clinical trial of early hospital discharge and home follow-up of very-low-birth-weight infants. *New England Journal of Medicine, 315*(15), 934–939.

Brown, S. A. (1991). Measurement of quality of primary studies for meta-analysis. *Nursing Research, 40*(6), 352–355.

Brown, S. A., & Grimes, D. E. (1995). A meta-analysis of nurse practitioners and nurse midwives in primary care. *Nursing Research, 44*(6), 332–339.

Bulechek, G. M., & McCloskey, J. C. (1994). Nursing interventions classification (NIC): Defining nursing care. In J. C. McCloskey & H. K. Grace (Eds.), *Current issues in nursing* (4th ed., pp. 129–135). St. Louis: Mosby-Year Book.

Burgess, A. W., Lerner, D. J., D'Agostino, R. B., Vokonas, P. S., Hartman, C. R., & Gaccione, P. (1987). A randomized control trial of cardiac rehabilitation. *Social Science and Medicine, 24*(4), 359–370.

Caldwell, L. M. (1994). Critique of the NIC taxonomy structure Iowa Intervention Project. *Nursing Scan in Research, 7*(2), 1–2.

Campbell, D. T., & Stanley, J. C. (1963). *Experimental and quasi-experimental designs for research.* Chicago: Rand McNally.

Cook, T. D., & Campbell, D. T. (1979). *Quasi-experimentation: Design and analysis issues for field settings.* Chicago: Rand McNally.

Cox, D. R. (1958). *Planning of experiments.* New York: Wiley.

Daly, J. M., McCloskey, J. C., & Bulechek, G. M. (1994). Nursing interventions classification use in long-term care. *Geriatric Nursing, 15*(1), 41–46.

Egan, E. C., Snyder, M., & Burns, K. R. (1992). Intervention studies in nursing: Is the effect due to the independent variable? *Nursing Outlook, 40*(4), 187–190.

Fetter, M. S., Fettham, S. L., D'Apolito, K., Chaze, B. A., Fink, A., Frink, B. B., Hougart, M. K., & Rushton, C. H. (1989). Randomized clinical trials: Issues for researchers. *Nursing Research, 38*(2), 117–120.

Fisher, R. A. (1935). *The design of experiments.* New York: Hafner.

French, J. F., & Kaufman, N. J. (1981). *Handbook for preven-*

tion evaluation: Prevention evaluation guidelines. Rockville, MD: National Institute on Drug Abuse.

Fridriksdottir, M., & McCarthy, D. O. (1995). The effect of caloric density of food on energy intake and body weight in tumor-bearing rats. *Research in Nursing & Health, 18*(4), 357–363.

Gilliss, C. L., & Kulkin, I. L. (1991). Monitoring nursing interventions and data collection in a randomized clinical trial. *Western Journal of Nursing Research, 13*(3), 416–422.

Gleit, C., & Graham, B. (1989). Secondary data analysis: A valuable resource. *Nursing Research, 38*(6), 380–381.

Gottlieb, L. N., & Bailles, J. (1995). Firstborns' behaviors during a mother's second pregnancy. *Nursing Research, 44*(6), 356–362.

Hanneman, S. K. G. (1994). Multidimensional predictors of success or failure with early weaning from mechanical ventilation after cardiac surgery. *Nursing Research, 43*(1), 4–10.

Harris, R. B., & Hyman, R. B. (1984). Clean vs. sterile tracheotomy care and level of pulmonary infection. *Nursing Research, 33*(2), 80–85.

Hashisaki, P., Swenson, T., Mooney, B., Epstein, B., & Bowcutt, C. (1984). Decontamination of urinary bags for rehabilitation. *Archives of Physical Medicine and Rehabilitation 65*(8), 474–476.

Henker, R., Bernardo, L. M., O'Connor, K., & Sereika, S. (1995). Evaluation of four methods of warming intravenous fluids. *Journal of Emergency Nursing, 21*(5), 385–390.

Iowa Intervention Project. (1992a). *Nursing interventions classification (NIC): Taxonomy of nursing interventions.* Iowa City: The University of Iowa, College of Nursing.

Iowa Intervention Project. (1992b). In J. C. McCloskey & G. M. Bulechek (Eds.), *Nursing interventions classification (NIC).* St. Louis: Mosby-Year Book.

Iowa Intervention Project. (1993). The NIC taxonomy structure. *Image: Journal of Nursing Scholarship, 25*(3), 187–192.

Iowa Intervention Project. (1995). Validation and coding of the NIC taxonomy structure. *Image: Journal of Nursing Scholarship, 27*(1), 43–49.

Johnson, M. (1995). Healing determinants in older people with leg ulcers. *Research in Nursing & Health, 18*(5), 395–403.

Kirchhoff, K. T., & Dille, C. A. (1994). Issues in intervention research: Maintaining integrity. *Applied Nursing Research, 7*(1), 32–46.

Lamb, K. (1979). Effect of positioning of postoperative fractured-hip patients as related to comfort. *Nursing Research, 28*(5), 291–294.

Lauver, D. (1989). Instructional information and breast self-examination practice. *Research in Nursing & Health, 12*(1), 11–19.

Lauver, D. (1992, October). *Promoting prompt care seeking for breast cancer symptoms in Caucasian and African-American women.* Paper presented at University of Illinois Conference: Reframing women's health: Multidisciplinary research and practice, Chicago, IL.

Lauver, D. (1994). Care-seeking behavior with breast cancer symptoms in Caucasian and African-American women. *Research in Nursing & Health, 17*(6), 421–431.

Lauver, D., & Tak, Y. (1995). Optimism and coping with a breast cancer symptom. *Nursing Research, 44*(4), 202–207.

Legault, M., & Goulet, C. (1995). Comparison of kangaroo and traditional methods of removing preterm infants from incubators. *Journal of Gynecologic and Neonatal Nursing, 24*(6), 501–506.

Lepczyk, M., Raleigh, E. H., & Rowley, C. (1990). Timing of preoperative patient teaching. *Journal of Advanced Nursing, 15*(3), 300–306.

Lewis, L. L. (1995). One year in the life of a woman with premenstrual syndrome: A case study. *Nursing Research, 44*(2), 111–116.

Ludington-Hoe, S., & Kasper, C. E. (1995). A physiologic method for monitoring premature infants. *Journal of Nursing Measurement, 3*(1), 13–29.

Mason-Hawkes, J., & Holm, K. (1989). Causal modeling: A comparison of path analysis and LISREL. *Nursing Research, 38*(5), 312–314.

McCain, L. J., & McCleary, R. (1979). The statistical analysis of the simple interrupted time-series quasi-experiment. In T. D. Cook & D. T. Campbell (Eds.), *Quasi-experimentation: Design and analysis issues for field settings* (pp. 233–293). Chicago: Rand McNally.

McCloskey, J. C., & Bulechek, G. M. (1993). Defining and classifying nursing interventions. In P. Moritz (Ed.), *Patient outcomes research: Examining the effectiveness of nursing practice: Proceedings of the state of the science conference* (NIH Publication No. 93-5411, pp. 63–69). Washington, DC: National Institute of Nursing Research.

McCloskey, J. C., & Bulechek, G. M. (1994a). Classification of nursing interventions: Implications for nursing research. In J. Fitzpatrick, J. Stevenson, & N. Polis (Eds.), *Nursing research and its utilization* (pp. 65–81). New York: Springer.

McCloskey, J. C., & Bulechek, G. M. (1994b). Standardizing the language for nursing treatments: An overview of the issues. *Nursing Outlook, 42*(2), 56–63.

Mirolo, B. R., Bunce, I. H., Chapman, M., Olsen, T., Eliadis, P., Hennessy, J. M., Ward, L. C., & Jones, L. C. (1995). Psychosocial benefits of postmastectomy lymphedema therapy. *Cancer Nursing, 18*(3), 197–205.

Moorhead, S. A., McCloskey, J. C., & Bulechek, G. M. (1993). Nursing interventions classification (NIC): A comparison with the Omaha system and the home health care classification. *Journal of Nursing Administration, 23*(10), 23–29.

Newman, M. A. (1986). *Health as expanding consciousness.* St. Louis: Mosby.

O'Flynn, A. I. (1982). Meta-analysis. *Nursing Research, 31*(5), 314–316.

Pohl, J. M., Boyd, C., Liang, J., & Given, C. W. (1995). Analysis of the impact of mother-daughter relationships on the commitment to caregiving. *Nursing Research, 44*(2), 68–75.

Prescott, P. A., Soeken, K. L., & Griggs, M. (1995). Identification and referral of hospitalized patients in need of home care. *Research in Nursing & Health, 18*(2), 85–95.

Quayhagen, M. P., Quayhagen, M., Corbeil, R. R., Roth, P. A., & Rodgers, J. A. (1995). A dyadic remediation program for care recipients with dementia. *Nursing Research, 44*(3), 153–159.

Reichardt, C. S. (1979). The statistical analysis of data from nonequivalent group designs. In T. D. Cook & D. T. Campbell (Eds.), *Quasi-experimentation: Design and analysis issues for field settings* (pp. 147–206). Chicago: Rand McNally.

Robinson, K. M., & Kaye, J. (1994). The relationship between spiritual perspective, social support, and depression in caregiving and noncaregiving wives. *Scholarly Inquiry for Nursing Practice: An International Journal, 8*(4), 375–396.

Shiao, S. P. K., Youngblut, J. M., Anderson, G. C., DiFiore, J. M., & Martin, R. J. (1995). Nasogastric tube placement: Effects on breathing and sucking in very-low-birth-weight infants. *Nursing Research, 44*(2), 82–88.

Spector, P. E. (1981). *Research designs.* Beverly Hills, CA: Sage.

Stewart, B. J., & Archbold, P. G. (1992). Nursing intervention studies require outcome measures that are sensitive to change, part 1. *Research in Nursing & Health, 15*(6), 477–481.

Stewart, B. J., & Archbold, P. G. (1993). Nursing intervention studies require outcome measures that are sensitive to change, part 2. *Research in Nursing & Health, 16*(1), 77–81.

Thomas, K. A. (1991). The emergence of body temperature biorhythm in preterm infants. *Nursing Research, 40*(2), 98–102.

Timm, M. M. (1979). Prenatal education evaluation. *Nursing Research, 28*(6), 338–342.

Tripp-Reimer, T., Woodworth, G., McCloskey, J. C., & Bulechek, G. (1996). The dimensional structure of nursing interventions. *Nursing Research, 45*(1), 10–17.

Tyzenhouse, P. S. (1981). Technical notes: The nursing clinical trial. *Western Journal of Nursing Research, 3*(1), 102–109.

United States Department of Health and Human Services (USDHHS) (1968). *The Framingham Study: An epidemiological investigation of cardiovascular disease.* Bethesda, MD: U.S. Department of Health and Human Services (RC667F813).

Van Rossum, E. V., Frederiks, C., Philipsen, H., Lierop, J. K., Mantel, A., Portengen, J., & Knipschild, P. (1991). Design of a Dutch study to test preventive home visits to the elderly. *Nursing Research, 40*(3), 185–188.

Waltz, C. F., & Bausell, R. B. (1981). *Nursing research: Design, statistics and computer analysis.* Philadelphia: Davis.

Whitney, J. D., Stotts, N. A., & Goodson, W. H., III. (1995). Effects of dynamic exercise on subcutaneous oxygen tension and temperature. *Research in Nursing & Health, 18*(2), 97–104.

Wikblad, K., & Anderson, B. (1995). A comparison of three wound dressings in patients undergoing heart surgery. *Nursing Research, 44*(5), 312–316.

Wilbur, J., Zoeller, L. H., Talashek, M., & Sullivan, J. A. (1990). Career trends of master's-prepared family nurse practitioners. *Journal of the American Academy of Nurse Practitioners, 2*(2), 69–78.

Woods, N. F. (1990). Testing theoretically based nursing care: Necessary modifications of the clinical trial. *Western Journal of Nursing Research, 12*(6), 777–782.

Yin, R. (1984). *Case study research: Design and methods.* Applied Social Research Methods Series, Vol. 5. Beverly Hills, CA: Sage.

Youssef, F. A. (1990). The impact of group reminiscence counseling on a depressed elderly population. *Nurse Practitioner, 15*(4), 32–38.

Zahr, L. K., & Balian, S. (1995). Responses of premature infants to routine nursing interventions and noise in the NICU. *Nursing Research, 44*(3), 179–185.

12 Sampling

One tends to enter the field of research with preconceived notions about samples and sampling, many of which are acquired through exposure to television advertisements, polls of public opinion, market researchers in shopping centers, and newspaper reports of research findings. The commercial boasts that four out of five doctors recommend their product; the newscaster announces that John Jones is predicted to win the senate election by a margin of 3 to 1; the newspaper reports that scientists have now shown that treatment of early breast cancer with lumpectomy and radiation is as effective as mastectomy.

All of the aforementioned examples use sampling techniques. However, some of the outcomes are more valid than others. The differences in validity are due, in part, to the sampling techniques used. In most instances, television, newspapers, and advertisements do not explain their sampling techniques. You may hold certain opinions about the adequacy of these techniques, but there is inadequate information from which to make a judgment.

In research, it is critical that the sampling component of the research process be carefully thought out and clearly described. This requires knowledge of the techniques of sampling and the reasoning behind them. With this knowledge, you can make intelligent judgments about sampling when critiquing studies or developing a sampling plan for your own study. This chapter examines sampling theory and concepts, sampling plans, probability and nonprobability sampling plans, sample size, and the process of acquiring a sample.

SAMPLING THEORY

Sampling involves selecting a group of people, events, behaviors, or other elements with which to conduct a study. A *sampling plan* defines the process of making the selections; *sample* denotes the selected group of people or elements. Sampling decisions have a major impact on the meaning and generalizability of the findings.

Sampling theory was developed to determine mathematically the most effective way to acquire a sample that would accurately reflect the population under study. The theoretical, mathematical rationale for decisions related to sampling emerged from survey research, though the techniques were first applied to experimental research by agricultural scientists. One of the most important surveys that stimulated improvements in survey techniques was the national census. The assumptions of sampling theory have been adopted by researchers and incorporated within the research process.

Key concepts of sampling theory include elements, populations, sampling criteria, representativeness, sampling errors, randomization, sampling frames, and sampling plans. The following sections explain the meaning of these concepts. In later sections, these concepts will be used to explain a variety of sampling techniques.

ELEMENTS AND POPULATIONS

The individual units of a population are called *elements*. An element can be a person, event, behavior, or any other single unit of a study. When elements are persons, they are referred to as *subjects*. The *population,* sometimes referred to as the *target population,* is the entire set of individuals or elements who meet the sampling criteria. An *accessible population* is the portion of the target population to which the researcher has reasonable access. The accessible population might be elements within a state, city, hospital, or nursing unit. The sample is obtained from the accessible population, and findings are generalized first to the accessible population and then, more abstractly, to the target population. Generalizing means that the findings can be applied more generally than just to the sample under study. Because of the importance of generalizing, there are risks to defining the accessible population too narrowly. For example, a narrow definition of the accessible population reduces the ability to generalize from the study and thus reduces the meaningfulness of the findings. Biases may be introduced that make generalization to the broader target population difficult to defend. If the accessible population is defined as individuals in a white upper-middle-class setting, one cannot generalize to nonwhite or lower income populations. These biases are similar to those that may be encountered in a nonrandom sample.

In some studies, the entire population is the target of the study. These studies are referred to as *population studies* (Barhyte, Redman, & Neill, 1990). In many of these studies, data used for the study is available in large databases such as the census data or other government maintained databases. Epidemiologists often use entire populations for their large database studies. In other studies, the entire population of interest in the study is very small and well defined. For example, one could conduct a study in which the defined population was all living heart transplant patients.

In some cases, a hypothetical population is defined. A hypothetical population assumes the presence of a population that cannot be defined according to sampling theory rules, which require a list of all members of the population. For example, individuals who successfully lose weight would be a hypothetical population. The number of individuals in the population, who they are, how much weight they have lost, how long they have kept it off, or how they achieved the weight loss is unknown. Some populations are elusive and constantly changing. For example, listing all women in active labor in the United States, all people grieving the loss of a loved one, or all people coming into an emergency room would be impossible.

SAMPLING CRITERIA

Sampling criteria list the characteristics essential for membership in the target population. The criteria are developed from the research problem, the purpose, the conceptual and operational definitions of the study variables, and the design. The sample is selected from the population that meets the sampling criteria. When the study is completed, the findings are generalized to this population. The sampling criteria may be designed to make the population as homogeneous as possible or to control for extraneous variables. In descriptive or correlational studies, the sampling criteria may be defined to insure a heterogeneous population with a broad range of values on the variables being studied. In quasi-experimental or experimental studies, the primary purpose of sampling criteria is to limit the effect of extraneous variables on the particular interaction between the dependent and independent variables. Subjects are selected to maximize the effects of the independent variable and minimize the effects of variation in other variables. The number of restrictions that can be imposed by the sampling criteria depends on the typical patient load in the selected setting.

Sampling criteria may include such characteristics as the ability to read, to write responses on the data collection instruments or forms, and to comprehend and communicate using the English language. Age limitations are often included, such as studying adults 18 years and older. Subjects may be limited to those not participating in any other study. Persons who are able to participate fully in the procedure for obtaining informed consent are often selected as subjects. If potential subjects have diminished autonomy or are unable to give informed consent, consent must be obtained from their legal representative. Thus, persons who are legally or mentally incompetent, terminally ill, or confined to an institution are more difficult to access as subjects. Sampling criteria can become so restrictive that an adequate number of subjects cannot be found. Narrow and restrictive sampling criteria will reduce the sample size or make obtaining a sample difficult.

Inclusion criteria and exclusion criteria may be

used to develop the desired sample. *Inclusion criteria* are characteristics that must be present for the element to be included in the sample. For example, for subjects to be included in the study, they must have been diagnosed with Stage II breast cancer within the previous three months. *Exclusion criteria* are exceptions to the inclusion criteria. For example, women who meet the inclusion criteria of diagnosis with Stage II breast cancer within the previous three months might be excluded if they had a previous diagnosis of breast cancer. The researcher needs to provide logical reasons for the inclusions and exclusions. Larson (1994) suggests that some groups such as women, ethnic minorities, the elderly, and the poor are unnecessarily excluded from many studies. A review of approved research protocols in one tertiary care center (1989–1990) revealed that 75% of studies listed exclusion criteria, many of which were not justified by the researchers. The most common exclusions for which no justification was provided were age, socioeconomic status, and race. Only 26.6% of nursing protocols included a justification for age. Exclusions limit generalizability and should be carefully considered.

Good (1995), in a study of the effects of jaw relaxation and music on postoperative pain, described their sampling criteria as follows.

◾

"The sampling frame included every eligible patient listed for elective abdominal surgery in two teaching and two community hospitals during a 7-month period. Patients were identified daily by the investigator from surgery lists, and eligibility was decided in consultation with office nurses. Inclusion criteria were: (a) aged 21 to 65 years, (b) scheduled for major abdominal surgery, (c) receiving intramuscular (IM) PRN analgesia, and (d) hospitalized 2 or more days postoperatively. Patients who had laparoscopic surgeries or psychosis or retardation were excluded. All eligible patients ($N = 126$) were contacted in the nursing unit, holding area, clinic, or by telephone. Of the 102 patients who consented and were assigned, 2 patients later withdrew and 16 were excluded from the analysis because of canceled surgery ($n = 4$), inability to ambulate after surgery ($n = 2$), unforseen patient-controlled analgesia ($n = 9$), or treatment error ($n = 1$). Thus, the sample consisted of 84 subjects, 25 men and 59 women aged 23 to 64 years." (p. 53) ◾

Note that the study excluded subjects over the age of 65 and provided no justification for this exclusion. It is left to the imagination of the reader to guess the reasons for the exclusions. One might guess that laparoscopic surgeries would not generally be classified as major abdominal surgery and might have a different pain trajectory than surgeries requiring an incision, or that providing instructions for relaxation and measuring differences in pain relief for patients with psychosis or retardation might require a different study design and different measurement methods.

REPRESENTATIVENESS

Representativeness means that the sample must be like the population in as many ways as possible. It is especially important that the sample be representative in relation to the variables being studied and to other factors that may influence the study variables. For example, if the study examined attitudes toward AIDS, the sample should be representative of the distribution of attitudes toward AIDS that exists in the specified population. In addition, a sample needs to be representative of such characteristics as age, gender, ethnicity, income, and education, which often influence study variables.

The accessible population must be representative of the target population. If the accessible population is limited to a particular setting or type of setting, the individuals seeking care at that setting may be different than those who would seek care for the same problem at other settings, or from those who choose to use self-care to manage their problems. Studies conducted in private hospitals usually exclude the poor. Other settings could exclude the elderly or the undereducated, while those who do not have access to care are usually excluded from studies. Subjects in research centers and the care they receive are different from patients and the care they receive in community hospitals, public hospitals, veterans' hospitals, or rural hospitals. Obese individuals who chose to enter a program to lose weight may differ from those who did not enter a program. All of these factors limit representativeness. This, in turn, limits our understanding of phenomena important to the nursing body of knowledge.

Representativeness is usually evaluated by comparing numerical values of the sample (a *statistic* such as the mean) with the same values from the target population. A numerical value of a population is called a *parameter*. We can estimate the population parameter by identifying the values obtained in previous studies examining the same variables. The accuracy with which the population parameters have been estimated within a study is referred to as *precision*. These statistical concepts are discussed further in Chapter 16. Precision in estimating parameters requires well-developed methods of measurement that are used repeatedly across studies. Parameters can be defined by conducting a series of descriptive and correlational studies, with each study examining a different segment of the target population. Meta-analysis can then be performed to estimate the population parameter.

Of major importance is whether the samples used to establish parameters were representative of the target population in terms of characteristics such as age, gender, ethnicity, educational level, and socioeconomic status. Assessment of this information may lead to redefining the target population for which we have a body of knowledge in a particular area of study.

SAMPLING ERROR

The difference between a sample statistic and a population parameter is called the *sampling error* (see Figure 12–1). A large sampling error means that the sample is not providing a precise picture of the population; it is not representative. Sampling error is usually larger with small samples and decreases as the sample size increases. Sam-

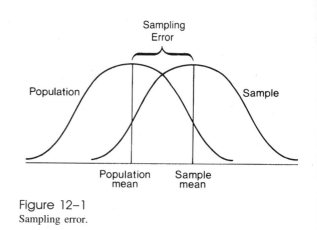

Figure 12–1
Sampling error.

pling error decreases the power to detect differences between groups or accurately describe the relationships between or among variables, and occurs as a result of random variation and systematic variation.

Random Variation

Random variation is the expected difference in values that occurs when one examines different subjects from the same sample. If the mean is used to describe the sample, the values of individuals in that sample will not all be exactly the same as the sample mean. Individual subject's values will vary from the value of the sample mean. The difference is random because the value of each subject is likely to vary in a different direction. Some values will be higher and others will be lower than the sample mean. Thus, the values will be randomly scattered around the mean. As the sample size becomes larger, overall variation in sample values decreases, with more values being close to the sample mean. As the sample size increases, the sample mean is also more likely to have a value similar to that of the population mean.

Systematic Variation

Systematic variation, or systematic bias, is a consequence of selecting subjects whose measurement values are different, or vary, in some specific way from the population. Because the subjects have something in common, their values tend to be similar to others in the sample but different in some way from those of the population as a whole. These values do not vary randomly around the population mean. Most of the variation from the mean is in the same direction; it is systematic. All the values in the sample may tend to be higher or lower than the population mean. For example, if all the subjects in a study examining some type of knowledge have an intelligence quotient (IQ) above 120, their scores will likely all be higher than the mean of a population that includes individuals with a wide variation in IQ. The IQs of the subjects have introduced a systematic bias. This could occur, for example, if all of the subjects were college students, which has been the case in the development of many measurement methods in psychology. Because of systematic variance, the sample mean is different from the population mean. The extent of the difference is the sampling error. Exclusion criteria tend to increase the systematic bias in the sample and thus, increase the sampling error. An extreme example of this problem is the highly restrictive sampling criteria used by clinical trials, resulting in a large sampling error and greatly diminished representativeness.

If the method of selecting subjects produces a sample with a systematic bias, increasing the sample size will not decrease the sampling error. When a systematic bias occurs in an experimental study, it can lead the researcher to think that the treatment has made a difference when, in actuality, the values would be different even without the treatment. This usually occurs because of an interaction of the systematic bias with the treatment. Systematic variation is most likely to occur when the sampling process is not random.

RANDOM SAMPLING

From a sampling theory point of view, each individual in the population should have a greater than zero opportunity to be selected for the sample. The method of achieving this opportunity is referred to as *random sampling*. In experimental studies in which a control group is used, subjects are randomly selected for placement in the control group and the experimental group as well as being randomly selected for participation in the study. The use of the term *control group* is limited to those studies using random sampling methods. If nonrandom methods are used for sample selection, the group not receiving a treatment is referred to as a *comparison group* since there is an increased possibility of pre-existing differences in the experimental and the comparison groups. The purpose of random sampling is to increase the extent to which the sample is representative of the target population. However, the random sampling must take place in an accessible population that is representative of the target population. Exclusion criteria limit true randomness. Thus, a study can use random sampling techniques, but have such restrictive sampling criteria that the study is not truly random. In any case, it is rarely possible to obtain a purely random sample for clinical nursing studies because of informed consent requirements. Those who volunteer to participate in a study may differ in important ways from those not willing to participate. Methods of achieving random sampling are described later in the chapter.

SAMPLING FRAMES

In order for each person in the target or accessible population to have an opportunity for selection in the sample, each person in the population must be identified. To accomplish this, a listing of every member of the population must be acquired, using the sampling criteria to define membership. This listing is referred to as the *sampling frame*. Subjects are then selected from the sampling frame using a sampling plan.

SAMPLING PLANS

A *sampling plan* describes the strategies that will be used to obtain a sample for a study. It is developed to increase representativeness, decrease systematic bias, and decrease the sampling error. To accomplish this task, sampling theory has devised strategies for optimal sample selection. The sampling plan may use probability (random) sampling methods or nonprobability (nonrandom) sampling methods. A *sampling method* is similar to a design; it is not specific to a study. The sampling plan provides detail about the use of a sampling method in a specific study. The sampling plan needs to be described in detail for purposes of critique, replication, and future meta-analyses.

PROBABILITY (RANDOM) SAMPLING METHODS

Probability sampling methods have been developed to ensure some degree of precision in accurately estimating the population parameters. Thus, probability samples reduce sampling error. The term *probability sample* refers to the fact that *every* member (element) of the population has a probability higher than zero of being selected for the sample. Inferential statistical analyses are based on the assumption that the sample from which data were derived have been obtained randomly. Thus, probability samples are often referred to as random samples. Such a sample is more likely to be representative of the population than a nonprobability sample. All the subsets of the population, which may differ from each other but contribute to the parameters of the population, have a chance to be represented in the sample. There is less opportunity for systematic bias if subjects are selected randomly although it is possible for a systematic bias to occur by chance. Using random sampling, the researcher cannot decide that person X will be a better subject for the study than person Y. In addition, researchers cannot exclude a subset of people from being selected as subjects because they do not agree with them, do not like them, or find them hard to deal with. Potential subjects cannot be excluded because they are too sick, not sick enough, coping too well, or not coping adequately. Researchers, who have a vested interest in their study could tend (con-

sciously or unconsciously) to select subjects whose conditions or behaviors are consistent with their hypothesis. It is tempting to exclude uncooperative or noncompliant individuals. Random sampling leaves the selection to chance and thus increases the validity of the study.

Theoretically, to obtain a probability sample, the researcher must identify every element in the population. A sampling frame must be developed, and the sample must be randomly selected from the sampling frame. Thus, according to sampling theory, it is not possible to select a sample randomly from a population that cannot be clearly defined. Four sampling designs have been developed to achieve probability sampling: simple random sampling, stratified random sampling, cluster sampling, and systematic sampling.

SIMPLE RANDOM SAMPLING

Simple random sampling is the most basic of the probability sampling methods. To achieve simple random sampling, elements are selected at random from the sampling frame. This can be accomplished in a variety of ways, limited only by the imagination of the researcher. If the sampling frame is small, names can be written on slips of paper, placed in a container, mixed well, and then drawn out one at a time until the desired sample size has been reached. Another technique is assigning a number to each name in the sampling frame. In large population sets, elements may already have assigned numbers. For example, numbers are assigned to medical records, organizational memberships, and licenses. Numbers then are selected randomly to obtain a sample.

There can be some differences in the probability for the selection of each element, depending on whether the selected element's name or number is replaced before the next name or number is selected. Selection with replacement, the most conservative random sampling approach, provides exactly equal opportunities for each element to be selected. For example, if the researcher draws names out of a hat to obtain a sample, each name must be replaced prior to drawing the next name to ensure equal opportunities for each subject. Selection without replacement gives each element differing levels of probability of selection. For example, if the researcher is selecting 10 subjects from a population of 50, the first name has a 1 in 5 chance, or a .2 probability, of being selected. If the first name is not replaced, the second name has a 9 in 49 chance, or a .18 probability, of being selected. As further names are drawn, the probability of being selected decreases.

There are many ways of achieving random selection. For example, a computer, bingo wheel, or roulette wheel could be used. The most common method of random selection is a table of random numbers. A section from a random numbers table is presented in Table 12–1. To use a table of random numbers, a pencil or the finger is placed on the random table with the eyes closed. That number is the starting place. Then moving up, down, right, or left, numbers are used in order until the desired sample size is obtained. If the pencil were initially placed on 58 in Table 12–1, which is in the 4th column from the left and 4th row down; if five subjects were to be selected from a population of 100; and if a decision were made to go across the column to the right, the subject numbers would be 58, 25, 15, 55, and 38. This particular table is only useful if the population number is less than 100. However, tables are available for larger populations. A larger random numbers table is available in Appendix A. With very large populations in which the sampling frame has been computerized, the simplest approach is to write a computer program to select subjects randomly.

Hart (1995) used random sampling in her study of pregnant women with Orem's self-care

deficit theory as a framework. She describes her sample selection as follows.

"A random sample of women over 18 years of age who could read, write and speak English was chosen from a tertiary hospital obstetric clinic, a health department clinic, and a private federally-funded clinic in south Georgia. Women were in at least their 30th week of pregnancy. It was felt that by this time the subjects would have established a prenatal care routine and would have established the foundations for dependent-care agency. The researcher reviewed the daily appointment book to determine the list of eligible participants. Using a flip of the coin, a list of potential subjects was generated. Subjects were approached individually in the waiting room and asked to participate in the study. Data were collected over a period of 7 months. A total of 147 pregnant women were asked to participate; 127 completed the questionnaires. Most refusals were due to lack of interest or time and dealing with their children in the waiting room. An adequate number of participants was determined based on power analysis described by Cohen (1988). In this study, the number of independent variables is equal to eight. Because R^2 cannot be estimated, Cohen (1988) suggests a medium effect size of $R^2 = .13$ as adequate for correlational research. The power selected was .80." (pp. 121–122) ∎

STRATIFIED RANDOM SAMPLING

Stratified random sampling is used in situations in which the researcher knows some of the variables in the population that are critical to achieving representativeness. Variables commonly used for stratification include age, gender, ethnicity, socioeconomic status, diagnosis, geographic region, type of institution, type of care, and site of care. The variable(s) chosen to stratify needs to be correlated with the dependent variables being examined in the study. Subjects within each stratum are expected to be more alike (homogeneous) in relation to the study variables than they are to be

Table 12–1
Section from a Random Numbers Table

06	84	10	22	56	72	25	70	69	43
07	63	10	34	66	39	54	02	33	85
03	19	63	93	72	52	13	30	44	40
77	32	69	58	25	15	55	38	19	62
20	01	94	54	66	88	43	91	34	28

like other age strata or the total sample. In stratified random sampling, the subjects are randomly selected based on their classification into the selected strata. For example, if a sample of 100 subjects were planned, the researcher might plan to obtain 25 subjects under the age of 20, 25 subjects in the age range of 20 to 39, 25 subjects in the age range of 40 to 59, and 25 subjects over the age of 60.

Stratification ensures that all levels of the identified variables will be adequately represented in the sample. Stratification allows the researcher to use a smaller sample size and achieve the same degree of representativeness as a large sample acquired through simple random sampling. Sampling error is decreased, power is increased, data collection time is reduced, and the cost of the study is lower using stratification.

One question that arises in relation to stratification is whether each stratum should have equivalent numbers of subjects in the sample (disproportionate sampling) or whether the numbers of subjects should be selected in proportion to their occurrence in the population (proportionate sampling). For example, if stratification were being achieved by ethnicity and the population was 60% Caucasian, 20% African American, 15% Mexican American, and 5% Asian, the researcher would have to decide whether to select equal numbers of each ethnic group or calculate a proportion of the sample. Good arguments exist for both approaches. Stratification is not as useful if one stratum contains only a small number of subjects. In the aforementioned situation, if proportions are used and the sample size is 50, the study would include only 2 Asians, hardly enough to be representative. If equal numbers of each group are used, each group will contain at least 12 subjects; however, the Caucasian group will be underrepresented. In this case, mathematically weighting the findings from each stratum can equalize the representation to ensure proportional contributions of each stratum to the total score of the sample. This procedure is described in most textbooks on sampling (Cochran, 1977; Friday, 1967; Hansen, Hurwitz, & Madow, 1953; Levy & Lemsbow, 1980; Sudman, 1974; Williams, 1978; Yates, 1981).

Princeton and Gaspar (1991) used stratified random sampling in their study, "First-line nurse administrators in academe: How are they prepared, what do they do, and will they stay in their jobs?" The following is their description of the sampling procedure.

■

"A random sample of 42 schools was drawn from the 114 nursing schools throughout the nation that were accredited by the National League for Nursing at the time, and that offered bachelor's degree and graduate nursing programs. The sample was stratified by geographic area and source of funding (public or private). The rationale for using these schools was that there was a high probability that they differentiated top-, mid-, and first-level administrative roles due to the size of the student population and the programs offered. This rationale was validated during the research project." (p. 82) ■

CLUSTER SAMPLING

Cluster sampling is used in two situations. The first situation is when a simple random sample would be prohibitive in terms of travel time and cost. Imagine trying to arrange personal meetings with 100 people, each in a different part of the United States. The second situation is in cases in which the individual elements making up the population are not known, thus preventing the development of a sampling frame. For example, there is no list of all the open-heart surgery patients in the United States. In these cases, it is often possible to obtain lists of institutions or organizations with which the elements of interest are associated.

In *cluster sampling,* a sampling frame is developed that includes a list of all the states, cities, institutions, or organizations with which elements of the identified population would be linked. States, cities, institutions, or organizations are selected randomly as units from which to obtain elements for the sample. In some cases, this random selection continues through several stages and is then referred to as multistage sampling. For example, the researcher might first randomly select states, then randomly select cities within the sampled states. Then hospitals within the randomly selected cities might be randomly selected. Within the hospitals, nursing units might be randomly selected. At this level, all the patients on the nursing unit who fit the criteria for the study might be included, or patients could be randomly selected.

Cluster sampling provides a means for obtaining a larger sample at a lower cost. However, there are some disadvantages. Data from subjects associated with the same institution are likely to be correlated and, thus, not completely independent. This can lead to a decrease in precision and an increase in sampling error. However, these disadvantages can be offset to some extent by a larger sample.

Mitchell, Woods, and Lentz (1994) used multistage cluster sampling in their study differentiating women with three perimenstrual symptom patterns. They describe their sampling procedure as follows.

■───────────────────────

"The community sample of healthy women participating in this study was obtained through a multistage sampling procedure commonly used in epidemiological studies. First, census block groups were selected using age, income, and ethnicity to facilitate the selection of a sample of menstruating women between the ages of 18 and 45 with a wide range of incomes. The ethnic mix was representative of the northwestern metropolitan area that was sampled. Second, street segments were identified and randomly ordered by computer from the selected census block groups. Third, residential telephone numbers for every household within the computer-generated street segments were obtained from a city directory. Finally, telephone contact was made with 5,755 households, and 1,135 women between the ages of 18 and 45 were identified.

Criteria for inclusion were as follows: age between 18 and 45, not currently pregnant, not being treated for a gynecological problem, having menstrual periods, and the ability to write and understand English. Women taking birth control pills (BCP) were included in the original data collection but were excluded from the analysis for this study to avoid confounding the sample selection and results with effects of exogenous hormones.

Six hundred fifty-six eligible women who satisfied all the inclusion criteria completed an in-home interview and received instructions about keeping the Washington Women's Health Diary (WWHD). Three hundred forth-three women returned at least one complete cycle of daily data. Of these 343 women, 47 were taking BCPs, leaving 296 women who were not on any ovarian hormones. A total of 142 of these women fell into one of the three subgroups of interest for this study. The remaining 154 women fell into one of 25 other possible symptom severity subgroups that were not part of this study." (pp. 26–27) ■

SYSTEMATIC SAMPLING

Systematic sampling can be conducted when an ordered list of all members of the population is available. The process involves selecting every kth individual on the list, using a starting point selected randomly. If the initial starting point is not random, it is not a probability sample. In order to use this design, the researcher must know the number of elements in the population and the size of the sample desired. The population size is divided by the desired sample size, giving k, the size of the gap between elements selected from the list. For example, if the population size was $N = 1200$ and the desired sample size was $n = 50$, then $k = 24$. Every 24th person on the list would be included in the sample. This value is obtained by dividing 1200 by 50. There is argument that this procedure does not truly give each element an opportunity to be included in the sample; it provides a random but not equal chance for inclusion.

Care needs to be taken to determine that the original list has not been set up with any ordering that could be meaningful in relation to the study. The assumption is being made that the order of the list is random in relation to the variables being studied. If the order of the list is related to the study, it would introduce a systematic bias. In addition to this risk, computation of the sampling error using this design is difficult. For additional information in systematic sampling, see Floyd (1993).

Stuifbergen (1995) may have used systematic sampling in her study, "Health-promoting behaviors and quality of life among individuals with multiple sclerosis." She described her sampling procedure as follows.

"In this descriptive correlational study, subjects were recruited through a mailing to 200 individuals on the mailing list of the local chapter of the National Multiple Sclerosis Society. To protect the privacy of respondents, the mailing labels on the envelopes were affixed by staff at the MS office. Individuals who were interested in receiving more information about the study and possibly participating were asked to return a card providing name and phone number to the investigator. Seventy-five postcards were returned. A target sample size of 60 that would allow correlations greater than .25 to be detected as statistically significant at the .05 level was chosen for this study (Glass & Stanley, 1970). Research staff contacted interested individuals by phone to explain study requirements and procedures. If the individual wished to participate, a data collection visit was scheduled at a mutually acceptable time at the investigator's research office. Calls continued until 61 subjects were recruited. Only two phone contacts declined to participate, one for transportation reasons; a second was too disabled to leave the home setting." (pp. 38–39) ∎

NONPROBABILITY (NONRANDOM) SAMPLING METHODS

In *nonprobability sampling,* not every element of the population has an opportunity for being included in the sample. Although this approach to sampling increases the possibilities of samples that

are not representative, it has been commonly used in nursing studies. In an analysis of nursing studies published in six nursing journals from 1977 to 1986, only 9% used random sampling (Moody et al., 1988). The majority of the studies examined were descriptive or correlational in nature. Only 30% of the nursing studies reported during this period used quasi-experimental or experimental designs likely to require assignment of subjects to groups.

Kraemer and Thiemann (1987) classify studies as exploratory or confirmatory. Confirmatory studies should be conducted only after a large body of knowledge has been gathered through exploratory studies. Confirmatory studies are expected to have large samples and to use random sampling techniques. These expectations are lessened for exploratory studies. Exploratory studies are not intended for generalization to large populations. They are designed to increase the knowledge of the field of study. For example, pilot or preliminary studies to test a methodology or provide estimates of an effect size are often conducted prior to a larger study. In other studies, the variables, not the subjects, are the primary area of concern. The same variables may be examined in several studies using different populations. In these types of studies, the specific population used may be somewhat incidental. Data from these studies may be used to define population parameters. This information can then be used to conduct confirmatory studies using large, randomly selected samples.

There are several types of nonprobability sampling designs. Each addresses a different research need. The five nonprobability designs included are convenience sampling, quota sampling, random assignment to groups, purposive sampling, and network sampling.

CONVENIENCE (ACCIDENTAL) SAMPLING

Convenience sampling is considered a poor approach to sampling because it provides little opportunity to control for biases. In *convenience sampling,* subjects are included in the study because they happened to be in the right place at the right time. Available subjects are simply entered into the study until the desired sample size is reached. Multiple biases may exist in the sample, some of which may be subtle and unrecognized. However, serious biases are not always present in convenience samples.

The researcher needs to identify and describe known biases in the sample. Carefully thinking through the characteristics of the population, the researcher can identify biases likely to occur. Steps can then be taken to increase the representativeness of the sample. For example, if you are studying home care management of patients with complex health care needs, educational level will be an important extraneous variable. One solution would be to redefine the sampling criteria to include only those individuals with a high school education. This would limit the extent of generalization. Another option would be to select a population known to include individuals with a wide variety of educational levels. Data could be collected on educational level, so that the description of the sample would include information on educational level. With this information, one could judge the extent to which the sample was representative in respect to educational level.

Decisions related to sample selection need to be carefully described to allow others to evaluate the possibility of biases. In addition, data need to be gathered to allow a thorough description of the sample. This information can be used to evaluate for possible biases. Data on the sample can be used to compare the sample with other samples and for estimating the parameters of populations through meta-analyses.

Many strategies are available for selecting a convenience sample. A classroom of students might be used. Patients who attend a clinic on a specific day, subjects who attend a support group, patients currently admitted to a hospital with a specific diagnosis or nursing problem, and every fifth person who enters the emergency room are examples of types of frequently selected convenience samples.

Convenience samples are inexpensive, accessible, and usually require less time to acquire than other types of samples. Convenience samples provide means to conduct studies on topics that could not be examined using probability sampling. They provide means to acquire information in unexplored areas. As Kerlinger (1986) stated: "Used with reasonable knowledge and care, it [convenience sampling] is probably not as bad as it has been said to be" (p. 120). Kerlinger recommends using this type of sampling only if there is no possibility of obtaining a sample by other means. Convenience sampling is useful for exploratory studies but, in most cases, is unacceptable for confirmatory studies.

Duffy (1994) used convenience sampling in her study, "Testing the theory of transcending options: Health behaviors of single parents." The following is a description of her sample selection.

"The participants were identified from the divorce records of three counties in Northern California. Selection criteria included the following: (a) the women had received their divorce within the previous 3 months; (b) they were divorced for the first time; (c) they had joint or sole physical custody of one or more children under the age of 18; and (d) they were single. Data were collected annually for 2 years because the women's psychological status and social support (independent variables) were expected to change as they adjusted to divorce.

The women were selected by reviewing the divorce records. Women with children were sent a letter explaining the study and the criteria for participation. A follow-up telephone call was made approximately 2 weeks after the mailing to receive permission to mail a packet of questionnaires. The power analysis indicated that 116 women would be sufficient, with 90% power to pick up a medium effect size for a multiple regression model with an alpha equal to .05 and five predictors (Cohen, 1977). Of the 252 women who participated at Time 1, 148 women (58.7%) remained single parents and completed the study. There were no significant differences at Time 1 on the major demographic variables—age, income, education, years married, and years single—between the women who completed the study and those who did not. The primary reasons for sample mortality were refusal to participate in subsequent years, inability to locate, and remarriage." (p. 195) ■

QUOTA SAMPLING

Quota sampling uses a convenience sampling technique with an added feature, a strategy to ensure the inclusion of subject types that are likely to be underrepresented in the convenience sample, such as women, minority groups, the aged, the poor, the rich, and the undereducated. It may also be used to mimic the known characteristics of the target population or to ensure adequate numbers of subjects in each strata for the planned statistical analyses. The technique is similar to that used in stratified random sampling. If necessary, mathematical weighting can be used to adjust sample values so that they are consistent with the proportion of subgroups found in the population. Quota sampling offers an improvement over convenience sampling and tends to decrease potential biases. In most studies in which convenience samples are used, quota sampling could be used and should be considered.

Gottlieb and Baillies (1995) used quota sampling in their study, "Firstborns' behaviors during a mother's second pregnancy." They described their sample selection as follows.

███████

"Eighty mothers and their only preschoolers agreed to participate. The study included four groups of 20 preschoolers: three groups of children of pregnant mothers (one each from the early, middle, and late phases of pregnancy); and a fourth group of children of non-pregnant mothers. Because the majority of pregnant women do not see a physician until the end of the first trimester, the study was begun at 12 weeks and extended to the 38th week, close to the birth.

The families were all intact families, and the preschoolers were their only children, 18 to 60 months of age. The mothers were employed less than 21 hours per week and had no intervening pregnancies between the first child and their participation in this study. To examine how behaviors differed as a function of a child's age and/or sex, each group was balanced for age (young: 18 to 36 months; old: 37 to 60 months) and sex. Thus, within each group, there were five young boys, five old boys, five young girls, and five old girls.

Families were recruited from the practices of obstetricians and pediatricians. Of the 72 eligible families expecting a second child, five families refused, and seven mothers did not complete the data collection schedule. The design called for 26 children per group for each age and sex to attain a power of .8 with alpha equal to .05 to detect a large effect size, $d = .4$ (Cohen, 1988). Preliminary analyses indicated significant effects with 20 per group; therefore, the sample was considered adequate. Children of the comparison group were recruited from the practices of pediatricians and nursery schools. The groups were compared for equivalency on all major background characteristics and, with the exception of mothers' and fathers' ages, did not differ significantly. Parents in the three pregnancy groups were younger than parents in the comparison group, $p < .05$. Families were predominantly white, middle-class, and well educated. Parents had been together an average of 7 years." (p. 357) ■

RANDOM ASSIGNMENT TO GROUPS

Random assignment is a procedure used to assign subjects to treatment or control groups randomly. Random assignment is most commonly used in nursing and medicine to assign subjects obtained through convenience sampling methods to groups for purposes of comparison. Random assignment used without random sampling is purported to decrease the risk of bias in the selection of groups. However, a meta-analysis by Ottenbacher (1992) examining the effect of random assignment versus nonrandom assignment on outcomes failed to reveal significant differences in these two sampling techniques. He suggests that previous assumptions regarding design strategies should be empirically tested.

Traditional approaches to random assignment involve the use of a random numbers table or flipping an unbiased coin to determine group assignment. However, these procedures can lead to unequal group sizes and thus a decrease in power. Hjelm-Karlsson (1991) suggests using what is referred to as a biased coin design to randomly assign subjects to groups. Using this technique, selection of the group to which a particular subject will be assigned is biased in favor of groups that have smaller sample sizes at the point of the assignment of a particular subject. This strategy is particularly useful when assignment is being made to more than two groups. Calculations for the sequencing of assignment to groups can be completed prior to initiation of data collection, thus freeing the researcher for other activities during this critical period of time. Hjelm-Karlsson (1991) suggests using cards to make group assignments. The subject number is placed on the card as well as the random group assignment. As each subject agrees to participate in the study, the next card is drawn, indicating that subject's number and group assignment.

Stout, Wirtz, Carbonari, and Del Boca (1994) suggest a similar strategy they refer to as urn randomization. "One would begin the study with two urns, each urn containing a red marble and a blue marble. There is one urn for each level of the stratifying variable; that is, in this example there is an urn for severely ill patients and another urn for the less severe patients. When a subject is ready for randomization, we determine whether or not he/she is severely ill and consult the corresponding urn. From this urn (say, for the severely ill group) we randomly select one marble and note its color. If the marble is red we assign the patient to Treatment A. Then we drop that marble back into the urn *and put a blue marble into the urn as well.* This leaves the 'severely ill' urn with one red and two blue marbles. The next time a severely ill patient shows up, the probability that he/she will be assigned to Group B will be ⅔ rather than ½, thus biasing the selection process toward

balance. A similar procedure is followed every time a severely ill subject presents for randomization. After each subject is assigned, the marble chosen from the urn is replaced together with a marble of the opposite color. The urn for the less severely ill group is not affected. If a low-severity patient presents for the study, that patient's probability of assignment to either treatment is not affected by the assignment of patients in the other stratum. To some extent, urn randomization can be tailored to maximize balancing or to maximize randomization" (p. 72). The authors also provide strategies for balancing several variables simultaneously during random assignment.

Brennan, Moore, and Smyth (1995) used random assignment in their study of "The effects of a special computer network on caregivers of persons with Alzheimer's disease." They describe their sampling procedure as follows.

"Caregivers of persons with Alzheimer's disease (N = 102) were recruited from three sources: A research registry for an Alzheimer's disease research center (n = 40); Alzheimer's Association Area Chapter support groups (n = 26); and self-referral, primarily in response to a letter from an area chapter inviting caregivers to participate in the study (n = 36). Eligibility criteria included: (a) primary responsibility as a family caregiver for a person with Alzheimer's disease who was living at home; (b) a local telephone exchange; and (c) the ability to read and write English.

Caregivers were randomly assigned to either the ComputerLink group (n = 51) or a comparison group (n = 51). Three subjects in the ComputerLink group were not able to have the computer terminal installed in their homes: two encountered technical installation difficulties, and one experienced a severe physical illness between recruitment into the study and installation of the computer. One additional caregiver asked to have the computer terminal removed from her home within the first 24 hours after installation, stating that 'it makes me nervous.' Thus, 47 caregivers had access to ComputerLink during the study period. Two subjects dropped out of the comparison group: one caregiver died before the end of the data collection period, and one could not be located at the second data collection timepoint. All other subjects participated for a 12-month period." (p. 167) ■

PURPOSIVE SAMPLING

Purposive sampling is sometimes referred to as judgmental sampling. Purposive sampling involves the conscious selection by the researcher of certain subjects or elements to include in the study. Efforts might be made to include typical subjects or typical situations. Examples of good care and poor care, good patients and bad patients might be used. This approach is often used in qualitative studies. Using insights gained from initial data collection, the qualitative researcher may decide to seek subjects with particular characteristics in order to increase theoretical understanding of some facet of the phenomenon being studied. For example, the researcher might find through subject interviews that a few subjects differed strikingly from the views of the group. The researcher might intentionally seek interviews with those individuals who differed. The strategy has been criticized because there is no way to evaluate the precision of the researcher's judgment. How does one determine that the patient or element was typical, good, bad, effective, or ineffective? However, this sampling method may be a way to get some beginning ideas about an area not easily examined using other sampling techniques. Sandelowski (1995) suggests that purposive samples can be too small to achieve informational redundancy or theoretical saturation or too large to perform the detailed analyses of data required in qualitative studies. Purposive sampling will be discussed in more detail in Chapter 20, Qualitative Research Methodology.

Villarruel (1995) used purposive sampling in her study of "Mexican-American cultural meanings, expressions, self-care and dependent-care actions associated with experiences of pain." Her description of sample selection is as follows.

"Mexican-Americans who worked or resided in the Hispanic community of a large midwestern city were selected purposefully for participation in this study. General and key informants were identified in the context of the investigator's participation at different community events and settings, including the waiting room of the major community health center. Identification and participation of informants was facilitated further by clinic staff, community residents, and by informants who had participated in the study. Criteria for informant selection included Mexican-American male and female adults and children who were willing to participate in the study and who had a recent experience with pain, or were living in the same household as a family member who had a recent pain experience. Efforts were made in the selection of informants to include family members, children, a wide range of pain experiences, a balance of males and females, and persons at high and low levels of acculturation.

Twenty key informants (male = 7; female = 13) ranging in ages from 10 to 67 years participated in this study. With the exception of 5 children, all key informants had a minimum of a high school education. While specific data about family income were not obtained, all families were determined to be of low to middle income on the basis of observation and other family data. Sociocultural orientation was conceptualized as Mexican-American cultural group membership and level of acculturation. The majority of informants (N = 15) were born in the United States and were either first or mixed second generation Mexican-Americans. The remainder of the informants were born in Mexico but had lived in the United States for over 10 years. Based on scores on the Short Acculturation Scale for Hispanics (SAS (Marín, Sabogal, Marín, Ortero-Sabogal, & Perez-Stable, 1987)), 12 informants were determined to be at a high level of acculturation, while 8 informants were determined to be at a low level of acculturation.

In addition, 14 general informants, including 5 persons who were family members of key informants, participated in the study. The focus of interactions with these informants was mainly to confirm information from key informants, as well as to confirm impressions, formulations, and findings. General informant characteristics including the nature and type of pain experiences, socio-economic factors, age, gender, and indicators of Hispanic ethnicity were similar to those of key informants." (pp. 428–429) ■

NETWORK SAMPLING

Network sampling, sometimes referred to as snowballing, holds promise for locating samples difficult or impossible to obtain in other ways. Network sampling takes advantage of social networks and the fact that friends tend to hold characteristics in common. When the researcher has found a few subjects with the needed criteria, the subjects are asked for their assistance in getting in touch with others with similar characteristics. This strategy is particularly useful for finding subjects in socially devalued populations such as alcoholics, prostitutes, child abusers, sex offenders, drug addicts, and criminals. These individuals are seldom willing to make themselves known to others. Other groups such as widows, grieving siblings, or those successful at lifestyle changes can be located using this strategy. These individuals are outside the existing health care system and are difficult to find. Obviously, there are biases built into the sampling process, since the subjects are not independent of each other.

Stevens (1995) used network sampling to obtain subjects for her study of "Structural and interpersonal impact of heterosexual assumptions on lesbian health care clients." She describes her sampling procedure as follows.

"Through community-based snowball sampling (Watters & Biernacki, 1989) in San Francisco, 45 lesbians were recruited to participate in the study during 1990 and 1991; 32 were interviewed individually and 13 were involved in three focus groups. Participants met the inclusion criteria: self-identified as lesbian, at least 21 years old, and conversant in English." (p. 26) ■

SAMPLE SIZE

One of the most frequent questions asked by beginning researchers is, "What size sample should I use?" Historically, the response to this question has been that a sample should contain at least 30 subjects. There is no logical reason for the selection of this number and, in most cases, 30 subjects will be inadequate as a sample size. Currently, the deciding factor in determining an adequate sample size for correlational, quasi-experimental, and experimental studies is power. *Power* is the capacity of the study to detect differences or relationships that actually exist in the population. Expressed another way, it is the capacity to correctly reject a null hypothesis. The minimum acceptable power for a study is .80. If a researcher does not have sufficient power to detect differences or relationships that exist in the population, one might question the advisability of conducting the study. Determining the sample size needed to obtain sufficient power is made by performing a power analysis. The statistical procedures used to perform power analyses is described in Chapter 16.

Nurse researchers have only recently begun using power analysis to determine sample size, and frequently fail to report the results of the power analyses in published results of the study. This is a particular problem in studies that fail to detect significant differences or relationships where the results might be due to an inadequate sample size rather than incorrect hypotheses. Polit and Sherman (1990) evaluated the sample size of 62 studies published in 1989 in *Nursing Research* and *Research in Nursing & Health.* The mean sample size for a group on which comparative data analysis was performed was 83. Two-thirds of the studies had group samples under 100. Most of the studies had inadequate sample sizes to make comparisons between groups. The studies needed an average of 218 subjects per group to have a power level of .80. Only one of these studies reported having performed a power analysis to determine the adequacy of their sample size. Beck (1994) reviewed the reporting of power analysis in three nursing research journals over the 5-year period of 1988–1992. "During this 5-year period, in only

8 studies published in *Nursing Research,* 9 studies in *Research in Nursing & Health,* and 3 studies in *Western Journal of Nursing Research* had the researcher specified that power analysis had been done and supplied the readers with the particulars of their analysis" (p. 78).

The adequacy of sample sizes needs to be more carefully evaluated in future nursing studies *prior to data collection.* Studies with inadequate sample sizes should not be approved for data collection unless they are preliminary pilot studies conducted prior to a planned larger study. If it is not possible to obtain a larger sample because of time or numbers of available subjects, the study should be redesigned so that the available sample is adequate for the planned analyses. If it is not possible to obtain a sufficient sample size, it is better not to conduct the study.

Large sample sizes are difficult to obtain in nursing studies, require long data collection periods, and are costly. Therefore, in developing the methodology for a study, it is important to evaluate the elements of the methodology that affect the required sample size. Kraemer and Thiemann (1987, p. 27) identify the following factors that need to be taken into consideration in determining sample size:

1. The more stringent the significance level (e.g., .001 vs .05), the greater the necessary sample size.
2. Two-tailed statistical tests require larger sample sizes than one-tailed tests. Tailedness of statistical tests is explained in Chapter 16.
3. The smaller the effect size, the larger the necessary sample size.
4. The larger the power required, the larger the necessary sample size.
5. The smaller the sample size, the smaller the power.

Other factors that need to be considered in making decisions about sample size (because they affect power) include the effect size, type of study, the number of variables, the sensitivity of the measurement tools, and the data analysis techniques.

EFFECT SIZE

Effect is the presence of a phenomenon. If a phenomenon exists, it is not absent and thus the null hypothesis is in error. However, effect is best understood when not considered in a dichotomous way—as present or absent. If a phenomenon exists, it exists to some degree. *Effect size* (ES) is the extent of the presence of a phenomenon. Effect in this case is used in a broader sense than that of "cause and effect." For example, you might examine the impact of distraction on the experience of pain during an injection. To examine this question, you might obtain a sample of subjects receiving injections and measure differences in the experience of pain in a group who were distracted compared to a group who were not distracted. The null hypothesis would be that there would be no difference in the amount of pain experienced by the two groups. If this were so, you would say that the effect of distraction on the experience of pain was zero. In another study, you might be interested in using the Pearson product moment correlation r to examine the relationship between coping and anxiety. Your null hypothesis would be that the population r would be zero. Coping would have no effect (in terms of relationship) with anxiety (Cohen, 1988).

It is easier in a study to detect large differences between groups than to detect small differences. Thus, smaller samples can detect large ESs; smaller effect sizes require larger samples. Broadly, a small effect size would be about .2, a medium effect size, .5, and a large effect size, .8. Effect size is smaller with a small sample and is thus more difficult to detect. Increasing the sample size also increases the effect size, making it more likely that the effect will be detected. Extremely small effect sizes may not be clinically significant. Knowing the effect size that would be considered important clinically allows us to limit the sample to the size needed to detect that level of ES (Kraemer & Thiemann, 1987). A result is clinically significant if the effect is sufficiently large to alter clinical decisions. For example, an effect size of .1° F in oral temperature when comparing glass thermometers with electronic thermometers is probably not important enough to influence selection of a particular type of thermometer.

Effect sizes vary based on the population being studied. Thus, we need to determine the ES for the particular effect being studied in a particular population. The most desirable source of this information is evidence from previous studies. Using such information as the mean and standard deviation, the ES can be calculated. This calculation, however, can be used only as an estimate of ES for your study. If you change the measure used, or the design or the population being studied, the ES will be altered. The best estimate of a population parameter of ES is obtained from a meta-analysis in which an estimated population effect size is calculated using statistical values from all studies included in the analysis (Polit & Sherman, 1990).

If few relevant studies have been conducted in the area of interest, small pilot studies can be performed and data analysis results used to calculate the effect size. If pilot studies are not feasible, dummy table analysis can be used to calculate the smallest effect size that would be sufficiently large to have clinical or theoretical value. Yarandi (1991) describes the process of calculating a dummy power table. If all else fails, ES can be estimated as small, medium, or large. Numerical values would be assigned to these estimates and the power analysis performed. Cohen (1988) has indicated the numerical values for small, medium, and large effects based on specific statistical procedures. In new areas of research, effect sizes are usually small (Polit & Sherman, 1990).

In the nursing studies examined by Polit and Sherman (1990), 52.7% of the effect sizes computed were small. They found that in nursing studies, for small effects, average power was under .30. Thus, there was less than a 30% probability that acceptance of the null hypothesis was correct. This was, in most cases, due to an insufficient sample size. Even when the effect size was moderate, the average power in the nursing studies examined was only .70. Only when the effect size was large did nursing studies reach an acceptable

level of power, and 11% of these studies were underpowered. Only 15% of the studies had sufficient power for all of their analyses.

TYPE OF STUDY

Qualitative studies and case studies tend to use very small samples. Comparisons between groups are not being performed, and problems related to sampling error and generalization have little relevance for these studies. A small sample size may better serve the researcher who is interested in examining the situation in depth from various perspectives. The qualitative researcher will stop seeking additional participants when theoretical saturation is achieved.

Descriptive studies, particularly those using survey questionnaires, and correlational studies often require very large samples. In these studies, multiple variables may be examined, and extraneous variables are likely to affect subject response(s) to the variables under study. Statistical comparisons are often made on multiple subgroups in the sample, requiring that an adequate sample be available for each subgroup being analyzed. In addition, subjects are likely to be heterogeneous in terms of demographic variables, and measurement tools are sometimes not adequately refined. Although target populations may have been identified, sampling frames may not be available, and parameters have not usually been well defined from previous studies. All of these factors lower the power of the study and require increases in sample size (Kraemer & Thiemann, 1987).

In the past, quasi-experimental and experimental studies often used smaller samples than descriptive and correlational studies. As control in the study increases, the sample size can decrease and still approximate the population. Instruments in these studies tend to be refined, thus increasing precision. However, sample size must be sufficient to achieve an acceptable level of power to reduce the risk of a Type II error (Kraemer & Thiemann, 1987).

The study design influences power, but the design with the greatest power may not always be the most valid design to use. The experimental design with the greatest power is the pretest–posttest design with a historical control group. However, this design may have questionable validity because of the historical control group. Can the researcher demonstrate that the historical control group is comparable to the experimental group? The repeated measures design will increase power if the trait being assessed is relatively stable over time. Designs that use blocking or stratification usually increase the total sample size required. The sample size increases in proportion to the number of cells included in the data analysis. Designs that use matched pairs of subjects have increased power and thus require a smaller sample. The higher the degree of correlation between subjects on the variable on which the subjects are matched, the greater the power (Kraemer & Thiemann, 1987).

Confirmatory studies such as those testing the effects of nursing interventions on patient outcomes or those testing the fit of a theoretical model require large sample sizes. Clinical trials are being conducted in nursing for these purposes. The power of these large, complex studies needs to be carefully analyzed (Leidy & Weissfeld, 1991). To obtain the large sample sizes needed, subjects are acquired at a number of clinical settings, sometimes in various parts of the country. Kraemer and Thiemann (1987) believe that these studies should not be performed until extensive information is available from exploratory studies. This should include meta-analysis and the definition of a population effect size.

NUMBER OF VARIABLES

As the number of variables under study increases, the needed sample size may increase. Adding variables such as age, gender, ethnicity, and education to the analysis plan (just to be on the safe side) can increase the sample size by a factor of 5 to 10 if the selected variables are uncorrelated with the dependent variable. In this case, instead of a sample of 50, you may need a sample of 500 if

you plan to use these variables in your statistical analyses. (Using them only to describe the sample does not cause a problem in terms of power.) However, if the variables are highly correlated with the dependent variable, the effect size will increase and the sample size can be reduced. Therefore, variables included in the data analysis need to be carefully selected. They should be essential to the research question or have a documented strong relationship to the dependent variable (Kraemer & Thiemann, 1987). A number of the studies analyzed by Polit and Sherman (1990) had sufficient sample size for the primary analyses but failed to plan for analyses involving subgroups, such as analyzing the data by age categories or by ethnic groups. The inclusion of multiple dependent variables also increases the sample size needed.

MEASUREMENT SENSITIVITY

Well-developed instruments measure phenomena with precision. A thermometer, for example, measures body temperature precisely. Tools measuring psychosocial variables tend to be less precise. However, a tool with strong reliability and validity tends to measure more precisely than a tool that is less well developed. Variance tends to be higher in a less well-developed tool than in one that is well developed. An instrument with a smaller variance is preferred because the power of a test is always decreased by increased within-group variance (Kraemer & Thiemann, 1987). For example, if anxiety were being measured and the actual anxiety score of several subjects was 80, the subjects' scores on a less well-developed tool might range from 70 to 90, whereas a well-developed tool would tend to show a score closer to the actual score of 80 for each subject. As variance in instrument scores increases, the sample size needed to gain an accurate understanding of the phenomenon under study increases.

The range of measured values influences power. For example, a variable might be measured in 10 equally spaced values, ranging from 0 to 9. Effect sizes will vary depending on how near the value is to the population mean. If the mean value is 5, effect sizes will be much larger in the extreme values and lower for values near the mean. If the researcher decides to use only subjects with values of 0 and 9, the effect size will be large and the sample could be small. However, the credibility of the study might be questionable since the values of most individuals would not be 0 or 9 but rather tend to be in the middle range of values. If a decision is made to include subjects who have values in the range of 3 to 6, excluding the extreme scores, the effect size would be small and a much larger sample would be required. The wider the range of values sampled, the larger the effect size (Kraemer & Thiemann, 1987). Each measure of response should be used in as sensitive a form as can be reliably measured. If measurement on a continuum is reliable, the measure should not be reduced to a scale or dichotomized since this will reduce the power. If an interval level measure is reduced to an ordinal or nominal level, a much larger sample size is required to achieve adequate power (Kraemer & Thiemann, 1987).

DATA ANALYSIS TECHNIQUES

Data analysis techniques vary in ability to detect differences in the data. Statisticians refer to this as the *power* of the statistical analysis. The most powerful statistical test appropriate to the data should be selected for data analysis. Overall, parametric statistical analyses are more powerful in detecting differences than nonparametric techniques if the data meet criteria for parametric analysis. However, in many cases, nonparametric techniques are more powerful if the assumptions of parametric techniques are not met. Parametric techniques vary widely in their capacity to distinguish fine differences in the data. Parametric and nonparametric analyses are discussed in Chapter 16.

There is also an interaction between the measurement sensitivity and the power of the data analysis technique. The power of the analysis technique increases as precision in measurement increases. Larger samples need to be used when the power of the planned statistical analysis is weak.

For some statistical procedures, such as the *t* test and ANOVA, equal group sizes will increase power because the effect size is maximized. The more unequal the group sizes are, the smaller the effect size. Therefore, in unequal groups, the total sample size needs to be larger (Kraemer & Thiemann, 1987).

Chi-square (χ^2) is the weakest of the statistical tests and requires very large sample sizes to achieve acceptable levels of power. As the number of categories increases, the sample size needed increases. Also, if there are small numbers in some of the categories, the sample size needs to be increased. Kraemer and Thiemann (1987) recommend that the chi-square test be used only when no other options are available. In addition, the number of categories should be limited to those essential to the study.

RECRUITING AND RETAINING SUBJECTS

Once a decision has been made about the size of the sample, the next step is to develop a plan for recruiting subjects. Recruitment strategies differ depending on the type of study and the setting. Special attention needs to focus on recruiting subjects who tend to be underrepresented in studies, such as minorities and women (Murdaugh, 1990). The sampling plan, initiated at the beginning of data collection, is almost always more difficult than is expected. Some researchers never obtain their planned sample size. Retaining acquired subjects is critical to the study and requires consideration of the effects of data collection strategies on subject mortality (loss of subjects to the study). Problems with retaining subjects increase as the data collection period lengthens.

RECRUITING SUBJECTS

Effective recruitment of subjects is crucial to the success of a study. Few studies have examined the effectiveness of various strategies of subject recruitment. Most information available to guide researchers comes from the personal experiences of skilled researchers. Schain (1994) suggests that factors that influence subjects' decisions to participate include self-protectiveness, a high need for personal control, time and travel constraints, and the nature of the informed consent. The initial approach to a potential subject usually strongly affects his or her decision about participating in the study. Therefore, the approach needs to be pleasant and positive. The importance of the study is explained, and the researcher makes clear exactly what the subject will be asked to do, how much time will be involved for the subject, and what the time range of the study will be. Subjects are valuable resources. The recognition of this value needs to be communicated to the potential subject. High pressure techniques, such as insisting that the subject make an instant decision to participate in a study, usually lead to resistance and increased refusals. The researcher accepts refusals to participate gracefully—in terms of body language as well as words. The actions of the researcher can influence the decision of other potential subjects who observe or who hear about the encounter. Studies in which a high proportion of individuals refuse to participate have a serious validity problem. The sample is likely to be biased, because usually only a certain type of individual has agreed to participate. Therefore, records are kept of the numbers of persons who refuse and, if possible, the reasons for refusal.

Recruiting minority subjects for a study can be particularly problematic. Minority individuals may be difficult to locate and are often reluctant to participate in studies because of feelings of being used while receiving no personal benefit from their involvement. Pletsch, Howe, and Tenney (1995) recommend using "feasibility analysis, developing partnerships with target groups and community members, using active face-to-face recruitment, and using process evaluation techniques" (p. 211).

If data collectors are being used in the study, the researcher needs to verify that they are following the sampling plan, especially in random sam-

ples. When the data collectors encounter difficult subjects or are unable to make contact easily, they may simply shift to the next person without informing the principal investigator. This behavior could violate the rules of random sampling and bias the sample. If data collectors do not understand or believe in the importance of randomization, their decisions and actions can undermine the intent of the sampling plan. Thus, data collectors need to be carefully selected and thoroughly trained. A plan needs to be developed for the supervision and follow-up of data collectors, increasing their sense of accountability.

When surveys are used, the researcher may never have personal contact with the subjects. In this case, the researcher will have to rely on the use of attention-getting techniques, persuasively written material, and strategies for following up on individuals who do not respond to the initial written communication. Because of the serious problems of low response rates in survey studies, strategies to increase the response rate are critical. We have received such things as a tea bag or packet of instant coffee with a questionnaire, with a statement in the letter to have a cup of coffee (or tea) on the researcher while you take a break from your work to complete the questionnaire. Creativity is required in the use of such strategies since they will tend to lose their effect on groups who receive questionnaires frequently (such as faculty). In some cases, small amounts of money (fifty cents to a dollar) are included with the letter. The letter may include a suggestion that you buy yourself a soft drink or that the money is a small offering for completing the questionnaire. This strategy imposes some sense of obligation on the recipient of the letter to complete the questionnaire but is not thought to be coercive (Baker, 1985). Avoid holidays or times of the year when workloads are high and the return rate might be reduced.

The letter to potential subjects needs to be carefully composed. This may be your only chance to persuade the subject to invest the time needed to complete the questionnaire. You need to sell the readers on the importance of your study and the importance of their response. The tone of your letter will be their only image of you as a person, and yet, for many subjects, it may be their response to the perception of you as a person that most influences their decision about completing the questionnaire. Seek examples of letters sent by researchers who had high response rates to questionnaires. Save letters you receive that you responded positively to. Pilot test your letter on individuals who can give you feedback on their reaction to the tone of the letter. Follow-up letters or cards have been repeatedly shown to increase response rates to surveys. The timing is important. If too long a period has lapsed, the questionnaire may have been discarded. Sending it too soon could be offensive. Baker (1985) describes her strategy for following up on questionnaires.

"Before the questionnaires were mailed, precise plans were made for monitoring the return of each questionnaire as a means of follow-up procedure. A bar graph was developed to record the return of each questionnaire as a means of suggesting when the follow-up mailing should occur (Babbie, 1973). Each square on the graph paper represented one questionnaire. Day 1 on the graph was the day on which the questionnaires were mailed. The cumulative number and percentage of responses were logged on the graph to reflect the overall data collection process. When the daily responses declined, a follow-up, first-class mailing was sent, containing another questionnaire, a modified cover letter, and a return envelope. Study participants and questionnaires were assigned the same code numbers, and nonrespondents were identified by checking the list of code numbers of unreturned questionnaires. A second follow-up questionnaire, with a further modified cover letter, and a return envelope were sent by certified mail. Should there still have been unreturned questionnaires, a dialogue was prepared for a final follow-up by telephone." (p. 119) ■

The factors involved in the decision to respond to a questionnaire are not well understood. One obvious factor is the time required to respond. This includes the time required to orient to the directions and the emotional energy to deal with the threats and anxieties generated by the questions. There is also a cognitive demand for thinking. Subjects seem to make a judgment about the relevance of the research topic and the potential for personal application of findings. Previous experience with mailed questionnaires is also a deciding factor (Baker, 1985).

To reduce costs, nurse researchers are now using the mail to collect far more extensive data than that of the simple questionnaire. In some cases, multiple scales will be mailed to subjects to be completed at home and returned. Recruitment strategies for these subjects may require some form of personal contact prior to mailing the material as well as telephone contact during the data collection period.

Traditionally, subjects for nursing studies have been sought in the hospital setting. However, access to these subjects is becoming more difficult—in part because of the increased numbers of nurses now conducting research (Cronenwett, 1986). Nurse researchers are now recruiting subjects from a variety of sources. An initial phase of recruitment may involve obtaining community and institutional support for the study. Support from other health professionals, such as nurses and physicians, may be critical to successful recruitment of subjects. Studies may also benefit from endorsement by community leaders. This may include individuals such as city officials and key civic leaders, and social, educational, religious, or labor groups. In some cases, these groups may be involved in planning the study, leading to a sense of community ownership of the project. Community groups may also assist in recruitment of subjects for the study. Sometimes, subjects who meet the sampling criteria will be found in the groups assisting with the study. Endorsement may involve letters of support and, in some cases, funding. These activities add legitimacy to the study and make involvement in the study more attractive to potential subjects (Diekmann & Smith, 1989).

Media support can be helpful in recruiting subjects. Advertisements can be placed in local newspapers and church and neighborhood bulletins.

Radio stations can make public service announcements. Members of the research team can speak to groups relevant to the study population. Posters can be placed in public places such as supermarkets, drugstores, and washaterias. With permission, tables can be placed in shopping malls with a member of the research team present to recruit subjects (Diekmann & Smith, 1989).

Lusk, Ronis, Kerr, and Atwood (1994) obtained a sample of 645 workers in a study testing the effectiveness of the health promotion model to explain workers' use of hearing protection using multiple recruitment strategies.

■

"A convenience sample of 645 workers (319 blue-collar, 209 skilled trades, and 117 white-collar) was recruited to complete written questionnaires. Supervisors were encouraged to give release time to workers who wished to participate. Posters, flyers, and the plant newsletter were used to publicize the study, and pairs of university football game tickets were offered as lottery prizes as an incentive for participation. To obtain sufficient power for analyses, data collection was designed to continue until at least 300 blue-collar, 200 skilled trades, and 100 white-collar subjects volunteered. The participants represented approximately 14.4% of the 4,473 workers employed at the plant (day and evening shifts only), in comparison to the 2 to 3% participation rate reported for other voluntary activities at the plant." (p. 153) ■

Recruitment of subjects for clinical studies requires a different set of strategies. For clinical trials, recruitment may be occurring simultaneously in several sites (perhaps in different cities). Many of these studies never achieve their planned sample size. The number of subjects meeting the sampling criteria who are available in the selected clinical site(s) may not be as large as anticipated. Researchers must often screen twice as many patients as are required for the study in order to obtain a sufficient sample size. Screening logs need to be kept during the recruiting period to record data on patients who met the criteria but were not

entered into the study. Researchers commonly underestimate the amount of time required to recruit subjects for a clinical study. In addition to defining the number of subjects and the time set aside for recruitment, it may be helpful to develop short-term or interim recruitment goals designed to maintain a constant rate of patient entry (Diekmann & Smith, 1989).

RETAINING SUBJECTS

One of the serious problems in many studies is subject retention. Often, subject loss cannot be avoided. Subjects move, die, or withdraw from treatment. If data must be collected at several points across time, subject mortality (loss of subjects from the study) can become a problem. Subjects who move frequently and those without telephones pose a particular problem. A number of strategies have been found to be effective in maintaining the sample. Names, addresses, and telephone numbers of at least two family members or friends need to be obtained when the subject is enrolled in the study. Consent may be sought from the subject to give the researcher access to unlisted phone numbers in the event that the subject changes the phone number. In some studies, the subject is reimbursed for participation. A bonus payment may be included for completing a certain phase of the study. Gifts can be used in place of money. Sending greeting cards for birthdays and holidays helps maintain contact. Rudy, Estok, Kerr, and Menzel (1994) compared the effect on recruitment and retention of money versus gifts. They found no differential effect on recruitment but found that money was more effective than gifts in retaining subjects in longitudinal studies. However, the researchers point out the moral issues related to providing monetary payment to subjects. This strategy can compromise the voluntariness of participation in a study and particularly has the potential of exploiting low-income persons.

Collecting data takes time. The researcher always keeps in mind that the subject's time is valuable and should be used frugally. During data collection, it is easy to begin taking the subject for granted. Taking time for social amenities with subjects may pay off. However, one needs to take care that these interactions do not influence the data being collected. Beyond that, nurturing subjects participating in the study is critical. In some situations, providing refreshments and pleasant surroundings is helpful. During the data collection phase, often there are others interacting with the subjects who also need to be nurtured. These may be volunteers, family, staff, students, or other professionals. It is important to maintain a pleasant climate for the data collection process, which will pay off in the quality of data collected and the retention of subjects.

Some longitudinal studies require the completion of forms repeatedly at various time intervals. Sometimes the forms are diaries requiring daily entries over a set period. These studies face the greatest risk of subject mortality.

Barnard, Magyary, Booth, and Eyres (1987) described the extensive sample maintenance procedures required for their longitudinal study.

◼

"Sometimes the researcher needs to invest a great deal of time and money in sample maintenance. For example, for the 13-month assessment point in our current study of high-social-risk mothers and children, a research assistant picks up the mother and child at home (a 45-minute drive), brings them to the clinic for testing, and then drives them home again. In addition, the mother is given up to $10 to cover babysitting costs for her other children and is sent a free copy of the videotape we make of her and her child. Without these elaborate arrangements, we feel that our attrition rate would be very high." (p. 47) ◼

Subjects who have a personal investment in the study are more likely to continue in the study. This investment occurs through interactions with and nurturing by the researcher. A combination of the subject's personal belief in the significance of the study and the nurturing of the subject during data collection by the researcher may diminish subject mortality (Killien & Newton, 1990).

Gordon and Stokes (1989) described strategies they used in a longitudinal study of stressors and the onset of illness in individuals 65 years and older that required subjects to complete a set of scales that were mailed to them every 3 months for 1 year. In addition, subjects kept a health diary. All materials were color-coded according to the quarter of the year. Oversized lettering was used on all forms. All forms were kept consistent throughout the year so that subjects became increasingly familiar with them. Subjects remained anonymous throughout the study. Thus, telephone contact by the researcher was impossible. Materials were returned to the researchers by mail quarterly using preaddressed stamped envelopes of the same color as the data forms. Eighty-seven individuals participated in the study. The response rate the first quarter was 91%, second quarter, 86%; third quarter, 79%; and fourth quarter, 81%.

◼

"Development of commitment began with the first letter sent to subjects. The letter emphasized the importance of the study to the health and well-being of people in the subject's age group. Subjects were told they would be providing an important service to their peers by participating in the study. All subsequent letters requesting data emphasized the importance of each individual's participation to successful completion of the study. . . . Furthermore, as the study continued, subjects were told of the high response rate among their peers, in order to augment the feeling of being part of a larger group. They were encouraged to keep up the good work.

Information regarding the use of data from the study was forwarded to the participants. For example, when the New York Times reported the study, a copy of the newspaper article was sent to each participant. They were informed of professional presentations, radio interviews, and grant proposals submitted for funding of related work.

Personalized materials have been shown to raise response rates between 7 and 8% (Andreasen, 1970). Each letter was hand signed. The letters were phrased in an informal style using language of the cohort group. Pictures of the researchers and the school of nursing were included so the subjects could see those with whom they were communicating and the location to which they were sending their materials." (p. 375) ■

■ SUMMARY

Sampling involves selecting a group of people, events, behaviors, or other elements with which to conduct a study. Sampling denotes the process of making the selections; sample denotes the selected group of elements. Sampling theory was developed to determine mathematically the most effective way of acquiring a sample that would accurately reflect the population under study. Important concepts in sampling theory include target population, elements of the population, randomization, sampling frame, accessible population, representativeness, statistics, parameters, precision, sampling errors, and systematic bias.

A sampling plan is developed to increase representativeness, decrease systematic bias, and decrease the sampling error. The two main types of sampling plans are probability sampling and nonprobability sampling. Probability sampling plans have been developed to ensure some degree of precision in accurately estimating the population parameters. Thus, probability samples reduce sampling error. To obtain a probability (random) sample, the researcher must know every element in the population. A sampling frame must be developed and the sample randomly selected from the sampling frame. Four sampling designs have been developed to achieve probability sampling: simple random sampling, stratified random sampling, cluster sampling, and systematic sampling.

In nonprobability (nonrandom) sampling, not every element of the population has an opportunity for selection in the sample. There is no sampling frame. Five nonprobability designs are included in this text: convenience sampling, random assignment to groups, quota sampling, purposive sampling, and network sampling.

A major concern in conducting a study is determining the size of a sample. Sample size is determined by power analysis. Sampling error decreases as sample size increases. Many published nursing studies have an inadequate sample size and a high risk of a Type II error. One examination of published studies found that a nursing study needed an average of 218 subjects per group to have an acceptable power level. Factors that must be considered in making decisions about sample size include the type of study, the number of variables, the sensitivity of the measurement tools, the data analysis techniques, and the expected effect size. Effect size is the extent to which the null hypothesis is false. Calculating sample size requires that one know the level of significance, power, and effect size.

Another concern in conducting a study is acquiring and retaining subjects in a study. This process is almost always more difficult than was expected. The problems encountered are usually associated with human interaction rather than with the sampling plan. Acquiring subjects effectively depends on the initial approach by the researcher. When surveys are used, the researcher may never have personal contact with the subjects. In this case, the researcher will have to rely on the use of attention-getting techniques, persuasively written material, and strategies for following up on individuals who do not respond to the initial written communication. Traditionally, subjects

continued

continued

for nursing studies have been sought in the hospital setting. However, access to these subjects is becoming more difficult, and nurse researchers are now recruiting subjects from a variety of sources. An initial phase of recruitment may involve obtaining community and/or institutional support for the study. Endorsement may be obtained from individuals, such as city officials and key civic leaders, and social, educational, religious, or labor groups.

Retaining acquired subjects is critical to the study and requires consideration of the effects of data collection on subject mortality. A number of strategies have been found to be effective in maintaining the sample. Names, addresses, and telephone numbers of family members or friends may be obtained. A bonus payment may be included for completing a certain phase of the study. If subjects have a personal investment in the study, they are more likely to continue. This investment is developed through interactions with and nurturing by the researcher.

References

Abdellah, F. G., & Levine, E. (1979). *Better patient care through nursing research.* New York: Macmillan.

Andreasen, A. R. (1970). Personalizing mail questionnaires. *Public Opinion Quarterly, 34*(2), 273–277.

Babbie, E. R. (1973). *Survey research methods.* Belmont, CA: Wadsworth.

Baker, C. M. (1985). Maximizing mailed questionnaire responses. *Image: Journal of Nursing Scholarship, 17*(4), 118–121.

Barhyte, D. Y., Redman, B. K., & Neill, K. M. (1990). Population or sample: Design decision. *Nursing Research, 39*(5), 309–310.

Barnard, K. E., Magyary, D. L., Booth, C. L., & Eyres, S. J. (1987). Longitudinal designs: Considerations and applications to nursing research. *Recent Advances in Nursing, 17,* 37–64.

Beck, C. T. (1994). Statistical power analysis in pediatric nursing research. *Issues in Comprehensive Pediatric Nursing, 17*(2), 73–80.

Borenstein, M., & Cohen, J. (1989). *Statistical power analysis.* Release: 1.00. Hillsdale, NJ: Lawrence Erlbaum Associates, Inc. (ISBN 0-8058-0222-3).

Brennan, P. F., Moore, S. M., & Smyth, K. A. (1995). The effects of a special computer network on caregivers of persons with Alzheimer's disease. *Nursing Research, 44*(3), 166–172.

Brent, E. E., Jr., Scott, J. K., & Spencer, J. C. (1988). Ex-Sample™: *An expert system to assist in designing sampling plans. User's guide and reference manual,* Version 2.0. Columbia, MO: The Idea Works, Inc. (100 West Briarwood, Columbia, Missouri 65203, phone [314] 445-4554).

Cochran, W. G. (1977). *Sampling techniques* (3rd ed.). New York: Wiley.

Cohen, J. (1988). *Statistical power analysis for the behavioral sciences.* (2nd ed). New York: Academic Press.

Cronenwett, L. R. (1986). Access to research subjects. *Journal of Nursing Administration, 16*(2), 8–9.

Diekmann, J. M., & Smith, J. M. (1989). Strategies for assessment and recruitment of subjects for nursing research. *Western Journal of Nursing Research, 11*(4), 418–430.

Duffy, M. E. (1994). Testing the theory of transcending options: Health behaviors of single parents. *Scholarly Inquiry for Nursing Practice: An International Journal, 8*(2), 191–205.

Floyd, J. A. (1993). Systematic sampling: Theory and clinical methods. *Nursing Research, 42*(5), 290–293.

Friday, F. A. (1967). *The elements of probability and sampling.* New York: Barnes & Noble.

Glass, G. V., & Stanley, J. C. (1970). *Statistical methods in education and psychology.* Englewood Cliffs, NJ: Prentice-Hall.

Good, M. (1995). A comparison of the effects of jaw relaxation and music on postoperative pain. *Nursing Research, 44*(1), 52–57.

Gordon, S. E., & Stokes, S. A. (1989). Improving response rate to mailed questionnaires. *Nursing Research, 38*(6), 375–376.

Gottlieb, L. N., & Baillies, J. (1995). Firstborns' behaviors during a mothers' second pregnancy. *Nursing Research, 44*(6), 356–362.

Hansen, M. H., Hurwitz, W. N., & Madow, W. G. (1953). *Sample survey methods and theory.* New York: Wiley.

Hart, M. A. (1995). Orem's self-care deficit theory: Research with pregnant women. *Nursing Science Quarterly, 8*(3), 120–126.

Hjelm-Karlsson, K. (1991). Using the biased coin design for randomization in health care research. *Western Journal of Nursing Research, 13*(2), 284–288.

Kerlinger, F. N. (1986). *Foundations of behavioral research* (3rd ed.). New York: Holt, Rinehart and Winston.

Killien, M., & Newton, K. (1990). Longitudinal research—The challenge of maintaining continued involvement of participants. *Western Journal of Nursing Research, 12*(5), 689–692.

Kraemer, H. C., & Thiemann, S. (1987). *How many subjects? Statistical power analysis in research.* Newbury Park, CA: Sage.

Larson, E. (1994). Exclusion of certain groups from clinical research. *Image: Journal of Nursing Scholarship, 26*(3), 185–190.

Leidy, N. K., & Weissfeld, L. A. (1991). Sample sizes and power computation for clinical intervention trials. *Western Journal of Nursing Research, 13*(1), 138–144.

Levy, P. S., & Lemsbow, S. (1980). *Sampling for health professionals.* Belmont, CA: Lifetime Learning.

Lusk, S. L., Ronis, D. L., Kerr, M. J., & Atwood, J. R. (1994). Test of the health promotion model as a causal model of workers' use of hearing protection. *Nursing Research, 43*(3), 151–157.

Marín, G., Sabogal, F., Marín, B., Ortero-Sabogal, R., & Perez-Stable, E. (1987). Development of a short acculturation scale for Hispanics. *Hispanic Journal of Behavioral Sciences, 9*(2), 183–205.

Mitchell, E. S., Woods, N. F., & Lentz, M. J. (1994). Differentiation of women with three perimenstrual symptom patterns. *Nursing Research, 43*(1), 25–30.

Moody, L. E., Wilson, M. E., Smyth, K., Schwartz, R., Tittle, M., & Van Cott, M. L. (1988). Analysis of a decade of nursing practice research: 1977–1986. *Nursing Research, 37*(6), 374–379.

Murdaugh, C. (1990). Recruitment issues in research with special populations. *Journal of Cardiovascular Nursing, 4*(4), 51–55.

Ottenbacher, K. (1992). Impact of random assignment on study outcome: An empirical examination. *Controlled Clinical Trials, 13*(1), 50–61.

Pletsch, P. K., Howe, C., & Tenney, M. (1995). Recruitment of minority subjects for intervention research. *Image: Journal of Nursing Scholarship, 27*(3), 211–215.

Polit, D. F., & Sherman, R. E. (1990). Statistical power in nursing research. *Nursing Research, 39*(6), 365–369.

Princeton, T. C., & Gaspar, T. M. (1991). First-line nurse administrators in academics: How are they prepared, what do they do, and will they stay in their jobs? *Journal of Professional Nursing, 7*(2), 79–87.

Rudy, E. B., Estok, P. J., Kerr, M. E., & Menzel, L. (1994). Research incentives: Money versus gifts. *Nursing Research, 43*(4), 253–255.

Sandelowski, M. (1995). Sample size in qualitative research. *Research in Nursing & Health, 18*(2), 179–183.

Schain, W. S. (1994). Barriers to clinical trials. Part II: Knowledge and attitudes of potential participants. *Cancer, 74*(9 Suppl), 2666–2671.

Stevens, P. E. (1995). Structural and interpersonal impact of heterosexual assumptions on lesbian health care clients. *Nursing Research, 44*(1), 25–30.

Stout, R. L., Wirtz, P. W., Carbonari, J. P., & Del Boca, F. K. (1994). Ensuring balanced distribution of prognostic factors in treatment outcome research. *Journal of Studies in Alcoholism, 12*(Suppl), 70–75.

Stuifbergen, A. K. (1995). Health-promoting behaviors and quality of life among individuals with multiple sclerosis. *Scholarly Inquiry for Nursing Practice: An International Journal, 9*(1), 31–55.

Sudman, S. (1974). *Applied sampling.* New York: Academic Press.

Villarruel, A. M. (1995). Mexican-American cultural meanings, expressions, self-care and dependent-care actions associated with experiences of pain. *Research in Nursing & Health, 18*(5), 427–436.

Watters, J. K., & Biernacki, P. (1989). Targeted sampling: Options for the study of hidden populations. *Social Problems, 36*(4), 416–430.

Williams, B. (1978). *A sampler on sampling.* New York: Wiley.

Yarandi, H. N. (1991). Planning sample sizes: Comparison of factor level means. *Nursing Research, 40*(1), 57–58.

Yates, F. (1981). *Sampling methods for censuses and surveys.* New York: Macmillan.

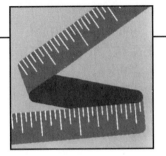

13

The Concepts
of Measurement

Measurement is the process of assigning "numbers to objects (or events or situations) in accord with some rule" (Kaplan, 1963, p. 177). The numbers assigned can indicate numerical values or categories. *Instrumentation,* a component of measurement, is the application of specific rules to develop a measurement device (instrument). The purpose of instrumentation is to produce trustworthy evidence that can be used in evaluating the outcomes of research.

The rules of measurement ensure that the assignment of values or categories will be performed consistently from one subject (or event) to another and, eventually, if the measurement strategy is found to be meaningful, from one study to another. The rules of measurement established for research are similar to those used in nursing practice. For example, when pouring a liquid medication, the rule is that the measuring container needs to be held at eye level. This insures accuracy and consistency in the dose of medication. When taking a patient's temperature, the patient must not have recently drunk ice water or smoked a cigarette, and the thermometer is left in place a given length of time. Using these rules, nurses have more confidence in the accuracy of the temperature measurement. When measuring the abdominal girth to detect changes in ascites, the skin on the abdomen is marked to be sure that the measure is always taken the same distance below the waist. Using this method, any change in measurement can be attributed to a change in ascites rather than an inadvertent change in the measurement site. Developing consistent measures of concepts important to nursing practice is a major focus of nursing research.

An understanding of the logic within measurement theory is important to the selection, utilization, and development of measurement instruments. As with most theories, measurement theory uses terms with meanings that can be understood only within the context of the theory. The following explanation of the logic of measurement theory includes definitions of directness of measurement, measurement error, levels of measurement, reference of measurement, reliability, and validity.

DIRECTNESS OF MEASUREMENT

Measurement begins by clarifying the object, characteristic, or element to be measured. Only then can strategies or techniques be developed to measure it. In some cases, identification of the measurement object and measurement strategies can be quite simple and straightforward, as when we are measuring concrete factors such as a person's height or wrist circumference. This is referred to as *direct measurement.* The technology of health care has made direct measures of concrete elements such as height, weight, temperature, time, space, movement, heart rate, and respiration familiar to us. Technology is available to measure many bodily functions and biological and chemical characteristics. The focus of measurement theory in these instances is in the precision of measurement. Nurses are also experienced in gathering direct measures of attribute variables such as age, gender, ethnic origin, diagnosis, marital status, income, and education.

However, in many cases in nursing, the characteristic to be measured is an abstract idea such as stress, caring, coping, anxiety, compliance, or pain. If the element to be measured is abstract, clarification is usually achieved through conceptual definition. The conceptual definition is then used to select or develop appropriate means of measuring the concept. The tool used in the study needs to match the conceptual definition. When abstract concepts are measured, the concept is not directly measured; instead, indicators or attributes of the concept are used to represent the abstraction. This is referred to as *indirect measurement.* For example, indicators of coping might be the frequency or accuracy of problem identification, the speed or effectiveness of problem resolution, level of optimism, and self-actualization behaviors. Rarely, if ever, can a single measurement strategy completely measure all the aspects of an abstract concept.

MEASUREMENT ERROR

There is no perfect measure. Error is inherent in any measurement strategy. *Measurement error* is the difference between what exists in reality and what is measured by a research tool. Measurement error exists in both direct and indirect measures and can be random or systematic. Direct measures, which are considered to be highly accurate, are subject to error. For example, the scale may not be accurate, the machine may be precisely calibrated but it may change with use, or the tape measure may not be held at exactly the same tightness.

There is also error in indirect measures. Efforts to measure concepts usually result in measuring only part of the concept or measures that identify an aspect of the concept but also include other elements that are not part of the concept. Figure 13–1 shows a Venn diagram of the concept A measured by instrument A-1. As can be seen, A-1 does not measure all of A. In addition, some of what A-1 measures is outside the concept of A. Both of these are examples of errors in measurement.

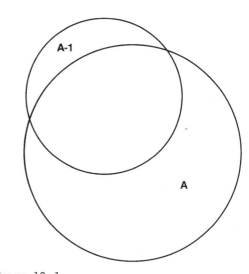

Figure 13–1
Measurement error when measuring a concept.

TYPES OF MEASUREMENT ERRORS

There are two types of errors that are of concern in measurement: random errors and systematic error. To understand these types of errors, we must first understand the elements of a score on an instrument or an observation. According to measurement theory, there are three components to a measurement score: the *true score* (T), the observed score (O), and the error score (E). The true score is what would be obtained if there were no error in measurement. Because there is always some measurement error, the true score is never known. The *observed score* is the measure obtained. The *error score* is the amount of random error in the measurement process. The theoretical equation of these three measures is:

$$O = T + E$$

This equation is a means of conceptualizing random error and not a basis for calculating it. Since the true score is never known, the random error is never known, only estimated. Theoretically, the smaller the E (error score), the more closely O (observed score) reflects T (true score). Therefore, using measurement strategies that reduce the error score increases the accuracy of the measurement.

A number of factors can occur during the measurement process that can result in random error. These include (1) transient personal factors such as fatigue, hunger, attention span, health, mood, mental set, and motivation; (2) situational factors such as a hot stuffy room, distractions, the presence of significant others, rapport with the researcher, and playfulness or seriousness of the situation; (3) variations in the administration of the measurement procedure, such as interviews in which wording or sequence of questions is varied, questions are added or deleted, or different coders code responses differently; and (4) processing of data, such as errors in coding, a subject accidentally marking the wrong column, punching the wrong key while entering the data into the computer, or totaling instrument scores incorrectly.

Random error causes individuals' observed scores to vary haphazardly around their true score. For example, with random error, one subject's observed score may be higher than his or her true score, whereas another subject's observed score may be lower than his or her true score. According to measurement theory, the sum of random errors is expected to be zero, and the random error (E) is not expected to be correlated with the true score (T). Thus, random error will not influence the direction of the mean but, rather, will increase the amount of unexplained variance around the mean. When this occurs, estimation of the true score is more diffuse.

If a variable were measured for three subjects and the random error was diagramed, it might appear as demonstrated in Figure 13–2. The differ-

ence between the true score of subject one (T_1) and the observed score (O_1) is two positive measurement intervals. The difference between the true score (T_2) and observed score (O_2) for subject two is two negative measurement intervals. The difference between the true score (T_3) and observed score (O_3) for subject three is zero. The random error for these three subjects is zero $(+ 2 - 2 + 0 = 0)$. In viewing this example, one needs to remember that this is only a means of conceptualizing random error.

Measurement error that is not random is referred to as *systematic error*. A weight scale that weighed subjects two pounds more than their true weights would result in systematic error. All of the weights would be higher and, as a result, the mean would be higher than it should be. Systematic error occurs because something else is being measured in addition to the concept. A conceptualization of systematic error is presented in Figure 13–3. Systematic error (represented by diagonal lines in the figure) is due to the part of A-1 that is outside of A. This part of A-1 measures factors other than A and will bias scores in a particular direction.

Systematic error is considered part of T (true

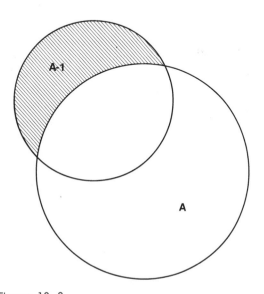

Figure 13–3
Conceptualization of systematic error.

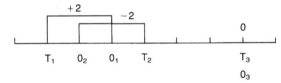

Figure 13–2
Conceptualization of random error.

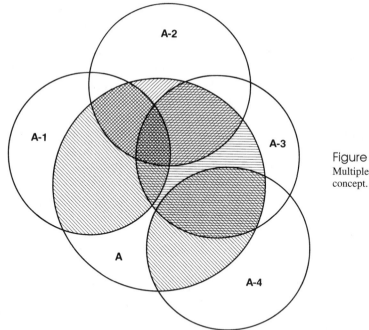

Figure 13–4
Multiple measures of an abstract
concept.

score) and reflects the true measure of A-1, not A. When the true score (with systematic error) is added to the random error (which is 0), it equals the observed score:

$$T + E = O$$

T (True Score with Systematic Error)
+ E (Random Error of 0) = O (Observed Score)

There will be some systematic error in almost any measure; however, a close link between the abstract theoretical concept and the development of the instrument will greatly decrease systematic error. Because of its importance in a study, researchers will spend considerable time and effort refining their measurement instruments in order to decrease systematic error.

Another effective means of diminishing systematic error is to use more than one measure of a concept and to compare the measures of one concept with comparable measures of the second concept. A variety of data collection methods,

such as interview and observation, are used, and the same measurement methods are used for each concept. This technique has been referred to as the *multimethod-multitrait technique* and was developed by Campbell and Fiske (1959). More recently, it is described as a version of methodological triangulation as discussed in Chapter 10. Using this technique, more dimensions of the abstract concept can be measured, and the effect of the systematic error on the composite observed score decreases. Figure 13–4 illustrates how more dimensions of concept A are measured by using instruments A-1, A-2, A-3, and A-4. The scores obtained from the four instruments are combined in such a way to give a single observed score for concept A.

For example, anxiety could be measured by (1) administering Taylor's Manifest Anxiety Scale, (2) recording blood pressure readings, (3) asking the subject about anxious feelings, and (4) observing the subject's behavior. The results of each of these measures would then be combined in some way to give a single observed score of anxiety for each subject. A second concept, relaxation, could be measured using (1) a scale of relaxation, (2) recording blood pressure readings, (3) asking the subject about feeling relaxed, and (4) observing the subject's behavior. These four measures are then combined to give a single observed score of relaxation for each subject. Thus, four methods and two traits (anxiety and relaxation) are being compared. A series of bivariate correlations are performed on the matrix of values obtained to examine relationships among the methods of measurement and the traits.

In some studies, instruments are used to examine relationships. Consider a hypothesis in which the relationship between concept A and concept B is being tested. In Figure 13–5, the true relationship between concepts A and B is represented by the area enclosed in the dark lines.

If two instruments (A-1 and B-1) were used to examine the relationship between concepts A and B, the part of the true relationship actually reflected by these measures is represented by diagonal lines in Figure 13–6. As the instruments (A-1 and B-1) provide a more accurate measure

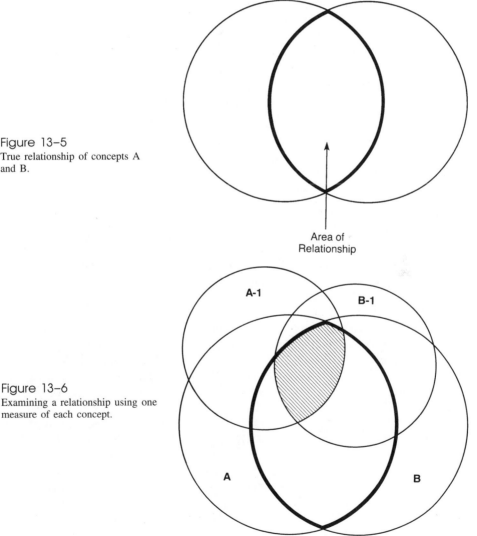

Figure 13–5
True relationship of concepts A and B.

Figure 13–6
Examining a relationship using one measure of each concept.

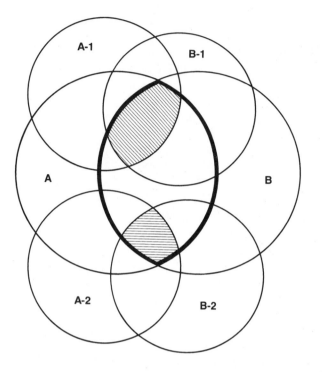

Figure 13–7
Examining a relationship using two
measures of each concept.

of concepts A and B, more of the true relationship between concepts A and B will be measured.

If additional instruments (A-2 and B-2) are used to measure concepts A and B, more of the true relationship might be reflected. Figure 13–7 demonstrates the parts of the true relationship that might be reflected using two instruments to measure concept A (A-1 and A-2) and two instruments to measure concept B (B-1 and B-2).

LEVELS OF MEASUREMENT

The traditional levels of measurement have been used for so long that the categorization system has been considered absolute law and inviolate. The system was developed by Stevens in 1946,

who organized the rules for assigning numbers to objects so that a hierarchy in measurement was established. The levels of measurement from lower to higher are nominal, ordinal, interval, and ratio.

In recent years, controversy has erupted over justification for the categories, leading to two factions in regard to the system: the fundamentalists and the pragmatists. Pragmatists consider measurement to occur on a continuum rather than by discrete categories, whereas fundamentalists adhere rigidly to the original system of categorization. The primary focus of the controversy is related to classification of data into the categories of ordinal and interval. The controversy developed because, according to the fundamentalists, many of the current statistical analysis techniques can be used only with interval data. Many pragmatists believe that if Stevens's rules were rigidly adhered to, few if any measures in the social sciences would meet the criteria to be considered interval-level data. They also believe that violating Stevens's criteria does not lead to serious consequences in the outcomes of data analysis.

NOMINAL-SCALE MEASUREMENT

Nominal-scale measurement is the lowest of the four measurement categories. It is used when data can be organized into categories of a defined property but the categories cannot be compared. Thus, one cannot say that one category is higher than another or that category A is closer to category B than to category C. The categories differ in quality but not quantity. Therefore, one cannot say that subject A possesses more of the property being categorized than does subject B. (Rule: The categories must be unorderable.) Categories must be established in such a way that a datum will fit into only one of the categories. (Rule: The categories must be exclusive.) All the data must fit into the established categories. (Rule: The categories must be exhaustive.)

Data such as gender, ethnicity, marital status, and diagnoses are examples of nominal data. When data are coded for entry into the computer, the categories are assigned numbers. For example, gender may be classified as 1 = male, 2 = female. The numbers assigned to categories in nominal measurement are used only as labels and cannot be used for mathematical calculations.

ORDINAL-SCALE MEASUREMENT

Data that can be measured at the *ordinal-scale level* can be assigned to categories of an attribute that can be ranked. There are rules for how one ranks data. As with nominal-scale data, the categories must be exclusive and exhaustive. With ordinal-scale data, the quantity of the attribute possessed can be identified. However, it cannot be demonstrated that the intervals between the ranked categories are equal. Therefore, ordinal data are

considered to have unequal intervals. Scales with unequal intervals are sometimes referred to as ordered metric scales.

Level of education is frequently used as an ordinal-scale measure. Many scales used in nursing research are ordinal levels of measure. For example, one could rank intensity of pain, degrees of coping, levels of mobility, ability to provide self-care, or daily amount of exercise on an ordinal scale. Using daily exercise, the scale could be 0 = no exercise; 1 = moderate exercise, no sweating; 2 = exercise to the point of sweating; 3 = strenuous exercise with sweating for at least 30 minutes per day; 4 = strenuous exercise with sweating for at least 1 hour per day. This type of scale may be referred to as a metric ordinal scale. In some cases, this type of ordinal scale may be treated as an interval scale.

INTERVAL-SCALE MEASUREMENT

Interval-scale measurements have equal numerical distances between intervals of the scale in addition to following the rules of mutually exclusive categories, exhaustive categories, and rank ordering. Interval scales are assumed to be a continuum of values. Thus, the magnitude of the attribute can be much more precisely defined. However, it is not possible to provide the absolute amount of the attribute because of the absence of a zero point on the interval scale.

Temperature is the most commonly used example of an interval scale. A difference between a temperature of 70° and one of 80° is the same as the difference between a temperature of 30° and one of 40°. Changes in temperature can be precisely measured. However, it is not possible to say that a temperature of 0° means the absence of temperature.

RATIO-LEVEL MEASUREMENT

Ratio-level measurements are the highest form of measure and meet all the rules of other forms of measures: mutually exclusive categories, exhaustive categories, rank ordering, equal spacing between intervals, and a continuum of values. In addition, ratio-level measures have absolute zero points. Weight, length, and volume are commonly used examples of ratio scales. All of these have absolute zero points at which a value of zero indicates the absence of the property being measured: zero weight means the absence of weight. In addition, because of the absolute zero point, one can justifiably say that object A weighs twice as much as object B, or that container A holds three times as much as container B.

STATISTICAL ANALYSES AND LEVELS OF MEASUREMENT

The level of measurement is associated with the types of statistical analyses that can be performed on the data. Therefore, it is advisable to obtain the highest level of measurement possible. For example, age can be grouped into categories such as 20 to 29, 30 to 39, and so on. However, more sophisticated analyses can be performed if the actual age of each subject is obtained. Mathematical operations are limited in the lower levels of measurement. With nominal levels of measurement, only summary statistics such as frequencies, percentages, and contingency correlation procedures can be used.

There is a controversy over levels of measurement related to the statistical operations that can justifiably be performed with scores from the various levels of measure (Armstrong, 1981, 1984; Knapp, 1984, 1990). For example, can one calculate a mean using ordinal data? Fundamentalists believe that appropriate statistical analysis is contingent upon the level of measurement. They disagree with the contention that the scaling procedures used for most psychosocial instruments provide interval-level data. For example, the Likert Scale (discussed in Chapter 14) uses a scale of strongly disagree, disagree, uncertain, agree, and strongly agree. Numerical values (e.g., 1, 2, 3, 4, 5) are assigned to these categories. Fundamental-

ists claim that equal intervals do not exist between these categories. It is not possible to prove that there is the same magnitude of feeling between uncertain and agree as there is between agree and strongly agree. Therefore, parametric analyses cannot be used. Pragmatists believe that with many measures taken at the ordinal level, such as scaling procedures, an underlying interval continuum is present that justifies the use of parametric statistics. Our position is more like that of the pragmatists than of the fundamentalists. However, many data in nursing research are obtained using crude measurement methods that can only be classified into the lower levels of measurement. Therefore, we have included the nonparametric procedures needed for their analysis in Chapter 18.

REFERENCE OF MEASUREMENT

Referencing involves comparing a subject's score against a standard. There are two types of testing that involve referencing: norm-referenced testing and criterion-referenced testing. *Norm-referenced testing* addresses the question, "How does the average person score on this test?" It involves the use of standardized tests that have been carefully developed over several years and have extensive reliability and validity data available. The best-known norm-referenced test is the MMPI (Minnesota Multiphasic Personality Inventory), which is commonly used in psychology and occasionally in nursing research. Many psychological tests are norm-referenced and must be ordered from a psychological testing company and returned to it after data collection for analysis. Usually, this service is provided for a fee.

Criterion-referenced testing asks the question, "What is desirable in the perfect subject?" It involves the comparison of a subject's score with a criterion of achievement that includes the definition of target behaviors. When these behaviors are mastered, the subject is considered proficient in the behavior. The criterion might be a level of knowledge or desirable patient outcome measures.

Criterion measures are not as useful in research as they might be in evaluation studies. Norm referencing will generally lead to higher levels of measurement and greater variability than will criterion-referenced testing and, thus, to increased possibility of achieving statistical significance.

RELIABILITY

Reliability represents the consistency of measure obtained. For example, if one were using a scale to obtain the weight of subjects, one would expect the scale to indicate the same weight if the subject stepped on and off the scale several times. A scale that did not show the same weight each time would be unreliable.

If two data collectors were observing the same event and recording their observations on a carefully designed data collection instrument, one would hope that the recordings would be comparable. The equivalence of their results would indicate the reliability of the measurement technique. In addition, if the same questionnaire is administered to the same individuals at two different times, one hopes that the individuals' responses to the items remain the same. If their responses vary each time the test is administered, there is a chance that the instrument is not reliable.

Reliability testing is considered a measure of the amount of random error in the measurement technique. It is concerned with such characteristics as dependability, consistency, accuracy, and comparability. Since all measurement techniques contain some random error, reliability exists in degrees and is usually expressed as a form of correlation coefficient, with a 1.00 indicating perfect reliability and .00 indicating no reliability. A reliability of .80 is considered the lowest acceptable coefficient for a well-developed measurement tool. For a newly developed instrument, a reliability of .70 is considered acceptable. Estimates of reliability are specific to the sample being tested. Thus, high-reported reliability values on an established instrument do not guarantee that reliability will be satisfactory in another sample or with a different population. Therefore, reliability testing needs to be performed on each instrument used in a study prior to performing other statistical analyses. These values need to be included in published reports of the study. Reliability testing focuses on three aspects of reliability: stability, equivalence, and homogeneity.

STABILITY

Stability is concerned with the consistency of repeated measures. This is usually referred to as *test-retest reliability*. This measure of reliability is generally used with physical measures, technological measures, and paper-and-pencil scales. Use of the technique requires an assumption that the factor to be measured remains the same at the two testing times and that any change in the value or score is a consequence of random error.

Physical measures and equipment can be tested and then immediately retested, or the equipment can be used for a period of time and then retested to determine the necessary frequency of recalibration. With paper-and-pencil measures, a period of 2 weeks to a month is recommended between the two testing times. After retesting, correlational analysis is performed on the scores from the two measures. A high correlation coefficient indicates high reliability.

Test-retest reliability has not proved to be as effective with paper-and-pencil measures as was originally anticipated. There are a number of problems with the procedure. Subjects may remember their responses at the first testing time, which will lead to overestimating the reliability. Subjects may actually be changed by the first testing and therefore respond to the second test differently, leading to underestimation. In tests that measure such factors as attitudes, the assumption that the attitude being measured does not change between the two measurement periods may not be justifiable. If the factor being measured does change, the test is not a measure of reliability. In fact, if the measures stay the same when the attitude has changed, it may be an indication of unreliability.

EQUIVALENCE

The focus of *equivalence* is on comparing two versions of the same paper-and-pencil instrument or two observers measuring the same event. When two observers are being compared, it is referred to as *interrater reliability.* When two paper-and-pencil instruments are being compared, it is referred to as *alternate forms,* or *parallel forms, reliability.* Alternate forms of instruments are of more concern in the development of normative knowledge testing. However, when repeated measures are part of the design, alternate forms of measurement, although not commonly used, would improve the design. Demonstrating that one is actually testing the same content in both tests is extremely complex and, thus, the procedure is rarely used in clinical research.

Determining interrater reliability is a more immediate concern in research and is used in many observational studies. Interrater reliability values need to be reported in any study in which observational data are collected or where judgments are made by two or more data gatherers. Two techniques determine interrater reliability. Both techniques require that two or more raters independently observe and record the same event using the protocol developed for the study or that the same rater observe and record an event on two occasions. To adequately judge interrater reliability, the raters need to observe at least ten subjects or events (Washington & Moss, 1988). Recording the same event on two occasions can be accomplished by videotaping the event. Every data collector utilized in the study needs to be tested for interrater reliability.

The first procedure for calculating interrater reliability requires a simple computation involving a comparison of the agreements obtained between raters on the coding form with the number of possible agreements. This calculation is performed using the following equation:

$$\frac{\text{number of agreements}}{\text{number of possible agreements}}$$

This formula tends to overestimate reliability, and this is a particularly serious problem when the rat-

ing requires only a dichotomous alternative. In this case, there is a 50% probability that the raters will agree on a particular item by chance alone. Appropriate correlational techniques can be used to provide a more accurate estimate of reliability. If more than two raters are involved, a statistical procedure to calculate coefficient alpha may be used. Analysis of variance may also be used as a means of testing for differences among raters. There is no absolute value below which interrater reliability is unacceptable. However, any value below .80 should generate serious concern about the reliability of the data. The value needs to be included in research reports.

When raters know they are being watched, their accuracy and consistency are considerably better than when they believe they are not being watched. Thus, interrater reliability declines (sometimes dramatically) when the raters are assessed covertly (Topf, 1988). Strategies can be used to monitor and reduce the decline in interrater reliability, but these may entail considerable time and expense.

The coding of data into categories has received little attention in regard to reliability. There are two types of reliability related to categorizing data: unitizing reliability and interpretive reliability. *Unitizing reliability* assesses the extent to which each judge (data collector, coder, researcher) consistently identifies the same units within the data as appropriate for coding. This is of concern in observational studies and those using text transcribed from interviews. In observational studies, the data collector needs to select particular units of what is being observed as appropriate to record and code. Of concern is the extent to which two data collectors observing the same event would select the same units to record. In studies using transcribed text from interviews, the researcher needs to select particular units of the transcribed text to code into preselected categories. To what extent would two individuals reading the same text select the same passages to code into categories? (Garvin, Kennedy, & Cissna, 1988)

In some studies, selection of units for coding is simple and straightforward. For example, a unit may begin when a person starts talking. However, in other studies, the identification of an appropriate unit for coding may require some degree of inference or judgment on the part of the rater. For example, if the unit began when the baby awakened, the rater would need to determine at what point the baby was indeed awake. Studies in which every event in the unit is coded require less inference than studies in which only select acts in the unit are to be coded. In all cases, reliability improves when the researcher clearly identifies the units to be coded rather than relying on the judgment of the coder (Washington & Moss, 1988). Unitizing reliability can be calculated using Guetzkow's (1950) index (U) (Garvin et al., 1988).

Interpretive reliability assesses the extent to which each judge assigns the same category to a given unit of data. Most studies using categories report only a global level of reliability in which the overall rate of reliability is examined. The most commonly used measure of global reliability is Guetzkow's (1950) P, which reports the extent to which the judges agree in the selection of categories. A more desirable method of calculating the extent of agreement between judges is Cohen's (1960) Kappa. However, global measures of interpretive reliability provide no information on the degree of consistency in assigning data to a particular category. Category-by-category measures of reliability include the assumption that some categories are more difficult to use than others, and thus, have a lower reliability. Using this method of evaluating reliability, the researcher needs to analyze statistically the reliability category by category, determine the equality of the frequency distribution across categories, and examine the possibility that coders may be systematically confusing some categories (Garvin et al., 1988).

HOMOGENEITY

Tests of instrument *homogeneity* are used primarily with paper-and-pencil tests and address the correlation of various items within the instrument. The original approach to determining homogeneity was *split-half reliability*. This strategy was a way of getting at test-retest reliability without administering the test twice. Rather, the instrument items were split in half, and a correlational procedure was performed between the two halves. The Spearman-Brown correlation formula has generally been used for this procedure. One of the problems with the procedure was that although items were usually split into odd-even items, it was possible to split them in a variety of ways. Each approach to splitting the items would yield a different reliability coefficient. Therefore, the researcher could continue to split the items in various ways until a satisfactorily high coefficient was obtained.

More recently, testing the homogeneity of all the items in the instrument has been seen as a better approach to determining reliability. Although the mathematics of the procedure are complex, the logic is simple. One way to view it is as though one conducted split-half reliabilities in all the ways possible and then averaged the scores to obtain one reliability score. This procedure examines the extent to which all the items in the instrument measure the same construct. It is a test of internal consistency. The statistical procedures used for this process are Cronbach's alpha coefficient and, when the data are dichotomous, K-R 20 (Kuder-Richardson formula).

If the coefficient value were 1.00, each item in the instrument would be measuring exactly the same thing. When this occurs, one might question the need for more than one item. A slightly lower coefficient (.8 to .9) indicates an instrument that will reflect more richly the fine discriminations in levels of the construct. Magnitude can then be discerned more clearly.

Other approaches to testing internal consistency include Cohen's Kappa statistic, which determines the percent of agreement with the probability of chance being taken out, correlating each item with the total score for the instrument, or correlating each item with each other item in the instrument. In this procedure, often used in instrument development, items that do not correlate highly may be deleted from the instrument. Factor analysis may also be used to develop reliability of instruments. After the factor analysis has been performed, instrument items with low factor weights can be deleted. After deleting these items, reliability scores on the instrument will be higher. If there is more than one factor, correlations can be performed between items and factor scores.

An instrument that has low reliability values cannot be valid since it is inconsistent in its measurement. An instrument that is reliable cannot be assumed to be valid for a particular study or population.

VALIDITY

The *validity* of an instrument is a determination of the extent to which the instrument actually reflects the abstract construct being examined. Validity has been discussed in the literature in terms of three primary types: content validity, predictive validity, and construct validity. Within each of these types, subtypes were identified. These multiple types of validity were very confusing, especially since the types were not discrete but interrelated.

Presently, validity is considered a single broad method of measurement evaluation referred to as construct validity (Berk, 1990; Rew, Stuppy, & Becker, 1988). All of the previously identified types of validity are now considered evidence of construct validity. New standards used to judge the evidence of validity were published in the *Standards for Educational and Psychological Testing* in 1985 by the American Psychological Association (APA). This important work greatly extends our understanding of what validity is and how to achieve it.

Validity, as well as reliability, is not an all-or-nothing phenomenon but rather a matter of degree. No instrument is completely valid. Thus, one determines the degree of validity of a measure rather than whether or not validity exists. Defining the validity of an instrument requires years of work. Many equate the validity of the instrument with the rigorousness of the researcher. The assumption is that since the researcher develops the instrument, the researcher also needs to develop the validity. However, this is to some degree an erroneous view, as pointed out by Brinberg and McGrath (1985).

■

"Validity is not a commodity that can be purchased with techniques. Validity, as we will treat it, is a concept designating an ideal state—to be pursued, but not to be attained. As the roots of the word imply, validity has to do with truth, strength, and value. The discourse of our field has often been in tones that seem to imply that validity is a tangible 'resource,' and that if one can acquire a sufficient amount of it, by applying appropriate techniques, one has somehow 'won' at the game called research. We reject this view. In our views, validity is not like money—to gain and lose, to count and display. Rather, validity is like integrity, character, or quality, to be assessed relative to purposes and circumstances." (p. 13) ■

In Figure 13–8, validity (the shaded area) is illustrated by the extent to which the instrument A-1 reflects concept A. As measurement of the concept improves, validity improves. The extent to which the measurement tool measures items other than the concept is referred to as *systematic error* (also identified in the figure). As systematic error decreases, validity increases.

Validity will vary from one sample to another and from one situation to another; therefore, validity testing actually validates the use of an instrument for a specific group or purpose, rather than being directed toward the instrument itself. An instrument may be very valid in one situation but not valid in another. Therefore, validity needs to be re-examined in each study situation. Although many instruments used in nursing studies were developed for use in other disciplines, it is important that the measure be valid in terms of nursing knowledge. Nagley and Byers (1987) give an example of a study in which a measure of cognitive function was used to measure confusion. However, the instrument did not capture the nursing meaning of confusion. Nurses consider persons confused who do not know their age or location.

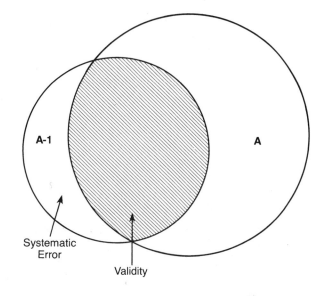

Figure 13–8
Representation of instrument validity.

The aforementioned measure of cognitive function does not categorize these individuals as confused.

Beck, Weissman, Lester, and Trexler (1974) developed a tool to measure hopelessness using hospitalized suicidal patients. Later, one of us (Burns, 1981) used the instrument in another study examining family members of cancer patients. One had to question whether a tool to measure hopelessness in the original population would be valid to measure hopelessness in family members of cancer patients. A computer search revealed that although the instrument had been used in 17 studies, none of the studies had re-examined the validity or reliability of the instrument. Further statistical analyses indicated that the instrument was indeed valid for both purposes.

CONTENT-RELATED VALIDITY EVIDENCE

Content-related validity evidence examines the extent to which the method of measurement includes all the major elements relevant to the construct being measured. This evidence is obtained from three sources: the literature, representatives of the relevant populations, and content experts.

Twenty years ago, the only type of validity addressed in most studies was referred to as *face validity,* which verified basically that the instrument *looked* like or gave the appearance of measuring the content. This approach is no longer considered acceptable evidence for validity. However, it is still an important aspect of usefulness of the instrument, since the willingness of subjects to complete the instrument is related to their perception that the instrument measures the content they agreed to provide (Lynn, 1986; Thomas, 1992).

Documentation of content-related validity evidence begins with instrument development. The first step of instrument development is to identify *what* is to be measured. This is referred to as the *universe* or *domain* of the construct. The domain may be determined through a concept analysis or an extensive literature search. Qualitative methods can also be used for this purpose. Macnee and Talsma (1995), in developing the Barriers to Cessation scale asked subjects to identify what made it most difficult for them to resist smoking. Their responses and the new scale were given to five individuals familiar with smoking cessation and with research. These individuals were asked to determine whether the subjective responses of the subjects could be considered examples of specific items in the scale. Of 38 responses, 29 were categorized as examples of an item in the scale. The remaining nine items could not be categorized and may need to be included in further development of the instrument.

The procedures used to develop or select items for the instrument that are representative of the domain of the construct need to be described. One helpful strategy commonly used is to develop a blueprint or matrix, such as is used in developing test items for an examination. However, before developing items, the blueprint specifications need to be submitted to an expert panel to validate that they are appropriate, accurate, and representative. Selection of at least five experts is recommended; however, a minimum of three experts is acceptable if it is not possible to locate additional individuals with expertise in the area (Lynn, 1986). These experts need to be given specific guidelines for judging the appropriateness, accuracy, and representativeness of the specifications. Berk (1990) recommends that the experts first make an independent assessment and then meet for a group discussion of the specifications. The specifications are then revised and resubmitted to the experts for a final independent assessment.

The researcher then needs to determine how the domain is to be measured. The item format, item content, and procedures for generating items need to be carefully described. Items are then constructed for each cell in the matrix or observational methods designated to gather data related to a specific cell. The researcher is expected to describe the specifications used in constructing items or selecting observations. Sources of content for items need to be documented. The items are then assembled, refined, arranged in a suitable order, and submitted to the content experts for evaluation. Specific instructions for evaluating each item and the total instrument need to be given to the experts.

A numerical value reflecting the level of content-related validity evidence can be obtained by using the index of content validity (CVI) developed by Waltz and Bausell (1981). Using this instrument, experts rate the content relevance of each item using a 4-point rating scale. Lynn (1986) recommends standardizing the options on

this scale to read: "1 = not relevant; 2 = unable to assess relevance without item revision or item is in need of such revision that it would no longer be relevant; 3 = relevant but needs minor alteration; 4 = very relevant and succinct" (p. 384). In addition to evaluating existing items, the experts need to be asked to identify important areas not included in the instrument. Berk (1990) suggests that judges also be asked to evaluate the items in terms of readability and possible offensiveness of the language to subjects or data gatherers.

Before sending the instrument to experts for evaluation, the researcher needs to determine the number of experts who must agree on each item and on the total instrument in order for the content to be considered valid. Items that do not achieve minimum agreement by the expert panel need to be eliminated from the instrument or revised.

With some modifications, this procedure can also be used with existing instruments, many of which have never been evaluated for content-related validity. With the author's permission, instrument revision could be implemented to improve the content-related validity (Lynn, 1986).

Berk (1990) describes the use of the foregoing procedure to obtain evidence of content-related validity for an instrument measuring the nursing care needs of patients with AIDS. The matrix used to develop items related to respiratory and circulatory function is shown in Table 13–1. Berk used four AIDS nurses, one each from hospital, ambulatory care, home care, and nursing home settings as experts. These nurses attended nine sessions of 2 to 3 hours for a total of 22.5 hours to assist in the development of this complex instrument.

Readability is an essential element of the validity and reliability of an instrument. Assessing the level of readability of an instrument is relatively simple and takes about 20 minutes. There are more than 30 readability formulas. These formulas use counts of language elements to provide an index of the probable degree of difficulty of comprehending the text. Evanoski (1990) used the Fog formula to calculate the level of readability of literature developed to provide health education

Table 13–1
Example of a Matrix Developed to Test Content-Related Validity

Indicator	Level 1	Level 2	Level 3	Level 4
A. Airway	Effective clearance	Congested, clears with coughing	Ineffective clearance requiring suction, chest PT	Obstruction threatening life
B. Breathing	Effective patterns with adequate gas exchange	SOB or DOE after moderate activity (e.g., climbing stairs); diminished or adventitious breath sounds (e.g., wheezing/rales/ronchi)	Dyspnea at rest or during ADL/minimal activity; impairment (e.g., retractions, nasal flaring)	Inadequate to meet survival needs (e.g., apnea periods)
C. Cardiovascular status	Unimpaired, normal pulse and BP	Fluctuates (e.g., decreased cardiac output and/or BP abnormality controlled by medication/diet); irregular heartbeat; abnormal heart sounds; chest pain	Decompensation as evidenced by poorly controlled arrhythmia, vertigo, syncope; poorly controlled BP or BP with orthostatic changes	Life-threatening abnormality in flow patterns or cardiac output (e.g., uncontrolled arrhythmia or BP)
D. Endurance	Sufficient	Fatigue, does not interfere with ADLs	Limited; affects ability to perform ADLs	Unable to perform ADLs

Revised Domain Specifications: Sample of Respiratory and Circulatory Function Subdomain (8. Respiratory and circulatory function revised: The body functions concerned with (a) the transfer of gases to meet ventilatory needs, and (b) the supply of blood to body tissues via the cardiovascular system).

(From Berk, R. A. [1990]. Importance of expert judgement in content-related validity evidence. *Western Journal of Nursing Research, 12*[5], 663. Reprinted by permission of Sage Publications, Inc. © 1990.)

Table 13–2
How to Find the Fog Index (Fog Formula)

1. Pick a sample of writing 100 to 125 words long. Count the average number of words per sentence. In counting, treat independent clauses as separate sentences. "In school we studied; we learned; we improved" is three sentences.
2. Count the words of three syllables or more. Do not count: (a) capitalized words; (b) combinations of short words like butterfly or manpower; or (c) verbs made into three syllables by adding "-es" or "-ed" such as trespasses or created. Divide the count of long words by the number of words in the passage to get the percentage.
3. Add the results from no. 1 (average sentence length) and no. 2 (percentage of long words). Multiply the sum by 0.4. Ignore the numbers after the decimal point.

The result is the years of schooling needed to understand the passage tested easily. Few readers have over 17 years' schooling, so give any passage higher than 17 a Fog Index of 17-plus.

(Adapted with permission from Gunning, R. [1968]. *The technique of clear writing* [rev. ed.]. New York: McGraw-Hill. © 1968 McGraw-Hill. "Fog Index" is a service mark of Gunning-Mueller Clear Writing Institute, Santa Barbara, California.)

for patients with ventricular tachycardia. Instructions for use of the Fog formula are presented in Table 13–2. Although readability has never been formally identified as a component of content validity, it should be. How valid is content that is incomprehensible? Miller and Bodie (1994) suggest that the reading comprehension level of the population to be studied be assessed directly before calculating readability using a formula. They indicate that the assumption that literacy is equivalent to the last grade level completed is likely to be erroneous. These authors recommend use of the Classroom Reading Inventory (CRI), which is based on the Flesch, Space, Dale, and Fry reading comprehension scales (Silvaroli, 1986). This instrument determines the level at which an individual can comprehend written material without assistance.

Ahijevych and Bernhard (1994), in discussing the use of the Health-Promoting Lifestyle Profile (HPLP), reported on a study of health-promoting behaviors of African American women.

"Readability of the HPLP instrument could have affected its reliability and validity. Anecdotal information with this sample is pertinent. Women asked the investigator the meaning of the HPLP items 'Enthusiastic and optimistic about life' and 'Like myself.' These were not among the terms clarified by Foster (1987) in her use of the HPLP with older African American adults, for whom she developed explanatory prompts. However, Kerr and Ritchey (1990) reported that Mexican American migrant farm workers frequently asked questions about several items, including 'Like myself.'

Analysis using RightWriter (RightSoft, Inc., Sarasota, FL) revealed the HPLP is written at a seventh-grade level, but there were 21 words readers may not understand, such as 'interpersonal.' Meade, Byrd, and Lee (1989) reported that educational grade level completion was a poor predictor of reading skill among subjects recruited at primary care clinics. They found that although subjects had a reported mean educational level of grade 11, their reading skills as estimated on the Wide Range Achievement Test were at grade 7. Since mean educational level in this study was 12.4 years and 28% of the women had completed 11 or fewer years of education, this may have influenced understanding of the HPLP.

The tool may have a middle-class bias that is inappropriate for poor people who have, for example, little or no time, desire, or energy to 'Attend educational programs on improving the environment,' one item on the scale. The item, 'Find my living environment pleasant and satisfying,' yielded comments such as 'Yes, when the doors are locked, I feel safe.' " (p. 89) ■

EVIDENCE OF VALIDITY FROM FACTOR ANALYSIS

Exploratory factor analysis can be performed to examine relationships among the various items of the instrument. Items that are closely related are clustered into a factor. The analysis may indicate the presence of several factors, which may indicate that the instrument reflects several constructs rather than a single construct. The number of constructs in the instrument can be validated through the use of confirmatory factor analysis. Items that do not fall into a factor (and thus do not correlate with other items) may be deleted. Factor analysis is further described in Chapter 19.

EVIDENCE OF VALIDITY FROM CONTRASTING GROUPS

Validity of the instrument can be tested by identifying groups that are expected to have contrasting scores on the instrument. Hypotheses are generated about the expected response of various groups to the construct. Samples are selected from at least two groups that are expected to have opposing responses to the items in the instrument. Hagerty and Patusky (1995) developed a measure of Sense of Belonging Instrument (SOBI). The instrument was tested on three groups: community college students, clients diagnosed with major depression, and retired Roman Catholic nuns.

"The community college sample was chosen for its heterogeneous mix of students and ease of access. Depressed clients were included based on the literature and the researcher's clinical experience that interpersonal relationships and feeling 'connected' are difficult when one is depressed. It was hypothesized that the depressed group would score significantly lower on the SOBI than the student group. The nuns were selected to examine the performance of the SOBI with a group that, in accordance with the theoretical basis of the instrument, should score significantly higher than the depressed and student groups." (p. 10). ■

EVIDENCE OF VALIDITY FROM EXAMINING CONVERGENCE

In many cases, other instruments are available to measure the same construct. For a number of possible reasons, the existing instruments may not be satisfactory for a particular purpose or a particular population. However, it is important to determine how closely these instruments measure the same construct as the newly developed instrument. Selecting instruments that used a variety of measurement strategies strengthens the test of validity. All of the selected instruments are administered to a sample concurrently. The results are examined using correlational analyses. If the measures are highly positively correlated, the validity of each instrument is strengthened.

EVIDENCE OF VALIDITY FROM EXAMINING DIVERGENCE

Sometimes, instruments can be located that measure a construct opposite to the construct measured by the newly developed instrument. For example, if the newly developed instrument was a measure of hope, a search could be made for an instrument that measured hopelessness. If possible, this instrument is administered at the same time as the instruments used to test convergent validity. Correlational procedures are performed with all the measures of the construct. If the divergent measure is negatively correlated with other measures, validity for each of the instruments is strengthened.

EVIDENCE OF VALIDITY FROM DISCRIMINANT ANALYSIS

Sometimes, instruments have been developed to measure constructs closely related to the construct measured by the newly developed instrument. If such instruments can be located, the validity of the two instruments can be strengthened by testing the extent to which the two instruments can finely discriminate between these related concepts. To test this discrimination, the two instruments are administered simultaneously to a sample and a discriminant analysis is performed. This procedure is described in Chapter 19.

EVIDENCE OF VALIDITY FROM PREDICTION OF FUTURE EVENTS

The ability to predict future performance or attitudes based on instrument scores adds to the validity of an instrument. For example, nurse researchers might determine the ability of a scale that measures health-related behaviors to predict the future health status of individuals. The future level of health of individuals might be predicted by examining reported stress levels of these individuals for the past 3 years. Validity of the Holmes and Rahe Life Events Scale could be tested in this manner. Miller (1981) discussed the validity and reliability of the Holmes and Rahe Life Events Scale in measuring stress levels in a variety of populations. The accuracy of predictive validity is determined by correlational analysis.

EVIDENCE OF VALIDITY FROM PREDICTING CONCURRENT EVENTS

Validity can be tested by examining the ability to predict the current value of one measure based on the value obtained on the measure of another concept. For example, one might be able to predict the self-esteem score of an individual who had a high score on an instrument to measure coping.

SUCCESSIVE VERIFICATION OF VALIDITY

After initial instrument development, other researchers begin using the instrument in unrelated studies. Each of these studies adds to the validity information on the instrument. Thus, there is a successive verification of the validity of the instrument across time.

RELIABILITY AND VALIDITY OF PHYSIOLOGIC MEASURES

Reliability and validity of physiologic and biochemical measures tend not to be reported in published studies. The assumption is made that routine physiologic measures are valid and reliable, an assumption that is not always correct. The most common physiologic measures used in nursing studies are blood pressure, heart rate, weight, and temperature. These measures are often obtained from the patient's record with no consideration given to their accuracy. It is important to consider the possibility of differences between the obtained value and the true value of physiologic measures. Thus, researchers using physiologic measures need to provide evidence of the validity of their measures (Gift & Soeken, 1988).

Evaluation of physiologic measures may require a slightly different perspective than behavioral measures in that standards for physiologic measures are defined by the National Bureau of Standards rather than the APA. The construct by which physiologic validity is judged is human physiology and the mechanics of physiologic equipment. However, the process is similar to that for behavioral measures and needs to be addressed (Gift & Soeken, 1988).

Gift and Soeken (1988) identify five terms that are critical to evaluation of physiologic measures: accuracy, selectivity, precision, sensitivity, and error.

ACCURACY

Accuracy is comparable to validity, in which evidence of content-related validity addresses the extent to which the instrument measured the domain defined in the study. For example, measures of pulse oximetry could be compared with arterial blood gas measures. Evidence of criterion-related validity can be demonstrated by indicating the degree to which instrument scores are correlated with a criterion measure taken concurrently or in the future. The researcher needs to be able to document the extent to which the measure is an effective predictive clinical tool. For example, peak expiratory flow rate can predict asthma episodes.

SELECTIVITY

Selectivity, an element of accuracy, is "the ability to identify correctly the signal under study and to distinguish it from other signals" (Gift & Soeken, 1988, p. 129). Because body systems interact, instruments need to be chosen that have selectivity for the dimension being studied. For example, electrocardiographic readings allow one to differentiate electrical signals coming from the myocardium from similar signals coming from skeletal muscles.

Content validity of biochemical measures can be determined by contacting experts in the laboratory procedure and asking them to evaluate the procedure used for collection, analysis, and scoring. They may also be asked to judge the appropriateness of the measure for the construct being measured. Contrasted groups techniques can be used by selecting a group of subjects known to have high values on the biochemical measures and comparing them with a group of subjects known to have low values on the same measure. In addition, the results of the test can be compared with results using a known, reliable method in order to obtain concurrent validity (DeKeyser & Pugh, 1990).

PRECISION

Precision is the degree of consistency or reproducibility of measurements using physiological instruments. Precision is comparable to reliability. The reliability of most physiologic instruments is determined by the manufacturer and is part of quality control testing. Because of fluctuations in most physiologic measures, test-retest reliability is inappropriate. Engstrom (1988) suggests that assessment of reliability for physiologic variables that yield continuous data needs to include "mean, minimal, and maximal differences; standard deviation of the net differences; technical error of measurement; and indices of agreement" (p. 389). She suggests displaying these differences graphically and recommends exploratory data analysis (EDA) techniques for summarizing differences. EDA techniques are described in Chapter 17. Correlation coefficients are not adequate tests of reliability of physiologic measures.

Two procedures are commonly done to determine precision of biochemical measures. One is the Levy-Jennings Chart. For each analysis method, a control sample is analyzed daily for 20 to 30 days. The control sample contains a known amount of the substance being tested. The mean, standard deviation, and the known value of the sample are used to prepare a graph of the daily test results. Only one value out of 22 is expected to be greater or less than 2 standard deviations from the mean. If two points or more are greater than 2 standard deviations from the mean, the method is unreliable in that laboratory. Another method of determining precision of biochemical measures is the duplicate measurements method. Duplicate measures are performed on randomly selected specimens for a specific number of days. Results will be the same each day if there is perfect precision. Results are plotted on a graph and the standard deviation is calculated based on difference scores. The use of correlation coefficients is not recommended (DeKeyser & Pugh, 1990).

SENSITIVITY

Sensitivity of physiologic measures is related to "the amount of change of a parameter that can be measured precisely" (Gift & Soeken, 1988, p. 130). If changes are expected to be very small, the instrument must be very sensitive in order to detect the changes. Thus, sensitivity is associated with effect size. With some instruments, sensitivity may vary at the ends of the spectrum. This is referred to as the frequency response. The stability of the instrument is also related to sensitivity. This may be judged in terms of the ability of the system to resume a steady state after a disturbance in input. For electrical systems, this is referred to as freedom from drift (Gift & Soeken, 1988).

ERROR

Sources of *error in physiologic measures* can be grouped into five categories: environment, user, subject, machine, and interpretation error. The environment affects both the machine and the subject. Environmental factors include temperature, barometric pressure, and static electricity. User er-

rors are caused by the person using the instrument and may be associated with variations by the same user, different users, changes in supplies, and/or procedures used to operate the equipment. Subject errors occur when the subject alters the machine or the machine alters the subject. In some cases, the machine may not be used to its full capacity. Machine error may be related to calibration or to the stability of the machine. Signals transmitted from the machine are also a source of error and can result in misinterpretation (Gift & Soeken, 1988).

Sources of error in biochemical measures are biologic, preanalytic, analytic, and postanalytic. Biological variability in biochemical measures is due to such factors as age, gender, and body size. Variability in the same individual is due to such factors as diurnal rhythms, seasonal cycles, and aging. Preanalytic variability is due to errors in collecting and handling specimens. These errors include sampling the wrong patients; using an incorrect container, preservative, or label; lysis of cells; and evaporation. Preanalytic variability may also be due to patient intake of food or drugs, exercise, or emotional stress. Analytic variability is associated with the method used for analysis and may be due to materials, equipment, procedures, and personnel used. The major source of postanalytic variability is transcription error. This source of error can be greatly reduced by entering the data directly into the computer (DeKeyser & Pugh, 1990).

OBTAINING VALIDITY IN QUALITATIVE RESEARCH

One of the most serious concerns related to qualitative research has been the lack of strategies to determine the validity of the measurements that led to the development of theory. Qualitative researchers tend to work alone. Biases in their work, which threaten validity, can easily go undetected. Miles and Huberman (1994) caution the qualitative researcher to be alert to the occurrence of the holistic fallacy. This occurs as the researcher becomes more and more sure that his or her conclusions are correct and that his or her model does in fact explain the situation. This feeling should arouse suspicion and alert the researcher to take action to validate the findings. Recently, Miles and Huberman (1994) described 12 strategies for examining the validity of qualitative measures.

1. *Checking for Representativeness.* Qualitative measurement can be biased by either the attention of the researcher or a bias in the people from whom they obtain their measures. To ensure that measures are representative of the entire population, a search is made for sources of data not easily accessible. The researcher assumes that observed actions are representative of actions that occur when the researcher is not present. However, efforts need to be made to determine whether this is so.

2. *Checking for Researcher Effects.* In many cases, the researcher's presence can alter behavior, leading to invalid measures. The researcher needs to remain on the site long enough to become familiar, use unobtrusive measures, and seek input from informants to avoid this effect.

3. *Triangulating.* The qualitative researcher needs to compare all the measures from different sources to determine the validity of the findings.

4. *Weighing the Evidence.* Qualitative research involves reducing large amounts of data during the process of coming to conclusions. In this process, some evidence is captured from this mass of data and is used in reaching conclusions. The researcher needs to review the strength of the captured data to validate the conclusions. The researcher determines the strength of the evidence from the source, circumstances of data collection, and researcher's efforts to validate the evidence. The researcher needs to search actively for reasons why the evidence should not be trusted.

5. *Making Contrasts/Comparisons.* Contrasts between subjects or events in relation to the study conclusions need to be examined. For example, if nursing supervisors consider an action to be very important but staff nurses consider it simply another administrative activity, this is a contrast. The two extreme positions need to be examined. Then a decision needs to be made about whether the difference is a significant one.

6. *Checking the Meaning of Outliers.* Exceptions to findings need to be identified and examined. These exceptions are referred to as outliers. The outliers provide a way to test the generality of the findings. Therefore, in selecting subjects, it may be important to seek out individuals who seem to be outliers.

7. *Using Extreme Cases.* Certain types of outliers, referred to as extreme cases, can be useful in confirming conclusions. The researcher can compare the extreme case with the theoretical model that was developed and determine the key factor that causes the model not to fit the case. Purposive sampling is often used to insure that extreme cases are included.

8. *Ruling Out Spurious Relations.* This strategy requires the examination of relationships identified in the model in order to consider the possibility of a third variable influencing the situation.

9. *Replicating a Finding.* Documenting the findings from several independent sources increases the dependability of the findings and diminishes the risk of the holistic fallacy. The findings can be tested with new data collected later in the study, or data from another site or data set. The second option is more rigorous.

10. *Checking Out Rival Explanations.* The qualitative researcher is taught to keep several hypotheses in mind and to constantly compare the plausibility of each with the possibility of one of the others being more accurate. However, near the end of data analysis, when the researcher is more emotionally wedded to one idea, it is useful to get someone not involved in the research to act as a devil's advocate. Questions need to be directed toward "What could disprove the hypothesis?" or, conversely, "What does the present hypothesis disprove?" Evidence that does not fit the hypothesis needs to be carefully examined.

11. *Looking for Negative Evidence.* This action

naturally flows from the search for outliers and the search for rival explanations. In this step, there is an active search for disconfirmation of what is believed to be true. The researcher goes back through the data, seeking evidence to disconfirm the conclusions. However, the inability to find disconfirming evidence never decisively confirms the conclusions reached by the researcher.

12. *Obtaining Feedback from Informants.* Conclusions need to be given to the informants, and feedback is sought from them about the accuracy of the causal network developed. Although researchers have been getting feedback from informants throughout the analysis period, feedback after completion of the model will provide a different type of verification of information.

■ SUMMARY

Measurement is the process of assigning numbers to objects, events, or situations in accord with some rule. The numbers assigned can indicate numerical values or categories. A component of measurement is instrumentation. Instrumentation is the application of specific rules to develop a measurement device or instrument. A variety of measurement strategies are necessary to examine the concrete and abstract concepts relevant to nursing.

Measurement theory and the rules within this theory have been developed to direct the measurement of abstract and concrete concepts. Measurement theory addresses the directness of measurement, measurement error, levels of measurement, reference of measurement, reliability, and validity. There is direct and indirect measurement. The technology of health care has made direct measures of concrete elements such as height, weight, heart rate, temperature, and blood pressure very familiar. Indirect measurement is used with abstract concepts, when the concepts are not measured directly, but when the indicators or attributes of the concepts are used to represent the abstraction. Measurement error is the difference between what exists in reality and what is measured by a research tool. Measurement exists in both direct and indirect measures and can be random or systematic. The levels of measurement from lower to higher are nominal, ordinal, interval, and ratio. Refer

encing involves comparing a subject's score against a standard. There are two types of testing that involve referencing: norm-referenced testing and criterion-referenced testing.

Reliability in measurement is concerned with how consistently the measurement technique measures the concept of interest. Reliability testing is considered a measure of the amount of random error in the measurement technique. Reliability testing focuses on three aspects of reliability: stability, equivalence, and homogeneity. The validity of an instrument is a determination of the extent to which the instrument actually reflects the abstract construct being examined. Validity, as well as reliability, is not an all-or-nothing phenomenon but rather a matter of degree. No instrument is completely valid. Validity is considered a single broad method of measurement evaluation referred to as construct validity. Validity testing validates the use of an instrument for a specific group or purpose, rather than being directed toward the instrument itself. An instrument may be very valid in one situation but not valid in another. Therefore, validity needs to be re-examined in each study situation.

There are a number of sources for obtaining evidence of the validity of an instrument. Content-related validity evidence examines the extent to which the method of measurement includes all the major elements

continued

continued

relevant to the construct being measured. This evidence is obtained from three sources: the literature, representatives of the relevant populations, and content experts. Exploratory factor analysis can be performed to examine relationships among the various items of the instrument. The validity of the instrument can be tested by identifying groups that are expected to have contrasting scores on the instrument. Other instruments can be compared with the instrument to determine how closely correlated the scores are.

Sometimes, instruments can be located that measure a construct opposite to the construct measured by the instrument. If the divergent measure is negatively correlated with values from the instrument, validity of the instruments is strengthened. Sometimes, instruments have been developed to measure constructs closely related to the construct measured by the instrument. If such instruments can be located, the validity of the two instruments can be strengthened by testing the extent to which the two instruments can finely discriminate between these related concepts. The ability to predict future performance or attitudes based on instrument scores adds to the validity of

an instrument. Validity can also be tested by examining the ability to predict the current value of one measure based on the value obtained on the measure of another concept. After initial instrument development, other researchers begin using the instrument in unrelated studies. Each of these studies adds to the validity information on the instrument. Thus, there is successive verification of the validity of the instrument across time.

Reliability and validity of physiologic and biochemical measures tend not to be reported in published studies. The assumption is erroneously made that routine physiologic measures are valid and reliable. Evaluation of physiologic measures requires a different perspective from that of behavioral measures. Five terms are critical to evaluation of physiologic measures: accuracy, selectivity, precision, sensitivity, and error.

One of the most serious concerns related to qualitative research has been the lack of strategies to determine the validity of the measurements that led to the development of theory. However, strategies are being identified to examine the validity of qualitative measures.

References

Ahijevych, K., & Bernhard, L. (1994). Health-promoting behaviors of African American women. *Nursing Research, 43*(2), 86–89.

American Psychological Association's Committee to Develop Standards. (1985). *Standards for educational and psychological testing.* Washington, DC: American Psychological Association.

Armstrong, G. D. (1981). Parametric statistics and ordinal data: A pervasive misconception. *Nursing Research, 30*(1), 60–62.

Armstrong, G. D. (1984). Parametric statistics [letter]. *Nursing Research, 33*(1), 54.

Beck, A., Weissman, A., Lester, D., & Trexler, L. (1974). The measurement of pessimism: The hopelessness scale. *Journal of Consulting and Clinical Psychology, 42*(6), 861–865.

Berk, R. A. (1990). Importance of expert judgment in content-related validity evidence. *Western Journal of Nursing Research, 12*(5), 659–671.

Brinberg, D., & McGrath, J. E. (1985). *Validity and the research process.* Beverly Hills, CA: Sage.

Burns, N. (1981). *Evaluation of a supportive-expressive group for families of cancer patients.* Unpublished doctoral dissertation, Texas Woman's University, Denton, TX.

Campbell, D. T., & Fiske, D. W. (1959). Convergent and discriminant validation by the multitrait-multimethod matrix. *Psychological Bulletin, 56*(2), 81–105.

Cohen, J. A. (1960). A coefficient of agreement for nominal scales. *Education and Psychological Measurement, 20*(1), 37–46.

DeKeyser, F. G., & Pugh, L. C. (1990). Assessment of the reliability and validity of biochemical measures. *Nursing Research, 39*(5), 314–317.

Engstrom, J. L. (1988). Assessment of the reliability of physical measures. *Research in Nursing & Health, 11*(6), 383–389.

Evanoski, C. A. M. (1990). Health education for patients with ventricular tachycardia: Assessment of readability. *Journal of Cardiovascular Nursing, 4*(2), 1–6.

Foster, M. (1987). A study of the relationships among perceived current health, health-promoting activities, and life satisfaction in older black adults. Unpublished doctoral dissertation, The University of Texas at Austin.

Garvin, B. J., Kennedy, C. W., & Cissna, K. N. (1988). Reliability in category coding systems. *Nursing Research, 37*(1), 52–55.

Gift, A. G., & Soeken, K. L. (1988). Assessment of physiologic instruments. *Heart & Lung, 17*(2), 128–133.

Guetzkow, H. (1950). Unitizing and categorizing problems in coding qualitative data. *Journal of Clinical Psychology, 6*(1), 47–58.

Gunning, R. (1968). *The technique of clear writing* (rev. ed.). New York: McGraw-Hill.

Hagerty, B. M. K., & Patusky, K. (1995). Developing a measure of sense of belonging. *Nursing Research, 44*(1), 9–13.

Kaplan, A. (1963). *The conduct of inquiry: Methodology for behavioral science.* New York: Harper and Row.

Kerr, M. J., & Ritchey, D. A. (1990). Health-promoting lifestyles of English-speaking and Spanish-speaking Mexican-American migrant farm workers. *Public Health Nursing, 7*(2), 80–87.

Knapp, T. R. (1984). Parametric statistics [letter]. *Nursing Research, 33*(1), 54.

Knapp, T. R. (1990). Treating ordinal scales as interval scales: An attempt to resolve the controversy. *Nursing Research, 39*(2), 121–123.

Lynn, M. R. (1986). Determination and quantification of content validity. *Nursing Research, 35*(6), 382–385.

Macnee, C. L., & Talsma, A. (1995). Development and testing of the Barriers to Cessation Scale. *Nursing Research, 44*(4), 214–219.

Meade, C., Byrd, J., & Lee, M. (1989). Improving patient comprehension of literature on smoking. *American Journal of Public Health, 79*(10), 1411–1412.

Miles, M. B., & Huberman, A. M. (1994). *Qualitative data analysis: A sourcebook of new methods* (2nd ed.). Beverly Hills, CA: Sage.

Miller, B., & Bodie, M. (1994). Determination of reading comprehension level for effective patient health-education materials. *Nursing Research, 43*(2), 118–119.

Miller, T. W. (1981). Life events scaling: Clinical methodological issues. *Nursing Research, 30*(5), 316–320A.

Nagley, S. J., & Byers, P. H. (1987). Clinical construct validity. *Journal of Advanced Nursing, 12*(5), 617–619.

Rew, L., Stuppy, D., & Becker, H. (1988). Construct validity in instrument development: A vital link between nursing practice, research, and theory. *Advances in Nursing Science, 10*(4), 10–22.

Silvaroli, N. J. (1986). *Classroom reading inventory* (5th ed.). Dubuque, IA: William C. Brown.

Stevens, S. S. (1946). On the theory of scales of measurement. *Science, 103*(2684), 677–680.

Thomas, S. (1992). Face validity. *Western Journal of Nursing Research, 14*(1), 109–112.

Topf, M. (1988). Interrater reliability decline under covert assessment. *Nursing Research, 37*(1), 47–49.

Waltz, C. W., & Bausell, R. B. (1981). *Nursing research: Design, statistics and computer analysis.* Philadelphia: Davis.

Washington, C. C., & Moss, M. (1988). Pragmatic aspects of establishing interrater reliability in research. *Nursing Research, 37*(3), 190–191.

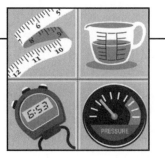

14

Measurement Strategies in Nursing

Nursing studies examine a wide variety of phenomena and thus require the availability of an extensive array of measurement tools. However, nurse researchers have often found that there were no available tools to measure phenomena central to the development of nursing science. Tools used in older nursing studies tended to be developed for a specific study and had little if any documentation of validity and reliability. In the early 1980s, development of valid and reliable tools to measure phenomena of concern to nursing was identified as a priority. The number and quality of measurement methods developed have greatly increased since the first edition of this text.

Knowledge of measurement methods in nursing is important at all levels of nursing. An adequate critique of a study requires that you have some knowledge not only of measurement theory, but also of the state of the art in developing measures to examine the phenomena included in the study. You might want to know whether the researcher was using an older tool that had been surpassed by a number of more recently developed instruments. It might help you to know that measuring a particular phenomenon has been a problem with which nurse researchers have struggled for a number of years. Your understanding of the successes and struggles in measuring nursing phenomena may stimulate your creative thinking as a nursing research user and eventually lead to a contribution of your own to the development of measurement approaches. Many nursing phenomena have not been examined because no one has thought of a way to measure them. This is a problem for clinical practice as well as for research.

This chapter describes the common measurement approaches used in nursing research, including physiologic measures, observations, interviews, questionnaires, and scales. Other methods of measurement discussed include Q methodology, visual analogue scales, Delphi technique, projective techniques, and diaries. This presentation is followed by discussions of the selection of an existing instrument, locating existing instruments, examining existing instruments, assessing the readability of existing instruments, and describing an instrument in a written report. The chapter also includes a description of the process of scale construction and issues related to translating an instrument into another language.

PHYSIOLOGIC MEASUREMENT

Much of nursing practice is oriented toward physiologic dimensions of health. Therefore, many of our questions require the measurement of these dimensions. Of particular importance are studies linking physiologic and psychosocial variables. In 1993, the National Institute of Nursing Research (NINR) expressed a need for increased numbers of physiologic based nursing studies, indicating that 85% of NINR funded studies involved nonphysiologic variables. According to NINR staff, a review of physiologic studies funded by NINR found that "the biological measurements used in the funded grants often were not state-of-the-science, and the biological theory underlying the measurements often was underutilized" (Cowan, Heinrich, Lucas, Sigmon, & Hinshaw, 1993, p. 4). This would suggest that there needs to be an increase, not only of the number of biologically based studies, but of the quality of measurements used in these studies. The Second Conference on Nursing Research Priorities identified biobehavioral studies as one of the five priority areas and proposed targeting the following biobehavioral foci: (1) assessment of the effectiveness of biobehavioral nursing interventions in HIV/AIDS, (2) development of biobehavioral and environmental approaches to remediating cognitive impairment, and (3) identification of biobehavioral factors related to immunocompetence (Pugh & DeKeyser, 1995).

Physiologic measures can be obtained using a variety of methods. The following sections describe obtaining physiologic measures by self-report, observation, direct or indirect measurement, laboratory tests, electronic monitoring, and creative development of new methods of measurement. The measurement of physiologic variables across time is also addressed. The section concludes with a discussion of selecting physiologic variables for a particular study.

OBTAINING PHYSIOLOGIC MEASURES BY SELF-REPORT

Self-report or paper-and-pencil scales can be used to obtain physiologic information. These means may be particularly useful when the subjects are not in a closely monitored setting such as a hospital. For example, Heitkemper, Jarrett, Bond, and Turner (1991) used self-report to obtain information on stool frequency and stool consistency for their study. Other phenomena of possible nursing research interest that could be measured by self-report are sleep patterns, patterns of daily activities, eating patterns, patterns of joint stiffness, variations in degree of mobility, and exercise patterns. For some variables, self-report may be the only means of obtaining the information. This may be the case, for example, when the physiologic phenomenon is experienced by the subjects but cannot be observed or measured by others. Nonobservable physiologic phenomena include pain, nausea, dizziness, indigestion, patterns of hunger or thirst, variations in cognition, visual phenomena, tinnitus, itching, and fatigue. Pope (1995) points out that sound is an essential and con-

stant component of the human condition but its importance to health has been little recognized. Although one can measure sounds, one cannot measure sound perception and sensitivity. Pope recommends the development of instruments to measure these responses, specifically pointing out the potential impact of these variables in settings such as critical care units. Rhodes, McDaniel, Hanson, Markway, and Johnson (1994) used self-report to obtain information on the sensory perceptions of cancer patients for their study.

"During development of the method of measurement, six patients reported their sensations before, during, and after chemotherapy. Subject descriptions were reviewed by a panel of experts. Questions related to each of the five senses were formulated from the subject descriptions. Definitions of each sensation were carefully constructed. The questions, designed for use in a telephone or personal interview, were worded to avoid biasing the subject's responses. The first question related to the senses was, 'What is the first thing that comes to mind when I ask you what your senses told you during your treatment?' This question was followed by a definition, descriptor, and question related to the sense that was first mentioned by the patient. For example: 'Touch can be a lot of different things. It can be what you feel on your skin; it can be what you feel inside your body. It can be various sensations such as a tickle, a caress, an itch, or a burning. Can you help me understand any sensations you felt inside or outside your body?' " (p. 47) ■

Using self-report measures may enable nurses to ask research questions not previously considered. This could be an important means to build knowledge in areas not previously explored. The insights gained could alter the nursing management of patient situations now considered problematic and improve patient outcomes.

OBTAINING PHYSIOLOGIC MEASURES USING OBSERVATION

Data on physiologic parameters are sometimes obtained using observational data collection measures and recording the results on a scale or index. The scale provides criteria for quantifying various levels or states of physiologic functioning. In addition to collecting clinical data, this method provides a means to gather data from the observations of caregivers. This source of data has been particularly useful in studies involving persons with Alzheimer's disease, advanced cancer, and the frail elderly living in the community. Studies based in home health agencies and hospices often use observation tools to record physiologic dimensions of patient status. These data are sometimes stored electronically and are available for large database analyses by researchers.

Grossman (1995) used the Injury Severity Score (ISS) in her study of critically-injured patients. She describes the ISS as follows.

▄▄▄▄▄▄

"The Injury Severity Score (ISS) is a quantitative measure of the severity of blunt and penetrating injuries. It predicts mortality by taking into account both the severity of the critical injury and the number of body areas involved. The ISS is derived from the Abbreviated Injury Scale (AIS) which gives a separate rating of the extent of injuries sustained by each body region: the head/neck, face, thorax, abdomen, extremities and external (skin). These ratings are made within 72 hours of injury and based on a 6-point Likert scale ranging from 1, minor injuries to 6, untreatable. The ISS is the sum of the squares of the highest AIS score in three different body regions. Injury severity scores between 1 and 4 are considered nil, 5 and 10, slight, 11 and 18, moderately severe, and, greater than 18, severe. This scale has been widely used in studies of critically-injured patients and has been shown to be a proven predictor of mortality and morbidity." (p. 16) ▄

OBTAINING PHYSIOLOGIC MEASURES DIRECTLY OR INDIRECTLY

Measurement of physiologic variables can be either direct or indirect. Direct measures are more

valid. Norman, Gadaleta, and Griffin (1991) used both direct and indirect measures of blood pressure in their study. The measurement of arterial pressure waveforms through an arterial catheter provides a direct measure of blood pressure whereas use of a stethoscope and sphygmomanometer provides an indirect measure. Keefe, Kotzer, Froese-Fretz, and Curtin (1996) used the Infant State Monitor to measure physiologic parameters of the preverbal infant. They describe the measurement as follows.

▄▄▄▄▄▄

"The Infant State Monitor has been described by Keefe, Kotzer, Reuss, and Sander (1989). Sensors embedded within a mattress monitor the infant's respiratory pattern and body movement continuously for up to 24 hours. The Sleep State Evaluation program (SSEP) reads the analog data stored on disk and uses a role-based algorithm to classify the activity pattern into the following primary infant states: quiet sleep, active sleep, awake, and indeterminate. In addition, the following additional sleep characteristics are summarized and reported: sleep transitions, sleep breaks, startles, sleep cycles, sleep periods, and noncyclic sleep sessions. In total, 62 variables reflecting the minimum, maximum, average, standard deviation, and totals of these sleep parameters are generated and reported by the SSEP software program. The concurrent validity of this system was assessed in a preliminary study (Keefe et al., 1988). In the current study, interrater reliability was assessed for a subset of 25 randomly selected records. Agreement between the computerized categorization of infant state and live reviewer scoring ranged from 67% to 94%. The overall average percentage of agreement was 78%." (p. 6) ▄

OBTAINING PHYSIOLOGIC MEASURES FROM LABORATORY TESTS

Biochemical measures, such as activated partial thromboplastin time must be obtained through invasive procedures. Sometimes these invasive procedures are part of the routine care of the patient and can be obtained from the patient's record. Although nurses are now performing some biochemical measures on the nursing unit, these often require laboratory analysis. When invasive procedures are not part of routine care but rather are performed specifically for a study, great care needs to be taken to protect the subjects and to follow guidelines for informed consent and institutional approval.

OBTAINING PHYSIOLOGIC MEASURES THROUGH ELECTRONIC MONITORING

The availability of electronic monitoring equipment has greatly increased the possibilities of physiologic measurement in nursing studies, particularly in intensive care environments. Understanding the processes of electronic monitoring can make the procedure less formidable to those critiquing published studies and those considering using the method for measurement. The Keefe and colleagues' (1996) study described above used electronic sensing.

To use electronic monitoring, sensors are usually placed on or within the subject. The sensors measure changes in bodily functions such as elec-

trical energy. For many sensors, an external stimulus is needed to trigger measurement by the sensor. Transducers convert the electrical signal. Electrical signals often include interference signals as well as the desired signal. An amplifier may be used to decrease interference and amplify the desired signal. The electrical signal is then digitized (converted to numerical digits or values) and stored on magnetic tape. In addition, it is immediately displayed using a monitor. The display equipment may be visual, auditory, or both. A writing recorder will provide a printed version of the data. One type of display equipment is an oscilloscope that displays the data as a waveform, and it may provide information such as time, phase, voltage, or frequency of the data. Some electronic equipment provides simultaneous recording of multiple physiologic measures that are displayed on a monitor. The equipment is often linked to a computer, which allows the review of data, and the computer often contains complex software for detailed analysis of the data and will provide a printed report of the analysis (De-Keyser & Pugh, 1991). Figure 14–1 illustrates the process of electronic measurement.

One disadvantage of using sensors to measure physiologic variables is that the presence of a transducer within the body can alter the reading. For example, the presence of a flow transducer in

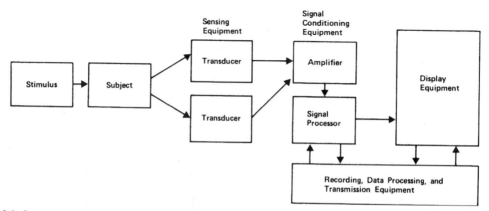

Figure 14–1

Process of electronic measurement. (From Waltz, C. F., Strickland, O. L., & Lenz, E. R. [1991]. *Measurement in Nursing Research.* Philadelphia: Davis, p. 389, with permission.)

the blood vessel can partially block the vessel and thus alter the flow. The reading, then, is not an accurate reflection of the flow.

Norman and colleagues (1991) used electronic sensing in their study evaluating three blood pressure methods in a stabilized acute trauma population, and described their instrumentation.

"A Littmann Classic II Medallion Combination Stethoscope (model 2100), 3M Medical-Surgical Division (St. Paul, Minnesota), was used for all indirect blood pressure readings. Bell and diaphragm values for K1, K4, and K5 were measured with a Hawksley random-zero (R) sphygmomanometer (W. A. Baum Company Inc., Copiague, NY). The RZ is a conventional mercury sphygmomanometer with calibrations from 0 to 300 mm Hg. The singular feature of this instrument is a zero shifting device that allows the mercury column to be stopped randomly between 0 and 20 mm Hg. According to the manufacturers, the zero shifting device effectively eliminates observer bias because true blood pressure values remain unknown until after auscultation (personal communication, November 1987).

Direct blood pressure was measured via radial arterial catheter. The catheters were connected to transducers which sent arterial pressure waveforms to Hewlett-Packard (H-P) four-channel monitors (#78534C). H-P monitors have strip chart recorders with frequency responses ranging from 0.05 to 100 Hz. Simultaneous EKG, pulmonary artery pressure, and arterial pressure waveforms were recorded from these monitors.

Procedure: Demographic information was obtained from patient charts. The catheter-tubing-transducer system was visually assessed for bubbles, and monitor waveforms were checked for damping. Phlebostatic axis was noted before leveling, calibrating, and flushing the pulmonary artery and radial arterial lines. Core body temperature, right atrial pressure, cardiac output, and heart rate were recorded for each subject.

The fidelity and accuracy of the radial catheter-tubing-transducer systems were assessed by calculating natural frequency (Fn) and damping coefficient (zeta) values using Gardner's formula (1981). Natural frequency (Fn) is the ability of a system to oscillate between fast and slow waves (Henneman & Henneman, 1989). Damping coefficient (zeta) refers to how quickly the system comes to rest. Specialists believe a lack of familiarity with natural frequency and damping coefficient calculations is a major reason for inconsistent blood pressure measurement (Gibbs & Gardner, 1988; Henneman & Henneman, 1989)." (p. 87) ∎

CREATIVE DEVELOPMENT OF PHYSIOLOGIC MEASURES

Some studies require imaginative approaches to measuring phenomena that are traditionally observed in clinical practice but not measured. The first step in this process is the recognition that the phenomenon being observed by the nurse could be measured. Once that idea has emerged, one can begin envisioning various means of measuring the phenomenon. Fahs and Kinney's (1991) innovative approach to measuring the extent of bruising illustrates creativity. They traced the outline of the bruise onto polyethylene wrap with a ballpoint pen. This outline was then traced onto a graph with carbon paper. The surface area of the bruise was calculated in units of millimeters squared.

Ziemer, Cooper, and Pigeon (1995) used photographic slides to measure the damage to nipple skin during the first week of breast-feeding. The following is their description of the measurement process.

"To optimize visualization of the nipple skin, serial photographic slides were obtained for later assessment of skin characteristics. The slides provided a magnified image of the nipple skin and areola, which could not be readily observed with the naked eye. To generate reliable documentation of nipple skin condition, the serial photographs were taken with a 35 mm camera fitted with a macro lens and a ring light flash and loaded with Eastman Kodak ASA 25 Kodachrome film. All film was purchased at the same time to ensure similarity of the film emulsions. To obtain consistent exposure distance from the film plate (approximately 10 in.), the automatic focus was disabled and the lens length maximized. This approach resulted in a 1:1 exposure of the film. The same laboratory was used for photographic development in an effort to ensure consistency and reduce variation in color tones. Slide images of nipple skin were assessed to identify the amount of surface area covered by eschar and to rate the severity of erythema and fissures visible on the nipple skin. Eschar was measured by projecting the image downward onto a 20 × 20-in. digitizing tablet with a magnification ratio of 1:22. Visible eschar was then traced and its area calculated." (p. 348) ∎

OBTAINING PHYSIOLOGIC MEASURES ACROSS TIME

Most studies using physiologic measures of interest in nursing are focused on a single point in time. However, there is insufficient information on normal variations on physiologic measures across time, much less changes in physiologic measures across time in individuals in abnormal physiologic states. In some cases, physiologic states demonstrate cyclic activity and are associated with circadian rhythms and day-night patterns. When a clinician observes variation in a physiologic value, it is important to know whether the variation is within normal ranges or is a signal of a change in the patient's condition. Studies need to be performed to describe patterns of physiologic function. Thomas (1995) lists findings from studies examining infant biorhythms in Table 14–1. Dunbar and Farr (1996) studied heart rate (HR), systolic blood pressure (SBP), and diastolic blood pressure (DBP) in cardiac and noncardiac patients over 65 years of age, and described the measurement process.

∎

"Heart rate (HR), systolic blood pressure (SBP, and diastolic blood pressure (DBP) were measured by the indirect automatic oscillometric technique with a Dinamap 8100T (Critikon). The validity of this noninvasive technique was established in several studies that compared BPs obtained with the Dinamap and intraarterial measures. Correlations ranged from $r = .97$ for SBP to $r = .90$ for DBP (Park & Menard, 1987; Ramsey, 1979). The Critikon Company reports the Dinamap 8100T to be accurate in measuring BP to a standard deviation range from 2.4 to 4.1 mm Hg, compared with the standard of direct aortic pressures. Appropriate cuff size was determined according to the circumference of the subject's upper arm.

Rate-pressure product (RPP) was calculated by multiplying HR × SBP at each time of measurement. RPP is considered a noninvasive index of myocardial oxygen consumption (mVO_2) (Amsterdam, Hughes, DeMaria, Zellis, & Mason, 1974). Correlations between direct measures of mVO_2 and RPP of $r = .83$ have been reported (Gobel, Nordstrom, Nelson, Jorgenson, & Wang, 1978) . . . .

For 4 consecutive days, HR, SBP, and DBP were measured when subjects woke in the morning and then every 2 hours while they were awake. Subjects were asked to maintain their normal routines during this period. If they awoke during the night, they were instructed to turn on their call light, and HR and BP measures were obtained. These procedures yielded approximately 36 to 48 measures per subject. HR and BP were taken after subjects assumed a sitting position for at least 5 minutes. Initial BP was measured in both arms, with all subsequent measures obtained from the arm with the highest BP." (p. 45) ∎

SELECTING A PHYSIOLOGIC MEASURE

The researcher designing a physiologic study has less assistance available in selecting methods of measurement than those conducting studies using psychosocial variables. There are multiple books discussing various means to measure psychosocial variables. In addition, numerous articles in nursing journals describe the development of psychosocial variables or discuss various means of measuring a particular psychosocial variable. Literature guiding the selection of physiologic variables is less available.

Table 14-1
Examples of Infant Biorhythms Research Findings

Author	Subjects	Findings
Abe et al., 1978[25]	118 subjects, 5 days PNA—adult	Adult-like temperature rhythm at 7 years; diurnal at 1 month; phase similar to adult at 10–11 months
Anders, 1975[20]		Sleep-wake diurnal at 16 weeks' PNA
Bamford et al., 1990[47]	174 term infants	Circadian pattern in sleep at 6 weeks' PNA
Brown et al., 1992[48]	30 infants, 2–26 weeks' PNA	1 hour periodic oscillations in temperature in 24 out of 30; amplitude 0.2°–0.3°C
Cornelissen et al., 1990[49]	Neonates, 1–7 days' PNA	Heart rate and blood pressure circadian, circaseptan, circannual present in first week of life
de Roquefeuil et al., 1993[50]	12 term infants	Sleep-wake circadian pattern at 4 months' PNA; sleep consolidation 6–7 months
Finley and Nugent, 1983[51]	11 term infants, 1 day–4 weeks' PNA	Periodicity of respiration and heart rate
Franks, 1967[52]	75 infants and children	Adult-like pattern of 17-hydroxycorticosteroid between 1–3 years
Gupta, 1986[13]	Infants and children	Melatonin diurnal rhythm at 3–9 months' PNA
Hellbrügge et al., 1964[10]	Infants and children	Body temperature and sleep-wake pattern diurnal at 2–3 weeks' PNA; heart rate diurnal at 4–20 weeks' PNA; circadian rhythms synchronized to day/night after 23 weeks' PNA
Mirmiran and Kok, 1991[53]	12 preterm infants, 26–32 weeks' GA, 29–35 weeks' PCA	No circadian rhythm in any variable in four infants; many variables with ultradian rhythms, number of subjects demonstrating circadian rhythms; temperature (7), heart rate (5), motor pattern (1)
Mirmiran et al., 1990[54]	Nine infants, 28–34 weeks' PCA	Five out of nine had circadian rhythm body temperature
Putet et al., 1990[37]	Seven preterm infants, mean GA 31 weeks, PNA mean 21.3 ± 11.7 days	Five out of seven had 3- to 4-hour cycle of oxygen consumption, meal frequency strong zeitgeber, handling with feeding a factor
Sankaran et al., 1989[55]	17 preterm infants, 26–41 weeks' GA, 3–4 days' PNA	Diurnal rhythm of beta-endorphin evident at mean GA 31.7 ± 4.8 weeks and mean PNA 3.3 ± 4.8 days
Sitka et al., 1994[56]	17 term infants at 2 days' PNA; 11 at 4 weeks' PNA	On day 2 of lift 12 out of 17 had circadian rhythm of systolic blood pressure and heart rate; 16 out of 17 had circadian skin temperature; 17 out of 17 had circadian rectal temperature
Sostek et al., 1976[46]	12 infants, 37–43 weeks' GA	Diurnal sleep/wake pattern by 8 weeks' PNA
Thomas, 1991[57]	Five preterm infants, 30–34 weeks' GA, 5–10 days PNA	Ultradian rhythm of temperature in 3 out of 5; period length 2–6 hours
Updike et al., 1985[58]	Six preterm infants, 34–37 weeks, 10–20 days' PNA	Circadian cycles of body temperature; $TcPO_2$ and respiratory pauses showed diurnal pattern
Vermes et al., 1980[59]	45 neonates–3-year-olds	Cortisol rhythm at 3 months' PNA
Wailoo et al., 1989[26]	Term infants, 3–4 months' PNA	Well-organized temperature endogenous rhythm at 4 months' PNA but not linked to time of day
Wu et al., 1990[60]	Term infants	Circaseptan and circannual rhythms present in first week of life; circannual acrophase in winter

GA = gestational age; PNA = postnatal age; PCA = postconceptional age. Superscript reference numbers apply to original source.
(From Thomas, K. A. [1995]. Biorhythms in infants and role of the care environment. *Journal of Perinatal and Neonatal Nursing, 9*[2], 68–69. Copyright © 1995, Aspen Publishers, Inc., with permission.)

A number of factors need to be considered in selecting a physiologic measure for a study. The first step is to identify the physiologic variables relevant to the study. Do the variables need to be measured continuously or at a particular point in time? Are repeated measures needed? Are there characteristics of the population under study that place limits on the measurement approaches that can be used?

The next step is to determine how that variable has been measured in previous research. This is a more difficult process for physiologic measures than for psychosocial measures. There are few books or articles that address available options for particular physiologic measures. The sources most commonly used are previous studies that have measured that variable. Literature reviews or meta-analyses can provide reference lists of relevant studies. Because the measure is likely to have been used in studies unrelated to the current research topic, it is usually necessary to examine the research literature broadly.

Physiologic measures need to be carefully linked conceptually with the framework of the study. The logic of operationalizing the concept in a particular way needs to be well thought out and expressed clearly. Triangulation of diverse physiologic measures of a single concept is often advisable to reduce the impact of extraneous variables that might affect measurement. The operationalization and its link to concepts in the framework need to be made explicit in the published report of the study.

The validity and reliability of physiologic measures need to be evaluated. Until recently, researchers commonly used information from the manufacturer of equipment to describe the accuracy of measurement. This information is useful but not sufficient to evaluate validity and reliability. Validity and reliability of physiologic measures are discussed in Chapter 13.

The researcher needs to consider problems that might be encountered in using various approaches to physiologic measurement. One factor of concern is the sensitivity of the measure. Will the measure detect differences finely enough to avoid a Type II error? Physiologic measures are usually norm-referenced. Thus, data obtained from a subject will be compared with a norm as well as with other subjects. The researcher needs to determine whether the norm used for comparison is relevant for the population under study. For example, if the norm is for healthy adults, is it relevant for chronically ill children? How labile is the measure? Some measures vary within the individual from time to time, even when conditions are similar. Circadian rhythms, activities, emotions, dietary intake, or posture can also affect physiologic measures. To what extent will these factors affect the ability to interpret measurement outcomes?

Many measurement strategies require the use of specialized equipment. In many cases, the equipment is available in the patient care area and is a part of routine patient care on that unit. Otherwise, the equipment may need to be purchased, rented, or borrowed specifically for the study. The researcher needs to be skilled in operating the equipment or obtain the assistance of someone who has these skills. Care is taken that the equipment operate in an optimal fashion and be used in a consistent manner. In some cases, the equipment needs to be recalibrated regularly to ensure consistent readings. Recalibration means that the equipment is reset to ensure precise measurements. For example, weight scales are recalibrated periodically to ensure that the weight indicated is accurate.

Table 14–2 lists the physiologic variables most frequently included in nursing studies from 1989 to 1993 in four nursing research journals: *Image: Journal of Nursing Scholarship, Nursing Research, Research in Nursing & Health,* and *Western Journal of Nursing Research.* In addition, a list of recent nursing publications related to physiologic measurement can be found in the appendices of the student study guide accompanying this text.

In publishing the results of a physiologic study, the measurement technique needs to be described in considerable detail. This allows adequate critique of the study, facilitates replication of the study by others, and promotes clinical application of the results. At present, few replications of physiologic studies have been reported in the

Table 14-2*
Physiologic Variables Most Frequently Included in Nursing Studies from 1989 to 1993

Blood pressure
Callow & Pieper, 1989
Folta et al., 1989
Genden et al., 1989
Hahn et al., 1989
Jones & Thomas, 1989
Lookinland, 1989
MacVicar et al., 1989
Rebensen-Piano et al., 1989
Storm et al., 1989
Brown & Tanner, 1990
Byra-Cook et al., 1990
Davis & Nomura, 1990
Kemp et al., 1990
Lu et al., 1990
Metzger & Therrien, 1990
Stevenson & Topp, 1990
Thomas & Friedman, 1990
Grossman, 1991
Marchette et al., 1991
Norman et al., 1991
Brunt & Love, 1992
Smyth & Yarandi, 1992
Weiss, 1992
Baker et al., 1993
Hahn et al., 1993a
Hahn et al., 1993b
Meek, 1993

Heart rate
Folta et al., 1989
Geden et al., 1989
Jones & Thomas, 1989
Lookinland, 1989
MacVicar et al., 1989
Storm et al., 1989
Brown & Tanner, 1990
Davis & Nomura, 1990
Deiriggi, 1990
Lu et al., 1990
Metzger & Therrien, 1990
Stevenson & Topp, 1990
Thomas & Friedman, 1990
Gundersen et al., 1991
Harrison et al., 1991
Margolius et al., 1991
Fuller et al., 1992
McCain, 1992
Paine et al., 1992 (Fetal)
Weiss, 1992
Baker et al., 1993
Buchanan et al., 1993
Medoff-Cooper et al., 1993
Meek, 1993
Miller & Anderson, 1993

Temperature
Bliss-Holtz, 1989
Mravinac et al., 1989
Neff et al., 1989
Beckman, 1990
Heidenreich & Guiffre, 1990
Heidenreich et al., 1990
Erickson & Yount, 1991
Hunter, 1991
Thomas, 1991
Caruso et al., 1991
Gift et al., 1991
McCarthy et al., 1991
Bliss-Holtz, 1992
Cole, 1992
McCarthy et al., 1992
Meek, 1992

Muscle strength
Brink et al., 1989
Dougherty et al., 1989
Sampselle et al., 1989
Dougherty et al., 1991
Sampselle & Delancey, 1992
Kasper et al., 1993
Kim et al., 1993
Maloni et al., 1993

Nutrition/weight
Aaronson & McNee, 1989
Heitkemper et al., 1989
Williams & Williams, 1989
Keithley et al., 1992
McCarthy & Daun, 1992
Smyth & Yarandi, 1992
Westfall & Heitkemper, 1992

Pulmonary artery pressure
Levin-Silverman, 1990
Lookinland & Appel, 1991
Stone et al., 1991

Cardiac output
Lookinland, 1989
Lookinland & Appel, 1991

Respiratory rate
Davis & Nomura, 1990
Weiss, 1992

Urinary laboratory reports
Stebor, 1989
Heitkemper et al., 1991
Wyman et al., 1993

Oxygen saturation
Gift, 1991
Harrison et al., 1991
Lookinland & Appel, 1991
Medoff-Cooper et al., 1993
Becker et al., 1993
Medoff-Cooper et al., 1993

Blood glucose
Pollack, 1989
Wakefield et al., 1989
Beckman, 1990
O'Connell et al., 1990
Pressley et al., 1990
Westfall & Heitkemper, 1992

Other blood laboratory reports
Cahill, 1989
Heitkemper et al., 1989
Pollock et al., 1990
Smith et al., 1990
Fahs & Kinney, 1991
Heitkemper et al., 1991
Levine, 1991
Jones, 1992
Keithley et al., 1992
McCarthy et al., 1992
Smyth & Yarandi, 1992
Brown et al., 1993
Estok et al., 1993
McCarthy et al., 1993

Sucking
Medoff-Cooper et al., 1989
Medoff-Cooper, 1991
Medoff-Cooper et al., 1991
deMonterice et al., 1992
Medoff-Cooper et al., 1993
Miller & Anderson, 1993

Gastric tube location
Metheny et al., 1989
Beckstrand et al., 1990
Metheny et al., 1993

Salivary laboratory reports
Ahevych & Wewers, 1993
Tombes & Gallucci, 1993

*alphabetic order by year; study may be cited more than once
(From: Push, L. C., & DeKeyser, F. G. [1995]. Use of physiologic variables in nursing research. *Image: Journal of Nursing Scholarship, 27*[4], 274, with permission.)

literature. The detailed description of physiologic measures in a research report includes the exact procedure followed and specifics of equipment used in the measurement. The examples used in this section can be used as models for describing the method used to obtain a physiologic measure.

OBSERVATIONAL MEASUREMENT

Although measurement by observation is most commonly used in qualitative research, it is used to some extent in all types of studies. Measurement in qualitative research is not distinct from analysis; rather, the two occur simultaneously. For more detail on measurement and analysis in qualitative research, refer to Chapter 20. Measurement of observations is not quite as simple as it sounds. One first needs to decide what is to be observed and then determine how to ensure that every variable is observed in a similar manner in each instance. Observation tends to be more subjective than other types of measurement and, thus, is often seen as less credible. However, in many cases, this is the only possible approach to obtain important data for nursing's body of knowledge.

As with any means of measurement, consistency is very important. Therefore, much attention needs to be given to training data collectors. If the measurement technique is complex, written instructions need to be provided. Opportunities for pilot testing of the technique are needed, and data on interrater reliability need to be generated.

UNSTRUCTURED OBSERVATIONS

Unstructured observation involves spontaneously observing and recording what is seen with a minimum of prior planning. Although unstructured observations give freedom to the observer, there is a risk of loss of objectivity and a possibility that the observer may not remember all the details of the observed event. If possible, notes are taken during observation periods. If not possible, the researcher needs to record the observations as soon afterward as possible. In some studies, the observation period is videotaped for extensive examination at a later time.

One type of unstructured observation is the chronolog. A *chronolog* provides a detailed description of an individual's behavior in a natural environment. Observational procedures used in a chronolog are designed to reduce the effect of the presence of an observer on the behavior being observed. The method of observation is intense. Therefore, the recommended maximal length of time for observation by one researcher is 30 minutes. If longer periods of observation are necessary, a team of observers may need to take turns observing. For details on the methodology of a chronolog, see Hodson (1986).

STRUCTURED OBSERVATIONS

The first step in structured observational measurement is to define carefully what is to be observed. From that point, the concern is with how the observations are to be made, recorded, and coded. In most cases, a category system is developed for organizing and sorting the behaviors or events being observed. The extent to which these categories are exhaustive varies with the study.

Category Systems

The observational categories should be mutually exclusive. If the categories overlap, the observer will be faced with making judgments as to what category should contain each observed behavior, and data collection may not be consistent. In some category systems, only the behavior that is of interest is recorded. Most category systems require some inference by the observer from the observed event to the category. The greater the degree of inference required, the more difficult the category system is to use. Some systems are developed to be used in a wide variety of studies, whereas others are specific to the study for which they were designed. The number of categories used varies considerably with the study. An optimal number for ease of use and therefore effectiveness of observation is 15 to 20 categories.

Checklists

Checklists are techniques of indicating whether or not a behavior occurred. In this case, tally marks are generally placed on a data collection form each time the behavior is observed. Behaviors other than those on the checklist are ignored. In some studies, multiple tally marks may be placed in various categories while one is observing a particular event. However, in other studies, the observer is required to select a single category by which to place the tally mark. Checklists can be used as self-report instruments. Jacobsen, Munro, and Brooten (1996) used the Multiple Affect Adjective Check List (MAACL) in their study of nurse specialist transitional care. They describe the instrument as follows: "The original checklist (MAACL) consists of 132 affect-connoting adjectives. The instructions ask subjects to check all the words that describe 'how are you now—today.' Subjects do not rate the adjectives; instead, each item is scored as either checked or not checked. The MAACL is routinely completed by subjects in about 5 minutes" (p. 57).

Rating Scales

Rating scales, which will be discussed in a later section of this chapter, can be used for observation as well as for self-report. A rating scale allows the observer to rate the behavior or event on a scale. This provides more information for analysis than the dichotomous data, which indicates only that the behavior either occurred or did not occur.

Keefe, Kotzer, Froese-Fretz, and Curtin (1996) used a rating scale in their study of irritable and nonirritable infants, and described the instrument.

"The Fussiness Rating Scale was originally adapted from the Intensity Rating Scale developed by Emde, Gauensbauer, and Harmon (1976). The scale defines fussiness as a state of irritability not easily explained, which may in-

clude crying, fussing, and restlessness. Parents are asked to rate their child's typical unexplained fussy behavior over the past week on the following three dimensions: amount of fussiness, intensity of fussiness, and hours of fussiness per day. For this study, parents were also asked the number of fussy episodes the infant had per week. Response options ranged from no episodes to every day of the week. Independent mother and father ratings of infant fussiness revealed interrater correlations ranging from $r = .91$ to $r = .72$." (p. 6) ■

INTERVIEWS

Interviews involve verbal communication between the researcher and the subject, during which information is provided to the researcher. Although this measurement strategy is most commonly used in qualitative and descriptive studies, it can be used in other types of studies. There are a variety of approaches to conducting an interview, ranging from a totally unstructured interview in which the content is completely controlled by the subject, to interviews in which the content is similar to a questionnaire, with the possible responses to questions carefully designed by the researcher.

Planning measurement by interview requires careful, detailed work and has almost become a science in itself. Many excellent books are available on the techniques of developing interview questions (Bedarf, 1986; Briggs, 1986; Converse & Presser, 1986; Dillman, 1978; Dillon, 1990; Fowler, 1990; Gorden, 1987; McCracken, 1988; McLaughlin, 1990; Mishler, 1986; Schuman, 1981). Researchers planning to use this strategy need to consult a text on interview methodology prior to designing their instrument. Because nurses frequently use interview techniques in nursing assessment, the dynamics of interviewing are familiar; however, using the technique for measurement in research requires greater sophistication.

UNSTRUCTURED INTERVIEWS

Unstructured interviews are used primarily in descriptive and qualitative studies. The researcher may be seeking to understand how the subject organizes ideas on a particular topic or to identify attitudes. In some cases, this type of interview may be used as a step in developing a more precise measurement tool in a particular area of study.

The interview may be initiated by asking a broad question such as, "Describe for me your experience with. . . ." After the interview is begun, the role of the interviewer is to encourage the subject to continue talking, using techniques such as nodding the head or making sounds that indicate interest. In some cases, the subject may be encouraged to further elaborate on a particular dimension of the topic of discussion.

STRUCTURED INTERVIEWS

Structured interviews include strategies that provide increasing amounts of control by the researcher over the content of the interview. Questions asked by the interviewer are designed by the researcher prior to the initiation of data collection, and the order of the questions is specified. In some cases, the interviewer is allowed to further explain the meaning of the question or modify the way in which the question is asked so that the subject can better understand the question. In more structured interviews, the interviewer is required to ask the question precisely as it has been designed. If the subject does not understand the question, the interviewer can only repeat the question. The subject may be limited to a range of responses previously developed by the researcher, similar to those in a questionnaire. If the possible responses are lengthy or complex, they may be printed on a card that is handed to the subject for selection of a response.

Designing Interview Questions

The development and sequencing of interview questions are similar to those used in questionnaires and will be elaborated on in the section on questionnaires. Briefly, questions progress from broad and general to narrow and specific. Ques-

tions are grouped by topic, with fairly "safe" topics being addressed first, and sensitive topics reserved until late in the interview process. Less interesting data, such as age, educational level, income, and other demographic information, are usually collected last. These data should not be collected in an interview if they can be obtained from another source such as a patient record. The wording of questions in an interview is dependent on the educational level of the subjects. The wording of certain questions may have a variety of interpretations by different subjects, and the researcher needs to anticipate this. After the interview protocol has been developed, feedback needs to be sought from an expert in interview technique and also from a content expert.

Pretesting the Interview Protocol

When the protocol has been satisfactorily developed, it needs to be pilot tested on subjects similar to those who will be used in the study. This allows the researcher to identify problems in the design of questions, sequencing of questions, or procedure for recording responses. It also allows an assessment of the reliability and validity of the interview instrument.

Training Interviewers

Developing skills in interviewing requires practice. Interviewers need to be very familiar with the content of the interview. They must anticipate situations that might occur during the interview and develop strategies for dealing with them. One of the most effective methods of developing a polished approach is role-playing. Playing the role of the subject can give the interviewer insight into the experience of a subject and thus facilitate an effective response to particular situations.

The interviewer needs to learn how to establish a permissive atmosphere in which the subject will be encouraged to respond to sensitive topics. Methods of maintaining an unbiased verbal and nonverbal manner must also be developed. The wording of a question, the tone of voice, raising an eyebrow, or shifting body position can all communicate a positive or negative reaction of the interviewer to the subject's responses. Positive as well as negative verbal or nonverbal communications can alter the data.

Preparing for an Interview

If the interview is to be lengthy, an appointment needs to be made. The researcher needs to be nicely dressed but not overdressed and should be prompt for the appointment. The site selected for the interview needs to be quiet, allow privacy for the interaction, and provide a pleasant environment. Instructions given to the subject about the interview are carefully planned prior to the interview. For example, the interviewer might say, "I am going to ask you a series of questions about. . . . Before you answer each question you need to . . . Select your answer from the following . . . and then you may elaborate on your response. I will record your answer and then, if it is not clear, I may ask you to explain some aspect further."

Probing

Probing is used by the interviewer to obtain more information in a specific area of the interview. In some cases, the question may be repeated. If the subject has said, "I don't know," the interviewer may press for a response. In other situations, the interviewer may further explain the question or ask the subject to explain statements that have been made. At a deeper level, the interviewer may pick up on a comment made by the subject and begin asking questions to obtain further meaning from the subject. Probes should be neutral to avoid biasing the subject's responses. Probing needs to be done within reasonable guidelines to prevent the subject from feeling that he or she is being cross-examined or grilled on a topic.

Recording Interview Data

Data obtained from interviews are recorded either during the interview or immediately following the interview. The recording may be in the form of handwritten notes or tape recordings. If notes are hand recorded, the interviewer needs to have skills in identifying key ideas (or capturing essential data) in an interview and concisely recording this information. The recording of data needs to be done without distracting the interviewee. In some situations, interviewees have difficulty responding if note-taking or taping is obvious. Sometimes, the interviewer may need to record data after completing the interview. Tape-recording requires the permission of the subject. Verbatim transcriptions of tapes are made prior to data analysis. Data from unstructured interviews are difficult to analyze. In some studies, content analysis is used to capture the meaning within the data.

ADVANTAGES AND DISADVANTAGES OF INTERVIEWS

Interviewing is a flexible technique that can allow the researcher to explore greater depth of meaning than can be obtained with other techniques. Interpersonal skills can be used to facilitate cooperation and elicit more information. There is a higher response rate to interviews than to questionnaires, leading to a more representative sample. Interviews allow collection of data from subjects unable or unlikely to complete questionnaires, such as the very ill or those whose reading, writing, and ability to express themselves are marginal.

Interviews are a form of self-report, and the researcher must assume that the information provided is accurate. Interviewing requires much more time than questionnaires and scales and thus is more costly. Because of time and costs, sample size is usually limited. Subject bias is always a threat to the validity of the findings, as is inconsistency in data collection from one subject to another.

Dzurec and Coleman (1995) used hermeneutics to study the experiencing of interviewing from the perspective of the interviewer. They found that there was an unspoken power gradient during an interview that made the process difficult for the interviewer. The insights from the interview process and the relating to the interviewee as a person made the process seem worthwhile. As respondents indicated, "You find out stuff you never even thought to ask" (p. 245). Recommendations emerging from the study included "(a) identifying one's agenda for conducting an interview and sharing it with interviewees in a way comfortable for the interviewer; (b) staying in touch with personal discomforts of the interviewer-interviewee relationship, for example, their disparate roles, knowledge levels, and health and social status; (c) allowing the interview to follow its own course, even if structured by an interview format; and (d) conducting retrospective analyses of interview data to guide subsequent interviews" (p. 245).

Interviewing children requires some special understanding of the art of asking children questions. The interviewer needs to use words that children tend to use to define situations and events, and understand the development of language at varying stages of development. Children view topics differently than adults do. Their perception of time, past and present, is also different. Holaday and Turner-Henson (1989) provide detailed suggestions for developing an interview guide or questionnaire appropriate for children.

Knafl, Pettengill, Bevis, and Kirchhoff (1988) used a structured telephone interview with subjects across the United States to study the role of the nurse researcher employed in a clinical setting. Interviews were recorded and transcribed verbatim. Development of the interview guide is described in the following excerpt.

"Throughout the instrument development process, the research team was guided by the literature on nurse researchers in clinical settings, Lofland's (1971) discussion of interview guide development and Dillman's (1978) guidelines for questionnaire construction.

The literature on nurse researchers, although limited and not research based, indicated that the following topics were salient for the study of clinical nurse researchers: their education, personality, and research experience; relationships of the clinical nurse researcher to others in the organization; ability of the clinical nurse researcher to meet the needs of the nursing department; and the range and nature of the clinical nurse researcher's activities. Once a list of topics consistent with the literature on clinical nurse researchers and with the proposed research questions had been generated, Lofland's general guidelines for interview guide construction were followed." (p. 31) ■

The resulting instrument contained elements characteristic of the qualitative intensive interviewing technique combined with more structured quantitative elements. Thus, method triangulation was used. A sample of the questions is shown in Table 14–3. Data collection, using the interview instrument, was described in the following excerpt.

"During the course of data collection, questions arose regarding the extent to which interviewers should be guided by the canons of flexibility associated with conducting intensive interviews or of standardization associated with much of survey research. Guidelines needed to be established regarding how much freedom individual interviewers had to vary the wording and sequencing of questions on the interview guide.

In the clinical nurse researcher study, interviews were conducted by five persons with variable experiences with conducting interviews. In order to fulfill the intent of the study, it was necessary to obtain comparable data across all subjects in general and clinical nurse researcher-chief nurse executive pairs in particular. This goal pulled the research team in the direction of standardization. At the same time, the investigators wanted to allow interviewers sufficient flexibility to follow up on interesting leads, probe for additional information as they judged appropriate, and interact naturally with subjects.

Regarding standardization of the use of the interview guide, it was decided that all questions would be asked in the order specified. If a subject addressed a question on the guide before it was asked, the question was still asked in sequence. When this happened, the interviewer acknowledged that the topic already had been

Table 14-3
Number and Examples of Highly, Moderately, and Minimally Structured Questions Used in Clinical Nurse Researcher and Chief Nurse Executive Interview Guides

Clinical Nurse Researcher Guide

Highly Structured Questions ($n = 2$)
   Example: We have talked about the activities in which you are involved. Can you tell me approximately what percentage of your time is spent in each type of activity?

Type of Activity	% Time
Administrative	
Staff development	
Research	
Other	

Moderately Structured Questions ($n = 5$)
   Example: Now I'd like to ask how you go about evaluating your performance. In general, what is your feeling about how well you are doing in your job?
   What criteria or cues do you use to decide how well you are doing?
   How do you think the clinical nurse researcher's contributions to an organization should be judged or evaluated?

Minimally Structured Questions ($n = 11$)
   Example: What advice would you have for a new clinical nurse researcher or someone considering taking a job as a clinical nurse researcher?

Chief Nurse Executive Guide

Highly Structured Questions (none)
Moderately Structured Questions ($n = 6$)
   Example: In general, what is your overall feeling about how well the clinical nurse researcher is doing in her or his job?
   What do you see as his or her major accomplishments?
   Are there things which you wanted the clinical nurse researcher to accomplish which he or she has not?
   How do you think a clinical nurse researcher's contribution to an organization should be judged or evaluated?

Minimally Structured Questions ($n = 8$)
   Example: What do you see as the advantages of having a clinical nurse researcher?

(From Knafl, K. A., Pettengill, M. M., Bevis, M. E., & Kirchhoff, K. T. [1988]. Blending qualitative and quantitative approaches to instrument development and data collection. *Journal of Professional Nursing,* 4[1], 30–37, with permission.)

addressed and prefaced the asking of the question in sequence with a statement such as, 'I know you've already talked a bit about this, but perhaps there's more you'd like to say.' This approach both communicated that the interviewer had been paying attention, gave the subject an opportunity to expand on what had been said originally, and precluded omission or cursory investigation of a question by the interviewer. Furthermore, it was agreed that interviewers were not to engage in major rewordings of the questions; when revisions were suggested these were negotiated during the weekly staff meetings of the research team.

In an effort to keep the use of the guide flexible, interviewers were encouraged to engage in 'minor' rewordings of the questions in order to make them more consistent with the interviewer's own style, thereby making the interview more conversational in nature. Interviewers also reworded questions when it was necessary to clarify their meaning to subjects. . . . In addition, interviewers were asked to follow up on any responses that they judged to be of interest but were not covered by a specific question in the guide and to probe for additional information and clarification as they thought appropriate. Probing was less frequent than minor rewordings and focused on asking for additional information (e.g., 'Are there other things you would like to mention?') or in clarifying data (e.g., 'Can you talk just a little more about that?')." (pp. 32–33) ■

QUESTIONNAIRES

A *questionnaire* is a printed self-report form designed to elicit information that can be obtained through written responses of the subject. The information obtained through questionnaires is similar to that obtained by interview, but the questions tend to have less depth. The subject is unable to elaborate on responses or ask for clarification of questions, and the data collector cannot use probe strategies. However, questions are presented in a consistent manner, and there is less opportunity for bias than in the interview.

Questionnaires can be designed to determine facts about the subject or persons known by the subject; facts about events or situations known by the subject; or beliefs, attitudes, opinions, levels of knowledge, or intentions of the subject. They can be distributed to very large samples, either directly or through the mail. The development and administration of questionnaires has been the topic of many excellent books focusing on survey techniques that can be helpful in the process of designing a questionnaire (Berdie, Anderson, & Niebuhr, 1986; Converse & Presser, 1986; Fox & Tracy, 1986; Kahn & Cannell, 1957; Sudman & Bradburn, 1982). Two nursing methodology texts (Shelley, 1984; Waltz, Strickland, & Lenz, 1991) provide detailed explanations of the questionnaire development procedure. Although questions on a questionnaire appear easy to design, the well-designed item requires considerable effort.

Like interviews, questionnaires can have varying degrees of structure. Some questionnaires ask open-ended questions, which require written responses from the subject. Others ask closed-ended questions, which have options selected by the researcher.

Data from open-ended questions are often difficult to interpret, and content analysis may be used to extract meaning. Open-ended questionnaire items are not advised when data are obtained from large samples. A recent modification is the use of computers to gather questionnaire data (Saris, 1991).

DEVELOPMENT OF QUESTIONNAIRES

The first step in either selecting or developing a questionnaire is to identify the information desired. For this purpose, a blueprint or table of specifications is developed. The blueprint identifies the essential content to be covered by the questionnaire, and the content needs to be at the educational level of the potential subjects. It is difficult to stick to the blueprint in designing the questionnaire because it is tempting to add "just one more question" that seems a "neat idea" or a question that someone insists "really should be included." As the questionnaire becomes longer, fewer subjects are willing to respond and more questions are left blank.

The second step is to search the literature for questionnaires or items in questionnaires that match the blueprint criteria. Sometimes published studies include questionnaires, but frequently you must contact the authors of a study in order to receive a copy of their questionnaire. Unlike scaling instruments, questionnaires are seldom copyrighted. Researchers are encouraged to use questions in exactly the same form as those in previous studies to facilitate comparing results between studies. However, questions that are poorly written need to be modified, even if it interferes with comparison with previous results.

For some studies, the researcher can find a questionnaire in the literature that matches the questionnaire blueprint that has been developed for a study. However, frequently the researcher must add items to or delete items from an existing questionnaire to accommodate the blueprint developed. In some situations, items from two or three questionnaires are combined to develop an appropriate questionnaire.

An item on a questionnaire has two parts: a lead-in question (or stem) and a response set. Each lead-in question needs to be carefully designed and clearly expressed. Problems include ambiguous or vague meaning of language, leading questions that influence the response of the respondent, questions that assume a pre-existing state of affairs, and double questions.

In some cases, the respondents will interpret terms used in the lead-in question in one way while the meaning to the researcher is different. For example, the researcher might ask how heavy the traffic is in the neighborhood in which the family lives. The researcher might be asking about automobile traffic but the respondent interprets the question in relation to drug traffic. The researcher might define *neighborhood* as a region composed of a three-block area whereas the respondent considered a neighborhood to be a much larger area. Family could be defined as those living in one house or all close blood relations (Converse & Presser, 1986). If a question includes a term with which the respondent may not be familiar or for which there are several meanings, the term needs to be defined.

Leading questions suggest the answer desired by the researcher. These types of questions often include value-laden words and indicate the bias of the researcher. For example, a question might ask, "Do you believe physicians should be coddled on the nursing unit?" or "All hospitals are bad places to work, aren't they?" These are extreme examples. Most leading questions are constructed more subtly than these. The degree of formality with which the question is expressed and the permissive tone of the question are, in many cases, important for obtaining a true measure. A permissive tone suggests the acceptableness of any of the possible responses.

Questions implying a pre-existing state of affairs lead the respondent to admit to a previous behavior regardless of how the question is answered. The favorite example of professors teaching questionnaire development is the question,

"When did you stop beating your wife?" Similar questions more relevant to our times are, "How long has it been since you used drugs?" or, to an adolescent, "Do you use a condom when you have sex?"

Double questions ask for more than one bit of information. For example, a question might ask, "Do you like intensive care nursing and working closely with physicians?" It would be possible for the respondent to be affirmative about working in intensive care settings and negative about working closely with physicians. In this case, the question would be impossible to answer. A similar question is, "Was the inservice program educational and interesting?"

Questions with double negatives are also difficult to answer. For example, one might ask, "Do you believe nurses should not question doctors' orders?" Yes or No. In this case, it is difficult to determine the meaning of a yes or no. Thus, the sample responses are uninterpretable.

Each item in a questionnaire has a *response set,* which provides the parameters within which the question is to be answered. This response set can be open and flexible, as it is with open-ended questions, or narrow and directive, as it is with closed-ended questions. For example, an open-ended question might have a response set of three blank lines. With closed-ended questions, the response set includes a specific list of alternatives from which to select.

Response sets can be constructed in a variety of ways. The cardinal rule is that there must be a response category for every possible answer. If the sample may include respondents who might not have an answer, include a response category of "don't know" or "uncertain." If the information sought is factual, this can be accomplished by including "other" as one of the possible responses. However, it must be recognized that the item "other" is essentially lost data. Even if the response is followed by a statement such as "Please explain," it is rarely possible to analyze the data meaningfully. If a large number of subjects (greater than 10%) select the alternative "other," the alternatives included in the response set might not be appropriate for the population studied.

The simplest response set is the dichotomous Yes/No option. Arranging responses vertically preceded by a blank will reduce errors. For example,

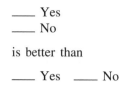

____ Yes
____ No

is better than

____ Yes   ____ No

since, in the latter, the respondent might not be sure whether to indicate Yes by placing a response before or after the Yes.

Response sets need to be mutually exclusive. This might not be the case in the following response set:

working full-time
full-time graduate student
working part-time
part-time graduate student

Burns (1986) used a questionnaire to examine smoking patterns of nurses in the state of Texas. Items from that questionnaire, which demonstrates a variety of response sets, are given in Figure 14–2.

Each question should clearly instruct the subject how to respond (i.e., choose one, mark all that apply), or instructions should be included at the beginning of the questionnaire. The subject needs to know whether to circle, underline, or fill in a circle as he or she responds to items. Clear instructions are difficult to construct and usually require several attempts, and each pilot should be tested with naive subjects who are willing and able to express their reactions to the instructions.

After the questionnaire items have been developed, the ordering of the items needs to be carefully planned. Questions related to a specific topic need to be grouped together. General items are included first, progressing to more specific items. More important items might be included first, progressing to items of lesser importance. Questions of a sensitive nature, or those that might be threatening, should appear last on the questionnaire. In some cases, the response to one item may influence the response to another. If so, their order

needs to be carefully considered. Any open-ended questions should be included last, because their responses will require more time than closed-ended questions. The general trend is to include demographic data about the subject at the end of the questionnaire.

In large studies, optical scanning sheets may be used to speed up data entry to the computer and to decrease errors. This decision needs to be carefully thought out, however, because subjects who are not familiar with these sheets may make errors in entering their responses (thus decreasing measurement validity), and fewer subjects may be willing to complete the questionnaire.

A cover letter needs to accompany the questionnaire, explaining the purpose of the study, the name of the researcher, the approximate amount of time required to complete the form, and organizations or institutions supporting the study. Instructions include an address to which the questionnaire can be returned. This address needs to be at the end of the questionnaire as well as on the cover letter and the envelope. Respondents will often discard both the envelope and the cover letter, and, after completion of the questionnaire, will not know where to send it. It is also wise to provide a stamped, addressed envelope for the subject to return the questionnaire.

A pilot test of the questionnaire needs to be performed to determine the clarity of questions, effectiveness of instructions, completeness of response sets, time required to complete the questionnaire, and success of data collection techniques. As with any pilot test, the subjects and techniques need to be as similar to those planned for the main study as possible. In some cases, some open-ended questions are included in a pilot test to obtain information for the development of closed-ended response sets for the main study.

QUESTIONNAIRE VALIDITY

One of the greatest risks in developing response sets is leaving out an important alternative or response. For example, if the questionnaire item addressed the job position of nurses working in a

Select the response that most accurately describes you and mark it on the attached Scantron sheet.

1. Do you currently smoke cigarettes?
   a. no
   b. yes

2. How old were you when you started smoking?
   a. under 15   e. 18 years   h. 21 years
   b. 15 years   f. 19 years   i. 22 years
   c. 16 years   g. 20 years   j. over 22 years
   d. 17 years

3. Before entering your basic (GENERIC) nursing education program, on the average, about how many cigarettes a day did you smoke?
   a. didn't smoke at all   d. 15–24 cigarettes/day
   b. didn't smoke every day   e. 25–39 cigarettes/day
   c. less than 15 cigarettes/day   f. 40 or more cigarettes/day

4. During your basic nursing (GENERIC) education program, on the average, about how many cigarettes a day did you smoke?
   a. didn't smoke at all   d. 15–24 cigarettes/day
   b. didn't smoke every day   e. 25–39 cigarettes/day
   c. less than 15 cigarettes/day   f. 40 or more cigarettes/day

5. How many organized programs have you attended to help you quit smoking?
   a. none   d. three   g. six
   b. one   e. four   h. seven
   c. two   f. five   i. more than seven

6. What is the longest single period you have stopped smoking?
   a. have never stopped   e. more than 1 month but less than 1
   b. less than a day   year
   c. less than a week   f. more than 1 year but less than 3
   d. less than a month   years
                            g. 3 years or more

7. Aside from what you think you actually could do, which would you most like to do?
   a. quit smoking   d. not sure at this time
   b. cut down   e. smoke as much as now
   c. cut down just a little

Figure 14–2
Example of items from a smoking questionnaire.

hospital and the sample included nursing students, a category must be included that indicates the student role. When seeking opinions, there is a risk of obtaining a response from an individual who actually has no opinion on the subject. When an item requests knowledge that the respondent does not possess, his or her guessing interferes with obtaining a true measure.

The response rate to questionnaires is generally lower than that with other forms of self-report, particularly if the questionnaires are mailed out. If the response rate is lower than 50%, the representativeness of the sample is seriously in question. The response rate for mailed questionnaires is usually small (25 to 30%), so the researcher is frequently unable to obtain a representative sample, even with randomization. Strategies that can increase the response rate include enclosing a stamped, addressed envelope, and sending a postcard two weeks after the questionnaire was mailed to those who have not returned it. Sometimes a phone call follow-up is made to increase the return rate of questionnaires (Baker, 1985). Gordon and Stokes (1989) were successful in maintaining an 80% response rate in a study in which subjects were followed quarterly for one year and asked to keep a diary. The impressive strategies they used to accomplish this high response rate are described in detail in their paper.

Commonly, respondents fail to mark responses to all the questions, which is especially a problem with long questionnaires. This can threaten the validity of the instrument. In some cases, responses will be written in if the respondent does not agree with the available choices, or comments may be written in the margin. Generally, these responses cannot be included in the analysis; however, a record needs to be kept of such responses. It is advisable to decide prior to distributing the questionnaires those questions that are critical to the research topic. If any of these questions is omitted in a questionnaire, it is not included in the analysis.

Consistency in the way that the questionnaire is administered is important to validity. For example, administering some questionnaires in a group setting and mailing out others is not wise. There should not be a mix of mailing to business addresses and home addresses. If questionnaires are administered in person, the administration needs to be consistent. Several problems in consistency can occur: (1) Some subjects may ask to take the form home to complete it and return it later, whereas others will complete it in the presence of the data collector; (2) some subjects may complete the form themselves, whereas others may ask a family member to write the responses that the respondent dictates; and (3) in some cases, the form may be completed by a secretary or colleague rather than by the individual. These situations lead to biases in responses that are unknown to the researcher and that alter the true measure of the variables.

ANALYSIS OF QUESTIONNAIRE DATA

The data from questionnaires are usually ordinal in nature, limiting analysis for the most part to summary statistics and nonparametric statistics. However, in some cases, ordinal data from questionnaires are treated as interval data, and t tests or analyses of variance (ANOVA) are used to test for differences between responses of various subsets of the sample. Discriminant analysis may be used to determine the ability to predict membership in various groups from responses to particular questions.

SCALES

Scales, a form of self-report, are a more precise means of measuring phenomena than are questionnaires. The majority of scales have been developed to measure psychosocial variables. However, self-reports can be obtained on physiologic variables, such as pain, nausea, or functional capacity, using scaling techniques. Scaling is based on mathematical theory, and there is a branch of science in which the primary concern is the development of measurement scales. From the point of view of scaling theory, considerable measurement error (random error) and systematic error are expected in a single item. Therefore, in most scales, the various items on the scale are summed to obtain a single score. These are referred to as summated scales. Less random error and systematic error exist when using the total score of a scale. Using several items in a scale to measure a concept is comparable to using several instruments to measure a concept (see Figure 13–7, p. 324). The various items in a scale increase the dimensions of the concept that are reflected in the instrument. The types of scales described include rating scales, the Likert scale, and semantic differentials.

RATING SCALES

Rating scales are the crudest form of measure using scaling techniques. A rating scale lists an ordered series of categories of a variable, assumed to be based on an underlying continuum. A numerical value is assigned to each category. The fineness of the distinctions between categories varies with the scale. Rating scales are commonly used by the general public. In conversations, one can hear statements such as "on a scale of one to ten,

I would rank that . . ." Rating scales are easy to develop; however, one needs to be careful to avoid end statements that are so extreme that no subject will select them. A rating scale could be used to rate the degree of cooperativeness of the patient or the value placed by the subject on the nurse-patient interactions. This type of scale is often used in observational measurement to guide data collection. Burns (1974) used the rating scale in Figure 14–3 (on pp. 364–365) to examine differences in nurse-patient communication of cancer patients and other medical-surgical patients.

LIKERT SCALE

The *Likert scale* is designed to determine the opinion or attitude of a subject and contains a number of declarative statements with a scale after each statement. The Likert scale is the most commonly used of the scaling techniques. The original version of the scale consisted of five categories. Values are placed on each response, with a value of 1 on the most negative response and a value of 5 on the most positive response (Nunnally, 1978).

Response choices in a Likert scale most commonly address agreement, evaluation, or frequency. Agreement options may include such statements as *strongly agree, agree, uncertain, disagree,* and *strongly disagree.* Evaluation responses ask the respondent for an evaluative rating along a good/bad dimension, such as positive to negative or excellent to terrible. Frequency responses may include statements such as *rarely, seldom, sometimes, occasionally,* and *usually.* The terms used are versatile and need to be selected for their appropriateness to the stem (Spector, 1992). Sometimes seven options are given, sometimes only four.

There has been controversy over the use of the uncertain or neutral category, which allows the subject to avoid making a clear choice of positive or negative statements. Thus, sometimes, only four or six options are offered, with the uncertain category omitted. This is referred to as a *forced choice* version. Sometimes, respondents will become annoyed at forced choice items and refuse to complete them. Researchers who use the forced choice version consider an item that is left blank as a response of "uncertain." However, responses of "uncertain" are difficult to interpret, and, if a large number of respondents select that option or leave the question blank, the data may be useless.

The phrasing of item stems depends on the type of judgment the respondent is being asked to make. Agreement items are declarative statements such as "Nurses should be held accountable for managing a patient's pain." Frequency items can be behaviors, events, or circumstances to which the respondent can indicate how often they occur. A frequency stem might be "You read research articles in nursing journals." An evaluation stem could be "The effectiveness of X drug for relief of nausea after chemotherapy." Items need to be clear, concise, and concrete (Spector, 1992).

An instrument using a Likert scale usually consists of 10 to 20 items addressing dimensions of a particular issue. Half the statements should be expressed positively and half negatively to avoid inserting a bias in the responses. Scale values of negatively expressed items must be reversed prior to analysis. Usually, the values obtained from each item in the instrument are summed to obtain a single score for each subject. Although the values of each item are technically ordinal-level data, the summed score is often treated as interval-level data, thus allowing more sophisticated statistical analyses. Some researchers now treat each item as interval-level data. The items (not actually part of a scale) in Figure 14–4 (on p. 366) indicate the types of statements commonly used in Likert scales.

Flaskerud (1988) reports difficulty using the Likert scale with some cultural groups. Hispanic and Vietnamese subjects had difficulty understanding the request to select one of four or five possible responses and insisted on responding to each item with a simple yes or no. Additional explanation did not sway them from this position. The reason for this difficulty is not understood.

SEMANTIC DIFFERENTIALS

The *semantic differential* was developed by Osgood, Suci, and Tannenbaum (1957) to measure attitudes or beliefs. A semantic differential scale

1. Nurses come into my room
   a. rarely
   b. sometimes
   c. whenever I call them
   d. frequently just to speak or check me
2. I would like nurses to come into my room
   a. rarely
   b. sometimes
   c. whenever I call them
   d. frequently just to speak or check me
3. When a nurse enters my room, she usually
   a. talks very little
   b. tries to talk about things I do not wish to discuss
   c. talks only about casual things
   d. is willing to listen or discuss what concerns me
4. When a nurse enters my room, I would prefer that she
   a. talk very little
   b. talk only when necessary
   c. talk only about casual things
   d. be willing to listen or discuss what concerns me
5. When a nurse talks with me she usually seems
   a. not interested
   b. in a hurry
   c. polite but distant
   d. caring for me as a person
6. When a nurse talks with me, I would prefer that she be
   a. not interested
   b. in a hurry
   c. polite but distant
   d. caring for me as a person
7. When a nurse talks with me she usually
   a. stands in the doorway
   b. stands at the foot of the bed
   c. stands at the side of the bed
   d. sits beside the bed
8. When a nurse talks with me I would prefer that she
   a. stand in the doorway
   b. stand at the foot of the bed
   c. stand at the side of the bed
   d. sit beside the bed
9. When a nurse talks with me, she is
   a. strictly business
   b. casual
   c. friendly but does not talk about feelings
   d. open to talking about things I worry or think about
10. When a nurse talks with me, I would prefer that she keep the conversation
    a. strictly business
    b. casual
    c. friendly but not talking about feelings
    d. open to talk about things I worry or think about

Figure 14–3
A rating scale used to measure the nature of nurse-patient communications.

11. Nurses talk with me about things important to me
    a. rarely
    b. sometimes
    c. frequently
    d. as often as I need to talk
12. I would <u>like</u> for the nurse to talk with me about things important to me
    a. rarely
    b. sometimes
    c. frequently
    d. as often as I need to talk
13. The nurse looks me in the eye when she talks with me
    a. rarely
    b. sometimes
    c. frequently
    d. very frequently
14. I would <u>prefer</u> that the nurse look me in the eye when she talks with me
    a. rarely
    b. sometimes
    c. frequently
    d. very frequently
15. When a nurse talks to me, she touches me
    a. rarely
    b. sometimes
    c. frequently
    d. very frequently
16. When a nurse talks with me, I would <u>prefer</u> that she touch me
    a. rarely
    b. occasionally
    c. frequently
    d. very frequently
17. My feelings about nurses talking to me are
    a. They should do their work well and otherwise leave me alone.
    b. They may talk if they need to; it does not bother me.
    c. I enjoy talking with the nurses.
    d. When the nurse lets me talk with her about things important to me, I feel that she cares for me as a person.

On question 18, please mark as many answers as you wish.
18. I would like to feel free to talk with the nurse about my
    a. illness
    b. future
    c. financial problems
    d. feelings about myself
    e. feelings about my family
    f. life up to this time

Figure 14–3 *Continued*

	Strongly Disagree	Disagree	Uncertain	Agree	Strongly Agree
People with cancer almost always die					
Chemotherapy is very effective in treating cancer					
We are close to finding a cure for cancer					
I would work next to a person with cancer					
I could develop cancer					
Nurses take good care of patients with cancer					

Figure 14–4

Example of items that could be included in a Likert scale.

consists of two opposite adjectives with a seven-point scale between them. The subject is to select one point on the scale that best describes his or her view of the concept being examined. The scale is designed to measure connotative meaning of the concept to the subject. Although the adjectives may not seem to be particularly related to the concept being examined, the technique can be used to distinguish varying degrees of positive and negative attitudes toward a concept. Figure 14–5 illustrates the form used for this type of scale.

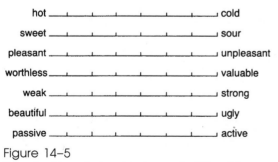

NURSING RESEARCH

hot _____ cold

sweet _____ sour

pleasant _____ unpleasant

worthless _____ valuable

weak _____ strong

beautiful _____ ugly

passive _____ active

Figure 14–5

Example of items in the original semantic differential.

Some semantic differentials use descriptive phrases, rather than the original adjectives used by Osgood and colleagues (1957) to develop the semantic differential instrument. Burns (1981, 1983) developed a semantic differential to measure beliefs about cancer that uses descriptive phrases. Figure 14–6 includes some of the descriptive phrases from a 23-item scale.

In the semantic differential, values are assigned to each of the spaces, from 1 to 7, with 1 being the most negative response and 7, the most positive. The placement of negative responses to the left or right of the scale should be randomly varied to avoid global responses (in which the sub-

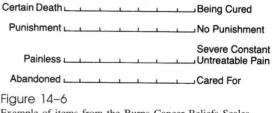

CANCER

Certain Death _____ Being Cured

Punishment _____ No Punishment

Painless _____ Severe Constant Untreatable Pain

Abandoned _____ Cared For

Figure 14–6

Example of items from the Burns Cancer Beliefs Scales.

ject places checks in the same column of each scale). Each line is considered one scale. The values for the scales are summed to obtain one score for each subject. Factor analysis is used to determine the factor structure, which is expected to reflect three factors or dimensions: evaluation, potency, and activity. The researcher needs to explain theoretically why particular items on the scale cluster together in the factor analysis. Thus, the development of the instrument contributes to theory development. Factor analysis is also used to evaluate the validity of the instrument. With some of these instruments, three factor scores, each representing one of the dimensions, are used to describe the subject's responses and are a basis for further analysis (Nunnally, 1978).

Q METHODOLOGY

Q methodology is a technique of comparative rating that preserves the subjective point of view of the individual (McKeown & Thomas, 1988). Cards are used to categorize the importance placed on various words or phrases in relation to the other words or phrases in the list. Each phrase is placed on a separate card. The number of cards should range from 40 to 100 (Tetting, 1988). The subject is instructed to sort the cards into a designated number of piles, usually 7 to 10 piles ranging from most to least important. However, the subject is limited in the number of cards that may be placed in each pile. If the subject must sort 59 cards, category 1 (of greatest importance) may allow only 2 cards; category 2, 5 cards; category 3, 10 cards; category 4, 25 cards; category 5, 10 cards; category 6, 5 cards; category 7 (the least important), 2 cards. Thus, the placing of the cards fits the patterns of a normal curve. The subject is usually advised to first select the cards that he or she wishes to place in the two extreme categories, then work toward the middle category, which contains the largest number of cards until they are satisfied with the results.

The Q-sort method can also be used to determine the priority of or most important items to include in the development of a scale. In the previ-

ously mentioned example, the behaviors sorted into categories 5, 6, and 7 might be organized into a 17-item scale. Correlational or factor analysis is used to analyze the data (Dennis, 1986; Tetting, 1988). Simpson (1989) suggests using the Q-sort for cross-cultural research, using pictures rather than words for nonliterate groups.

Wyers, Grove, and Pastorino (1985) used the Q-sort technique to reduce 75 job behaviors of the clinical nurse specialist (CNS) to 40 essential behaviors. In a pilot study, these investigators identified 75 behaviors from the literature and from interviews with nursing administrators, nursing educators, and CNSs. These 75 behaviors were sorted into 7 categories by 24 subjects (7 nursing administrators, 8 nursing educators, and 9 CNSs) to identify 40 essential behaviors of the CNS role.

VISUAL ANALOGUE SCALES

One of the problems of concern in scaling procedures is the difficulty in obtaining fine discrimination of values. A recent effort to resolve this problem is the *visual analogue scale,* sometimes referred to as magnitude scaling (Gift, 1989). This technique seems to provide interval-level data, and some researchers argue that it provides ratio-level data (Sennott-Miller, Murdaugh, & Hinshaw, 1988). It is particularly useful in scaling stimuli (Lodge, 1981). This scaling technique has been used to measure mood, anxiety, alertness, craving for cigarettes, quality of sleep, attitudes toward environmental conditions, functional abilities, and severity of clinical symptoms (Wewers & Lowe, 1990, p. 229).

The stimuli must be defined in a way that is clearly understandable to the subject. Only one major cue should appear for each scale. The scale is a line 100 mm in length with right angle stops at each end. The line may be horizontal or vertical. Bipolar anchors are placed beyond each end of the line. The anchors should *not* be placed underneath or above the line before the stop. These end anchors should include the entire range of sensations possible in the phenomenon being measured. Examples include "all" and "none," "best" and

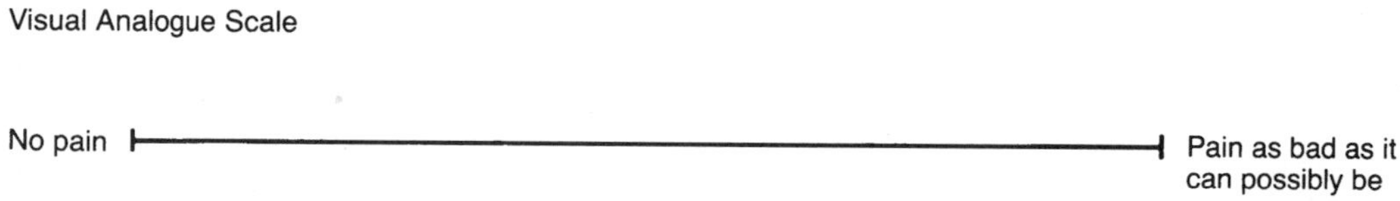

Visual Analogue Scale

No pain ├──┤ Pain as bad as it
can possibly be

Figure 14–7
Example of a visual analogue scale.

"worst," "no pain" and "pain as bad as it could possibly be." These scales can be developed for use with children by using pictorial anchors at each end of the line rather than words (Lee & Kieckhefer, 1989).

The subject is asked to place a mark through the line to indicate the intensity of the stimulus. A ruler is then used to measure the distance between the left end of the line and the mark placed by the subject. This measure is the value of the stimulus. The scale is designed to be used while the subject is seated. Whether use of the scale from the supine position influences the results by altering perception of the length of the line has yet to be determined (Gift, 1989).

Wewers and Lowe (1990) have published an extensive evaluation of the reliability and validity of visual analogue scales, though reliability is difficult to determine. Since most of the variables measured using the tool are labile, test-retest is not appropriate, and since a single measure is obtained, examination of internal consistency is not possible. The visual analogue scale is much more sensitive to small changes than numerical and rating scales and can discriminate between two dimensions of pain. Comparisons of the scale with other instruments measuring the same construct have had varying results and are difficult to interpret. An example of a visual analogue scale is shown in Figure 14–7.

DELPHI TECHNIQUE

The *Delphi technique* is used to measure the judgments of a group of experts, assess priorities, or make forecasts. It provides a means to obtain the opinion of a wide variety of experts across the country to provide feedback without the necessity of meeting together. Using the Delphi technique, the opinions of individuals cannot be altered by the persuasive behavior of a few people at a meeting.

To implement the technique, a panel of experts is identified. A questionnaire is developed that addresses the topics of concern. Although most responses are closed-ended questions, there are usually opportunities on the questionnaire for open-ended responses by the expert. The questionnaires are then returned to the researcher, and results are summarized. The outcome of the statistical analysis is returned to the panel of experts, along with a second questionnaire. Respondents with extreme responses to the first round of questions may be asked to justify their responses. The second round of questionnaires is returned to the researcher for analysis. This procedure is repeated until data reflect a consensus among the panel. A model of the Delphi technique was developed by Couper (1984) and is presented in Figure 14–8.

Goodman (1987) identified several potential problems that could be encountered in the use of the Delphi technique. There has been no documentation that the responses of "experts" are different from those one would receive from a random sample of subjects. Because the panelists are anonymous, there is no accountability for their responses. They could make hasty, ill-considered judgments knowing that there will be no negative feedback as a result. Feedback on the consensus of the group tends to centralize opinion, and the traditional analysis using means and medians may mask the responses of those who are resistant to the consensus. Thus, conclusions could be misleading.

Lindeman (1975) conducted a Delphi survey

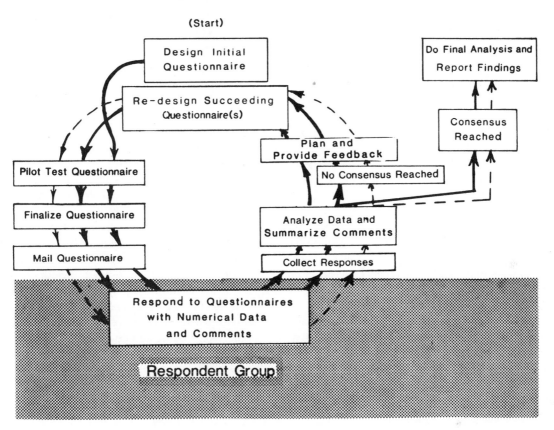

Experimenter

(Start)

Design Initial Questionnaire

Re-design Succeeding Questionnaire(s)

Do Final Analysis and Report Findings

Consensus Reached

Plan and Provide Feedback

No Consensus Reached

Pilot Test Questionnaire

Finalize Questionnaire

Mail Questionnaire

Analyze Data and Summarize Comments

Collect Responses

Respond to Questionnaires with Numerical Data and Comments

Respondent Group

Figure 14–8

Delphi technique sequence model. (From Couper, M. R. [1984]. The Delphi technique: Characteristics and sequence model. Reported from *Advances in Nursing Science,* Vol. 7, No. 1, p. 75, with permission of Aspen Publishers, Inc. Gaithersburg, MD.)

to determine research priorities in clinical nursing research. She used a panel of 433 experts, both nurses and non-nurses, with a wide range of interests. Four rounds of a 150-item questionnaire were sent to the panel. The report, published in *Nursing Research,* had an important influence on the directions of research program development in nursing.

PROJECTIVE TECHNIQUES

Projective techniques are based on the assumption that the responses of individuals to unstructured or

ambiguous situations reflect the attitudes, desires, personality characteristics, and motives of the individual. The technique is most frequently used in psychology and includes such techniques as the Rorschach Inkblot Test, Machover's Draw-A-Person Test, word association, sentence completion, role-playing, and play techniques. The technique is an indirect measure of data that is unlikely to be obtained directly. Analysis of the data requires that inferences be made about the meaning and thus is subjective. Many of the tests require extensive training for administration and interpretation and thus have not been frequently used in nursing research. However, with the increased frequency of interdisciplinary research, their use in nursing studies may increase. At present, the technique is used in nursing primarily in studying children (Waltz, Strickland, & Lenz, 1991). Johnson (1990) provides an excellent explanation of the techniques used to interpret children's drawings.

DIARIES

A recent approach to obtaining information that must be collected over time is to ask the subjects to keep a record or *diary* of events. The data in this diary can then be collected and analyzed by researchers. A diary, which allows recording shortly after an event, is more accurate than obtaining the information through recall at an interview, the reporting level of incidents is higher, and one tends to capture the participant's perception of situations.

This technique provides a means to obtain data on topics of particular interest within nursing that have not been accessible by other means. Some potential topics for diary collection include expenses related to a health care event (particularly out-of-pocket expenses), self-care activities (fre-

quency and time required), incidence of symptoms, eating behaviors, exercise behaviors, and care provided by family members in a home care situation. Although diaries have been used primarily with adults, they are also an effective means of data collection with school-age children. Butz and Alexander (1991) report an 88% completion rate in a study of children with asthma, with most children (72.3%) keeping the diary without assistance from their parents.

Health diaries have been used to document health problems, responses to symptoms, and efficacy of responses. Diaries may also be used to determine how people spend their days; this could be particularly useful information in managing the care needs of individuals with chronic illnesses. In experimental studies, diaries may be used to determine subjects' responses to experimental treatments. There are two types of health diaries: a ledger in which different types of events are recorded, such as the occurrence of a symptom, and a journal, where daily entries are made related to specific topics. An example of a ledger is shown in Figure 14-9 and an example of a journal is shown in Figure 14-10. Validity and reliability have been examined by comparing the results to data obtained through interviews and have been

Date	What symptom did you have?	Did you talk with a family member or friend about the symptom?		Did you talk with a health professional about it?		Did you take any pills or treatments for the symptom?	
		No	Yes	No	Yes	No	Yes, Specify

Figure 14-9
Sample ledger diary. (From Burman, M. E. [1995]. Health diaries in nursing research and practice. *Image: Journal of Nursing Scholarship, 27*[2], 148, with permission.)

Date _____/_____/_____

1. Did you have any symptoms today?

    1. NO → Go to question 5
    2. YES, Please specify _____

    _____

    _____

2. Did you talk to a family member about the symptom(s)?
    1. NO

    2. YES

3. Did you talk to a health care professional about the symptom(s)?
    1. NO

    2. YES

4. Did you take any pills for the symptom(s)?

    1. NO → Go to question 5
    2. YES, Please specify _____

    _____

    _____

5. How would you rate your health today?

Excellent _____ Poor

Figure 14–10

Sample journal diary. (From Burman, M. E. [1995]. Health diaries in nursing research and practice. *Image: Journal of Nursing Scholarship, 27*[2], 148, with permission.)

found to be acceptable. Participation in studies using health diaries has been very good and attrition rates are reported as low. Adequate instructions related to completing the diary and arranging for pick-up are critical (Burman, 1995).

Burman (1995, p. 151) makes some recommendations regarding the general use of health diaries.

1. Critically analyze the phenomenon of interest to ensure that it can be adequately captured using a diary. Infrequent major events, very minor health events or behaviors, and vague symptoms are less likely to be reported than more frequent, definable acute problems. The use of a diary should be evaluated in light of other data collection approaches such as interviews and mail surveys, that may lead to higher data quality depending on the specific phenomenon of interest.

2. Determine which format—ledger or journal—should be used to decrease participant burden while minimizing missing data. The ledger format may be less burdensome but evaluation of missing data is more complicated.

3. Evaluate whether closed- or open-ended questions will result in clearer reporting. Closed-ended questions reduce respondent burden, but may result in overreporting of symptoms.

4. Pilot test any new or refined diary with the target population of interest to identify possible problems, to ensure that the phenomenon can be recorded with this approach, and to evaluate the ability of participants to complete diaries. Participation rates in diary studies vary, although those with high incomes and

education levels, and better writing skills may be overrepresented. However, diaries have been used successfully with ill and general-community populations.

5. Determine the diary period that is necessary to adequately record changes and fluctuations in the phenomenon of interest, balancing this with respondent burden. Typical diary periods are 2 to 4 weeks.

6. Provide clear instructions to all participants on the use of a diary before participation begins to enhance data quality. Participants need to know how to use the diaries, what types of events are to be reported, and how to contact the investigator or clinician with questions.

7. Use follow-up procedures during data collection to enhance completion rates. Telephone contacts enhance completion rates. Diaries may be mailed; however, returning diaries through the mail may result in somewhat lower completion rates.

8. Plan analysis procedures during diary development or refinement to be sure the data are in the appropriate form for the analyses. Diary data are very dense and rich, carefully prepared plans can minimize problems.

Problems related to the diary method include costs, subject cooperation, quality of the data, conditioning effects of keeping a diary on the subject, and the complexity of data analysis. Costs include interview time, mail and telephone expenses, and remuneration to subjects. Costs are higher than single face-to-face interviews but lower than repeated interviews. Costs are lowest when diaries are used with telephone interviews and highest when diaries are used with repeated face-to-face interviews. Costs are lower when diaries are mailed in rather than picked up. Most subject non-cooperation occurs in the first month with only a 1 to 2% subject loss after that point. Diary completion rates are higher (80 to 88%) than other data collection methods such as surveys. Picking up the diary increases the completion rate (Butz & Alexander, 1991).

There are, however, some disadvantages to using diaries. Keeping the diary may, in some cases, alter the behavior or events under study. For ex-

ample, if a person were keeping a diary of the nursing care that he or she was providing to patients, that care might be changed based on the insights he or she gained from recording the information in the diary. Subjects can become more sensitive to items (such as symptoms or problems) reported in the diary. This can result in overreporting. Subjects may also become bored with keeping the diary and become less thorough in recording items. This leads to underreporting (Butz & Alexander, 1991).

Oleske, Heinze, and Otte (1990) used a diary in a study designed to understand the quality of life of persons with cancer receiving home nursing care. The home care agency was offered $10 for each patient in the agency who completed the diary. Patients who completed the diary were offered $5 by the researcher and were allowed to keep the organizer that contained the diary. The authors describe the diary as follows.

"This study employed a diary as a data collection instrument, which was enclosed in a medical At-a-Glance organizer. The front cover was labeled, Client Diary Health Record. The 'assurance-of-confidentiality statement' was also affixed to the front cover. The organizer contained a calendar diary on which to record health problems; a patient information sheet; a consent form; an 8–1/2 × 11-inch pad of lined paper; general instructions for writing in the diary; sample recordings of diary entries.

The sample recordings and instructions indicated that if a health problem occurred, 4 pieces of information were also to be recorded on the calendar: (a) the person contacted, (b) whether the contact was by phone or visit, (c) the date of the contact, and (d) whether or not needed help was received. There was no standard 'lists of problems' from which patients could choose a condition pertaining to themselves. This was done in order to avoid 'suggesting' problems in patients, and thus creating a bias. The patient was instructed to write his or her health problems in the diary, even if unsure whether it was appropriate to record it. The individual was asked to document who was con-

The following samples are provided as a guide to keeping your diary. <u>Every day</u> when you write in the diary, please:

1. Record any <u>health problem</u> or problems you had (for example: constipation, skin rash on back, need bandages for surgery wound).

2. For each health problem, list the type of contact and person you contacted outside your home (such as nurse, doctor, social worker, pharmacist, or family member) and the place or agency (name of the hospital, agency or facility, for example: Visiting Nurse Association).

3. Check (✓) whether you made the contact by telephone or in person for each contact.

4. Record the date of each contact. If you visited or called the same place at different times list each contact separately.

5. Identify, "yes" or "no", if the visit or telephone call helped you with your health problem.

6. Record the <u>health problem</u> even if you did not contact someone outside your home for help with it.

Sample Patient Diary

What <u>health problem</u> did you have?	What person and place did you contact for this health problem?	What type of contact did you make? Check ✓ one		When did you call/visit? (Record date)	Did you receive the help you needed?	
		Telephone call	Visit		Yes	No
skin irritation on back	Nurse, St. Jude Hospital	✓		Dec. 6, 1980	✓	
needed cold pack for leg pain	Pharmacist Mitchel's Pharmacy		✓	Jan. 6, 1981		✓
difficulty in walking, needed a cane	Counselor, American Cancer Society	✓		Jan. 26, 1981	✓	
feeling depressed	Minister, St. Paul's Church		✓	Jan 26, 1981	✓	

Figure 14-11
Patient diary reports of home nursing. (From Oleske, D. M., Heinze, S., & Otte, D. M. [1990]. The diary as a means of understanding the quality of life of persons with cancer receiving home nursing care. *Cancer Nursing, 13*[3], 161, with permission.)

tacted for the problem as a means of verifying the event and assisting in recall of the problem." (p. 160) ■

A sample of the diary is shown in Figure 14–11.

SELECTION OF AN EXISTING INSTRUMENT

Selecting an instrument for measurement of the variables in a study is a critical process in research. The method of measurement must closely fit the conceptual definition of the variable. An extensive search of the literature may be required to identify appropriate methods of measurement. In many cases, instruments will be found that measure some of the needed elements but not all, or the content may be related but somehow different from that needed for the study being planned. Instruments found in the literature may have little or no documentation of the validity and reliability of the instrument.

The initial reaction of the beginning researcher is that no methods of measurement exist and a tool must be developed by the researcher. At the time, this seems to be the simplest solution, since the researcher has a clear idea of what needs to be measured. This solution, however, should not be used unless all else fails. The process of tool development is lengthy and requires considerable research sophistication. Using a new instrument in a study without first evaluating its validity and reliability is unacceptable.

LOCATING EXISTING INSTRUMENTS

Locating existing measurement methods has become easier in recent years. A relatively new computer data base, the Health and Psychological Instruments Online (HAPI) is available in many libraries and can search for instruments that measure a particular concept or for information on a particular instrument. The Measurement Appendix at the end of your Student Study Guide lists some of the recent publications in nursing journals related to instrument development.

Many reference books have compiled published measurement tools, some that are specific to instruments used in nursing research. The measurement appendices at the end of your student study guide list some of these sources. Dissertations often contain measurement tools that have never been published, so a review of *Dissertation Abstracts* might be helpful. *Dissertation Abstracts* is now online on the World Wide Web (WWW).

Another important source of recently developed measurement tools is word-of-mouth communication between researchers. Information on tools is often presented at research conferences years before publication. There are often networks of researchers conducting studies on similar nursing phenomena. These researchers are often associated with a nursing organization and keep in touch through newsletters, correspondence, telephone, electronic mail, computer bulletin boards, and World Wide Web pages. Thus, questioning available nurse researchers can lead to a previously unknown tool. These researchers are often easily contacted by telephone or letter and are usually willing to share their tools in return for access to the data to facilitate work on developing validity and reliability information. The Sigma Theta Tau *Directory of Nurse Researchers* provides address and phone information of nurse researchers.

In addition, it lists nurse researchers by category according to their area of research.

EVALUATING EXISTING INSTRUMENTS

You need to examine several instruments to find the one most appropriate for your study. The selection of an instrument for research requires careful consideration of how the instrument was developed, what the instrument measures, and how to administer it. The following questions need to be addressed when examining an instrument.

1. Does this instrument measure what you want to measure?
2. Is the instrument reflective of your conceptual definition of the variable?
3. Is the instrument well constructed?
4. Does your population resemble populations previously studied using the instrument?
5. Is the readability level of the instrument appropriate for your population?
6. How sensitive is the instrument in detecting small differences in the phenomenon being measured (what is the effect size)?
7. What is the process for obtaining, administering, and scoring the instrument?
8. What skills are required to administer the instrument?
9. How are the scores interpreted?
10. What is the time commitment for the subjects and researcher for administration of the instrument?
11. What evidence is available related to reliability and validity of the instrument?

ASSESSING READABILITY LEVELS OF INSTRUMENTS

The readability level of an instrument is a critical factor in selecting an instrument for a study. Regardless of how valid and reliable the instrument is, it cannot effectively be used in a study if the items are not understandable to the subjects. Calculating readability is relatively easy and can be performed in about 20 minutes. Many word processing programs and computerized grammar checkers will report the readability level of written material. The Fog formula described in Chapter 13 provides a quick and easy way to assess readability.

CONSTRUCTING SCALES

Scale construction is a complex procedure that should not be undertaken lightly. However, in many cases, measurement methods have not been developed for phenomena of concern to nurse researchers. Measurement tools that have been developed may be poorly constructed and have insufficient evidence of validity to be acceptable for use in studies. It is possible for the researcher to carry out instrument development procedures on an existing scale prior to using it in a study. Neophyte nurse researchers could assist researchers in carrying out some of the field studies required to complete the development of a scale. The procedures for developing a scale have been well defined. The following discussion describes this theory-based process and the mathematical logic underlying it.

The theories on which scale construction is most frequently based include classical test theory (Nunnally, 1978), item response theory (Hulin, Drasgow, & Parsons, 1983), multidimensional scaling (Davison, 1983; Kruskal & Wish, 1990), and unfolding theory (Coombs, 1950). Most existing instruments used in nursing research have been developed using classical test theory, which assumes a normal distribution of scores.

CONSTRUCTING A SCALE USING CLASSICAL TEST THEORY

Using classical test theory, the following process is used to construct a scale.

1. **Define the Concept.** A scale cannot be constructed to measure a concept until the nature of the concept has been delineated. The more clearly the concept is defined, the easier it is to write items to measure it (Spector, 1992). Concept definition is achieved through concept analysis, a procedure discussed in Chapters 4 and 7.

2. **Design the Scale.** Items should be constructed to reflect the concept as fully as possible. The process of construction will differ somewhat depending on whether the scale is a rating scale, Likert scale, or semantic differential scale. Items previously included in other scales can be used if they have been shown empirically to be good indicators of the concept (Hulin et al., 1983). A blueprint may be helpful in ensuring coverage of all elements of the concept. Each item needs to be stated clearly and concisely and express only one idea. The reading level of items needs to be identified and considered in terms of potential respondents. The number of items constructed needs to be considerably larger than that planned for the completed instrument since items will be discarded during the item analysis step of scale construction. Nunnally (1978) suggests developing an item pool at least twice the size of that desired for the final scale.

3. **Seek Item Review.** As items are constructed, it is advisable to ask qualified individuals to review them. Crocker and Algina (1986, p. 71) recommend asking for feedback in relation to accuracy, appropriateness, or relevance to test specifications, technical item-construction flaws, grammar, offensiveness or appearance of bias, and level of readability. Revise items based on the critique.

4. **Conduct Preliminary Item Tryouts.** While items are still in draft form, it is helpful to test the items on a limited number of subjects (15–30) representative of the target population. Observe reactions of respondents during testing, noting such behaviors as long pauses, answer-changing, or other indications of confusion about specific items. After testing, a debriefing session needs to be held during which respondents are invited to comment on items and offer suggestions for improvements. Descriptive

and exploratory statistical analyses are performed on data from these tryouts, noting means, response distributions, items left blank, and outliers. Revise items based on this analysis and comments from respondents.

5. **Perform a Field Test.** Administer all of the items in their final draft form to a large sample of subjects representative of the target population. Spector (1992) recommends a sample size of 100 to 200 subjects. However, the sample size needed for the statistical analyses to follow is dependent somewhat on the number of items. Some recommend including 10 subjects for each item being tested. If the final instrument was expected to have 20 items, and 40 items were constructed for the field test, this could require as many as 400 subjects.

6. **Conduct Item Analyses.** The purpose of item analyses is to identify those items that form an internally consistent scale and eliminate those items that do not meet this criterion. Internal consistency implies that all of the items measure the same concept. Prior to these analyses, negatively worded items need to be reverse scored. The analyses examine the extent of intercorrelation among the items. The only statistical computer program currently providing (as a package) the set of statistical procedures needed to perform item analyses is SPSS and SPSS/PC. This package performs item-item correlations and item-total correlations. In some cases, the value of the item being examined is subtracted from the total score and an item-remainder coefficient is calculated. This latter coefficient is the most useful in evaluating items for retention in the scale.

7. **Select Items to Retain.** Based on the number of items desired in the final scale, those items with the highest coefficients are retained. Alternatively, a criterion value for the coefficient (e.g., .40) can be set and all items over this value retained. The greater the number of items retained, the smaller the item-remainder coefficients can be and still have an internally consistent scale. Following this selection process, coefficient alpha is calculated for the scale. This value is a direct function of the number of items and the magnitude of intercorrelation. Thus, one can increase the value of coefficient alpha by increasing the number of items or raise the intercorrelations through inclusion of more highly intercorrelated items. Values of coefficient alpha range from 0 to 1. The alpha value should be at least .70 to indicate sufficient internal consistency (Nunnally, 1978). An iterative process of removing and/or replacing items, recalculating item-remainder coefficients, and then recalculating the alpha coefficient is repeated until a satisfactory alpha coefficient is obtained. Deleting poorly correlated items will raise the alpha coefficient but decreasing the number of items will lower it (Spector, 1992).

The initial attempt at scale development may not achieve a sufficiently high coefficient alpha. In this case, additional items will need to be written, more data collected, and the item analysis redone. This is most likely to occur when too few items were developed initially or when many of the initial items were poorly written. It may also be a consequence of attempts to operationalize an inadequately defined concept (Spector, 1992).

8. **Conduct Validity Studies.** When scale development is judged to be satisfactory, studies must be performed to evaluate the validity of the scale. Refer to the discussion of validity in Chapter 13. These studies require the collection of additional data from large samples. As part of this process, scale scores need to be correlated with scores on other variables proposed to be related to the concept being put into operation. Hypotheses need to be generated regarding variations in the mean values of the scale in different groups. Exploratory and then confirmatory factor analysis (discussed in Chapter 19) is usually performed as part of establishing the validity of the instrument. As many different types of evidence of validity should be collected as possible (Spector, 1992).

9. **Evaluate the Reliability of the Scale.** Various statistical procedures need to be performed to determine the reliability of the scale. These

analyses can be performed using the data collected to evaluate validity. (See Chapter 13 for a discussion of the procedures performed to examine reliability.)

10. **Compile Norms on the Scale.** The determination of norms requires the administration of the scale to a large sample representative of the groups to which the scale is likely to be given. Norms should be acquired for as many diverse groups as possible. Data acquired during validity and reliability studies can be included for this analysis. In order to obtain the very large samples needed for this purpose, many researchers give permission to others to use their scale with the condition that data from their studies be provided for compiling norms.

11. **Publish the Results of the Scale Development.** Scales are often not published for a number of years after the initial development because of the length of time required to validate the instrument. Some researchers never publish the results of this work. Studies using the scale are published, but the instrument development process may not be available except by writing to the author. This information needs to be added to the body of knowledge, and instrument developers need to be encouraged by their colleagues to complete the work and submit it for publication (Lynn, 1989; Norbeck, 1985).

CONSTRUCTING A SCALE USING ITEM RESPONSE THEORY

Using item response theory to construct a scale proceeds initially in a similar fashion to that of classical test theory. There is an expectation of a well-defined concept to operationalize. Initial item writing is similar to that previously described, as are item tryouts and field testing. However, with the initiation of item analysis, the process changes. The statistical procedures used are more sophisticated and complex than those used in classical test theory. Using data from field testing, item characteristic curves (ICCs) are calculated using logistic regression models (Hulin et al., 1983). After selecting an appropriate model based on information obtained from the analysis, item parameters are estimated. These parameters are used to select items for the scale. This strategy is used to avoid problems encountered with classical test theory measures.

Scales developed using classical test theory are very effective in measuring the characteristics of subjects near the mean. Statistical procedures used assume a linear distribution of scale values. Items reflecting responses of subjects closer to the extremes tend to be discarded because of the assumption that scale values should approximate the normal curve. Therefore, scales developed in this manner often do not provide a clear understanding of subjects at the high or low end of values.

One of the purposes of item response theory is to choose items in such a way that estimates of characteristics at each level of the concept being measured are accurate. This is accomplished by using maximum likelihood estimates. A curvilinear distribution of scale values is assumed. Rather than choose items based on the item-remainder coefficient, the researcher specifies a test information curve (TIC). The scale can be tailored to have a desired measurement accuracy. Comparing a scale developed by classical test theory to one developed from the same items using item response theory, one would find differences in some of the items retained. Biserial correlations would be lower in the scale developed using item response theory than using classical test theory. Item bias is lower in scales developed using item response theory. Item bias occurs when respondents from different subpopulations having the same amount of an underlying trait have different probabilities of responding to an item positively (Hulin, Drasgow, & Parsons, 1983, p. 152).

CONSTRUCTING A SCALE USING MULTIDIMENSIONAL SCALING

Multidimensional scaling is used when the concept being operationalized is actually a very abstract construct believed to be most accurately represented by multiple dimensions. The scaling techniques used allow the researcher to uncover the hidden structure in the construct. The analysis techniques use proximities among the measures as input. The outcome of the analysis is a spatial representation, a geometric configuration of data points, that reveals the hidden structure. The procedure tends to be used to examine differences in stimuli rather than differences in people. Thus, differences in perception of light or of pain might be examined. Scales developed using this procedure are effective in revealing patterns among items. The procedure is used in the development of rating scales and semantic differentials (Kruskal & Wish, 1990).

CONSTRUCTING A SCALE USING UNFOLDING THEORY

During construction of a scale using unfolding theory, subjects are asked to respond to the items in the rating scale. Then they are asked to rank the various response options in relation to the response option they selected for that item. This procedure is followed for each item in the scale. Using this procedure, the underlying continuum for each scale item is "unfolded." As an example, suppose you developed the following item:

My favorite ice cream flavor is

1. Chocolate
2. Vanilla
3. Strawberry
4. Butter Pecan

You would ask subjects to select their response to the item. Then they would be asked to rank the other options according to the proximity to their choice. The subject might choose strawberry as no. 1, vanilla as no. 2, butter pecan as no. 3, and chocolate as no. 4. Although preferences of other subjects would differ, the results can be plotted to reveal patterns of an underlying continuum. Items selected for the scale would be those with evidence of a pattern of responses.

TRANSLATING A SCALE TO ANOTHER LANGUAGE

Contrary to expectations, translating an instrument from the original language to a target language is a complex process. The goal of translating a scale is to allow comparisons of concepts among respondents of different cultures. This requires that one first infer and then validate that the conceptual meaning in which the scale was developed is the same in both cultures. This process is highly speculative and conclusions about the similarities of meanings in a measure must be considered tentative (Hulin et al., 1983).

Four types of translations can be performed: pragmatic translations, aesthetic-poetic translations, ethnographic translations, and linguistic translations. The purpose of pragmatic translations is to communicate accurately in the target language the content from the source language. The primary concern is the information conveyed. An example of this type of translation is the use of translated instructions for assembling a computer. The purpose of aesthetic-poetic translations is to evoke moods, feelings, and affect in the target language identical to those evoked by the original material. In ethnographic translation, the purpose is to maintain meaning and cultural content. In this case, translators must be very familiar with both languages and cultures. Linguistic translations strive to present grammatical forms with equivalent meanings. Translating a scale is generally done in the ethnographic mode (Hulin et al., 1983).

One strategy to translate scales is to translate from the original language to the target language and then to back-translate from the target language to the original language using translators not involved in the original translation. Discrepancies are identified and the procedure repeated until troublesome problems are resolved. Following this procedure, the two versions are administered to bilingual subjects and scored using standard procedures. The resulting sets of scores are examined to determine the extent to which the two versions yield similar information from the subjects. This procedure assumes that the subjects are equally skilled in both languages. One problem with this strategy is that bilingual subjects may interpret meanings of words differently from monolingual subjects. This is a serious concern since the target subjects for most cross-cultural research are monolingual (Hulin et al., 1983).

Hulin and colleagues (1983) suggest the use of item response theory procedures to address some of the problems of translation. These proce-

dures can provide direct evidence about the meanings of items in the two languages. Item characteristic curves (ICCs) for an item in the two languages can be compared, and also scale scores in the two languages. This procedure eliminates the need for bilingual samples. It also eliminates the need for the two populations to be equivalent in terms of the distributions of their scores on the trait being measured.

SUMMARY

Common measurement approaches that are used in nursing research include physiologic measures, observations, interviews, questionnaires, and scales. Specialized measurements include the Q-sort, visual analogue scale, Delphi technique, projective techniques, and diaries. Much of nursing practice is oriented toward the physiologic dimensions of health. Therefore, many of our questions require the measurement of these dimensions. Measurements of physiologic variables can be either direct or indirect. Many physiologic measures require the use of specialized equipment. Some require laboratory analysis. In publishing the results of a physiologic study, the measurement technique must be described in great detail.

Measurement of observations requires that one first decide what is to be observed and then determine how to ensure that every variable is observed in a similar manner in each instance. Careful attention is given to training data collectors. Observational measurement may be unstructured or structured. In structured observational studies, category systems must be developed. Checklists or rating scales are developed from the category systems and are used to guide data collection.

Interviews involve verbal communication between the researcher and the subject, during which information is provided to the researcher. Approaches range from a totally un-

structured interview in which the content is completely controlled by the subject to interviews in which the content is similar to a questionnaire, with the possible responses to questions carefully designed by the researcher. Interview questions are grouped by topic, with fairly safe topics being addressed first and sensitive topics reserved until late in the interview process. Interviewers need to be trained in the skills of interviewing, and the interview protocol needs to be pretested.

A questionnaire is a printed self-report form designed to elicit information through written responses of the subject. The information obtained through questionnaires is similar to that obtained by interview, but the questions tend to have less depth. The subject is unable to elaborate on responses or ask for clarification of questions, and the data collector cannot use probe strategies. Like interviews, questionnaires can have varying degrees of structure. An item on a questionnaire has two parts: a lead-in question and a response set. Each lead-in question needs to be carefully designed and clearly expressed to avoid influencing the response of the respondent.

Scales, a form of self-report, are a more precise means of measuring phenomena than are questionnaires. The majority of scales have been developed to measure psychosocial variables. However, self-reports can be obtained on physiologic variables, such as pain, nausea,

continued

continued

or functional capacity, using scaling techniques. Rating scales are the crudest form of measure using scaling techniques. A rating scale lists an ordered series of categories of a variable, assumed to be based on an underlying continuum. A numerical value is assigned to each category. The Likert scale is designed to determine the opinion or attitude of a subject and contains a number of declarative statements with a scale after each statement. A semantic differential scale consists of two opposite adjectives with a seven-point scale between them. The subject is to select one point on the scale that best describes his or her view of the concept being examined. The scale is designed to measure connotative meaning of the concept to the subject.

One of the problems of concern in scaling procedures is the difficulty in obtaining fine discrimination of values. A recent effort to resolve this problem is the visual analogue scale, sometimes referred to as magnitude scaling. It is particularly useful in scaling stimuli. The scale is a line 100 mm in length with right angle stops at each end. Bipolar anchors are placed beyond each end of the line. These end anchors should include the entire range of sensations possible in the phenomenon being measured.

The Delphi technique is used to measure the judgments of a group of experts, assess priorities, or make forecasts. It provides a means to obtain the opinion of a wide variety of experts across the country without the necessity of meeting. Projective techniques are based on the assumption that the responses of individuals to unstructured or ambiguous situations reflect the attitudes, desires, personality characteristics, and motives of the individuals.

The technique is most frequently used in psychology and includes such techniques as the Rorschach Inkblot Test, Machover's Draw-A-Person Test, word association, sentence completion, role-playing, and play techniques.

A recent approach to obtaining information that must be collected over time is to ask the subjects to keep a record or diary of events. The data in this diary can then be collected and analyzed by researchers. A diary, which allows recording shortly after an event, is more accurate than obtaining the information through recall at an interview, the reporting level of incidents is higher, and one tends to capture the participant's perception of situations.

The choice of tools for use in a particular study is a critical decision that will have a major impact on the significance of the study. The researcher first needs to conduct an extensive search for existing tools. When tools are found, they need to be carefully evaluated. Tools that are selected for a study need to be described in great detail in the proposal or publication. Scale construction is a complex procedure that should not be undertaken lightly. Theories on which scale construction is most frequently based include classical test theory, item response theory, multidimensional scaling, and unfolding theory. Most existing instruments used in nursing research have been developed using classical test theory.

Translating a scale to another language is a complex process. The goal of translating is to allow comparisons of concepts among respondents of different cultures. Item response theory can be useful in evaluating the effectiveness of translated scales.

References

Amsterdam, E. A., Hughes, J. L., DeMaria, A. M., Zellis, R., & Mason, D. T. (1974). Indirect assessment of myocardial oxygen consumption in the evaluation of mechanisms and therapy of angina pectoris. *American Journal of Cardiology, 33*(6), 737–743.

Baker, C. M. (1985). Maximizing mailed questionnaire responses. *Image: Journal of Nursing Scholarship, 17*(4), 118–121.

Bedarf, E. W. (1986). *Using structured interviewing techniques.* Washington, DC: Program Evaluation and Methodology Division, United States General Accounting Office.

Berdie, D. R., Anderson, J. F., & Niebuhr, M. A. (1986). *Questionnaires: Design and use.* Metuchen, NJ: Scarecrow Press.

Briggs, C. L. (1986). *Learning how to ask: A sociolinguistic appraisal of the role of the interview in social science research.* Cambridge, UK: Cambridge University Press.

Burman, M. E. (1995). Health diaries in nursing research and practice. *Image: Journal of Nursing Scholarship, 27*(2), 147–152.

Burns, N. (1974). *Nurse-patient communication with the advanced cancer patient.* Unpublished master's thesis, Texas Woman's University, Denton, TX.

Burns, N. (1981). *Evaluation of a supportive-expressive group for families of cancer patients.* Unpublished doctoral dissertation, Texas Woman's University, Denton, TX.

Burns, N. (1983). Development of the Burns cancer beliefs scale. *Proceedings of the American Cancer Society Third West Coast Cancer Nursing Research Conference,* 308–329.

Burns, N. (1986). *Research in progress.* American Cancer Society, Texas Division.

Burns, N., & Carney, K. (1985). The caring aspect of hospice: A study. In L. F. Paradis (Ed.), *Hospice handbook: A guide for managers and planners* (pp. 249–279). Rockville, MD: Aspen.

Butz, A. M., & Alexander, C. (1991). Use of health diaries with children. *Nursing Research, 40*(1), 59–61.

Converse, J. M., & Presser, S. (1986). *Survey questions: Handcrafting the standardized questionnaire.* Newbury Park, CA: Sage.

Coombs, C. H. (1950). Psychological scaling without a unit of measurement. *Psychological Review, 57*(3), 145–158.

Couper, M. R. (1984). The Delphi technique: Characteristics and sequence model. *Advances in Nursing Science, 7*(1), 72–77.

Cowan, M. J., Heinrich, J., Lucas, M., Sigmon, H., & Hinshaw, A. S. (1993). Integration of biological and nursing sciences: A 10-year plan to enhance research and training. *Research in Nursing & Health, 16*(1), 3–9.

Crocker, L., & Algina, J. (1986). *Introduction to classical modern test theory.* New York: Holt, Rinehart and Winston.

Davison, M. L. (1983). *Multidimensional scaling.* New York: Wiley.

DeKeyser, F. G., & Pugh, L. C. (1991). Approaches to physiologic measurement. In C. F. Waltz, O. L. Strickland, & E. R. Lenz (Eds.), *Measurement in nursing research* (2nd ed., pp. 387–412). Philadelphia: Davis.

Dennis, K. E. (1986). Q methodology: Relevance and application to nursing research. *Advances in Nursing Science, 8*(3), 6–17.

Dillman, D. (1978). *Mail and telephone surveys: The total design method.* New York: Wiley.

Dillon, J. T. (1990). *The practice of questioning.* New York: Routledge.

Dunbar, S. B., & Farr, L. (1996). Temporal patterns of heart rate and blood pressure in elders. *Nursing Research, 45*(1), 43–49.

Dzurec, L. C., & Coleman, P. A. (1995). A Hermeneutic analysis of the process of conducting interviews. *Image: Journal of Nursing Scholarship, 27*(3), 245.

Emde, R. M., Gauensbauer, T. J., & Harmon, R. J. (1976). The early postnatal period: Unexplained fussiness. Emotional expression in infancy: A bio-behavioral study. *Psychological Issues, 10*(37), 80–85.

Fahs, P. S. S., & Kinney, M. R. (1991). The abdomen, thigh, and arm as sites for subcutaneous sodium heparin injections. *Nursing Research, 40*(4), 204–207.

Flaskerud, J. H. (1988). Is the Likert scale format culturally biased? *Nursing Research, 37*(3), 185–186.

Fowler, F. J. (1990). *Standardized survey interviewing: Minimizing interviewer-related error.* Newbury Park, CA: Sage.

Fox, J. A., & Tracy, P. E. (1986). *Randomized response: A method for sensitive surveys.* Beverly Hills: Sage.

Gardner, R. M. (1981). Direct blood pressure measurement—dynamic response requirements. *Anesthesiology, 54*(3), 227–236.

Gibbs, N. C., & Gardner, R. M. (1988). Dynamics of invasive monitoring systems: Clinical and laboratory evaluation. *Heart & Lung, 17*(1), 43–51.

Gift, A. G. (1989). Visual analogue scales: Measurement of subjective phenomena. *Nursing Research, 38*(5), 286–288.

Gobel, F. L., Nordstrom, L. A., Nelson, R. R., Jorgenson, C. R., & Wang, Y. (1978). The rate-pressure product as an index of myocardial oxygen consumption during exercise in patients with angina pectoris. *Circulation, 57*(3), 549–556.

Goodman, C. M. (1987). The Delphi technique: A critique. *Journal of Advanced Nursing, 12*(6), 729–734.

Gorden, R. L. (1987). *Interviewing: Strategy, techniques, and tactics.* Chicago: Dorsey Press.

Gordon, S. E., & Stokes, S. A. (1989). Improving response rate to mailed questionnaires. *Nursing Research, 38*(6), 375–376.

Grossman, M. (1995). Received support and psychological adjustment in critically-injured patients and their family. *Journal of Neuroscience Nursing, 27*(1), 11–23.

Heitkemper, M., Jarrett, M., Bond, E. F., & Turner, P. (1991). GI symptoms, function, and psychophysiological arousal in dysmenorrheic women. *Nursing Research, 40*(1), 20–26.

Henneman, E. A., & Henneman, P. L. (1989). Intricacies of blood pressure measurement: Reexamining the ritual. *Heart & Lung, 18*(31), 263–271.

Hodson, K. E. (1986). Research in nursing education and practice: The ecological methods perspective. *Western Journal of Nursing Research, 8*(1), 33–48.

Holaday, B., & Turner-Henson, A. (1989). Response effects in surveys with school-age children. *Nursing Research, 38*(4), 248–250.

Hulin, C. L., Drasgow, F., & Parsons, C. K. (1983). *Item response theory: Application to psychological measurement*. Homewood, IL: Dow Jones-Irwin.

Jacobsen, B. S., Munro, B. H., & Brooten, D. A. (1996). Comparison of original and revised scoring systems for the Multiple Affect Adjective Check List. *Nursing Research, 45*(1), 57–60.

Johnson, B. H. (1990). Children's drawings as a projective technique. *Pediatric Nursing, 16*(1), 11–17.

Kahn, R., & Cannell, C. F. (1957). *The dynamics of interviewing*. New York: Wiley.

Keefe, M. R., Kotzer, A. M., Froeser-Fretz, A., & Curtin, M. (1996). A longitudinal comparison of irritable and nonirritable infants. *Nursing Research, 45*(1), 4–9.

Keefe, M. R., Kotzer, A. M., Reuss, J. L., & Sander, L. W. (1989). Development of a system for monitoring infant state behavior. *Nursing Research, 38*(6), 344–347.

Keefe, M. R., Pepper, G., & Stoner, M. (1988). Toward research-based nursing practice: The Denver Collaborative Research Network. *Applied Nursing Research, 1*(3), 109–115.

Knafl, K. A., Pettengill, M. M., Bevis, M. E., & Kirchhoff, K. T. (1988). Blending qualitative and quantitative approaches to instrument development and data collection. *Journal of Professional Nursing, 4*(1), 30–37.

Kruskal, J. B., & Wish, M. (1990). *Multidimensional scaling*. Newbury Park, CA: Sage.

Lee, K. A., & Kieckhefer, G. M. (1989). Measuring human responses using visual analogue scales. *Western Journal of Nursing Research, 11*(1), 128–132.

Lindeman, C. A. (1975). Delphi survey of priorities in clinical nursing research. *Nursing Research, 24*(6), 434–441.

Lodge, M. (1981). *Magnitude scaling: Quantitative measurement of opinions*. Beverly Hills, CA: Sage.

Lofland, H. (1971). *Analyzing social settings: A guide to qualitative observation and analysis*. Belmont, CA: Wadsworth.

Lynn, M. R. (1989). Instrument reliability: How much needs to be published? *Heart & Lung, 18*(4), 421–423.

McCracken, G. D. (1988). *The long interview*. Newbury Park, CA: Sage.

McKeown, B., & Thomas, D. (1988). *Q methodology*. Newbury Park, CA: Sage.

McLaughlin, P. (1990). *How to interview: The art of asking questions* (2nd ed.). North Vancouver, BC: International Self-Counsel Press.

Mishler, E. G. (1986). *Research interviewing: Context and narrative*. Cambridge, MA: Harvard University Press.

Norbeck, J. S. (1985). What constitutes a publishable report of instrument development? *Nursing Research, 34*(6), 380–381.

Norman, E., Gadaleta, D., & Griffin, C. C. (1991). An evaluation of three blood pressure methods in a stabilized acute trauma population. *Nursing Research, 40*(2), 86–89.

Nunnally, J. C. (1978). *Psychometric theory* (2nd ed.). New York: McGraw-Hill.

Oleske, D. M., Heinze, S., & Otte, D. M. (1990). The diary as a means of understanding the quality of life of persons with cancer receiving home nursing care. *Cancer Nursing, 13*(3), 158–166.

Osgood, C. E., Suci, G. J., & Tannenbaum, P. H. (1957). *The measurement of meaning*. Urbana, IL: University of Illinois Press.

Park, M. K., & Menard, S. M. (1987). Accuracy of blood pressure measurement by the Dinamap monitor in infants and children. *Pediatrics, 79*(6), 907–914.

Pope, D. S. (1995). Music, noise, and the human voice in the nurse-patient environment. *Image: Journal of Nursing Scholarship, 27*(4), 291–296.

Pugh, L. C., & DeKeyser, F. G. (1995). Use of physiologic variables in nursing research. *Image: Journal of Nursing Scholarship, 27*(4), 273–276.

Ramsey, M. (1979). Noninvasive automatic determination of mean arterial pressure. *Medical and Biological Engineering and Computing, 17*(1), 11–18.

Rhodes, V. A., McDaniel, R. W., Hanson, B., Markway, E., & Johnson, M. (1994). Sensory perception of patients on selected antineoplastic chemotherapy protocols. *Cancer Nursing, 17*(1), 45–51.

Saris, W. E. (1991). *Computer-assisted interviewing*. Newbury Park, CA: Sage.

Schuman, H. (1981). *Questions and answers in attitude surveys: Experiments on question form, wording, and context*. New York: Academic Press.

Sennott-Miller, L., Murdaugh, C., & Hinshaw, A. S. (1988). Magnitude estimation: Issues and practical applications. *Western Journal of Nursing Research, 10*(4), 414–424.

Shelley, S. I. (1984). *Research methods in nursing and health*. Boston: Little, Brown.

Simpson, S. H. (1989). Use of Q-sort methodology in cross-cultural nutrition and health research. *Nursing Research, 38*(5), 289–290.

Spector, P. E. (1992). *Summated rating scale construction: An introduction*. Newbury Park, CA: Sage.

Sudman, S., & Bradburn, N. (1982). *Asking questions: A practical guide to questionnaire design*. San Francisco: Jossey-Bass.

Tetting, D. W. (1988). Q-sort update. *Western Journal of Nursing Research, 10*(6), 757–765.

Thomas, K. A. (1995). Biorhythms in infants and role of the care environment. *Journal of Perinatal and Neonatal Nursing, 9*(2), 61–75.

Waltz, C. F., Strickland, O. L., & Lenz, E. R. (1991). *Measurement in nursing research*. Philadelphia: Davis.

Wewers, M. E., & Lowe, N. K. (1990). A critical review of visual analogue scales in the measurement of clinical phenomena. *Research in Nursing & Health, 13*(4), 227–236.

Wyers, M. E., Grove, S. K., & Pastorino, C. (1985). Clinical nurse specialist: In search of the right role. *Nursing & Health Care, 6*(4), 202–207.

Ziemer, M. M., Cooper, D. M., & Pigeon, J. G. (1995). Evaluation of a dressing to reduce nipple pain and improve nipple skin condition in breast-feeding women. *Nursing Research, 44*(6), 347–351.

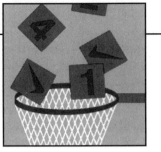

15

Collecting and Managing Data

The initiation of data collection is one of the most exciting parts of research. After all the planning, writing, and negotiating, you are getting to the real part of research—the doing part. There is a sense of euphoria and excitement—an eagerness to get on with it. But before you jump into data collection, spend some time carefully planning this adventure. It may save you some headaches later. Consider problems you might encounter during data collection and develop strategies for addressing those problems. You need to make careful plans for managing data as you collect it. This chapter is divided into three sections to assist you in planning data collection, collecting data, and managing data for quantitative studies. Data collection strategies for qualitative studies is described in Chapter 20.

PLANNING DATA COLLECTION

A *data collection plan* details how the study will be implemented. The data collection plan is specific to the study being conducted and requires consideration of some of the more prosaic elements of research. Elements that need to be planned include the procedures to be used to collect data, the time and costs of data collection, developing data collection forms that facilitate data entry, and developing a codebook.

PLANNING DATA COLLECTION PROCEDURES

To plan the process of data collection, the researcher needs to determine step by step how and in what sequence data will be collected from a single subject. The timing of this process also needs to be determined. For example, how much time will be required to identify potential subjects, explain the study, and obtain consent? How much time is needed for such activities as completing questionnaires or obtaining physiologic measures? Next, one needs to envision the overall activities that will be occurring during data collection. At what point are subjects assigned to groups? Will data be collected from more than one subject at a time, or is it necessary to focus attention on one subject at a time? How many subjects per day can be accessed for data given the study design and the setting? It might be helpful to conduct a trial run by collecting data from two or three subjects to get a better feel for the process. Developing a data collection tree to illustrate the process of collecting data can be helpful. An example of such a tree is shown in Figure 15–1 (on p. 384).

DECISION POINTS

Decision points that occur during data collection need to be identified and all options considered. Decisions might include such things as whether potential subjects meet the sampling criteria, whether a subject understands the information needed to give informed consent, what group the subject will be assigned to, whether the subject comprehends instructions related to providing data, and whether the subject has provided all of the data needed. Each point at which a decision is made should be indicated in your data collection tree.

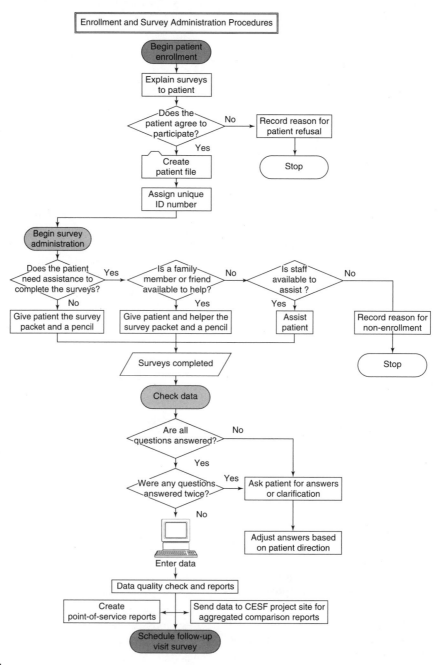

Figure 15-1

Data collection tree. (From Alles, P. [1995]. CESF medical outcomes research project: Implementing outcomes research in a clinical setting. *Wisconsin Medical Journal, 94*[1], 27–31, with permission.)

CONSISTENCY

Consistency in data collection across subjects is critical. If more than one data collector is used, consistency among data collectors (interrater reliability) is also necessary. Identify situations in your study that might interfere with consistency and develop a plan that will maximize consistency. The specific days and hours of data collection may influence the consistency of the data collected and thus need to be carefully considered. For example, the energy level and state of mind of subjects from whom data are gathered in the morning may differ from that of subjects from whom data are gathered in the evening. Visitors are more likely to be present at certain times of day and may interfere with data collection or influence subject responses. Patient care routines vary with time of day. In some studies the care recently received or the care currently being provided may alter the data you gather. Subjects who are approached to participate in the study on Saturday may differ from subjects approached on weekday mornings. Subjects seeking care on Saturday may have a full-time job, whereas those seeking care on weekday mornings may be either unemployed or too ill to work.

Decisions regarding who collects the data also need to be made. Will the data all be collected by the researcher, or will data collectors be employed for this purpose? Can data collectors be nurses working in the area? Researchers have experienced difficulties in studies in which they expected nurses providing patient care to also be data collectors. Patient care will take priority over data collection, leading to missing data or missed subjects.

If data collectors are used, they need to be informed of the research project, introduced to the instruments to be used, and provided equivalent training in the data collection process. In addition to training, written guidelines are necessary for the data collectors that indicate which instruments to use, the order to introduce the instruments, how to administer the instruments, and a time frame for the data collection process (Gift, Creasia, & Parker, 1991).

Following training, data collectors must be evaluated to determine their consistency in the data collection process. Washington and Moss (1988) suggest that a minimum of 10 subjects need to be rated with the complete instrument before interrater reliability can be adequately assessed. The data collectors' interrater reliability is usually assessed intermittently throughout data collection to assure consistency. Data collectors also need to be encouraged to identify and record any problems or variations in the environment that effect the data collection process.

TIME FACTORS

The time required for data collection is often inadequately estimated when planning a study. Data collection often requires two to three times longer than anticipated. It is helpful to write out a time plan for the data collection period. A pilot study can be conducted to refine the data collection process and to determine the time required to collect data from a subject.

Events during the data collection period are sometimes not under the control of the researcher. Such events as a sudden heavy workload of staff may make data collection temporarily difficult or impossible, or the number of potential subjects might be reduced for a period of time. In some situations, approval for data collection stipulates that the physician's approval must be obtained for each subject prior to collecting data on that subject. Activities required to meet this stipulation, such as contacting physicians, explaining the study, and obtaining approval require extensive time. In some cases, many potential subjects are lost before the approval can be obtained, thus extending the time required to obtain the necessary number of subjects.

COST FACTORS

Cost factors must also be examined in planning a study. Measurement tools, such as Holter monitors, spirometers, infrared thermometers, pulse oximeters, or glucometers used in physiological studies may cost money to rent or purchase. If questionnaires or scales must be ordered, there may be a fee for the scale and a fee for analyzing the data. Data collection forms must be typed and duplicated. In some cases, there are printing costs related to materials that are to be distributed during data collection, such as teaching materials, questionnaires, or scales. In some studies, there are postage costs. There may be costs involved in coding the data for entry into the computer and for conducting data analyses. Consultation with a statistician early in the development of a research project and during data analysis must also be budgeted. Sometimes it is necessary to hire a typist for the final report.

In addition to these direct costs, there are also indirect costs. The researcher's time is a cost, and there are costs for traveling to and from the study site and for meals eaten out while working on the study. The expense of presenting the research project at conferences also needs to be estimated and included in a budget. To prevent unexpected costs from delaying the study, costs need to be examined in an organized manner during the planning phase of the study. A budget is best developed early in the planning process and revised as plans are modified (see Chapter 26 for a sample budget). Seeking funding for at least part of the study costs can facilitate the conduct of a study. See Conducting Research on a Shoestring in Chapter 26.

Neophyte researchers have difficulty making reasonable estimates of time and costs related to a study. We advise validating the time and cost estimates with an experienced researcher. If the cost and time factors are prohibitive, the study can be simplified so fewer variables are measured, fewer instruments are used, the design is made less complex, and fewer agencies are used for data collection. These are serious changes in a study and their impact must be thoroughly examined before the revisions are made. If time or cost estimates go beyond expectations, the time schedules and budget can be revised with a new projection for completing the study.

DEVELOPING DATA COLLECTION FORMS

Before data collection begins, the researcher may need to develop or modify forms on which to record data. These forms can be used to record demographic data, information from the patient record, observations, or values from physiologic measures. The demographic variables commonly collected in nursing studies include age, gender, race, education, income or socioeconomic status, employment status, diagnosis, and marital status. Other data that may be either extraneous or confounding need to be collected, and might include such variables as the subject's physician, stage of illness, length of illness or hospitalization, complications, date of data collection, time of day and day of week of data collection, and any untoward events that occur during the data collection period. In some cases, the length of time required of individual subjects for data collection may be a confounding variable and needs to be recorded. If it is necessary to contact the subject at a later time, his or her address and telephone number need to be obtained, but only with the subject's awareness and permission. Names and phone numbers of family members may also be useful if the subjects are likely to move or be difficult to contact. The importance of each piece of data and the amount of subject's time required to collect it needs to be considered. If the data can be obtained from patient records or any other written sources, the subject should not be asked to provide this information.

Data collection forms need to be designed to allow ease in recording during data collection and for easy entry into the computer. A decision must be made about whether data are collected in raw form or coded at the time of collection. *Coding* is the process of transforming data into numerical symbols that can be easily entered into the computer. For example, the measurement of variables such as gender, ethnicity, and diagnoses produces data that can be categorized and given numerical labels. Gender has two categories, female and male, and the female category could be identified by a 1, and the male category by a 2. The variable of ethnicity might include four categories: Caucasian, African American, Hispanic, and other. The Caucasian category could be represented by the numerical label of 1, African American by a 2, Hispanic by a 3, and other by a 4.

The coding categories developed for a study must be mutually exclusive but exhaustive, which means that the value for a specific variable fits into only one category but each observation must fit into a category. For example, the salary ranges would not be mutually exclusive if they were categorized as (1) $30,000 to 35,000; (2) $35,000 to 40,000; (3) $40,000 to 45,000; (4) $45,000 to 50,000; and (5) $50,000 and over. These categories overlap, so a subject with a $45,000 income could mark category 3, 4, or both. For many items, a code for "other" should be included for unexpected classifications of variables such as marital status or ethnicity.

There are a number of response styles that can be selected for use on the data collection form. The person completing the form (subject or data collector) might be asked to check a blank space before or after the terms male or female, to circle the word male or female, or to write a 1 or a 2 in a blank space before or after the term selected. If codes are used, the codes should be indicated on the collection forms for easy access by the individual completing the form.

The placement of data on data collection forms is important for ease in completing the form and locating responses for computer entry. Placement of blanks on the left side of the page seems to be most efficient for data entry, but may be problematic when subjects are completing the forms. The least effective is the placement of data irregularly on the form. In this case, the risk of data being missed during data entry is high. Subjects' names should not be on the data collection forms; only the subject's identification number should appear. A master list of subjects and associated coding numbers can be kept separately by the researcher.

An example data collection form is provided in Figure 15–2 (on pp. 388–389). This data collection form includes four items that could be problematic in terms of coding and/or data analyses. The blank used to enter the Surgical Procedure Performed will lead to problems devising effective ways to enter the data into a computerized data set. Because multiple surgical procedures could have been performed, developing codes for the various surgical procedures would be difficult and time-consuming. In addition, the same surgical procedure could be recorded using different wording. It may be necessary to tally the surgical procedures by hand. Unless this degree of specification of procedures is important to the study, an alternative would be to develop larger categories of procedures prior to data collection, placing the categories on the data collection form. A category of other might be useful for less commonly performed procedures. This method would require the data collector to make a judgment as to which category was appropriate for a particular surgical procedure. Another option would be to write in the category code number for a particular surgical procedure after the data collection form is completed but before data entry. Similar problems occur with the items Narcotics Ordered After Surgery and Narcotic Administration. Unless these data are to be used in statistical analyses, it might be advisable to manually categorize this information for descriptive purposes. If these items are needed for planned statistical procedures, careful thought will be required to develop appropriate codes. In this study, the researcher might be interested in determining differences in the amounts of narcotics administered in a given period of time in relation to weight and height. Recording the treatment groups on the data collection form may be problematic because the information could influence the data recorded by the data collector.

DEVELOPING A CODEBOOK FOR DATA DEFINITIONS

A *codebook* identifies and defines each variable in your study and includes an abbreviated variable name (limited to 6–8 characters), a descriptive variable label, and the range of possible numerical values of every variable entered in a computer file.

DATA COLLECTION FORM

Demographics

____ Subject Identification Number

____ Age

____ Gender

   1. Male

   2. Female

____ Weight (in pounds)

____ Height (in inches)

_____ Surgical Procedure Performed

__/__/__ Surgery Date (Month/Day/Year)

__/__/__ Surgery Time (Hour/Minute/AM or PM)

Narcotics Ordered After Surgery _____

                                _____

Narcotic Administration

	Date	Time	Narcotic	Dose
1.				
2.				
3.				
4.				
5.				

Instruction on Use of Pain Scale

__/__/__ Date (Month/Day/Year)

__/__/__ Time (Hour/Minute/AM or PM)

Comments:

____ Treatment Group

   1. TENS

   2. Placebo–TENS

   3. No-treatment Control

Treatment Implemented

__/__/__ Date (Month/Day/Year)

__/__/__ Time (Hour/Minute/AM or PM)

Comments:

Figure 15-2

Example of a data collection form.

Dressing Change

__/__/__ Date (Month/Day/Year)

__/__/__ Time (Hour/Minute/AM or PM)

____ Hours since surgery

Comments:

Measurement of Pain

____ Score on Visual Analogue Pain Scale

__/__/__ Date Pain Measured (Month/Day/Year)

__/__/__ Time Pain Measured (Hour/Minute/AM or PM)

Comments:

____ Data Collector Code

Comments:

Figure 15-2 *Continued*

Some codebooks also identify the source of each datum, thus linking your codebook with your data collection forms and scales. The codebook keeps you in control and provides a safety net for you in accessing the data later. Some computer programs, such as SPSS for Windows, will allow you to print out your data definitions after setting up a database. Figure 15–3 (on pp. 390–393) is an example of data definitions from SPSS for Windows. Another example of coding is presented in Figure 15–4 (on p. 393).

Developing a logical method of abbreviating variable names can be challenging. For example, you might use a Quality of Life (QOL) questionnaire in your study. It will be necessary for you to develop an abbreviated variable name for each item in the questionnaire. For example, the fourth item on a quality of life (QOL) questionnaire might be given the abbreviated variable name QOL4. A question asking the last time you visited your mother might be abbreviated Lstvisit. Although abbreviated variable names usually seem quite logical at the time the name is created, it is easy to confuse or forget these names unless they are documented clearly.

It is advisable to develop your codebook before initiating data collection. This provides a means for you to identify places in your forms that might prove to be a problem during data entry because of lack of clarity. Also, you may find that a single question contains, not one, but five variables. For example, an item might ask if the subject received support from her or his mother, father, sister, brother, or other relatives and be asked to circle those who provided support. You might think that you could code mother as 1, father as 2, sister as 3, brother as 4, and other as 5. However, because the individual can circle more than one, each relative must be coded separately. Thus, mother is one variable and would be coded 1 if circled and 0 if not circled. The father would be coded similarly as a second variable, etc. Identifying these items before data collection may allow you to restructure the item on the questionnaire or data collection form to facilitate easier entry into the computer.

20 Feb 96 SPSS for MS WINDOWS Release 6.1 Page 1

— SYSFILE INFO —

File a:\mxco2.sav
Created: 25 Jan 96 15:18:39–241 variables and 151 cases

File Type: SPSS Data File

N of Cases: 151
Total # of Defined Variable Elements: 241
Data Are Not Weighted
Data Are Compressed
File Contains Case Data

Variable Information:

Name **Position**

STUDY-ID STUDY ID NUMBER 1
Format: F3

RACE RACE 2
Format: F1
Value Label
1 white
2 black
3 Hispanic
4 Asian
5 other

EDUC EDUCATION 3
Format: F1
Value Label
1 CURRENTLY ENROLLED IN HIGH SCHOOL
2 CURRENTLY ENROLLED IN COLLEGE
3 PREVIOUS COLLEGE WORK
4 COLLEGE GRADUATE
5 CURRENTLY ENROLLED GRAD STUDENT

GENDER GENDER 4
Format: F1
Value Label
1 MALE
2 FEMALE

AGE AGE 5
Format: F1
Value Label
1 16–18 YEARS
2 19–21 YEARS
3 22–25 YEARS
4 31–40 YEARS
5 41–50 YEARS
6 51–60 YEARS
7 OVER 60 YEARS

Figure 15–3
Example of data definitions from SPSS for Windows.

Name   **Position**

INCOME   ANNUAL INCOME   6
  FORMAT: F1
  Value   Label
   1   <$10,000
   2   $10,000–$19,999
   3   $20,000–$29,999
   4   $30,000–$39,999
   5   $40,000–$49,999
   6   >$50,000

AHEALTH   OVERALL HEALTH STATUS   55
  Format: F1
  Value   Label
   1   EXCELLENT
   2   GOOD
   3   FAIR
   4   POOR

AEXP1   EXPECT PRE 1 EXPECT MEXICANS TO BE FRIENDLY   56
FORMAT: F1
  Value   Label
   0   NO
   1   YES

AEXP2   EXPECT PRE 2 EXPECT TO USE PUBLIC TRANSPORTATION   57
Format: F1
  Value   Label
   0   NO
   1   YES

AEXP3   EXPECT PRE 3 EXPECT TO MAKE FRIENDS WITH MEXICANS   58
  Format: F1
  Value   Label
   1   YES
   2   NO

AEXP4   EXPECT PRE 4 EXPECT TO UNDERSTAND MEXICAN HUMOR   59
  Format: F1
  Value   Label
   0   NO
   1   YES

AEXP5   EXPECT PRE 5 EXPECT MEXICANS TO BE POLITE/HELPFUL   60
  Format: F1
  Value   Label
   0   NO
   1   YES

Figure 15–3 *Continued*

Name	Position

SOCMID1   SOC SIT MID 1 FRIENDS   78
Format: F1
Value   Label
    1   NEVER EXPERIENCED
    2   NO DIFFICULTY
    3   SLIGHT DIFFICULTY
    4   MODERATE DIFFICULTY
    5   GREAT DIFFICULTY
    6   EXTREME DIFFICULTY

SOCMID2   SOC SIT MID 2 SHOPPING   79
Format: F1
Value   Label
    1   NEVER EXPERIENCED
    2   NO DIFFICULTY
    3   SLIGHT DIFFICULTY
    4   MODERATE DIFFICULTY
    5   GREAT DIFFICULTY
    6   EXTREME DIFFICULTY

SOCMID3   SOC SIT MID 3 PUB TRANSPORTATION   80
Format: F1
Value   Label
    1   NEVER EXPERIENCED
    2   NO DIFFICULTY
    3   SLIGHT DIFFICULTY
    4   MODERATE DIFFICULTY
    5   GREAT DIFFICULTY
    6   EXTREME DIFFICULTY

SOCMID5   SOC SIT MID 5 MAKING MEXICAN FRIENDS   82
Format: F1
Value   Label
    1   NEVER EXPERIENCED
    2   NO DIFFICULTY
    3   SLIGHT DIFFICULTY
    4   MODERATE DIFFICULTY
    5   GREAT DIFFICULTY
    6   EXTREME DIFFICULTY

SOCMID12   SOC SIT MID 12 BEING WITH OLDER MEXICAN PEOPLE   89
Format: F1
Value   Label
    1   NEVER EXPERIENCED
    2   NO DIFFICULTY
    3   SLIGHT DIFFICULTY
    4   MODERATE DIFFICULTY
    5   GREAT DIFFICULTY
    6   EXTREME DIFFICULTY

Figure 15–3 *Continued*

Name   **Position**

SOCMID13   SOC SIT MID 13 MEETING STRANGERS/NEW PEOPLE   90
   Format: F1
   Value   Label
     1   NEVER EXPERIENCED
     2   NO DIFFICULTY
     3   SLIGHT DIFFICULTY
     4   MODERATE DIFFICULTY
     5   GREAT DIFFICULTY
     6   EXTREME DIFFICULTY

Figure 15–3 *Continued*

The codebook with its data definitions should be given to the individual(s) who will enter your data into the computer *before initiating data collection* as well as the following information:

1. Copies of all scales, questionnaires, and data collection forms to be used in the study.
2. Information on the location of every variable on scales, questionnaires, or data collection forms.
3. Information on the statistical package to be used for analysis of the data.
4. The database in which the data will be entered.
5. Information related to receiving the data, for example, whether you will deliver the data in batches or wait until all the data have been gathered before delivering it.
6. Estimated number of subjects.
7. Planned date for delivering the data.

Using this information, the assistant can develop the database in preparation for receiving the data for entry. Preparation of the database will require an average of 16 hours of concentrated work. Approximate dates for completion of the data entry work and/or analyses need to be negotiated before beginning data collection. If you have a deadline for completion or a presentation of results at a conference, this information should be shared with those performing data entry/analysis.

COLLECTING DATA

Data collection is the process of selecting subjects and gathering data from these subjects. The actual steps of collecting the data are specific to each

Variable Name	Variable Label	Source	Value Labels	Valid Range	Missing Data	Comments
A1 to A5	Family Apgar	Q2Family Apgar	1 = never 2 = hardly ever 3 = some of the time 4 = almost alwys 5 = always	1 – 5	9	Code as is (CAI)
MF3	Mother's feeling, Day 3	Tuesday diary, mother	1 = poor 6 = good	1 – 6	9	Code 1 to 6 left to right

Figure 15–4

Example of coding. (From Lobo, M. L. [1993]. Code books—A critical link in the research process. *Western Journal of Nursing Research, 15*[3], 380. Reprinted by permission of Sage Publications, © 1993.)

study and are dependent on the research design and measurement methods. Data may be collected on subjects by observing, testing, measuring, questioning, and/or recording. The researcher is actively involved in this process either by collecting data or supervising data collectors. Effective people management and problem-solving skills are used constantly as data collection tasks are implemented, kinks in the research plan are resolved, and support systems are utilized.

DATA COLLECTION TASKS

In both quantitative and qualitative research, the investigator performs four tasks during the process of data collection. These tasks are interrelated and occur concurrently rather than in sequence. The tasks include selecting subjects, collecting data in a consistent way, maintaining research controls as indicated in the study design, and solving problems that threaten to disrupt the study. Selecting subjects is discussed in Chapter 12. Data collection tasks for qualitative studies are discussed in more detail in Chapter 20.

Collecting Data

Collecting data may involve administering written scales, asking subjects to complete data collection forms, or recording data from observations or from the patient record. Sometimes subjects are asked to enter data on scantron sheets that can be directly entered into the computer by optic scanner (Dennis, 1994). This speeds up the process of entering data and reduces errors related to data entry. However, subjects may be reluctant to use the scantron sheets, and some inaccuracies in the data may occur because of subject error in completing these sheets.

With the advent of microcomputers, data collectors can code data directly into a microcomputer at the data collection site. If a computer is used for data collection, a program must be written for entering the data. If a computer programmer is hired for this purpose, there is, of course, a fee involved. A microcomputer enables collection of large amounts of data with few errors. Questionnaires might be placed within the micro-

computer so that the subject could enter responses directly into the computer. Small data collection machines are also available to allow the researcher to code data into the machine from observations as they occur.

The advancement of technology has made it possible to interface bioinstruments with computers for data collection. The advantages of using computers for acquisition and storage of physiological data from bioinstruments are listed by Harrison (1989).

1. Increased accuracy and reliability are achieved by reducing errors that may occur when manually recording or transcribing physiologic data from patient monitors or other clinical instruments.
2. Linking microcomputers with biomedical instruments (e.g., cardiac, respiratory, blood pressure, or oxygen saturation monitors) permits more frequent acquisition and storage of larger amounts of data (e.g., once or more per second) than is practical with manual recording procedures.
3. Once established, computerized data acquisition systems save researcher time during both the data collection and analysis phases of research.
4. Even though the initial cost of equipment may be high, over the long run computerized data collection systems are less expensive, more efficient, and more reliable than hiring and training multiple human data collectors. (p. 131)

There are also disadvantages to using computers for data collection. The microcomputer and the equipment to interface it with the bioinstruments take up space in an already crowded clinical setting. Purchasing the equipment, setting it up, and installing the software can be time-consuming and expensive at the start of the research project. Another concern is that the nurse researcher will focus mainly on the machine and will neglect observing and interacting with the patient. The most serious disadvantage is the possibility of measurement error that can occur with equipment malfunctions and software errors, although these problems can be reduced with regular maintenance and reliability checks of the equipment and software.

Lookinland and Appel (1991) used a microcomputer interfaced with bioinstruments to collect data for their study of "Hemodynamic and oxygen transport changes following endotracheal suctioning in trauma patients." (p. 133)

■

"Data from the transcutaneous oxygen sensor and the pulse oximeter were obtained via the analogue interfaces of the instruments. The voltage was converted by a specially designed 16-channel analogue to digital conversion board installed in a NEC PCII microcomputer. Custom database software was used for acquisition and storage of data at specified intervals. Data were then available for retrieval and display in numeric or graphic form by a variety of commercially available software packages. Use of analogue interfaces allowed continuous monitoring during the suction episodes." (p. 135) ■

Maintaining Controls

Maintaining consistency and controls during subject selection and data collection protects the integrity or validity of the study. Research controls were built into the design to minimize the influence of intervening forces on study findings. Maintenance of these controls is essential. These controls are not natural in a field setting and letting them slip is easy. In some cases, these controls slip without the researcher realizing it. In addition to maintaining the controls identified in the plan, the researcher needs to continually watch for previously unidentified extraneous variables that might have an impact on the data being collected. These variables are often specific to a study and tend to become apparent during the data collection period. The extraneous variables identified during data collection must be considered during data analysis and interpretation. These variables also need to be noted in the research report to allow future researchers to control them.

Problem Solving

Problems can be perceived either as a frustration or as a challenge. The fact that the problem occurred is not as important as the success of problem resolution. Therefore, the final and perhaps most important task of the data collection period may be problem resolution. Little has been written about the problems encountered by nurse researchers. The research reports often read as though everything went smoothly. The implication is that if you are a good researcher, you will have no problems, which is not true. Research journals generally do not provide sufficient space to allow description of problems encountered, and this gives a false impression to the inexperienced researcher. A more realistic picture can be obtained by personal discussions with researchers about the process of data collection. Some of the common problems experienced by researchers are discussed in the following section.

DATA COLLECTION PROBLEMS

Murphy's law (If anything can go wrong, it will, and at the worst possible time) seems to prevail at times in research as in other dimensions of life. For example, data collection frequently requires more time than was anticipated, and collecting the data is often more difficult than was expected. Sometimes changes must be made in the way that the data are collected, in the specific data collected, or in the timing of data collection. People react to the study in unpredicted ways. Institutional changes may force modifications in the research plan, or unusual or unexpected events may occur. The researcher must be as consistent as possible in data collection but must also be flexible in dealing with unforeseen problems. Sometimes, sticking with the original plan at all costs is a mistake. Skills in finding ways to resolve problems that will protect the integrity of the study can be critical.

In preparation for data collection, possible problems need to be anticipated, and possible solutions for these problems need to be explored.

In the following discussion, some of the common problems and concerns are described, and possible solutions are presented. Problems that tend to occur with some regularity in studies have been categorized as people problems, researcher problems, institutional problems, and event problems.

People Problems

Unfortunately, nurses cannot place a subject in a test tube in a laboratory, instill one drop of the independent variable, and then measure the effect. Nursing studies are conducted by examining the subjects in interaction with their environments. When research involves people, nothing is completely predictable. People, in their complexity and wholeness, have an impact on all aspects of nursing studies. Researchers, potential subjects, family members of subjects, health professionals, institutional staff, and others ("innocent bystanders") interact within the study situation. These interactions need to be closely observed and evaluated by the researcher for their impact on the study.

Problems Selecting a Sample

The first step in initiating data collection—selecting a sample—may be the beginning of people problems. The researcher may find that few available people fit the sample criteria or that many of those approached refuse to participate in the study, even though the requests seem reasonable. Appropriate subjects, who were numerous a month previously, seem to have disappeared. Institutional procedures may change, which might result in many potential subjects becoming ineligible for participation in the study. The sample criteria may have to be reevaluated or additional sources for potential subjects sought. In research institutions that provide care for the indigent, patients tend to be reluctant to participate in research. This lack of participation might be due to exposure to frequent studies, a feeling of being manipulated, or a misunderstanding of the research. Patients may feel that they are being used or are afraid that they will be harmed.

Subject Mortality

After a sample has been selected, certain problems might cause subject mortality (a loss of the subjects from the study). For example, some subjects may agree to participate but then fail to follow through. Some may not complete needed forms and questionnaires or may fill them out incorrectly. Researcher supervision while the subjects complete essential documents reduces these problems. Some subjects may not return for a second interview or may not be home for a scheduled visit. Although time has been invested in data collection with these subjects, their data may have to be excluded from analysis because of incompleteness.

Sometimes subjects must be dropped from the study because of changes in health status. For example, the patient may be transferred out of intensive care where the study is being conducted; the patient's condition may worsen, so he or she may no longer meet sample criteria; or the patient may die. Clinic patients may be transferred to another clinic or discharged from the service. In the community, subjects may choose to discontinue services; or the limits of third-party reimbursement may force discontinuation of services that are being studied.

Subject mortality occurs, to some extent, in all studies. One way to deal with this problem is to anticipate the mortality rate and increase the planned number of subjects to ensure a minimally desired number of subjects who will complete the study. If subject mortality is higher than expected, the researcher may consider continuing data collection for a longer period of time to achieve an adequate sample size. Completing the study with a smaller than expected sample size may become necessary. If so, the effect of a smaller sample on the power of planned statistical analyses needs to be considered, because the smaller sample may not be adequate to test the hypotheses.

Subject as an Object

The quality of interactions between the researcher and subjects during the study is a critical dimension for maintaining subject participation. When there is pressure to complete a study, people can be treated as objects rather than as subjects. In addition to being unethical, this also alters interactions, diminishes the subject's satisfaction in serving as a subject, and increases subject mortality. Subjects are scarce resources and must be treated with care. The researcher's treatment of the subject as an object can lead to similar treatment by other health care providers, which results in poor quality of care. In this case, participation in the study becomes detrimental to the subject.

External Influences on Subject Responses

People interacting with the subject, researcher, or both can have an important impact on the data collection process. Family members may not agree to the subject's participation in the study or may not understand the study process. These people will, in most cases, influence the subject's decisions related to the study. In many studies, time needs to be invested in explaining the study to and seeking the cooperation of family members. Family cooperation is essential when the potential subject is critically ill and unable to give informed consent.

Family members or other patients may also influence the subject's responses to questionnaires or interview questions. In some cases, subjects may ask family members, friends, or other patients to complete study forms for them. Questions asked on the forms may be discussed with whomever happens to be in the room. When this occurs, subjects' real feelings may not be those recorded on the questionnaire. If interviews are conducted while other persons are in the room, the subject's responses may be dependent on his or her need to respond in ways expected by the other persons. Sometimes, questions addressed verbally to the patient may be answered by a family member. Thus, the setting where a questionnaire is completed or an interview is conducted may determine the extent to which the answers are a true reflection of the subject's feelings. If the privacy af-

forded by the setting varies from one subject to another, the subjects' responses may also vary.

Usually the most desirable setting is a private area away from distractions. If this is not possible, the presence of the researcher at the time that the questionnaire is completed may decrease the influence of others. If the questionnaire is to be completed later or taken home and returned at a later time, the probability of influence by others increases and the return of questionnaires greatly decreases. The impact of this on the integrity of the study depends on the nature of the questionnaire.

Passive Resistance

Health professionals and institutional staff working with the subject may affect the data collection process. Some professionals will verbalize strong support for the study and yet passively interfere with data collection. For example, nurses providing care may fail to follow guidelines agreed upon for providing specific care activities being studied, or information needed for the study may be left off patient records. The researcher may not be informed of the admission of a potential subject, and a physician who has agreed that his or her patients can be study subjects may decide as each patient is admitted that this one is not quite right for the study. In addition, the physician might become unusually unavailable to the researcher.

Nonprofessional staff may not realize the impact of the data collection process on their work patterns until the process is initiated. Their beliefs about how care should be provided (and has been provided for the last 20 years) may be violated by the data collection process. If ignored, their resistance can lead to the complete undoing of a carefully designed study. For example, research on skin care may disrupt a nursing aide's bathing routine, so he or she continues the normal routine regardless of the study protocol and invalidates the study findings.

Because of the potential impact of these problems, the researcher needs to maintain open communication and nurture positive relationships with other professionals and staff during data collection. Problems that are recognized early and dealt with promptly have fewer serious consequences for the study than those that are ignored. However, not all problems can be resolved. Sometimes it is necessary to find creative ways to work around an individual or to counter the harmful consequences of passive resistance.

Researcher Problems

Some problems are a consequence of the interaction of the researcher with the study situation or lack of skill in data collection techniques. These problems are often difficult to identify because of the personal involvement of the researcher. However, their effect on the study can be serious.

Researcher Interactions

The researcher can become so involved in interactions with people involved in the study that data collection on the subject is not completed. Researcher interactions can also interfere with data collection in interview situations. If the researcher is collecting data while surrounded by familiar professionals with whom he or she typically interacts socially and professionally, it is sometimes difficult to completely focus on the study situation. This lack of attention usually leads to loss of data.

Lack of Skill in Data Collection Techniques

The researcher's skill in using a particular data collection technique can affect the quality of data collected. The researcher who is unskilled at the beginning of data collection might practice the data collection techniques with the assistance of an experienced researcher. A pilot study to test the data collection techniques can be helpful. If data collectors are being used, they also need opportunities to practice data collection techniques before the study is initiated. If skill is developed in the study itself, as skill increases the data being col-

lected may change, confounding the study findings and threatening the validity of the study. If more than one data collector is used, changes in skill can occur more frequently than if the researcher is the data collector. The skills of data collectors need to be evaluated during the study to detect any changes in their data collection techniques.

Researcher Role Conflict

The professional nurse conducting clinical research often experiences a conflict between the researcher role and the clinician role during data collection. As a researcher, one is observing and recording events. In some cases, involvement of the researcher in the event, such as providing physical or emotional care to a patient during an interview, could alter the event and thus bias the results. It would be difficult to generalize the findings to other situations in which the researcher was not present to intervene. However, in some situations, the needs of patients must take precedence over the needs of the study. The dilemma is to determine when the needs of patients are great enough to warrant researcher intervention.

Some patient situations are life threatening, such as respiratory distress and changes in cardiac function, and require immediate action by anyone present. Other patient needs are simple, are expected of any nurse available, and are not likely to alter the results of the study. Examples of these interventions include giving the patient a bedpan, informing the nurse of the patient's need for pain medication, or assisting the patient in opening food containers. These situations seldom cause a dilemma. Other situations, however, do not have as easy a solution.

Suppose, for example, that the study involved examining emotional responses of patients' family members during and immediately after the patients' operations. The study included an experimental group that received a treatment of one 30-minute family support session before and during the patients' operations and a control group that received no treatment. Both sets of families are being followed for one week after the surgeries, measuring their levels of anxiety and coping strategies. The researcher is currently collecting data on the control group. The data consist of demographic information and scales measuring anxiety and coping. One of the family members is in great distress. After completing the demographic information, she verbally expresses her fears and the lack of support she has received from the nursing staff. Two other subjects from different families hear the expressed distress and concur, moving closer to the conversation and looking to the researcher. In this situation, supportive responses from the researcher are likely to modify the results of the study, because these responses are part of the treatment to be provided to the experimental group. This is likely to narrow the difference between the two groups and thus decrease the possibility of showing a significant difference between the two groups. How should the researcher respond? Is there an obligation to provide support? To some extent almost any response by the researcher will be supportive. One alternative is to provide the needed support and not include these family members in the control group. Another alternative is to recruit the help of a nonprofessional to collect the data from the control group. However, one must recognize that most people will provide some degree of support in the described situation, even though their skills in supportive techniques may vary.

Other dilemmas include witnessing unethical behaviors that interfere with patient care or witnessing subjects' unethical or illegal behaviors (Field & Morse, 1985). These dilemmas need to be anticipated prior to data collection whenever possible. Pilot studies can be helpful in identifying dilemmas likely to occur in a study and strategies can be built into the design to minimize or avoid these dilemmas. However, some dilemmas cannot be anticipated and must be responded to spontaneously. There is no prescribed way to handle difficult dilemmas; each case must be dealt with individually. We recommend discussing unethical and illegal behaviors with colleagues, members of ethics committees, or legal advisors. After the dilemma is resolved, it is wise to reexamine the situation for its effect on study results and to consider options in case the situation arises again.

Maintaining Perspective

Data collection includes both joys and frustrations. Researchers need to be able to maintain some degree of objectivity during the process and yet not take themselves too seriously. A sense of humor is invaluable. One must be able to feel the emotions experienced and then move to being the rational problem solver. Management skills and mental health are invaluable to a lifetime researcher.

Institutional Problems

Institutions are in a constant state of change. They will not stop changing for the period of a study, and these changes often affect data collection. The nurse who has been most helpful in the study may be promoted or transferred. The unit on which the study is conducted may be reorganized, moved, or closed during the study. An area used for subjects' interviews may be transformed into an office or a storeroom or may be torn down. Patient record forms may be revised, omitting data that were being collected. The record room personnel may be reorganizing their files and be temporarily unable to provide needed charts.

These problems are, for the most part, completely outside the control of the researcher. It is helpful to keep an ear to the internal communication network of the institution for advanced warning of impending changes. Contacts within the administrative decision-making system of the institution could facilitate communication about the impact of proposed changes on an ongoing study. However, in many cases, data collection strategies might have to be modified to meet the newly emerging situation. Again, flexibility while maintaining the integrity of the study may be the key to continuing successful data collection. Byers (1995) suggests that the home setting may be more desirable in the future as a data collection site than institutions and that the response rate in this setting is better than that in institutions. The disadvantage is that home visits are time intensive and the subject may not be home at the agreed upon appointment time.

Event Problems

Unpredictable events can be a source of frustration during a study. Research tools ordered from a testing company may be lost in the mail. The duplicating machine may break down just before 500 data collection forms were to be copied, or a machine to be used in data collection may break down and require 6 weeks for repair. A computer ordered for data collection may not arrive when promised, a tape recorder may become jammed in the middle of an interview, or after an interview, the data collector may discover that the play button on the recorder had been pushed rather than the record button, leaving no record of the interview. Data collection forms may be misplaced, misfiled, or lost.

Local, national, or world events and nature can also influence subjects' responses to a study. For example, one of our graduate students was examining patients' attitudes toward renal dialysis. She planned to collect data for 6 months. Three months into data collection, three patients died as a result of a dialysis machine malfunction in the city where the study was being conducted. The event made national headlines. Obviously, this event could be expected to modify subjects' responses. In attempting to deal with the impact of the event on the study, the graduate student could have modified the study and continued collecting data to examine the impact of news such as this on attitudes. However, the emotional climate of the clinics participating in the study was not conducive to this option. She chose to wait 3 months before collecting additional data, examining the data before and after the event for statistically significant differences in responses. Since there were none, she could justify using all the data for analysis.

Other less dramatic events can also have an impact on data collection. If data collection for the entire sample is planned for a single time, a snowstorm or a flood may require canceling the meeting or clinic. Weather may decrease attendance far below that expected at a support group or series of teaching sessions. A bus strike can disrupt transportation systems to such an extent that subjects can no longer get to the data collection site. A new health agency may open in the city, which may decrease demand for the care activities being studied. On the other hand, an external event can also increase attendance at clinics to such an extent that existing resources are stretched and data collection is no longer possible. These events are also outside the control of the researcher and are impossible to anticipate. In most cases, however, restructuring the data collection period can salvage the study. In order to do this, it is necessary to examine all possible alternatives for collecting the study data. In some cases, data collection can simply be rescheduled; in other situations, the changes needed may be more complex.

SERENDIPITY

Serendipity is the accidental discovery of something useful or valuable. During the data collection phase of studies, researchers often become aware of elements or relationships not previously identified. These aspects may be closely related to the study being conducted or have little connection with it. They come from increased awareness and close observation of the study situation. Because the researcher is focused on close observation, other elements in the situation can come into clearer focus and take on new meaning. This is similar to the open context discussed in Chapter 4. The researcher's perspective shifts, and new gestalts are formed.

Serendipitous findings are important to the development of new insights in nursing theory. They can be important in understanding the totality of the phenomenon being examined. Additionally, they lead to areas of research that generate new knowledge. Therefore, it is essential to capture these insights as they occur. These events need to be carefully recorded, even if their impact or meaning is not understood at the time. Sometimes, when these notes are reexamined at a later time, patterns begin to emerge.

Serendipitous findings can also lead the researcher astray. Sometimes researchers forget the original plan and move right into examining the newly discovered dimensions. Although modifying data collection to include data related to the new discovery may be valid, the researcher must remember that there has not been time to plan carefully a study related to the new findings. Examination of the new data should only be an offshoot of the initial study. Data collected as a result of serendipitous findings can guide future studies, and need to be included in presentations and publications related to the study. Although the meaning of the discovery may not be understood, sharing the information may lead to insights by researchers studying related phenomena.

HAVING ACCESS TO SUPPORT SYSTEMS

The researcher must have access to individuals or groups who can provide support and consultation during the data collection period. Support systems themselves have been the subject of much study in recent years. In some cases, support systems can be the source of both stress and support. However, current theorists propose that to be classified as support, the individual or group must enhance the ego strength of the individual. Three dimensions of support have been identified: (1) physical assistance; (2) provision of money or other concrete needs, such as equipment or information; and (3) emotional support. These types of support can usually be obtained from academic committees; institutions serving as research settings; and colleagues, friends, and family.

Support of Academic Committees

Although thesis and dissertation committees are basically seen as stern keepers of the sanctity of the research process, they also serve as support systems for neophyte researchers. In fact, committee members need to be selected from faculty who are willing and able to provide the needed support. Experienced researchers among faculty are usually more knowledgeable about the types of support needed. Because they are directly involved in research, they tend to be sensitive to the needs of neophyte researchers.

Institutional Support

A support system within the institution where the study is being conducted is also important. Support might be provided by people serving on the institutional research committee or by nurses working on the unit where the study is to be conducted. These people often have knowledge of how the institution functions, and their closeness to the study can increase their understanding of the problems experienced by the researcher and subjects. Their ability to provide useful suggestions and assistance must not be overlooked. Resolution of some of the problems encountered during data collection may be dependent on having someone within the power structure of the institution who can intervene.

Personal Support

In addition to professional support, it is helpful to have at least one significant other with whom one can share the joys, frustrations, and current problems of data collection. A significant other can often serve as a mirror to allow you to see the situation clearly and perhaps more objectively. Through personal support, feelings can be shared and released, allowing the researcher to achieve distance from the data collection situation. Discussions of alternatives for problem resolution can then occur. Data collection is a demanding but rewarding time that increases the confidence and expertise of the neophyte researcher.

MANAGING DATA

When data collection begins, the researcher will have to handle large quantities of paper. The situation can quickly grow to a state of total confusion unless careful plans are made before data collection begins. Plans need to be made to keep all data from a single subject together until analysis is begun. The subject code number is written on each form, and the forms for each subject are checked to ensure they are all present. Researchers have been known to sort their data by form, such as putting all the scales of one kind together, only to realize afterwards that they had failed to code the forms with subject identification numbers first. They then had no idea which scale belonged to which subject, and valuable data were lost.

Space needs to be allotted for storing forms. File folders could be purchased, and a labeling method could be designed to allow easy access to data, and color coding is often useful. For example, if multiple forms are being used, the subject's demographic sheet could be one color, with different colors for the visual analogue scale, the pain questionnaire, the physiological data sheet with blood pressure, pulse, and respiration readings, and the interview notes. Envelopes can be used to hold small pieces of paper or note cards that might fall out of a file folder. Plans need to be made to code data and enter them into the computer as soon as possible after data collection to help reduce the loss or disorganization of data.

PREPARING DATA FOR COMPUTER ENTRY

Data needs to be carefully checked and problems corrected before data entry is initiated. The data entry process should be essentially automatic and require no decisions regarding the data. This will reduce the number of data entry errors and markedly decrease the time required for entry. It is not sufficient to establish general rules for those entering data such as "in this case always do X." This action still requires the data enterer to recognize a problem, refer to a general rule, and correct the data before entering them. Anything that alters the rhythm of data entry increases errors. The researcher needs to examine carefully each datum,

searching for the following problems and resolving them prior to data entry:

1. *Missing data.* Provide the data if possible or determine the impact of the missing data on your analysis. In some cases, the subject must be excluded from at least some of the analyses. This requires that you determine what data are essential.

2. *Items in which the subject provided two responses when only one was requested.* For example, if the item asked the subject to mark the most important in a list of ten items and the subject selected two, you must decide how to resolve this; do not leave the decision to an assistant who is entering the data. On the form, indicate how the datum is to be coded.

3. *Items in which the subject has marked a response between two options.* This problem commonly occurs with Likert-type scales, particularly those using forced choice options. Given four options, the subject places a mark on the line between response 2 and response 3. On the form, indicate how the datum is to be coded.

4. *Items that ask the subject to write in some information such as occupation or diagnosis.* Items such as this are the data enterer's nightmare. A list of codes need to be developed by the researcher for entering such data. Rather than leaving it up to the assistant to determine which code matches the subject's written response, this code should be indicated by the researcher before turning the data over for entry. After the data have been checked and needed codes written in, it is prudent to make a copy rather than turning over the only set of your data to an assistant.

THE DATA ENTRY PERIOD

If you are entering your own data, develop a rhythm to your entry. Avoid distractions while entering data. Limit your data entry periods to two hours at a time to reduce errors. A backup of the database should be made after each data entry period and stored on a floppy disk or backup tape. It is possible for the computer to crash, losing your data. If an assistant is entering your data, make yourself as available as possible to respond to questions and address problems. After entry, the data should be checked for accuracy. Data checking is discussed in Chapter 16 in the section Preparation of the Data for Analysis.

Storage and Retrieval of Data

Storage of data from a study is relatively easy in this time of floppy disks and backup tapes. One decision which must be made is how long to store the data. The original data forms need to be stored as well as the database. Storage of data serves several purposes. The data can be used for secondary analyses of data. For example, individuals who are participating in a research program related to a particular research focus may pool data from various studies for access by all members of the group. The data are available to document the validity of your analyses and the published results of your study. Because of nationally publicized incidences of researchers inventing data from which multiple publications were developed, you are wise to preserve documentation that your data were obtained as you claim. Issues that have been raised include how long data should be stored, the need of institutional policy regarding storage of data, and whether graduate students who conduct a study should leave a copy of their data at the university. Thomas (1992) surveyed 153 researchers to determine their responses to these questions. She found the length of data storage varied greatly, with 29% storing their data 5 years, 31% storing it 10 years, and 21% storing it forever. Most researchers stored their data in their office (84%), and a few used a central location (12%) or a laboratory (4%). The forms of data storage devices preferred were disk (54%), tape (47%), and paper/raw data (32%). Some researchers indicated a preference for more than one storage device for their data. The majority of the researchers (86%) indicated that their institutions did not have a policy for data storage, and most graduate students (74%) did not leave a copy of their data at the university.

SUMMARY

The initiation of data collection is one of the most exciting parts of research. But some time needs to be spent carefully planning this adventure. A data collection plan details how the study will be implemented. To plan the process of data collection, the researcher needs to determine step by step how and in what sequence data will be collected and the timing of the process. Decision points that occur during data collection need to be identified and all options considered.

Consistency in data collection across subjects is critical and so is consistency among data collectors if more than one data collector is used. Decisions regarding who collects the data also need to be made. If data collectors are used, they need to be informed of the research project, introduced to the instruments to be used, and provided equivalent training in the data collection process. Following training, data collectors must be evaluated to determine their consistency.

The time required for data collection is often inadequately estimated in conducting a study. It is helpful to write out a time plan for the data collection period. Cost factors must also be examined in planning a study. Neophyte researchers have difficulty making rea-

continued

continued

sonable estimates of time and costs related to a study and might wish to validate estimates with an experienced researcher.

Before data collection begins, the researcher may need to develop forms on which to record data. Data collection forms need to be developed for easy recording during data collection and for easy entry into the computer. A decision must be made about whether data are collected in raw form or coded at the time of collection. Coding is the process of transforming qualitative data into numerical symbols that can be easily entered into the computer.

A codebook documents the variable name, abbreviated variable name, and possible values of every variable entered in a computer file. It is advisable to develop the codebook before initiating data collection. This provides a means to identify places in data collection forms that might prove to be a problem during data entry. If the data are being given to an assistant for data entry, information on the data should be provided to the assistant before data entry. Using this information, the assistant can develop the database in preparation for receiving the data for entry.

Data collection is the process of selecting subjects and gathering data from these subjects. Data collection involves five tasks: selecting subjects, collecting data in a consistent way, maintaining research controls, and solving problems that threaten to disrupt the study. Some of the common problems encountered by researchers during data collection include problems selecting a sample, subject mortality, treating the subject as an object, external influences on subject responses, passive resistance, researcher interactions, lack of skill in data collection techniques, research role conflicts, and maintaining perspective.

Serendipity is the accidental discovery of something useful or valuable. During the data collection phase of studies, researchers often become aware of elements or relationships not previously identified. Serendipitous findings are important to the development of new insights in nursing and can lead to areas of research that generate new knowledge.

During data collection, the researcher needs access to individuals or groups who can provide support and consultation. Support needs to be available from academic committees, involved institutions, and significant others.

When data collection begins, the researcher will have to handle large quantities of papers. Plans need to be made for organizing and storing the data as they are gathered. Data need to be carefully checked and problems corrected before data entry is initiated. Storage of data after the study is completed must also be considered. The original data forms as well as the database needs to be stored. Because of nationally publicized incidences of researchers inventing data from which multiple publications were developed, you are wise to preserve documentation that your data were obtained as you claim.

References

Alles, P. (1995). CESF medical outcomes research project: Implementing outcomes assessment in a clinical setting. *Wisconsin Medical Journal, 94*(1), 27–31.

Bostrom, J., Dibble, S., & Rizzuto, C. (1995). Data collection as an educational process. *Journal of Continuing Education in Nursing, 22*(6), 248–253.

Byers, V. L. (1995). Overview of the data collection process. *Journal of Neuroscience Nursing, 27*(3), 188–193.

Dennis, K. E. (1994). Managing questionnaire data through optical scanning technology. *Nursing Research, 43*(6), 376–378.

Field, P. A., & Morse, J. M. (1985). *Nursing research: The application of qualitative approaches* (pp. 65–90). Rockville, MD: Aspen.

Gift, A. G., Creasia, J., & Parker, B. (1991). Utilizing research assistants and maintaining research integrity. *Research in Nursing & Health, 14*(3), 229–233.

Harrison, L. L. (1989). Interfacing bioinstruments with computers for data collection in nursing research. *Research in Nursing & Health, 12*(2), 129–133.

Lobo, M. L. (1993). Code books—A critical link in the research process. *Western Journal of Nursing Research, 15*(3), 377–385.

Lookinland, S., & Appel, P. L. (1991). Hemodynamic and oxygen transport changes following endotracheal suc-

tioning in trauma patients. *Nursing Research, 40*(3), 133–138.

Thomas, S. P. (1992). Storage of research data: Why, how, where? *Nursing Research, 41*(5), 309–311.

Washington, C. C., & Moss, M. (1988). Methodology corner: Pragmatic aspects of establishing interrater reliability in research. *Nursing Research, 37*(3), 190–191.

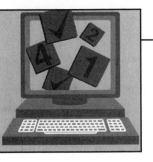

16

Concepts of Statistical Theory

The period of data analysis is probably the most exciting part of research. During this period, one finally obtains answers to the questions that initially generated the research activity. And yet, nurses probably experience greater anxiety about knowledge of this phase of the research process than any other, whether the knowledge is needed in order to critique published studies or to conduct research. To critique a quantitative study, the nurse needs to be able to (1) identify the statistical procedures used; (2) judge whether these statistical procedures were appropriate to the hypotheses, questions, or objectives of the study and to the data available for analysis; (3) comprehend the discussion of data analysis results; (4) judge whether the author's interpretation of the results is appropriate; and (5) evaluate the clinical significance of the findings.

The neophyte researcher performing a quantitative study is confronted with many critical decisions related to data analysis that require statistical knowledge. Information relevant to these needs will continue in Chapters 17, 18, and 19. This chapter begins with a discussion of some of the more pragmatic aspects of quantitative data analysis: the purposes of statistical analysis, the process of performing data analysis, choosing appropriate statistical procedures for a study, and resources for statistical analysis. The latter portion of the chapter provides a review of statistical concepts and logic.

PURPOSES OF STATISTICAL ANALYSIS

Statistics can be used for a variety of purposes: to (1) summarize, (2) explore the meaning of devia-

tions in the data, (3) compare or contrast descriptively, (4) test the proposed relationships in a theoretical model, (5) infer that the findings from the sample are indicative of the entire population, (6) examine causality, (7) predict, or (8) infer from the sample to a theoretical model. Statisticians such as John Tukey (1977) divide the role of statistics into two parts: exploratory data analysis and confirmatory data analysis. *Exploratory data analysis* is performed to get a preliminary vision of the nature of the data and to search the data for hidden structure or models. *Confirmatory data analysis* involves traditional inferential statistics that assist the researcher to make an inference about a population or a process based on evidence from the study sample.

THE PROCESS OF DATA ANALYSIS

There are several stages to quantitative data analysis: (1) preparation of the data for analysis; (2) description of the sample; (3) testing the reliability of measurement; (4) exploratory analysis of the data; (5) confirmatory analyses guided by the hypotheses, questions, or objectives; and (6) post hoc analyses. Although not all of these stages are equally reflected in the final published report of the study, they all contribute to the insights that can be gained from analysis of the data. Many novice researchers do not plan the details of data analysis until the data are collected and they are confronted with the analysis task. This is a poor research technique and often leads to the collection of unusable data or the failure to collect data needed to answer the research questions. Plans for data analysis need to be made during the development of the methodology.

PREPARATION OF THE DATA FOR ANALYSIS

Except in very small studies, computers are almost universally used for data analysis. The use of computers for analysis has increased as personal computers (PCs) have become more accessible and easy-to-use data analysis packages have become available. When computers are used for analysis, the first step of the process is entering the data into the computer.

Prior to entering data into the computer, the computer file that will hold the data needs to be carefully prepared using information from the codebook described in Chapter 15. The location of each variable in the computer file needs to be identified. Each variable needs to be labeled in the computer so that variables involved in a particular analysis will be clearly designated in the computer printouts. The researcher needs to develop a systematic plan for data entry designed to reduce errors during the entry phase, and data need to be entered during periods of time in which there are few interruptions. However, entering data for long periods of time without respite results in fatigue and an increase in errors. If the data are being stored in a PC hard disk drive, a backup needs to be made on a floppy disk each time more data are entered. It is wise to keep a second floppy disk of the data filed at a separate, carefully protected site. If the data are stored on a mainframe computer, request that a tape backup be made that you can keep in your possession, or download the data onto a floppy disk. After data entry, store the original data in locked files for safekeeping.

Cleaning the Data

Print the data file. When the data size allows, cross-check every piece of datum on the printout with the original datum for accuracy. Otherwise, randomly check the accuracy of data points. Cor-

rect all errors found in the computer file. Computer analysis of frequencies of each value of every variable is performed as a second check of the accuracy of the data. Search for values outside the appropriate range of values for that variable. See Chapter 15 for more information on computerizing and cleaning data.

Identifying Missing Data

Identify all missing data points. Determine whether the information can be obtained and entered into the data file. If there are missing data on a large number of subjects in relation to specific variables, a judgment needs to be made regarding the availability of sufficient data to perform analysis using those variables. In some cases, subjects must be excluded from the analysis because of missing essential data.

Transforming Data

In some cases, data must be transformed prior to initiating data analyses. Items in scales are often arranged so that the location of the highest values on the item are varied. This prevents a global response by the subject to all items in the scale. To reduce errors, the values on these items need to be entered into the computer exactly as they appear on the data collection form. Values on the items are then reversed using computer commands.

Skewed, or nonlinear, *data* that do not meet the assumptions of parametric analyses can sometimes be transformed in such a way that the values are expressed in a linear fashion. Various mathematical operations are used for this purpose. Examples of these operations include squaring each value, or calculating the square root of each value. These operations may allow the researcher insights into the data not evident from the raw data.

Calculating Variables

Sometimes, a variable used in the analysis is not collected but calculated from other variables. For example, if data are collected on the number of patients on a nursing unit and on the number of nurses on a shift, one might calculate a ratio of nurse to patient for a particular shift. The data will be more accurate if this calculation is performed by the computer rather than manually. The results can then be stored in the data file as a variable, rather than being recalculated each time the variable is used in an analysis.

Making Data Backups

When the data cleaning process is complete, backups need to be made again; labeled as the complete, cleaned data set; and carefully stored. Data cleaning is a time-consuming process one does not wish to repeat unnecessarily.

DESCRIPTION OF THE SAMPLE

The next step is to obtain as complete a picture of the sample as possible. Begin with frequencies of descriptive variables related to the sample. Calculate measures of central tendency and measures of dispersion relevant to the sample. If the study is composed of more than one sample, comparisons of the various groups need to be performed. Relevant analyses might include examination of age, educational level, health status, gender, ethnicity, or other features for which data are available. If information is available on estimated parameters of the population from previous research or meta-analyses, measures in the present study need to be compared with these estimated parameters. If the samples are not representative of the population, or two groups being compared are not equivalent in ways important to the study, a decision will need to be made regarding the justification of continuing the analysis.

TESTING THE RELIABILITY
OF MEASUREMENT

Examine the reliability of the methods of measurement used in the study. Reliability of observational measures or physiological measures may

have been obtained during the data collection phase but needs to be noted at this point. Additional evaluation of the reliability of these measures may be possible at this point. If paper and pencil scales were used in data collection, alpha coefficients need to be performed. The value of the coefficient needs to be compared with values obtained for the instrument in previous studies. If the coefficient is unacceptably low, a decision must be made regarding the justification of performing analysis using data from the instrument.

EXPLORATORY ANALYSIS
OF THE DATA

Examine all the data descriptively, with the intent of becoming as familiar as possible with the nature of the data. This step is often omitted by neophyte researchers, who tend to jump immediately into analysis designed to test their hypotheses, questions, or objectives. However, they do this at the risk of missing important information in the data and of performing analyses using data inappropriate for the analysis. The researcher needs to examine data on each variable using measures of central tendency and dispersion. Is the data skewed or normally distributed? What is the nature of variation in the data? Are there outliers with extreme values that seem unlike the rest of the sample? The most valuable insights from a study often come from careful examination of outliers (Tukey, 1977).

The methods of EDA (exploratory data analysis) described in Chapter 17 provide simple, easy-to-use techniques for an exploratory examination of your data. In many cases, as a part of exploratory analysis, inferential statistical procedures are used to examine differences and associations within the sample. From an exploratory perspective, these analyses are relevant only to the sample under study. There should be no intent to infer to a population. If group comparisons are made, effect sizes need to be determined for the variables involved in the analyses.

In many nursing studies, the purpose of the study is exploratory analysis. In such studies, often the sample sizes are small, power is low, measurement is crude, and the field of study is relatively new. If treatments are tested, the procedure is approached as a pilot study. The most immediate need is tentative exploration of the phenomena under study. Confirming the findings of these studies will require more rigorously designed studies with much larger samples. Unfortunately, many of these exploratory studies are reported in the literature as confirmatory studies and attempts are made to infer to larger populations. Because of the unacceptably high risk of a Type II error in these studies, negative findings should be viewed with caution.

Using Tables and Graphs for Exploratory Analyses

Although tables and graphs are commonly thought of as a way of presenting the findings of a study, these tools may be even more useful in providing a means for the researcher to become familiar with the data. Tables and graphs need to be made that illustrate the descriptive analyses being performed, even though these will likely never be included in a research report. They are only for the benefit of the researcher; they assist in identifying patterns in the data and in interpreting exploratory findings. Visualizing the data in various ways can greatly increase the insights regarding the nature of the data (see Chapter 17).

CONFIRMATORY ANALYSES

As the name implies, confirmatory analysis is performed to confirm expectations regarding the data that are expressed as hypotheses, questions, or objectives. The findings are inferred from the sample to the population. Thus, inferential statistical procedures are used. The design of the study, the methods of measurement, and the sample size must be sufficient for this confirmatory process to be justified. A written analysis plan needs to clearly describe the confirmatory analyses that will be performed to examine each hypothesis, question, or objective. The following steps need to be

followed for each analysis used in performing a systematic confirmatory analysis:

1. Identify the level of measurement of data available for analysis related to the research objective, question, or hypothesis.
2. Select statistical procedure(s) appropriate to the level of measurement that will respond to the objective, answer the question, or test the hypothesis.
3. Select the level of significance that you will use to interpret the results.
4. Choose a one-tailed or two-tailed test if this is appropriate to your analysis.
5. Determine the sample size available for the analysis. If several groups will be used in the analysis, the size of each group needs to be identified.
6. Evaluate the representativeness of the sample.
7. Determine the risk of a Type II error for the analysis by performing a power analysis.
8. Develop dummy tables and graphics to illustrate the methods you will use to display your results in relation to your hypotheses, questions, or objectives.
9. Determine the degrees of freedom for your analysis.
10. Perform the analysis, manually or with a computer.
11. Compare the statistical value obtained to the table value using the level of significance, tailedness of the test, and degrees of freedom previously identified. If you have performed your analysis on a computer, this information will be provided on the computer printout.
12. Reexamine the analysis to ensure that the procedure was performed using the appropriate variables and that the statistical procedure was correctly specified in the computer program.
13. Interpret the results of the analysis in terms of the hypothesis, question, or objective.
14. Interpret the results in terms of the framework.

POST HOC ANALYSES

Post hoc analyses are commonly performed in studies with more than two groups when the analysis indicates that the groups are significantly different but does not identify which groups are different. This situation occurs, for example, in chi-square analyses and in analysis of variance (ANOVA). In other studies, the insights obtained through the planned analyses generate further questions that can be examined with the available data. These analyses may be tangential to the initial purpose of the study but may be fruitful in providing important information and in generating questions for further research.

STORING COMPUTER PRINTOUTS FROM DATA ANALYSIS

Computer printouts tend to accumulate rapidly during data analysis. Results of data analyses can easily become lost in the mountain of computer paper. These printouts need to be systematically stored to allow easy access later when theses or dissertations are being written or research papers are being prepared for publication. We recommend storing the printouts by time sequence. Most printouts identify the date (and even the hour and minute) the analysis was performed. Some mainframe computers also assign a job number to each printout, which can be recorded. This makes it easy to distinguish earlier analyses from those performed later. Sometimes printouts can be sorted by variable or by hypothesis and then arranged within those categories by time.

When papers describing the study are being prepared, the results of each analysis reported in the paper need to be cross-indexed with the computer printout for reference as needed, listing job number, date, time, and page number in the printout. This needs to include a printout of the program used for the analysis. As interpretation of results proceeds and you attempt to link various findings, you may question some of the results. They may not seem to fit with the rest of the results, or they may not seem logical. You may find that you have failed to include some statistical information that is needed. When rewriting the paper, you may decide to report results not originally included. The search for a particular data analysis printout can be time-consuming and frustrating if

the printouts have not been carefully organized. It is easy to lose needed results and have to repeat the analysis.

After the paper has been submitted for publication (or to a thesis or dissertation committee), we recommend storing a copy of the page from the printout for each statistical value reported with the text. This copy needs to provide sufficient detail to allow you to gain access to the entire printout if needed. Thesis and dissertation committees and journal reviewers often recommend including additional information related to statistical procedures prior to acceptance. You often have only a short time frame within which to obtain the information and modify the paper to meet deadlines. Even after the paper is published, we have had requests from readers for validation of our results. If this request is made months (or years) after the study is complete, finding the information can be a nightmare if you have failed to store your printouts carefully.

RESOURCES FOR STATISTICAL ANALYSES

COMPUTER PROGRAMS

Packaged computer analyses programs, such as SPSS (Statistical Packages for the Social Sciences), SAS (Statistical Analysis System), and BMDP (Biomedical Data Processing), are available on the mainframe computers of many universities. A variety of data analysis packages, such as SAS, SPSS, ABSTAT, and NCSS (Number Cruncher Statistical System) are also available for the PC. Table 16–1 lists sources of data analysis packages for the PC. The emergence of more powerful, high-speed PCs has made it relatively easy to conduct most analyses on the PC. Although the mathematical formulas needed to conduct analyses using a packaged program have been written as part of the computer program, one needs to know how to instruct the computer program to perform the selected analysis. Manuals, available for each program, demonstrate how to perform the analyses and provide a detailed discussion of the mathemat-

Table 16–1
Sources of Data Analysis Packages for the PC

NCSS (Number Cruncher Statistical System)
Dr. Jerry L. Hintze
329 North 1000 East
Kaysville, Utah 84037
Phone (801) 546-0445
FAX (801) 546-3907
SPSS/PC
SPSS, Inc.
444 N. Michigan Avenue
Chicago, Illinois 60611
Phone (312) 329-3500
FAX (312) 329-3668
SAS
SAS Institute, Inc.
SAS Circle, Box 8000
Cary, NC 27512-8000
Phone (919) 467-8000
ABSTAT
Anderson-Bell
11479 S. Pine Drive
Suite 400-M
Parker, Colorado 80134
Phone (303) 841-9755
Telex: 499-4230

ical logic behind each type of analysis. The researcher needs to understand this logic, even though the computer will perform the analysis. Most manuals suggest up-to-date and comprehensive sources related to each type of analysis that may be helpful in further understanding the logic of the procedure.

Packaged computer programs can perform your data analysis and provide you with the results of the analysis in a computer printout. However, an enormous amount of information is provided in a computer printout and its meaning can easily be misinterpreted. In addition, computers conduct analysis on whatever data are provided. If the data entered into the computer are garbage (e.g., numbers from the data are typed in incorrectly or data are typed into the wrong columns), the computer output will be garbage. If the data are inappropriate for the particular type of analysis selected, the computer program is often unable to detect that error and will proceed to perform the analysis. The results will be meaningless, and the researcher's conclusions will be completely in error (Hinshaw & Schepp, 1984).

STATISTICAL ASSISTANCE

Programmers assist in writing the programs that give commands to the computer to implement the mathematical processes selected. Programmers are skilled in the use of computer languages but are not statisticians; thus, they do not interpret the outcomes of analyses. Computer languages are the messages used to give detailed commands to the computer. Even when packaged programs are being used, a programmer skilled in the use of common software packages can be of great help in selecting the appropriate programs, writing them according to guidelines, and speeding up the debugging process. In universities, computer science students are often available for programming services.

A statistician has an educational background that qualifies him or her as an expert in statistical analyses. Statisticians vary in their skills related to specific statistical procedures, and usually charge an hourly fee for services. However, some may contract to perform an agreed-upon analysis for a set fee. Although the extent of need for statistical consultation is dependent on the educational background of the researcher, most nurse researchers will benefit from statistical consultation. However, the researcher remains the content expert and must be the final authority in interpreting the meaning of the analyses in terms of the discipline's body of knowledge. Therefore, it is not acceptable to abdicate the total responsibility for data analyses to the statistician. The nurse researcher remains accountable for understanding the statistical procedures used and for interpreting these procedures to various audiences when the results of the study are communicated.

THE CONCEPTS OF STATISTICAL THEORY

One reason that nurses tend to avoid statistics is that many were taught only the mathematical mechanics of calculating statistical formulas, with little or no explanation of the logic behind the analysis procedure or the meaning of the results. This

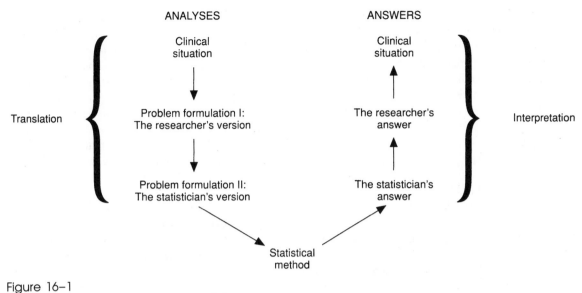

ANALYSES   ANSWERS

Clinical   Clinical
situation   situation

Translation   Problem formulation I: The researcher's   Interpretation
                   The researcher's version   answer

                   Problem formulation II: The statistician's
                   The statistician's version   answer

                          Statistical
                           method

Figure 16–1
Process of translation and interpretation in statistics.

mechanical process is usually performed by computer, and information about it is of little assistance in making statistical decisions or explaining results. We will approach data analysis from the perspective of enhancing the reader's understanding of the meaning underlying statistical analysis. This understanding can then be used either to critique or to perform data analyses.

As is common in many theories, theoretical ideas related to statistics are expressed using unique terminology and logic that is unfamiliar to many. Research ideas, particularly data analysis, expressed in the language of the clinician and the researcher are perceived by statisticians to be relatively imprecise and vague because they are not expressed in the formal language of the professional statistician. To resolve this language barrier, developing a plan for data analysis requires translation from the common language (or even general research language) to the language of statisticians. When the analysis is complete, the results must be translated from the language of the statistician back to the language of the researcher and the clinician. Thus, explanation of the meaning of the results is a process of interpretation (Chervany, 1977). Figure 16–1 illustrates this process of translation and interpretation.

The ensuing discussion presents an explanation of some of the concepts commonly used within statistical theory. The logic of statistical theory is embedded within the explanations of these concepts. The concepts presented include probability theory, decision theory, inference, the theoretical normal curve, sampling distributions, sampling distribution of a statistic, statistics and parameters, samples and populations, estimation of parameters, degrees of freedom, tailedness, Type I and Type II errors, level of significance, power, clinical significance, parametric and nonparametric statistical analyses, causality, and relationships.

PROBABILITY THEORY

Probability theory addresses statistical analysis from the perspective of the extent of a relationship or the probability of accurately predicting an event. Probability theory is deductive in nature. Using probability theory, the researcher might be interested in examining the amount of variation in the data that could be explained using a particular analysis. The meaning attributed to the results is dependent on the interpretation of the researcher, who is most familiar with the field of study. A finding that would have little meaning in one field of study might be an important finding in another (Good, 1983). You might be interested in the probability of a particular nursing outcome, or the probability that your sample is representative of a larger population. Probability is expressed as a lower case *p,* with values expressed as percentages or as a decimal value ranging from 0 to 1. If the exact probability is known, for example, to be .23, this would be expressed as $p = .23$.

DECISION THEORY AND HYPOTHESIS TESTING

Decision theory is inductive in nature and is based on assumptions associated with the theoretical normal curve. This approach is used when testing for differences between groups with the expectation that all of the groups are members of the same population. This expectation (or assumption) is expressed as a null hypothesis. See Chapter 8 for an explanation of null hypothesis. To test the assumption, a cutoff point is selected prior to data collection. This cutoff point, referred to as alpha (α), or the level of significance, is the point on the normal curve at which the results of statistical analysis indicate a statistically significant difference between the groups. Decision theory requires that the cutoff point be absolute. Absolute means that even if the value obtained is only a fraction above the cutoff point, the samples are considered to be from the same population and no meaning can be attributed to the differences. Thus, it is inappropriate using this theory to make a statement that "the findings approached significance at the .051 level" if the alpha level was set at .05. Using decision theory rules, this finding indicates that the groups tested are not significantly different and the null hypothesis is not rejected. On the other hand, if the analysis reveals a significant difference of .001, this result is not more significant than the .05 originally proposed (Slakter, Wu, & Suzuki-Slakter, 1991).

INFERENCE

Statisticians use the term *inference* or *infer* in somewhat the same way a researcher uses the term *generalize.* Inference requires the use of inductive reasoning. One infers from a specific case to a general truth, from a part to the whole, from the concrete to the abstract, from the known to the unknown. Using inferential reasoning, you can never prove things; you can never be certain. However, one of the reasons for the rules that have been established related to statistical procedures is to increase the probability that inferences are accurate. Inferences are made cautiously and with great care.

THE NORMAL CURVE

The theoretical *normal curve* is an expression of statistical theory. It is a theoretical frequency distribution of all *possible* scores. No real distribution exactly fits the normal curve. The idea of the normal curve was developed by an 18-year-old mathematician, Johann Gauss, in 1795. He found that data measured repeatedly in many samples from the same population, using scales based on an underlying continuum, can be combined into one large sample. From this very large sample, one can develop a more accurate representation of the pattern of the curve in that population than is possible with only one sample. Surprisingly, in most cases, the curve is similar, regardless of the specific data that have been examined or the population being studied.

This theoretical normal curve is symmetrical and unimodal and has continuous values. The mean, median, and mode (summary statistics) are equal (see Figure 16–2). The distribution is completely defined by the mean and standard deviation. The measures in the theoretical distribution have been standardized using Z scores. These terms are explained further in Chapter 17. Note Z scores and standard deviations in Figure 16–2. The proportion of scores that may be found in a particular area of the normal curve has been identified. In the normal curve, 68% of the scores will be within 1 standard deviation or 1 Z score above or below the mean, 95% will be within 2 standard deviations above or below the mean, and more than 99% will be within 3 standard deviations above or below the mean. Even when statistics,

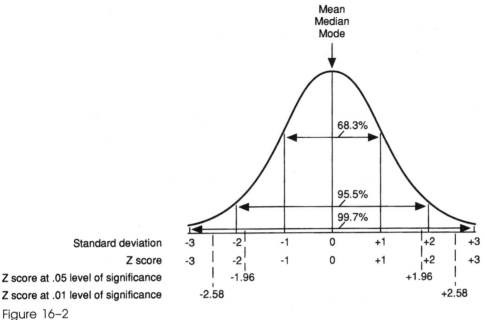

Figure 16–2
The normal curve.

such as means, come from a population with a skewed (asymmetrical) distribution, the sampling distribution developed from multiple means obtained from that skewed population will tend to fit the pattern of the normal curve. This phenomenon is referred to as the central limit theorem. One requirement for the use of parametric statistical analyses is that the data be normally distributed—*normal* meaning that the data approximately fit the normal curve. Because many statistical measures from skewed samples also fit the normal curve because of the *central limit theorem,* some statisticians feel that it is justifiable to use parametric statistical analyses even with data from skewed samples if the sample is large enough (Volicer, 1984).

SAMPLING DISTRIBUTIONS

A *sampling distribution* is developed using statistical values (such as the means) of many samples obtained from the same population. The mean of this type of distribution is referred to as the *mean*

of means (μ). Sampling distributions can also be developed from standard deviations. Other values, such as correlations between variables, scores obtained from specific measures, and scores reflecting differences between groups within the population, can yield values that can be used to develop sampling distributions.

The purpose of the sampling distribution is to allow us to measure sampling error. *Sampling error* is the difference between the sample statistic used to estimate a parameter and the actual but unknown value of the parameter. If we know the sampling distribution of a statistic, it allows us to measure the probability of making an incorrect inference. One should never make an inference without being able to calculate the probability of making an incorrect inference.

SAMPLING DISTRIBUTION OF A STATISTIC

Just as it is possible to develop distributions of summary statistics within a population, it is possible to develop distributions of inferential statistical outcomes. For example, if one repeatedly obtained two samples of the same size from the same population and tested for differences in the means using a *t* test, a sampling distribution could be developed from the resulting *t* values using probability theory. Using this approach, a distribution could be developed for samples of many varying sizes. This has, in fact, been done using *t* values. A table of the *t* distribution is available in Appendix C. Tables have been developed using this strategy to organize the statistical outcomes for many statistical procedures from various sample sizes. Because listing all possible outcomes would require many pages, most tables include only those values that have a low probability of occurring in the present theoretical population. These probabilities are expressed as *alpha* (α), commonly referred to as the *level of significance,* and as beta (β), the probability of a Type II error.

Using the appropriate sampling distribution, one could determine the probability of obtaining a specific statistical result if two samples being studied were really from the same population. Statistical analysis makes an inference that the samples being tested can be considered part of the population from which the sampling distribution was developed. This inference is expressed as a null hypothesis.

STATISTICS AND PARAMETERS, SAMPLES AND POPULATIONS

The use of the terms *statistic* and *parameter* can be confusing because of the various populations referred to in statistical theory. A *statistic* ($\overline{X}$) is a numerical value obtained from a sample. A *parameter* is a true (but unknown) numerical characteristic of a population. For example, μ is the population mean or arithmetical average. The mean of the sampling distribution (mean of samples' means) can be shown to also be equal to μ. Thus, a numerical value that is the mean of the sample is a statistic; a numerical value that is the mean of the population is a parameter (Barnett, 1982).

Relating a statistic to a parameter requires an inference as one moves from the sample to the

sampling distribution and then from the sampling distribution to the population. The population referred to is in one sense real (concrete) and in another sense abstract. These ideas are illustrated thusly:

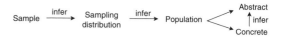

For example, perhaps you are interested in the cholesterol level of women in the United States. Your population is women in the United States. Obviously, you cannot measure the cholesterol level of every woman in the United States; therefore, you select a sample of women from this population. Since you wish your sample to be as representative of the population as possible, you obtain your sample using random sampling techniques. In order to determine whether the cholesterol levels in your sample are like those in the population, you must compare the sample with the population. One strategy would be to compare the mean of your sample with the mean of the entire population. Unfortunately, it is highly unlikely that you *know* the mean of the entire population. Therefore, you must make an estimate of the mean of that population. You need to know how good your sample statistics are as estimators of the parameters of the population.

First, you make some assumptions. You assume that the mean scores of cholesterol levels from multiple randomly selected samples of this population would be normally distributed. Implied by this assumption is another assumption: that the cholesterol levels of the population will be distributed according to the theoretical normal curve—that difference scores and standard deviations can be equated to those in the normal curve.

If you assume that the population in your study is normally distributed, you can also assume that this population can be represented by a normal sampling distribution. Thus, you infer from your sample to the sampling distribution, the mathematically developed theoretical population made up of parameters such as the mean of means and the standard error. The parameters of this theoretical population are those measures of the dimensions identified in the sampling distribution. You can then infer from the sampling distribution to the population. You have both a concrete population and an abstract population. The concrete population are all of those individuals that meet your sampling criteria. The abstract population are those individuals that will meet your sampling criteria in the future or those groups addressed theoretically by your framework.

ESTIMATION OF PARAMETERS

There are two approaches to estimating the parameters of a population: point estimation and interval estimation.

Point Estimation

A statistic that produces a value as a function of the scores in a sample is called an *estimator*. Much of inferential statistical analysis involves the use of *point estimation* to evaluate the fit between the estimator (a statistic) and the population parameter. A point estimate is a single figure that estimates a related figure in the population of interest. The best point estimator of the population mean is the mean of the sample being examined. However, the mean of the sample rarely equals the mean of the population. In addition to the mean, other commonly used estimators include the median, variance, standard deviation, and correlation coefficient.

Interval Estimation

When sampling from a continuous distribution, the probability of the sample mean being exactly equal to the population mean is zero. Therefore, we know we are going to be in error if we use point estimators. The difference between the sample estimate and the true but unknown parameter value is sampling error. The source of sampling error is the fact that we did not count every individual in the population. Sampling error is due to chance and chance alone. It is not due to some flaw in the researcher's methodology. Interval estimation is an attempt to overcome this problem

by controlling the initial precision of an estimator. An interval procedure that gives a 95% confidence will produce a set of intervals 95% of which will include the true value of the parameter. Unfortunately, after a sample is drawn and the estimate is calculated, there is no way to tell whether the interval contains the true value of the parameter.

An *interval estimate* is a segment of a number line (or range of scores) where the value of the parameter is thought to be. For example, using a sample with a mean of 40 and a standard deviation of 5, one might use the range of scores between 2 standard deviations below the mean to 2 standard deviations above the mean (30,50) as the interval estimation. This provides a set of scores rather than a single score. However, there is no absolute certainty that the mean of the population lies within that range. Therefore, it is necessary to determine the probability that this interval estimate contains the population mean.

This need to determine probability brings us back to the sampling distribution. We know that 95% of the means in the sampling distribution lies within 2 standard deviations of the mean of means (the population mean). If these scores are converted to Z scores, the unit normal distribution table can be used to determine how many standard deviations out from the mean of means one must go to ensure a specified probability (e.g., 70%, 95%, or 99%) of obtaining an interval estimate that includes the population parameter that is estimated.

Examining the normal distribution (see Figure 16–2), one finds that 2.5% of the area under the normal curve lies below a Z score of -1.96, or $\mu - (1.96\ SD/\sqrt{N})$, and 2.5% of the area lies above a Z score of 1.96, or $\mu + (1.96\ SD/\sqrt{N})$, where μ is the mean of means, SD is the standard deviation and N is the sample size. The probability is .95 that a randomly selected sample would have a mean within this range. The calculation of confidence intervals is explained in Chapter 17.

DEGREES OF FREEDOM

The concept of *degrees of freedom* (*df*) is a product of statistical theory and is easier to calculate than it is to explain because of the complex mathematics involved in demonstrating the justification for the concept. Degrees of freedom involves the freedom of a score's value to vary given the other existing scores' values and the established sum of these scores.

A simple example may provide beginning insight into the concept. Suppose difference scores are obtained from a sample of 4 and the mean is 4. The difference scores are -2, -1, $+1$, and $+2$. As with all difference scores, the sum of these scores is 0. As a result, if any three of the difference scores are calculated, the value of the fourth score is not free to vary. Its value will depend on the values of the other three in order to maintain a mean of 4 and a sum of 0. The degree of freedom in this example is three, since only three scores are free to vary. In this case and in many other analyses, degree of freedom is the sample size (N) minus 1 ($N - 1$).

$$df = N - 1$$

In this example, $df = 4 - 1 = 3$ (Roscoe, 1969, p. 162). In some analyses, determination of levels of significance on tables of statistical sampling distributions requires knowledge of the degrees of freedom.

TAILEDNESS

On the normal curve, extremes of statistical values can occur at either end of the curve. Because this is true, the 5% of statistical values that are considered statistically significant according to decision theory must be distributed between the two extremes of the curve. The extremes of the curve are referred to as *tails*. If the hypothesis is nondirectional and assumes that an extreme score can occur in either tail, the analysis is referred to as a *two-tailed test of significance* (see Figure 16–3).

In a *one-tailed test of significance*, the hypothesis is directional, and extreme statistical values that occur on a single tail of the curve are of interest. Developing a one-tailed hypothesis requires sufficient knowledge of the variables and their interaction on which to base a one-tailed test. Otherwise, the one-tailed test is inappropriate. This knowledge may be theoretical or from previous research. (Refer to Chapter 8 for formulating hypotheses.) One-tailed tests are uniformly more

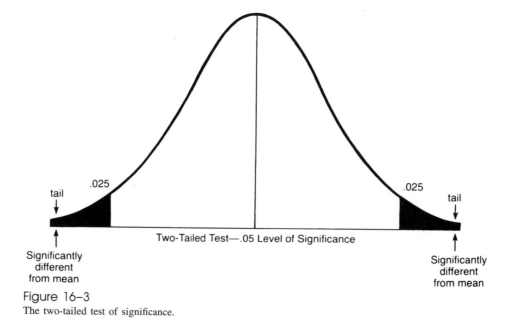

Figure 16–3

The two-tailed test of significance.

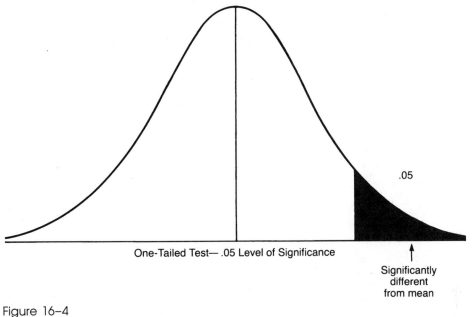

.05

One-Tailed Test— .05 Level of Significance

Significantly
different
from mean

Figure 16–4
The one-tailed test of significance.

powerful than two-tailed tests, increasing the possibility of rejecting the null hypothesis. In this case, extreme statistical values occurring on the other tail of the curve are not considered significantly different. In Figure 16–4, which is a one-tailed figure, the portion of the curve where statistical values will be considered significant is in the right tail of the curve.

TYPE I AND TYPE II ERRORS

According to decision theory, two types of error can occur in making decisions about the meaning of a value obtained from a statistical test: Type I errors and Type II errors. A *Type I error* occurs when the null hypothesis is rejected when it is true. This error is possible because even though statistical values in the extreme ends of the tail of the curve are rare, they do occur within the population. In viewing Table 16–2, remember that the null hypothesis states that there is no difference or no association between groups.

There is a greater risk of a Type I error with a .05 level of significance than with a .01 level of significance. As the level of significance becomes more extreme, the risk of a Type I error decreases, as illustrated in Figure 16–5. For example, suppose you studied the effect of a treatment in an experimental study using two groups and found that the difference between the two groups was relatively equivalent in magnitude to the standard error. The sampling distribution of the difference between group means tells you that even if there is no real difference between the groups, a difference as large or larger than the one you detected would occur by chance about once in every three times. That is, the difference that you found is just what you could expect to occur if the true treatment effect were zero. This does not mean that the true difference is zero, but that on the basis of the results of the study, you would not be justified in claiming there is a real difference between the groups. The data from your samples do not establish a case for the position that a true treatment effect exists.

Suppose, on the other hand, that you find that the difference in your groups is over twice its stan-

Table 16–2
Occurrence of Type I and Type II Errors

Data Analysis Indicates	In Reality the Null Hypothesis Is	
	True	*False*
results significant null rejected	Type I error	correct decision (power)
results not significant null not rejected	correct decision	Type II error

dard error (Z score > 1.96). (Examine the Z scores in Figure 16–2.) A treatment difference of this magnitude would occur by chance less than one time in 20, and we say that these results are statistically significant at the .05 level. A difference of more than 2.6 times the standard error would occur by chance less than one time in 100, and we say that the difference is statistically significant at the .01 level. Cox (1958) states, "Significance tests, from this point of view, measure the adequacy of the data to support the qualitative conclusion that there is a true effect in the direction of the apparent difference" (p. 159). Thus, the decision is a judgment and can be in error. The level of statistical significance attained is an indication of the degree of uncertainty in taking the position that the difference between the two groups is real.

A *Type II error* occurs when the null hypothe-

sis is regarded as true when, in fact, it is false. This type of error occurs because in some cases there is some degree of overlap between the values of different populations, so that a value with a greater than 5% probability of being within one population may in fact be within the dimensions of another population (see Figure 16–6).

As the risk of a Type I error decreases (by setting a more extreme level of significance), the risk of a Type II error increases. When the risk of a Type II error is decreased (by setting a less extreme level of significance), the risk of a Type I error increases. It is not possible to decrease both types of error simultaneously without a corresponding increase in sample size. Therefore, the researcher needs to decide which risk poses the greatest threat within a specific study. In nursing research, many studies are conducted with small

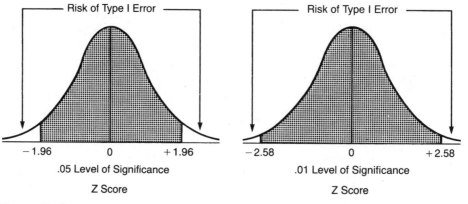

Risk of Type I Error

−1.96   0   +1.96

.05 Level of Significance

Z Score

Risk of Type I Error

−2.58   0   +2.58

.01 Level of Significance

Z Score

Figure 16–5
Risk of Type I error.

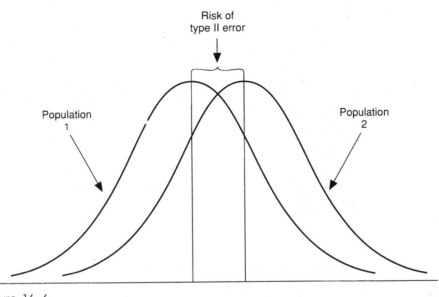

Figure 16–6
Risk of Type II error.

samples and instruments that are not precise measures of the variables under study. In many nursing situations, multiple variables also interact to lead to differences within populations. However, when one is examining only a few of the interacting variables, small differences can be overlooked, leading to a false conclusion of no differences between the samples. In this case, the risk of a Type II error is a greater concern, and a more lenient level of significance is in order.

As an example of the concerns related to error, consider the following problem. If you were to obtain three samples using the same methodology, each sample would have a different mean. Yet you need to make a decision to accept or reject the null hypothesis. The null hypothesis states that the population mean is 50 and that the three samples below are all from the same population. Assume you obtain the following results:

Sample Size	Sample Mean
$N = 50$ subjects	$\bar{X} = 52.0$
$N = 50$ subjects	$\bar{X} = 60.5$
$N = 50$ subjects	$\bar{X} = 52.2$

How much evidence would it take to convince you to switch from believing the null hypothesis to believing the alternate hypothesis? Will you choose correctly or will you make a Type I or a Type II error?

LEVEL OF SIGNIFICANCE— CONTROLLING THE RISK OF A TYPE I ERROR

The formal definition of the *level of significance* (α) is the probability of making a Type I error when the null hypothesis is true. The level of significance, developed from decision theory, is the cutoff point used to determine whether the samples being tested are members of the same population or from different populations. The decision criteria are based on the selected level of significance and the sampling distribution of the mean. For this, the assumption is made that the sampling distribution of the mean is normally distributed. As mentioned previously, 68% of the means from samples in a population will fall within 1 standard deviation from the mean of means (μ), 95% will fall within 2 standard deviations, 99% within 3 standard deviations, and 99.9% within 4 standard deviations. This decision theory explanation of the expected distribution of means is equivalent to the confidence interval explanation described previously. It is simply expressed differently. In keeping with decision theory, the level of significance sought in a statistical test must be established prior to conducting the test. In fact, the significance level needs to be established prior to collecting the data. In nursing studies, the level of significance is usually set at .05 or .01. However, in preliminary studies, it might be prudent to select a less stringent level of significance, such as .10.

If one wishes to predict with a 95% probability of accuracy, the level of significance would be $p \leq 1 - .95$ or $p \leq .05$. The mathematical symbol $\leq$ means "less than or equal to." Thus, $p \leq .05$ means there is a probability less than or equal to 5% of getting a test statistic at least as extreme as the calculated test statistic if the null hypothesis is true.

In computer analysis, the observed level of significance (p-value) obtained from the data is frequently provided on the printout. For example, the actual level of significance might be $p \leq .03$ or $p \leq .07$. This level of significance should be provided in the research report as well as the level of significance set prior to the analysis. This allows other researchers to make their own judgment of the significance of your findings.

POWER—CONTROLLING THE RISK OF A TYPE II ERROR

Power is the probability that a statistical test will detect a significant difference that exists. Often, reported studies failing to reject the null hypothesis (in which power is unlikely to have been examined) will have only a 10% power level to detect a difference if one exists. An 80% power level is desirable. Until recently, the researcher's primary interest was in preventing a Type I error. Therefore, great emphasis was placed on the selection of a level of significance but little on power. This

point of view is changing as we recognize the seriousness of a Type II error in nursing studies.

A Type II error occurs when the null hypothesis is not rejected by the study even though a difference actually exists between groups. If the null hypothesis assumes no difference between the groups, the difference score in the measure of the dependent variable between groups would be zero. In a two-sample study, this would be expressed mathematically as $A - B = 0$. The research hypothesis would be stated as $A - B \neq 0$ where ($\neq$) means "not equal to." A Type II error occurs when the difference score is not zero but is small enough that it is not detected by the statistical analyses. In some cases, the difference is negligible and not of interest clinically. However, in other cases, the difference in reality is greater than is indicated. This undetected difference is often due to research methodology problems.

Type II errors can occur for three reasons: (1) a stringent level of significance, (2) a small sample size, and (3) a small difference in measured effect between the groups. Difference in measured effect is due to a number of factors, including a large variation in scores on the dependent variable within groups, crude instrumentation that does not measure with precision (e.g., does not detect small changes in the variable and thus leads to a small detectable effect size), and/or confounding or extraneous variables that mask the effects of the variables under study.

You can determine the risk of a Type II error through *power analysis* and modify the study to decrease the risk if necessary. Cohen (1988) has identified four parameters of power: (1) significance level, (2) sample size, (3) effect size (ES), and (4) power. If three of the four are known, the fourth can be calculated using power analysis formulas. Significance level and sample size are fairly straightforward. *Effect size* is "the degree to which the phenomenon is present in the population, or the degree to which the null hypothesis is false" (Cohen, 1988, pp. 9–10). For example, if one were measuring changes in anxiety levels, measured first when the patient is at home and then just prior to surgery, effect size would be large if a great change in anxiety was expected.

If only a small change in the level of anxiety was expected, the effect size would be small.

Small effect sizes require larger samples to detect these small differences. If the power is too low, it may not be worthwhile conducting the study unless a large sample can be obtained because statistical tests are unlikely to detect differences that exist. Deciding to conduct a study in these circumstances is costly in time and money, cannot add to the body of nursing knowledge, and can actually lead to false conclusions. Power analysis can be used to determine the sample size necessary for a particular study. This use of power analysis is discussed in Chapter 12. Power analysis can be calculated using a program in NCSS (Number Crunchers Statistical System) called PASS (Power Analysis and Sample Size). Sample size can also be calculated by a program called EX-SAMPLE produced by Idea Works, Inc. (Brent, Scott, & Spencer, 1988). SPSS for Windows also now has the capacity to perform power analyses. Yarandi (1994) provides the commands needed to perform power analyses for comparing two binomial proportions using SAS.

The power analysis should be reported in studies that fail to reject the null hypothesis. Results of power analysis should be presented in the results section of the study. If power is high, it strengthens the meaning of the findings. If power is low, the researcher needs to address this in the discussion of implications. The modifications in the research methodology that resulted from the use of power analysis also need to be reported.

CLINICAL SIGNIFICANCE

The findings of a study can be statistically significant but may not be clinically significant. For example, one group of patients might have a body temperature .1°F higher than that of another group. Data analysis might indicate that the two groups are statistically significantly different. However, the findings have no clinical significance. In studies, it is often important to know the magnitude of the difference between groups. However, a statistical test that indicates significant differences between groups (as in a *t*-test) provides no information on the magnitude of the difference. The extent of the level of significance (.01 or .0001) tells you nothing about the magnitude of the difference between the groups. These differences can best be determined through descriptive or exploratory analysis of the data (see Chapter 17).

PARAMETRIC AND NONPARAMETRIC STATISTICAL ANALYSES

The most commonly used statistical analyses are *parametric statistics*. The analyses are referred to as parametric because the findings are inferred to the parameters of a normally distributed population. These approaches to analysis emerged from the work of Fisher and require meeting the following three assumptions before they can justifiably be used: (1) The sample was drawn from a population for which the variance can be calculated. The distribution is usually expected to be normal or approximately normal (Conover, 1971). (2) Because most parametric techniques deal with continuous variables rather than discrete variables, the level of measurement should be interval data or ordinal data with an approximately normal distribution. (3) The data can be treated as random samples (Box, Hunter, & Hunter, 1978).

Nonparametric, or distribution-free, techniques can be used in studies that do not meet the first two assumptions just listed. However, the data still need to be treated as random samples. Most nonparametric techniques are not as powerful as their parametric counterparts. In other words, nonparametric techniques are less able to detect differences and have a greater risk of a Type II error if the data meet the assumptions of parametric procedures. However, if these assumptions are not met, nonparametric procedures are more powerful. The techniques can be used with cruder forms of measurement than are required for parametric analyses. In recent years, there has been a greater tolerance to using parametric techniques when some of the assumptions were not met, recognizing that the analyses were robust to moderate violation of the assumptions. Robust means that the analysis will yield accurate results even if some of the assumptions are violated by the data used for the analysis. However, one needs to carefully think through the consequences of violating the assumptions of a statistical procedure. The validity of the results diminishes as the violation of assumptions becomes more extreme.

CAUSALITY AND RELATIONSHIPS

Correlational analyses provide important information about relationships within samples and populations. In addition to clarifying the relationships among theoretical concepts, correlational analyses can assist in identifying causal relationships that can then be tested using inferential analyses. In any situation involving causality, a relationship will exist between the factors involved in the causal process. Therefore, the first clue to the possibility of a causal link is the existence of a relationship. But a relationship does not mean causality. Two variables can be highly correlated but have no causal relationship whatsoever. However, as the strength of a relationship increases, the possibility of a causal link increases. The absence of a relationship precludes the possibility of a causal connection between the two variables being examined, given adequate measurement of the variables and the absence of other variables that might mask the relationship. Thus, a correlational study can be the first step in determining the dynamics important to nursing practice within a particular population. The best-known example of this case is the multitude of studies relating smoking to cancer. Determining these dynamics can allow us to increase our ability to predict and control the situation studied, whether or not we can ever clearly prove definite causal links (Kenny, 1979). However, correlation cannot be used alone to demonstrate causality.

■ SUMMARY

To critique a study, the nurse needs to be able to identify the statistical procedures used; judge whether these statistical procedures were appropriate to the hypotheses, questions, or objectives of the study and to the data available for the analysis; comprehend the discussion of data analysis results; judge whether the author's interpretation of the results is appropriate; and evaluate the clinical significance of the findings. The neophyte researcher performing a quantitative study is confronted with multiple critical decisions related to data analysis that require statistical knowledge. Statistics can be used for a variety of purposes, including to (1) summarize, (2) explore the meaning of deviations in the data, (3) compare or contrast descriptively, (4) test the proposed relationships in a theoretical model, (5) infer that the findings from the sample are indicative of the entire population, (6) examine causality, (7) predict, or (8) infer from the sample to a theoretical model.

The role of statistics can be divided into two parts: exploratory data analysis and confirmatory data analysis. Exploratory data analysis is performed to get a preliminary vision of the nature of the data and to search the data for hidden structure or models. Confirmatory data analysis involves traditional inferential statistics that assist the researcher to make an inference about a population or a process based on evidence from the study sample. There are several stages to quantitative data analysis: (1) preparation of the data for analysis; (2) description of the sample; (3) testing the reliability of measurement; (4) exploratory analysis of the data; (5) confirmatory analyses guided by the hypotheses, questions, or objectives; and (6) post hoc analyses.

The selection of a statistical procedure to

continued

continued

analyze a particular set of data in relation to a specific hypothesis, question, or objective is not straightforward. Rarely can one identify a single procedure that is the only right approach to analyzing a particular set of data. Knowledge of statistical procedures and their assumptions regarding the data is necessary for the selection of appropriate statistical procedures.

The procedures of statistical analyses are based on statistical and mathematical theory. As is common in many theories, theoretical ideas related to statistics are expressed using unique terminology and logic that is unfamiliar to many. Evaluating the results of published research, developing a data analysis plan, and interpreting the results of a study require that you understand the language and logic of statistics. Inductive logic is used by statisticians to make inferences about the data. Probability theory addresses analyses from the perspective of explaining the likelihood of an event or the degree of a relationship. Decision theory is used when testing for differences between groups. A cutoff point is identified that will guide the decision of whether or not the groups are members of the same population. The cutoff point is the level of significance or alpha (α).

The theoretical normal curve, a product of mathematical theory, is symmetrical, unimodal, and has continuous values. The mean, median, and mode are equal. A sampling distribution is developed using statistical values of many samples obtained from the same population. The mean of a sampling distribution of means is referred to as the mean of means (μ). The purpose of the sampling distribution is to allow us to measure sampling error, which is the difference between the sample statistic used to estimate a parameter and the actual but unknown value of the parameter. Just as it is possible to develop distributions

of summary statistics within a population, it is possible to develop distributions of inferential statistical outcomes. For example, a sampling distribution could be developed by testing for differences in the means using a *t* test.

Standardized scores have been developed to facilitate comparison of a score in one distribution with a score in another distribution. Raw scores are transformed into standard scores to allow an easy conceptual grasp of the meaning of the score.

A statistic like $\overline{X}$ is a numerical value obtained from a sample. The parameter (μ) refers to that same true (but unknown) value within a population. Relating a statistic to a parameter requires an inference as one moves from the sample to the sampling distribution and then from the sampling distribution to the population.

A statistic that produces a value as a function of the scores in a sample is called an estimator. Much of inferential statistical analysis involves the use of point estimation to evaluate the fit between the estimator (a statistic) and the population parameter. A point estimate is a single figure that estimates the related figure in the population of interest. Three characteristics of the estimator are considered important: (1) unbiasedness, (2) consistency, and (3) relative efficiency. The mean of the sample is the most unbiased estimator. When sampling from a continuous distribution, that is, one with either an interval or ratio scale, the probability of the sample mean being exactly equal to the population mean is equal to zero. Therefore, we know we are going to be in error if we use point estimators. Interval estimation is an attempt to overcome this problem by controlling the initial precision of an estimator. An interval estimate is a segment of a number line where the value of the parameter is thought to be.

The concept of degrees of freedom (*df*) in-

continued

continued

volves the freedom of a score's value to vary given the other existing scores' values and the established sum of these scores. On the normal curve, extremes of statistical values can occur at either end of the curve. Because this is true, the 5% of statistical values that are considered statistically significant must be distributed between the two extremes of the curve. The extremes of the curve are referred to as tails. If the hypothesis is nondirectional and assumes that an extreme score can occur in either tail, the analysis is referred to as a two-tailed test of significance. In a one-tailed test of significance, the hypothesis is directional, and extreme statistical values that occur in a single tail of the curve are of interest.

Two types of error can occur in making decisions about the meaning of a value obtained from a statistical test: Type I errors and Type II errors. A Type I error occurs when the researcher concludes that the samples tested are from different populations (there is a significant difference between groups) when, in fact, the samples are from the same population (there is no significant difference between groups). A Type II error occurs when the researcher concludes that the samples are from the same population when, in fact, they are from different populations. As the risk of a Type I error decreases (by setting a more extreme level of significance), the risk of a Type II error increases. When the risk of a Type II error is decreased (by setting a less extreme level of significance), the risk of a Type I error increases. It is not possible to decrease both types of error simultaneously without increasing the sample size. Therefore, the researcher needs to decide which risk poses the greatest threat within a specific study.

The formal definition of the level of significance or alpha (α) is the probability of making a Type I error when the null hypothesis is true. The level of significance, developed from decision theory, is the cutoff point used to determine whether the samples being tested are members of the same population or from different populations. Power is the probability that a statistical test will detect a significant difference that exists. Many studies do not have the power to detect differences resulting in a Type II error. The strategy used to determine the Type II error risk is power analysis.

When a statistical test determines that there are significant differences between groups, the researcher has no information on the magnitude of the difference. Magnitude estimation is a strategy to estimate the degree of difference between groups.

Both parametric and nonparametric techniques are valuable methods to analyze data. The choice of technique is determined by the type of data available for analysis. The most commonly used procedures are parametric statistics. The three assumptions of parametric statistics are (1) the sample was drawn from a population for which the variance can be calculated, (2) the level of measurement should provide interval data or ordinal data with an approximately normal distribution, and (3) random sampling techniques were used to obtain the sample. Nonparametric techniques are not as powerful as parametric techniques but can be used with cruder forms of measurement that yield nominal or ordinal data. Correlational analyses provide important information about relationships within samples and populations. In addition to clarifying the relationship among theoretical concepts, correlational analyses can assist in identifying causal relationships that can then be tested using inferential analyses.

References

Barnett, V. (1982). *Comparative statistical inference.* New York: Wiley.

Box, G. E. P., Hunter, W. G., & Hunter, J. S. (1978). *Statistics for experimenters.* New York: Wiley.

Brent, E. E., Jr., Scott, J. K., & Spencer, J. C. (1988). *Ex-Sample™: An expert system to assist in designing sampling plans. User's guide and reference manual,* Version 2.0. The Idea Works, Inc., 100 West Briarwood, Columbia, Missouri 65203.

Chervany, N. L. (1977). *The logic and practice of statistics.* Written materials provided with a presentation at the Institute of Management Science. Bloomington, MN, Dec. 15, 1977.

Cohen, J. (1988). *Statistical power analysis for the behavioral sciences* (2nd ed.). New York: Academic Press.

Conover, W. J. (1971). *Practical nonparametric statistics.* New York: Wiley.

Cox, D. R. (1958). *Planning of experiments.* New York: Wiley.

Good, I. J. (1983). *Good thinking: The foundations of probability and its applications.* Minneapolis: University of Minnesota Press.

Hinshaw, A. S., & Schepp, K. (1984). Problems in doing nursing research: How to recognize garbage when you see it! *Western Journal of Nursing Research, 6*(1), 126–130.

Kenny, D. A. (1979). *Correlation and causality.* New York: Wiley.

Roscoe, J. T. (1969). *Fundamental research statistics for the behavioral sciences.* New York: Holt, Rinehart and Winston.

Slakter, M. J., Wu, Y. B., & Suzuki-Slakter, N. S. (1991). *, **, and ***, statistical nonsense at the .00000 level. *Nursing Research, 40*(4), 248–249.

Tukey, J. W. (1977). *Exploratory data analysis.* Reading, MA: Addison-Wesley.

Volicer, B. J. (1984). *Multivariate statistics for nursing research.* New York: Grune & Stratton.

Yarandi, H. N. (1994). Using the SAS system to estimate sample size and power for comparing two binomial proportions. *Nursing Research, 43*(2), 124–125.

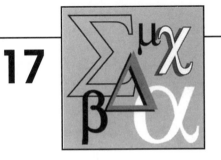

17

Descriptive and Exploratory Analyses

Data analysis begins with descriptive statistics in any study in which the data are numerical, including some qualitative studies. *Descriptive statistics* allow the researcher to organize the data in ways that give meaning and facilitate insight, to examine a phenomenon from a variety of angles in order to understand more clearly what is being seen. Theory development and generation of hypotheses can emerge from descriptive analyses. For some descriptive studies, descriptive statistics will be the only approach to analysis of the data. This chapter will describe two approaches to descriptive analysis: summary statistics and exploratory data analysis (EDA). Summary statistics presented include frequency distributions, measures of central tendency, measures of dispersion, the shape of distributions, standardized scores, and confidence intervals. EDA techniques described include stem-and-leaf displays, identification and analysis of residuals, plots of relationship, Q-plots, box-and-whiskers plots, and symmetry plots.

SUMMARY STATISTICS

FREQUENCY DISTRIBUTIONS

Frequency distributions are usually the first strategy used to organize the data for examination. In addition, frequency distributions are used to check for errors in coding and computer programming. There are two types of frequency distributions: ungrouped frequency distributions and grouped frequency distributions. In addition to providing a means to display the data, these distributions may

influence decisions concerning further analysis of the data.

Ungrouped Frequency Distribution

Most studies have some categorical data that are presented in the form of ungrouped frequency distributions. To develop an ungrouped frequency distribution, list all categories of that variable on which you have data and tally each datum on the listing. For example, the categories of pets in the homes of elderly clients might include dogs, cats, birds, and rabbits. A tally of the ungrouped frequencies would have the following appearance:

Dogs   ~~////~~ ~~////~~ ~~////~~ ////
Cats   ~~////~~ ~~////~~ ~~////~~ ~~////~~ ~~////~~ ///
Birds   ~~////~~ ~~////~~ ///
Rabbits //

The tally marks are then counted, and a table is developed to display the results. This approach is generally used on discrete rather than continuous data. Examples of data commonly organized in this manner include gender, ethnicity, marital status, and diagnostic category. Continuous data, such as test grades or scores on a data collection instrument, could be organized in this manner; however, if the number of possible scores is large, it is difficult to extract meaning from examination of the distribution.

Grouped Frequency Distribution

Some method of grouping is generally necessary when continuous variables are being examined.

Age, for example, is a continuous variable. Many measures taken during data collection are continuous, including income, temperature, vital lung capacity, weight, scale scores, and time. Grouping requires that the researcher make a number of decisions that will be important to the meaning derived from the data.

Any method of grouping results in loss of information. For example, if age is being grouped, a breakdown of under 65–over 65 will provide considerably less information than grouping by 10-year spans. The grouping should be made to provide the greatest possible meaning in terms of the purpose of the study. If the data are to be compared with data in other studies, groupings should be similar to those of other studies in that field of research.

The first step in developing a grouped frequency distribution is to establish a method of classifying the data. The classes that are developed must be exhaustive; each datum must fit into one of the identified classes. The classes must be mutually exclusive; each datum can fit into only one of the established classes. A common mistake is to list ranges that contain overlaps. The range of each category must be equivalent. In the case of age, for example, if 10 years is the range, each category must include 10 years of ages. The first and last categories may be open-ended and worded to include all scores above or below a specified point. The precision with which the data will be reported is an important consideration. For example, data might be listed only in whole numbers, or decimals may be used. If decimals are used, you will need to decide at how many decimal places rounding off will be performed.

Percentage Distributions

Percentage distributions indicate the percent of the sample whose scores fall in a specific group as well as the number of scores in that group. Percentage distributions are particularly useful in comparing the present data with findings from other studies that have varying sample sizes. A cumulative distribution is a type of percentage distribution in which the percentages and frequencies

Table 17–1
Example of a Cumulative Frequency Table

Score	Frequency	Percent	Cumulative Frequency (f)	Cumulative Percent
1	4	8	4	8
3	6	12	10	20
4	8	16	18	36
5	14	28	32	64
7	8	16	40	80
8	6	12	46	92
9	4	8	$N = 50$	100

of scores are summed as one moves from the top of the table to the bottom (or the reverse). Thus, the bottom category would have a cumulative frequency equivalent to the sample size and a cumulative percentage of 100 (see Table 17–1). Frequency distributions can be displayed using tables, diagrams, or graphs. Four types of illustrations are commonly used: pie diagrams, bar graphs, histograms, and frequency polygons. Some examples of diagrams and graphs are presented in Chapter 23. Frequency analysis and graphic presentation of the results can be performed on the computer.

MEASURES OF CENTRAL TENDENCY

A *measure of central tendency* is frequently referred to as an average. The term *average* is a lay term not commonly used in statistics because of its vagueness. The measures of central tendency are the most concise statement of the location of the data. The three measures of central tendency commonly used in statistical analyses are the mode, median, and mean.

Mode

The *mode* is the numerical value or score that occurs with greatest frequency; it does not necessarily indicate the center of the data set. The mode can be determined by examination of an ungrouped frequency distribution of the data. In Table 17–1, the mode is the score of 5, which occurred 14 times in the data set. The mode can be used to describe the typical subject, or to identify the most frequently occurring value on a scale item. The mode is the appropriate measure of central tendency for nominal data and is used in the calculation of some nonparametric statistics. Otherwise, it is seldom used in statistical analyses. A data set can have more than one mode. If two modes exist, the data set is referred to as bimodal. More than two would be multimodal.

Median

The *median* is the score at the exact center of the ungrouped frequency distribution. It is the 50th percentile. The median is obtained by rank ordering the scores. If there are an uneven number of scores, exactly 50% of the scores are above the median, and 50% are below the median. If there are an even number of scores, the median is the average of the two middle scores. Thus, the median may not be an actual score in the data set. The median is not considered to be as precise an estimator of the population mean when sampling from normal populations as is the sample mean. In most other cases, it is actually the preferred choice because in these cases it is a more precise measure of central tendency. The median is not affected by extreme scores in the data (outliers), as is the mean. The median is the most appropriate measure of central tendency for ordinal data and is frequently used in nonparametric analyses.

Mean

The most commonly used measure of central tendency is the mean. The *mean* is the sum of the scores divided by the number of scores being summed. Thus, like the median, the mean may not be a member of the data set. The formula for calculating the mean is listed below.

$$\overline{X} = \frac{\Sigma X}{N}$$

where:

$\overline{X}$ = the mean
Σ = sigma (the statistical symbol for the process of summation)
X = a single raw score
N = number of scores being entered in the calculation

The mean was calculated for the data provided in Table 17–1.

$$\overline{X} = \frac{4 + 18 + 32 + 70 + 56 + 48 + 36}{50} = \frac{264}{50} = 5.28$$

The mean is an appropriate measure of central tendency for approximately normally distributed populations. This formula will be found repeatedly within more complex formulas of statistical analyses.

MEASURES OF DISPERSION

Measures of dispersion, or variability, are measures of individual differences of the members of the population and sample. They give some indication of how scores in a sample are dispersed around the mean. These measures provide information about the data not available from measures of central tendency. They indicate how different the scores are—the extent to which individual scores deviate from one another. If the individual scores are similar, measures of variability are small and the sample is relatively *homogeneous* in terms of those scores. *Heterogeneity* (wide variation in scores) is important in some statistical procedures, such as correlation. Heterogeneity is determined by measures of variability. The measures most commonly used are modal percentage, range, difference scores, sum of squares, variance, and the standard deviation.

Modal Percentage

The *modal percentage* is the only measure of variability appropriate for use with nominal data. It

Table 17–2
Data for Calculation of Mean and Standard Deviation

Score X	Frequency (f)	fX	fX^2	
1	4	4	4 (1) =	4
3	6	18	6 (9) =	54
4	8	32	8 (16) =	128
5	14	70	14 (25) =	350
7	8	56	8 (49) =	392
8	6	48	6 (64) =	384
9	4	36	4 (81) =	324
	$N = 50$	$\Sigma X = 264$	$\Sigma X^2 = 1636$	

indicates the relationship of the number of data scores represented by the mode to the total number of data scores. To determine the modal percentage, the frequency of the modal scores is divided by the total number of scores. For example, in Table 17–2, the mode is 5, 14 of the subjects scored 5, and the sample size is 50; thus, 14/50 = .28. The result of that operation is then multiplied by 100 to convert it to a percentage. In the example given, the modal percentage would be 28%, which means that 28% of the sample is represented by the mode. The complete calculation would be 14/50(100) = 28%. This strategy allows comparison of the present data with other data sets.

Range

The simplest measure of dispersion is the *range*. The range is obtained by subtracting the lowest score from the highest score. The range for the scores in Table 17–2 is calculated as follows: 9 − 1 = 8. The range is a difference score, which uses only the two extreme scores for the comparison. It is a very crude measure and is sensitive to outliers. Outliers are subjects with extreme scores that are widely separated from scores of the rest of the subjects. The range is generally reported but is not used in further analyses. It is not a very useful method of comparing the present data with that from other studies.

Difference Scores

Difference scores are obtained by subtracting the mean from each score. Sometimes a difference score is referred to as a deviation score since it indicates the extent to which a score deviates from the mean. The difference score will be positive when the score is above the mean and negative when the score is below the mean. Difference scores are the basis for many statistical analyses and can be found within many statistical equations. The sum of difference scores is zero, making the sum a useless measure. The formula for difference scores is:

$$X - \overline{X}$$

The Sum of Squares

A common strategy used to allow meaningful mathematical manipulation of difference scores is to square them. These squared scores are then summed. The mathematical symbol for the operation of summing is Σ. When negative scores are squared, they become positive. Because of this, the sum will no longer equal zero. This mathematical maneuver is referred to as the *sum of squares* (*SS*). In this case, the *SS* is actually the sum of squared deviations. The equation for *SS* is:

$$SS = \Sigma(X - \overline{X})^2$$

The larger the value of *SS*, the greater the variance. Because the value of *SS* is dependent on the measurement scale used to obtain the original scores, comparison of *SS* with the sum of squares obtained in other studies is limited to studies using similar data. The sum of squares is a valuable measure of variance and is used in many complex statistical equations. The *SS* importance is due to the fact that when deviations from the mean are squared, the sum is smaller than the sum of squared deviations from any other value in a sample distribution. This is referred to as the *least-squares principle* and is important in mathematical manipulations.

Variance

The *variance* is another measure commonly used in statistical analyses. The equation for variance (*V*) is:

$$V = \frac{\Sigma(X - \bar{X})^2}{N - 1}$$

As can be seen, the variance is the mean or average of the sum of squares. Again, because the result is dependent upon the measurement scale used, it has no absolute value and can be compared only with data obtained using similar measures. However, in general, the larger the variance, the larger the dispersion of scores (Shelley, 1984).

Standard Deviation

The *standard deviation* (*SD*) is simply the square root of the variance. This is an important step mathematically because squaring mathematical terms changes them in some important ways. Obtaining the square root reverses this change. The equation for obtaining the *SD* is:

$$SD = \sqrt{\frac{\Sigma(X - \bar{X})^2}{N - 1}}$$

Although this equation clarifies the relationships among difference scores, sum of squares, and variance, using it requires that all these measures in turn be calculated. If the *SD* is being calculated directly by hand (or with the use of a calculator), the following computational equation is easier to use. The data from Table 17–2 were used to calculate the *SD*:

$$SD = \sqrt{\frac{\Sigma X^2 - (1/N)\,(\Sigma X)^2}{N - 1}}$$

$$SD = \sqrt{\frac{1636 - (1/50)(264)^2}{50 - 1}}$$

$$SD = \sqrt{\frac{1636 - 1393.92}{49}}$$

$$SD = \sqrt{4.94}$$

$$SD = 2.22$$

Just as the mean is the "average" score, the standard deviation is the "average" difference (deviation) score. The standard deviation provides a measure of the average deviation of a score from the mean in that particular sample. It indicates the degree of error that would be made if the mean alone were used to interpret the data. Standard deviation is an important measure, both in understanding dispersion within a distribution and in interpreting the relationship of a particular score to the distribution. Descriptive statistics (mean, median, mode, and standard deviation) are usually calculated using the computer.

THE SHAPES OF DISTRIBUTIONS

The shape of the distribution provides important information about the data being studied. The outline of the distribution shape is obtained using a histogram. Then, within this outline, the mean, median, mode, and standard deviation can be graphically illustrated (see Figure 17–1 on p. 434). This visual presentation of combined summary statistics provides increased insight into the nature of the distribution. As the sample size becomes larger, the shape of the distribution will more accurately reflect the shape of the population from which the sample was taken.

Symmetry

Several terms are used to describe the shape of the curve (and thus the nature of a particular distribution). The shape of a curve is usually discussed in terms of symmetry, skewness, modality, and kurtosis. A symmetrical curve is one in which the left side of the curve is a mirror image of the right side. (See discussion of normal curve in Chapter 16.) In these curves, the mean, median, and mode are equal and are the dividing point between the left and right side of the curve (see Figure 17–1).

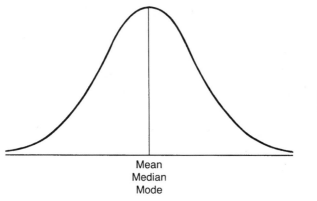

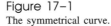

Mean
Median
Mode

Figure 17–1
The symmetrical curve.

Skewness

Any curve that is not symmetrical is referred to as skewed or asymmetrical. *Skewness* may be exhibited in the curve in a variety of ways (see Figure 17–2). A curve may be positively skewed, which means that the largest portion of data is below the mean. For example, the data on length of enrollment in hospice are positively skewed. The majority of the people die within the first 3 weeks of enrollment, with increasingly smaller numbers surviving over a period of months. A curve can also be negatively skewed, which means that the largest portion of data is above the mean. For example, the data on the occurrence of chronic illness in a population are negatively skewed, with the majority of chronic illnesses occurring in older age groups.

In a skewed distribution, the mean, median, and mode are not equal. Skewness interferes with the validity of many statistical analyses; therefore, statistical procedures have been developed to measure the skewness of the distribution of the sample being studied. Very few samples will be perfectly symmetrical; however, as the deviation from symmetry increases, the seriousness of the impact on statistical analyses increases. A popular skewness measure is expressed in the following equation:

$$\text{skewness} = \frac{\Sigma(X - \overline{X})^3}{N(SD^3)}$$

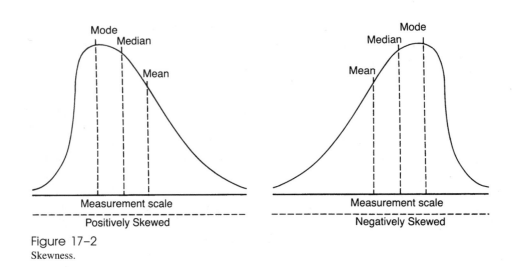

Figure 17–2
Skewness.

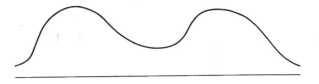

Figure 17–3
Biomodal distribution.

Using the equation, a result of zero indicates a completely symmetrical distribution; a positive number indicates a positively skewed distribution; and a negative number indicates a negatively skewed distribution. Statistical analyses conducted by computer will often automatically measure skewness, which is then indicated in the computer printout. Skewness values greater than 0.2 or less than −0.2 are sufficiently severe to affect statistical results (Hildebrand, 1986). Strongly skewed distributions must often be analyzed using nonparametric techniques, which make no assumptions of normally distributed samples. In a positively skewed distribution, the mean will be greater than the median, which will be greater than the mode. In a negatively skewed distribution, the mean will be less than the median, which will be less than the mode.

Modality

Another characteristic of distributions is their *modality*. Most curves found in practice are unimodal, which means that there is one mode and frequencies progressively decline as they move away from the mode. Symmetrical distributions are usually unimodal. However, curves can also be bimodal (see Figure 17–3) or multimodal. When you find a bimodal sample, it usually means that you have not sufficiently identified your populations of interest.

Kurtosis

Another term used to describe the shape of the distribution curve is *kurtosis*. Kurtosis explains the degree of peakedness of the curve, which is related to the spread or variance of scores. An extremely peaked curve is referred to as *leptokurtic;* an intermediate degree of kurtosis as *mesokurtic;* and a relatively flat curve is termed *platykurtic* (see Figure 17–4). Extreme kurtosis can affect the validity of statistical analyses because there is little variation in scores. Many computer programs analyze kurtosis prior to conducting statistical analyses. A common equation used to measure kurtosis is:

$$kurtosis = \frac{\Sigma(X - \overline{X})^4}{N(SD^4)} - 3$$

A kurtosis of zero indicates the curve is mesokurtic. Values above zero indicate a leptokurtic curve

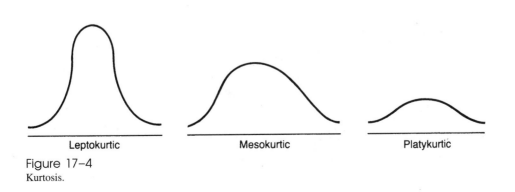

Leptokurtic   Mesokurtic   Platykurtic

Figure 17–4
Kurtosis.

and values below zero indicate a platykurtic curve. (Box, Hunter, & Hunter, 1978).

STANDARDIZED SCORES

Because of differences in the characteristics of various distributions, comparing a score in one distribution with a score in another distribution is difficult. For example, if you were comparing test scores from two classroom examinations and one test had a high score of 100 while the other had a high score of 70, the scores would be difficult to compare. To facilitate this comparison, a mechanism has been developed to transform raw scores into standard scores. Numbers that make sense only within the framework of measurements used within a specific study are transformed to numbers *(standard scores)* that have a more general meaning. Transformation to standard scores allows an easy conceptual grasp of the meaning of the score.

A common standardized score is called a *Z score*. It expresses deviations from the mean (difference scores) in terms of standard deviation units. The equation for a *Z* score is:

$$Z = \frac{X - \overline{X}}{SD}$$

A score that falls above the mean will have a positive *Z* score, whereas a score that falls below the mean will have a negative *Z* score (see Figure 17–1). The mean expressed as a *Z* score is zero. The standard deviation of *Z* scores is 1. Thus, a *Z* score of 2 indicates that the score from which it was obtained is 2 standard deviations above the mean. A *Z* score of −.5 indicates that the score was .5 standard deviations below the mean. The larger the absolute value of the *Z* score, the less likely the observation is to occur. For example, a *Z* score of 4 would be extremely unlikely. The cumulative normal distribution expressed in *Z* scores is given in Appendix B.

CONFIDENCE INTERVALS

When the probability of including the value of the parameter within the interval estimate is known

(as described in Chapter 16), it is referred to as a *confidence interval*. Calculating the confidence interval involves using two formulas to identify the upper and lower ends of the interval. The formula for a 95% confidence interval for a population when sampling from a population with a known standard deviation or a normal population with the sample size greater than 30 is:

$$\overline{X} - 1.96 \, SD/\sqrt{N} \quad \overline{X} + 1.96 \, SD/\sqrt{N}$$

If one had a sample with a mean of 40, a standard deviation of 5, and an *N* of 50, a confidence interval could be calculated.

$$40 - 1.96 \left(\frac{5}{\sqrt{50}}\right) = 40 - 1.386 = 38.6$$

$$40 + 1.96 \left(\frac{5}{\sqrt{50}}\right) = 40 + 1.386 = 41.4$$

Confidence intervals are usually expressed as (38.6, 41.4), with 38.6 being the lower end of the interval and 41.4 being the upper end of the interval. Theoretically, we can produce a confidence interval for any parameter of a distribution. It is a generic statistical procedure. For example, confidence intervals can also be developed around correlation coefficients (see Glass & Stanley, 1970, pp. 264–268). Estimation can be used for a single population or for multiple populations. In estimation, we are inferring the value of a parameter from sample data and have no preconceived notion of the value of the parameter. In contrast, in hypothesis testing we have an a priori theory about the value of the parameter or parameters or some combination of parameters.

EXPLORATORY DATA ANALYSIS

Although the use of summary statistics has been the traditional approach to describing data or describing the characteristics of the sample prior to inferential statistical analysis, it is limited as a means of understanding the nature of data. For example, using measures of central tendency, particularly the mean, to describe the nature of the data obscures the impact of extreme values or of deviations in the data. Thus, significant features in the data may be concealed or misrepresented. Often anomalous, unexpected, problematic data and discrepant patterns are seen but regarded as not meaningful (Ferketich & Verran, 1986; Fox, 1990).

Ferketich and Verran (1986) contend that there has been a tremendous push in nursing toward the use of inferential statistics. However, they consider the confirmatory approach to data analysis to be inefficient.

"When one basic hypothesis, the null, is tested we know only what is not supported in a study. The rejection or failure to reject a null hypothesis, which is all the statistical test can provide, is insufficient use of often rich data bases. For example, a null hypothesis that states there is no difference between groups on a particular parameter is the usual approach. However, through good exploratory techniques, it might be discovered that part of each group is similar to the corresponding part of the other group; but for the extremes of the group, differences are profoundly manifested. These extremes might have been missed if only summary statistics were used but could be discovered by various resistant statistics of EDA. The most efficient use of the data base is to discover alternate hypotheses and to explore many instead of one single path. EDA provides such exploration without concern for restrictive model assumptions." (pp. 465–466) ∎

Exploratory data analysis (EDA), developed by Tukey (1977) and more recently expanded by Fox and Long (1990), is designed to detect the unexpected in the data and to avoid overlooking crucial patterns that may exist. In nursing, identification and explanation of patterns is considered critical to both theory and practice. The procedures also facilitate comparison of groups. The outcome of EDA may be theory generation or the development of hypotheses for confirmatory data analysis. Graphic analysis of data, central to EDA, requires an element of subjective interpretation. However, when a series of visual displays continues to show evidence of the same pattern, subjectivity is minimized. There is a building of evidence to support the discovery of a basic pattern in the data (Ferketich & Verran, 1986). Using graphics as an element of data analysis is a relatively new strategy. More commonly, graphics have been used to present the results of data analysis. With EDA, the purpose of graphic displays is discovery. Even numeric summaries are presented in such a way that the researcher can visualize patterns in the data. Although EDA is a relative newcomer, most mainframe and PC data analysis programs perform the statistical procedures and graphic techniques of EDA.

The techniques of EDA use new terms and require different logical processes and a different mind-set in the researcher than those of summary statistics. The researcher must be flexible, open to the unanticipated, and sensitive to patterns that are revealed as the analysis proceeds. Tukey (1977) suggests that "exploratory data analysis is detective work" (p. 1); it is a search for clues and evidence. When using EDA, it is important for the researcher to get a feel for what the data are like. During analysis, the researcher will move back and forth among the techniques of numeric summaries, graphic displays of the data, pattern identification, and theoretical exploration of the meaning of discoveries (Ferketich & Verran, 1986).

Tukey's (1977) procedures make analyses fun, rather than mysterious. EDA is somewhat akin to playing with numbers. It captures the right brain's playful, creative portion of the intellect as well as the logical, deductive practical left-brain portion. Tukey (1977) has even given the procedures playful, imaginative names. And yet EDA provides a depth of understanding not possible with previous approaches to data analysis. The following section describes some of the initial approaches to EDA. If you are interested in exploring some of the more advanced procedures of EDA, we refer you to Tukey (1977) and Fox and Long (1990).

STEM-AND-LEAF DISPLAYS

The *stem-and-leaf display* is a visual presentation of numbers that may provide important insights. It is useful for batches of data values from approximately 20 to 200 (Fox, 1990). To develop the display, the numbers are organized by lines. Each line of the display is a stem. Each piece of information on the stem is a leaf. To develop a stem-and-leaf display, the last digit (or in some cases, the last two digits) of the number is used as the leaf; the rest of the number is the stem. An example is provided in the following sections.

Distribution

Assume we have a batch of numbers with the values shown in Table 17–3. There are 43 values with a mean of 57 and a standard deviation of 6. However, these summary statistics would not be the primary interest of Tukey. He would want to see what the data looked like.

Stem-and-Leaf

In a stem-and-leaf display, the stem is the first digit of each number and is placed to the left of the bar as in Table 17–4. Adding the leaves to the display, the last digit of each number is placed on the appropriate line of the stem. The first row includes the values of 12, 14, 16, and 18. The stem for the first row is 1 and the leaves are 2, 4, 6, and 8.

Median

The distribution in Table 17–4 appears positively skewed. This is validated by the difference in the mean (57) and the median (52). Determining the

Table 17–3
Sample Data Set

12, 83, 59, 43, 26, 61, 66, 55, 84, 39, 75, 16, 125, 22, 65, 89, 28, 66, 40, 163, 73, 38, 21, 78, 35, 50, 42, 96, 32, 33, 59, 54, 47, 172, 18, 14, 68, 73, 52, 43, 49, 76, 25.

Table 17–4
Stem-and-Leaf Display

Stem	Leaf
1	2 4 6 8
2	1 2 5 6 8
3	2 3 5 8 9
4	0 2 3 3 7 9
5	0 2 4 5 9 9
6	1 5 6 6 8
7	3 3 5 6 8
8	3 4 9
9	6
11	
12	5
13	
14	
15	
16	3
17	2

median from a stem-and-leaf display is relatively easy. The median is either the single middle value or the mean of the two middle values (Tukey, 1977, p. 29). The equation for the position of the median from the ends of the distribution is $1/2(1 + N)$. In this set of 43 numbers, $1/2(1 + 43) = 1/2(44) = 22$. The median is the 22nd number to the right of the bar, or 52.

Ranking

Values in the distribution may be ranked from the lowest value to the highest value, or from the highest value to the lowest value. Depth can also be ranked, with the median being the greatest rank and the extremes being 1. Depth is the number of values between the median and one of the extremes. These three rankings are illustrated in Table 17–5.

Extreme Values

The extreme values are also of interest. In the distribution shown in Table 17–5, the upper extreme value (UE) is 172. The lower extreme value (LE) is 12.

Hinges

Hinges (H) are determined by calculating the value halfway from each extreme to the median.

Table 17–5
Ranked Values

Upward Rank	Value	Downward Rank	Depth
1	12 (LE)	43	1
2	14	42	2
3	16	41	3
4	18	40	4
5	21	39	5
6	22	38	6
7	25	37	7
8	26	36	8
9	28	35	9
10	32	34	10
11	33	33	11
12	35	32	12
13	38	31	13
14	39	30	14
15	40	29	15
16	42	28	16
17	43	27	17
18	43	26	18
19	47	25	19
20	49	24	20
21	50	23	21
22	52 (MD)	22	22
23	54	21	21
24	55	20	20
25	59	19	19
26	59	18	18
27	61	17	17
28	65	16	16
29	66	15	15
30	66	14	14
31	68	13	13
32	73	12	12
33	73	11	11
34	75	10	10
35	76	9	9
36	78	8	8
37	83	7	7
38	84	6	6
39	89	5	5
40	96	4	4
41	125	3	3
42	163	2	2
43	172 (UE)	1	1

LE, lower extreme value; MD, median; UE, upper extreme value.

A hinge is calculated in the same manner as the median. Thus, $1/2(1 + 22) = 11.5$. However, Tukey (1977) drops the .5, preferring the simplicity of whole numbers, and the hinges will be the 11th value from each extreme. In our distribution, the lower hinge (LH) is 33 and the upper hinge (UH)

is 73. To allow you to see the positioning of the values more clearly, they are presented in folded form in Figure 17–5 (on p. 440), in which the angle of the values changes at the hinge. These values may also be expressed as a 5-number summary, as shown in Table 17–6 (on p. 440).

Values that describe the spread of the distribution can also be expressed. The LH-LE spread in our distribution is 21, obtained by subtracting 12 (LE) from 33 (LH). The LH-MD spread is 19. The UH-MD spread is 21 and the UE-UH spread is 99. The low spread (LS) is the spread between LE and MD; midspread (MS) is the spread between LH and UH (sometimes referred to as the hinge spread or H-spread); and high spread (HS) is the spread between MD and UH. These values can all be placed in a table that is referred to as the median hinge number summary (see Table 17–7 on p. 440). These values can be used in other displays to illustrate the shape of the distribution (Verran & Ferketich, 1987a).

If the distribution is symmetrical, the distance between LE and LH should be equal to the distance between UH and UE. Distances between the median and the two hinges should also be equal, as should the distances between the hinges and the extremes. The distances between the median and the two hinges should be smaller than the distances between the extremes and the hinges. The LS should be equal to the HS (Verran & Ferketich, 1987a). Clearly, the sample presented in Table 17–7 is not symmetrical.

Fences

Two sets of fences, upper (Uf) and lower (Lf) and inner and outer, are used to identify outliers. These fences are defined by *steps*. A step is $1.5 \times MS$ (midspread). The inner fences (f) are one step beyond the hinges. This can be calculated using the following equation:

$$Uf = UH + 1.5 \times MS$$
$$Lf = LH - 1.5 \times MS$$

In our sample, the upper inner fence (Uf) is 133. The lower inner fence (Lf) is -27.

```
                            52(MD)
     12(LE)             50  54
        14            49    55                172(UE)
        16           47     59                163
        18          43      59                125
        21          43      61                 96
        22         42       65                 89
        25        40        66                 84
        26      39          66               83
        28    38            68              76
        32  35               73  75
          33(LH)              73 (UH)
```

Figure 17–5
Data distribution in folded form.

Table 17–6
Five-Number Summary Table of Data Distribution

12	33	52	73	172
(LE)	(LH)	(MD)	(UH)	(UE)

LE, lower extreme value; LH, lower hinge; MD, median; UH, upper hinge; UE, upper extreme value.

Outer fences (F) are two steps beyond the hinges and can be calculated using the following equation:

$$UF = UH + 3 \times MS$$
$$LF = LH - 3 \times MS$$

In our sample, the upper outer fence (UF) is 193. The lower outer fence (LF) is −87. Values beyond the inner fence are referred to as *outside,* whereas values beyond the outer fence are referred to as *far out.* However, Fox (1990) points out that "outside—and even far-outside—values are not necessarily 'outliers,' in the sense of not belonging with the rest of the data" (p. 75). They are displayed individually because they are unusual and should be looked at closely.

The decision regarding what to do about outliers is specific to the particular study. The researcher needs to be aware of their presence and their possible effect on outcomes of planned statistical analyses. In some cases, outliers are judged not to be representative of the population under study and are removed from the analyses. In others, specific analyses are planned to examine outliers. Information on outliers needs to be included in the research report since they can provide valuable insights into the phenomenon under study.

WHAT CAUSES OUTLIERS?

Outliers, or extreme values, occur for four main reasons (Slinkman, 1984). The first three reasons were identified by Barnett and Lewis (1978) and include inherent variability, measurement error, and execution error. *Inherent variability* means that in data you can naturally expect a few random observations to be in the extreme ends of the tail. For example, if you had 1,000 observations from

Table 17–7
Median Hinge Number Summary

12		33		52		73		172
(LE)		(LH)		(MD)		(UH)		(UE)
	21		19		21		99	
	(LH-LE)		(MD-LH)		(UH-MD)		(UE-UH)	
		40		40		120		
		(LS)		(MS)		(HS)		

a normally distributed population, you could expect to find 2.6 observations to be more than three standard deviations from the mean. Outliers also occur because of *measurement error.* This was discussed in Chapter 13. If you can determine that the outlier is, in fact, caused by measurement error, the observation should be removed from the data set since it will have a negative influence on statistical analyses. *Execution errors* occur because of a defect in the data collection procedure. These erroneous observations, when detected, should also be removed from the data set.

However, the most important cause of outliers from the point of view of data analysis is *error in identifying the variables,* important in explaining the nature of the phenomenon under study (Weisberg, 1977). In this case, the summary statistics, the regression line, or the path analysis results (see Chapter 19) do not turn out as expected and the outlier provides new and unexpected information. This unexpected information is central to the discovery of new knowledge.

RESIDUALS

Most statistical procedures focus on measures of central tendency, which Tukey (1977) refers to as the *fit.* For any expression of fit that summarizes the data as a whole, there is a residual. For example, the result of regression analysis is a "line of best fit," which is drawn on a graph showing a plot of the individual values (see Chapter 18). For each point on that line (the fit) there are also individual values that vary from the fit. If the fit is the mean, then the difference (or deviation) values would be the residuals. Combined, these variations are the residuals for that data set. This can be expressed as

$$\text{RESIDUALS} = \text{DATA} - \text{FIT}$$

These residuals are the main tool of EDA. "They are to the data analyst what powerful magnifying glasses, sensitive chemical tests for bloodstains, and delicate listening devices are to a story-book detective" (Tukey, 1977, p. 125). Displays illustrating residuals are as important as displays of

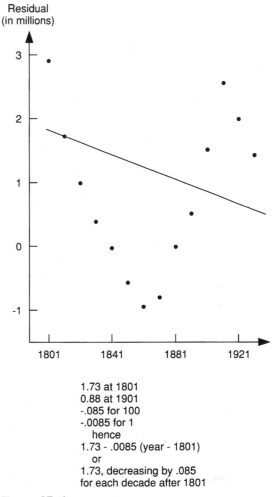

1.73 at 1801
0.88 at 1901
-.085 for 100
-.0085 for 1
   hence
1.73 - .0085 (year - 1801)
   or
1.73, decreasing by .085
for each decade after 1801

Figure 17–6
Example of a residual plot. (From Tukey, J. W. [1977]. *Exploratory data analysis.* Copyright © 1977 Addison-Wesley Publishing Company, Inc. Reprinted by permission of Addison-Wesley Longman Publishing Company, Inc.)

raw data or of the fit. Tukey (1977, p. 136) provides mathematical calculations for plotting residual values. These plots can provide evidence of hidden structure or of unusual values (Verran & Ferketich, 1987c). Figure 17–6 is an example of such a plot.

PLOTS OF RELATIONSHIP

In exploratory data analysis, displays of the data such as plots are an important part of the process of analysis. They help the researcher get a feel for

D

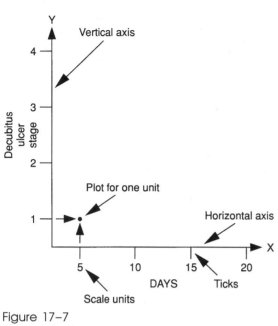

Figure 17–7
Structure of a plot.

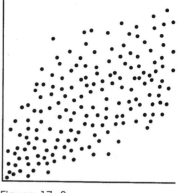

Figure 17–8
Example of a scatter plot.

the data. A plot of relationship is a common way to illustrate graphically the relationship of two variables (Verran & Ferketich, 1987b). To develop a plot of relationship, you must first determine the units you will use for the horizontal and vertical scales. For example, if you are using time for one scale, your units on the horizontal (or x) axis might be 1 day, 5 days, or 10 days. The vertical (or y) axis might be the occurrence and stage of a decubitus ulcer. The units are selected to provide the best image of the data. Scale units are indicated on the graph by marks or ticks along the axes. Units must be equal across the axes to avoid distorting the data. The marks (or ticks) along the axes are used to plot the points on the graph and to provide perspective to the information within the graph. Ticks should be sufficient to orient the viewer without distracting attention from the data presentation within the graph (see Figure 17–7).

The variables are usually expressed as x and y. The plot is constructed using a scale for the values of each variable, with the scale for y being placed vertically and the scale for x, horizontally. For each unit or subject, there is a value for x and

a value for y. The plot illustrates the relationship between these two values. In one type of plot, a scatter plot, the point at which each value of x and of y intersect is plotted on the graph (see Figure 17–8). In other cases, a single line on the graph expresses the results of a statistical analysis summarizing the best fit for the overall data (see Figure 17–9). Usually, the scatter plot and the line of best fit are overlaid (see Figure 17–10).

The structure of the graph should be carefully planned to facilitate the visual impact of the presentation of the data. Graphs are for looking at the

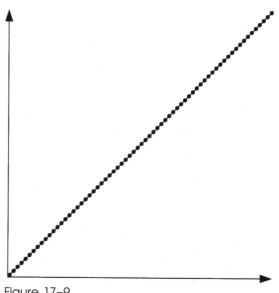

Figure 17–9
Best fit line.

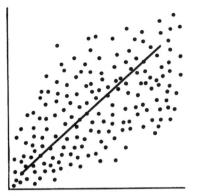

Figure 17–10
Overlay of scatter plot and best fit line.

Table 17–8
Actual Values and Quantile Values

Upward Rank	Value	Quantile
1	12	.0116 (LE)
2	14	.0349
3	16	.0581
4	18	.0814
5	21	.1047
6	22	.1279
7	25	.1512
8	26	.1744
9	28	.1977
10	32	.2209
11	33	.2442 (LH)
12	35	.2674
13	38	.2907
14	39	.3140
15	40	.3372
16	42	.3605
17	43	.3837
18	43	.4070
19	47	.4302
20	49	.4535
21	50	.4767
22	52	.5 (MD)
23	54	.5233
24	55	.5465
25	59	.5698
26	59	.5930
27	61	.6163
28	65	.6395
29	66	.6628
30	66	.6860
31	68	.7093
32	73	.7326
33	73	.7558 (UH)
34	75	.7791
35	76	.8023
36	78	.8256
37	83	.8488
38	84	.8721
39	89	.8953
40	96	.9186
41	125	.9419
42	163	.9651
43	172	.9884 (UE)

data, they are not stores of quantitative information. The graph should be constructed to keep the viewer's eyes on the points. Symbols should be large enough to stand out; if more than one kind are used, each should be clearly different and equally noticeable. The graph should be constructed to facilitate the viewer's ability to see the behavior of the data. In exploring the data, plots of y against x may help even "when we know nothing about the logical connection from x to y—even when we do not know whether or not there is one—even when we know that such a connection is impossible" (Tukey, 1977, p. 131).

Q-PLOTS

Q-plots display values in the distribution by quantile. A quantile shows the location of the score within the distribution, similar to that obtained by ranking the scores. However, it goes a step beyond ranking the scores. If i symbolizes the rank of a particular score, the quantile may be calculated using the following formula:

$$(i - .5)/n$$

For example, in our sample of 43, rank 1 is calculated as $(1 - .5)/43 = .0116$. Use of this calculation yielded the values for our distribution shown in Table 17–8. Using the actual value as y and the quantile value as x, a bivariate plot can be created (see Figure 17–11). These plots reveal a pattern in the data (Verran & Ferketich, 1987a).

BOX-AND-WHISKER PLOTS

Box-and-whisker plots give a fast visualization of some of the major characteristics of the data, such as the spread, symmetry, and outliers. The median (MD) and upper (UH) and lower hinges (LH) are illustrated by the box in Figure 17–12. The whiskers (lines extending from the box) extend to the

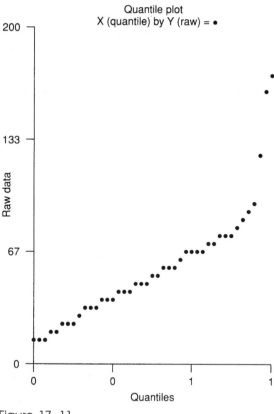

Figure 17–11
Example of a Q-plot.

SYMMETRY PLOT

A *symmetry plot* is designed to determine the presence of skewness in the data. Since symmetrical distributions are equally balanced for each value above and below the median, if values in the same position above and below the median are plotted against each other, a straight line will result. This then can be a measure of symmetry. To develop the plot, one must first compute the distances from the median to the next lower and next higher values. These distances are then plotted against each other (Verran & Ferketich, 1987a). In our sample, the median is 52. The next lower value is 50; therefore, the distance between them is 2. The distance between the median and the next higher value is 2. Thus, 2 on the horizontal axis and 2 on the vertical axis will be plotted against each other. This procedure continues until all of the values have been plotted. The results are illustrated in Figure 17–13. Although a line can be seen, some skewness is evident in the graph.

most extreme value within one midspread of the hinge. Open circles represent values from 1 to 1.5 midspread (MS) beyond the whisker. There are two open circles in this display. Extreme values or outliers (beyond 1.5 MS) are often represented by closed circles or asterisks. There are no extreme values in our data set.

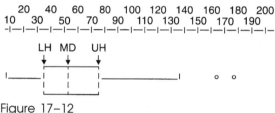

Figure 17–12
A box-and-whiskers plot.

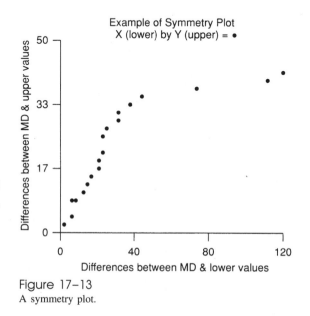

Figure 17–13
A symmetry plot.

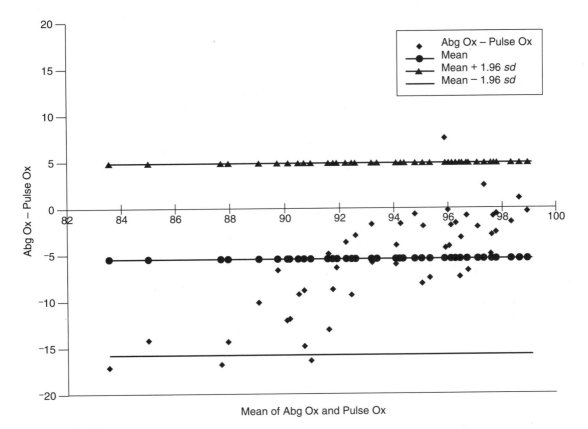

Figure 17–14
Example of a Bland and Altman plot.

BLAND AND ALTMAN PLOT

The *Bland and Altman plot* is a method of examining the extent of agreement between two measurement techniques. Generally, it is used to compare a new technique to an established one. It has been used primarily with physiologic measures. For example, one might wish to compare pulse oximeter values with arterial blood gas values (Figure 17–14). The method was developed by Bland and Altman (1986) and statistical programs to perform the plots are not yet available in the commonly used statistical packages but may be ordered from Med-Calc Software (Broekstratt 52, 9030 Mariakerke, Belgium). A World Wide Web page discussing the procedure is available at http://allserv.rug.ac.be/~fschoonj/

In the plot, the difference between the mea-sures of the two methods can be plotted against the average of the two methods. Thus, for each pair, the difference between the two values would be calculated and an average of the two values would be calculated. These values are then plotted on a graph displaying a scatter diagram of the differences plotted against the averages. Three horizontal lines are displayed on the graph showing the mean difference, the mean difference plus 1.96 times the standard deviation of the differences, and the mean difference minus 1.96 times the standard deviation of the differences. The purpose of the plot is to reveal the relationship between the differences and the averages, to look for any systematic bias, and to identify outliers. In some cases, two measures may be closely related near the mean, but may become more divergent as they move away from the mean. This has been the case with measures of pulse oximetry and arterial blood gases (see Figure 17–14). Traditional methods of comparing measures such as correlation procedures will not identify such problems. Interpretation of the results is based on whether the differences are clinically important (Bland & Altman, 1986).

The repeatability of a single method of measurement may also be examined with this analysis technique. Using the graph, one can examine whether the variability or precision of a method is related to the size of the characteristic being measured. Since the same method is being repeat-edly measured, the mean difference should be zero. A coefficient of repeatability (CR) can be calculated using the following formula. MedCalc can perform this computation of CR (Schoonjans, 1993–1995).

$$CR = 1.96 \times \sqrt{\frac{\Sigma (d_2 - d_1)^2}{n - 1}}$$

where:

d = the value of a measure

SUMMARY

Data analysis begins with descriptive statistics in any study in which the data are numerical, including some qualitative studies. Descriptive statistics allow the researcher to organize the data in ways that give meaning and facilitate insight. Descriptive statistics include summary and exploratory procedures. Summary statistics include measures of central tendency and measures of dispersion. Frequency distributions are usually the first strategy used to organize the data for examination. There are two types of frequency distributions: ungrouped and grouped. Frequency distributions are often displayed using tables or graphs.

The measures of central tendency are the most concise statement of the nature of the data. The three measures of central tendency commonly used in statistical analyses are the mode, the median, and the mean. The mode is the numerical value or score that occurs with greatest frequency. The median is the score at the exact center of the ungrouped frequency distribution. The mean is the sum of the scores divided by the number of scores being summed.

Measures of dispersion, or variability, are measures of individual differences of the members of the population and sample. They give some indication of how scores in a sample are dispersed around the mean. The measures most commonly used are modal percentage, range, difference scores, sum of squares, variance, and the standard deviation. The modal percentage indicates the relationship of the number of data scores represented by the mode to the total number of data scores. The range is obtained by subtracting the lowest score from the highest score. Difference scores are obtained by subtracting the mean from each score. Sum of squares is the sum of squared difference scores. Variance is the mean or average of the sum of squares. The standard deviation is the square root of the variance.

The shape of the distribution provides important information about the data being studied. The outline of the distribution shape is obtained using the histogram. Then, within this outline, the mean, median, mode, and standard deviation can be graphically illustrated. A symmetrical curve is one in which the left side of the curve is a mirror image of the right side. In these curves, the mean, median, and mode are equal and are the dividing

continued

continued

point between the left and right sides of the curve.

Any curve that is not symmetrical is referred to as skewed or asymmetrical. A curve may be positively skewed, which means that the largest portion of data is below the mean. The curve can also be negatively skewed, which means that the largest portion of data is above the mean. In a skewed distribution, the mean, median, and mode are not equal.

Another characteristic of distributions is their modality. Symmetrical distributions are usually unimodal. Kurtosis explains the degree of peakedness of the curve, which is related to the spread or variance of scores. Standardized scores are sometimes used in distributions to allow an easy conceptual grasp of the meaning of the score. A common standardized score is a Z score.

Exploratory data analysis (EDA) is designed to detect the unexpected in the data and to avoid overlooking crucial patterns that may exist. Probably the most important strategy in EDA for identifying patterns is the visual or graphic examination of the data. EDA should begin by getting a general feel for what the numbers are like. The median of the distribution is calculated. Values in the distribution may be ranked. Extreme values are also of interest. Hinges are determined by calculating the value halfway from each extreme to the median. Values that describe the spread of the distribution can also be expressed. These values can all be placed in a table referred to as the median hinge number summary. Two sets of fences are used to identify outliers: the inner fences and the outer fences.

One way of looking at data more closely is to examine residuals in the data. Residuals are essentially difference (or deviation) values. Displays illustrating residuals are as important as displays of raw data or of the fit.

The stem-and-leaf display is a visual presentation of numbers that may provide insights into the data. Scatter plots are also used. Box-and-whisker plots give a fast visualization of some of the major characteristics of the data, such as the spread, symmetry, and outliers. The median and the upper and lower hinges are illustrated on the figure and the whiskers extend to the most extreme value within one midspread of the hinge. A symmetry plot is designed to determine the presence of skewness in the data. Since symmetrical distributions are equally balanced for each value above and below the median, if values in the same position above and below the median are plotted against each other a straight line will result. This then can be a test of symmetry.

References

Barnett, V., & Lewis, T. (1978). *Outliers in statistical data.* New York: Wiley.

Bland, J. M., & Altman, D. G. (1986). Statistical methods for assessing agreement between two methods of clinical measurement. *The Lancet I*(8476), 307–310.

Box, G. E. P., Hunter, W. G., & Hunter, J. S. (1978). *Statistics for experimenters.* New York: Wiley.

Ferketich, S., & Verran, J. (1986). Exploratory data analysis—Introduction. *Western Journal of Nursing Research, 8*(4), 464–466.

Fox, J. (1990). Describing univariate distributions. In J. Fox & J. S. Long (Eds.), *Modern methods of data analysis* (pp. 58–125). Newbury Park, CA: Sage.

Fox, J., & Long, J. S. (1990). *Modern methods of data analysis.* Newbury Park, CA: Sage.

Glass, G. V., & Stanley, J. C. (1970). *Statistical methods in education and psychology.* Englewood Cliffs, NJ: Prentice-Hall.

Hildebrand, D. K. (1986). *Statistical thinking for behavioral scientists.* Boston: Duxbury.

Schoonjans, F. (1993–1995). MedCalc, Broekstratt 52, 9030 Mariakerke, Belgium.

Shelley, S. I. (1984). *Research methods in nursing and health.* Boston: Little, Brown.

Slinkman, C. W. (1984). *An empirical comparison of data analytic regression model building procedures.* Unpublished dissertation, University of Minnesota.

Tukey, J. W. (1977). *Exploratory data analysis.* Reading, MA: Addison-Wesley.

Verran, J. A., & Ferketich, S. L. (1987a). Exploratory data analysis—Examining single distributions. *Western Journal of Nursing Research, 9*(1), 142–149.

Verran, J. A., & Ferketich, S. L. (1987b). Exploratory data analysis—Comparisons of groups and variables. *Western Journal of Nursing Research, 9*(4), 617–625.

Verran, J. A., & Ferketich, S. L. (1987c). Testing linear model assumptions: Residual analysis. *Nursing Research, 36*(2), 127–130.

Weisberg, S. (1977). *MULTREG user's manual* (Technical Report No. 298). St. Paul, MN: School of Statistics, University of Minnesota.

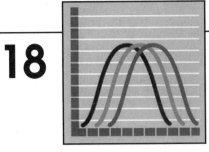

18

Bivariate Inferential Data Analyses

Those critiquing a study and those planning a study are confronted with a similar dilemma: determining the suitability of various statistical procedures for a particular study. The decision is a complex one, and not straightforward. Regrettably, there is not usually one right statistical procedure for a particular study. In addition, the number of statistical procedures from which to choose has increased dramatically in recent years. Judging suitability in a critique requires not only that you be familiar with the statistical procedure used in the study and the theoretical assumptions on which the statistical procedure is based, but that you compare that procedure with others that could have been used, perhaps to greater advantage. You must judge whether the procedure was performed appropriately and the results interpreted correctly.

Neophyte researchers must integrate all the aspects of a planned study that influence the selection of statistical procedures with their knowledge of the statistical procedures and a recognition of what is realistic in their situation. Using this information, they must select statistical procedures for their study, though their choice is made with a higher degree of uncertainty than that of the experienced researcher because of their limited knowledge of statistical procedures.

This chapter is designed to assist those critiquing research and neophyte researchers in judging, choosing, and using statistical procedures in relation to particular studies. The first section presents the factors involved in determining the suitability of a statistical procedure. The second section includes a variety of statistical procedures. The procedures presented are by no means exhaustive, but rather include those most commonly used in nursing studies.

CHOOSING APPROPRIATE STATISTICAL PROCEDURES FOR A STUDY

Multiple factors are involved in determining the suitability of a statistical procedure for a particular study. Some of these are related to the nature of the study, some to the nature of the researcher, and others to the nature of statistical theory. These include (1) the purpose of the study; (2) hypotheses, questions, or objectives; (3) design; (4) level of measurement; (5) previous experience in statistical analyses; (6) statistical knowledge level; (7) availability of statistical consultation; (8) financial resources; and (9) access to computers. Using items 1 to 4, statistical procedures that meet the requirements of the study are identified. The options may then be further narrowed through the process of elimination based on items 5 through 9.

One approach to selecting an appropriate statistical procedure or judging the appropriateness of an analysis technique for a critique is to use a decision tree. A decision tree directs your choices by gradually narrowing your options through the decisions you make. A simplified decision tree focusing on level of measurement, independence of measurement, and number of variables is included on the inside back cover of this book and directs you to the corresponding page number where appropriate statistical procedures are discussed. Two other decision trees that have been helpful in selecting statistical procedures are presented in Figures 18–1 and 18–2.

One disadvantage of decision trees is that if

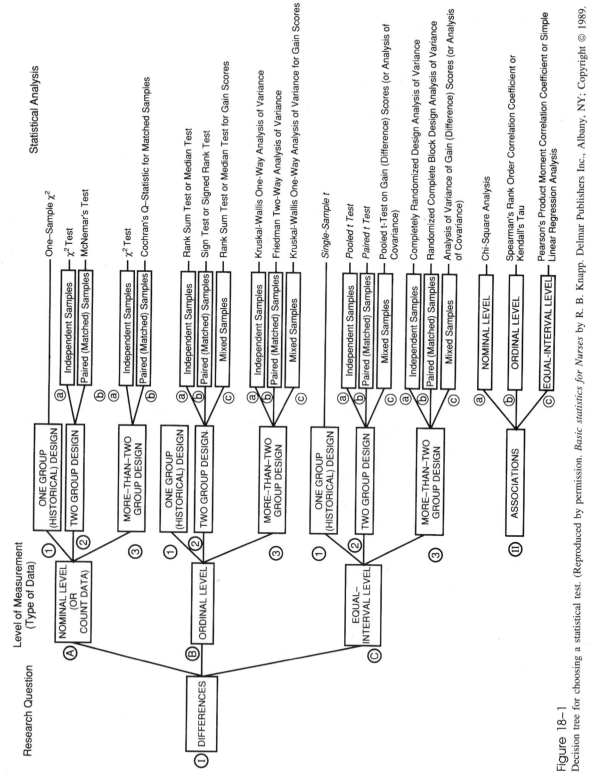

Figure 18-1

Decision tree for choosing a statistical test. (Reproduced by permission. *Basic statistics for Nurses* by R. B. Knapp. Delmar Publishers Inc., Albany, NY; Copyright © 1989.

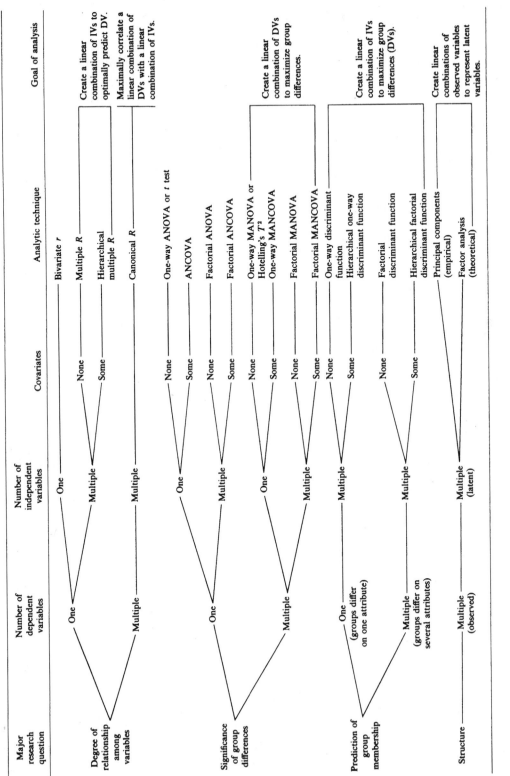

Figure 18–2
Choosing among statistical techniques. (Tabachnick, B. G., & Fidell, L. S. [1983]. *Using multivariate statistics*. New York: Harper & Row, with permission.)

you make an incorrect or uninformed decision (guess) you can be led down a path by which you might select an inappropriate statistical procedure for your study. Decision trees are often constrained by space and therefore do not include all of the information needed to make an appropriate selection. The most extensive decision tree we have found is presented in *A Guide for Selecting Statistical Techniques for Analyzing Social Science Data* by Andrews, Klem, Davidson, O'Malley, and Rodgers (1981). The following examples of questions designed to guide the selection or evaluation of statistical procedures were extracted from this book.

1. How many variables does the problem involve?
2. How do you want to treat the variables with respect to scale of measurement?
3. What do you want to know about the distribution of the variable?
4. Do you want to treat outlying cases differently from others?
5. What is the form of the distribution?
6. Is a distinction made between a dependent and an independent variable?
7. Do you want to test whether the means of the two variables are equal?
8. Do you want to treat the relationship between variables as linear?
9. How many of the variables are dichotomous?
10. Is the dichotomous variable a collapsing of a continuous variable?
11. Do you want to treat the ranks of ordered categories as interval scales?
12. Do the variables have the same distribution?
13. Do you want to treat the ordinal variable as if it were based on an underlying normally distributed interval variable?
14. Is the interval variable dependent?
15. Do you want a measure of the strength of the relationship between the variables or a test of the statistical significance of differences between groups?
16. Are you willing to assume that the intervally scaled variable is normally distributed in the population?
17. Is there more than one dependent variable?
18. Do you want to remove statistically the linear effects of one or more covariates from the dependent variable?
19. Do you want to treat the relationships among the variables as additive?
20. Do you want to analyze patterns existing among variables or among individual cases?
21. Do you want to find clusters of variables that are more strongly related to one another than to the remaining variables?

Each question confronts you with a decision. The decision you make narrows the field of available statistical procedures. Decisions must be made regarding the following:

1. Number of variables (1, 2, more than 2).
2. Type of measurement (nominal, ordinal, interval).
3. Type of variable (independent, dependent, research).
4. Distribution of variable (normal, non-normal).
5. Type of relationship (linear, nonlinear).
6. What you want to measure (strength of relationship, difference between groups).
7. Nature of groups (equal or unequal in size, matched or unmatched, dependent or independent).
8. Type of analysis (descriptive, classification, methodological, relational, comparison, predicting outcomes, intervention testing, causal modeling, examining changes across time).

As you can see, selecting and evaluating statistical procedures requires that you make a number of judgments regarding the nature of the data and what you want to know. Knowledge of the statistical procedures and their assumptions is necessary to the selection of appropriate statistical procedures. One must weigh the advantages and disadvantages of various statistical options. Access to a statistician can be invaluable in selecting the appropriate procedures.

INFERENTIAL STATISTICAL PROCEDURES

This section has been organized to present approaches to analysis according to the nature of the groups under study and the level of measurement available for analysis. Procedures for analyses are categorized according to whether the data for analysis are being treated as nominal, ordinal, or interval. Within those categories, procedures have been further categorized according to the number of groups and whether the groups under study are independent or dependent. In *independent groups,* the selection of one subject is totally unrelated to the selection of other subjects. For example, if subjects were randomly assigned to treatment and control groups, the groups would be independent. In *dependent groups,* subjects or observations selected for data collection are, in some way, related to the selection of other subjects or observations. For example, if subjects serve as their own control by using the pretest as a control, the observations (and therefore the groups) are dependent. Also, if matched pairs of subjects are used for control or treatment groups, the observations are dependent. For example, when studying twins, one might be placed in the control group and another in the treatment groups. Since they are twins, they are *matched* on several variables. The presentation of each statistical procedure includes a discussion of the purpose of the procedure, the mathematical assumptions on which the analysis is based, the method of calculation, and interpretation of the results.

INDEPENDENT GROUPS— NOMINAL DATA

Nominal data are frequently organized using contingency tables. *Contingency tables,* or cross-tabulation, allow visual comparison of summary data output related to two variables within the sample. This is a useful preliminary strategy for examining large amounts of data. In most cases, the data are in the form of frequencies or percent-

Table 18–1
The Relationship Between Parents' Reports of Impact on Family Life and Outside Help

| | Parents' Reports | | |
Outside Help	*Neutral*	*Negative*	*Total*
No*	18	7	25
Yes†	16	21	37
Total	34	28	62

* Includes cases from "Alone" category.
† Combines cases from "Some Help" and "Delegation" categories.
$p < 0.05$; $\chi^2 = 4.98$; $df = 1$.
(Modified from Knafl, K. A. [1985]. How families manage a pediatric hospitalization. *Western Journal of Nursing Research, 7*[2], 163.)

ages. Using this strategy, one can compare two or more categories of one variable with two or more categories of a second variable. The simplest version is referred to as a 2 × 2 table (two categories of two variables). Table 18–1 shows an example of a 2 × 2 contingency table from Knafl's (1985) study of how families manage a pediatric hospitalization.

The data are generally referenced in rows and columns. The intersection between the row and column in which a specific numerical value is inserted is referred to as a *cell.* The upper left cell would be row 1, column 1. In the example in Table 18–1, the cell of row 1, column 1 has the value of 18, and the cell of row 1, column 2 has the value of 7 and so on. The output from each row and each column is summed, and the sum is placed at the end of the row or column. In the example, the sum of row 1 is 25; the sum of row 2, 37; the sum of column 1, 34; and the sum of column 2, 28. The percent of the sample represented by that sum can also be placed at the end of the row or column. The row sums and the column sums total to the same value, which is 62 in the example.

Although contingency tables are most commonly used to examine nominal or ordinal data, they can be used with grouped frequencies of interval data. However, one must recognize that information about the data will be lost when this is

Table 18–2 Independent Groups—Nominal Data		
Chi-square	Contingency coefficient C	
Phi	Lambda	
Cramer's V		

done with interval data. This usually causes a loss of statistical power, that is, the probability of failing to reject a false null hypothesis is greater than if an appropriate parametric procedure could be used. Therefore, it is not generally the technique of choice. A contingency table is sometimes useful when an interval level measure is being compared with a nominal or ordinal level measure.

In some cases, the contingency table is presented and no further analysis is conducted. The table is presented as a form of summary statistics. However, in many cases, statistical analysis of the relationships or differences between the cell values is performed. The most familiar analysis of cross-tabulated data is the use of the chi-square statistic. Chi-square (χ^2) is designed to test for significant differences between cells. Some statisticians prefer to examine chi-square from a probability framework, using it to detect possible relationships (Goodman & Kruskal, 1954, 1959, 1963, 1972). Many correlational techniques can be used to analyze nominal data for independent groups (see Table 18–2).

Computer programs are also available to analyze data from cross-tabulation tables (contingency tables). These programs can generate output from chi-square and many correlational techniques and indicate the level of significance for each technique. One should know which statistics are appropriate for one's data and how to interpret the outcomes from these multiple analyses. The information presented on each of these tests provides guidance in the selection of a test and interpretation of the findings.

Chi-Square Test of Independence

The *chi-square test* of independence tests whether the two variables being examined are independent

or related. Chi-square is designed to test for differences in frequencies of observed data and compare them with the frequencies that could be expected to occur if the data categories were actually independent of each other. If differences are indicated, the analysis will not identify where these exist within the data.

Assumptions

One assumption of the test is that there is only one entry of data for each subject in the sample. Therefore, if repeated measures from the same subject are being used for analysis, such as pretests and post-tests, chi-square is not an appropriate test. Another assumption is that, for each variable, the categories are mutually exclusive and exhaustive. No cells may have an expected frequency of zero. However, in the actual data, the observed cell frequency may be zero. Until recently, each cell was expected to have a frequency of at least 5, but this requirement has been mathematically demonstrated not to be necessary. However, no more than 20% of the cells should have less than 5 (Conover, 1971). The test is distribution-free, or nonparametric, which means that there is no assumption of a normal distribution of values in the population from which the sample was taken.

Calculation

The formula is relatively easy to calculate manually and can be used with small samples, making it a popular approach to data analysis. The first step in the calculation of chi-square is to categorize the data, record the observed values in a contingency table, and sum the rows and columns. Next, the expected frequencies are calculated for each cell. The expected frequencies are those frequencies that would occur if there were no group differences; these are calculated from the row and column sums using the following formula:

$$E = \frac{(Tr)(Tc)}{N}$$

where:

E = expected cell frequency
Tr = row total for that cell
Tc = column total for that cell
N = total number of subjects in the sample

Thus, the expected frequency for a particular cell is obtained by multiplying the row total by the column total and dividing by the sample size. When the expected frequencies have been calculated for all the cells, the sum should be equivalent to the total sample size. The calculations of the expected frequencies for the four cells in Table 18–2 follow; they total 62 (sample size).

Cell 1, 1	Cell 1, 2
$E = \dfrac{(25)(34)}{62} = 13.71$	$E = \dfrac{(25)(28)}{62} = 11.29$

Cell 2, 1	Cell 2, 2
$E = \dfrac{(37)(34)}{62} = 20.29$	$E = \dfrac{(37)(28)}{62} = 16.71$

Using this same example, a contingency table could be constructed of the observed and expected frequencies (see Table 18–3). The chi-square statistic is then calculated using the following formula:

$$\chi^2 = \Sigma \frac{(O - E)^2}{E}$$

where:

O = observed frequency
E = expected frequency

Note that the formula includes difference scores between the observed frequency for each cell and the expected frequency for that cell. These difference scores are squared, divided by the expected frequency, and summed for each cell. The chi-square value was calculated using the observed and expected frequencies in Table 18–3.

Table 18–3
Contingency Table of Observed and Expected Frequencies

	Parents' Reports	
Outside Help	*Neutral*	*Negative*
No	O = 18	O = 7
	E = 13.71	E = 11.29
Yes	O = 16	O = 21
	E = 20.29	E = 16.71

O = observed frequencies.
E = expected frequencies.

$$\chi^2 = \frac{(18 - 13.71)^2}{13.71} + \frac{(7 - 11.29)^2}{11.29}$$

$$+ \frac{(16 - 20.29)^2}{20.29} + \frac{(21 - 16.71)^2}{16.71} = 4.98$$

$$df = 1; p < .05$$

With any chi-square analysis, the degrees of freedom (df) must be calculated to determine the significance of the value of the statistic. The following formula is used for this calculation:

$$df = (R - 1)(C - 1)$$

where:

R = number of rows
C = number of columns

In the example presented previously, the chi-square value was 4.98, and the df was 1, which was calculated as follows:

$$df = (2 - 1)(2 - 1) = 1$$

Interpretation of Results

The chi-square statistic is compared with the chi-square values in the table in Appendix E. The table includes the critical values of chi-square for specific degrees of freedom at selected levels of significance (usually .05 or .01). A critical value is the value of the statistic that must be obtained to indicate that a difference exists in the two populations represented by the groups under study. If the value of the statistic is equal to or greater than the value identified in the chi-square table, there is a significant difference between the two variables. If the statistic remains significant at more extreme probability levels, the largest p value at which significance is achieved is reported. The analysis indicates that there are group differences in the categories of the variable and that those differences are related to changes in the other variable. Although a significant chi-square indicates difference, the magnitude of the difference is not revealed by the analysis. If the statistic is not significant, we cannot conclude that there is a difference in the distribution of the two variables, and they are considered independent (Siegel, 1956).

Interpretation of the results is dependent on the design of the study. If the design was experimental, causality can be considered and the results can be inferred to the associated population. If the design was descriptive, differences identified are associated only with the sample under study. In either case, the differences found are related to differences among all the categories of the first variable and all the categories of the second variable. The specific differences among variables and categories of variables cannot be identified with this analysis. Often, in reported research, the researcher will visually examine the data and discuss differences in the categories of data as if they had been demonstrated to be statistically significantly different. These reports must be viewed with caution by the reader. Partitioning, the contingency coefficient C, the phi coefficient, or Cramer's V can be used to examine the data statistically, to determine in exactly which categories the differences lie. The last three strategies can also shed some light on the magnitude of the relationship between the variables. These strategies are discussed later in this chapter.

In reporting the results, contingency tables are generally presented only for significant chi-square analyses (refer to Table 18-2). The value of the statistic is given, including the *df* and *p* values. Data in the contingency table are sufficient to allow other researchers to repeat the chi-square analyses and thus check the accuracy of the analyses.

Partitioning of Chi-Square

Partitioning involves breaking up the contingency table into several 2 × 2 tables and conducting chi-square analyses on each table separately. Partitioning can be performed on any contingency table greater than a 2 × 2 with more than one degree of freedom. The number of partitions that can be conducted is equivalent to the degrees of freedom. The sum of the chi-square values obtained by partitioning is equal to the original chi-square value. There are some rules that must be followed during partitioning to prevent inflating the value of chi-square. The initial partition can include any four cells as long as two values from each variable are used. The next 2 × 2 must compress the first four cells into two cells and include two new cells. This process can continue until no new cells are available. Using this process, it is possible to determine which cells have contributed to the significant differences found.

Phi

The *phi coefficient* (ϕ) is used to describe relationships in dichotomous, nominal data. It is also used with the chi-square test to determine the location of difference(s) among cells. Phi is used only with 2 × 2 tables (see Table 18-4).

Table 18-4
Framework for Developing a 2 × 2 Contingency Table

| Variable Y | Variable X | | |
	0	*1*	*Totals*
0	A	B	A + B
1	C	D	C + D
Totals	A + C	B + D	N

Calculation

If chi-square (χ^2) has been calculated, the following formula can be used to calculate phi. Using the data presented in Table 18–1, the following phi coefficient was calculated. The chi-square analysis indicated a significant difference, and the phi coefficient indicated the magnitude of effect.

$$\text{Phi} = \sqrt{\frac{\chi^2}{N}} \qquad \text{Phi}(\phi) = \sqrt{\frac{4.98}{62}} = \sqrt{.0803} = .283$$

where:

N = the total frequency of all cells

Alternatively, phi can be calculated directly from the 2 × 2 table, using the following formula (Siegel, 1956). Again, the data from Table 18–1 are used to calculate the phi coefficient.

$$\text{Phi} = \frac{AD - BC}{\sqrt{(A + C)(B + D)(A + B)(C + D)}}$$

$$= \frac{(18)(21) - (7)(16)}{\sqrt{(34)(28)(25)(37)}} = .283$$

Interpretation of Results

The phi coefficient can be compared with Pearson's product-moment correlation coefficient (r), discussed later in this chapter, except that two dichotomous variables are involved. Phi values range from -1 to $+1$, with the magnitude of the relationship decreasing as the coefficient nears zero. The results show the strength of the relationship between the two variables.

Cramer's V

Cramer's V is a modification of phi used for contingency tables larger than 2 × 2. It is designed for use with nominal data. The value of the statistic ranges from zero to one.

Calculation

The formula can be calculated from the chi-square statistic. Using the data presented in Table 18–1, Cramer's V was calculated.

$$V = \sqrt{\frac{\chi^2}{N(L - 1)}} \qquad V = \sqrt{\frac{4.98}{62(7 - 1)}}$$

$$= \sqrt{.01334} = .115$$

where:

L = the smaller of either the number of columns or rows

N = total frequency of all cells

The Contingency Coefficient

The *contingency coefficient* (C) is used with two nominal variables and is the most commonly used of the three chi-square-based measures of association.

Calculation

The contingency coefficient can be calculated with the following formula, which uses the data presented in Table 18–1:

$$C = \sqrt{\frac{\chi^2}{\chi^2 + N}} \qquad C = \sqrt{\frac{4.98}{4.98 + 62}}$$

$$= \sqrt{.07435} = .273$$

The relationship demonstrated by C cannot be interpreted on the same scale as Pearson's r, phi, or Cramer's V because it does not reach an upper limit of one. The formula does not consider the number of cells, and the upper limit varies with the size of the contingency table. With a 2 × 2 table, the upper limit is .71; with a 3 × 3 table, the upper limit is .82; and with a 4 × 4 table, the upper limit is .87. Contingency coefficients from separate analyses can be compared only if the table sizes are the same.

Lambda

Lambda measures the degree of association (or relationship) between two nominal level variables. The value of lambda can range from zero to one. Two approaches to analysis are possible: asymmetrical and symmetrical. The asymmetrical approach indicates the capacity to predict the value of the dependent variable given the value of the independent variable. Thus, when asymmetrical lambda is used, it is necessary to specify a dependent and an independent variable. Symmetrical lambda measures the degree of overlap (or association) between the two variables and makes no assumptions regarding which variable is dependent and which is independent (Waltz & Bausell, 1981).

INDEPENDENT GROUPS— ORDINAL DATA

The statistical tests commonly used to analyze ordinal data are presented in Table 18–5.

Mann-Whitney *U* Test

The *Mann-Whitney* U *test* is the most powerful of the nonparametric tests, with 95% of the power of the *t* test to detect differences between groups of normally distributed populations. If the assumptions of the *t* test are violated, such as a non-normal distribution or ordinal-level data, the Mann-Whitney *U* test is more powerful. Although ranks are used for the analysis, ties in ranks have little effect on the outcome of the analysis.

Calculation

Prior to calculation, the scores from the two samples must be combined and ranked, with the lowest score assigned the rank of 1. Each score should also be identified as to group membership. If one had two groups (males and females) and the males scored 50, 55, 62, and 70 on an anxiety tool and the females scored 45, 58, 75, 76, and 77 on the same tool, these scores could be combined and ranked. The groups, scores, and ranks of these scores are presented in Table 18–6. The formula for calculating the Mann-Whitney *U* test follows. The *U* statistic was calculated using the data presented in Table 18–6.

$$\hat{U} = n_1 n_2 + \frac{n_1(n_1 + 1)}{2} - R_1$$

$$U' = n_1 n_2 - \hat{U}$$

where:

n_1 = number of observations in the smallest group

n_2 = number of observations in the largest group

R_1 = sum of ranks assigned to n_1

U = the smaller value of $\hat{U}$ or U'

$$\hat{U} = (4)(5) + \frac{4(4 + 1)}{2} - (2 + 3 + 5 + 6)$$

$$= 20 + 10 - 16 = 14$$

$$U' = (4)(5) - 14 = 20 - 14 = 6$$

Table 18–5
Tests for Independent Groups— Ordinal Data

Mann-Whitney *U*
Kolmogorov-Smirnov two-sample test
Wald-Wolfowitz runs test
Spearman rank-order correlation
Kendall's tau

Table 18–6
Ranked Scores from Two Groups

Group	F	M	M	F	M	M	F	F	F
Score	45	50	55	58	62	70	75	76	77
Rank	1	2	3	4	5	6	7	8	9

Interpretation of Results

The equations for both $\hat{U}$ and $\acute{U}$ must be calculated. Two tables are available to determine the significance of U. If n_2 is less than or equal to 8, the tables in Appendix F are used. If n_2 is between 9 and 20, the table in Appendix G is used. In the example, $U = 6$, $n_1 = 4$, and $n_2 = 5$. The probability (that the samples are from two different populations rather than one) listed in the table in Appendix F is .206, which is not significant. If n_2 is greater than 20, the Z statistic is calculated using the following equation. The normal distribution (see Appendix B) is used to determine the level of significance.

$$Z = \frac{U - n_1 n_2/2}{\sqrt{\dfrac{(n_1 n_2)(n_1 + n_2 + 1)}{12}}}$$

Kolmogorov-Smirnov Two-Sample Test

The Kolmogorov-Smirnov two-sample test is a nonparametric test used to determine whether two independent samples have been drawn from the same population. This test uses the cumulative frequency from two samples for analysis. Either grouped or ungrouped frequencies can be used. If groupings are used, the same intervals must be used for developing the distribution of each sample. Larger numbers of groups lead to a more meaningful analysis. For example, if age were being used, 5-year age spans would provide more meaningful analysis than 20-year spans. The test is sensitive to any differences in the distributions of the two samples, including differences in measures of central tendency, dispersion, or skewness. There is less risk of a Type II error with this test than with chi-square when small samples are being examined.

Calculation

The scores within two groups are ranked separately. The cumulative relative frequency is calculated for each rank by dividing the ranking by the number in the sample. In Table 18–7, a score of 2 is ranked 1 in a sample of 9; therefore, the relative

Table 18–7
Ranking of Scores for the Kolmogorov-Smirnov Two-Sample Test

| Sample 1 ($n = 10$) | | Sample 2 ($n = 9$) | | |
Scores	Cumulative Probability	Scores	Cumulative Probability	Absolute Value of the Difference
	.00	2	$^1/_9$ = .11	.11
	.00	3	$^2/_9$ = .22	.22
	.00	5	$^3/_9$ = .33	.33
	.00	6	$^4/_9$ = .44	.44
	.00	9	$^5/_9$ = .56	.56
	.00	10	$^6/_9$ = .67	.67*
11	$^1/_{10}$ = .10		.67	.57
12	$^2/_{10}$ = .20	12	$^7/_9$ = .78	.58
13	$^3/_{10}$ = .30		.78	.48
14	$^4/_{10}$ = .40		.78	.38
15	$^5/_{10}$ = .50	15	$^8/_9$ = .89	.39
18	$^6/_{10}$ = .60	18	$^9/_9$ = 1.00	.40
19	$^7/_{10}$ = .70		1.00	.30
21	$^8/_{10}$ = .80		1.00	.20
23	$^9/_{10}$ = .90		1.00	.10
25	$^{10}/_{10}$ = 1.00		1.00	.00

* The largest difference score.

frequency is $1/9 = .11$. A difference score is obtained for each point on the distribution by subtracting the smaller relative frequency from the larger relative frequency. For the score of 2, sample 1 had no scores that low, so the cumulative probability was .00 and the difference score was $.11 - .00 = .11$. The largest difference score in the example is indicated with an asterisk in Table 18–7.

Interpretation of Results

One difficulty with the Kolmogorov-Smirnov two-sample test is that one cannot determine whether the difference is in central tendency, dispersion, or skewness; therefore, conclusions must be broad. The test compares the cumulative distributions of the two samples with the assumption that if they are from the same population, differences in the distribution will be only random deviations. If the deviation is large enough, it is considered evidence for rejecting the null hypothesis.

The largest difference score is identified and used to compare with the tabled values in Appendix H. If the difference score is equal to or greater than the table value, the test indicates a significant difference. In the example in Table 18–7, the largest difference score, .67, compared with the table value of .578 at the .05 level for a two-tailed test, indicates that the samples are significantly different at the .05 level.

Wald-Wolfowitz Runs Test

The *Wald-Wolfowitz runs test*, a nonparametric test, is used to determine differences between two populations. The null hypothesis is false if the two populations differ in any way, including central tendency, variability, or skewness.

Calculation

The scores from the two samples are merged and ranked. The group membership of each score is recorded with the rank. Then the number of runs in the ranked series of scores is determined. A run is any sequence of scores from the same sample.

In the following example given, sample 1 is coded as A, and sample 2 is coded as B. The merged scores from samples A and B are presented below. Using this example, 6 runs were identified.

2	3	5	6	9	10	11	11	12	13	14	15
B	B	B	B	B	B	A	A	B	B	A	A
			1				2		3		4

16	17	18	19	21	23	25
B	B	A	A	A	A	A
	5			6		

Interpretation of Results

The runs test assumes that if the samples are from the same population, the scores will be well mixed. Therefore, r, the number of runs, will be large. When the null hypothesis is false, r is small. The table for the runs test is found in Appendix I. For the samples in the example, the table value of r is 5, which means that the number of runs must be equal to or less than 5 to be significant. Since there are 6 runs in the example, the null hypothesis is accepted.

The Spearman Rank-Order Correlation Coefficient (RHO)

The *Spearman rho,* a nonparametric test, is an adaptation of Pearson's product-moment correlation, discussed later in this chapter. This test is used when the assumptions of Pearson's analysis cannot be met. For example, the data may be ordinal, or the scores may be skewed.

Calculation

The data must be ranked in order to conduct the analysis. Therefore, if scores from measurement scales are used to perform the analysis, the scores must be converted to ranks. As with all correlational analyses, there must be a score (or value) on each of two variables (variable x and variable y) for each subject in the analysis. The scores on each variable are ranked separately. Rho is calculated based on difference scores between a subject's ranking on the first set of scores and its ranking on the second set of scores. The formula for this calculation is:

$$D = x - y$$

As in most statistical analyses, difference scores are difficult to use directly in equations because negative scores tend to cancel out positive scores; therefore, the scores are squared for use in the analysis. The formula is as follows:

$$\text{rho} = 1 - \frac{6 \sum D^2}{N^3 - N}$$

where:

rho = Spearman correlation coefficient (derived from Pearson's r)
D = difference score between the ranking of a score on variable x and the ranking of a score on variable y
N = number of paired ranked scores

Interpretation of Results

When the equation is used on data that meet the assumptions of Pearson's correlational analysis, the results are equivalent or slightly lower than Pearson's r, discussed later in this chapter. If the data are skewed, rho has an efficiency of 91% in detecting an existing relationship. The significance of rho must be tested as with any correlation; the formula used is presented below. The t distribution is presented in Appendix C, and the $df = N - 2$.

$$t = \text{rho} \sqrt{\frac{N - 2}{1 - \text{rho}^2}}$$

Kendall's Tau

Kendall's tau is a nonparametric measure of correlation used when both variables have been measured at the ordinal level. It can be used with very small samples. The statistic tau reflects a ratio of the actual concordance obtained between rankings with the maximal concordance possible. Marascuilo and McSweeney's (1977) explanation of this analysis technique is used in this text.

Calculation

To calculate tau, rank the scores on each of the two variables independently. Arrange the paired scores by subject, with the lowest ranking score on variable x at the top of the list and the ranking score on variable y for the same subject in the same row. An example of the ranking of scores for 5 subjects on variables x and y is presented in Table 18–8.

Next, comparisons are made of the relative ranking position between each pair of subjects on variable y, shown in the last column in the table. (It is not necessary to compare rankings on variable x, because the data have been arranged in order by rank.) If the comparison is concordant, the ranking of the score below will be higher than

---

Table 18–8
Ranking of Scores for Calculation of Kendall's Tau

Subject	Score on Variable x	Ranking on Variable x	Score on Variable y	Ranking on Variable y
A	3	1	4	2
B	5	2	2	1
C	6	3	6	3
D	9	4	8	5
E	12	5	7	4

Table 18-9
Calculation of Concordant–Discordant States in Kendall's Tau

Comparison Subjects	Value for x	Value for y	State
AB	+1	−1	Discordant
AC	+1	+1	Concordant
AD	+1	+1	Concordant
AE	+1	+1	Concordant
BC	+1	+1	Concordant
BD	+1	+1	Concordant
BE	+1	+1	Concordant
CD	+1	+1	Concordant
CE	+1	+1	Concordant
DE	+1	−1	Discordant

the ranking of the score above and is assigned a value of +1. If the comparison is discordant, the ranking of the score below will be lower than the ranking of the score above and is assigned a value of −1. In Table 18–9, the comparisons are identified as concordant (+1) or discordant (−1) for the ranked scores identified in Table 18–8. In this example, the number of discordant pairs is two; the number of concordant pairs is eight. The statistic S is then calculated using the following equation:

$$S = N_c - N_d \quad \text{Example: } S = 8 - 2 = 6$$

where:

N_c = number of concordant pairs
N_d = number of discordant pairs

At this point, tau is calculated using the following equation:

$$\text{Tau} = \frac{2S}{n(n-1)}$$

$$\text{Example: Tau} = \frac{(2)(6)}{5(5-1)} = .6$$

where:

n = number of paired scores

Interpretation of Results

If the ranking of values of x is not related to the ranking of values of y, any particular rank ordering of y is just as likely to occur as any other. The sample tau can be used to test the hypothesis that the population tau is 0. The significance of tau can be tested using the following equation for the Z statistic. The Z statistic was calculated using the previous example.

$$Z = \frac{\text{tau} - \text{mean}}{SD_{\text{tau}}}$$

$$Z = \frac{.6 - 0}{\sqrt{\dfrac{2(10 + 5)}{(9)(5)(5 - 1)}}} = \frac{.6}{.408} = 1.47$$

where:

$$\text{mean} = \mu_{\text{Tau}} = 0$$

$$SD_{\text{tau}} = \sqrt{\frac{2(2n + 5)}{9n(n - 1)}}$$

The Z values are approximately normally distributed and therefore the table of Z scores available in Appendix B can be used. The Z score for the example was 1.47, which is nonsignificant at the .05 level.

INDEPENDENT GROUPS— INTERVAL DATA

The common parametric tests used to analyze interval data for independent groups are presented in Table 18–10.

Table 18-10
Tests for Independent Groups— Interval Data

t Test—independent group
Pearson's correlation
Analysis of variance
Simple regression

t Test for Independent Samples

One of the most common parametric analyses used to test for significant differences between statistical measures of two samples is the *t test*. The *t* test uses the standard deviation of the sample to estimate the standard error of the sampling distribution. The ease in calculating the formula is attractive to researchers who wish to conduct their analyses by hand. This test is particularly useful when only small samples are available for analysis. The *t* test being discussed here is for independent samples. The *t* test for related samples is described on page 475.

The *t* test is frequently misused by researchers who use multiple *t* tests to examine differences in various aspects of data collected in a study. When this is done, there is an escalation of significance that results in a greatly increased risk of a Type I error. The *t* test can be used only one time during analysis to examine data from the two samples in a study. *Bonferroni's procedure,* which controls for the escalation of significance, can be used if various *t* tests must be performed on different aspects of the same data. A Bonferroni adjustment is easily done by hand; you simply divide the overall significance level by the number of tests and use the resulting number as the significance level for each test. Analysis of variance is always a viable alternative to the pooled *t* test and is preferred by many researchers who have become wary of the *t* test because of its frequent misuse. Mathematically, the two approaches are the same when only two samples are being examined.

Use of the *t* test involves the following assumptions:

1. Sample means from the population are normally distributed.
2. The dependent variable is measured at the interval level.
3. There is equal variance in the two samples.
4. There is independence of all observations within each sample.

The *t* test is *robust* to moderate violation of its assumptions. Robustness means that the results of analysis can still be relied upon to be accurate when one of the assumptions has been violated. The *t* test is not robust with respect to the between-samples or within-samples independence assumptions, nor is it robust with respect to extreme violation of the normality assumption unless the sample sizes are extremely large. Sample groups do not have to be equal for this analysis— the concern is, rather, for equal variance. A variety of *t* tests have been developed for various types of samples. Independent samples means that the two sets of data were not taken from the same subjects and that the scores in the two groups are *not* related.

Calculation

The *t* statistic is relatively easy to calculate. The numerator is the difference scores of the means of the two samples. The test uses the pooled standard deviation of the two samples as the denominator, which gives a rather forbidding appearance to the formula:

$$t = \frac{\overline{X}_a - \overline{X}_b}{\sqrt{\dfrac{\sum X_a^2 - \dfrac{(\sum X_a)^2}{n_a} + \sum X_b^2 - \dfrac{(\sum X_b)^2}{n_b}}{(n_a + n_b - 2)} \left(\dfrac{1}{n_a} + \dfrac{1}{n_b}\right)}}$$

$\overline{X}_a$ = mean of sample 1
$\overline{X}_b$ = mean of sample 2
n_a = number of subjects in sample 1
n_b = number of subjects in sample 2
$\sum X_a^2$ = sum of Group a squared deviation scores
$\sum X_b^2$ = sum of Group b squared deviation scores

$$df = n_a + n_b - 2$$

In the following example, the *t* test was used to examine the difference between a control group and an experimental group. The independent variable administered to the experimental group was a form of relaxation therapy. The dependent variable was pulse rate. The pulse rates for the experi-

Table 18–11
Data and Computations for the _t_ Test

Pulse Rate (Control Group)

X_a	Frequency (f)	fX_a	X_a^2	fX_a^2
70	1	70	4900	4900
72	2	144	5184	10,368
76	5	380	5776	28,880
82	3	246	6724	20,172
84	1	84	7056	7056
$n_a = 12$	$\overline{X}_a = 77$	$\Sigma X_a = 924$		$\Sigma X_a^2 = 71376$

Pulse Rate (Experimental Group)

X_b	Frequency (f)	fX_b	X_b^2	fX_b^2
64	1	64	4096	4096
66	2	132	4356	8712
70	5	350	4900	24500
72	3	216	5184	15552
78	1	78	6084	6084
$n_b = 12$	$\overline{X}_b = 70$	$\Sigma X_b = 840$		$\Sigma X_b^2 = 58944$

mental and control groups are presented in Table 18–11 with the calculations for the _t_ test.

$$t = \frac{77 - 70}{\sqrt{\frac{71,376 - \frac{(924)^2}{12} + 58,944 - \frac{(840)^2}{12}}{(12 + 12 - 2)}\left(\frac{1}{12} + \frac{1}{12}\right)}}$$

$$= \frac{7}{\sqrt{\frac{(71,376 - 71,148 + 58,944 - 58,800)(.1667)}{22}}}$$

$$= \frac{7}{1.679} = 4.169$$

$$df = 12 + 12 - 2 = 22$$

Interpretation of Results

To determine the significance of the _t_ statistic, the degrees of freedom must be calculated. The value of the _t_ statistic is then found on the table for the sampling distribution. If the sample size is 30 or less, the _t_ distribution is used; a table of this distribution can be found in Appendix C. For larger sample sizes, the normal distribution may be used; a table of this distribution can be found in Appendix B. The level of significance and the degrees of freedom are used to identify the critical value of _t_. This value is then used to obtain the most exact _p_ value possible. The _p_ value is then compared with the significance level. In the example presented in Table 18–11, the calculated $t = 19.55$, and the $df = 22$. This _t_ value was significant at the .001 level.

Bivariate Correlation

Bivariate correlation measures the extent of linear relationship between two variables. Multiple correlation, a more complex analysis technique that examines linear relationships among three or more variables, will be discussed in Chapter 19. Bivariate correlational analysis is generally performed on data collected from a single sample. Measures of the two variables to be examined must be available for each subject in the data set. Less commonly, data are obtained from two related subjects, such as blood lipid levels in father and son. Correlational analysis provides two pieces of information about the data: the nature of a linear relationship (positive or negative) between the two variables, and the magnitude (or strength) of the linear relationship. The outcomes of correlational analyses are symmetrical rather than asymmetrical. Symmetrical means that there is no indication from the analysis of the direction of the linear relationship. One cannot say from the analysis that variable *A* leads to or causes variable *B*.

Scatter diagrams provide useful preliminary information about the nature of the linear relationship between the variables and can be used in planning correlational analyses. The statistical analysis techniques used will depend on the type of data available. Correlational techniques are available for nominal, ordinal, or interval types of data. Many of the correlational techniques (gamma, Somers' D, Kendall's tau, contingency coefficient, phi, and Cramer's *V*) are used in conjunction with contingency tables. The correlational technique for interval data described here is the Pearson's product-moment correlation coefficient.

In a *positive linear relationship,* the scores being correlated vary together (in the same direction). When one score is high, the other score tends to be high; when one score is low, the other score tends to be low. In a *negative linear relationship,* when one score is high, the other score tends to be low. A negative linear relationship is sometimes referred to as an *inverse linear relationship.* These linear relationships can be plotted as a straight line on a graph. In some cases, the outcome is not linear, but *curvilinear.* In this case, a linear relationship plot will appear as a curved line, rather than a straight one. Analyses designed to test for linear relationships, such as Pearson's correlation, cannot detect a curvilinear relationship.

Pearson's Product-Moment Correlation Coefficient (*r*)

Pearson's correlation was the first of the correlation measures developed and is the most commonly used. All other correlation measures have been developed from Pearson's equation and are adaptations designed to control for violation of the assumptions that must be met in order to use Pearson's equation. These assumptions are:

1. Interval measurement of both variables
2. Normal distribution of at least one variable
3. Independence of observational pairs
4. Homoscedasticity

Data that are *homoscedastic* are evenly dispersed both above and below the regression line, which indicates a linear relationship on a scatter diagram (plot). Homoscedasticity is a reflection of equal variance of both variables. A *regression line* is the line that best represents the values of the raw scores plotted on a scatter diagram.

Calculation

Numerous formulas can be used to compute Pearson's *r*. With small samples, Pearson's *r* can be generated fairly easily with a calculator using the following formula:

$$r = \frac{n(\sum XY) - (\sum X)(\sum Y)}{\sqrt{[n(\sum X^2) - (\sum X)^2][n(\sum Y^2) - (\sum Y)^2]}}$$

where:

r	= Pearson's correlation coefficient
n	= number of paired scores
X	= score of the first variable
Y	= score of the second variable
XY	= product of the two paired scores

An example is presented that demonstrates the calculation of Pearson's *r*. The correlation between the two variables of functioning and coping was calculated. The functional variable (variable *X*) was operationalized using Karnofsky's scale, and coping was operationalized using a family coping tool. Karnofsky's scale ranges from 1 to 10; 1 is normal function, and 10 is moribund (fatal processes progressing rapidly). The family coping tool (variable *Y*) was developed using nursing di-

Table 18-12
Data and Computations for Pearson's *r*

Subjects	X	Y	XY	X²	Y²
1	10	4	40	100	16
2	7	3	21	49	9
3	3	2	6	9	4
4	6	3	18	36	9
5	1	1	1	1	1
6	5	2	10	25	4
7	2	2	4	4	4
8	9	4	36	81	16
9	4	1	4	16	1
10	8	4	32	64	16
Sums	55	26	172	385	80

agnosis terminology and ranges from 1 to 4, with 1 being effective family coping; 2 is ineffective family coping, potential for growth; 3 is ineffective family coping, compromised; 4 is ineffective family coping, disabling. The data for these two variables using 10 subjects are presented in Table 18–12. Usually, correlations are conducted on larger samples; this example serves only to demonstrate the process of calculating Pearson's *r*.

$$r = \frac{(10)(172) - (55)(26)}{\sqrt{[10(385) - (55)^2][10(80) - (26)^2]}}$$

$$= \frac{1720 - 1430}{\sqrt{(3850 - 3025)(800 - 676)}}$$

$$= \frac{290}{\sqrt{102,300}} = \frac{290}{319.844} = .907$$

Interpretation of the Results

The outcome of the Pearson product-moment correlation analysis is an *r* value of between −1 and +1. This *r* value indicates the degree of linear relationship between the two variables. A score of zero indicates no linear relationship.

−1 ——————— 0 ——————— +1

A −1 indicates a perfect negative (inverse) correlation. In a negative linear relationship, a high score on one variable is related to a low score on the other variable. A +1 indicates a perfect positive linear relationship. In a positive linear relationship, a high score on one variable is associated with a high score on the other variable. A positive correlation also exists when a low score on one variable is related to a low score on the other variable. As the negative or positive values of *r* approach zero, the strength of the linear relationship decreases. Traditionally, an *r* of .1 to .3 is considered a weak linear relationship, .3 to .5 a moderate linear relationship, and above .5 a strong linear relationship. However, this interpretation depends to a great extent on the variables being examined and the situation within which they were observed. Therefore, interpretation requires some judgment on the part of the researcher. In the example provided, the *r* value was .907, which indicates a strong positive linear relationship between the Karnofsky's scale and the family coping tool in this sample.

When Pearson's correlation coefficient is squared (r^2), the resulting number is the *percent of variance* explained by the linear relationship. In the preceding computation based on data in Table 18–12, $r = .907$, and $r^2 = .822$. In this case, the linear relationship explains 82% of the variability in the two scores. Except for perfect correlations, r^2 will always be lower than *r*. This *r* value is very high. Results in most nursing studies will be much lower.

There has been a tendency to disregard weak correlations in nursing research. However, there is a serious possibility of ignoring a linear relationship that may have some meaning within nursing knowledge when examined in the context of other variables. This is similar to a Type II error. This situation commonly occurs for three reasons. First, many nursing measurements are not powerful enough to detect fine discriminations, and some instruments may not detect extreme scores. In this case, the linear relationship may be stronger than indicated by the crude measures available. Second, correlational studies must have a wide range of variance for linear relationships to be detected. If the study scores are homogeneous or if the sample is small, linear relationships that exist in the population will not show up as clearly in the sample. Third, in many cases, bivariate analysis does not provide a clear picture of the dynamics in the situation. A number of variables can be linked through weak correlations, but together they provide increased insight into situations of interest. Therefore, although one should not overreact to small Pearson's coefficients, the information must be recorded for future reference. If the linear relationship is intuitively important, one may have to plan better designed studies and reexamine the linear relationship.

Testing the Significance of a Correlation Coefficient

In order to infer that the sample correlation coefficient applies to the population from which the sample was taken, statistical analysis must be performed to determine whether the coefficient is significantly different from zero (no correlation). In other words, we can test the hypothesis that the population Pearson correlation coefficient is 0. The test statistic used is the t, distributed according to the t distribution, with $n - 2$ degrees of freedom. The formula for calculating the t statistic follows. This formula was used to calculate the t value for the example where $r = .907$.

$$t = \frac{r\sqrt{n-2}}{\sqrt{1-r^2}} \qquad t = \frac{.907\sqrt{10-2}}{\sqrt{1-(.907)^2}}$$

$$= \frac{2.565}{\sqrt{.177}} = \frac{2.565}{.421} = 6.09$$

where:

r = Pearson's product-moment correlation coefficient

n = sample size of paired scores

$df = n - 2$

The significance of the t obtained from the formula is determined using the t distribution table in Appendix C. With a small sample, a very high correlation coefficient (r) can be nonsignificant.

With a very large sample, the correlation coefficient can be statistically significant when the degree of association is too small to be clinically significant. Therefore, in judging the significance of the coefficient, one must consider both the size of the coefficient and the significance of the t test. The t value calculated in the example was 6.09, and the df for the sample was 8. This t value was significant at the .001 level. When reporting the results of a correlation coefficient, both the r value and the p value should be reported.

One-Way Analysis of Variance

Analysis of variance (ANOVA) tests for differences between means. Expressed another way, it determines whether the samples under consideration were drawn from the same population and thus have the same population mean. As previously mentioned, the pooled variance t test is simply a specialized version of ANOVA in which only two means are examined. Although one-way ANOVA is a bivariate analysis, it is more flexible than other analyses in that it can examine data from two or more groups. This is accomplished by using group membership as one of the two variables under examination and a dependent variable as the second variable. ANOVA has been considered a much more rigorous approach to statistical analysis than regression analysis (which is often mistakenly equated with correlation analysis). However, statistically, ANOVA is simply a specialized version of regression analysis (Volicer, 1984).

ANOVA compares the variance within each group with the variance between groups. The outcome of the analysis is a numerical value for the F statistic, which will be used to determine if the groups are significantly different. The variance within each group is a result of individual scores in the group varying from the group mean and is referred to as the *within-group variance*. This variance is determined in the same way that variance was calculated earlier in this text (p. 433). The amount of variation about the mean in each group is assumed by ANOVA to be equal. The group means also vary around the grand mean (the mean of the total sample), which is referred to as the *between-groups variance*. One could assume that if all the samples were drawn from the same population, there would be little difference in these two sources of variance. The variance from within and between the groups explains the total variance in the data. When these two types of variance are combined, they are referred to as the total variance. Assumptions involved in ANOVA include:

1. Homogeneity of variance
2. Independence of observations
3. Normal distribution of the populations from which the samples were drawn, or random samples
4. Interval level data

Calculation

Several calculation steps are required for AN-OVA because the value of each source of variance must be determined and then compared with other sources of variance. ANOVA is usually calculated using a computer. However, ANOVA is not difficult to calculate by hand with small groups. It is important to understand the process of calculation and the terms used for each step of the analysis. The mathematical logic follows easily from the formulas previously presented. To clarify this connection, the conceptual formulas are used to explain the process.

To begin calculations, scores are separated by group and summed, and a mean is calculated for each group. Then scores from all groups are combined and summed, and a mean is obtained for all scores. This mean is referred to as the *grand mean*. Next, three different sums of squares are calculated: (1) the total sum of squares, (2) the sum of squares within, and (3) the sum of squares between. The sum of squares within and the sum of squares between will equal the total sum of squares. As with any sum of squares, difference scores are used for the calculation. The formula for the *total sum of squares* for three groups is:

$$SS_T = \Sigma(X_1 - \bar{\bar{X}})^2 + \Sigma(X_2 - \bar{\bar{X}})^2 + \Sigma(X_3 - \bar{\bar{X}})^2$$

where:

SS_T = total sum of squares
X_1 = single score from group 1
X_2 = single score from group 2
X_3 = single score from group 3
$\bar{\bar{X}}$ = grand mean

This formula indicates that the total sum of squares is obtained by summing the sum of squares from each group in the study. The formula for *sum of squares within* (or error) for three groups is:

$$SS_W = \Sigma(X_1 - \bar{X}_1)^2 + \Sigma(X_2 - \bar{X}_2)^2 + \Sigma(X_3 - \bar{X}_3)^2$$

where:

SS_W = sum of squares within
X_1 = single score from group 1
$\bar{X}_1$ = mean from group 1
X_2 = single score from group 2
$\bar{X}_2$ = mean from group 2
X_3 = single score from group 3
$\bar{X}_3$ = mean from group 3

The formula for *sum of squares between* for these groups is:

$$SS_B = n_1(\bar{X}_1 - \bar{\bar{X}})^2 + n_2(\bar{X}_2 - \bar{\bar{X}})^2 + n_3(\bar{X} - 3\bar{\bar{X}})^2$$

where:

SS_B = sum of squares between
n_1 = number of scores in group 1
n_2 = number of scores in group 2
n_3 = number of scores in group 3

Following these calculations, degrees of freedom are determined for the total, within, and between using the following formulas:

$$df_T = N - 1$$

$$df_W = N - k$$

$$df_B = k - 1$$

where:

k = number of groups
N = total number of scores

Using the sum of squares and the degrees of freedom, the mean square between (MS_B) and the mean square within (MS_W) are calculated using the following formulas:

$$MS_B = \frac{SS_{between}}{k - 1}$$

$$MS_W = \frac{SS_{within}}{N - k}$$

From these equations (MS_B and MS_W), the F statistic is calculated as follows:

$$F = \frac{MS_{between}}{MS_{within}}$$

Researchers who perform analysis of variance on their data frequently record the results in an ANOVA summary table. Popkess (1981) examined self-image scores between two groups (obese and nonobese). The two variables studied were self-image and group membership. An ANOVA was performed on the data; a summary table of the results is presented in Table 18–13. In this example, the mean square between (MS_B), mean

square within (MS_W), and F value were calculated as follows:

$$MS_B = \frac{776.69}{1} = 776.69$$

$$MS_W = \frac{11,228.74}{141} = 79.64$$

$$F = \frac{776.69}{79.64} = 9.75$$

Interpretation of Results

The test for ANOVA is always one-tailed. The critical region is in the upper tail of the test. The F distribution for determining the level of significance of the F statistic can be found in Appendix D. Use of the table requires knowledge of the degrees of freedom of MS_B and MS_W as well as the desired level of significance. If the F statistic (or ratio) is equal to or greater than the appropriate table value, there is a significant difference between the groups. In the example, the df for MS_B was 1, the df for MS_W was 141, and the F value was 9.75, which is significant at the .002 level.

If only two groups are being examined, the location of a significant difference is clear. However, if there are more than two groups under study, it is not possible to determine from the ANOVA exactly where the significant differences lie. One cannot assume that all the groups examined are significantly different. Therefore, post hoc analyses are conducted to determine the location of the differences among groups. There are several

Table 18–13
One-Way Analysis of Variance of Weight Groups and Self-Image

Source	df	SS	MS	F	F Probability
Between groups	1	776.69	776.69	9.75	.002
Within groups	141	11,228.74	79.64		
Total	142	12,005.43			

(From Popkess, S. A. [1981]. Assessment scales for determining the cognitive-behavioral repertoire of the obese subject. *Western Journal of Nursing Research, 3*[2], 199. © 1981. Reprinted by permission of Sage Publications, Inc.)

options for conducting post hoc analyses. When ANOVA has been conducted using a computer, the computer usually automatically conducts several post hoc analyses and includes their levels of significance on the computer printout. The implications of each analysis must be understood in order to interpret accurately the meaning attached to the outcomes.

POST HOC ANALYSES. One might wonder why a researcher would conduct a test that failed to provide the answer sought—namely, where the significant differences were in a data set. It would seem more logical to perform *t* tests or ANOVAs on the groups in the data set in pairs, thus clearly determining whether there is a significant difference between those two groups. However, when this is done with three groups in the data set, the risk of a Type I error increases from 5% to 14%. As the number of groups increases (and with the increase in groups, an increase in the number of necessary comparisons), the risk of a Type I error increases strikingly.

Post hoc tests have been developed specifically to determine the location of differences after ANOVA. These tests were developed to reduce the incidence of a Type I error. The frequently used post hoc tests are Bonferroni's procedure, the Newman-Keuls test, the Tukey HSD test, the Scheffé test, and Dunnett's test. When these tests are calculated, the alpha level is reduced in proportion to the number of additional tests required to locate statistically significant differences. As the alpha level is decreased, reaching the level of significance becomes increasingly more difficult.

The Newman-Keuls test compares all possible pairs of means and is the most liberal of the post hoc tests considered acceptable by publication editors. Liberal means that the alpha level is not as severely decreased. The Tukey HSD test computes one value with which all means within the data set are compared. It is considered more stringent than the Newman-Keuls test and requires approximately equal sample sizes in each group. The Scheffé test is the most conservative of the post hoc tests and has a good reputation among researchers. However, one must keep in mind that a test that is very conservative increases the risk

of a Type II error. Dunnett's test requires a control group for its use. The mean for each experimental group is then compared with the control group. The test does not require a reduction of alpha and thus is advisable to use when the conditions for the test are met.

Simple Linear Regression

Simple linear regression provides a means to estimate the value of a dependent variable based on the value of an independent variable. The regression equation is a mathematical expression of a causal proposition emerging from a theoretical framework. This linkage between the theoretical statement and the equation should be made clear prior to the analysis.

Simple linear regression is an effort to explain the dynamics within the scatter plot by drawing a straight line (the line of best fit) through the plotted scores. This line is drawn to provide the best explanation of the linear relationship between two variables. Knowing that linear relationship, we can, with some degree of accuracy, use regression analysis to predict the value of one variable if we know the value of the other variable. In addition, the following assumptions need to be met:

1. The presence of homoscedasticity—equal scatter of values of *y* above and below the regression line at each value of *x* (constant variance).
2. The dependent variable is measured at the interval level.
3. The expected value of the residual error is zero.

Calculation

Simple linear regression is a method of determining parameters *a* and *b*. The formula is developed mathematically based on the requirement that the squared deviation values (squared difference scores) be minimized. When squared deviation values are minimized, variance from the line of best fit is minimized. To understand the mathematical process, it is helpful to recall the algebraic equation for a straight line:

$$y = a + bx$$

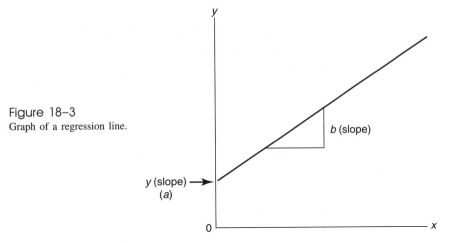

Figure 18–3
Graph of a regression line.

In regression analysis, the straight line is usually plotted on a graph, with the horizontal axis representing x (the independent, or predictor, variable) and the vertical axis representing y (the dependent, or predicted, variable). The value represented by the letter a is referred to as the y *intercept*. This is the point where the regression line crosses (or intercepts) the y axis. At this point on the regression line, $x = 0$. The value represented by the letter b is referred to as the *slope,* or the coefficient of x. The slope determines the direction and angle of the regression line within the graph. The slope expresses the extent to which y changes for every one unit change in x. Figure 18–3 is a graph of these points.

In simple, or bivariate, regression, predictions are made using two variables. The score on variable y (dependent variable) is predicted based on the same subject's known score on variable x (independent variable). The predicted score (or estimate) is referred to as $\hat{y}$ (expressed y-hat) or occasionally as y' (expressed y-prime).

No single regression line can be used to predict with complete accuracy every y value from every x value. In fact, one could draw an infinite number of lines through the scattered paired values. However, the purpose of the regression equation is to develop the line to allow the highest degree of prediction possible—the line of best fit. The procedure for developing the line of best fit is the *method of least squares*.

To explain the method of least squares, we must return to difference scores. In a real sample in which values on both x and y are known, the regression line is plotted subject by subject, using both values to determine the placement of each point. The multiple subjects who have a single value on x can have various values on y. Only the mean of these y values is located on the regression line. Therefore, at each point on the x axis, one can determine difference scores from the mean on the y axis. From these difference scores, a sum of squares can be calculated. There can, then, be a sum of squares for each point on the x axis. The sum of squares of all difference scores is an indicator of how good a fit the regression line is to the data.

The equations to estimate the regression line have been developed in such a way that the value of the sum of squares will be minimized, thus decreasing the variance and maximizing the predictive power of the resulting equation. The three equations for the method of least squares are:

$$b = \frac{n(\sum xy) - (\sum x)(\sum y)}{n(\sum x^2) - (\sum x)^2}$$

$$a = \bar{y} - b\bar{x}$$

$$\hat{y} = a + bx$$

where:

b = slope
n = number of paired values
x = known value of x
a = y intercept
$\hat{y}$ = predicted value of y

The coefficient of x, which is b, can be determined from the analysis of raw data or from the analysis of Z scores. When the slope is determined from Z scores, it is no longer the coefficient of x but the coefficient of the Z score-transformed x. If b is determined from Z scores, it is referred to as *beta*. Beta is preferred when comparisons are made with the results of other analyses. Computer analyses usually provide both values.

Interpretation of Results

The outcome of analysis is the regression coefficient R. When R *is* squared, it indicates the amount of variance in the data that is explained by the equation. A null regression hypothesis states that the population regression slope is 0, which indicates that there is no useful linear relationship between x and y. (There are regression analyses that test for nonlinear relationships.) The test statistic used to determine the significance of a regression coefficient is t. However, the test uses a different equation than the t test used to determine significant differences between means. In determining the significance of a regression coefficient, t tends to become larger as b moves farther from zero. However, if the sum of squared deviations from regression is large, the t value will decrease. Small sample sizes also decrease the t value.

In reporting the results of a regression analysis, the equation is expressed with the calculated coefficient values. The R^2 value and the t values are also documented. The format for reporting the results of regression is as follows:

$$\begin{array}{cc} y \text{ intercept} & b(\text{slope}) \\ \downarrow & \downarrow \\ \hat{y} = 3.45 + 8.72x & \quad R^2 = .63 \\ (2.79) \quad (4.68) & \leftarrow t \text{ value} \end{array}$$

Table 18–14
Predicted Values of y from Known Values of x Using Regression Analysis

Value of x	Predicted value of y
0	3.45 (y Intercept)
1	12.17 (y Intercept + b)
2	20.89 (+ b)
3	29.61 (+ b)
4	38.33 (+ b)

The figures in parentheses are not always t values. They may be the standard error of the estimate. Therefore, the report must indicate which values are being reported. If t values are being used, the t value that indicates significance should also be reported. A t value equal to or greater than the table value (Appendix C) indicates significance. From these results, a graph can be developed to illustrate the outcome. Additionally, a table can be developed indicating the changes that are predicted to occur in the value of y with each increase in the value of x. Names are usually given to identify the variables of x and y. Using the example in which the y intercept = 3.45 and b = 8.72, a table (see Table 18–14) of x and y values was developed. These values are graphed in Figure 18–4.

After a regression equation has been developed, the equation is tested against a new sample to determine its accuracy in prediction. This is called *cross-validation*. In some studies, data are collected from a hold-out sample obtained at the initial data collection period but not included in the initial regression analysis. The regression equation is then tested against this sample. Some "shrinkage" of R^2 is expected, because the equation was generated to fit best the sample from which it was developed. However, an equation is most useful if it maintains its ability to predict accurately across many and varied samples. The first test of an equation against a new sample should use a sample very similar to the initial sample.

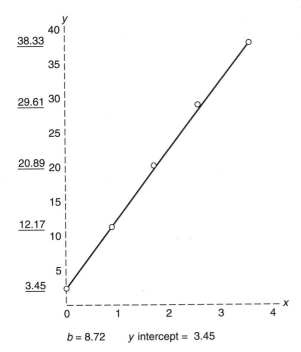

b = 8.72   y intercept = 3.45

Figure 18–4
Regression line developed from values in Table 18–14.

TWO DEPENDENT GROUPS— NOMINAL DATA

Dependent groups implies that the measures taken from the two groups are related in some way. For example, measures may be taken on the same subject at two time periods, such as a pretest and a post-test. If the pretest scores are considered one group and the post-test scores are considered another group, the two sets of scores (and thus the groups) are related. This situation violates the assumptions of many statistical tests and requires the use of tests developed specifically for these situations. The nonparametric McNemar test is described in this section.

McNemar Test for Significance of Changes

The *McNemar test* analyzes changes that occur in dichotomous variables using a 2 × 2 table. This

Table 18–15			
2 × 2 Contingency Table for the McNemar Test			

| | | Post-Test | |
		−	+
Pretest	+	A	B
	−	C	D

nonparametric test is particularly appropriate for before and after or pretest/post-test designs in which the subjects serve as their own control and the data are nominal. For example, one might be interested in determining the number of nurses in a sample who changed from hospital nursing to home health care and vice versa. The two work places in the aforementioned example are nominal, because there is no way to rank one as being better than the other. Pluses and minuses are used to indicate the two conditions, and the assigning of a plus or minus to a variable is at the discretion of the researcher. Data are placed in a 2 × 2 contingency table as exemplified in Table 18–15.

Subjects whose scores changed from positive to negative are tallied in cell A. In the example, those nurses who changed from home health care to hospital nursing were tallied in cell A; there were five nurses. Those who changed from negative to positive are tallied in cell D. If the score remained negative, the subject is tallied in cell C, and if the score remained positive, the subject is tallied in cell B. Only subjects whose scores changed are included in the analysis; therefore, only the tally marks in cells A and D are considered. The null hypothesis is that the population probability of changing from negative to positive is the same as the population probability of changing from positive to negative.

If one were to study the nurses who changed from home health care to hospital nursing, the data might appear as presented in Table 18–16. Cell A contains the number of nurses that changed from home health nursing to hospital nursing; there were five nurses in this category. Fifteen (cell D)

Table 18-16
Example of 2 × 2 Contingency Table for McNemar Test

Pretest		Post-Test −	Post-Test +
	+	A 5	B 5
	−	C 3	D 15

nurses changed from hospital nursing to home health care. Five nurses (cell B) stayed in home health nursing, and three nurses (cell C) remained in hospital nursing.

Calculation

If $\frac{1}{2}(A + D)$ is 5 or less, the binomial distribution is used to determine the level of probability. Otherwise, the chi-square (χ^2) test with the correction for continuity is used to test the hypothesis. The χ^2 value is calculated for the data presented in Table 18-16.

$$\chi^2 = \frac{(|A - D| - 1)^2}{A + D}$$

$$\chi^2 = \frac{(|5 - 15| - 1)^2}{5 + 15} = \frac{(10 - 1)^2}{20}$$

$$= \frac{81}{20} = 4.05$$

Interpretation of Results

The significance of the χ^2 value with $df = 1$ is determined from the χ^2 table in Appendix E. If the value is equal to or greater than the table value, the two groups are considered significantly different. In the example, the χ^2 value was 4.05, and the $df = 1$; the χ^2 value is significant at the .05 level.

TWO DEPENDENT GROUPS— ORDINAL DATA

The sign test and the Wilcoxon matched-pairs signed-ranks test are described in this section.

Sign Test

The *sign test* is a nonparametric test that was developed for data for which it is difficult to assign numerical values. However, the data can be ranked on such dimensions as agree-disagree, easier-harder, earlier-later, more-less, higher-lower.

The sign test acquired its name from the use of the + sign and the − sign to rank or place value on the variables under study. The test makes no assumptions about the shape of the underlying distribution or that all subjects are from the same population. The null hypothesis states that the population probability of changing from negative to positive is the same as the population probability of changing from positive to negative.

Calculation

To conduct the sign test, the pretest/post-test or matched-pairs values are examined to determine whether there was a positive or negative change from the first observation to the second observation. Subjects in whom no change was observed are dropped from the analysis, and the N is reduced accordingly. N is the number of pairs of observations. The number of pluses and minuses for these paired observations is counted. If N is 25 or less, the binomial distribution is consulted for the level of probability. If N is greater than 25, the Z statistic is calculated using the following equation:

$$Z = \frac{(x + 0.5) - \frac{1}{2}N}{\frac{1}{2}\sqrt{N}}$$

where:

x = the smaller of either the sum of pluses or the sum of minuses

N = number of paired values retained for analysis

For a two-tailed test, a Z score of 1.96 indicates significance at the .05 level. For a one-tailed test, a Z score of 1.643 indicates significance at the .05 level. The table for the Z distribution (cumulative normal distribution) can be found in Appendix B.

Wilcoxon Matched-Pairs Signed-Ranks Test

The *Wilcoxon matched-pairs signed-ranks test,* like the sign test, is a nonparametric test that examines changes that occur in pretest/post-test measures or matched-pairs measures. It is more powerful than the sign test, because it examines both the direction and the magnitude of change that occurs. A pair of scores in which a greater amount of change has occurred is given more weight than a pair in which very little change has occurred. This test requires that the researcher be able to assess the magnitude of a change between the first and second observation. When no change has occurred between the first and second observation, the subject or pair is dropped from the analysis and the sample size is decreased.

Calculation

Initially, a difference score (*d*) is calculated for each pair of scores. If the difference score is zero, the pair is omitted. The plus or minus sign associated with each difference score must be retained. Ignoring the plus and minus signs, the difference scores are ranked, with the lowest difference score ranked 1. If some of the difference scores are tied, the ranks of the tied scores are averaged. For example, if ranks 3, 4, and 5 had the same difference score, the ranks would be summed and divided by the number of ranks [(3 + 4 + 5)/3 = 4], and the resulting rank would be assigned to each of the pairs. The next difference scores would then be assigned the rank of 6.

In the second step of analysis, the sign of the difference score is affixed to each rank. This indicates which ranks resulted from a negative change and which ranks resulted from a positive change. If the two groups being examined are not differ-

ent, the positive and negative ranks should be relatively interspersed, with the greatest difference scores occurring equally among positive and negative ranks. The third step in analysis is to sum the ranks having positive signs and to sum the ranks having negative signs. If there is no difference in the two groups, these two sums should be similar.

Interpretation of Results

The smallest value of the two sums (*T*) and the number of pairs (*N*) are used to determine the significance of the difference in the two sums. If *N* is 25 or less, the Wilcoxon matched-pairs signed-ranks table in Appendix J is used to determine significance. If *T* is equal to or less than the table value, the null hypothesis that there is no difference in the values of the two sums is rejected. If *N* is greater than 25, the Z score is calculated using the following equation:

$$Z = \frac{T - \dfrac{N(N+1)}{4}}{\sqrt{\dfrac{N(N+1)(2N+1)}{24}}}$$

where:

T = the smallest value of the two sums
N = number of matched pairs retained for
    analysis

In a two-tailed test, a Z score of 1.96 or less indicates a level of significance of .05. For a one-tailed test, a Z score of 1.68 or less indicates a level of significance of .05. The table for the Z distribution is in Appendix B.

TWO DEPENDENT GROUPS— INTERVAL DATA

t Tests for Related Samples

When samples are related, the formula used to calculate the *t* statistic is different from the formula described on page 463. Samples may be related because matching has been performed as part of the design or because the scores used in the analysis were obtained from the same subjects under different conditions (e.g., pretest and post-test). This test requires that the differences between the paired scores be independent and normally or approximately normally distributed.

Calculation

The following formula assumes that scores in the two samples are, in some way, correlated (dependent).

$$t = \frac{\bar{d}}{\sqrt{\dfrac{\Sigma d^2}{n(n-1)}}}$$

where:

$\bar{d}$ = the mean difference between the paired scores

Σd^2 = sum of squared deviation difference scores

n = number of paired scores

df = $n - 1$

Interpretation of Results

Results of the analysis are interpreted in the same way as those of the independent t test described earlier in the chapter.

THREE OR MORE INDEPENDENT GROUPS—NOMINAL DATA

The chi-square (χ^2) test of independence can be used with two or more groups. In this case, group membership is used as the independent variable. The χ^2 statistic is calculated using the same formula presented on page 454. If there are more than two categories of the dependent variable, differences in both central tendency and dispersion are tested by the analysis.

THREE OR MORE INDEPENDENT GROUPS—ORDINAL DATA

The Kruskal-Wallis One-Way Analysis of Variance by Ranks

The *Kruskal-Wallis test* is the most powerful non-parametric test for examining three independent groups. It has 95% of the power of the F statistic to detect existing differences between groups. The technique tests the null hypothesis that all samples are from the same population. The main assumption with this test is that there is an underlying continuous distribution.

Calculation

The initial step in analysis is to rank all scores from all samples together, with the smallest score being assigned a rank of 1. N is equal to the largest rank or the total number of observations from all samples. Next, the ranks from each sample are summed. The Kruskal-Wallis test determines whether the sum of ranks from each group is different enough that we can reject the hypothesis that the samples come from the same population. The statistic used in the Kruskal-Wallis test is H, and the following formula is used to calculate this statistic.

$$H = \frac{12}{N(N+1)} \sum \frac{R_j^2}{n_j} - 3(N+1)$$

where:

j = number assigned to each sample

n_j = number of scores in j sample

N = total number of scores across all samples

R_j = sum of ranks from j sample

$\sum \dfrac{R_j^2}{n_j}$ indicates that $\dfrac{R_j^2}{n_j}$ is to be calculated separately for each sample and the results are to be summed

Interpretation of Results

If there are more than five subjects in each group, the chi-square table in Appendix E can be used to determine levels of significance. Degrees of freedom (df) is calculated as the number of samples minus 1. If the value obtained for H is equal to or greater than the table value, the groups are considered statistically significantly different. If there are three samples and each sample contains fewer than five subjects, exact probabilities for these samples can be found in Appendix K.

THREE OR MORE DEPENDENT GROUPS—NOMINAL DATA

The Cochran Q Test

The *Cochran Q test* is an extension of the McNemar test for two related samples. The Cochran Q test can be used in such situations as (1) when subjects have been matched and several levels of treatment have been administered, (2) when more than one matched control group has been used for comparison, or (3) for repeated measures of the dependent variable across time. Measures of the dependent variable must be coded dichotomously. For example, 1 could be coded if an event occurred, 0 if it did not occur; 1 could be coded for yes, 0 for no; + for a positive change, − for a negative change.

Calculation

Data are arranged in a contingency table where k is equal to the number of columns and N is equal to the number of rows. The null hypothesis is that there is no difference in frequency or proportion of responses by category in each column except

that of chance. The computational equation is as follows:

$$Q = \frac{(k - 1)[k\Sigma G_j^2 - (\Sigma G_j)^2]}{k\Sigma L_i - \Sigma L_i^2}$$

where:

i = number assigned to each row
j = number assigned to each column
k = number of columns
G_j = total number of positive responses (yes, 1 or +) in each column
L_i = total number of positive responses (yes, 1 or +) in each row

Interpretation of Results

The value of Q is compared with the chi-square table in Appendix E using $df = k - 1$. If the value of Q is greater than or equal to the table value, the frequency or proportion of subjects coded as positive differs significantly among the samples. The power efficiency of Cochran's Q is not known, because there are no parametric tests with which it can be compared.

THREE OR MORE DEPENDENT GROUPS—ORDINAL DATA

The Friedman Two-Way Analysis of Variance by Ranks

The *Friedman two-way ANOVA* by ranks may be used with matched samples or in repeated measures. The null hypothesis is that the samples come from the same population. The Friedman test considers magnitude of differences and therefore is more powerful than the Cochran Q test in rejecting a false null hypothesis, given the same data.

SCORE TOTALS

	Condition			
	I	II	III	IV
Group 1	22	16	8	2
Group 2	41	26	8	12
Group 3	2	8	36	44

ROW RANKS

	Condition			
	I	II	III	IV
Group 1	4	3	2	1
Group 2	4	3	1	2
Group 3	1	2	3	4
R_j	9	8	6	7
R_j^2	81	64	36	49

$(R_j)^2 = 81 + 64 + 36 + 49 = 230$

Figure 18–5
Example of contingency tables for the Friedman test.

Calculation

Data are placed in a contingency table with N rows and k columns. Rows represent groups of subjects, columns represent conditions being studied. Scores within each cell are summed and ranked by row. In Figure 18–5, the scores and the row ranks for these scores are presented in contingency tables. The value of the Friedman test statistic χ_r^2 can be calculated using the following equation:

$$\chi_r^2 = \frac{12}{Nk(k+1)} \Sigma(R_j)^2 - 3N(k+1)$$

where:

N	=	number of rows
k	=	number of columns
j	=	column number
R_j	=	sum of ranks in j column
$\Sigma (R_j)^2$	=	instructs to sum the squares of R_j over all columns

The χ_r^2 value was calculated for the data presented in Figure 18-5.

$$\chi_r^2 = \frac{12}{3(4)(4+1)}[(9)^2 + (8)^2 + (6)^2 + (7)^2]$$
$$- (3)(3)(4+1) = \frac{12}{60}(230) - 45$$
$$= (.2)(230) - 45 = 1.0$$

Interpretation of Results

The value of the χ_r^2 statistic is compared with the values in Appendix L. If the value of the test statistic is equal to or greater than the table value for the selected level of significance (e.g., .05), the ranks in the various columns differ significantly; therefore, the value of a score depends on the condition. In the example, the $\chi_r^2 = 1.0$, which is not significant, and the null hypothesis would be accepted. If k (number of columns) is greater than 4, the χ_r^2 statistic is compared with the chi-square distribution in Appendix E. The power efficiency to reject the null is equivalent to the F statistic when alpha is .05, and 85% of the F statistic when alpha is .01.

SUMMARY

Bivariate analysis involves the comparison of summary values from two groups on the same variable or of two variables within a group. Selection of the statistical analysis will depend on the level of measurement (nominal, ordinal, interval, or ratio) of the data. In independent groups, the selection of one subject is totally unrelated to the selection of other subjects. In dependent groups, subjects or observations selected for data collection are, in some way, related to the selection of other subjects or observations.

The common tests used to analyze nominal data for independent groups are chi-square, phi, Cramer's *V*, contingency coefficient *C*, and lambda. Nominal data are frequently organized using contingency tables. Contingency tables, or cross-tabulation, allow visual comparison of summary data output related to two variables within the sample. Using this strategy, one can compare two or more categories of one variable to two or more categories of a second variable. The simplest version is referred to as a 2×2 table.

Magnitude estimation is a strategy to estimate the degree of difference between groups. Magnitude estimation of differences between groups when the dependent variable is continuous is commonly obtained using Pearson's product-moment correlation coefficient. Squaring the statistic *r* will indicate the amount of variance in the variable scores explained by group membership. Degrees of freedom (*df*) involves the freedom of a score's value to vary given the other existing scores' values and the established sum of these scores.

The statistical tests commonly used to analyze ordinal data are the Mann-Whitney *U*, Kolmogorov-Smirnov two-sample test, Wald-Wolfowitz runs test, Spearman rank-order correlation, and Kendall's tau. The Mann-Whitney *U* test is the most powerful of the nonparametric tests, with 95% of the power of the *t* test to detect differences between groups. If the assumptions of the *t* test are violated, the Mann-Whitney *U* test is more powerful.

The common parametric tests used to analyze interval data for independent groups are the *t* test for independent groups, Pearson's correlation, analysis of variance, and simple regression. One of the most common parametric analyses used to test for significant differences between statistical measures of two samples is the *t* test. The *t* test is frequently misused by beginning researchers, who use multiple *t* tests to examine differences in various aspects of data collected in a study. When this is done, there is an escalation of significance that results in a greatly increased risk of a Type I error. Use of the *t* test involves the following assumptions: (1) sample means from the population are normally distributed, (2) the dependent variable is measured at the interval level, and (3) equal variance exists in the two samples.

Pearson's correlation is the most commonly used of the correlation measures. The assumptions of Pearson's correlation are (1) interval measurement of both variables, (2) normal distribution of variables, (3) independent distribution of variables, and (4) homoscedasticity. Homoscedastic data are evenly dispersed both above and below the regression line, which indicates a linear relationship. Homoscedasticity is a reflection of equal variance of both variables.

Analysis of variance (ANOVA) tests for differences between means. ANOVA compares the variance within each group with the variance between groups. The assumptions of ANOVA include (1) homogeneity of variance, (2) independence of observations, (3) normal distribution of the populations from which the samples were drawn, and (4) interval level data. If only two groups are being examined, the location of a significant difference is clear.

continued

continued

However, if there are more than two groups under study, it is not possible to determine from the ANOVA exactly where the significant differences lie. One cannot assume that all the groups examined are significantly different. Therefore, post hoc analyses are conducted to determine the location of the differences among groups.

Dependent groups implies that the measures taken from the two groups are related in some way. For example, measures may be taken on the same subject at two time periods, such as a pretest and a post-test. If the pretest scores are considered one group and the post-test scores are considered another group, the two sets of scores (and thus the groups) are related. The test used for two dependent groups with nominal data is the McNemar test for significance of changes. The tests used for two dependent groups with ordinal data are the sign test and the Wilcoxon matched-pairs signed-ranks test. The test used for two dependent groups with interval data is the t test for related samples.

The chi-square test of independence can be used with more than two groups with nominal data. Three or more independent groups with ordinal data can be tested using the Kruskal-Wallis test. The Kruskal-Wallis test is the most powerful nonparametric test for examining three independent groups. This test has 95% of the power of the F statistic to detect existing differences between groups. The Cochran Q test is an extension of the McNemar test for two related samples and can be used in dependent groups of three or more with nominal data. Three or more dependent groups with ordinal data can be tested using the Friedman two-way analysis of variance by ranks.

References

Andrews, F. M., Klem, L., Davidson, T. N., O'Malley, P. M., & Rodgers, W. L. (1981). *A guide for selecting statistical techniques for analyzing social science data* (2nd ed.). Ann Arbor, MI: Survey Research Center, Institute for Social Research, The University of Michigan.

Conover, W. J. (1971). *Practical nonparametric statistics.* New York: Wiley.

Goodman, L. A., & Kruskal, W. H. (1954). Measures of association for cross classifications. *Journal of the American Statistical Association, 49,* 732–764.

Goodman, L. A., & Kruskal, W. H. (1959). Measures of association for cross classifications, II: Further discussion and references. *Journal of the American Statistical Association, 54*(285), 123–163.

Goodman, L. A., & Kruskal, W. H. (1963). Measures of association for cross classifications, III: Approximate sampling theory. *Journal of the American Statistical Association, 58*(302), 310–364.

Goodman, L. A., & Kruskal, W. H. (1972). Measures of association for cross classifications, IV: Simplification of asymptotic variances. *Journal of the American Statistical Association, 67*(338), 415–421.

Goodwin, L. D. (1984). The use of power estimation in nursing research. *Nursing Research, 33*(2), 118–120.

Knafl, K. A. (1985). How families manage a pediatric hospitalization. *Western Journal of Nursing Research, 7*(2), 151–176.

Knapp, R. G. (1985). *Basic statistics for nurses* (2nd ed.). New York: Wiley.

Marascuilo, L. A., & McSweeney, M. (1977). *Nonparametric and distribution-free methods for the social sciences.* Monterey, CA: Brooks/Cole.

Popkess, S. A. (1981). Assessment scales for determining the cognitive-behavioral repertoire of the obese subject. *Western Journal of Nursing Research, 3*(2), 199–215.

Siegel, S. (1956). *Nonparametric statistics for the behavioral sciences.* New York: McGraw-Hill.

Tabachnick, B. G., & Fidell, L. S. (1983). *Using multi-variate statistics.* New York: Harper & Row.

Volicer, B. J. (1984). *Multivariate statistics for nursing research.* New York: Grune & Stratton.

Waltz, C., & Bausell, R. B. (1981). *Nursing research: Design, statistics and computer analysis.* Philadelphia: Davis.

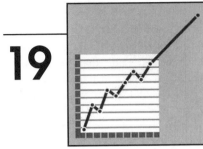

19

Advanced Statistical Analyses

Many of the phenomena of concern to nurse researchers are complex in nature and require use of advanced statistical procedures. Although use and interpretation of these analyses require a statistical sophistication not usually acquired before the doctoral level, important studies using the techniques are appearing with increasing frequency in the nursing literature. In this text, our approach is to provide sufficient information to allow the beginning researcher and the nursing research consumer to read, comprehend, and perform a beginning critique of published studies using these analyses. The explanation will assist in understanding the terminology, the process of analysis, and the results of analysis.

To perform a critique, the reader needs to determine whether the analysis was properly performed and interpreted, and whether the analysis was appropriate to the study. Appropriateness is judged in relation to the purpose of the study and the fit between the design, the measurements, and the statistical analysis. Making this type of judgment requires an understanding of the logic on which the analysis is based and of alternative analyses that could have been used to achieve the same purpose.

This chapter presents an explanation of the following statistical procedures: multiple regression, factorial analysis of variance, analysis of covariance, factor analysis, discriminant analysis, canonical correlation, structural equations modeling, time-series analysis, and survival analysis. Two computer programs not previously discussed in this text, LISREL and EQS, are used to perform a number of these analyses. LISREL, developed

in 1966 by Jöreskog, maximizes the capacity to explain interactions among multiple variables by developing a covariance structure model (Long, 1983a, 1983b). Use of the programs in LISREL requires considerable sophistication in statistical logic and computer-based statistical analyses. The mathematical model for EQS was developed in 1979 by Bentler and Weeks to analyze linear structural equation systems. The computer program was developed by Bentler in 1985. EQS, which performs all of the analyses in LISREL, has a simplicity and coherence that makes it easier to learn and apply than LISREL (Bentler, 1989). Although LISREL must be performed on a mainframe computer, EQS is available for use on 386-type personal computers (PCs) as well as the mainframe computer.

MULTIPLE REGRESSION

Multiple regression analyses have become the most frequently used multivariate analyses in nursing studies, replacing the ANOVA models so popular a few years ago. This change is a reflection of the move in nursing away from decision theory reasoning to the logic of probability. Multiple regression is an extension of the simple linear regression described in Chapter 18. However, in multiple regression, more than one independent variable is entered into the analysis. The purpose of a regression analysis is to predict or explain as much of the variance in the value of the dependent variable as possible. In some cases, the analysis is exploratory and the focus is prediction. In others, variables are selected based on a theoretical position and the purpose is explanation, to confirm the theoretical position.

ASSUMPTIONS

The assumptions of multiple regression analysis are:

1. The variables (dependent and independent) were measured without error.
2. Variables can be treated as interval-level measures.
3. The residuals are not correlated.
4. Dependent variable scores come from a normal distribution.
5. Scores are homoscedastic (equally dispersed about the line of best fit); thus, there is a normal distribution of Y scores at each value of X.
6. Y scores have equal variances at each value of X; thus, difference scores (residuals or error scores) are random and have homogeneous variance.

Determining whether or not these assumptions have been violated in a data set is difficult. Therefore, a set of statistical procedures, residual analyses, has been developed to test for violation of the assumptions (Verran & Ferketich, 1987). The results of residual analysis need to be included in the research report.

Many versions of regression analyses are used in a variety of research situations. Some versions have been developed particularly for situations in which some of the foregoing assumptions are violated.

The typical multiple regression equation is expressed as:

$$Y = a + bX_1 + bX_2 + \cdots bX_i$$

The dependent variable (or predicted variable) is represented by Y in the regression equation. The independent variables (or indicators) are represented by X_i in the regression equation. The i indicates the number of independent variables in the equation. The coefficient of the independent variable, b, is a numerical value that indicates the amount of change that occurs in Y for each change in the associated X and can be reported as a b weight (based on raw scores) or a beta weight (based on Z scores). These two weights are discussed in Chapter 18.

The outcome of a multiple regression is an R^2 value. The significance of the R^2 is reported as well as the significance of b for each independent variable. Regression, unlike correlation, is one way the independent variables can predict the values of the dependent variable, but the dependent variable cannot be used to predict the values of the independent variables. If the b is not significant, that independent variable is not an effective predictor of the dependent variable using that set of independent variables. In this case, the researcher may remove variables with nonsignificant coefficients from the equation and repeat the analysis. This action will often increase the amount of variance explained by the equation and thus raise the R^2 value. To be effective predictors, independent variables selected for the analysis should have strong correlations with the dependent variable but only weak correlations with other independent variables in the equation.

The significance of an R^2 value is tested using an F test. The procedure is similar to that used in ANOVA. A significant F value indicates that the regression equation has been effective in predicting variation in the dependent variable and that the R^2 value is not a random variation from an R^2 value of zero.

TYPES OF INDEPENDENT VARIABLES

The variables in a regression equation can take many forms. Traditionally, as with most multivariate analyses, variables are measured at the interval level. However, categorical or dichotomous measures (referred to as *dummy variables*), multiplicative terms, and transformed terms are also used. A mixture of types of variables may be used in a single regression equation. The following discussion describes the various terms used as variables in regression equations.

Dummy Variables

To use categorical variables in regression analysis, a coding system is developed to represent group membership. Categorical variables of interest in nursing that might be used in regression analysis include gender, income, ethnicity, social status, level of education, and diagnosis. If the variable is dichotomous, such as gender, members of one category are assigned the number 1, and all others are assigned the number 0. In this case, for gender, the coding could be:

$$1 = \text{female}$$
$$0 = \text{male}$$

If the categorical variable has three values, two dummy variables are used; for example, social class could be classified as lower class, middle class, or upper class. The first dummy variable (X_1) would be classified as:

$$1 = \text{lower class}$$
$$0 = \text{not lower class}$$

The second dummy variable (X_2) would be classified as:

$$1 = \text{middle class}$$
$$0 = \text{not middle class}$$

The three social classes would then be specified in the equation in the following manner:

lower class	$X_1 = 1, X_2 = 0$
middle class	$X_1 = 0, X_2 = 1$
upper class	$X_1 = 0, X_2 = 0$

When more than three categories define the values of the variable, increased numbers of dummy vari-

ables are used. The number of dummy variables is always one less than the number of categories.

Time Coding

Time is commonly expressed in a regression equation as an interval measure. However, in some cases, codes may need to be developed for time periods. Using this strategy, time is coded in a categorical form and used as an independent variable. For example, if 5 years of data were available, the following system could be used to provide dummy codes for the time variable:

$$-2 = \text{subjects cared for in the first year}$$
$$-1 = \text{subjects cared for in the second year}$$
$$0 = \text{subjects cared for in the third year}$$
$$+1 = \text{subjects cared for in the fourth year}$$
$$+2 = \text{subjects cared for in the fifth year}$$

Effect Coding

Effect coding is similar to dummy coding but is used when the effects of treatments are being examined by the analysis. Each group of subjects is assigned a code. The code numbers used are 1, 0, and -1. The codes are assigned in the same way as dummy codes. While using dummy codes, one category will be assigned 0, in effect coding one group in each set will be assigned -1, one group will be assigned 1, and all others will be assigned 0 (Pedhazur, 1982).

Multiplicative Terms

The multiple regression model $Y = a + b_1X_1 + b_2X_2 + b_3X_3$ assumes that the independent variables have an additive effect on the dependent variable. This means that each independent variable has the same relationship with the dependent variable at each value of the other independent variables. Thus, if variable X_1 increased as X_2 increased in lower values of X_2, X_1 would be expected to continue to increase at the same rate at higher values of X_2. However, in some analyses, this does not prove to be the case. For example, in a study of hospice care conducted by one of the authors (Burns & Carney, 1986), minutes of care (*MC*) was used as the dependent variable. Duration (*DUR*), or number of days of care, and age (*AGE*) were included as independent variables. When duration was short, minutes of care increased as age increased. However, when duration was long, minutes of care decreased as age increased.

In this situation, better prediction can occur if multiplicative terms are included in the equation. In this case, the regression model takes the following form:

$$Y = a + b_1X_1 + b_2X_2 + b_3X_1X_2$$

The last term ($b_3X_1X_2$) takes the form of a multiplicative term and is the product of the first two variables (X_1 multiplied by X_2). This term expresses the joint effect of the two variables. For example, duration (*DUR*) might be expected to interact with the subject's age (*AGE*). The third term would show the combined effect of the two variables (*DURAGE*). The example equation would then be expressed as:

$$MC = a + b_1DUR + b_2AGE + b_3DURAGE$$

This procedure is similar to multivariate ANOVA, in which main effects and interaction effects are considered. Main effects are the effects of a single variable. Interaction effects are the multiplicative effects of two or more variables.

Transformed Terms

The typical regression model assumes a linear regression in which the relationship between X and Y can be illustrated on a graph as a straight line. However, in some cases, the relationship is not linear but curvilinear. The fact that the scores are curvilinear can sometimes be demonstrated by graphing the values. In these cases, deviations from the regression line will be great and predictive power will be low; the F ratio will not be significant and R^2 will be low, resulting in a Type

II error. Adding another independent variable to the equation, a transformation of the original independent variable obtained by squaring the original variable, may accurately express the curvilinear relationship. This strategy will improve the predictive capacity of the analysis. An example of a mathematical model that includes a squared independent variable is:

$$Y = a + b_1X + b_2X^2$$

This equation states that Y is related to both X and X^2 in such a way that changes in Y's values are a function of both X and X^2. The nonlinearity analysis can be extended beyond the squared term to add more transformed terms; thus, such values as X^3, X^4, and so on can be included in the equation. Each term adds another curve in the regression line. Using this strategy, very complicated relationships can be modeled. However, small samples can lead incorrectly to a perfect fit. For these complex equations, the researcher needs a minimum of 30 observations per term (Cohen & Cohen, 1983). If the complex equation provides better prediction, the R^2 will be increased and the F ratio will be significant.

RESULTS

The outcome of regression analysis is referred to as a *prediction equation*. This equation is similar to that described for simple linear regression except that making a prediction is more complex. Consider the following sample equation:

DURATION =

10.6 + .3 AGE + 2.4 INCOME + 3.5 COPING
(4.56) (2.78)   (4.43)   (7.52)

$R^2 = .51$ $n = 350$ $F = 1.832$ $p < .001$

If duration were measured in the number of days that the patient received care, the Y intercept would be 10.6 days. (This value is not meaningful apart from the equation.) For each increase of 1 year in age, the patient would receive .3 days more of care. For each increase in income level, the patient would receive an additional 2.4 days of care. For each increase in coping ability measured on a scale, the patient would receive an additional 3.5 days of care. In this example, $R^2 = .51$, which means that these variables explain 51% of the variance in the duration of care. The regression analysis of variance indicates that the equation is significant at a $p \leq .001$ level.

Relating these findings to real situations requires additional work. First, it is necessary to know how the variables were coded for the analysis; for example, one would need to know the range of scores on the coping scale, the income classifications, and the range of ages in the sample. Then, possible patient situations would be proposed and duration of care would be predicted for a patient with those particular dimensions of each independent variable. For example, suppose a patient is 64 years of age, in income level 3, and in coping level 5. In this case, the patient's predicted duration would be 10.6 + (64 × .3) + (3 × 2.4) + (5 × 3.5), or 54.5 days of care.

The results of a regression analysis are not expected to be sample specific. The final outcome of a regression analysis is a model from which values of the independent variables can be used to predict and perhaps explain values of the dependent variable in the population. If so, the analysis can be repeated in other samples with similar results. The equation is expected to have predictive validity. Knapp (1994) has listed the essential elements of a regression analysis that need to be included in a publication.

CROSS-VALIDATION

To determine the accuracy of the prediction, the predicted values are compared with actual values obtained from a new sample of subjects or values from a sample obtained at the time of the original data collection but held out from the initial analysis. This analysis is conducted on the difference scores between predicted values and the means of actual values. Thus, in the new sample, the num-

ber of days of care for all patients 64 years of age, in income level 3, and in coping level 5, would be averaged, and the mean would be compared with 54.5 days of care. Each possible case within the new sample would be compared in this manner. An R^2 is obtained on the new sample and compared with the original sample. In most cases, the R^2 will be lower in the new sample, because the original equation was developed to predict most precisely scores in the original sample. This is referred to as the *shrinkage of* R^2. Shrinkage of R^2 is greater in small samples and when multicollinearity (see next section) is great.

Mischel, Padilla, Grant, and Sorenson (1991) performed a cross-validation procedure to test the uncertainty in illness theory by replicating a study examining the mediating effects of mastery and coping. They describe their methodology as follows.

"To compare the results of this study with those of the prior research, regression equations were compared for consistency in variables entering the equations and for percent of variance explained. Additionally, the unstandardized regression coefficients were compared by using a 95% confidence interval to determine the comparability of the two models. For comparability to exist, the regression coefficients for this study should fall within the confidence interval calculated for those from previous research (Verran & Reid, 1987).

Prescott (1987) notes that with highly homogeneous samples, the cross-validation procedure is likely to result in substantially similar findings. Thus, if the goal of the replication is to determine the limits of the supported relationships and the population and contextual variability under which the relationships hold, then some heterogeneity in the sample and setting are desirable. To determine the heterogeneity of the samples, a series of chi-square and *t* test analyses were run on the demographic variables. The first sample had a significantly larger number of elderly subjects (above 70 years of age), more subjects with ovarian cancer, a greater number of ovarian cancer patients in Stages III and IV, and a greater number of subjects receiving chemotherapy as compared with the sample for the replication testing.

Differences between the samples on the major predictor and dependent variables were explored through two MANOVA analyses. . . . Significant differences were found on all variables in this analysis. . . . The difference between the samples on the measures was not in a consistent direction, but supported that the two samples were not homogeneous." (p. 237)

"Regression analysis was used to test the mediating effects of mastery and coping following the procedure described by Baron and Kenny (1986) and applied in the initial test of the model (Mischel & Sorenson, 1991). To test for mediating effect of each mediator, three regression equations were run. The mediator was regressed on the independent variable, the dependent variable was regressed on the independent variable, and the dependent variable was regressed on both the independent variable and the mediator. In order to have the appropriate conditions to test the mediation effect of a variable, the independent variable must have a significant relationship with the mediating variable and with the dependent variable, plus the mediator must significantly account for variation in the dependent variable. When both the independent variable and mediating variable are entered on the dependent variable, the strength of the relationship between the independent and dependent variables should decrease. The ideal case is a reduction in the magnitude of the beta so that the path is insignificant. . .

Results of the model tests demonstrated significant relationships to be the same and in the same direction for uncertainty to mastery, mastery to danger, danger to an emotion-focused coping strategy, danger to emotional distress, the emotion-focused coping strategy to emotional distress, opportunity appraisal to a problem-focused coping strategy, and the problem-focused coping strategy to emotional distress. In considering the mediating function of mastery, mastery consistently reduced the strength of the impact of uncertainty on danger and opportunity but was inconsistent in its strength as a mediator in the relationship between uncertainty and opportunity. Both mastery and the emotion-focused coping strategy of wishful thinking were significant mediators in both tests of the model, although the mediation effect of wishful thinking was very small and not substantively meaningful." (p. 239)

"Although there were selected paths that replicated across testing with different samples, there was sufficient lack of fit between the two models to lead to speculation about moderating variables to explain the divergence. The finding that subjects differed in appraisal due to their location at data collection has some possible clinical implications. If the appraisal of uncertainty is held in abeyance during hospitalization or clinic visits, then it is an ideal time for the nurse to work with the patient to influence the course of uncertainty appraisal." (p. 240) ■

MULTICOLLINEARITY

Multicollinearity occurs when the independent variables in a regression equation are strongly correlated. In nursing studies, some multicollinearity is inevitable; however, it can be minimized by careful selection of independent variables. Multicollinearity does not affect predictive power (the capacity of the independent variables to predict values of the dependent variable in that specific sample), but rather causes problems related to generalizability. The equation will not have predictive validity. The amount of variance explained by each variable in the equation is inflated. The *b* values will not remain consistent across samples when cross-validation is performed because multicollinearity leads to the following problems:

1. It decreases the power of significance tests for the partial regression coefficients by increasing the sampling error of the coefficients. The values of *b* obtained in the analysis will not be found to be significant when, in reality, they are significant—a Type II error.
2. It sometimes causes the signs of the coefficients to be wrong.
3. It may adversely affect the accuracy of poorly written computer programs.
4. The removal of a single observation may cause a large change in the calculated coefficients.

5. The R^2 of the estimated regression will be large but all the coefficients may be insignificant.

The first step in the identification of multicollinearity is the examination of correlations among the independent variables. Therefore, usually, the researcher performs multiple correlation analyses prior to conducting the regression analyses. The correlation matrix is carefully examined for evidence of multicollinearity. Most researchers consider multicollinearity to exist if the bivariate correlation is greater than .65. However, some researchers use a correlation of .80 or greater as an indication of multicollinearity (Schroeder, 1990).

The *coefficient of determination* (R^2), computed from a matrix of correlation coefficients, provides important information on multicollinearity. This value indicates the degree of linear dependencies among the variables. As the value of the determinant approaches zero, the degree of linear dependency increases. Thus, it is preferable that this R^2 be large. Identifying the extent of multicollinearity is important in selecting regression procedures and interpreting results. Therefore, Schroeder (1990) describes additional procedures that researchers use to diagnose the extent of multicollinearity.

The extent of multicollinearity in the data needs to be examined by the researcher as part of the analysis procedure and reported in publication of the study. An example from Braden (1990) follows.

"A correlation matrix of model variables showed no evidence of multicollinearity in the multiple regression equations used to answer the research questions. Gordon's (1968) criteria of $r \leq .65$ for correlation of variables entered in the same equation was used." (p. 44) ∎

EXPLORATORY REGRESSION ANALYSIS

A wide variety of regression analysis procedures are available. Selection of a particular procedure is based on the purpose of the study, the type of data available, and the experience of the researcher in performing regression procedures. Regression analyses can be broadly categorized into exploratory and confirmatory procedures. *Exploratory regression analysis* is the most commonly used strategy in nursing studies. In an exploratory mode, the researcher may not have sufficient information to determine which independent variables are effective predictors of the dependent variable. There may be no theoretical justification for the selection of variables or for considering one variable as a more important predictor than another. In this case, many variables may be entered into the analysis simultaneously. During the analysis, the program enters variables into the equation and/or removes them, based on the amount of variance the variable explains relative to other variables in the equation. An example of an exploratory procedure is stepwise regression.

Stepwise Regression

In *stepwise regression,* the independent variables are entered into or removed from the analysis one at a time. Although the researcher can control the sequence of movement of variables, it is most commonly done by the computer program, based on the amount of additional variance of the dependent variable explained by that particular independent variable. In *forward stepwise regression,* independent variables are entered into the analysis one at a time, and an analysis is made of the effect of including that variable on R^2. Thus, the computer printout indicates the increase in R^2 with the addition of the new variable and the statistical significance (F value) of the change. In *backward stepwise regression,* all the independent variables are initially included in the analysis. Then, one variable at a time is removed from the equation and the effect of that removal on R^2 is evaluated.

During the process of stepwise regression analysis, the amount of variance of Y explained by X_1 is removed from the analysis before the variance explained by X_2 is analyzed. This procedure, referred to as *partialing out* the variance, continues throughout the analysis. Each additional variable included in the analysis will tend to explain a smaller additional amount of the variance in Y. As more variables are included, the increase in R^2 is less and the degrees of freedom decrease, making it more difficult to obtain a significant F statistic for the increase in R^2.

Kammer (1994) used stepwise regression in her study of stress and coping of family members responsible for nursing home placement of an older adult. She described her data analysis as follows.

"Multiple regression analysis, using a backward elimination procedure (Pedhazur, 1982), was done to examine the relationship between 16 person-environment characteristics as independent variables and stress appraisal as the dependent variable. A second regression analysis using the same procedure with person-environment characteristics and stress appraisal as independent variables and coping as the dependent factor also was conducted. Stress appraisal, coping, and eight of the person-environment characteristics were entered as interval data. The remaining person-environment characteristics were coded as: (a) gender—male = 1, female = 2; (b) religions—Jewish = 1, other = 2; (c) employment—yes = 1, no = 2; (e) resident well health, considering age—yes = 1, no = 2; (f) resident physical impairment—yes = 1, no = 2; (g) resident mental impairment—yes = 1, no = 2; and (h) mutual admission decision—yes = 1, no = 2. The backward elimination procedure was chosen to determine the maximum R^2 that could be achieved when all variables were entered. The adjusted R^2 value is reported because of the exploratory nature of this study and the number of predictor variables. The maximum number of predictor variables remaining in any regression was seven; guidelines ($n \geq 10\ v$) given by Marascuilo and Levin (1983). A probability level of .10 was set as the significance level for retaining a variable in the equations in order to see trends." (p. 92) ■

The results of the first regression are presented below. The results of the second regression can be found in Kammer's paper.

"Person-environment characteristics significantly contributed to variance in stress appraisals as shown in Table 19–1. Higher *harm* appraisals were associated with more frequent visiting, higher satisfaction with nursing home resident relationship prior to admission, lack of mutual admission decision, lower present satisfaction with nursing home resident relationship, younger respondent age, and fewer number of respondent children at home. These six variables accounted for 23% of the variance in harm appraisals. Higher *benefit* appraisals were associated with younger respondent age, well older adult health status, less frequent visiting, and no respondent employment (16% variance). Higher *threat* appraisals were associated with more frequent visiting, respondents being employed, fewer children at home, and nursing home resident mental impairment (20% variance). Higher *challenge* appraisals were associated with not being employed, higher present satisfaction with nursing home resident relationship, well resident health status, no resident physical impairments and younger respondent age (24% variance).

Comparing the effect of person-environment variables across all stress appraisal categories showed *visit frequency* was the only variable significantly related to all appraisal. *Younger age* was associated with higher harm, benefit and challenge appraisals. *Fewer children at home* was associated with both harm and threat appraisals. Well nursing home resident *health* was associated with higher challenge and benefit appraisals. Being *employed* was associated with higher threat, while not being employed was associated with higher benefit and challenge appraisals." (pp. 93–94) ■

The discussion related to these findings can be found in Kammer's paper.

There are several problems to be considered in using stepwise regression. First, the strategy is somewhat akin to fishing in the data to find whatever significance is there. This is similar to conducting t tests between each two variables in a data set that includes many variables. With both strategies, researchers run a great risk of detecting significant differences present in the data that are the result of random error. This greatly increases

Table 19–1
Final Step Regression for Person-Environment Characteristics with Stress Appraisals as Dependent Variables (N = 89)

Variables	Beta	SE Beta	r	Partial r	t Value
Harm appraisal					
Visits	.23	.10	.27	.25	2.32**
Mutual decision[a]	.17	.09	.22	.19	1.79*
Prior relationship	.27	.11	.10	.26	2.45**
Now relationship	−.31	.10	−.25	−.32	−3.02***
Age	−.33	.11	−.17	−.30	−2.88***
Child at home	−.20	.11	−.08	−.20	−1.89**
	Multiple R = .53	Adj. R^2 = .23	$F(6,82)$ = 5.25****		
Benefit appraisal					
Visits	−.33	.10	−.34	−.34	−3.32****
Employed[a]	.21	.11	.12	.21	1.92*
Resident health well[a]	−.17	.10	−.20	−.18	−1.70*
Age	−.19	.11	−.11	−.19	−1.73*
	Multiple R = .44	Adj. R^2 = .16	$F(4,84)$ = 5.08****		
Threat appraisal					
Visits	.28	.10	.28	.30	2.89***
Mental impairment[a]	−.17	.10	−.16	−.19	−1.74*
Employed[a]	−.28	.10	−.17	−.30	−2.84***
Child at home	−.30	.10	−.28	−.32	−3.07***
	Multiple R = .49	Adj. R^2 = .20	$F(4,84)$ = 6.53****		
Challenge appraisal					
Visits	−.20	.10	−.15	−.22	−2.03**
Employed[a]	.34	.11	.19	.33	3.19***
Resident health well[a]	−.41	.11	−.34	−.39	−3.82****
Now relationship	.18	.10	.13	.20	1.87*
Age	−.32	.11	−.13	−.31	−2.97***
Physical impairment[a]	−.22	.11	.04	−.21	−1.90*
	Multiple R = .54	Adj. R^2 = .24	$F(6,82)$ = 5.59****		

[a] Dummy coding: yes = 1, no = 2.
* $p < .10$. ** $p < .05$. *** $p < .01$. **** $p < .001$.
(From Kammer, C. H. [1994]. Stress and coping of family members responsible for nursing home placement. *Research in Nursing & Health*, *17*[2], 94. Copyright © 1994. Reprinted with permission of John Wiley & Sons, Inc.)

the risk of a Type I error. The shrinkage of R^2 when cross-validation is conducted is likely to be great; thus, the value of R^2 in stepwise regression is likely to be inflated. Also, stepwise regression is very sample-specific. If the data are collinear, then small changes in data values will cause changes in the independent variables selected by the analysis. A good description of some of the difficulties with stepwise regression can be found in Aaronson (1989).

Second, in forward stepwise regression, the first variable to be included in the equation is the one that explains the greatest amount of variance in the dependent variable. This first step limits the possibility of inclusion of other variables that initially explain a lesser portion of the variance but if joined with a different combination of variables would explain a greater portion of the variance.

Third, the variables selected in the procedure may be effective in *predicting* values of the dependent variable, but not very effective in *explaining* the variance in the dependent variable. From a theoretical point of view, this is not satisfactory. Knowing why part of the variance of the dependent variable is explained by a particular independent variable is important, because your ability to explain changes in values of the dependent variable is a prerequisite to controlling those values.

CONFIRMATORY REGRESSION ANALYSES

Regression analysis procedures designed to achieve confirmatory purposes assume a theoretically proposed set of variables. The purpose of the *confirmatory regression analysis* is to test the validity of a theoretically proposed statement expressed as a regression equation. This equation is the hypothesis of the study. A number of regression procedures are used for this purpose. Procedures presented below include simultaneous regression, hierarchical regression, and logistic regression.

Simultaneous Regression

In simultaneous regression, all independent variables are entered at the same time into a single analysis. A theoretical justification for the selected independent variables is presented by the author and expressed as a hypothesis prior to describing the analysis. Several simultaneous equations may be used as hypotheses for a study.

Hierarchical Regression

Sometimes fully testing the theoretically proposed ideas requires a series of linked regression equations. This is referred to as hierarchical regression. Suppose the researcher had a set of four independent variables (age, education, attitudes about cancer, and social support) thought to explain variation in the dependent variable (coping). Nursing actions can have little effect on age and education, but perhaps the literature review indicates that these two variables are important predictors of coping. The researcher is interested in knowing if, given the effects of age and education, attitudes and support also influence coping. One strategy for examining this question is to first determine the amount of variance explained by age and education using regression analysis, and then determine if adding attitudes and support will increase the amount of variance in coping that can be explained. The series of equations would be expressed as follows.

$$Y = X_1$$
$$Y = X_1 + X_2$$
$$Y = X_1 + X_2 + X_3$$
$$Y = X_1 + X_2 + X_3 + X_4$$

The second equation controls for the variance explained by X_1 before testing the effect of X_2. If there is an increased amount of variance explained by adding X_2 to the equation, it will be reflected by an increase in R^2. Additional variables are added, either one at a time or as a set, testing for their effect on R^2.

This technique can be extended to test the effect of the same set of independent variables on several dependent variables of interest in a particular area of study. An analysis might include three linked dependent variables designated Y_1, Y_2, and Y_3. The set of independent variables would be designated X_1, X_2, X_3, X_4. The independent variables may be entered into analysis one at a time, or some may be entered as a set. The entire set of hierarchical equations might have the following appearance:

$$Y_1 = X_1$$
$$Y_1 = X_1 + X_2$$
$$Y_1 = X_1 + X_2 + X_3$$
$$Y_1 = X_1 + X_2 + X_3 + X_4$$
$$Y_2 = X_1$$
$$Y_2 = X_1 + X_2$$
$$Y_2 = X_1 + X_2 + X_3$$
$$Y_2 = X_1 + X_2 + X_3 + X_4$$
$$Y_3 = X_1$$
$$Y_3 = X_1 + X_2$$
$$Y_3 = X_1 + X_2 + X_3$$
$$Y_3 = X_1 + X_2 + X_3 + X_4$$

Wu (1995) suggests the use of hierarchical regression to conduct multilevel data analyses. In *multilevel analysis,* the researcher is examining two or more units simultaneously. For example, the study might include a number of nursing homes as well as the nurses employed within the nursing homes. Each nursing home would be one unit of measure and each nurse another unit of measure. Using hierarchical regression, the re-

Table 19–2
Summary Descriptive Statistics of Healing Determinants

Category of Variable	N	M (Mode)	SD
Independent Variables			
Physiologic			
Edema	155	1.2(1)	.94
Hyperpigmentation	155	1.1(0)	1.30
Liposclerosis	155	.61(0)	.89
Wound status	155	2.5(2)	.65
Initial ulcer area	156	637	868
Clot history	153	0.2(0)	.42
Pain on mobility	152	1.4(1)	.78
Therapeutic			
Diuretics	150	0.5(1)	.50
Ankle compression	152	29.2	19.0
Limb positioning			
elevated	145	.87	2.7
horizontal	145	13.01	4.44
dependent	145	6.2	4.2
Dressing	145	32.07	8.77
Psychosocial			
Social support	134	22.25	10.09
Self-efficacy	145	5.7	3.08
Dependent Variable			
Healing rate	140	−.12	.94

(From Johnson, M. [1995]. Healing determinants in older people with leg ulcers. *Research in Nursing & Health, 18*[5], 399. Copyright © 1995. Reprinted with permission of John Wiley & Sons, Inc.)

searcher can examine the random variation at both the individual and organizational level.

Johnson (1995) provided an excellent presentation of hierarchical regression in her study of healing determinants in older people with leg ulcers. This study was also used as an example of a predictive correlational design in Chapter 11. A summary of descriptive statistics of all independent and dependent variables in Johnson's study is presented in Table 19–2. She describes her use of hierarchical analysis as follows.

"Each predictor variable was assessed to determine the best parameterization possible; nonmetric data (diuretic usage, clot history, and liposclerosis) were converted to dummy codings (absence, mild = 0; moderate, severe = 1) (Hair, Anderson, Tatham, & Black, 1992). Violations to statistical assumptions of multiple regression were examined using normal probability plots of the residuals (the difference between the observed and the predicted values for the dependent variable) versus the predictor variables for all models (Hair et al., 1992). The dependent variable, healing rate, was normally distributed. No evidence of curvilinear relationships were demonstrated in partial plots of the dependent and independent variables. Examination of standardized residuals identified one outlier, which was removed. Multicollinearity was also assessed with correlations between independent variables ranging from $r = .006$ to $= .57$. Similarly, variance inflation factors (1.0–1.02), and tolerances (.97–.99) were within acceptable limits (Hair et al., 1992). In the initial analysis, the level of significance for entry into the model was $\leq .10$; this was raised to .05 in the final reduced models.

Hierarchical multiple regression procedures were applied to examine how much variance in healing rate was explained for each set of variables—physiologic, therapeutic, and psychosocial—and allowed for comparison with other studies that examined physiologic factors in venous subjects only. It was also important to identify variables significant (.05) in the venous-only sample and apply these to other disease groups not studied thus far. Data losses in individual variables have resulted in subject losses in these groups throughout the regression procedures. . .

Physiologic factors were the first set of variables entered into the venous disease model at step 1. . . . Hyperpigmentation was positively correlated with liposclerosis ($r = .51$) and was not included. Pain on mobility and moderate and severe liposclerosis were related to poorer healing, while improved wound status scores were associated with increased healing rates; these variables explained 41% of the variance in the healing rate, adj. $R^2 = .36$, $F = 7.04$, $p \geq .001$. A history of leg clots, initial ulcer areas, and edema were not significant. Therapeutic variables were included in the second step and did not significantly contribute to healing, although increased limb hours in horizontal positions were related to poorer healing rates (adj. $R^2 = .39$). Hours with limbs elevated was negatively correlated with horizontal position hours ($r = -.57$), and was not included in the model. . . . Psychosocial factors were entered on the third step, and did not significantly contribute to the model (adj. $R^2 = .37$).

Social support and self-efficacy beliefs were not significant.

All variables involved in this model explained 49% of the variance in the healing rate, $F = 4.31$, $p < .0001$. In order to produce a simpler model, significant variables, $p \leq .05$–.10, were combined in one step and resulted in only four variables remaining significant at the .05 level: increased pain on mobility, $\beta = .46$, $p < .0001$, higher wound status scores, $\beta = -.33$, $p = .0007$, moderate or severe liposclerosis, $p = .003$, and increased hours in a horizontal position, $\beta = .24$, $p = .02$. These four variables explained 40% of the variance in the healing rate, $F = 11.74$, $p < .001$." (pp. 398–399) ∎

Logistic Regression

Logistic regression (sometimes called logit analysis) is used in studies in which the dependent variable is categorical. Although most regression analysis procedures are based on a least-squares approach to estimating parameters, logistic regression uses maximum likelihood estimation. The procedure estimates the likelihood of the fit of a theoretical model proposing the probability of various outcomes. It calculates the odds of one outcome occurring rather than other possible outcomes (Yarandi & Simpson, 1991). Because of the current clinical interest in predicting outcomes of nursing practice, this procedure is expected to become increasingly important to nursing research.

A less theoretical alternative to logistic regression is discriminant analysis (described later) which is used to predict group membership.

Albers, Lydon-Rochelle, and Krulewitch (1995) used logistic regression in their study of maternal age and labor complications in healthy primigravidas at term. They describe their analysis as follows.

"Multivariate analysis using logistic regression was used to assess predictors of labor complications for the study sample. This technique tests the effect of each variable in the model on the risk of labor complications, with simultaneous control of all other variables. A forward selection strategy was used to sequentially add one control variable at a time to a model containing only maternal age. Variables were added to the model based on statistical significance ($p < .05$) until no further variables were contributory.

Table 19–3 shows the results of logistic regression for predictors of cesarean section with simultaneous control of the other potential confounding factors. The odds ratios for the age/cesarean relationship are inflated compared with the risk ratios in stratified analysis. In most cases the odds ratio for maternal age in the final model are decreased slightly from the results of stratified analysis. This suggests minimal confounding in the simultaneous adjustment for epidural anesthesia

Table 19–3
Logistic Regression Analysis of Risk for Primary Cesarean Section—Odds Ratio (95% Confidence Interval)

Model	Age 20–29	Age 30+	Epidural	Adequate PNC
C/S = age	1.4 (1.1–2.0)	3.0 (2.1–4.4)	——	——
C/S = age + epidural	1.3 (0.9–1.8)	2.5 (1.7–3.7)	3.5 (2.6–4.5)	——
C/S = age + epidural + adequate PNC	1.2 (0.9–1.7)	2.3 (1.4–3.4)	3.4 (2.6–4.5)	1.3 (1.0–1.8)

*Reference group = age <20.
PNC, prenatal care; C/S, cesarean section.
(Reprinted by permission of Elsevier Science, Inc. from Albers, L. L., Lydon-Rochelle, M. T., & Krulewitch, C. J. [1995]. Maternal age and labor complications in healthy primigravidas at term. *Journal of Nurse-Midwifery, 40*[1], 10. Copyright © 1995 by The American College of Nurse-Midwives.)

and receipt of adequate prenatal care. Highly significant predictors of cesarean delivery in this sample of healthy primigravidas were maternal age ≥ 30 and epidural anesthesia." (pp. 7–8) ■

FACTORIAL ANALYSIS OF VARIANCE

Mathematically, *factorial analysis of variance* is simply a specialized version of multiple regression. A number of types of factorial ANOVAs have been developed to analyze data from specific experimental designs. These include two-way ANOVA developed for studies with two independent variables, multifactorial ANOVA for studies with more than two independent variables, randomized block ANOVA, repeated measures ANOVA, and multivariate ANOVA for studies with more than one dependent variable (MANOVA). The following assumptions can be made:

1. The dependent variable is treated as an interval-level measure.
2. At least one independent variable must have values that are categorical rather than continuous.
3. The variance of the dependent variable must be equal in the various groups included in the analysis.
4. Subjects should be randomly selected.
5. The sample size in each group should be equal or approximately equal.
6. There is no measurement error.

ANOVA is generally robust to violation of its assumptions. However, it is relatively sensitive to variations in sample sizes between groups. This becomes an increasing problem as the complexity of the design increases and, with it, the number of groups. Although computerized forms of ANOVA have included modifications of the analysis to control for different group sizes, there remains a problem of interpreting interaction effects when group sizes vary. In these cases, it may be advisable to use regression analysis with dummy variables.

In each type of ANOVA, the mathematical equations differ slightly. However, one element is

characteristic of them all: a partitioning of the sum of squares. The result of this partitioning is a lessening of the error term, or the amount of unexplained (within-group) variance. With the decrease in the unexplained (within-group) variance comes an increased probability of detecting existing differences between groups in the variables under study. Additionally, the partitioning provides the opportunity to examine interactions between variables, which may illustrate effects not initially considered.

Two types of effects are considered in interpreting the results of a factorial ANOVA. Main effects are the effects of a single factor. Interaction effects are the multiplicative effects of two or more factors. In complex designs, the interaction effects can be difficult to interpret, particularly when they are the combined effect of three or more variables.

The summary table is used to report both main effects and interaction effects, the F value of each, and the level of significance of the F value. Interaction effects are evaluated prior to consideration of main effects, because interaction effects may render main effects meaningless.

Jadack, Hyde, and Keller (1995) conducted a multivariate analysis of variance (MANOVA) in their study of gender and knowledge about HIV, risky sexual behavior, and safer sex practices. The analysis procedure allowed them to incorporate a number of variables considered important in explaining sexual practices. They reported their results as follows.

■

"In general, respondents demonstrated accurate knowledge of the likelihood of transmission from various sexual behaviors. For example, persons reported that having vaginal intercourse without using a condom with a person infected with HIV, having multiple sexual partners, and having unprotected anal intercourse with a person infected with HIV carried risk of transmission.

The hypothesis that predicted no gender differences in knowledge about HIV transmission was not supported for sexual and needle injection routes. Counter to theoretical predictions, a

Table 19–4
Mean Ratings (*SD*) and Univariate *F* Tests of the Perceived Likelihood of Becoming Infected with HIV from Selected Behaviors

	Women (*n* = 141)	Men (*n* = 131)	*F*(1, 270)
Having vaginal intercourse without using a condom with a person infected with HIV	1.07 (.26)	1.28 (.62)	12.83**
Having anal intercourse without using a condom with a person infected with HIV	1.19 (.43)	1.15 (.40)	.42
Having multiple sexual partners	1.37 (.54)	1.83 (.75)	34.56**
Having sexual intercourse with prostitutes	1.39 (.57)	1.64 (.65)	11.60**
Having homosexual sexual relationships	1.52 (.63)	1.58 (.65)	.65
Having bisexual sexual relationships	1.54 (.61)	1.78 (.72)	9.33**
Having oral sex with a person infected with HIV	1.72 (.81)	2.04 (.85)	10.65**
Open mouth kissing with a person infected with HIV	3.20 (.88)	3.29 (.79)	.85
Donating blood	3.46 (.83)	3.68 (.67)	6.04*
Receiving a blood transfusion	2.75 (.96)	3.17 (.87)	14.01**
Using intravenous drugs	1.93 (.98)	2.20 (.99)	5.11*
Sharing needles with other intravenous drug users	1.19 (.43)	1.36 (.56)	7.81*

Ratings were made on 4-point scales (1 = very likely; 2 = somewhat likely; 3 = somewhat unlikely; 4 = very unlikely).
* *p* < .01. ** *p* < .001.
(From Jadack, R. A., Hyde, J. S., & Keller, M. L. [1995]. Gender and knowledge about HIV, risky sexual behavior, and safer sex practices. *Research in Nursing & Health, 18*[4], 318. Copyright © 1995. Reprinted with permission of John Wiley & Sons, Inc.)

MANOVA testing for gender differences on multiple variables measuring knowledge about sexual routes of transmission indicated a significant overall effect for gender, *F*(8,263) = 8.11, *p* < .001. Univariate results are shown on Table 19–4. For most of the sexual behaviors listed, men reported less likelihood of transmission of HIV from risky sexual behaviors than women. That is, men were more likely to downplay the likelihood of transmission in comparison to women." (p. 317) ■

ANALYSIS OF COVARIANCE

Analysis of covariance (ANCOVA) is designed to reduce the error term (or the variance within groups) using a somewhat different strategy than that of factorial ANOVA. ANCOVA partials out the variance resulting from a confounding variable by performing regression analysis prior to performing ANOVA. This strategy removes the effect of differences between groups that are due to a confounding variable. The procedure is actually a general linear regression model with a mixture of dummy and nondummy independent variables.

This technique is sometimes used as a method of statistical control, which is an alternative to design control. ANCOVA allows the researcher to examine the effect of the treatment apart from the effect of the confounding variable; for example, such variables as age, education, social class, or anxiety level may appear to explain initial differences between groups in a study. These variables, which can affect subjects' responses to a treatment, can be partialed out using ANCOVA. However, whenever possible, it is better to use a randomized block design than to use analysis of covariance.

ANCOVA is a useful approach to analysis in pretest–post-test designs in which differences occur in groups on the pretest. For example, individuals who achieve low scores on a pretest will tend to have lower scores on the post-test than those whose pretest scores were higher, even if the treatment had a significant effect on post-test scores. Conversely, if an individual achieves a high pretest score, it is doubtful that the post-test will indicate a strong change as a result of the treatment. ANCOVA maximizes the capacity to detect differences in such cases.

By using multiple regression, it is also possible to partial out the effects of several covariates. For each covariate, a degree of freedom is lost, somewhat decreasing the possibilities of achieving significance, especially with small samples. Therefore, researchers need to be cautious in their use of multiple covariates. ANCOVA can be used with the more advanced types of ANOVA, in analyses of studies using complex designs such as factorial designs and repeated measures designs.

The assumptions on which ANCOVA is based are:

1. randomization
2. homogeneity of within-group regression
3. statistical independence of covariate and treatment
4. fixed covariate values that are error-free
5. linearity of within-group regression
6. normality of conditional criterion scores
7. homogeneity of variance of conditional criterion scores
8. fixed treatment levels (Huitema, 1980, cited in Wu & Slakter, 1989).

Violating one or more of these assumptions will cause alpha (the level of significance) to deviate from the value it would have if the assumptions had been met. The assumption of greatest concern is that the regression slopes for each treatment group are expected to be equal. The results, however, are relatively robust unless the deviation from equal slopes is extreme. In studies using ANCOVA, design strategies should at least include random assignment and preferably total randomization. Subjects should be treated independently within groups. The covariate must be measured before the treatment is implemented since the treatment must not affect the covariate. In quasi-experimental studies in which randomization is not possible, ANCOVA needs to be interpreted with caution (Wu & Slakter, 1989).

Tollett and Thomas (1995) used analysis of covariance in their examination of a theory-based nursing intervention to instill hope in homeless veterans. They described the analysis as follows.

"The hypothesis that there is greater hope, self-efficacy, and self-esteem and less depression in subjects receiving a specific nursing intervention to instill hope than in subjects who receive the usual and customary treatment was tested using an analysis of covariance (ANCOVA) procedure with pretest scores as the covariate. There was a significant difference in levels of hope between the control and treatment groups ($F = 8.93$, $p = .006$). There were no other significant differences between the groups on the dependent variables; however, the scores on each of the other variables changed in the hypothesized direction." (p. 87) ■

FACTOR ANALYSIS

Factor analysis is mathematically related to regression analysis. In both analyses, equations are developed that are linear combinations of the variables. Regression analysis tests hypotheses involving dependent and independent variables. Factor analysis examines interrelationships among large numbers of variables and disentangles those relationships to identify clusters of variables that are most closely linked together. These closely related variables are grouped together into a *factor*. Several factors may be identified within a data set. Sample sizes must be large for a factor analysis. Nunnally (1978) recommends ten observations for each variable. Arrindell and van der Ende (1985) suggest that a more reliable determination is a sample size of 20 times the number of factors.

Once the factors have been identified mathematically, the researcher explains why the variables are grouped as they are. Thus, factor analysis aids in the identification of theoretical constructs. Factor analysis is also used to confirm the accuracy of a theoretically developed construct. For example, a theorist might state that the concept "hope" consisted of the elements (1) anticipation of the future, (2) belief that things will work out for the best, and (3) optimism. Ways could be developed to measure these three elements, and a factor analysis could be conducted on the data to determine whether subject responses clustered into these three groupings.

Factor analysis is frequently used in the process of developing measurement instruments, particularly those related to psychological variables such as attitudes, beliefs, values, or opinions. The instrument operationalizes a theoretical construct. The method can also be used with physiologic data. For example, Woods, Lentz, and Mitchell (1993) identified a large pool of symptoms commonly experienced during the perimenstruum. Based on daily ratings of severity of these symptoms by subjects, premenstrual symptom patterns were identified. The validity of these patterns were tested using factor analysis resulting in the selection of 33 symptoms used to classify women as having LS (low severity symptom pattern), PMS (premenstrual syndrome pattern), or PMM (premenstrual magnification pattern). The analysis revealed that these patterns (factors) were consistent across menstrual cycle phases and had internal consistency reliability estimates above .70 (Woods, Mitchell, & Lentz, 1995). Factor analysis can be used as a data reduction strategy in studies examining large numbers of variables. It can also be used to attempt to sort out meaning from large numbers of items on survey instruments.

There are two types of factor analysis: exploratory and confirmatory. *Exploratory factor analysis* is similar to stepwise regression, in which the variance of the first factor is partialed out before analysis is begun on the second factor. It is performed when the researcher has few prior expectations about the factor structure. *Confirmatory factor analysis* is more closely related to ordinary least-squares regression analysis or path analysis. It is based on theory and tests a hypothesis about the existing factor structure. In confirmatory factor analysis, statistical significance of the analysis outcomes is determined and the parameters of the population are estimated. Confirmatory factor analysis is usually conducted after examination of the correlation matrix or after initial development of the factor structure through exploratory factor analysis.

EXPLORATORY FACTOR ANALYSIS

The first step in exploratory factor analysis is the development of a correlation matrix of the scores on all variables to be included in the factor analysis. This matrix is usually developed automatically by the computer program conducting the analysis. Although there are multiple procedures for the actual factor analysis, the procedure described here is the one most commonly reported in the nursing literature.

The second step is a *principal components analysis,* which provides preliminary information needed by the researcher in order for decisions to be made prior to the final factoring. The computer printout of the principal components analysis will give (1) the eigenvalues, (2) the amount of variance explained by each factor, and (3) the weight for each variable on each factor. The weights (loadings) express the extent to which the variable is correlated with the factor. The weightings on the variables from a principal components factor analysis are essentially uninterpretable and are generally disregarded (Nunnally, 1978).

Eigenvalues are the sum of the squared weights for each factor. The researcher examines the eigenvalues to decide how many factors will be included in the factor analysis. To decide the number of factors to include, the researcher determines the minimal amount of variance that must be explained by the factor to add significant meaning. This decision is not straightforward and has resulted in some criticism of the analysis as being subjective. Several strategies have been proposed for determining the number of factors to be included in a construct. One approach is to select factors that have an eigenvalue of 1.00 or above. Another strategy used is the scree-test. Scree is a geological term that refers to the debris that collects at the bottom of a rocky slope. This test, which is considered by some to be the most reliable, requires that the eigenvalues be graphed (see Figure 19–1).

From this graph, one can see a change in the angle of the slope. A steep drop in value from one factor to the next indicates a large difference score between the two factors and an increase in the

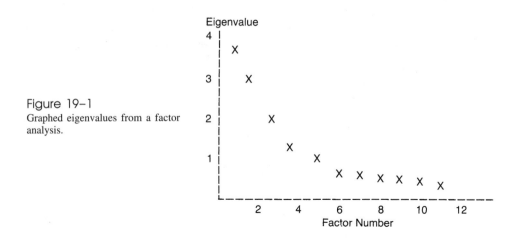

Figure 19–1
Graphed eigenvalues from a factor analysis.

amount of variance explained. When the slope begins to become flat, indicating small difference scores between factors, little additional information will be obtained by including more factors. In Figure 19–1, the slope begins to flatten at factor six; therefore, six factors would be extracted to explain the construct.

The third step in exploratory factor analysis is *factor rotation*. The purpose of factor rotation is to simplify the factor structure. The procedure most commonly used is referred to as the *varimax rotation*. In the varimax rotation, the factors are rotated for the best fit (best factor solution), and the factors are uncorrelated. An *oblique rotation* results in correlated factors.

The process of factor analysis is actually a series of multiple regression analyses (Kim & Mueller, 1978a, 1978b). The equation for a factor could be expressed as:

$$F = b_1X_1 + b_2X_2 + b_3X_3 + \cdots b_kX_k$$

where:

F = factor score
X_k = original variables from the matrix
b_K = weights of the individual variables in the factor. If the scores used are standardized, b is a beta weight.

In exploratory factor analysis, regression analysis is performed for the first factor. Then, the variance of each variable explained by the first factor is partialed out. Next, a second regression analysis is performed for the second factor on the residual variance. The variance from that analysis is then partialed out, and a regression is performed for the third factor. This process is continued until all the factors have been developed. The computer printout will include a rotated factor matrix that will contain information similar to that in Table 19–5 (on p. 498).

Factor Loadings

A factor loading is actually the regression coefficient of the variable on the factor. In Table 19–5, the factor loading indicates the extent to which a single variable is related to the cluster of variables. On variable 1, the factor loading is .76 on Factor I and .27 on Factor II. Squaring the factor loadings ($[0.76]^2 = .578$, and $[.27]^2 = .073$) will give the amount of variance in variable 1, which explains Factors I and II.

Communality

Communality (h^2) is the squared multiple regression coefficient for each variable and is closely

		Factors		
	Variable	I	II	h^2
	1	.76*	.27	.65
	2	.91*	.03	.83
	3	.64*	.29	.49
	4	.14	.67*	.47
	5	.22	.59*	.40
	6	.07	.77*	.60
Sum of shared loadings		1.89	1.55	
Variance		.22	.13	Total = .35

Table 19-5
Factor Loadings and Variance for Two Factors

* Indicates the variables to be included in each factor.

related to the R^2 in regression. Thus, the communality coefficient describes the amount of variance in a single variable that is explained across all the factors in the analysis. The communality for a variable can be obtained by summing the squared factor loadings on the variable for each factor. In Table 19–5, the communality coefficient for variable 1 is $(.76)^2 + (.27)^2 = .65$.

Identifying the Relevant Variables in a Factor

Only variables with factor loadings that indicate that a meaningful portion of the variable's variance is explained within the factor are included as elements of the factor. A cut-off point is selected for the purpose of identifying these variables. The minimum cutoff point that is acceptable is .30. In Table 19–5, the factor loadings with asterisks indicate the variables that will be included in each factor. In this example, which uses a .50 cutoff, variables 1, 2, and 3 would be included in Factor I, and variables 4, 5, and 6 would be included in Factor II. Ideally, a variable will *load* (have a factor loading above the selected cutoff point) on only one factor. If the variable does have high loadings on two factors, the lowest loading is referred to as a *secondary loading*. When many secondary loadings occur, it is not considered a clean factoring, and the researcher reexamines the variables included in the analysis. Sometimes, re-

searchers will attempt to set the cutoff point high enough to avoid secondary loadings of a variable.

"Naming" the Factor

At this point, the mathematics of the procedure takes a back seat, and the theoretical reasoning of the researcher takes over. The researcher examines the variables that have clustered together in a factor and explains that clustering. Variables with high loadings on the factor must be included, even if they do not fit the preconceived theoretical notions of the researcher. The purpose is to identify the broad construct of meaning that has caused these particular variables to be so strongly intercorrelated. Naming this construct is a very important part of the procedure, because the naming of the factor provides theoretical meaning.

Factor Scores

After the initial factor analysis, additional studies are conducted to examine changes in the phenomenon in various situations and to determine the relationships of the factors with other concepts. Factor scores are used during data analysis in these additional studies. To obtain factor scores, the variables included in the factor are identified, and the scores on these variables are summed for each subject. Thus, each subject will have a score for each factor in the instrument. Because some variables explain a larger portion of the variance of the factor than others, additional meaning can be added by multiplying the variable score by the weight (factor loading) of that variable in the factor. Using the example in Table 19–5, variable 1 had a factor loading of .76 on Factor I. If the subject score on variable 1 were 7, the score would be weighted by multiplying the variable score by the factor loading as follows:

$$7 \times .76 = 5.32$$

These weighted scores can be generated using the computer. If comparisons between studies are to be made, standardized (Z) scores (for variable scores) and beta weights (for factor loadings) are used. Once analysis is complete, factor scores can be used as independent variables in multiple regression equations.

Woods and colleagues (1995) used factor analysis in a study examining social pathways to premenstrual symptoms. Women were recruited for the study through advertisements in local newspapers. They describe their study as follows.

■

"Multiple indicators of the major constructs, feminine socialization, menstrual socialization, expectation of symptoms, stress, and support need, were included in the study. For purposes of data reduction, prior to comparing women with the LS (low symptom), PMS (premenstrual syndrome), and PMM (premenstrual magnification syndrome) symptom patterns, data from these indicators, obtained from all women who participated in the initial interview ($N = 488$), were included in a principal components factor analysis with a varimax rotation. This procedure yielded five factors with eigenvalues exceeding 1.0. . . Socialization as a woman reflects the ways in which women were socialized about the roles of women in society, including in the workplace and their families. . . . Socialization for menstruation reflected what women had learned about menstruation through exposure to their mothers and sisters and through teaching about the effects of menstruation. Menstrual socialization was

indicated by the respondent's rating of her mother's perimenstrual symptoms, a sister's symptoms, and the respondent's recollection of her menarcheal preparation. Expectations about menstrual symptoms reflected how women expected to experience menstruation and symptoms. . . Respondents also were asked two single items, one from the Menstrual Attitudes Scale tapping whether women could anticipate menses by their symptoms, the other whether they perceived they had PMS. Stress was measured using indicators of major life events and daily stressors. Life events were assessed with Norbeck's (1984) woman-oriented revision of the Sarason Life Events Scale (LES). . .

Factor analysis results are presented in Table 19–6 (on p. 500). Factor 1 (stress) included four variables: family-related stress, negative life events (LES scores), how stressed each woman felt over the past 3 months, and her rating of personal stress. Factor 2 (feminine socialization) included ratings of familism and attitudes toward women. High scores on this factor reflected more contemporary attitudes toward women and their roles vis-à-vis their families. Factor 3 (support needed) included women's ratings of need for more affirmation, advice, access to a confidant, and someone to share fun and relax with them, and someone to help them. Factor 4 (symptom expectation) included three variables: anticipating symptoms, self-perceived PMS, and attitudes toward menstruation as debilitating. Low scores indicated high expectation of symptoms. Factor 5 (menstrual socialization) included exposure to a mother and/or sister with perimenstrual symptoms and having been taught negative effects of menstruation. Of all the indicators analyzed, none had factor loadings of .40 or greater on any other factor. Each factor had an eigenvalue exceeding 1.0." (Woods, Mitchell, & Lentz, pp. 229–231) ■

CONFIRMATORY FACTOR ANALYSIS

Confirmatory factor analysis is a fairly recent development and is extremely complex mathematically. The procedure is usually performed using LISREL or EQS. Interpretation of results requires

Table 19–6
Factor Loadings for Indicators of Stress, Feminine Socialization, Support Need, Symptom Expectation, and Menstrual Socialization (N = 488)

Variables	Factors				
	1	*2*	*3*	*4*	*5*
Stress					
Negative life events	.70	−.01	.09	.07	.09
Stress, family	.70	−.03	−.10	−.19	.04
Stress, amount	.67	−.02	.21	−.09	−.08
Stress, personal	.64	.04	.23	−.01	.06
Feminine socialization					
Attitudes, women	.01	.90	.04	.03	−.07
Familism	−.01	.89	.04	.12	−.07
Support need					
Advice	.20	−.10	.63	.09	.15
Affirmation	.17	−.04	.62	−.09	−.04
Need relax	−.04	.16	.57	.14	.14
Confidant	.38	.17	.54	−.10	.09
Help	−.06	−.03	.52	−.34	−.18
Expectation of symptoms[a]					
Have PMS	.23	.04	−.09	−.73	.19
Anticipate symptoms	.03	.04	−.06	.67	.04
Not debilitating	−.06	.34	−.06	.60	−.29
Menstrual socialization					
Menstrual effects	.01	.02	−.02	−.04	.65
Mother's symptoms	.04	−.15	−.15	−.00	.64
Sister's symptoms	−.01	−.02	−.02	−.13	.62
Eigenvalues	2.85	2.18	1.35	1.26	1.16
% variance	16.8	12.8	7.9	7.4	6.8

[a] High scores = low symptom expectation.
(From Woods, N. F., Mitchell, E. S., & Lentz, M. J. [1995]. Social pathways to premenstrual symptoms. *Research in Nursing & Health, 18*[3], 230. Copyright © 1995. Reprinted with permission of John Wiley & Sons, Inc.)

a high level of sophistication in statistical analyses. In confirmatory factor analysis, the researcher develops hypotheses about the factor structure. Because the elements of each factor are set in the analysis, factor rotation and partialing out of variance are not performed. Cutoff points for representation within the factor may also be preset and included in the analysis. As an outcome of the analyses, estimation of the population parameters for the factor structure is made. The statistical significance of the results of the analyses is tested.

Wineman, Durand, and McCulloch (1994) used confirmatory factory analysis to examine the factor structure of the Ways of Coping Questionnaire with clinical populations. The original instrument

was based on the responses of undergraduate psychology students. The researchers describe their work as follows.

"The original Ways of Coping Checklist (WCCL) (Folkman & Lazarus, 1980) contained 68 items rated with a simple 'yes or no' format. Scale items were categorized as emotion-focused or problem-focused coping based on expert judgment. This rating scale did not measure the frequency with which coping behaviors were used and was thus revised (Folkman & Lazarus, 1988). The newer version, now called the Ways of Coping Questionnaire (Folkman & Lazarus, 1988), includes 66 items measured in a 4-point Likert-type format. Potential responses include 0 (does not apply and/or not used), 1 (used somewhat), 2 (used quite a bit), and 3 (used a great deal). The factor structure of this revised scale was analyzed using data from two separate community samples (Folkman & Lazarus, 1985; Folkman et al., 1986). The 1986 study formed the basis for the information reported in the 1988 *Ways of Coping Manual* because it used a community sample experiencing diverse stressful encounters. Eight coping scales were identified using alpha and principal factoring with oblique rotation (Folkman et al., 1986). Reliability estimates for the eight scales ranged from alpha coefficients of .61 to .79 (M = .70). Folkman and Lazarus (1988) contended that construct validity was supported because results were consistent with theoretical predictions about the coping process. That is, both problem-focused and emotion-focused strategies were used to cope with almost all stressful situations, and coping strategies changed in relation to situational demands (Folkman & Lazarus, 1988). . .

The eight-factor structure guided initial scale construction (Wineman et al., 1994). Cronbach's alpha coefficients were less than .74 for all eight scales, with four of these less than .60. . . These findings, consistent with the evidence of reliability insufficiency in the literature, led to the decision to compute an exploratory factor analysis (EFA).

An EFA with orthogonal rotation (quartimax) was done to obtain the simplest factor structure possible (Nunnally, 1978). . . Examination of the scree plot and eigenvalues suggested that two factors accounted for the covariation among the measured variables (Kim & Mueller, 1978a). The selection of items with factor loadings of .30 or greater on one factor (Nunnally, 1978) resulted in retention of 46 of the original 65 items (71%). Thirty-three items loaded on a problem-focused coping (PFC) scale and 13 items on an emotion-focused coping (EFC) scale. These scales supported coping theory that defines PFC as behaviors used to change a stressful situation and EFC as behaviors used to manage distressing feelings (Folkman et al., 1986). Acceptable reliability estimates were obtained: .90 for PFC and .76 for EFC. . .

Recent reports note that traditional factor analysis (EFC) does not allow for the specification of an exact factor structure, and that confirmatory factor analysis (CFA) with linear structural equation modeling provides the necessary control for testing theoretical expectations of the underlying relations among the variables (Long, 1983a; Youngblut, 1993). In other words, with CFA one can specify a priori which items (or measured indicators) are related to specific latent concepts (or factors). . .

In evaluating the goodness-of-fit of a model to observed data, no single statistic is sufficient for determining the adequacy of the fit (Raykov, Tomer, & Nesselroade, 1991). Four measures of overall fit were used to judge models in the present study: the chi-square statistic (χ^2), the goodness-of-fit index (GFI), the adjusted goodness-of-fit index (AGFI), and the root mean-squared residual (RMSR) (Jöreskog & Sörbom, 1989). An acceptably small χ^2 value was determined by obtaining the ratio of the χ^2 value to its degrees of freedom (*df*). Ratios of 3:1 or less supported a good fit (Carmines & McIver, 1981). The GFI and the AGFI, which assess the relative amount of variance and covariance jointly explained by the model, were considered acceptable if values were .90 or greater (Boyd et al., 1988). The RMSR, a measure of the average of the fitted residuals, was acceptable if close to zero (Jöreskog & Sörbom, 1989). The aim of this study was to reach a consensus of acceptable fit across all indicators of fit.

A CFA with LISREL version 7.20, a structural equation modeling program ((Jöreskog & Sörbom, 1988–1992), was performed to test the fit of data to the original hypothesized eight-factor structure (Folkman et al., 1986). Results indicated that the hypothesized factor structure did not provide a good fit to the data. . . These findings indicated that the eight-factor coping model developed in a well community-residing sample (Folkman et al., 1986) was inadequate for describing coping in a community sample of individuals with a non-life-threatening chronic illness or disability. Because it was reasonable to assume that coping behaviors required to manage life with a chronic illness or disability would be quite different from those needed in daily living situations of well individuals, alternative models of the coping factor structure based on a more conservative approach were examined, rather than pursuing modifications based only on empirical parameter estimates within the structural equation modeling framework.

The investigation of an alternative coping factor structure was conducted by randomly dividing the total study population into two samples and following a two-step procedure. This procedure generally consists of an initial EFA performed on one portion of the sample (1/3 of 655, $n = 218$) to derive an initial structure, followed by a CFA with the remaining sample (2/3 of 655, $n = 437$) to validate this structure. . .

In the following factor analyses, the two-step procedure described above was used twice to derive the best-fitting alternative factor structure. Using all 65 items, an EFA with a varimax rotation was performed on the smaller sample ($n = 218$). Selecting, as a more conservative estimate, a factor loading of .40 or greater (Nunnally, 1978), five factors were identified, with at least three items loading on each factor. If an item loaded on more than one factor it was not included. Twenty-five of the original 65 items were retained. To validate this 25-item, five-factor solution, a CFA with the remaining sample ($n = 437$) was used. The fit was not acceptable ($\chi^2 = 680.42$, $p < .01$, $df = 265$; $\chi^2/df = 2.57$; GFI = .89; AGFI = .86; RMSR = .06). Next, the model was modified slightly by omitting items with lambda y loadings of $< .40$, resulting in a 21-item, five-factor model. A CFA was then used to confirm this modified five-factor model. The fit improved, but was still slightly less than desirable ($\chi^2 = 429.54$, $p < .01$, $df = 179$; $\chi^2/df = 2.40$; GFI = .91; AGFI = .89; RMSR = .05). Because the modification indices indicated that one item loaded on four of the five factors, the next CFA was performed with this item omitted. An acceptable fit was obtained with this 20-item, five-factor solution ($\chi^2 = 325.94$, $p < .01$, $df = 160$; $\chi^2/df = 2.04$; GFI = .93; AGFI = .91; RMSR = .04).

Cronbach's alpha coefficients were acceptable for three of the five factors (.76, .709, and .69), but unacceptable for the other two (.55 and .61). Therefore, a final 14-item, three-factor model was tested using CFA, resulting in an acceptable fit ($\chi^2 = 149.16$, $p < .01$, $df = 74$; $\chi^2/df = 2.02$; GFI = .95; AGFI = .94; RMSR − .04). All standardized lambda y values were $> .40$ with the exception of one item that was .38. All but one of the goodness-of-fit indicators for this final three-factor model of coping were improved over earlier models." (Wineman, Durand, & McCulloch, pp. 269–271)

(From Wineman, N. M., Durand, E. J., & McCulloch, B. J. [1994]. Examination of the factor structure of the Ways of Coping Questionnaire with clinical populations. *Nursing Research 43*[5], 268–273. Used with permission of Lippincott–Raven Publishers, Philadelphia, PA.) ∎

Figure 19–2 shows the final results of the confirmatory factor analysis.

DISCRIMINANT ANALYSIS

Discriminant analysis is designed to allow the researcher to identify characteristics associated with group membership and to predict group membership. The dependent variable is membership in a particular group. The independent variables (discriminating variables) measure characteristics on which the groups are expected to differ. Discriminant analysis is closely related to both factor analysis and regression analysis. However, in discriminant analysis, the dependent variable values are categorical in form. Each value of the dependent variable is considered a group. When the dependent variable is dichotomous, multiple regression is performed. However, when there are more than two groups, analysis becomes much more complex. The dependent variable in discriminant analysis is referred to as the *discriminant function*. It is equivalent in many ways to a factor (Edens, 1987).

Two similar data sets are required for a complete analysis. The first data set must contain measures on all the variables to be included in the analysis and the group membership of each subject. The purpose of the analysis of the first data set is to identify variables that most effectively discriminate between groups. Variables are selected for the analysis based on the researcher's expectation that they will be effective in this regard. The variables selected for the discriminant function are then tested on a second set of data to determine their effectiveness in predicting group membership (Edens, 1987).

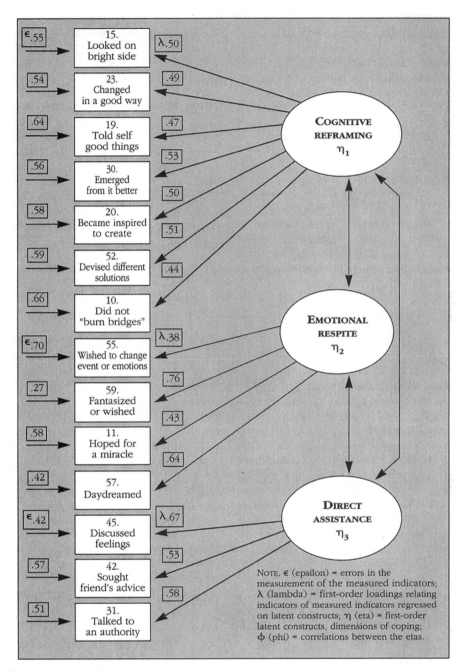

Figure 19-2

Results of the Confirmatory Factor Analysis for the Three-Factor Model of Coping. (From Wineman, N. M., Durand, E. J., & McCulloch, B. J. [1994]. Examination of the factor structure of the Ways of Coping Questionnaire with clinical populations. *Nursing Research, 43*[5], 260.)

The following are the assumptions of discriminant analysis:

1. The research problem must define at least two cases per group. The total sample size should be at least two or (preferably) three times the number of discriminating variables used.
2. The number of discriminating variables to be included in the analysis cannot exceed the total number of cases minus two $(n - 2)$, nor should they be fewer than the number of groups being compared.
3. Variables can be treated as interval-level measures.
4. No discriminating variable can be a linear combination of other discriminating variables.
5. The covariance matrices for the groups must be equal.
6. Each group must be drawn from a population with a multivariate normal distribution on the discriminating variables. (Edens, 1987, p. 257)

The first step in the analysis is to determine whether the groups can be differentiated based on the discriminating variables. If significant group differences exist, further analyses are performed to determine the number of dimensions on which the groups differ and which variables are effective in defining group membership. An effort is made in the analysis to maximize between-group variance while minimizing within-group variance. Variables that are expected to achieve this maximization and minimization of variance are selected for the discriminant function (Edens, 1987).

Discriminant function analysis is then performed. The variables can be entered in a stepwise manner if desired. During the procedure, variables are added and/or eliminated and the procedure repeated until the best subset of discriminating variables is obtained. The outcomes of this procedure are linear discriminant functions (LDFs). Several variables may be associated with one LDF or there may be as many LDFs as there are variables. Similar to the selection of factors in factor analysis, the LDFs are arranged according to the amount of between-group variance they explain. This is determined by examination of eigenvalues, the canonical correlation associated with each LDF, and/or tests of significance. The goal is to select LDFs that can achieve maximal group separation. The researcher eliminates LDFs that contribute little to group separation (Edens, 1987).

The results of the analysis must then be interpreted. This process is similar to that of explaining the variables that load on a factor in factor analysis. The researcher needs to determine the relative contribution of variables within the LDFs to effective discrimination among groups. Illustrating the LDFs graphically can provide useful insights. The coefficients associated with each LDF are also examined. There are two types of coefficients: (1) standardized coefficients, and (2) structured coefficients. Standardized coefficients are similar to the beta weights in regression analysis and allow the researcher to examine the relative contribution of each variable to an LDF. This examination is more difficult if multicollinearity exists. In this case, structured coefficients become important in the interpretation. Structured coefficients are correlations between each variable and each LDF (Edens, 1987).

To predict group membership using the LDFs developed in this analysis, one must move from the exploratory mode to the confirmatory mode. First, the researcher needs to determine the power of the LDFs to predict group membership. This is accomplished through cross-validation. Statistical procedures are then used to determine classifications. This involves examining the distance between each individual case and each group. From this examination, the probabilities of each case being identified as a member of each group are calculated. Using these probabilities, each case is classified. Classification can be based on each group having an equal chance of having a case classified, or it may be based on the knowledge that a certain percent of a population are members of a particular group. In some cases, discrimination is low or groups overlap. The researcher may need to determine whether each case must be assigned to one of the identified groups even when discrimination is low (Edens, 1987).

Woods and colleagues (1995) performed a discriminant analysis as a component of their study of premenstrual symptoms, which was described in the section on factor analysis. The purpose of the discriminant analysis was to "differentiate women with an LS, PMS, or PMM symptom pattern with respect to their feminine and menstrual socialization, expectations about menstrual symptoms, stressful life context, and resources for responding to stressors" (p. 228). Factor scores from the factor analysis described in the section on factor analysis in the chapter were entered as follows.

___

"(Factor scores were entered) along with indicators of health perception, health practices, depressed mood, pregnancies, income, education, and age into three 2-group discriminant function analyses to differentiate women with LS versus PMS, LS versus PMM, and PMS versus PMM patterns. Structure coefficients (discriminant loadings) represent the simple correlation of a vari-

able with the discriminant function and are not affected by multicollinearity. The square of the structure coefficient indicates the proportion of the variance in the function attributable to that variable. Canonical correlations (described below), which indicate the amount of variance accounted for by the function, are provided as a basis for judging the substantive value of the function. (Dillon & Goldstein, 1984)

The function differentiating women with LS and PMS patterns included six variables with a structure coefficient near or exceeding .3 (Dillon & Goldstein, 1984) (Table 19–7). Expectation of symptoms, depressed mood, stress, confirmed pregnancies, health perception, and education differentiated the two groups. Women with PMS had greater expectation of having perimenstrual symptoms, higher depression scores, more stress in their lives, and more pregnancies, rated themselves as less healthy, and had less formal education than women with the LS pattern. Although the structure coefficient was less than .3, men-

Table 19–7
Discriminant Analyses Differentiating Women with LS, PMS, and PMM Symptom Patterns

LS vs. PMS (n = 109)		LS vs. PMM (n = 133)		PMS vs. PMM (n = 168)	
Factor/Variable	**Structure Coefficient**	**Factor/Variable**	**Structure Coefficient**	**Factor/Variable**	**Structure Coefficient**
Symptom expectation (4)[a]	.68*	Symptom expectation (4)	.70*	Depression	.76*
Depression	−.36	Depression	−.63*	Symptom expectation (4)	−.62*
Stress (1)	−.33*	Stress (1)	−.36*	Stress (1)	.40*
Confirmed pregnancy	−.32*	Health perception	.31*	Menstrual socialization (5)	.31*
Health perception	.29	Menstrual socialization	−.27*	Income	−.29*
Education	.28*	Age	.19*	Health perception	−.27
Menstrual socialization (5)	−.24*	Income	.16*	Health practices	−.24
Health practices	.17	Education	.13	Feminine socialization (2)	.18*
Support need (3)	−.09*	Confirmed pregnancy	−.11*	Age	−.18
Income	.07	Health practices	.10	Support need (3)	.11
Feminine socialization (2)	.06*	Support need (3)	−.05*	Education	−.11
Age	−.01	Feminine socialization (2)	.01	Confirmed pregnancy	.00
Canonical correlation	.73	Canonical correlation	.72	Canonical correlation	.53
Centroids		Centroids		Centroids	
LS	.74	LS	.96	PMS	−.47
PMS	−1.49	PMM	−1.10	PMM	.81

LS = low symptom; PMS = premenstrual syndrome; PMM = premenstrual magnification.
[a] Number in parentheses refers to factor number.
* *p* < .05.
(From Woods, N. F., Mitchell, E. S., & Lentz, M. J. [1995]. Social pathways to premenstrual symptoms. *Research in Nursing & Health, 18*[3], 233. Copyright © 1995. Reprinted with permission of John Wiley & Sons, Inc.)

strual socialization also contributed significantly to this function, such that women with a PMS pattern had more negative menstrual socialization. This function explained 73% of the variance. Eighty-five percent of the women were correctly classified with similar prediction for the LS and PMS groups (LS = 85%; PMS = 86%).

Expectation of symptoms, depressed moods, stress, health perception, and menstrual socialization differentiated the women with LS and PMM patterns. Those with PMM demonstrated greater expectation of perimenstrual symptoms, higher depression scores, more negative health ratings, and higher stress levels, and were exposed to more negative socialization about menstruation (Table 19–7) than the women with an LS pattern. This function explained 72% of the variance and correctly classified 85% of the women (PMS = 73%; PMM = 74%).

Depressed mood, expectation of symptoms, stress, and menstrual socialization differentiated the women with a PMS and a PMM pattern. Women with a PMS pattern had lower scores on the depression scale, fewer expectations of symptoms, less stress, less negative menstrual socialization, and higher incomes than women with the PMM pattern. The function explained only 53% of the variance and correctly classified 73% of the women, with a similar classification of the women with a PMS pattern (73% vs. 74%).

These analyses provide support for inclusion of social as well as behavioral and biologic factors in a model distinguishing women who experience premenstrual symptoms (those with a PMS or PMM pattern) from those who do not (LS pattern). The ability to distinguish women with PMS and PMM patterns using the proposed model is limited. This may be a function of limited power, given the relatively modest sample sizes in these two groups, or it may reflect common social pathways for both symptom patterns." (pp. 232–234) ∎

The results of this discriminant analysis are also reported in Mitchell, Woods, and Lentz (1994).

Discriminant analysis is also a useful strategy in clinical physiologic studies where understanding the variables important in explaining patient outcomes has become increasingly more critical.

Hanneman (1994) used discriminant analysis in a study of multidimensional predictors of success or failure with early weaning from mechanical ventilation after cardiac surgery. They describe their study as follows.

■

"Empirically, postoperative cardiac surgery patients either fail early weaning attempts or have such attempts delayed for one or more of the following reasons: (a) hemodynamic instability, (b) poor gas exchange, and (c) poor pulmonary mechanics. The inadequate performance of weaning predictors may be explained by the inability of the dimensions to predict weaning outcome independently. Thus, the purpose of this study was to determine the interdependent contributions of hemodynamics, gas exchange, and pulmonary mechanics to the prediction of weaning outcome in cardiac surgery patients. Furthermore, given the desirability of predictors that can be used widely, a secondary purpose was to test common variables that are readily available to clinicians in all settings.

One hundred sixty-five adult patients admitted to the cardiovascular critical care unit of a 950-bed tertiary private nonprofit teaching hospital in Houston were selected for study. . . Three cases were discarded because the patients expired before a spontaneous ventilation trial. . . One hundred thirty-four (83%) patients were weaned and extubated within 24 hours of unit admission and constituted the success group. Twenty-eight (17%) patients were not weaned from mechanical ventilation within 24 hours of unit admission; they constituted the failure group. Chi-square demonstrated no significant differences between success and failure groups in gender, admitting diagnosis, type of surgery, cardiac rhythm, and weaning technique." (p. 5) ∎

Variables used in the study are shown in Table 19–8. Variables were measured at two points postoperatively: 2 hours after admission to the unit while the patient was on mechanical ventilation (MV), and during a spontaneous ventilation trial (SVT).

Table 19–8
Cardiopulmonary Study Variables on Mechanical Ventilation and During Spontaneous Ventilation Trial

On Mechanical Ventilation (MV)

Frequency of breaths (MVF)	Level of consciousness (LOC)
Tidal volume (MVVT)	Mixed venous oxygen saturation ($S\bar{v}O_2$)
Peak inspiratory pressure (MVPIP)	Cardiac index (CI)
Dynamic compliance (CMPDYN)	Capillary wedge pressure (PCW)
Airways resistance (RAW)	Mean pulmonary artery pressure (PAM)
Static compliance (CMPST)	Central venous pressure (CVP)
Positive end-expiratory pressure (PEEP)	Heart rate (MVHR)
Fraction of inspired oxygen (FIO_2)	Systolic arterial blood pressure (MVSBP)
Pressure support (PS)	Diastolic arterial blood pressure (MVDBP)
pH of the arterial blood (MVpH)	Mean arterial blood pressure (MVMAP)
Arterial carbon dioxide tension ($MVPaCO_2$)	Oximeter oxygen saturation (MVPOX)
Arterial oxygen tension ($MVPaO_2$)	Cardiac rhythm (CR)
Arterial oxygen saturation ($MVSaO_2$)	Ratio of arterial oxygen tension to fraction
Ratio of frequency to tidal volume (f/VT)	of inspired oxygen (PaO_2/FIO_2)

During Spontaneous Ventilation Trial (SVT)

Vital capacity (VC)	Diastolic arterial pressure (SVTDBP)
Negative inspiratory force (NIF)	Carbon dioxide tension ($SVTPaCO_2$)
Frequency of breaths (SVTF)	Arterial oxygen tension ($SVTPaO_2$)
Tidal volume (SVTVT)	Arterial oxygen saturation ($SVTSaO_2$)
Spontaneous minute volume (VES)	Cough effort (CE)
Total minute volume (VET)	Extubation date and time (EXTTIME)
Fraction of inspired oxygen ($SVTFIO_2$)	Mechanical ventilation time (MVTIME)
Heart rate (SVTHR)	Number of SVT trials (TRIAL)
Pulse oximeter oxygen saturation (SVTPOX)	Reason for SVT trial failure (FAIL)
Systolic arterial blood pressure (SVTSBP)	Arterial pH (SVTpH)
Mean arterial blood pressure (SVTMAP)	Ratio of arterial oxygen tension to fraction
Ratio of frequency to tidal volume (f/VT)	of inspired oxygen (PaO_2/FIO_2)

(From Hanneman, S. K. G. [1994]. Multidimensional predictors of success or failure with early weaning from mechanical ventilation after cardiac surgery. *Nursing Research, 43*[1], 6.)

"Given the consequences of erroneous prediction, the alpha was set at .01. Standard formulas (Griner, Mayewski, Mushlin, & Greenland, 1981; Yang & Tobin, 1991) were used to calculate the sensitivity (true positives/(true positives + false negatives)), specificity (true negatives/(true negatives + false positives)), positive predictive value (true positives/(true positives + false positives)), and negative predictive value (true negatives/(true negatives + false negatives)). Diagnostic accuracy (Krieger, Ershowsky, Becker, & Gazeroglu, 1989) was calculated by the following formula: (true positives + true negatives)/ (true positives + true negatives + false positives + false negatives).

A greater percentage of the failure group (82%) had a depressed level of consciousness postoperatively than the success group (42%; χ^2 = 15.3, df = 2, p = .0005). Strength of cough was different between groups (χ^2 = 17, df = 2, p = .0002), with the failure group demonstrating a weaker voluntary cough effort. The number of weaning attempts in the early postoperative period was greater in failure patients (M = 4.4) than in successful patients (M = 1.4; t = −10.11, df = 159, p < .001). Reasons for failing SVT attempts also were different between success and failure groups (χ^2 = 34, df = 8, p = .00005). Hemodynamic instability was prevalent in the failure group and prevented weaning within 24 hours, whereas depressed level of consciousness, carbon dioxide retention, and bleeding were dominant reasons in the success group but did not prevent weaning within 24 hours. Only 21 (13%) of the patients had left-atrial or pulmonary artery catheters. Therefore, the variables of venous oxygen saturation, cardiac index, pulmonary capillary wedge pressure, and pulmonary artery mean pressure were eliminated from the analysis. . .

The ratios during mechanical ventilation and spontaneous ventilation trials were included in the discriminant analysis. Half of the data cases ($n = 82$) were randomly selected for the analysis phase to examine the multivariate differences between success and failure groups, and half of the cases ($n = 80$) were left to test the predictive accuracy of the discriminant function variables. The proportion of variation in the discriminant function explained by the groups was 53% (canonical correlation = 0.733).

Examination of the magnitude of the standardized coefficients showed that the greatest contributions were made by arterial pH during SVT, vital capacity standardized by weight (VCKG), and arterial pH during MV. Using a correlation coefficient of > .30 to denote strength of relationship, the structure coefficients having the most in common with the discriminant function were: pH during SVT and mean arterial pressure and pH during mechanical ventilation. VCKG and PaO_2/FIO_2 had less in common with the discriminant function. The classification results, adjusted for prior probabilities, are shown in Table 19–9. Sensitivity was .98, specificity .71, positive predictive value .94, and negative predictive value .87, yielding a diagnostic accuracy of .93 for the predictor set of variables. Eleven (7%) of the 162 cases were misclassified using the discriminant score to predict group membership." (pp. 6–7) ∎

CANONICAL CORRELATION

Canonical correlation is an extension of multiple regression in which there is more than one dependent variable. Researchers using the technique need to be very familiar with both regression analysis and factor analysis. The purpose of the test is to analyze the relationships between two or more dependent variables and two or more independent variables. The least squares principle is used to partition and analyze variance. Two linear composites are developed: one associated with the dependent variables, and the other associated with the independent variables. The relationship between the two linear composites is then examined and expressed by the value RC. The square of this canonical correlation coefficient indicates the proportion of variance explained by the analysis. When there is more than one source of covariation, more than one canonical correlation can be identified. A more detailed explanation of canonical analysis can be found in Wikoff and Miller (1991).

Olson (1995) used canonical correlation in her study examining relationships between nurse-expressed empathy, patient-perceived empathy, and patient distress. Olson described the study as follows.

Table 19–9
Adjusted Classification Results for Analysis and Validation Samples

	Actual Group	Number of Cases	Predicted Group 1	Predicted Group 2
Analysis sample[a]				
Success	1	67	66 (99%)	1 (1%)
Failure	2	15	3 (20%)	12 (80%)
Validation sample[b]				
Success	1	67	65 (97%)	2 (3%)
Failure	2	13	5 (38%)	8 (62%)

[a] 95% correctly classified ($n = 82$).
[b] 92% correctly classified ($n = 80$).
(From Hanneman, S. K. G. [1994]. Multidimensional predictors of success or failure with early weaning from mechanical ventilation after cardiac surgery. *Nursing Research, 43*[1], 8.)

"A correlational study examined relationships between nurse-expressed empathy and two patient outcomes: patient-perceived empathy and patient distress. Subjects ($N = 140$) were randomly selected from RNs and patients on medical and surgical units in two urban, acute care hospitals. Nurse-subjects ($N = 70$) completed two measures of nurse-expressed empathy: the Behavioral Test of Interpersonal Skills and the Staff-Patient Interaction Response Scale. Patient-subjects ($N = 70$) completed the profile of Mood

Table 19-10
Canonical Between a Set of Empathy Variables and a Set of Patient Distress Variables

Variables	Factor Loadings
Empathy Variables	
Nurse Expressed Empathy (BTIS Feeling)	.68
Nurse Expressed Empathy (BTIS Content)	.62
Nurse Expressed Empathy (BTIS Don't Feeling)	−.42
Patient Perceived Empathy (BLRI)	.85
Patient Distress Variables	
POMS Anxiety	−.89
POMS Depression	−.90
POMS Anger	−.68
MAACL Anxiety	−.72
MAACL Depression	−.88
MAACL Anger	−.63
First Canonical Correlation	
$^a R_c$ = .71386^a	
p = .0002	

$^a R_c$ = the canonical correlation coefficient or the maximal correlation that can be developed between two linear functions of variables. (From Olson, J. K. [1995]. Relationships between nurse-expressed empathy, patient-perceived empathy and patient distress. *Image: Journal of Nursing Scholarship, 27*[4], 319, with permission.)

States, the Multiple Affect Adjective Checklist, and the Barrett-Lennard Relationship Inventory.

Nurse-expressed empathy is understanding what a patient is saying and feeling then communicating this understanding verbally to the patient. Patient-perceived empathy is the patient's feeling of being understood and accepted by the nurse. Patient distress is a negative emotional state. Three hypotheses were developed: (a) There will be negative relationships between measures of nurse-expressed empathy and measures of patient distress, (b) there will be negative relationships between patient-perceived empathy and measures of patient distress, and (c) there will be positive relationships between measures of nurse-expressed empathy and patient-perceived empathy.

Hypotheses one and two were tested together using one canonical correlation. The canonical correlation was generated to analyze the relationships between a set of empathy variables and a set of patient-distress variables. The empathy set included the measures of nurse-expressed empathy and the patient-perceived empathy score. The patient distress set included

measures of patient distress. The overall relationship between the two sets of variables was significant beyond the .001 alpha level (χ^2 (30) = 65.54, p = .001) using Bartlett's test of Wilk's lambda. Canonical correlations are reported in Table 19-10. The first canonical correlation is .71 (p = .0002), representing 50% of the variance for the first pair of canonical variates. This means that 50% of the variation in patient distress scores can be accounted for by a combination of the factors that make up nurse-expressed empathy on the BTIS and patient-perceived empathy. The first pair of canonical variates, therefore, accounted for significant relationships between the two sets of variables. The remaining three canonical correlations were effectively zero and are not included in the table. Correlations (factor loadings) above .40 are reported. . . Overall, patients of nurses who had high scores on nurse-expressed empathy . . . and who were rated by their patients as highly empathic (patient-perceived empathy) were less likely to be distressed (low scores on anxiety, depression, and anger)." (pp. 319–320) ∎

Olson points out that this study is one of the first to link behavioral measures of nurse empathy to patient outcomes.

STRUCTURAL EQUATION MODELING

Structural equation modeling is designed to test theories. In a theory, all of the concepts are expected to be interrelated. The web of relationships in a theory is often expressed as a conceptual map, as discussed in Chapter 7. Testing the structure of relationships within the theory as a whole provides much more information about the validity of the theory than testing only specific propositions. This can be achieved using structural equation modeling. The researcher hopes that the model derived from the structural equations is consistent with the proposed theory. Of course, this consistency does not prove the accuracy of the theory but does support it.

In any theory, elements external to the theory are related to variables within the theory and explain some of the variance within the theory.

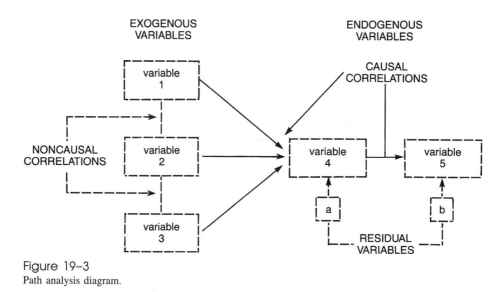

Figure 19-3
Path analysis diagram.

These elements are referred to as residual or exogenous variables and are important to structural equation modeling. Residual variables are not explained by the theory and yet they introduce a source of error into the analyses. Thus, understanding the residual variance is important to interpreting the results of structural equation modeling and to validating the theory.

In a sample map initially described in Chapter 11 (see Figure 19-3), variables 1, 2, and 3 are proposed to be causally related to variable 4. Variable 4 is proposed to be a cause of variable 5. The map demonstrates unidirectional causal flow; variable 5 would not be considered a cause of variable 4. Because the causal relationships will not explain all the variance in the model, residual variables (shown here as *a* and *b*) are introduced to indicate the effect of variables not included in the analysis. Noncausal relationships such as those between variables 1 and 2, 1 and 3, and 2 and 3 are not included in the causal model.

Structural equation modeling requires that the following assumptions be made:

1. The relationships examined in the model are causal, linear, and additive.
2. The residual variables are not correlated with other residual variables or with variables being examined in the model.

3. Causal pathways are unidirectional.
4. Variables can be treated as interval-level measures.

Testing a theory using structural equation modeling occurs in stages and can be categorized into exploratory stages and the confirmatory stage. Initially, the researcher will seek information on beta weights concerning specific relationships between concepts from previous research. In the early exploratory period, correlational analyses are performed and a covariance matrix is obtained. A series of regression analyses may be performed as the researcher gets a feel for the data.

Reliability and validity of measures used in the analysis are critical to the validity of the model. When possible, it is desirable to use multiple indicators of parameters. As with regression analysis, a large sample is desirable, with at least 30 subjects for each variable being considered. Larger samples are more likely to yield statistically significant path coefficients needed to validate the model, thus reducing the risk of a Type II error. Because of the importance of model building to theory development, a Type II error is a serious concern.

Data need to be carefully cleaned prior to analysis. Accuracy of the data is carefully checked. Subjects with missing data are removed. Outliers are identified and examined. Some statistical procedures will automatically exclude outliers from the analysis. The decision to retain or exclude outliers is a difficult one. The outliers may represent an important segment of the population under study, and yet the inclusion of a small amount of very divergent data can greatly alter the outcomes of the analysis.

In the exploratory stage, a path analysis is performed using a series of regression analyses. In the analysis, a *path coefficient* indicates the effect of an independent variable on the dependent variable. The symbol for a path coefficient is P with two subscripts. The first subscript indicates the dependent variable; the second subscript indicates the independent variable. For example, the direct effect of variable 4 on variable 5 would be symbolized as P_{54}. Path coefficients are usually expressed in the form of beta weights. (Beta weights were discussed in the section on simple linear regression.)

The map in Figure 19–3 would require two regression analyses to identify the path coefficients. In the first analysis, path coefficients would be obtained by regressing variable 4 on variables 1, 2, and 3. Then, variable 5 would be regressed on variable 4. In interpreting the results, the weight of the coefficient and its level of statistical significance are considered. A large coefficient that is highly significant validates the causal pathway.

Confirmatory structural equation modeling is performed using LISREL or EQS. Using these procedures, the assumptions of regression are relaxed: all relevant variables are not assumed to be included in the model; perfect measurement is not assumed. The analysis is concerned with the identification of latent variables—operationalizations of concepts that are not measurable by direct observation. Thus, one concept might be represented by the combination of several measures. In structural equation modeling, there are multiple dependent as well as independent variables. Using information obtained from previous studies and exploratory analyses, the researcher specifies the nature of the relationships and provides an initial estimation of the model as a starting point for the analysis. The analysis is an iterative procedure progressing in stages to a final estimation of the model (Mason-Hawkes & Holm, 1989).

Analysis involves three steps: specification, estimation, and assessing goodness of fit. In the specification step, the researcher specifies the parameters of the model, including variables and interrelationships (or paths). This is similar to developing a conceptual map. The variance (or covariance) of some parameters of the model is specified (or held constant at a selected value). This value is selected based on previous studies and exploratory analyses. These parameters are referred to as *fixed*. All other variables are referred to as *free*. The analysis procedure has rules that govern the selection of parameters to be fixed or free.

In the estimation step, the free parameters are estimated by computer analysis. The results, including fixed parameters and estimated parameters, are then assessed for goodness of fit. Initially, the resulting model is examined in relation to the data. If the model is not a good fit, parameters can be added or dropped. The values of fixed parameters may be modified and the analysis rerun to achieve a better fit. This is referred to as *respecification*. There is some judgment involved in determining what makes the model a fit. The initial evaluation is based on the statistical significance of each path proposed by the original model. Parameters that do not achieve significance in the analysis are carefully considered. Were measures used to examine the parameter adequate? Was the sample size sufficient? Is it possible that the original theory is incorrect? Should the parameter be omitted from the map of the theory? How important is the parameter in explaining the phenomenon? In some cases, because of their theoretical importance, parameters may be retained in the model in spite of failing to achieve statistical significance. Validation of the final model is achieved by conducting further analyses using data from new samples.

Neuberger, Kasal, Smith, Hassanein, and De-Viney (1994) used structural equation modeling to test their theoretical causal model of exercise and aerobic fitness in outpatients with arthritis.

"Factors that influenced exercise behaviors and aerobic fitness were identified in 100 outpatients with rheumatoid arthritis or osteoarthritis. Data included perceived health status, benefits of and barriers to exercise, and impact of arthritis on health; demographic and biologic characteristics; and past exercise behavior. Exercise measures included range-of-motion and strengthening exercises, 7-day activity recall, and the exercise subscale of the Health-Promoting Lifestyle Profile. An aerobic fitness level was obtained on each subject by bicycle ergometer testing. . .

To determine if rheumatoid arthritis ($n = 63$) subjects differed from osteoarthritis subjects ($n = 37$), the two groups were compared on the study variables using the t-statistic or chi-square. No statistically significant differences were found in the two groups on any of the study variables. Therefore, data on rheumatoid arthritis and osteoarthritis subjects were combined for analysis. . .

To simplify data analysis, a composite score of self-reported exercises was calculated by a principal component factor analysis of the four measures of exercise (ROM score, strengthening exercise score, MET score, and exercise subscale score) and calculating a factor score by the regression technique. To determine if the theoretical model predicted the composite exercise scores and the resulting aerobic fitness levels of the subjects, path analysis was conducted based on the causal model. The analysis for the path model was done by a set of ordinary least squares regression equations. The first set of three equations had perceived health status, perceived benefits, and perceived barriers as predicted variables. The independent variables in the equations were the modifying factors in Stage I (Figure 19–4). The three predicted variables were in turn used to predict participation in exercise. The last equation in the model was level of fitness predicted by participation in exercise. The standardized parameters from each equation were used as path coefficients to derive the indirect effects with the model.

The theoretical model proposed that the eight modifying factors would produce direct effects on the cognitive-perceptual factors and that the modifying factors would affect exercise behaviors (composite exercise scores) and the resulting aerobic fitness levels indirectly through their effects on the cognitive perceptual factors of perceived health status, perceived benefits of exercise, and perceived barriers to exercise. As seen in (Figure 19–4), three modifying factors—impact of arthritis on health status, duration of arthritis, and age—had significant ($p = .05$) direct effects on perceived health status. Higher impact of arthritis scores and longer duration of arthritis were significantly ($p = .05$) associated with poorer perceived health status scores. Older age was associated ($p = .05$) with better perceived health status. When path coefficients of .10 and above are considered, education level, income level, and pain scores also affected perceived health status. Fewer years of education and high pain scores were related to poorer perceived health status, while higher income levels were associated with better perceived health status. The total variance in perceived health status scores accounted for by the eight modifying factors was 26% (adj. $R^2 = .26$).

Subjects' scores on the eight modifying factors accounted for 18.4% of the variance in perceived benefits of exercise scores. Higher impact of arthritis scores were significantly ($p = .05$) associated with lower scores of perceived benefits of exercise. Previous exercise was significantly ($p = .05$) associated with higher perceived benefits of exercise scores. Longer duration of arthritis ($\beta = .098$), higher impact of arthritis scores ($\beta = .170$), higher body mass index scores ($\beta = .124$), and fewer years of education ($\beta = .122$) were related to lower perceived barriers to exercise. . .

The total amount of variance in composite exercise scores accounted for by the model was 20%. Perception of more benefits of exercise was positively associated ($\beta = .438$, $p = .05$) with exercise participation. Poorer perceived health status ($\beta = -.012$) and higher perceived barriers to exercise scores ($-.049$) were weakly ($\beta < .10$) associated with lower participation in exercise. As seen in Stage IV of the path model (Figure 19–4), regression of the aerobic fitness levels on composite exercise scores failed to predict any variance in aerobic fitness levels." (pp. 15–16) ∎

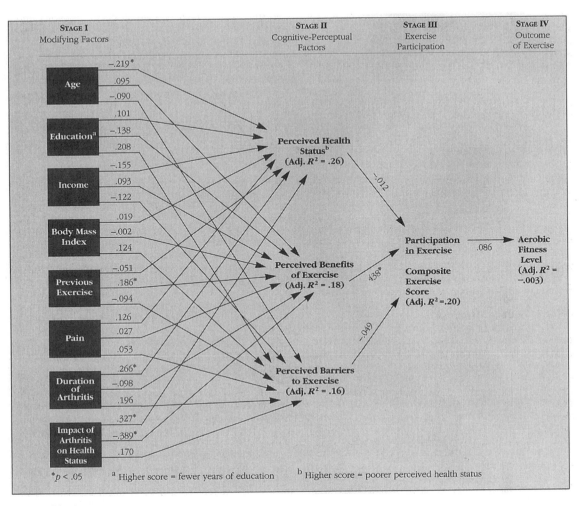

Figure 19-4
Path Coefficients of Model Testing Determinants of Exercise. (From Neuberger, G. B., Kasal, S., Smith, K. V., Hassanein, R., & DeViney, S. [1994]. Determinants of exercise and aerobic fitness in outpatients with arthritis. *Nursing Research, 43*[1], 12.)

TIME-SERIES ANALYSIS

Time-series analysis is a technique designed to analyze changes in a variable across time and thus to uncover pattern in the data. Multiple measures of the variable collected at equal intervals are required. There is growing interest in nursing in these procedures because of the interest in understanding pattern. For example, wave and field pattern is one of the themes of Martha Rogers's

(1986) theory. Pattern is also an important component of Margaret Newman's (1979) nursing theory. Pattern has been conceptually defined by Crawford (1982) as "the configuration of relationships among elements of a phenomenon" (qtd. in Taylor, 1990, p. 256). Taylor has expanded this definition to incorporate time into the study of patterns and defines pattern as "repetitive, regular, or continuous occurrences of a particular phenomenon. Patterns may increase, decrease, or maintain a stable state by oscillating up and down in degree of frequency. In this way, the structure of a pattern incorporates both change and stability, concepts which are important to the study of human responses over time" (Taylor, 1990, p. 256).

Although certainly the easiest strategy for analyzing time-series data is to graph the raw data, this approach to analysis misses some important information. Important patterns in the data are often missed because of residual effects in the data. Therefore, various statistical procedures have been developed to analyze the data.

In the past, the analysis of time-series data has been problematic because computer programs designed for this purpose were not easily accessible. The most common approach to analysis was ordinary least squares multiple regression. However, this approach has been unsatisfactory for the most part. Better approaches to analyzing this type of data are now available (Box & Jenkins, 1976; Glass, Willson, & Gottman, 1975; Gottman, 1981). With easier access to computer programs designed to conduct time-series analysis, information in the nursing literature on these approaches has been increasing (Jirovec, 1986; Lentz, 1990a, 1990b; Metzger & Schultz, 1982; Taylor, 1990; Thomas, 1987, 1990).

One approach to the analysis of time-series data was developed and described by McCain and McCleary (1979), McCleary and Hay (1980), and McDowall, McCleary, Meidinger, and Hay (1980). The most commonly used time-series analysis model is the *autoregressive integrated moving average (ARIMA) model,* which is based on work by Box and Jenkins (1976). A model is an equation or series of equations that explains a naturally occurring process (McCain & McCleary, 1979).

ARIMA modeling is based on the following four-step procedure: (1) identification, (2) estimation, (3) diagnostic checking, and (4) forecasting, with a feedback loop built into the process as shown in Figure 19–5.

The terminology and the problems that must be dealt with in time-series analysis are different from those that we are more familiar with in analyzing conventional data. A time series has two components: the deterministic component, and the

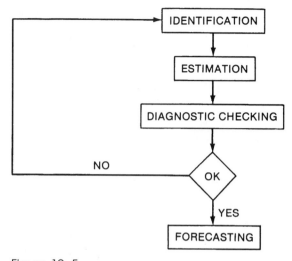

Figure 19–5
Steps of ARIMA modeling.

stochastic component. The *deterministic component* represents all the parameters of time series that are not dependent on error (or random variation in the data). However, this parameter cannot perfectly predict the values in a time series, because even though the underlying process may be systematic, a single observation will deviate from the expected value. The *stochastic component* describes what is referred to as *noise* (or random variance) in the data. There are two parts to the stochastic component, the systematic part and the unsystematic part. The systematic part is related to the autocorrelation inherent in time-series data. Autocorrelations, as the term implies, are repeated occurrences in the data that are systematic and to some extent patterned. Each one of these events is correlated with both past and future occurrences of the same event. The unsystematic part is the typical error variance that leads to differences from measures of central tendency found in all data. The unsystematic part is the element in time series from which such measures as standard deviations are calculated.

The ARIMA models describe time series as stochastic or noise processes. The null hypothesis is that only the noise component is present and that no change has occurred. There are three parameters to an ARIMA model: *p, d,* and *q.* The integer values of these parameters are identified through a simple statistical analysis called *identification.* However, first it is important to understand the parameters.

STATIONARITY

To use an ARIMA (*p, d, q*) model, the data must be either stationary or nonstationary in a homogeneous sense. The noise in a time series drifts up and down across time. If the data are stationary, it means that there is no decrease or increase in the level of the series as it drifts. However, most data in the social sciences are nonstationary. Nonstationary in the homogeneous sense means that differencing can be used to make the data stationary. To accomplish this, difference scores are calculated between the sequences in the time series. The value of the first observation is subtracted from the second, the value of the second is subtracted from the third, and so on. For example, consider the following series of numbers as a time series:

$$2, 4, 6, 8, 10, 12. \ldots$$

This series is nonstationary. But note the effect of differencing the series:

$$4 - 2 = 2$$
$$6 - 4 = 2$$
$$8 - 6 = 2$$
$$10 - 8 = 2$$

Now the series is stationary:

$$2, 2, 2, 2, 2, 2, \ldots 2.$$

Fortunately, most social science data can be differenced to achieve stationarity. Differencing has no effect on the deterministic parameters of the model, which will be used in the analysis to detect changes. The model parameter *d* indicates the number of times a series must be differenced be-fore it becomes stationary. A zero in the model (ARIMA [*p*, 0, *q*]) indicates that the time series is stationary and does not require differencing.

AUTOREGRESSIVE MODELS

The parameter *p* indicates the autoregressive order of the model. There are two elements in the parameter *p:* 0_1 and a_t. The 0_1 is a correlation coefficient that describes the degree of dependency between observations. If there is a direct relationship between adjacent observations, the value of *p* exceeds zero. This direct relationship between observations means that the observations are dependent. If they are dependent, the current value can be predicted based on the previous value in the series, and the present value can be used to predict future values. The *p* parameter of the model indicates the number of autoregressive terms included in the model. The a_t is the error term and describes what is referred to as white noise or random shock. This is the unsystematic element in the stochastic component of the model. In equations calculating this parameter, the 0_1 and a_t are summed.

MOVING AVERAGE MODELS

The *q* parameter in the ARIMA (*p, d, q*) model is an indication of the moving average order. In some time series, there is persistence of a random shock beyond a single observation. This persistence is similar to the effect of dropping a pebble in water. If this occurs, *q* exceeds zero. The statistic φ (phi) is a correlation coefficient that expresses the extent to which the current time-series observation can be predicted from preceding random shocks. Phi (φ) is used as the weight in a weighted term in a prediction equation. In some models, more than one weighted term may be used.

NOISE MODEL IDENTIFICATION

The systematic part of the stochastic component in an ARIMA (*p, d, q*) model is identified by using two functions: the autocorrelation function (ACF), and the partial autocorrelation function (PACF). When a likely model has been identified, the parameters are estimated using special nonlinear computer software. Then the ACF and PACF are used to diagnose the adequacy of the model. If the model is inadequate, a new ARIMA (*p, d, q*) model is identified, the parameters are estimated, and the residuals are diagnosed. This procedure continues until an adequate model is generated.

FORECASTING

When the first three steps of the modeling strategy—identification, estimation, and diagnosis—have been satisfactorily completed, the model can be used for forecasting. An ARIMA model could forecast such variables as infant mortality as a function of past infant mortality. The model cannot be used to explain causality. Three types of change can be detected by the model: abrupt, constant change; gradual, constant change; and abrupt, temporary change. In an adequate model, the residuals act like white noise, allowing the model to detect differences between the white noise and the effects of change.

Although the analysis process itself does not require extreme degrees of statistical sophistication, it will require some changes in the way that studies are designed in nursing. If a care process is being examined, each element of that care is an observation. Each behavioral response of the patient is an observation. Thus, the process of observation may require that the situation be broken down into very discrete elements (McCain & McCleary, 1979; McCleary & Hay, 1980; McDowall et al., 1980; Metzger & Schultz, 1982).

Nursing studies using time-series analysis techniques have only recently begun appearing in the nursing literature. Taylor (1994) describes a study evaluating therapeutic change in symptom severity at the level of the individual woman experiencing severe PMS.

"The purpose of this interrupted time-series study was to determine the effectiveness of a multi-model nursing intervention aimed at relieving the symptom severity and distress associated with PNA (perimenstrual negative affect), and to describe the occurrence of individual patterns of PNA symptoms and symptom pattern change. The use of a time-series design and methodology as an alternative to a cross-sectional group design allowed examination of individual responses over time, as well as an examination of the change in symptom patterns after treatment.

In this interrupted time-series design, each woman is considered as one experiment and serves as her own control. Internal validity is achieved in this design by accounting for the extraneous variables by multiple measures and planning for a stable baseline of data collection before introducing the independent variable (Gottman, 1984; Kazdin, 1982; Mitchell, 1988). Daily and weekly measures were collected across seven complete menstrual cycles in five women meeting restrictive sampling criteria. The baseline phase included three complete menstrual cycles followed by a seven-week intervention phase and a post-intervention phase of three menstrual cycles. Previous research had indicated that two complete menstrual cycles provide an adequate baseline (Mitchell, Woods, & Lentz, 1985, 1991; Taylor, 1986). Generalizability is achieved through systematic replication of the design in additional women.

The experimental treatment is a system of non-pharmacologic strategies involving self-monitoring, personal choice, self-regulation and self/environmental modification, administered within a group format of peer support and professional guidance. The purpose of the multi-modal approach is to provide a therapeutic environment for women to incorporate non-pharmacologic treatments, adhere to difficult treatment plans and to provide a milieu to model behavioral, cognitive and environmental change strategies.

A group format (two hours weekly for seven weeks) included formal presentations by a nurse-facilitator. The formal presentations provided the knowledge base for the individual treatments which have been suggested as non-pharmacologic remedies for PMS: (a) specific dietary changes (decreased caffeine and sugar, increased complex carbohydrates, small frequent meals); (b) PMS-formula vitamin supplementation perimenstrually; (c) aerobic and relaxation/stretching exercises; (d) behavioral stress reduction techniques (stress identification, thought stopping, affirmations, self-esteem enhancement); and (e) lifestyle alterations and environmental control (time and role management, communication and social competency training). Demonstration and practice sessions allowed the women to try out the therapies and discussion sessions provided a means for the women to express their unique treatment concerns. A personalized treatment plan was developed for each woman at the end of the seven weeks. . .

The analysis proceeded in two phases: within-individual, time-series analysis of pre-treatment baseline behavior and response; and an interrupted time-series analysis of treatment effect. For the baseline or pretreatment analysis, 90 data points were available for each woman for PNA symptom severity data. Examination of the shape and significance of the baseline PNA pattern permitted the analysis of symptom fluctuation within the menstrual cycle as well as confirmation of the initial classification of severe PNA. In the application of the interrupted time-series analysis to examine treatment effects, 120 daily data points were available for the post-treatment time-series. Simply, the time-series was 'interrupted' by the intervention. The pretreatment (or baseline) time-series data were analyzed for shape, structure and statistical significance, and compared with the shape, structure and statistical significance of the post-treatment time-series data (Abraham & Neundorfer, 1990; Gottman, 1984; Woods & Catanzaro, 1988).

The auto-correlation function (ACF) was used to identify significant patterns within each woman's daily symptom data. The ACF measures the correlation between observations and can be defined as the shared variance of one observation and each successive observation taken from the same individual. In this case, each woman had approximately 200 daily symptom severity data points. . . Since it was predicted that symptom severity would follow a menstrual cycle pattern, a 'lag' of 28 to 30 days was used for the ACF (depending on each individual menstrual cycle). For example, using a lag of 30 days, each daily symptom value was correlated, or 'lagged,' with the symptom severity value 30 days later (day one correlated with day 30). The ACF assumes serial dependency of the data points, since each data point is drawn from the same person.

Each woman's symptom time-series was divided into a baseline time-series (90 days of symptom data) and a post-treatment time-series (120 days of symptom data) and analyzed as an interrupted time-series using the ACF. The auto-correlations were examined for their structure, pattern and significance. Analysis of the 'shape' of the correlogram (plot of the auto-correlations), along with examination of significant auto-correlations, can reveal deterministic patterns which recur within the whole time-series and between the baseline and post-treatment time-series (Gottman, 1984; Taylor, 1990). Auto-correlations greater than two times the standard deviation of the auto-correlation, called the Bartlett Band of significance, were considered statistically significant at the $p = .05$ level (Gottman, 1984).

As expected by the use of careful sampling, a menstrual cycle pattern of PNA symptom severity was found in the baseline correlograms, but only in four of the five women. Due to space limitations, Figure 19–6 represents the baseline pattern found in participant No. 1, No. 2, and No. 4 (e.g., similar patterns were found in each of the three women). Figure 19–7 represents the menstrual cycle pattern found in participant No. 3. One woman (No. 5) did not demonstrate a menstrual cycle pattern in the baseline correlogram (Figure 19–8). The ACF was applied to all five baseline time-series, allowing the determination of both pattern structure and statistical significance for each individual baseline time-series. The shape of the correlogram for the first four women revealed a menstrual cycle pattern (Figure 19–6 and Figure 19–7) with positive auto-correlations at lag 1 to 5 days and lag 27 to 32 days representing the menstrual and premenstrual phases. Negative auto-correlations occur at lag 10 to 21 representing the mid-cycle of the menstrual cycle. In both baseline patterns in (Figure 19–6) and (Figure 19–7), the auto-correlations fall outside the Bartlett Band of statistical significance indicating that these menstrual cycle patterns would not be found by chance at $p = .05$.

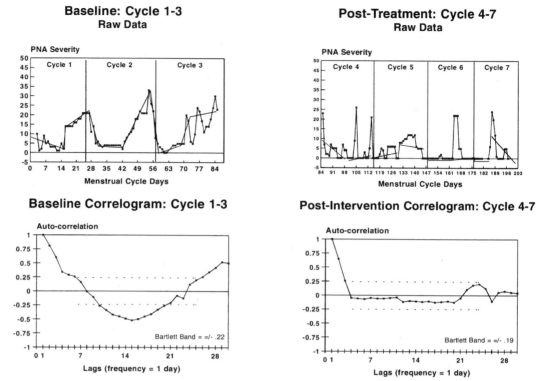

Figure 19–6

"Normalizing" Treatment Effect Pattern: PNA Severity (Participant No. 1, No. 2, No. 4). (From Taylor, D. L. [1994]. Evaluating therapeutic change in symptom severity at the level of the individual woman experiencing severe PMS. *Image: Journal of Nursing Scholarship, 26*[1], 28, with permission.)

Thus, four of the five women had confirmed PNA that followed a menstrual cycle pattern in the baseline phase. . .

In participant No. 1 and No. 2, the cyclic pattern of PNA changed significantly ($p = .05$) after treatment as represented by the interrupted time-series analyses (Figure 19–6). Perimenstrual negative affect was reduced in level and duration and postmenstrual negative affect was almost non-existent after the treatment. Average PNA severity levels dropped sharply during the treatment period (cycle three to four) and remained low during the post-treatment phase (cycle five to seven). The average PNA severity score ranged from 0.0 to 4.6 postmenstrually (mean severity = 1.9), and from 4.7 to 8.1 perimenstrually (mean severity = 5.9). The menstrual cycle patterning the baseline correlogram was dampened after the intervention, and significant

auto-correlations ($r = \pm.19$) were not apparent. There was a suggestion of a weak periodic process in the post-intervention series (day 23) which reflects the recurrence of low-intensity PNA in the premenstruum. For participants No. 1 and No. 2, the intervention clearly reduced the severity of cyclic PNA. The PNA symptom pattern became predictable and regular, with dramatic modification of symptom intensity, frequency, and duration. This pattern of therapeutic response was labeled a 'normalized' response pattern, whereby a high severity PNA pattern subsides to become a 'normal' menstrual cycle symptom pattern.

In participant No. 4, PNA severity decreased during the third baseline cycle and there were many zero scores which mediated the cycle phase differences in symptom scores as well as the treatment effect. Mean PNA severity levels

Baseline: Cycle 1-3
Raw Data

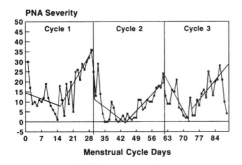

Post-treatment: Cycle 4-6
Raw Data

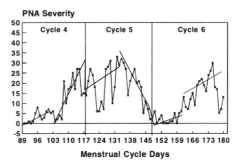

Baseline Correlogram: Cycle 1-3

Post-Intervention Correlogram: Cycle 4-6

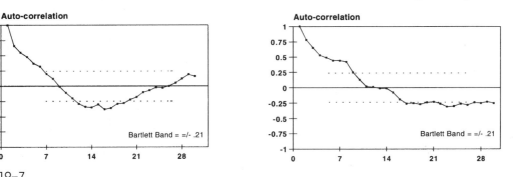

Figure 19–7

"Unstable" Treatment Effect Pattern: PNA Severity (Participant No. 3). (From Taylor, D. L. [1994]. Evaluating therapeutic change in symptom severity at the level of the individual woman experiencing severe PMS. *Image: Journal of Nursing Scholarship, 26*[1], 29, with permission.)

in the premenstruum were low after treatment (1.7 – 3.5), as were the postmenstrual PNA severity levels (mean severity = .75 – 4.2). A weak, non-significant pattern emerged at day 31 to 33 ($r = \pm.19$) in the post-treatment correlogram. It is notable that the improvement in PNA severity was very rapid, indicating that treatment effects occurred prior to treatment onset. Because of the rapid response soon after the first baseline cycle, this therapeutic response pattern was also considered as a 'normalized' pattern. PNA symptom severity declined during the second and third baseline period and remained low during the post-intervention period, indicating a 'normal' menstrual symptom pattern.

The intervention had little effect on PNA severity for participant No. 3, and the PNA pattern remained disorganized and unpredictable

across the post-treatment cycles (Figure 19–7). While peri- and postmenstrual negative affect symptom severity was moderate to high in the three cycles comprising the baseline period (mean severity = 16.8 to 40 for three phases), only post-menstrual negative affect declined after treatment (mean severity = 4.4 to 20 for three phases). Perimenstrual negative affect severity remained high (16.8 to 18.0) with little respite from symptom frequency or intensity due to the intervention. The auto-correlations suggested little change in PNA severity after the intervention. Unlike the baseline correlogram, the shape of the auto-correlations did not reflect a menstrual cycle pattern after the intervention, and there were no significant auto-correlations after lag 8. This response pattern was labeled an 'unstable' therapeutic response, whereby PNA se-

Baseline Correlogram: Cycle 1-3

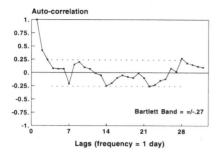

Post-Intervention Correlogram: Cycle 4-6

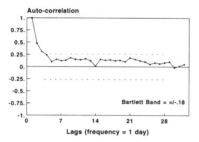

Figure 19–8

"Non-Menstrual cycle" Treatment Effect Pattern: PNA Severity (Participant No. 5). (From Taylor, D. L. [1994]. Evaluating therapeutic change in symptom severity at the level of the individual woman experiencing severe PMS. *Image: Journal of Nursing Scholarship, 26*[1], 30, with permission.)

verity did not decline to regular, low severity in the post-intervention period.

In participant No. 5, no menstrual cyclicity of PNA severity emerged before or after the treatment (Figure 19–8). PNA severity did not conform to a predictable pattern within cycles or across menstrual cycle phase (premenstrual PNA severity = 2.1 to 9.3; postmenstrual PNA severity = 4.3 to 9.7). After the intervention, the seven-day cyclic pattern in PNA severity became nonexistent and the shape of the correlogram revealed a non-cyclic PNA symptom pattern without statistical significance. This symptom pattern was labeled as a 'non-menstrual cycle' response pattern, whereby the shape of the auto-correlations did not resemble any cyclic pattern after the intervention.

Clear delineation of PMS and perimenstrual symptom clusters has plagued investigators attempting to understand the phenomena of symptoms that appear to follow a menstrual cycle pattern (Abplanalp, 1988). Certainly part of

the problem has been the reliance on aggregate data that obscures individual differences. Furthermore, when individual differences are wildly diverse, conventional analytic strategies are not able to find significant differences without large sample sizes." (pp. 26–30)
(From Taylor, D. L. [1994]. Evaluating therapeutic change in symptom severity at the level of the individual woman experiencing severe PMS. *Image: Journal of Nursing Scholarship, 26*[1], 25–33, with permission.) ∎

SURVIVAL ANALYSIS

Survival analysis is a set of techniques designed to analyze repeated measures from a given time (e.g., the beginning of the study, onset of a disease, the beginning of a treatment, the initiation of a stimulus) until a certain attribute (e.g., death, treatment failure, recurrence of a phenomenon) occurs. The determinants of various lengths of survival can be identified. The risk (hazard or probability) of an event occurring at a given point in time for an individual can be analyzed.

A common feature in survival analysis data is the presence of censored observations. These data come from subjects who have not experienced the outcome attribute being measured. They did not die, the treatment continued to work, the phenomenon did not recur, or they were withdrawn from the study for some reason. Because of censored observations and the frequency of skewed data in studies examining such outcomes, common statistical tests may not be appropriate.

The distribution of survival times is explained by three functions: (1) the survivorship function, $S(t)$; (2) the density function, $f(t)$; and the hazard function, $h(t)$. Survivorship function, $S(t)$, is the probability that a specific individual's time (T) is greater than a specified time (t). Density function, $f(t)$, is the probability that the individual fails in a specific small interval of time. Thus, density reflects the failure rate. Hazard function, $h(t)$, is the conditional failure rate. It is the probability of failure within a specific small interval of time given that the individual has survived until that point. The results of survival analysis are often plotted on graphs. For example, one might plot the period between the initiation of cigarette smoking and the occurrence of smoking-related diseases such as cancer (Allison, 1984; Gross & Clark, 1975; Hintze, 1990; Lee, 1984; Nelson, 1982).

Survival analysis has been used most frequently in medical research. When a cancer patient asks what his or her chances of cure are from a specific treatment, the information the physician provides was probably obtained using survival analysis. The procedure has been used less commonly in nursing research. However, because of further development of the statistical procedures and their availability in statistical packages such as NCSS for the PC, one can expect to see this analysis procedure more commonly in the nursing literature in the 1990s.

With use of the procedure, it is possible to study many previously unexamined facets of nursing practice. Possibilities include the effectiveness of various pain relief measures, length of breast feeding, maintenance of weight loss, abstinence from smoking, recurrence of decubitus ulcers, urinary tract infection after catheterization, and rehospitalization for the same diagnosis within the 60-day period in which Medicare will not provide reimbursement. The researcher could examine variables that are effective in explaining recurrence within various time intervals or characteristics of various groups who have received differing treatments.

■ SUMMARY

Advanced statistical procedures are being used with greater frequency in nursing research. These procedures are presented with sufficient detail to allow the beginning researcher and the nursing research consumer to read, comprehend, and perform a beginning critique of published studies using these analyses. The explanation will assist in understanding the terminology, the process of analysis, and the results of analysis. To perform a critique, the reader determines whether the analysis was properly performed and interpreted, and whether the analysis was appropriate to the study.

Multiple regression is an extension of simple linear regression in which more than one independent variable is entered into the analysis. The purpose of a regression analysis is to predict and/or explain as much of the variance in the values of the dependent variable as possible. In some cases, the analysis is exploratory and the focus is prediction. In others, variables are selected based on a theoretical position and the purpose is explanation, to confirm the theoretical position. The variables in a regression equation can take many forms. Traditionally, as with most multivariate analyses, variables are measured at the interval level. However, categorical or dichotomous measures (referred to as dummy variables), multiplicative terms, and transformed terms are also used. A mixture of types of variables may be used in a single regression equation.

The outcome of regression analysis is referred to as a prediction equation. The results of a regression analysis are not sample-specific. The final outcome is a model from which values of the independent variables can be used to predict and perhaps explain values of the dependent variable in the population. Thus, one can repeat the analysis in other samples and obtain similar results. The equation needs to have predictive validity. To determine the accuracy of the prediction, the predicted values are compared with actual values obtained from a new sample of subjects or values from a sample obtained at the time of the original data collection but held out from the initial analysis. In most cases, the R^2 will be lower in the new sample, because the original equation was developed to predict scores in the original sample most precisely. This is referred to as the shrinkage of R^2. Shrinkage of R^2 is greater in small samples and when multicollinearity is great. Multicollinearity occurs when the independent variables in a regression equation are strongly correlated.

continued

continued

A wide variety of regression analysis procedures are available. Selection of a particular procedure is based on the purpose of the study, the type of data available, and the experience of the researcher. Regression analyses can be broadly categorized into exploratory and confirmatory procedures. The exploratory mode is the most commonly used strategy in nursing studies. The most common approach to regression analysis in nursing research is stepwise regression. Confirmatory regression analysis procedures include logistic regression and hierarchical regression.

Factorial analysis of variance is simply a specialized version of multiple regression that has been developed to analyze data from specific experimental designs. Two types of effects are considered in interpreting the results of a factorial ANOVA. Main effects are the effects of a single factor. Interaction effects are the multiplicative effects of two or more factors. Interaction effects are evaluated prior to consideration of main effects, because interaction effects may render main effects meaningless.

Analysis of covariance (ANCOVA) is designed to reduce the error term (or the variance within groups) by partialing out the variance resulting from a confounding variable. This is accomplished by performing regression analysis prior to performing ANOVA. This strategy removes the effect of differences between groups that is due to a confounding variable.

Factor analysis is mathematically related to regression analysis. In both analyses, equations are developed that are linear combinations of the variables. Factor analysis examines interrelationships among large numbers of variables and disentangles those relationships to identify clusters of variables that are most closely linked together. These closely related variables are grouped together into a factor. Several factors may be identified within a data set. There are two types of factor analysis: exploratory and confirmatory. Exploratory factor analysis is similar to stepwise regression in which the variance of the first factor is partialed out before analysis is begun on the second factor. Confirmatory factor analysis is based on theory and tests a hypothesis about the existing factor structure.

Discriminant analysis is closely related to both factor analysis and regression analysis. However, in discriminant analysis, the dependent variable values are categorical in form. The dependent variable in discriminant analysis is referred to as the discriminant function. The purpose of the analysis is to identify variables that most effectively discriminate between groups.

Canonical correlation is an extension of multiple regression in which there is more than one dependent variable. The purpose of the test is to analyze the relationships between two or more dependent variables and two or more independent variables.

Structural equation modeling is designed to test theories. In a theory, all of the concepts are expected to be interrelated. Testing the structure of relationships within the theory as a whole provides much more information about the validity of the theory than testing only specific propositions. Testing a theory using structural equation modeling occurs in stages and can be categorized into exploratory stages and the confirmatory stage. In the exploratory stage, a path analysis is performed using a series of regression analyses. Using information from the path analysis, confirmatory structural equation modeling is performed. Analysis involves three steps: specification, estimation, and assessing goodness of fit.

Time-series analysis is a technique designed to analyze changes in a variable across time and thus to uncover pattern in the data. Multiple measures of the variable collected at

continued

continued

equal intervals are required. There is growing interest in nursing in these procedures because of the interest in understanding pattern. Although certainly the easiest strategy for analyzing time-series data is to graph the raw data, with this approach important patterns in the data are often missed because of residual effects in the data. The most commonly used time-series analysis model is the autoregressive integrated moving average (ARIMA) model. ARIMA modeling is based on the fol-lowing four-step procedure: (1) identification, (2) estimation, (3) diagnostic checking, and (4) forecasting.

Survival analysis is a set of techniques designed to analyze repeated measures from a given time until a certain attribute occurs. The determinants of various lengths of survival can be identified. Using the procedure, it is possible to examine many facets of nursing practice not previously examined.

References

Aaronson, L. S. (1989). A cautionary note on the use of stepwise regression. *Nursing Research, 38*(5), 309–311.

Abplanalp, J. (1988). Psychosocial theories. In Keye, W. R. (Ed.), *The premenstrual syndrome* (pp. 94–112). Philadelphia: Saunders.

Abraham, I. L., & Neudorfer, M. M. (1990). The design and analysis of time-series studies. In L. E. Moody (Ed.), *Advancing nursing science research* (Vol. 2, pp. 145–175). Newbury Park, CA: Sage.

Albers, L. L., Lydon-Rochelle, M. T., & Krulewitch, C. J. (1995). Maternal age and labor complications in healthy primigravidas at term. *Journal of Nurse-Midwifery, 40*(1), 4–12.

Allison, P. D. (1984). *Event history analysis: Regression for longitudinal event data.* Beverly Hills, CA: Sage.

Arrindell, W. A., & van der Ende, J. (1985). An empirical test of the utility of the observations-to-variables ratio in factor and components analysis. *Applied Psychological Measurement, 9*(2), 165–178.

Baron, R. M., & Kenny, D. A. (1986). The moderator-mediator variable distinction in social psychological research: Conceptual, strategic and statistical considerations. *Journal of Personality & Social Psychology, 51*(6), 1173–1182.

Bentler, P. M. (1989). *EQS: Structural equations program manual.* Los Angeles: BMDP Statistical Software, 1440 Sepulveda Boulevard, Suite 316, Los Angeles, CA 90025; Telephone: (213) 479–7799, Fax: (213) 312–0161.

Bentler, P. M., & Bonett, D. G. (1980). Significance tests and goodness of fit in the analysis of covariance structures. *Psychological Bulletin, 88*(3), 588–606.

Bentler, P. M., & Weeks, D. G. (1979). Interrelations among models for the analysis of moment structures. *Multivariate Behavioral Research, 14*(2), 169–185.

Box, G. E. P., & Jenkins, G. M. (1976). *Time-series analysis: Forecasting and control* (rev. ed.). San Francisco: Holden-Day.

Boyd, C. J., Frey, M. A., & Aaronson, L. S. (1988). Structural equation models and nursing research . . . LISREL: Part I. *Nursing Research, 37*(4), 249–252.

Braden, C. J. (1990). A test of the self-help model: Learned response to chronic illness experience. *Nursing Research, 39*(1), 42–47.

Burns, N., & Carney, N. (1986). Patterns of hospice care—the RN role. *The Hospice Journal, 2*(1), 37–62.

Carmines, E. G., & McIver, J. P. (1981). Analyzing models with unobserved variables: Analysis of covariance structures. In G. W. Bohrnstedt & E. F. Borgatta (Eds.), *Social measurement: Current issues* (pp. 65–115). Beverly Hills, CA: Sage.

Cohen, J., & Cohen, P. (1983). *Applied multiple regression/correlation analysis for the behavioral sciences.* Hillsdale, NJ: Lawrence Erlbaum.

Crawford, G. (1982). The concept of pattern in nursing: Conceptual development and measurement. *Advances in Nursing Science, 5*(1), 1–6.

Dillon, W., & Goldstein, M. (1984). *Multivariate analysis: Methods and applications.* New York: Wiley.

Edens, G. E. (1987). Discriminant analysis. *Nursing Research, 36*(4), 257–262.

Folkman, S., & Lazarus, R. S. (1985). If it changes it must be a process: Study of emotion and coping during three stages of a college examination. *Journal of Personality and Social Psychology, 48*(1), 150–170.

Folkman, S., & Lazarus, R. S. (1988). *Manual for the ways of coping questionnaire.* Palo Alto, CA: Consulting Psychologists Press.

Folkman, S., Lazarus, R. S., Dunkel-Schetter, C., DeLongis, A., & Gruen, R. J. (1986). Dynamics of a stressful encounter: Cognitive appraisal, coping, and encounter outcomes. *Journal of Personality and Social Psychology, 50*(5), 992–1003.

Glass, G. V., Willson, V. L., & Gottman, J. M. (1975). *Design and analysis of time-series experiments.* Boulder: Colorado University Associated Press.

Gottman, J. M. (1981). *Time-series analysis: A comprehensive introduction for social scientists.* Cambridge: Cambridge University Press.

Gottman, J. M. (1984). Time-series analysis. Cambridge: Cambridge University Press.

Griner, P. F., Mayewski, R. J., Mushlin, A., & Greenland, P. (1981). Selection and interpretation of diagnostic tests and procedures: Principles and applications. *Annals of Internal Medicine, 94,* 553–600.

Gross, A. J., & Clark, V. (1975). *Survival distributions: Reliability applications in the biomedical sciences.* New York: Wiley.

Hair, J. F., Anderson, R. E., Tatham, R. L., & Black, W. C. (1992). *Multivariate data analysis with readings.* New York: Macmillan.

Hanneman, S. K. G. (1994). Multidimensional predictors of success or failure with early weaning from mechanical ventilation after cardiac surgery. *Nursing Research, 43*(1), 4–10.

Hintze, J. L. (1990). *Survival analysis. Number cruncher statistical system version 5.5.* Kaysville, UT: Hintze.

Jadack, R. A., Hyde, J. S., & Keller, M. L. (1995). Gender and knowledge about HIV, risky sexual behavior, and safer sex practices. *Research in Nursing & Health, 18*(4), 313–324.

Jirovec, M. M. (1986). Time-series analysis in nursing research: ARIMA modeling. *Nursing Research, 35*(5), 315–319.

Johnson, M. (1995). Healing determinants in older people with leg ulcers. *Research in Nursing & Health, 18*(5), 395–403.

Jöreskog, K. G., & Sörbom, D. (1988–1992). *LISREL* [Computer Program]. Mooresville, IN: Scientific Software.

Jöreskog, K. G., & Sörbom, D. (1989). *LISREL 7: A Guide to the program and applications* (2nd ed.). Chicago: SPSS.

Kammer, C. H. (1994). Stress and coping of family members responsible for nursing home placement. *Research in Nursing & Health, 17*(2), 89–98.

Kazdin, A. (1982). *Single-case research designs.* New York: Oxford University Press.

Kim, J., & Mueller, C. W. (1978a). *Introduction to factor analysis: What it is and how to do it.* Beverly Hills, CA: Sage.

Kim, J., & Mueller, C. W. (1978b). *Factor analysis: Statistical methods and practical issues.* Beverly Hills, CA: Sage.

Knapp, T. R. (1994). Regression analyses: What to report. *Nursing Research, 43*(3), 187–189.

Krieger, B. P., Ershowsky, P. F., Becker, D. A., & Gazeroglu, H. B. (1989). Evaluation of conventional criteria for predicting successful weaning from mechanical ventilatory support in elderly patients. *Critical Care Medicine, 17*(9), 858–861.

Lee, E. T. (1984). *Statistical methods for survival data analysis.* Belmont, CA: Wadsworth.

Lentz, M. J. (1990a). Time series—Issues in sampling. *Western Journal of Nursing Research, 12*(1), 123–127.

Lentz, M. J. (1990b). Time-series analysis–Cosinor analysis: A special case. *Western Journal of Nursing Research, 12*(3), 408–412.

Long, J. S. (1983a). *Confirmatory factor analysis.* Beverly Hills, CA: Sage.

Long, J. S. (1983b). *Covariance structure models: An introduction to LISREL.* Beverly Hills, CA: Sage.

Marascuilo, L. A., & Levin, J. R. (1983). *Multivariate statistics in the social sciences.* Monterey, CA: Brooks/Cole.

Mason-Hawkes, J., & Holm, K. (1989). Causal modeling: A comparison of path analysis and LISREL. *Nursing Research, 38*(5), 312–314.

McCain, L. J., & McCleary, R. (1979). The statistical analysis of the simple interrupted time-series quasi-experiment. In T. D. Cook & D. T. Campbell (Eds.), *Quasi-experimenta-tion: Design and analysis issues for field settings* (pp. 233–293). Chicago: Rand McNally.

McCleary, R., & Hay, R. A., Jr. (1980). *Applied time-series analysis for the social sciences.* Beverly Hills, CA: Sage.

McDowall, D., McCleary, R., Meidinger, E. E., & Hay, R. A., Jr. (1980). *Interrupted time-series analysis.* Beverly Hills, CA: Sage.

Metzger, B. L., & Schultz, S., II. (1982). Time-series analysis: An alternative for nursing. *Nursing Research, 31*(6), 375–378.

Mischel, M. H., Padilla, G., Grant, M., & Sorenson, D. S. (1991). Uncertainty in illness theory: A replication of the mediating effects of mastery and coping. *Nursing Research, 40*(4), 236–240.

Mischel, M. H., & Sorrenson, D. S. (1991). Coping with uncertainty in gynecological cancer: A test of the mediating functions of mastery and coping. *Nursing Research, 40*(3), 167–170.

Mitchell, E., Woods, N., & Lentz, M. (1985). Methodologic issues in the definition of perimenstrual symptoms. *Proceedings of the Society for Menstrual Cycle Research.* Chicago: Chicago University Press.

Mitchell, E., Woods, N., & Lentz, M. (1991). Distinguishing among menstrual cycle symptom severity patterns. In D. Taylor & N. Woods (Eds.), *Menstruation, health and illness* (pp. 89–101). Washington, DC: Hemisphere.

Mitchell, E. S., Woods, N. F., & Lentz, M. J. (1994). Differentiation of women with three perimenstrual symptom patterns. *Nursing Research, 43*(1), 25–30.

Mitchell, P. H. (1988). Designing small sample studies. In N. F. Woods & M. Catanzaro (Eds.). *Nursing Research: Theory and Practice.* St. Louis, MO: Mosby.

Nelson, W. B. (1982). *Applied life data analysis.* New York: Wiley.

Neuberger, G. B., Kasal, S., Smith, K. V., Hassanein, R., & DeViney, S. (1994). Determinants of exercise and aerobic fitness in outpatients with arthritis. *Nursing Research, 43*(1), 11–17.

Newman, M. A. (1979). *Theory development in nursing.* Philadelphia: Davis.

Norbeck, J. (1984). Modification of life event questionnaires for use with female respondents. *Research in Nursing & Health, 7*(1), 61–71.

Nunnally, J. C. (1978). *Psychometric theory* (2nd ed.). New York: McGraw-Hill.

Olson, J. K. (1995). Relationships between nurse-expressed empathy, patient-perceived empathy and patient distress. *Image: Journal of Nursing Scholarship, 27*(4), 317–322.

Pedhazur, E. J. (1982). *Multiple regression in behavioral research: Explanation and prediction* (2nd ed.). New York: Holt, Rinehart and Winston.

Prescott, P. A. (1987). Multiple regression analysis with small samples: Cautions and suggestions. *Nursing Research, 36*(2), 130–133.

Raykov, T., Tomer, A., & Nesselroade, J. R. (1991). Reporting structural equation modeling results in *Psychology and Aging:* Some proposed guidelines. *Psychology and Aging, 6*(4), 499–503.

Rogers, M. (1986). Science of unitary human beings. In V. M. Malinski (Ed.), *Exploration on Martha Rogers' Science of Unitary Human Beings* (pp. 3–8). Norwalk, CT: Appleton-Century-Crofts.

Schroeder, M. A. (1990). Diagnosing and dealing with multicollinearity. *Western Journal of Nursing Research, 12*(2), 175–187.

Taylor, D. (1986). Perimenstrual symptoms: Typology development. *Communicating Nursing Research, 19,* 168.

Taylor, D. (1990). Use of autocorrelation as an analytic strategy for describing pattern and change. *Western Journal of Nursing Research, 12*(2), 254–261.

Taylor, D. L. (1994). Evaluating therapeutic change in symptom severity at the level of the individual woman experiencing severe PMS. *Image: Journal of Nursing Scholarship, 26*(1), 25–33.

Thomas, K. A. (1987). Exploration in time: Issues in studying response patterns. In *Communicating nursing research* (Vol. 20). Boulder, CO: Western Interstate Commission on Higher Education.

Thomas, K. A. (1990). Time-series analysis—Spectral analysis and the search for cycles. *Western Journal of Nursing Research, 12*(4), 558–562.

Tollett, J. H., & Thomas, S. P. (1995). A theory-based nursing intervention to instill hope in homeless veterans. *Advances in Nursing Science, 18*(2), 76–90.

Verran, J. A., & Ferketich, S. L. (1987). Testing linear model assumptions: Residual analysis. *Nursing Research, 36*(2), 127–130.

Verran, J. A., & Reid, P. J. (1987). Replicated testing of the nursing technology model. *Nursing Research, 36*(3), 190–194.

Wikoff, R. L., & Miller, P. (1991). Canonical analysis in nursing research. *Nursing Research, 40*(6), 367–370.

Wineman, N. M., Durand, E. J., & McCulloch, B. J. (1994). Examination of the factor structure of the Ways of Coping Questionnaire with clinical populations. *Nursing Research, 43*(5), 268–273.

Woods, N. F., & Catanzaro, M. (1988). *Nursing research: Theory and practice.* St. Louis, MO: Mosby.

Woods, N. F., Lentz, M.J., & Mitchell, E. S. (1993). *Prevalence of perimenstrual symptoms.* Unpublished report to National Center for Nursing Research.

Woods, N. F., Mitchell, E. S., & Lentz, M. J. (1995). Social pathways to premenstrual symptoms. *Research in Nursing & Health, 18*(3), 225–237.

Wu, Y. B. (1995). Hierarchical linear models: A multilevel data analysis technique. *Nursing Research, 44*(2), 123–126.

Wu, Y. B., & Slakter, M. J. (1989). Analysis of covariance in nursing research. *Nursing Research, 38*(5), 306–308.

Yang, K. L., & Tobin, M. J. (1991). A prospective study of indexes predicting the outcome of trials of weaning from mechanical ventilation. *New England Journal of Medicine, 324*(21), 1445–1450.

Yarandi, H. N., & Simpson, S. H. (1991). The logistic regression model and the odds of testing HIV positive. *Nursing Research, 40*(6), 372–373.

Youngblut, J. M. (1993). Comparison of factor analysis options using the home/employment orientation scale. *Nursing Research, 42*(2), 122–124.

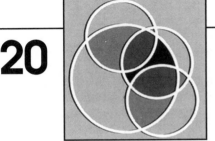

20

Qualitative Research Methodology

The researcher conducting a qualitative study will need to use methods of data collection and analyses that may be unique to qualitative research, although some of the techniques described in previous chapters, particularly methods of observation and interviewing as described in Chapter 14 may be useful. Qualitative data analysis occurs concurrently with data collection rather than sequentially as is true in quantitative research. Therefore, the researcher is attempting simultaneously to gather the data, manage a growing bulk of collected data, and interpret the meaning of the data. Qualitative analysis techniques use words rather than numbers as the basis of analysis. However, the same careful skills in analytic reasoning are needed by the qualitative researcher as those required by quantitative analysis. In qualitative analysis, the flow of reasoning moves from concreteness to increasing abstraction. This reasoning process guides the organization, reduction, and clustering of the findings and leads to the development of theoretical explanations.

This chapter describes some of the frequently used approaches to collection and analysis of qualitative data. Methods specific to the six qualitative approaches presented in Chapter 4 will be described, and detailed examples of published studies are provided to facilitate understanding of the techniques. The information in this chapter is sufficient to allow you to understand the process and to envision what the experience would be like if you chose to conduct this type of research. However, if you elect to conduct a qualitative study, we suggest that you seek additional sources of guidance for the process of collecting and analyzing qualitative data. Mentorship with someone experienced in the type of qualitative analysis you wish to perform is still the most useful approach to learning these skills.

DATA ANALYSIS ISSUES

The researcher is confronted with several decisions regarding the approach to qualitative data analysis that will be used for a particular study. Will the analysis be performed manually or will computers be used? Will documentation be recorded of decisions related to the data analysis process? Will the researcher adhere to the methodology of a particular qualitative research approach or mix methodologies from several approaches? The following section will discuss these issues.

USING THE COMPUTER FOR QUALITATIVE ANALYSIS

Traditionally, qualitative data collection and analysis has been performed manually. The researcher recorded the data on small bits of paper or note cards which were then carefully coded, organized, and filed at the end of a day of data gathering. Analysis requires cross-checking each bit of data with all the other bits of data on little pieces of paper. It is easy to lose data in the mass of paper. Keeping track of connections between various bits of data requires meticulous record keeping. This method was developed because of the importance of the qualitative researcher maintaining a close link with—or being immersed in—the data being analyzed.

Some qualitative researchers believe that using

the computer can make analysis of qualitative data quicker and easier without the researcher losing touch with the data (Anderson, 1987b; Miles & Huberman, 1994; Taft, 1993). Taft (1993) suggests that, because of the ease of coding and recoding, the researcher feels more free to play with the data and experiment with alternate ways of coding. This fosters analytic insight and thus facilitates data analysis. Researchers can also search for codes that tend to occur together. Because of easy access to the data, team research is facilitated. However, Taft expresses concern over the dark side of computer technology for qualitative researchers. The researcher may be tempted to study larger samples and sacrifice depth for breadth. Meaningful understanding of the data may also be sacrificed. Sandelowski (1995a) expresses concern that the use of computers will alter the aesthetics of qualitative research and suggests that the key motivation for using computer technology in qualitative research is to legitimate the claim that qualitative researchers are doing science. She states "computer technology permits qualitative researchers to have computer printouts of data (with the veneer of objectivity they confer) comparable to their quantitative counterparts whose claims to doing science are often not questioned. Even so-called *soft* data can become *hard* when produced by *hard*ware. Qualitative work can now have the look and feel, or aesthetic features, of science" (p. 205).

The computer offers assistance in such activities as processing, storage, retrieval, cataloging, and sorting, and leaves the analysis activities up to the researcher. Anderson (1987b) points out that "the computer does not perform the thinking, reviewing, interpretative, and analytic functions that the researcher must do for himself or herself. Rather, the computer makes the researcher more efficient and effective in those high-level functions, and eases some of the tedious 'mindless' tasks that otherwise consume so much time and energy" (pp. 629–630). However, Sandelowski (1995a) argues that replacing and streamlining the cutting and pasting activities may be seen as desirable by some because they are uncomfortably reminiscent of childhood play. She argues against the

claim that machine technology saves human labor, suggesting that it may actually increase labor since storage and retrieval of more data can occur and that once the data are stored, it must all be accounted for in the report of results.

Computer use has several advantages over the more traditional methods of recording and storing data. Multiple copies can be made with ease, and files can be copied onto backup disks and stored at another site without the need for a large amount of storage space. Blocks of data can also be moved around in the file or copied to another file when data are being sorted by category. The same block of data could be inserted within several categories, if this is desired. At the same time, interviews or descriptions of observations can be kept intact for reference as needed. In addition, most word processing programs can perform sort operations and can search throughout a text file for a selected word or a string of words. Files in a word processing program can be transferred to a database spreadsheet such as dBase or Lotus 1-2-3 to organize the data into matrices.

A number of computer programs have been developed specifically to perform qualitative analyses. One of the earliest attempts was described by Podolefsky and McCarty (1983). This program, Computer Assisted Topical Sorting (CATS), allowed the insertion of codes, designated as numbers, into a text file. A mainframe text editor provided the capacity to search for strings of characters such as words or phrases. Weitzman and Miles (1995) provide an evaluation of the currently available software used to assist in the analysis of qualitative data.

AUDITABILITY

The credibility of qualitative data analysis has been seriously questioned in some cases by the larger scientific community. The concerns expressed are related to the inability to replicate the outcomes of a study, even when using the same data set.

Miles and Huberman (1994) describe the problem as follows.

"Most qualitative researchers work alone in the field. Each is a one-person research machine: defining the problem, doing the sampling, designing the instruments, collecting the information, reducing the information, analyzing it, interpreting it, writing it up. A vertical monopoly. And when we read the reports, they are most often heavy on the 'what' (the findings, the descriptions) rather than on the 'how' (how you got to the 'what'). We rarely see data displays—only the conclusions. In most cases, we don't see a procedural account of the analysis, explaining just how the researcher got from 500 pages of field notes to the main conclusions drawn. So we don't know how much confidence we can place in them. Researchers are not being cryptic or obtuse. It's just that they have a slim tradition to guide their analytic moves, and few guidelines for explaining to their colleagues what they did, and how." (p. 262) ■

To respond to this concern, some qualitative researchers have attempted to develop strategies by which other researchers, using the same data, can follow the logic of the original researcher and arrive at the same conclusions. Guba and Lincoln (1982) refer to this strategy as auditability.

Auditability requires that the researcher establish decision rules for categorizing data, arriving at ratings, or making judgments. A decision rule might say, for example, that a datum would be placed in a specific category if it met specified criteria. Another decision rule might say that an observed interaction would be considered an instance of an emerging theoretical explanation if it met specific criteria. A record is kept of all decision rules used in the analysis of data. All raw data are stored so that they are available for review if requested. As the analysis progresses, the researcher documents the data and the decision rules on which each decision was based and the reasoning that entered into each decision. Thus, evidence is retained to support the study conclusions and the emerging theory and is made available on request (Burns, 1989). Marshall (1984, 1985), however, cautioned against undermining the strengths of qualitative research by overly mechanistic data

analysis. Marshall and Rossman (1989) express concern that efforts to increase validity will "filter out the unusual, the serendipitous—the puzzle that if tended to and pursued would provide a recasting of the entire research endeavor" (p. 113).

METHOD MIXING

Some studies are appearing in the literature in which the researchers have combined portions of various qualitative methodologies extracted from the philosophical bases for which the methodologies were developed. Morse (1989) expresses concern about the justification of this strategy, stating, "Such mixing, while certainly 'do-able,' violates the assumptions of data collection techniques and methods of analysis of all the methods used. The product is not good science; the product is a sloppy mishmash" (p. 4). It is likely that in this evolving research field, new qualitative methodologies will continue to emerge, some combining portions of previous methodologies. However, in qualitative research, the philosophy underlying the study is as important as the framework in a quantitative study and directs the interpretation of results. Therefore, it is essential that the researcher make the philosophical base of the study explicit and that methodologies used be compatible with the philosophical base.

DATA COLLECTION METHODS

Because data collection is occurring simultaneously with data analysis, the process is complex. The procedure of collecting data is not a mechanical process that can be carefully planned prior to initiation. The researcher as a whole person is totally involved—perceiving, reacting, interacting, reflecting, attaching meaning, recording. This is the case whether the study involves observing and participating in social situations as would occur in phenomenological, grounded theory, ethnographic, or critical social theory research or with written communications of persons as might occur in phenomenological, historical, philosophical, or critical social theory studies. For a particular study, the researcher may need to address data collection issues related to the relationships between the researcher and the participants, the reflections of the researcher upon the meanings obtained from the data, and the management and reduction of large volumes of data.

RESEARCHER–PARTICIPANT RELATIONSHIPS

One of the important differences between quantitative and qualitative research is the nature of relationships between the researcher and the individuals being studied. The nature of these relationships has an impact upon the data collected and its interpretation. In many qualitative studies, the researcher observes social behavior and may participate in social interactions with those being studied. Field and Morse (1985) identify four types of participant-observation: (1) *complete participation,* in which the observer becomes a member of the group and conceals the researcher role, (2) *participant-as-observer,* in which participants are aware of the dual roles of the researcher, (3) *observer-as-participant,* in which most of the researcher's time is spent observing and interviewing and less in the participation role, and (4) *complete observer,* in which the researcher is passive and has no direct social interaction in the setting.

In varying degrees, the researcher influences the individuals being studied and, in turn, is influenced by them. The mere presence of the researcher may alter behavior in the setting. This involvement, considered a source of bias in quantitative research, is thought by qualitative researchers to be a natural and necessary element of the research process. The researcher's personality is a key factor in qualitative research. Skills in empathy and intuition are cultivated. The researcher needs to become closely involved in the subject's experience in order to interpret it. It is necessary for the researcher to be open to the perceptions of the participants, rather than to attach his or her own meaning to the experience. Individuals being studied often participate in determining research questions, guiding data collection, and interpreting results.

The interface between the participant-observer role and the nurse role of the researcher is a concern. Because of the possible impact of the nursing role on the study, Robinson and Thorne (1988) claim that the nurse researcher has an obligation to explain in the study report the influence her or his professional perspective had on the process and outcomes of the study. In some studies, the researcher is expected to interact with participants but to stay in the role of researcher and avoid relating to participants as a nurse. Some insist that the nurse researcher must always relate first as a nurse and second as a researcher (Cooper, 1988; Fowler, 1988). Connors (1988) suggests that the qualitative researcher must be authentic and engaged as a whole person, rather than just as a researcher or as a nurse.

In addition to the role one takes in the relationship, expectations of the study must be carefully considered. Munhall (1988) points out that, ethically, it is essential that the qualitative researcher think through both the aims and the means of the study and determine whether those aims and means are consistent with those of the participants. For example, if the researcher's desire is to change the behavior of the participants, this needs also to be a desire of the participants. During the study, a level of trust develops between the researcher and the participant, who may provide information labeled as secret. Field and Morse (1985, pp. 72–73) describe the situations with which the researcher may be confronted. "For example, [participants] may state that this is 'Just between you and me . . .' or 'Don't put this in your report, but. . . .' 'Alternatively, informants may provide information that is later regretted. They will state, 'I shouldn't have told you that yesterday. . . .' As the researcher's first responsibility is to the informant, the informant has the right to retract information or to request that the information not be used in the report, and the researcher must respect the informant's wishes."

Establishing relationships with participants can cause harm that must be carefully considered. Participant observation requires a close relationship that invades the privacy of the individual. Although participants may experience confidence, commitment, and friendship from the encounter, they may also experience disappointment, perceived betrayal, and desertion as the researcher functions in the researcher role and then leaves (Munhall, 1988). The relationship can also cause harm to the researcher. Cowles (1988) described emotional pain and difficulty sleeping as she collected data from family members of murdered individuals. She frequently required support and opportunities to explore her feelings with colleagues during the process.

REFLEXIVE THOUGHT

The qualitative researcher needs to think through critically the dynamic interaction between the self and the data occurring during analysis. This interaction occurs whether the data are communicated person-to-person or through the written word. The critical thinking used to examine this interaction is referred to as *reflexive thought* or reflexivity (Lamb & Huttlinger, 1989). During this process, the researcher explores personal feelings and experiences that may influence the study and integrates this understanding into the study. The process requires a conscious awareness of self.

Drew (1989), in a paper describing her experiences in conducting a phenomenological study of caregiving behaviors, describes the impact of relationships on her study.

"A session with a person who had been willing to talk about his or her experiences with caregivers, and who had invested energy into the interview session, often generated for me a sense of doing something worthwhile, as well as a feeling that I would be competent to analyze the transcribed material in a meaningful way. This sense of competency dispelled any doubts about being an intruder. I became relaxed, unself-conscious, and

more self-assured. However, an encounter with a person with blunt affect, abrupt answers, and a paucity of responses left me feeling awkward and self-conscious. A sense of doubt about the validity of my project encroached as I attempted to elicit that person's thoughts. At the time, my immediate reaction was to think that I had obtained nothing from these individuals, when in fact, as I was to discover later, the 'nothing' was something important that I was as yet unable to see.

It was at the point of discouragement about my interviewing skills that I became aware that I was mentally classifying interviews as either 'good' or 'bad,' depending on my emotional response to the subjects. Good interviews were those in which I felt effective as an interviewer and was able to facilitate the person's recounting of experiences with caregivers. I enjoyed the interaction and felt that we connected on some level that produced meaningful discussion about the topic of relationships between patient and caregiver.

Bad interviews, on the other hand, were those in which I could not seem to get subjects to talk about how they had experienced their caregivers. There seemed to be no questions that I could devise with which to explore feelings, either positive or negative, with them. They gave no indications of awareness of their feelings, or of feelings in others. Whereas the subjects of the good interviews were people I experienced as open, curious, and thoughtful, those of the bad interviews were experienced as distrustful and elicited in me a sense of anxiety and frustration; it seemed I could not get through to them. I felt inadequate as an interviewer and was ready to discard these interviews. Frustration and anxiety arose because I felt that I was not getting the information that I needed for the study.

Subsequently, I discovered that my feelings of frustration and inadequacy were causing me to overlook data and that when I could put them aside, new data that were rich in meaning became apparent . . . This discovery was a powerful experience for me, affecting my approach to subsequent interviews and influencing analysis of data thereafter." (pp. 433–434) ∎

In some phenomenological research, especially for researchers using Husserl's interpretation of phenomenology, this critical thinking leads to bracketing, which is used to help the researcher avoid misinterpreting the phenomenon as it is being experienced by the individual. *Bracketing* is suspending or laying aside what is known about the experience being studied (Oiler, 1982). Other phenomenologists, especially those using Heideggerian phenomenology, do not bracket. But they do identify beliefs, assumptions, and preconceptions about the research topic. These are put in writing at the beginning of the study for self-reflection and external review. These procedures are intended to facilitate openness and new insights.

DATA MANAGEMENT AND REDUCTION

Data collected during a qualitative study may be narrative descriptions of observations, transcripts from tape recordings of interviews, entries in the researcher's diary reflecting on the dynamics of the setting, or notes taken while reading written documents. In the initial phases of data analysis, you need to become very familiar with the data as you gather them. This may involve reading and rereading notes and transcripts, recalling observations and experiences, listening to tapes, viewing videotapes, until you have become immersed in the data. Tapes contain more than words; they contain feeling, emphasis, nonverbal communications. These are at least as important to the communication as the words. In phenomenology this immersion in the data is referred to as *dwelling with the data.*

Because of the volumes of data acquired in a qualitative study, initial efforts at analysis focus on reducing the volume of data to facilitate examination, a process referred to as *data reduction.* During data reduction, you begin attaching meaning to elements in your data. You will discover classes of things, persons, and events, and discover properties that characterize things, persons, and events, You will also note regularities in the setting or the people. These discoveries will lead to classifying elements in your data. In some cases, you may use the classification scheme used by participants or authors. In other cases, you may wish to construct your own classification scheme.

According to Sandelowski (1995b), "Although data preparation is a distinctive stage in qualitative work where data are put into a form that will permit analysis, a rudimentary kind of analysis often begins when the researcher proofs transcripts against the audiotaped interviews from which they were prepared. Indeed, the proofing process is often the first time that a researcher gets a sense of the interview as a whole; it is, occasionally, the first time investigators will hear something said, even though they conducted the interview. During the proofing process, researchers will often underline key phrases, simply because they make some as yet inchoate impression on them. They may jot down ideas in the margins next to the text that triggered them, just because they do not want to lose some line of thinking" (p. 373).

Transcribing Interviews

If you have tape-recorded interviews, they are generally transcribed word for word. Field and Morse (1985) provide the following instructions for transcribing a tape-recorded interview.

"Pauses are denoted in the transcript with dashes, while series of dots indicate gaps or prolonged pauses. All exclamations, including laughter and expletives, are included. Instruct the typist to type interviews single-spaced with a blank line between speakers. A generous margin on both sides of the page permits the left margin to be used for coding and the researcher's own critique of the interview style, and the right margin to be used for comments regarding the content . . . Start a new paragraph each time a topic is changed . . . Ensure that all pages are numbered sequentially and that each page is coded with the interview number and the informant's number." (pp. 97–99) ∎

Sandelowski (1994) indicates that the researcher must choose what about the interview to preserve in print. These choices directly influence the nature and direction of the analysis. Once the interview is transcribed, the transcript takes on an independent reality and becomes the researcher's raw data. Sandelowski suggests that the process of transcription alters reality. The text is "many transformations removed from the so-called unadulterated reality it was intended to represent" (p. 312). She recommends asking the following questions regarding transcription:

1. Is a transcript necessary to achieve the research goals?
2. If a transcription is required, what features of the interview event should be preserved (if at all possible) and what features can be safely ignored?
3. What notation system should be used?
4. What purposes besides investigator analysis per se will the transcript serve? (pp. 312–313)

Sandelowski points out that transcriptions require about 3½ hours for each 1 hour of interview time. The cost for this work may be as high as $20/hour for an experienced typist.

After transcriptions are completed, Field and Morse (1985) advise making at least three copies of transcripts and keeping the original separate from copies. One set of copies should be locked in a separate location to insure against fire damage or loss. If the researcher is working in the field, one copy should be mailed home separately. Placing all data from your study in one suitcase when traveling is inviting disaster.

Listen to tape recordings as soon after the interview as possible. Listen carefully to voice tone, inflection, and pauses of both researcher and participant as well as to the content. These may indicate that the topic is very emotional or very important. While you are listening, read the written transcript of the tape. Make notations of your observations on the transcript (Field & Morse, 1985).

Codes and Coding

Coding is a means of categorizing. A code is a symbol or abbreviation used to classify words or phrases in the data. Codes may be placed in the data at the time of data collection, when entering data into the computer, or during later examination of the data. Through the selection of categories, or codes, the researcher is defining the domain of the study. Therefore, it is important that the codes be consistent with the philosophical base of the study. Organization of data, selection of specific elements of the data for categories, and naming these categories will reflect the philosophical base used for the study. Later in the study, coding may progress to the development of a taxonomy. For example, you might develop a taxonomy of types of pain, types of patients, or types of patient education.

Field and Morse (1985) suggest that, in selecting elements of the data to code, you note:

1. the kinds of things that are going on in the context being studied;
2. the forms a phenomenon takes; and
3. any variations within a phenomenon. (p. 104)

Such characteristics as "acts (one-shot events), activities (ongoing events), verbal productions that direct actions (meanings), participation of the actors, interrelationships among actions and the setting of the study [might be included] . . . In the anthropological tradition, the history, social structure, recurring events, economy, authority, beliefs, and values of a community may constitute the initial list of universal categories used to organize data" (Field & Morse, 1985, p. 104). Although a classification system can identify the elements of interest and name them, it cannot identify processes.

Initial categories should be as broad as possible but categories should not overlap. As more data are collected in relation to a particular category, the major category can be sectioned into smaller categories. Field and Morse (1985) find that "it is difficult during the initial data coding stage to work with more than ten major codes" (p. 101).

Field and Morse (1985) also suggest several innovative strategies for coding data. One approach is to use highlighter pens, with a different color for each major category. Another strategy, developed by Murdock (1971), is to assign each major category a number. The number is inserted in the computerized text. Using this approach, a word or phrase in the text could easily have several codes indicated by numbers. Anthropologists use McBee cards, which have holes punched in the top. The holes are used to sort data by category. Knafl and Webster (1988) suggest using colored markers, colored paper clips, colored index cards, or Post-it stickers to identify categories of data. Codes are often written in the margins. Then data can be sorted by cutting the pages into sections according to codes. Each section can be taped or pasted onto an index card for filing. This procedure can just as easily be performed using the computer programs for qualitative analysis in which broad margins are available for coding. In this case, computerized data can be sorted by code into a separate file for each code while retaining identification by such identifiers as data and source.

Field and Morse (1985) color code each page of a transcript in the left margin. One colored stripe is used for each participant and another for the interviewing sequence. When the pages are cut up according to topical codes, identification of the participant and the interviewing sequence is left intact.

Knafl and Webster (1988) described their coding process as follows.

"In order to develop coding categories, the co-principal investigators (PIs) and research staff independently read through a sample of interview transcripts, taking notes on the major topics discussed in the interviews. The PIs and staff then met to compare and revise the categories individually arrived at and to determine 'semifinal' coding categories. Each category was assigned a number. Next, using the number system, the PIs and research staff independently applied the categories to a second sample of interview transcripts. The PIs and staff again met to compare their individual applications of the categories. The purpose of this second comparison was to identify ambiguities, overlap, and lack of clarity in the categories.

During the entire process of developing coding categories, a record was maintained of criteria used in applying coding categories to the data. From this record, a codebook was developed in order to ensure consistent application of final coding categories. The codebook included the criteria for applying each category and a brief excerpt of data exemplifying each category.

All data subsequently were coded by indicating the number of the appropriate category or categories in the margin of the interview transcript. Each of the PIs worked with one of the research assistants in coding the data. In order to enhance consistency in application of the coding categories, each member of a PI-research assistant pair coded data independently and then met to compare application of the categories and resolve any differences. In addition, the PIs and research assistants met as a group on a regularly scheduled basis to discuss issues and questions regarding coding.

After completing the coding, the research assistant transferred the data to index cards. This was accomplished by photocopying the interview transcripts, cutting up the copies (with care taken to preserve wholeness and meaning of content) and taping the cut-up portions on 5 × 8 index cards. A color code system was devised, so that different categories of data were taped to different colored index cards." (pp. 200–201) ∎

There are three types of codes: descriptive, interpretative, and explanatory. *Descriptive codes* classify elements of the data using terms that describe how the researcher is organizing the data. It is the simplest method of classification and is commonly used in the initial stages of data analysis. Descriptive codes remain close to the terms used by the participant being interviewed. For example, if you were reading a transcribed interview in which a participant was describing experiences in the first days after surgery, you might use descriptive codes such as PAIN, MOVING, FEAR, REST.

Interpretative codes are usually developed

later in the data-collecting process as the researcher gains some insight into the processes occurring. These codes are used when the researcher begins to move beyond simply sorting statements, using the participant's terms to attach meanings to these statements. For example, in a study of postoperative experiences, you might begin to recognize that the participant was investing much energy in seeking relief of symptoms and seeking information about how the health care providers believed he or she is doing. These might be classified using interpretative codes of RELIEF and INFO.

Explanatory codes are developed late in the data-collecting process after theoretical ideas from the study have begun to emerge. The explanatory codes are part of the researcher's attempt to unravel the meanings inherent in the situation. These codes connect the data to the emerging theory, and the codes used may be specific to the theory or more general, such as PATT (pattern), TH (theme), or CL (causal link). Typically, codes will not stay the same throughout the study. Some codes will have to be divided down into subclassifications. Other codes may be discontinued because they do not work.

Reflective Remarks

While the notes are being recorded, thoughts or insights often emerge into the consciousness of the researcher. These thoughts are generally included within the notes and are separated from the rest of the notes by ((double parentheses)). Later, they may need to be extracted and used for memoing (Miles & Huberman, 1994).

Marginal Remarks

As the notes are being reviewed, observations about the notes need to be written immediately. These remarks are usually placed in the right-hand margin of the notes. The remarks often connect the notes with other parts of the data or suggest new interpretations. Reviewing notes can become boring, which is a signal that thinking has ceased.

Making marginal notes assists the researcher in "retaining a thoughtful stance" (Miles & Huberman, 1994).

Memoing

A *memo* is developed by the researcher to record insights or ideas related to notes, transcripts, or codes. Memos move the researcher toward theorizing and are conceptual rather than factual. They may link pieces of data together or use a specific piece of data as an example of a conceptual idea. The memo may be written to someone else in the study or may be just a note to oneself. The important thing is to value one's ideas and to get them written down quickly. Whenever an idea emerges, even if it is vague and not well thought out, it needs to be written down immediately. One's initial feeling is that the idea is so clear in one's mind that it can be written later. However, the thought is soon forgotten and often cannot be retrieved again. As one becomes immersed in the data, these ideas will occur at odd times, such as 2 a.m., or when one is driving, or when one is preparing a meal. Therefore, it is advisable to keep paper and pencil handy. If one is awakened with an idea, it should be written down immediately; it may be gone by morning. Memos need to be dated, titled with the key concept discussed, and connected by codes with the field notes or forms that generated the thoughts (Miles & Huberman, 1994).

Developing Propositions

As the study progresses, relationships among categories, participants, actions, and events will begin to emerge. You will develop hunches about relationships that can be used to formulate tentative propositions. If the study is being conducted by a team of researchers, everyone involved in the study can participate in the development of propositions. Statements or propositions can be written on index cards and sorted into categories or entered into the computer. A working list can then be printed and shared among the researchers, generating further discussion (Miles & Huberman, 1994).

DISPLAYING DATA FOR ANALYSIS AND PRESENTATION

Displays contain highly condensed versions of the outcomes of qualitative research. They are equivalent to the summary tables of statistical outcomes developed in quantitative research and allow the researcher to get across the main ideas of the research succinctly. The strategies for achieving displays are limited only by the imagination of the researcher. Some suggested ideas follow. Displays can be relatively easily developed using computer spreadsheets, graphics programs, or desktop publishing programs. Miles and Huberman (1994) provide very helpful guidelines for the development of displays of qualitative data.

Marsh (1990) used a process-oriented matrix to test conclusions and an emergent theory from a qualitative study examining positive health lifestyle changes. Seven individuals who had made or were making lifestyle changes were interviewed. The interview focused on the process of lifestyle change. The emergent theory describing the process of lifestyle change is as follows.

■

"An individual, aware of the need and desiring to alter his or her lifestyle, makes one or more attempts to change over time. The attempts result in relapse. A self-monitoring process mediates between awareness of the individual's need to change and his or her relapses in the process of change. At some point tension mounts over the need to change. This tension, labeled 'readiness,' is characterized by a combination of personal and environmental variables, such as low self-esteem or support from significant others. Following readiness, the individual experiences a profound self-revelation. The revelation is characterized by a dramatic self-insight, a coming to as if shaken by a new understanding of reality. The revelation is followed by a belief system change about personal power, following which the individual makes and sustains a health lifestyle change. An individual who experiences no revelation remains in the initial pattern of attempted change and relapse. Revelation appeared to be the emerging core variable of the lifestyle change process." (p. 45) ■

To evaluate the trustworthiness of the emergent theory, all the data were examined for their fit in a matrix. Categories for the matrix were developed and decision rules established for inclusion of data within a category. Every subject was represented in the matrix. When a subject had made more than one lifestyle change, each change was represented separately in the matrix. The matrix is presented in Table 20–1 (on pp. 538–539).

Subjects 1, 2, and 4 experienced revelations related to overeating. This revelation had been followed by a belief system change. Each of these individuals had a weight loss of 60 to 75 pounds that had been maintained for 4.5 months to 1 year. The third subject experienced no revelation and had no success in weight loss. Patterns in the data that might have been overlooked were revealed by the matrix. For example, Marsh assumed that the belief-system change that occurred was a change in health beliefs. The matrix illustrated that the change was rather one of personal empowerment and involved beliefs about self, not about health.

CRITICAL INCIDENT CHART

In some studies, the researcher, in an effort to gain increased insight into the dynamics of a process, identifies critical incidents occurring in the course of that process. The researcher can then compare these critical incidents in various subgroups of participants. The critical incidents and the subgroups can then be placed in a matrix listing the critical incidents in relation to time. Examination of the matrix can facilitate comparison of critical incidents in terms of timing and variation across participants or subgroups.

CAUSAL NETWORK

As the data are collected and analyzed, the researcher gains increasing understanding of the dynamics involved in the process under study. This understanding might be considered a tentative theory. The first tentative theories are vague and poorly pieced together. In some cases, they are altogether wrong. The best way to verify a tentative theory is to share it with others, particularly informants in the study situation. Informants have their own tentative theories, which have never been clearly expressed. The tentative theory needs to be expressed as a map. Developing a good map of the tentative theory is difficult and requires some hard work. The development of a tentative theory and an associated map is discussed in Chapter 7.

The validity of predictions developed in a tentative theory must be tested. However, finding effective ways to achieve this is difficult. Predictions are usually developed near the end of the study. Since the findings are often context-specific, the predictions must be tested on the same sample or on a sample that is very similar. One strategy suggested is to predict outcomes expected to occur 6 months after the completion of the study. Six months later, these predictions can be sent to informants who participated in the study. The informants can be asked to respond to the accuracy of (1) the predictions and (2) the explanation of why the prediction was expected to occur (Miles & Huberman, 1994).

DRAWING AND VERIFYING CONCLUSIONS

Unlike the case in quantitative research, conclusions are formed throughout the data analysis process. Conclusions are similar to the findings in a quantitative study. Miles and Huberman (1994) have identified 12 tactics used to draw and verify conclusions.

COUNTING

Qualitative researchers have tended to avoid any use of numbers. However, when judgments of qualities are made, counting is occurring. The researcher states that a pattern occurs "frequently" or "more often." Something is considered "important" or "significant." These judgments are made in part by counting. If the researcher is counting, it should be recognized and planned. Counting can help researchers see what they have; it can help verify a hypothesis; and it can help keep one intellectually honest. Qualitative researchers work by insight and intuition; however, their conclusions can be wrong. It is easier to see confirming evidence than to see disconfirming evidence. Comparing insights with numbers can be a good method of verification (Miles & Huberman, 1994).

NOTING PATTERNS, THEMES

People easily identify patterns, themes, and gestalts from their observations—almost too easily. The difficulty is in seeking real additional evidence of that pattern while remaining open to disconfirming evidence. Any pattern that is identified should be subjected to skepticism—that of the researcher and that of others (Miles & Huberman, 1994).

"The researcher must distinguish between representative cases and anecdotal cases. Representative cases appear with regularity and encompass the range of behaviors described within a category. The anecdotal case appears infrequently and depicts a small range of events which are atypical of the larger group. . . . Negative cases are those episodes that clearly refute an emergent theory or proposition. Negative cases are important as they help to clarify additional causal properties which influence the phenomena under study." (Field & Morse, 1985, p. 106) ■

Table 20–1
Process-Oriented Matrix of Life-Style Change

Subject No.	Life-Style Change	Problem Awareness	Relapse	Readiness	Revelation	Belief-System Change	Behavioral Outcome	Predicted Future Outcome
1	Overeating*	In 8th grade, I was conscious of being overweight. I need to do something for myself	I have no time to care for. I have character defects. I didn't want to commit and fail	My husband was supportive. I got friend to go to meeting with me. People at group were honest. I want to live. Success of others in group was inspirational	I can use my power along with God's power to conquer demon, overeating	I have strength in working with God; this gives me power and I can use it	60-lb weight loss sustained for 4.5 months, confident of continued success	Will sustain
2	Overeating*	I feel uncomfortable and short of breath	I tried all new diets. My spouse supported my failure, both have poor will power	I got help from spouse. I got help from group	I realized, if that woman can do it, so can I	I no longer need to eat to be happy	75-lb weight loss sustained over 1 year	Will sustain
	Alcohol	None	None	I got support from spouse. I have low self-esteem. I got group support—I went willingly, with no expectations	It suddenly hit: "I didn't like *me* anymore"	I have personal power. I find support in group	Alcohol abstinence	Will sustain
	Smoking	I have a bad cough	I made two failed attempts	My father's health was bad. I had a bad cough. I really wanted to quit	None	I can do it by myself (strength from alcohol problem)	Sustained smoking cessation for several years	Will sustain
3	Overeating*	Eating is a sin—I love it, I hate it. At a group I was obsessive/compulsive over food	I had many, many failures. Food controls me. I have little control. I tried groups; I like the support but can't keep with it	I have low self-esteem. I am concerned for my child. Group gives me hope and strength. I have been depressed, I hate my life. When I'm okay, everything else is	None	None	Repeated relapses	Escalation of readiness

4	Overeating*	I was a fat slob and an introvert since I was a small child	I wanted a magic cure with no responsibility	I felt depressed and suicidal I have low life satisfaction I'm a miserable, hurting person not in touch with self I have low self-esteem I joined group from fear of death I felt group inspiration, I'm not alone	I realized I can control my life and it's okay to seek guidance from others "All of a sudden everything was pulled together"	Asked my higher power for strength and help (higher power = God = inner self) Food controlled me, now I can control it. I'm proud of me	Sustained 65-lb loss 8 months. Still needs group support, seeks reinforcement from others	Success if group support continued
5	Smoking*	I was tired of it It was a hassle	I have no one to share problem with, no pats on back, no group support I'm a failure None	I'm joining groups to meet people in similar situation	None	None	Never got the group support sought Another relapse	Success with right group
	Alcohol	I was sneaking I was hiding problem from family	None	I feel concern and love from little sister	I was shaken by my little sister's concern I suddenly knew I needed help	I want help at any cost Group support will help; joined group 3–4 years old I'm making written commitment	Reformed alcoholic, no backsliding, 3 years of sustained change	Will sustain
6	Smoking*	I was thinking about change I feel scared, angry I need a focus My body and health are changing It's filthy I'm ambivalent	I made it convenient I quit in past, started again I want others to help	I am grasping a focus, letting others know once you start you need to keep going	None	None	Smoking cessation for 4 days Has not told family or friends, is afraid of failure	Relapse
7	Smoking*	It's expensive It's filthy I risk getting cancer of the mouth	I've made many attempts I'm angry I don't want to give it up	I want group help Support of my son helps I'm concerned for effect of my smoking on my granddaughter and son	None	None	Relapse	Continued relapse
	Alcohol	I was hiding bottles I was a closet drinker	I tried quitting for 6 years	I have low self-esteem	I realized no one could do it for me. I could do it by myself	I only have myself to blame I'm the only one who can do anything about it	Alcohol abstinence 6 years	Will sustain

* Change currently being made. (Reprinted from *Advances in Nursing Science*, Vol. 12, No. 3, pp. 51–52, with permission of Aspen Publishers, Inc. © 1990.)

SEEING PLAUSIBILITY

Often during analysis, a conclusion is seen as plausible. It seems to fit; it "makes good sense." When asked how one arrived at that point, the researcher may state that it "just feels right." These intuitive feelings are important in both qualitative and quantitative research. However, plausibility cannot stand alone. After plausibility must come systematic analysis. First, intuition occurs, then careful examination of the data to verify the validity of that intuition (Miles & Huberman, 1994).

CLUSTERING

Clustering is the process of sorting elements into categories or groups. It is the first step in inductive theorizing. In order to cluster objects, people, or behavior into a group, one must first conceptualize them as having similar patterns or characteristics. Clusters, however, like patterns, must be viewed with caution and verified. There may be alternative ways to cluster that would be more meaningful (Miles & Huberman, 1994).

MAKING METAPHORS

Miles and Huberman (1994) suggest that qualitative researchers should think and write metaphorically. A metaphor uses figurative language to suggest a likeness or analogy of one kind of idea used in the place of another. Metaphors provide a strong image with a feeling tone that is powerful in communicating meaning. For example, stating rationally and logically that you are in a heavy work situation does not provide the emotional appeal and meaning that you could express by saying, "I am up to my ears in work!" Miles and Huberman also believe that metaphors add meaning to the findings and use the example of the mother's separation anxiety, a phrase "which is less appealing, less suggestive, and less theoretically powerful than the empty nest syndrome"

(p. 221). The phrase "empty nest syndrome" communicates images loaded with meaning far beyond that conveyed by the words alone.

Metaphors are also *data-reducing devices* that involve generalizing from the particulars. They are *pattern-making devices* that place the pattern into a larger context. Metaphors are also effective *decentering devices*. They force the viewer to step back from the mass of particular observations to see the larger picture. Metaphors are also ways of *connecting findings* to theory. They are what initiates the researcher to thinking in more general terms. A few suggestions about developing metaphors: (1) It is unwise to look for metaphors early in the study. (2) In order to develop metaphors, one must be cognitively playful, moving from the denotative to the connotative. Interacting with others in a cognitively playful environment can be useful. (3) Metaphors can be taken too far in terms of meaning; therefore, one must know when to stop.

SPLITTING VARIABLES

Qualitative research is strongly oriented toward integrating concepts. However, in some cases, researchers must recognize the need for differentiation. They must have the courage to question; Miles and Huberman refer to this early integration as *premature parsimony*. Splitting variables is particularly important during the initial stages of the analysis to allow more detailed examination of the processes that are occurring. It also often occurs with the development of matrices. During theorizing, if the variable does not seem to relate well with the rest of the framework, it may have to be split to allow a more coherent, integrated model to be developed (Miles & Huberman, 1994).

SUBSUMING PARTICULARS INTO THE GENERAL

This process is similar to clustering, in that it involves the clumping of things together. Clustering tends to be intuitive and is similar to coding. Subsuming particulars into the general is a move from the specific and concrete to the abstract and theoretical.

FACTORING

The idea of factoring is taken from the quantitative procedure of factor analysis. If one has a list of characteristics, are there general themes within the list that allow one to explain more clearly what is going on? As with factor analysis, when clusters have been identified, they must be named. Factoring can occur at several levels of abstraction in the data. The important consideration is that they make a meaningful difference in clarity (Miles & Huberman, 1994).

NOTING RELATIONS BETWEEN VARIABLES

The development of relationships between variables was discussed previously. However, at this point, it is important to go beyond verifying that, in fact, a relationship exists to explain the relationship. The relationships described in Chapter 7 can be used to describe qualitative findings. Some relationships that might occur follow.

"1. A+, B+ (both are high, or both low at the same time)
2. A+, B− (A is high, B is low, or vice versa)
3. A↑, B↑ (A has increased, and B has increased)
4. A↑, B↓ (A has increased, and B has decreased)
5. A↑ then → B↑ (A increased first, then B increased)
6. A↑ then → B↑ then A↑ (A increased, then B increased, then A increased some more)." (Miles & Huberman, 1994, p. 257) ∎

FINDING INTERVENING VARIABLES

In some cases, the researcher believes that two variables should go together; however, findings do not verify this thinking. In other cases, two variables are found during data analysis to go together, but their connection cannot be explained. In both of these situations, a third variable may be responsible for the confusion. Therefore, the third variable must be identified. The matrices described earlier can be very useful in the search for this variable, and the search often requires some careful detective work. Finding an intervening variable is easiest when there are multiple cases of the two-variable relationship to examine (Miles & Huberman, 1994).

BUILDING A LOGICAL CHAIN OF EVIDENCE

At first glance, this would seem to be the same activity described earlier that resulted in the development of a tentative theory; however, this activity assumes the prior development of a tentative theory. Building a logical chain of evidence involves testing that theory. The researcher must go back and carefully trace evidence from the data through the development of the tentative theory; then, the elements, relationships, and propositions of the theory are tested against new data. The researcher looks for cases that closely fit the theory and for those that clearly do not fit the theory. The theory may then be modified.

This process is referred to as *analytic induction* and uses two interlocking cycles. The first cycle is *enumerative induction,* in which a number and variety of instances are collected that verify the model. The second cycle, *eliminative induction,* requires that the hypothesis be tested against alternatives. The researcher is required to check carefully for limits to the generalizability of the theory. The process of constant comparisons used in grounded theory is related to eliminative induction (Miles & Huberman, 1994).

MAKING CONCEPTUAL/ THEORETICAL COHERENCE

The previous steps have described a gradual move from empirical data to a conceptual overview of the findings. Inferences have been made as the analysis moved from the concrete to the more abstract. The steps then moved from metaphors to interrelationships, then to constructs, and from there to theories. The theory must now be connected with other existing theories in the body of knowledge. In order to accomplish this step, one must develop a familiarity with a wide variety of theories that could be used to explain the current phenomenon. If connections can be made with other theories, it further strengthens the present theoretical explanation (Miles & Huberman, 1994).

RESEARCH METHODOLOGY OF SPECIFIC QUALITATIVE APPROACHES

PHENOMENOLOGICAL RESEARCH METHODS

In phenomenological studies, several strategies can be used for data collection, and it is possible to use combinations of strategies. In order to conduct these data collection strategies, the researcher involves his or her personality and uses intuiting. *Intuiting* is the process of actually looking at the phenomenon. During intuiting, the researcher focuses all awareness and energy on the subject of interest to allow an increase in insight. Thus, this process requires absolute concentration and complete absorption with the experience being studied (Oiler, 1982). Intuiting is a strange idea to those of us in the Western world. It is a more common practice in

Eastern thought and is related to meditation practices and the directing of personal energy forces.

Data Collection Strategies

In one data collection strategy, participants are asked to describe verbally their experiences of a phenomenon. These verbal data need to be collected in a relaxed atmosphere with sufficient time allowed to facilitate a complete description by the respondent. Alternatively, informants can be asked to provide a written description of their experiences. Ruffing-Rahal (1986) recommends the use of personal documents, particularly autobiographical accounts, as a source of data.

Another strategy requires that the researcher be more directly involved in the experience. During the participant's experience, the researcher simultaneously observes verbal and nonverbal behavior, the environment, and his or her own responses to the situation. Written notes may be used, or the experience may be tape-recorded or videotaped. When observed behavior is being recorded, the researcher describes, rather than evaluates, observations.

There are several variations to analysis of phenomenological data. The methods of Van Kaam, Giorgi, and Colaizzi are most commonly used. In Table 20–2, Beck (1994) compares the three methods. Within nursing, Parse has developed a methodology that is now being used in phenomenological nursing studies.

Van Kaam

Van Kaam (1966) suggests classifying data and ranking the classifications according to the frequency of occurrence. This ranking is verified by a panel of judges. The number of categories is then reduced to eliminate overlapping, vague, or intricate categories, and again, agreement of the panel of judges is sought. Hypotheses are developed to explain the categories theoretically, and these hypotheses are tested on a new sample. This process is continued until no new categories emerge.

Table 20–2
Comparison of Three Phenomenological Methods

Colaizzi	Giorgi	Van Kaam
1. Read all of the subjects' descriptions in order to acquire a feeling for them.	1. One reads the entire description in order to get a sense of the whole.	1. Listing and preliminary grouping of descriptive expressions which must be agreed upon by expert judges. Final listing presents percentages of these categories in that particular sample.
2. Return to each protocol and extract significant statements.	2. Researcher discriminates units from the participants' description of the phenomenon being studied. Researcher does this from within a psychological perspective and with a focus on the phenomenon under study.	2. In reduction the researcher reduces the concrete, vague, and overlapping expressions of the participants to more precisely descriptive terms. There again, intersubjective agreement among judges is necessary.
3. Spell out the meaning of each significant statement, known as formulating meanings.	3. Researcher expresses the psychological insight contained in each of the meaning units more directly.	3. Elimination of these elements that are not inherent in the phenomenon being studied or which represent a blending of this phenomenon with other phenomena that most frequently accompany it is done.

4. Organize the formulated meanings into clusters of themes.
  a. Refer these clusters of themes back to the original protocols in order to validate them.
  b. At this point discrepancies may be noted among and/or between the various clusters. Researchers must refuse temptation of ignoring data or themes which do not fit.
	4. Researcher synthesizes all of the transformed meaning units into a consistent statement regarding the participant's experiences. This is referred to as the structure of the experience and can be expressed on a specific or a general level.	4. A hypothetical identification and description of the phenomenon being studied is written.

5. Results so far are integrated into an exhaustive description of phenomenon under study.		5. The hypothetical description is applied to randomly selected cases of the sample. If necessary, the hypothesized description is revised. This revised description must be tested again on a new random sample of cases.
6. Formulate the exhaustive description of the investigated phenomenon in as unequivocal a statement of identification as possible.		6. When operations described in previous steps have been carried out successfully, the formerly hypothetical identification of the phenomenon under study may be considered to be a valid identification and description.
7. A final validating step can be achieved by returning to each subject asking about the findings so far.		

(Beck, C. T. [1994]. Reliability and validity issues in phenomenology. *Western Journal of Nursing Research, 16*[3], 254–267. Reprinted by permission of Sage Publications, © 1994.)

Table 20-3
**Application of Giorgi's Method of Analysis
of Phenomenological Data**

Step No.	Theoretical Process	Pragmatic Process Used in Example
One	Reading of the entire disclosure of the phenomenon straight through to obtain a sense of the whole.	Reading and rereading the first three transcripts looking for emerging themes. Establishing the coding process and decision rules for coding.
Two	Rereading the same disclosure again in a purposeful manner to delineate each time that a transition in meaning occurs. This is done with the intention of discovering the essence of the phenomenon under study. The end result is a series of meaning units or themes.	Reading and coding each of the 20 transcripts for themes by each member of the research team. Weekly meetings of the coders to review the coding process and to reach consensus where questions or discrepancies had arisen. Intrarater and interrater reliability was established during this step.
Three	Examining the previously determined meaning units for redundancies, clarification, or elaboration by relating meaning units to each other and to a sense of the whole.	The meaning units or themes were examined and categories were developed which represented a higher level of abstraction. Themes not related to the research questions were categorized appropriately. The result was an extensive listing of data by categories.
Four	Reflecting upon the meaning units (still expressed essentially in the language of the subject) and extrapolating the essence of the experience for each subject. A systematic interrogation of each unit is undertaken for what it reveals about the phenomenon under study for each subject. During this process, each unit is transformed into the language of psychological science when relevant.	After reflecting upon the categories, such as thoughts, feelings, and responses of the subjects, a narrative was formulated for each subject capturing the essence of the phenomenon of an encounter with a suicide attempter. It was during this time that the true richness of the phenomenological method was realized.
Five	Formalizing a consistent description of the structure of the phenomenon under study across subjects, by synthesizing and integrating the insights achieved in the previous steps.	Decisions wre made as to what to accept as the common experience for the phenomenon. Responses offered by 25% or more of the subjects were accepted as the structure of the phenomenon of an encounter with a suicide attempter.

(Reprinted from Pallikkathayil, L., & Morgan, S. A. [1991]. Phenomenology as a method for conducting clinical research. *Applied Nursing Research, 4*[4], 197, with permission.)

Giorgi

Giorgi (1970) recommends a similar process but prefers to maintain more of the sense of wholeness. Although individual elements of the phenomenon are identified, their importance to the phenomenon is not established by the frequency of their occurrence but rather by the intuitive judgment of the researcher. Giorgi considers it important to identify the relationships of the units to each other and to the whole. In Table 20–3, Pallikkathayil and Morgan (1991) illustrate the steps of Giorgi's method of analysis using examples from their study of suicide attempters.

Colaizzi

Colaizzi (1978) has developed a method that involves observing and analyzing human behavior within its environment to examine experiences that cannot be communicated. This strategy is useful in studying phenomena such as behaviors of preverbal children, subjects with Alzheimer's disease, combative behavior of the unconscious patient, and body motion of subjects with new amputations.

Parse

Parse (1990) has described a research methodology specific to the Man-Living-Health theory. This methodology involves dialogical engagement, in which the researcher and respondent participate in an unstructured discussion about a lived experience. The experience is described as an I-Thou intersubjective *being with* the participant during the discussion. "The researcher, in true presence with the participant, engages in a dialogue surfacing the remembered, the now, and the not-yet all at once. Before the dialogue with the participant, the researcher 'dwells with' the meaning of the lived experience, centering self in a way to be open to a full discussion of the experience as shared by the participant. The discussion is audio and video tape-recorded (when possible), and the dialogue is transcribed to typed format for the extraction-synthesis process. Extraction-synthesis is a process of moving the descriptions from the language of the participants up the levels of abstraction to the language of science" (p. 11).

The researcher contemplates the phenomenon under study while listening to the tape, reading the transcribed dialogue, and viewing the videotape. Thus the researcher is multisensorily immersed in the data. According to Parse (1990), the details of this process include the following.

"1. Extracting essences from transcribed descriptions (participant's language). An extracted essence is a complete expression of a core idea described by the participant.
2. Synthesizing essences (researcher's language). A synthesized essence is an expression of the core idea of the extracted essence conceptualized by the researcher.
3. Formulating a proposition from each partici-

pant's description. A proposition is a non-directional statement conceptualized by the researcher joining the core idea of the synthesized essences from each participant.
4. Extracting core concepts from the formulated propositions of all participants. An extracted core concept is an idea (written in a phrase) that captures the central meaning of the propositions.
5. Synthesizing a structure of the lived experience from the extracted concepts. A synthesized structure is a statement conceptualized by the researcher joining the core concepts. The structure as evolved answers the research question: 'What is the structure of this lived experience?' " (p. 11) ∎

The results of this analysis are then moved up another level of abstraction to represent the meaning of the lived experience at the level of theory. The findings are interpreted in terms of the principles of Parse's theory.

Outcomes

Findings are often described from the orientation of the participants studied, rather than being translated into scientific or theoretical language. For example, the actual words used by the participants to describe an experience will often be used when reporting the findings. The researcher identifies themes found in the data. From these themes, a structural explanation of the findings is developed.

Phenomenological Nursing Study

One of the most significant nursing studies conducted using the phenomenological method is Benner's (1984) work from which emerged the critical description of nursing practice presented in her book, *From Novice to Expert*. This study was funded by a grant from the Department of Health and Human Services, Division of Nursing, at a time when external funding for qualitative research was almost unheard of. In Benner's study, the phenomenon to be explored was the experience of clinical practice. Benner's research question asked if there were "distinguishable, characteristic differences in the novice's and expert's descriptions of the same clinical incident. If so, how could these differences, if identifiable from the nurses' descriptions of the incidents, be accounted for or understood?" (p. 14)

Benner conducted paired interviews with beginning nurses and nurses recognized for their expertise. Twenty-one pairs of nurses were selected from three hospitals where preceptors were used to orient new graduates. Each member of the pair, one a preceptor and one a new graduate, was interviewed separately about patient care situations they had experienced together. In addition to these pairs, interviews and participant-observations were conducted with additional nurses, including 51 experienced nurse clinicians, 11 new graduates, and 5 senior nursing students. Individual interviews, small group interviews, and participant-observation were conducted at six hospitals. Before the interviews, participants were given written explanations of the kinds of clinical descriptions the researchers were interested in. Interviews were tape-recorded and transcribed.

Benner's data analysis was an interpretative strategy based on Heideggerian phenomenology. She describes the procedure as follows.

"The interviews and participant/observer records were read independently by the research team members, and interpretations of the data were compared and consensually validated. Each interpretation was accepted only if there was agreement in labeling and interpreting the major competency demonstrated and only if it was effective in describing skilled practice." (p. 16) ∎

Benner's structural explanation of her findings was presented as five stages of gaining experience in clinical practice, which describes the nurse in a particular clinical situation as novice, advanced beginner, competent, proficient, or expert.

Stage I: Novice

"Beginners have had no experience of the situations in which they are expected to perform. To give them entry to these situations and allow them to gain the experience so necessary for skill development, they are taught about the situations in terms of objective attributes such as weight, intake and output, temperature, blood pressure, pulse, and other such objectifiable, measurable parameters of a patient's conditions—features of the task that can be recognized without situational experiences. Novices are also taught context-free rules to guide action in respect to different attributes." (pp. 20–21)

Stage 2: Advanced Beginner

"Advanced beginners are ones who can demonstrate marginally acceptable performance, ones who have coped with enough real situations to note (or to have pointed out to them by a mentor) the recurring meaningful situational components . . . Aspects, in contrast to the measurable, context-free attributes or the procedural lists of things to do that are learned and used by the beginner, require prior experience in actual situations for recognitions. Aspects include overall, global characteristics that can be identified only through prior experience." (p. 22)

Stage 3: Competent

"Competence, typified by the nurse who has been on the job in the same or similar situations two to three years, develops when the nurse begins to see his or her actions in terms of long-range goals or plans of which he or she is consciously aware. The plan dictates which attributes and aspects of the current and contemplated future situation are to be considered most important and those which can be ignored. Hence, for the competent nurse, a plan establishes a perspective, and the plan is based on considerable conscious, abstract, analytic contemplation of the problem." (p. 26)

Stage 4: Proficient

"Characteristically, the proficient performer perceives situations as wholes rather than in terms of aspects, and performance is guided by maxims. (Maxims are cryptic instructions passed on by experts. Maxims make sense only if the person already has a deep understanding of the situation.

(p. 10)) Perception is the key word here. The perspective is not thought out but 'presents itself' based upon experience and recent events. Proficient nurses understand a situation as a whole because they perceive its meaning in terms of long-term goals." (p. 27)

Stage 5: Expert

"The expert performer no longer relies on an analytic principle (rule, guideline, maxim) to connect her or his understanding of the situation to an appropriate action. The expert nurse, with an enormous background of experience, now has an intuitive grasp of each situation and zeroes in on the accurate region of the problem without wasteful consideration of a large range of unfruitful, alternative diagnoses and solutions." (p. 32) ■

Benner (1984) also identified seven domains of practice: (1) the helping role, (2) the teaching-coaching function, (3) the diagnostic and patient-monitoring function, (4) effective management of rapidly changing situations, (5) administering and monitoring therapeutic interventions and regimens, (6) monitoring and ensuring the quality of health care practices, and (7) organizational and work-role competencies. Nursing competencies representative of each domain were identified.

GROUNDED THEORY METHODOLOGY

Data collection for a grounded theory study is referred to as field work. Participant-observation is a commonly used technique. The focus of observation is social interactions within the phenomenon of interest. Interviews may also be conducted to obtain the perceptions of participants. Data are coded in preparation for analysis that begins with the initiation of data collection. Stern (1980) and Turner (1981) have described the methodology used for grounded theory analysis.

1. **Category Development.** Categories, derived from the data, are identified and named. These categories are used as codes for data analysis. This is the beginning stage of the development of a tentative theory.

2. **Category Saturation.** Examples of the identified categories are collected until the characteristics of items that fit into the category become clear to the researcher. The researcher then examines all instances of the category in the data to determine whether they fit the emerging pattern of characteristics identified by the researcher.

3. **Concept Development.** The researcher formulates a definition of the category (now properly referred to as a concept) using the characteristics verified in step 2.

4. **Search for Additional Categories.** The researcher continues to examine the data and collect additional data to search for categories that were not immediately obvious but seem to be essential to understanding the phenomenon under study.

5. **Category Reduction.** Categories, which at this point in the research may have become numerous, are clustered by merging them into higher-order categories.

6. **Search for Negative Instances of Categories.** The researcher continually seeks instances that contradict or otherwise do not fit the characteristics developed to define a category.

7. **Linking of Categories.** The researcher seeks to understand relationships among categories. To accomplish this, data collection becomes more selective as the researcher seeks to determine conditions under which the concepts occur. Hypotheses are developed and tested using available data or selecting additional interviews or observations specifically to examine proposed links among the categories. A narrative presentation of the emerging theory, including the concepts, conceptual definitions, and relationships, is developed. The narrative is rewritten repeatedly to achieve an explanation of an emerging theory that is clearly expressed, logically consistent, reflective of the data, and compatible with the knowledge base of nursing. A conceptual map may be provided to clarify the theory (Burns, 1989).

8. **Selective Sampling of the Literature.** Unlike the case in traditional research, the literature is not extensively searched at the beginning of the study in order to avoid development of a sedimented view. At this point in the research, the literature is examined to determine the fit of findings from earlier studies and existing theory with present findings.

9. **Emergence of the Core Variable.** Through the aforementioned activities, the concept most important to the theory emerges. This concept, or core variable, becomes the central theme or focus of the theory.

10. **Concept Modification and Integration.** This step is a wrapping-up process in which the theory is finalized and is again compared with the data. "As categories and patterns emerge, the researcher must engage in the critical act of challenging the very pattern that seems so apparent. The researcher must search for other, plausible explanations for the data and the linkages among them" (Marshall & Rossman, 1989, p. 119). Sometimes, there is a poor fit between the data and the emerging theory. This can occur because the identification of patterns in the data has occurred before the researcher can logically fit all of the data within the emerging framework. In this case, the relationships proposed among the phenomena may be spurious. Miles and Huberman (1994) suggest that plausibility is the opiate of the intellectual. If the emerging schema makes good sense and fits with other theorists' explanations of the phenomena, the researcher locks into it prematurely. This is why it is so critical to test the schema by rechecking the fit between the emerging theory and the original data.

Grounded Theory Study

One significant study using a grounded theory approach that is relevant to clinical nursing practice is Fagerhaugh and Strauss's (1977) study of the politics of pain management. This study emerged from the previous work of Glaser and Strauss in the care of the dying (Glaser & Strauss, 1965,

1968; Strauss & Glaser, 1970) and chronic illness care (Strauss, 1975; Strauss, Corbin, Fagerhaugh, Glaser, Maines, Suczek, & Wiener, 1984). The study of pain involved five researchers and 2 years of systematic observations in 20 wards, 2 clinics, and 9 hospitals. The purposes of the study were twofold: to develop an approach to pain management that was radically different from established approaches, and to develop a substantive theory about "what happens in hospitals when people are confronted with pain and attempt to deal with it" (Fagerhaugh & Strauss, 1977, p. 13). The research questions were, "Under what conditions is pain encountered by staff?" and "How will it be handled?"

In the pain study, the researchers wished to observe a variety of situations in which pain was a common phenomenon. The areas studied included an intensive care unit for severe burns, a cardiac care unit, an obstetrics ward, a physical rehabilitation unit, a neurology and neurosurgery unit, a routine surgery unit, a medical ward, a radiology department, an emergency department, a kidney transplant unit, and a cancer ward. The following excerpt is from the report of the grounded theory study on pain. It focuses on a description of the sampling process and demonstrates the care and detailed thought that must go into the development of sampling categories.

"On all these wards we made 'internal comparisons' along the theoretical dimensions. That is, we continued our theory-directed sampling: for instance, high-pain regimens versus low-pain regimens; experienced inflicters of regimen pain versus new inflicters; delivering mothers who had the fathers supporting their efforts to endure pain versus those who had no such supporting or controlling agents. Meanwhile, we were also looking at an activity that spanned separate wards and which would maximize variables as they related to pain infliction. We followed a number of personnel who drew blood from patients. We observed some who were very experienced, some who were not; some who were able to work in a leisurely fashion, some who were not; some who met 'first-time' patients, others who met patients very experienced at this particular procedure; some who encountered patients with much ongoing pain and some who did not; some who had recently had experiences with accusations of incompetence and some who had not." (Fagerhaugh & Strauss, 1977, p. 308) ■

In the pain study, the core categories that evolved were pain work, pain trajectories, legitimation, balancing, and accountability. Pain work was further classified into relief of pain, the handling of pain expression, diagnosing the meaning of pain, inflicting pain, minimizing or preventing pain, patients enduring pain, and the staff members' controlling their own reactions to the patient's response to pain. The patient's cooperation in the pain work and negotiation between the staff and the patient were identified as important factors. An example of negotiation is described by Glaser (1973).

■

"This won't take long, I said to her . . . It's not going to hurt . . . I think I can inject it right into the IV tubing and not have to stick you. She looked unconvinced.

Honestly I won't stick you unless I have to." (p. 130) ■

Pain trajectories were divided into expected and unexpected trajectories. For example, an expectant mother would have a very different pain trajectory than a person with intractable back pain.

■

"An unexpected trajectory—unexpected for a given ward, that is—carries a potential for staff and patient disturbance and ward upset. Both the sentimental order and the work order of the ward are threatened . . . Patients with an unexpected or atypical trajectory tend to be labeled as 'uncooperative' or 'difficult,' and relations between them and the staff are likely to grow progressively worse." (Fagerhaugh & Strauss, 1977, pp. 22–23) ■

The researchers also concluded that the pain trajectory was influenced by the patients' illnesses, their previous experience with pain, the medical care they were receiving, and their social history. They observed that the nursing and medical staff seldom know anything about the patient's pain trajectory other than what is currently occurring.

Assessing and legitimizing pain was also identified as an important factor. Staff often suspected patients of claiming more pain than they had or of claiming pain when they had none. This left patients in the position of attempting to convince the staff that they were actually having the pain they claimed to have (legitimizing). The staff and patients were often involved in the process of balancing priorities during pain work. Decisions were based on what was considered to be the most important by staff.

■

"The staff members may not always agree among themselves, and the balancing done by the patient may not agree with the staff's. Patient and staff may even opt for opposite choices, disagreeing over the value of living a bit longer versus enduring terrible pain. They may be balancing quite different considerations. The staff may be balancing more work versus quicker pain relief, while the patient may be balancing pride in not complaining about pain versus difficulty of enduring it without more medication." (Fagerhaugh & Strauss, 1977, p. 25) ■

In terms of accountability, the researchers found that pain work was not a major priority of staff. Staff tended to be more responsible for controlling the patient's expression of pain than controlling the experience of pain. Fagerhaugh and Strauss (1977) drew the following conclusions from their study.

"Genuine accountability concerning pain work could only be instituted if the major authorities on given wards or clinics understood the importance of that accountability and its implications for patient care. They would then need to convert that understanding into a commitment that would bring about necessary changes in written and verbal communication systems. This kind of understanding and commitment can probably come about only after considerable nationwide discussion, such as now is taking place about terminal care, but that kind of discussion seems to lie far in the future." (p. 27) ■

ETHNOGRAPHIC METHODOLOGY

Gaining Entrance

One of the critical steps in any study is gaining entry into the area being studied. The mechanics of this process may vary greatly, depending on whether one is attempting to gain entrance to another country or into a specific institution. The researcher is responsible at this point for explaining the purposes and methods of the study to those with the power to grant entrance.

Acquiring Informants

In order to understand the culture, the researcher seeks out individuals who are willing to interpret the culture to them. These people (who are usually members of the culture) will not be research subjects in the usual sense of the word, but rather colleagues. The researcher must have the support and confidence of these individuals in order to complete the research. Therefore, maintaining these relationships is of utmost importance. Not only will the informants answer questions, they may also have to help formulate the questions, since they understand the culture better than the researcher.

Immersion in the Culture

The ethnographic researcher must become very familiar with the culture being studied, by living in it (active participation) and by extensive questioning. The process of becoming *immersed* in the culture involves gaining increasing familiarity with such things as language; sociocultural norms; traditions; and other social dimensions such as family, communication patterns (verbal and nonverbal), religion, work patterns, and expression of emotion. Immersion also involves gradually increasing acceptance of the researcher into the culture.

Gathering Data (Elicitation Procedures)

The activity of collecting data is referred to as *field research* and requires the taking of extensive notes. The quality of these notes will depend on the expertise of the researcher. A skilled researcher, experienced in qualitative research techniques, will be able to discern more easily what observations need to be noted than will a less experienced researcher or assistant. During observations, the researcher will be bombarded with information. Intuition plays an important role in determining which data to collect. Although researchers must be actively involved in the culture they are studying, they must avoid "going native," which will interfere with both data collection and analysis. In *going native,* the researcher becomes a part of the culture and loses all objectivity, and, with it, the ability to observe clearly.

Analysis of Data

Analysis of data is essentially analysis of the field notes and interviews. The notes themselves may be superficial. However, during the process of analysis, the notes are clarified, extended, and interpreted. The abstract thought processes (intuition, introspection, and reasoning discussed in Chapter 1) are involved in analysis. Interpretations are checked out with the informants. The data are then formed into categories and relationships developed between categories. Patterns of behavior are identified.

Outcomes

The analysis process in ethnography is used to provide detailed descriptions of cultures. These descriptions may be applied to existing theories of cultures. In some cases, the findings may lead to the development of hypotheses and/or the development of theory. The results are tested by whether another ethnographer, using the findings of the first ethnographic study, can accurately anticipate human behavior in the studied culture. Although the findings are not usually generalized from one culture or subculture to another, a case may be made for some degree of generalization to other similar cultures (Germain, 1986).

Ethnographic Study

Johnson (1993) used an ethnographic analysis and discourse analysis in her study of nurse practitioner-patient discourse to "uncover the voice of nursing in primary care practice." Discourse analysis was used to "uncover the forms and functions guiding conversation." Ethnographic analysis was used "to discover the beliefs guiding conversation and to establish a context for the NP-patient dialogue" (p. 143). Although a number of studies have documented the effectiveness of nurse practitioner (NP) outcomes compared to those of the physician, the process of NP care has not been examined. She sees the heart of the provider-patient relationship in primary care to be in the office visit. The focus of her study was "uncovering processes and skills used by NPs that could help expand understanding of their successful outcomes" (p. 143).

The study was conducted over a period of 1 year. During this period, Johnson sought to acquire knowledge of the culture of the unit, including its organizational structure. In relation to the discourse analysis, Johnson states, "The words (text) do not stand in isolation, rather they are a reflection of the values and beliefs of the individ-

ual, as well as of the organization. An interpretive approach for analyzing text was used, drawing on the model of Halliday and Hasan (1976) and Mishler's (1984) adaptation of the model for his study of physician-patient interaction" (p. 144). Johnson used field notes from observations and taped interviews as data sources. She asked the following research questions: "Do NP-patient communication strategies differ from those described in the literature as occurring during MD-patient interaction? To the degree that these differences are present, can they be explained by differences in the health care ideology between nursing and medicine?" (p. 144). Following is the context for the study.

Medicine and Nursing Ideology

"Mishler (1984) contends that one must understand the ideology or belief system that guides practice. Each profession has an ideology to which it socializes new members; adherence to these beliefs influences practice.

Medicine concerns itself with people as biologic systems. The biomedical model deals with disease as an entity independent of social behavior and views behavioral aberrations as somatic processes. Thus, the biomedical model entails reductionism and mind-body dualism (Engel, 1977).

Nursing places emphasis on the person's response to disease and maintenance of health. The nursing model includes biologic factors as well as psychological, social, and cultural concerns. This holistic valuing of mind, body, and spirit is evident in the writings of past and current nursing leaders (Henderson, 1964; Nightingale, 1860; Watson, 1985).

Lynaugh and Bates (1973) describe the results of the differing medical and nursing perspectives. The physician tends to emphasize structure, whether normal or diseased; the nurse is more concerned with function. This translates to a disease orientation for physicians and a person orientation for nurses. The development of NP education, a blending of knowledge and skills in the medical management of patient problems, has increased the potential for nurses to incorporate traditionally held medical skills into the nursing perspective. Understanding how these perspectives co-exist and how they are actualized in the NP's practice was part of the purpose of this study.

In studying MD-patient conversation, Mishler (1984) discusses two distinct voices in the dyad—the voice of medicine and the voice of the lifeworld. The concept of voice is used to specify underlying frameworks of meaning. The lifeworld represents the 'common-sense' natural attitude of everyday living, interpreting events with reference to one's own experience rather than by the scientific attitude of detached observation. The voice of medicine strips the illness experience of its subjective, biographical content to make it 'context free,' consistent with the scientific approach (Todd, 1989). The voice of the lifeworld represents illness as a personal experience.

Various strategies are used by the health care provider to maintain a focus consistent with his/her philosophy. For example, Mishler (1984) and Todd (1989) indicate that use of closed-ended questions by physicians controls the conversation and keeps the technologic aspect of the patient's condition in focus, whereas open-ended questions that would encourage subjectively meaningful descriptions of illness related to the lived experience of the patient are avoided. Other researchers of MD-patient interaction concur with these findings and interpret frequent questioning and interrupting of the patient as gestures of dominance to control the flow of conversation in a desired direction (Fisher, 1986; Fisher & Todd, 1983; West, 1984).

Brykczynski (1989) found in her research that NPs attended to contextual and situational aspects in provider-patient interactions. One would then anticipate that the voice of the lifeworld would be evident in NP-patient discourse. This study attempts to illuminate the *how* of this interactive process by analysis of NP-patient conversation. The connection of discourse to disciplinary ideology (belief system) is also a focus of this inquiry." (pp. 144–145) ∎

The setting of the study was an outpatient medical clinic in a large medical center that served as a clinical site for medical residents. Three full-time NPs with at least 2 years experience participated in the study; two having worked 5–10 years in the setting, the third 2 years. There were 22 women patients (women because of the researchers' general interest in woman-to-woman talk) who participated in the study. Patients were informed of the study by their NP who answered any questions; 76% agreed to participate and signed a consent form.

The sources of data for the study consisted of observations, NP-patient conversations, and interviews with each NP.

"Each NP was observed in the following situations: (1) on days when she was scheduled to see patients; (2) when she worked with a house staff group; (3) when care management was discussed (via the telephone) with patients; and (4) during consultation with colleagues. Interactions with other professional and administrative staff were also observed. This field work comprised 100 hours of observation which served to establish a comfort level with staff and patients prior to audiotaping and provided a context for the NP conversations." (p. 146) ∎

Field notes were made of all observations. Twenty-four NP-patient conversations were taped. It is not clear from the description whether the researcher was present and observed the NP-patient conversation or whether the NP taped the encounter for the researcher's later review. A 1½- to 2-hour audiotaped interview with each NP focused on her beliefs and expectations about patient care and practice. All audiotaped data were transcribed.

"Analysis of the texts proceeded in stages. NP-patient audiotapes were listened to as verbatim transcripts were proofed. Voice tone, work emphasis, and pauses were noted. Each NP-patient transcript was read several times, and memos kept on impressions of the interactions. The visit was divided into four sequences reflecting the major activities of an office encounter. Content of conversation was explored to look for patterns of communication strategies key to each sequence. Textual, interpersonal, and ideational functions of language were used to interpret the text (Halliday & Hasan, 1976; Mishler, 1984).

Textual function is the way in which coherence and continuity of discourse is maintained. This is determined by examining the type of questions asked, utterances used, and the transitions between speakers. For example, is the NP attentive to patient dialogue? Do her transitional comments maintain continuity and cohesion across the speakers, either by use of the patient's own words in a question, by responding directly to the meaning of the patient's inquiry, or by a transitional phrase which explains/introduces a shift? Interpersonal function refers to the role relationship of patient and NP and how this is expressed in speech. These roles are assumed to emanate from the beliefs of the individual and the discipline. The ideational function refers to content of conversation, its meaning and significance. What are the permissible topics in an NP-patient encounter? How is shared meaning established so the NP and patient understand each other?

Field notes were reviewed to develop descriptive narrative about the unit and to identify contextual factors relevant to the NP-patient conversations. The NP-researcher interviews were studied for values and expectations regarding practice in primary care. Both data sources were analyzed for perceived ideological differences between nursing and medicine." (p. 146) ■

Johnson organized the major activities of an office visit into four categories: establishing the agenda, eliciting information from the patient, conducting the physical exam, and developing a plan of care. These categories could then be used as a framework for her analysis. The published report of her study includes an excerpt of the NP-patient encounter for each category. An interpretation of the meanings extracted from the dialog follows, and a brief example is provided.

"The NP-patient encounters were by appointment with a specific reason for the visit emanat-

ing either from the patient or the provider. In the first few minutes of each encounter, a pattern was evident for a *negotiable agenda*. This process was initiated by the NP and is illustrated in the following text:

1. NP: So, how are you doing?
2. Pt: Not bad.
3. NP: Not bad. That's good. Let's see, the last time we saw you,
4. You had back pain that had gone away and neck pain, right?
5. Pt: Yeh.
6. NP: Okay. Did you have anything that you were particularly
7. concerned about today?
8. Pt: No.
9. NP: Not really huh? Okay, I think what we're supposed to do
10. today is your physical, right?
11. Pt: Yeh.
12. NP: Well let's do that while you are here today. How are
13. things going at home?
14. Pt: Still rough.
15. NP: Still rough?

The conversation begins with an open-ended question—'So, how are you doing?'—allowing the patient to establish the focus for discussion. The patient responds with a brief remark—'not bad.' The NP then *repeats* the words of the client 'not bad.' Repetition serves many purposes. Here it acknowledges that the nurse is attentive and listening to the patient. It also serves as a transition to her next query (line 4), a tag question. The NP recalls her understanding of the patient's condition on her previous visit and looks for validation from the patient with the interrogative— right? A tag question usually favors a response in a particular direction but it also indicates that the NP wants a response from the patient. Thus far, the open-ended and tag question yield little response. The NP's next question is direct—'Did you have anything that you were particularly concerned about?' When the patient says 'no' the NP uses repetition again—'not really, huh' and states the agenda for the visit (line 10), again using a tag question—'a physical exam (PE), right?' The patient is in agreement. Prior to the PE the woman is asked 'How are things going at home?' The question is predicated on past discussions with this woman. The patient responds 'still rough' and the NP again repeats the words of the woman 'still rough?' acknowledging that she heard, and encouraging further elaboration from the client. The woman proceeds to discuss life problems in her blended family since her last visit. About 10 minutes are spent on the topic before proceeding to the identified reason for the visit, a physical exam.'' (pp. 147–148).

''The majority of patients seen by the NPs were of long standing; a few were new to the practice. The identified purpose of the visit was generally apparent to the NPs, yet their opening remarks allowed the patient to either refocus the agenda, to make overt a hidden agenda, and/ or to elicit follow-up on previously discussed concerns related to the patient's health.'' (p. 148)

"The NPs considered nursing to be the umbrella for their practice. Physical assessment and medical management enabled them to be better nurses. Developing rapport with patients was considered primary. It was considered important to get to know each patient. As one NP stated: 'getting to know the patient's rest of his life-support, living arrangements, social issues, philosophy of life and goals, and what makes them happy; that's what will help me more effectively deal with a diabetic.' " (p. 154)

"The relationship between the NP and patient was viewed as a partnership. The bond established through collaboration 'gives the NP license to look at other areas of the person's life.' An element of camaraderie was viewed as positive and *not* in opposition to maintaining a professional stance.

The idea of NPs being physician extenders or mini-docs was viewed negatively. As one practitioner remarked:

'We're not mini-docs but teaching residents to be mini-NPs—they may not view it that way but we're teaching them the psychosocial skills they didn't learn in medical school; that is the essence of nursing.' " (p. 155) ■

The following are from Johnson's (1993) observations of the nurse practitioner's practice.

■

"Each of the NPs observed saw six to eight patients in a 4-hour clinic session. Between each visit, NPs triaged patient concerns, informed patients and physicians of test results, consulted with physicians and other colleagues, and linked patients with community resources. Much effort

went into unraveling the mystery of the patient's medication regimen—what was ordered versus what was changed versus what the patient was really taking. The knowledge these practitioners had about the personal lives of the patients, in addition to their medical problems, was impressive. They personalized their approach to the individual. For example, accommodating to the slow speech patterns of the frail elderly or athetoid speech of persons with cerebral palsy by allowing them time to express themselves. As busy as the NPs were, their busyness was not conveyed to the patient. Transcript review also made the researcher aware of the importance of voice tone. One practitioner had a calming quality evident in her work with a very anxious patient; all displayed empathy through voice tones. Although not the focus of this study, it is a strategy that needs to be further explored." (pp. 155–156)

"A mutual respect existed between the NPs and the medical residents. The relationship was viewed as non-hierarchical and the NPs believed they had authority to direct the residents on appropriate patient protocol. On the other hand, a disparity existed with the attending physicians' perspective on the purpose of the clinic and on the focus of patient care. The clinic exists to educate medical residents; all decisions regarding the clinic are made with this in mind. While the NPs see this education as important, they believe patient care should be top priority and that residents would benefit educationally by being involved in a model program. The focus of patient care by physicians is disease, whereas the 'whole person' orientation of the NPs places emphasis on prevention and continuity of care. The former was perceived by NPs as receiving higher priority from administration, reflecting the dominance of medicine within the institution and the acceptance of the medical model as norm." (p. 156) ■

HISTORICAL RESEARCH METHODOLOGY

Historical researchers spend considerable time refining their research questions prior to the initiation of data collection. Then sources of data relevant to the research question are identified. Sources of data are often remote from the researcher, who will need to make travel plans to obtain access to the data. In many cases, the researcher must obtain special written permission of the relevant library to obtain access to needed data. The validity and reliability of the data are an important concern in historical research.

Clarifying Validity and Reliability of Data

The validity and reliability concerns in historical research are related to the sources from which data are collected. The most valued source of data is the primary source. A primary source is material most likely to shed true light on the information being sought by the researcher. For example, material written by a person who experienced an event or letters and other mementos saved by the person being studied are primary source material. A secondary source is written by those who have previously read and summarized the primary source material. History books and textbooks are secondary source materials. Primary sources are considered more valid and reliable than secondary sources. "The presumption is that an eyewitness can give a more accurate account of an occurrence than a person not present. If the author was an eyewitness, he is considered a primary source. If the author has been told about the occurrence by someone else, the author is a secondary source. The further the author moves from an eyewitness account, the less reliable are his statements" (Christy, 1975, p. 191). Historiographers use primary sources whenever possible.

The historical researcher must consider the validity and reliability of primary sources used in the study. In order to determine this, the researcher uses principles of historical criticism.

"One does not merely pick up a copy of Grandmother's diary and gleefully assume that all the things Grandma wrote were the unvarnished facts. Grandmother's glasses may at times have been clouded, at other times rose-colored. The well-prepared researcher will scrutinize, criticize, and analyze before even accepting its having been written by Grandma! And even after the validity of the document is established, every attempt is made to uncover bias, prejudice, or just plain exaggeration on Grandmother's part. Healthy skepticism becomes a way of life for the serious historiographer." (Christy, 1978, p. 6) ■

Two strategies have been developed to determine the authenticity and accuracy of the source; these strategies are external and internal criticism.

External criticism determines the validity of source material. The researcher needs to know where, when, why, and by whom a document was written. This may involve verifying the handwriting or determining the age of the paper on which it was written. Christy (1975) describes some difficulties she experienced in establishing the validity of documents.

"An interesting problem presented by early nursing leaders was their frugality. Nutting occasionally saved stationery from hotels, resorts, or steamship lines during vacation trips and used it at a later date. This required double checking as to her exact location at the time the letter was written. When she first went to Teachers College in 1907, she still wrote a few letters on Johns Hopkins stationery. I found this practice rather confusing in early stages of research." (p. 190) ■

Internal criticism involves examination of the reliability of the document. The researcher must determine possible biases of the author. To verify the accuracy of a statement, the researcher should have two independent sources that provide the same information. In addition, the researcher should ensure that he or she understands the statements made by the writer, since words and their meanings change across time and across cultures. It is also possible to read into a document meaning not originally intended by the author. This is most likely to happen when one is seeking to find a particular meaning. Sometimes, words can be taken out of context (Christy, 1975).

Developing a Research Outline

The research outline is a guide for the broad topics to be examined and also serves as a basis for a filing system for classifying collected data. For example, data may be filed by time period. The materials may be cross-referenced for easy access. One piece of data may be filed under several classifications, and the researcher places a note in one file referring to data stored in another file. The research outline provides a checkpoint for the investigator during the process of data collection and can be used to easily identify gaps in the data collection process.

Data Collection

Data collection may require months or years of dedicated searching for pertinent material. Sometimes, one small source may open a door to an entire new field of facts. In addition, there is no clear, obvious end to data collection. By examining the research outline, the researcher must make the decision to discontinue collection of data. These facets of data collection are described by Newton (1965).

■

"The search for data takes the researcher into most unexpected nooks and corners and adds facet after facet to the original problem. It may last for months or years or a decade. Days and weeks may be fruitless and endless references may be devoid of pertinent material. Again, one minor reference will open the door to the gold mine of facts. The search becomes more exciting when others know of it and bring possible clues to the investigator. The researcher cultivates persistence, optimism, and patience in his long and sometimes discouraging quest. But one real 'find' spurs him on and he continues his search. Added to this skill is the training in the most meticulous recording of data with every detail complete,

and the logical classification of the data." (p. 23) ■

Analysis of Data

Analysis of data involves the synthesis of all the data collected. Data must be sifted and choices made about which to accept and which to reject. Matejski (1986) describes an investigation of Salem witches that contained a reference to *goody nurses.* One might infer that the term was a nickname or a reference to nurses. However, further investigation indicated that *goody* was short for *goodwife,* a term reserved for married women of middle social status within the Puritan community. Sometimes interesting data that do not contribute to the questions of the study are difficult to discard. Also, conflicting evidence must be reconciled. For example, if two primary sources give opposite information about an incident, the researcher will seek to interpret the differences and determine, as nearly as possible, what actually occurred.

Outcomes

Interpreting the outcomes of a historical study is influenced by the perspective of the researcher. Competing explanations can be created from the same data set. Evidence for conclusions is always partial because of missing data. Historical interpretation is not about describing the progress of events but of ascribing meaning to them. Thus, the responsibilities of interpreting historical data are great. Lynaugh and Reverby (1987, p. 4) suggest that "historical scholarship is judged on its ability to assemble the best facts and generate the most cogent explanation of a given situation or period."

Developing a Writing Outline

Before proceeding to write the research report, the researcher must decide the most appropriate means of presenting the data. Some options include a biography, a chronology, and a paper organized to focus on issues. If the outline has been well organized and detailed, the writing that follows should flow easily and smoothly.

Writing the Research Report

Historical research reports do not follow the traditional formalized style of much research. The studies are designed to attract the interest of the reader and may appear deceptively simple. The untrained eye may not recognize the extensive work required to write the paper. As explained by Christy (1975, p. 192), "The reader is never aware of the painstaking work, the careful attention to detail, nor the arduous pursuit of clues endured by the writer of history. Perhaps that is why so many nurses have failed to recognize historiography as a legitimate research endeavor. It looks so easy."

PHILOSOPHICAL STUDIES

The purpose of philosophical research is to clarify meanings, make values manifest, identify ethics, and study the nature of knowledge (Ellis, 1983). The philosophical researcher is expected to consider a philosophical question from all perspectives by examining conceptual meaning, raising further questions, proposing answers, and suggesting the implications of those answers. The data source for most philosophical studies is written materials and verbally expressed ideas relevant to the topic of interest. The researcher critically examines the text or the ideas for flaws in logic. A key element of the analysis is the posing of philosophical questions. The data are then searched for information relevant to the question. Ideas or values implied in the text are an important source of information since many philosophical analyses address very abstract topics. The researcher attempts to maintain an objective distance from perspectives in the data in order to abstractly examine the logic of the idea. Ideas, questions, answers, and consequences are often explored and/or debated with colleagues during the analysis phase.

There are three types of philosophical studies:

foundational inquiry, philosophical analyses, and ethical analyses.

Foundational Inquiries Methodology

Foundational inquiries are critical and exploratory. The researcher asks questions that reveal flaws in the logic with which the ideas of the science were developed. This may be an ambiguity, a discrepancy, or a puzzle in the way those within the science speak, think, and act. Generally, this knowledge is not seen as having logic problems by those within the science. The knowledge questioned could be in the form of ideas, concepts, facts, theories, or even various sorts of experiences and ways of doing things (Manchester, 1986). For example, one might question whether adaptation is a desired outcome of nursing action consistent with nursing's definition of health.

Outcomes

Foundational studies provide critical analyses of ideas and thought within a discipline, facilitating further development of the body of knowledge. The critique of studies within the science is guided by the outcomes of foundational studies, using the five traditional criteria for scientific thinking of accuracy, consistency, scope, simplicity, and fruitfulness (Manchester, 1986).

Example of a Foundational Study

By far the best-known foundational inquiry in nursing is Carper's (1978) study of the ways of knowing in nursing. This study was her doctoral dissertation and only a portion of it has been published. In conducting the study, Carper examined nursing textbooks and journals from 1964 to 1974. She identified four ways of knowing in nursing: empirical, esthetic, personal, and ethical.

EMPIRICAL KNOWING. Through this examination of the literature, Carper found that, beginning with the 1950s, there had been a sense of urgency regarding developing a body of empirical knowledge specific to nursing. There was no single conceptual structure with which nursing science could identify. The developing conceptual structures that did exist provided a perspective for considering the phenomena of health and illness in relation to human life processes. Carper suggested that these perspectives should be legitimized as discoveries of the discipline of nursing. Nursing science was at the stage of describing and classifying phenomena ascertainable by direct observation and inspection. However, she found increasing theoretical analysis directed toward explanations of empirical observations. She found a shift in the vocabulary of nursing from observational to theoretical, with terms that had distinct meanings and definitions within the context of explanatory theory.

ESTHETIC KNOWING. In addition to the development of empirical knowing, Carper found evidence that nursing was, in part, an art. There was a reluctance by nursing to acknowledge this esthetic way of knowing, perhaps due to efforts of nursing to move away from an apprentice-type of educational system. Carper (1978) suggested that this expressive element of nursing was essential and was reflected in the capacity for empathy. The design of nursing care, emerging from this expressive element, "must be controlled by the perception of the balance, rhythm, proportion, and unity of what is done in relation to the dynamic integration and articulation of the whole" (p. 18).

PERSONAL KNOWING. Carper considers nursing an interpersonal process, which requires that the nurse be skilled in the therapeutic use of self. This use of self requires personal knowledge, "the knowing, encountering, and actualizing of the concrete, individual self" (p. 18). From this position of knowing, the nurse stands in relation to another human being and confronts that human being as a person. It is a reciprocal relationship that cannot be described or experienced, it can only be actualized.

ETHICAL KNOWING. Nurses must make difficult personal choices within the practice of nursing. These choices raise questions about what is morally right and wrong action in connection with care. Moral dilemmas occur when the consequences of one's actions are difficult to predict. Carper (1978) suggests that the "moral code which guides the ethical conduct of nurses is based on the primary principle of obligation embodied in the concepts of service to people and respect for human life" (p. 20). This code requires an ethical way of knowing that guides the nurse in what ought to be done and includes judgments of moral value.

Philosophical Research

The primary purpose of philosophical analysis is to examine meaning and to develop theories of meaning. This is usually accomplished through concept analysis or linguistic analysis (Rodgers, 1989). Concept analyses have become common exercises for graduate nursing students, although most have not been performed using philosophical research strategies. Many of these have been published and are providing an important addition to the body of knowledge in nursing. One of the best known analyses, Smith's idea of health (1986), was performed using philosophical inquiry.

Example of Philosophical Inquiry

Smith searched the literature for fundamental concepts on the nature of health. Regardless of how health was defined, it was considered one extreme on a continuum of health and illness. Health was a relative term. A person was judged healthy when measured against some ideal of health. Who was considered healthy was based on the particular ideal of health being used. Smith identified four models (or ideals) of health: the eudaimonistic model, the adaptive model, the role-performance model, and the clinical model.

EUDAIMONISTIC MODEL. The eudaimonistic model suggests that the idea of health is associated with general well-being and self-realization. The writings of Maslow (1971) express this ideal. Thus, becoming healthy involves aspiring to achieve one's potential. Illness is any condition that impedes or prevents self-actualization. The cure of a physiological condition does not achieve health. The health extreme of the continuum is exuberant well-being. The illness extreme is enervation and languishing debility. The responsibility of the health professional is to assist the person toward self-fulfillment.

THE ADAPTIVE MODEL. The adaptive model relates health to effective interaction of an organism with the physical and social environment. The goal is adaptive behavior. Disease is a failure in adaptation, a breakdown in the capacity of the organism to cope with environmental changes. Medical treatment is directed toward restoring the ability to adapt. Even when persons are free of disease, they may not have achieved health. They may have difficulties with social functioning or be confronted with a hostile environment with which they cannot cope. The health extreme of this model is flexible adaptation. The illness extreme is alienation from the environment and failure of self-corrective measures. These ideas emerged from the writings of Dubos (1980).

ROLE-PERFORMANCE MODEL. The role-performance model, emerging from the writings of Talcott Parsons (1924) and others within medical sociology, suggests that sickness is the incapacity of a person to fulfill social roles (or do his or her job). If nothing impedes effective performance, the person is considered healthy. The relevant role seems to be the one through which the person receives income. However, a person has many roles and may experience role conflicts. The health extreme of this model is maximum performance of expected social roles. The illness extreme is failure to perform one's roles. In this model, a person could be physically ill but still able to perform social roles. From the perspective of this model, that person would be considered healthy.

THE CLINICAL MODEL. The clinical model emerged from the ideas of modern medicine. A person who consults a physician is in pain or experiencing some abnormal condition of the body or mind. The physician's response is to alleviate or eliminate the pain and free the patient of derange-

ments or malfunctioning of body organs. When relief is achieved and symptoms of disease are no longer present, the patient is restored to "health." In this model, the health extreme is the absence of signs and symptoms of disease or disability. The presence of signs and symptoms is the illness extreme.

This analysis has proven useful in exploring many issues related to nursing, including differing expectations of clients in relation to their health. An instrument has been developed to put this concept into operation, which will allow it to be examined in relation to a number of variables important to nursing (Smith, 1986).

Ethical Analysis

In ethical inquiry, the researcher identifies principles to guide conduct based on ethical theories. Problems in ethics are related to obligation, rights, duty, right and wrong, conscience, justice, choice, intention, and responsibility. Using a selected ethical theory, an analysis is performed. The actions prescribed by the analysis may vary with the ethical theory used. The ideas are submitted to colleagues for critique and debate. Conclusions are associated with rights and duties rather than preferences.

Example of Ethical Analysis

An ethical analysis of an elder's treatment is an example of ethical research (Kayser-Jones, Davis, Wiener, & Higgins, 1989). This case study was part of a 3-year project investigating the sociocultural factors likely to influence the evaluation and treatment of nursing home residents.

"Three research strategies were used to obtain data: participant observation; extensive interviews with nursing home residents, their families, nursing staff, and physicians (100 in each category); and event analysis. During the course of one year we followed 215 residents who developed an acute illness, describing in detail their treatment and the management of their care.

Mrs. M., an 85-year-old widow who had Alzheimer's disease and arthritis, had been in the nursing home for four years. Despite the diagnosis of Alzheimer's disease, she was socially active and functionally independent. She participated in social activities, enjoyed outings, and had developed a close friendship with a male resident. Mrs. M. was ambulatory, needed minimal assistance with her care, could converse with others, and was alert but confused at times. Her only relative, a son, lived in a nearby suburb.

On a Saturday morning, Mrs. M.'s condition suddenly changed. She complained of a sore throat. It was difficult for her to talk and swallow, and she could take only a small amount of food and liquids. The nurse called the physician to notify him of Mrs. M.'s condition, including her fever of 37.8°C (100°F) rectally. The physician prescribed oral erythromycin, 250 mg. four times a day for 6 days and Tylenol, gr. 10, every 4 hours for a fever of 37.8°C (100°F) and above." (p. 267)

"On Sunday morning, Mrs. M. refused breakfast and medications, saying she could not swallow; her temperature was 38.9°C (102°F). The physician was called. He advised the nurses to encourage her to drink, and said he would visit Mrs. M. the following day. By Sunday evening, Mrs. M. was restless; her chest was congested, and she refused all food. The nurses called the physician, who ordered her transferred to an acute hospital. Five minutes later he canceled the transfer, saying the family did not agree to the move.

By Monday, Mrs. M. was short of breath. The physician visited for the first time on Tuesday. The family was notified of her condition. On Wednesday, purulent secretions were draining from Mrs. M.'s mouth. The physician, called again by the nurses, stated that the family did not want any 'heroic measures.' On Thursday, the nurses notified the physician that Mrs. M. could not swallow her antibiotic. He prescribed penicillin by injection.

On Wednesday evening, a research assistant, who was a doctoral nursing student, learned of Mrs. M.'s condition. On visiting her, she found her in a septic condition. When she asked why intravenous fluids had not been started for hydration and antibiotics, she was told that the family did not want 'heroic measures.' The research assistant called the principal investigator, who visited on Thursday morning. 'At this time Mrs. M. did not respond to verbal stimuli, the right side of her face was swollen, and she appeared to be in pain.' Mrs. M. died on Friday.

Following the patient's death, the nursing staff, the physician, and Mrs. M.'s son were interviewed. When interviewing the staff development nurse (SDN), we learned that Thursday, the day before Mrs. M. died, the administrator, the DNS, the social worker, and the SDN held a conference. According to the SDN, she and the social worker expressed concern that not enough was being done for the patient, but the DNS was primarily concerned about the possibility of litigation, and remarked, 'We don't have to worry about this patient. The family does not care for her. The family is not going to sue us.' At one point the DNS reportedly said, 'Look, my God, this patient is almost 90. It is time for her to die.'

The SDN confided that she was upset when she saw Mrs. M.'s condition on Friday, the day she died. Mrs. M. was clearly in pain; she was moaning and lay in a fetal position. She had not received any morphine sulfate since it had been prescribed, six days earlier. The SDN was horrified to find Mrs. M. lying in a pool of urine. Further, she apparently had not received mouth care; purulent, bloody secretions were draining from her dry, encrusted mouth.

When interviewed, the physician said he had thought the patient had parotitis and initially believed she should be transferred. He spoke with the son, however, who said that his mother no longer recognized him, that she was 'just sort of existing,' and that there was 'nothing to save.' " (p. 268) ∎

Using this information, the ethics of the case were analyzed. There are two ethical principles of interest in this case: nonmaleficence and beneficence (doing good). Nonmaleficence is the most basic duty and means that above all we do no harm. "Harm can be defined in several ways, but usually means physical damage, including pain, disability, and death. Specifically, the emphasis here focuses on intending, causing, or permitting death; or creating the risk of death. Nonmaleficence also requires that we act in a thoughtful, careful manner;

harm or risk of harm is not always intentional" (Kayser-Jones, et al., 1989, p. 269).

The ethical questions posed for analysis included:

1. Did she receive reasonable care?
2. Was the duty of care met?
3. Did she receive the care that an ordinary, prudent person would provide under the same conditions?
4. Was harm done?

The first step of the analysis is to review the literature for relevant facts. Mrs. M. falls into a vulnerable category—elderly, institutionalized, mentally impaired, and as such devalued by society. When a person is devalued, we may act toward them in unethical ways and thus do harm. In addition, a person in a health care facility has a basic right to adequate care.

From this examination, further questions arise. The son did not want heroic measures. But what is meant by heroic measures and who is to define them? Can antibiotics be thought of as a heroic measure? Can not giving antibiotics be justified in this case? Is harm being done by giving antibiotics or by not giving antibiotics? The nurses accepted the physician's prescription of oral antibiotics knowing that the patient could not swallow, so that the patient's infection was not treated for five days. Are these nursing actions in line with the son's request for no heroics? Are these nursing actions in the best interest of the patient? What constitutes the best interest of Mrs. M.? Was this lack of treatment a harm to Mrs. M.? In addition to the patient's right to basic care, there is a question of relief of her pain. No pain medication was administered until the day she died.

■

Conclusions

"The principal variables at play in the course of events seem to be the patient's age, the inability to make her wishes known, her mental status, the family's desire for no heroics, and the lack of re-

sponsibility for care on the part of physicians and nurses. . . .

The argument can be made that this woman was allowed to die, not because her life was meaningless, albeit not as meaningful as a younger noninstitutionalized person's, but because the nurses and physician confused heroics with reasonable therapeutic care. . . ." (p. 269)

"The medical decision to limit treatment does not relieve the nursing staff of its obligation to provide adequate nursing care; it does introduce the possibility of abandonment. . . .

There is, therefore, no ethical justification for not providing nursing care to a patient in this setting. Do no harm, as an ethical principle, can come to mean that we either overtreat or do not treat when we should. But treatment is not at issue here; the issue is nursing care. One response to this question of providing basic nursing care may be that professional nurses themselves usually do not give this care, auxiliary personnel do. But this does not ethically justify what happened to Mrs. M. The professional nurse is responsible for the quality of care, and when she does not assume this responsibility, the potential for doing harm exists.

Allowing a reason such as not being sued to be the only guide for action is unprofessional. Such reasoning can lead us to be self-serving instead of putting the patient at the center of our professional actions.

The nursing care provided Mrs. M. was not of an acceptable standard, and the nurses' behavior suggests that they did not care for the patient. Caring calls for a philosophy of moral commitment to protect human dignity and preserve humanity, and for an underlying moral commitment to care, a will to care, and actions based on knowledge." (p. 270) ■

Critical Social Theory Methodology

The research process of critical social theory requires using oppositional thinking to perform a critique of the social situation under study, using the following four steps: (1) critically examining the implicit rules and assumptions of the situation under study in a historical, cultural, and political context; (2) using reflection to identify the conditions that would make uncoerced knowledge and action possible; (3) analyzing the constraints on communication and human action to develop a theoretical framework that uses causal relationships to explain distortions of communications and repression. The theoretical framework is then tested against individual cases (Hedin, 1986). The researcher then (4) participates in dialogue with those oppressed individuals within the social situation. Dialogue leads to collective consciousness raising and identification of ways to take action against oppressive forces. The action for change must come from the groups and communities rather than the researcher. The groups and communities must consider "(a) their common interests; (b) the risks they are willing to undergo; (c) the consequences they can expect; and (d) their knowledge of the circumstances of their own lives" (Hedin, 1986, p. 146).

As with most qualitative research methodologies, it is difficult to separate the steps. Dialogue is used both to collect and to interpret the data, and there is a constant movement back and forth between collection and interpretation. Dialogue, which uses some of the techniques of phenomenology, includes conversations between the researcher and persons within the society, and requires a relationship of equality and active reciprocity. In addition, the researcher dialogues with the data while collecting, analyzing, and interpreting it, using reflection and insight. "New meanings emerge, and phrases that have always been ignored suddenly come alive and demand explanation" (Thompson, 1987, p. 33). The process "exposes ways in which the self has been formed (or deformed) through the influence of coercive power relations. The work of critical scholarship is to make these power relations transparent, for these relations lose power when they become transparent" (Thompson, 1987, p. 33). Knowledge is created which furthers autonomy and responsibility by enlightening individuals about how they may rationally act to realize their own best interests (Holter, 1988).

Example of Critical Social Theory (Feminist) Study

Stevens (1995) conducted a study examining the structural and interpersonal impact of hetero-

sexual assumptions on lesbian health care clients. "In this feminist narrative study using in-depth interviews and focus groups, a racially and economically diverse sample of 45 lesbians describe their access to and experience with health care" (p. 25). Stevens describes the problem as follows.

"The existence of lesbians calls into question the universality of normative societal ideology about women. Many of society's institutions are based on heterosexual assumptions that reinforce the gender division of labor, sustain the secondary status of women wage earners, compel women's economic and emotional dependence on men, and confine women's identity to narrowly configured roles within traditional nuclear families (Allen, 1986; Jaggar, 1988; Rich, 1980). . . . Limited investigatory attention has been paid to the structural environments and interactional conditions in health that may act as barriers to help seeking by lesbian clients (Stevens, 1992b). Empirical efforts have generally focused on understanding the processes of how lesbians 'come out' (inform others that they are lesbian) in health care contexts (Hitchcock & Wilson, 1992; Smith, Johnson, & Guenther, 1985; Stevens & Hall, 1988). These projects have also documented the risks entailed by such actions. Disclosure of lesbian identity is known to evoke a wide array of reactions from health care providers, ranging from embarrassment to overt hostility. Reported responses include fear, ostracism, refusal to treat, cool detachment, shock, pity, voyeuristic curiosity, demeaning jokes, avoidance of physical contact, insults, invasions of privacy, rough physical handling, and breaches of confidentiality." (Stevens, 1992a) ∎

The feminist narrative study was designed to examine how lesbians experience clinical encounters. Stevens poses two research questions:

1. How do health care structures (i.e., economic, political, and social environments) affect lesbians' access to health care?
2. How do interpersonal interactions with health care providers affect lesbians' access to health care?

The sample was obtained through community-based snowball sampling. Informed consent was obtained from all subjects. Data collection involved open-ended, in-depth interviews and focus groups designed to elicit stories about health care experiences. The stories were invited with the question "What has it been like for you to get health care? I would like to hear about health care that has not gone so well." Probes and reflective statements were used to encourage experiential specificity. Interviews lasted about 2 hours. Focus groups lasted about 3 hours.

■

"All interviews and focus groups were audiotaped, as were field notes documenting environmental circumstances, participant characteristics, nonverbal behaviors, affect, communication processes, rapport, power dynamics, impressions, and any problems. (Briggs, 1986; Mishler, 1986)

Audiotapes of individual interviews, focus groups, and field notes were transcribed to create a textual database. Adherence to standards of rigor in feminist interpretive research, including dependability, reflexivity, credibility, coherence, consensus, and complexity (Hall & Stevens, 1991) supported the scientific adequacy of the project.

A multistaged narrative analysis was devised to explore the macrolevel and microlevel conditions uniquely faced by lesbians in obtaining health care. In the first stage, the boundaries of each data-based story were demarcated (Bell, 1988). The story was operationalized as the relating of a single interactional encounter in health care. To designate text as story, specific elements were necessary, including orientation, plot, evaluation, and resolution (Labov & Waletzky, 1967). In the process, 332 health care stories were identified and became the units of analyses. In stage two, story events and participants' interpretations of them were analyzed. An adequate paraphrase (Polanyi, 1985) of each story was constructed to highlight the structural and interpersonal contexts in which actions occurred. The third stage involved searching for story similarities and differences among individual participants and among ethnic/racial, socio-economic, and health status subgroups in the sample. While distinguishing the diversity of health care circumstances and meanings across the differently situated individuals in the study (Potter & Wetherell, 1987), patterns of shared experience were identified (Richardson, 1988).

In the fourth stage, health care narratives were analyzed in their entirety. Narrative was operationalized as the whole scheme of stories an individual woman related about her health care experiences. All of the health care stories told by each individual were taken into account to determine the pattern of structural environments and interpersonal interactions faced by each participant over time. Individual patterns were compared to analyze variability and identify larger patterns that represented the experiences of the entire sample.

Narrative analysis revealed that at the macrolevel, heterosexist structuring of health care delivery was obstructive to lesbians' seeking health care, their knowledge about health, and their behaviors. At the micro, or individual level, health care providers' heterosexual assumptions competed against potentially supportive interactions with lesbian clients.

A major constraint that disrupted lesbians' attempts to obtain health care was the heterosexist structuring of delivery systems. Heterosexist structuring meant that health care services were designed and distributed with the operating premise that heterosexuality is universal, superior, natural, and/or required for women. It seemed to participants that clinical and health education practices and policies were constructed around the unquestioned assumptions that all female clients are heterosexual and that women's health needs are primarily reproductive in nature. They pointed out how preventive services for women are located almost exclusively in birth control and obstetrical clinics and outreach to lesbian communities is largely nonexistent, leaving lesbians invisible, uninformed, and alienated from the health care process." (p. 26)

"Social and political environments in which health care was delivered also betrayed the heterosexism. Bias was apparent in written forms, health brochures and posters, and comments by auxiliary staff. It existed in advertisements for clientele, reading materials in the waiting rooms, and pictures on the walls. For instance, participants described how intake forms routinely require women to identify themselves as married, divorced, widowed, or single and go on to ask about spouse's income, occupation, health insurance, and where he can be reached. Inquiries about partnership status as it related to heterosexual marriage, and opportunities to provide information about one's significant other only through questions about husbands' activities, leave lesbians without the option to communicate their own circumstances." (p. 27)

The following quote illustrates some of the problems lesbians encounter in seeking health care:

"Every time I went to the HMO, I was asked the same questions about birth control. They wouldn't let up when I said, no, I didn't need birth control. So, sometimes I would come out as a lesbian, just to get them to move on to other things. The doctors would fumble around and say something like, 'Oh . . . uh . . . I'm sorry.' It was so awkward. I hadn't given them the responses they were expecting, so then they were not prepared with any follow-up questions.

There are questions providers should be asking us when they are taking our histories. But if their standard questions no longer fit once we say we are lesbian, they just stop the assessment cold. They simply skip the next 15 questions because they don't apply. But they don't have an alternate set of questions." (p. 28) ■

CONTENT ANALYSIS

Content analysis is designed to classify the words in a text into a few categories chosen because of their theoretical importance. Because content analysis uses counting, it is not considered a qualitative analysis technique by many qualitative researchers. Content analysis is frequently used in historical research. It is the primary approach to analysis used by Kalisch, Kalisch, and colleagues (1977, 1982, 1983, 1985) in their series of studies examining the image of nursing as reflected in news media and prime-time television.

The technique provides a systematic means of measuring the frequency, order, or intensity of occurrence of words, phrases, or sentences. Initially, the specific characteristics of the content to be

measured must be defined, then rules are developed by the researcher for identifying and recording these characteristics. The researcher first selects a specific unit of analysis, which may be individual words, word combinations, or themes. This unit of analysis is considered a symbolic entity and is often an indicator of an abstract concept.

To perform content analysis, text is divided into units of meaning (idea categories). These units are then quantified according to specific rules. The construction of idea categories and the selection of words considered representative of these idea categories is a crucial phase of content analysis. In more complex studies, more than one categorizing scheme may be used. One common approach to categorization is the use of a dictionary to identify terms and delineate their meaning (Kelly & Sime, 1990).

In some studies, the researcher is searching for latent meaning within the text. In these studies, the text cannot be analyzed using direct observation or identification of specific terms. Meaning may have to be inferred by more indirect means. The researcher may be looking for relationships among ideas, reality, and language (Kelly & Sime, 1990).

Brennan, Moore, and Smyth (1995) used content analysis as a component of their study of the effects of a special computer network on caregivers of persons with Alzheimer's disease (AD). Caregivers could access ComputerLink 24 hours a day at no charge. Special keys on the terminal keyboard were programmed to allow caregivers to connect easily with the central computer. ComputerLink provided three functions to caregivers: information, decision support, and communication. Communication included private mail, a public bulletin board known as the Forum, and an anonymous question and answer segment. During a 1-year study period, AD caregivers averaged two encounters per week with ComputerLink for sessions lasting an average of 13 minutes.

"Caregivers accessed the functions of the communications area most often and spent more time in this feature than in any other. They used the Forum more extensively than they used the private mail features. Caregiver behavior in the communication function included reading messages of others and posting messages to others; posting outnumbered reading by greater than 5 to 1." (p. 170)

"A content analysis of the 622 messages posted by the caregivers on the Forum was completed using a categorization designed by Toseland and Rossiter (1989) in their review of

themes present in support groups for caregivers of older persons with dementia. The frequency of these themes in the ComputerLink messages was as follows: group and its members as a mutual support group system (37%); information about the care recipient's situation (24%); emotional impact of caregiving (19%); development and use of support systems outside the group (13%); problematic interpersonal relationships (4%); self-care (3%); and home-care skills (2%)." (p. 170) ■

■ SUMMARY

Qualitative data analysis occurs concurrently with data collection rather than sequentially as is true in quantitative research. Therefore, the researcher is attempting simultaneously to gather the data, manage a growing bulk of collected data, and interpret the meaning of the data. Qualitative analysis techniques use words rather than numbers as the basis of analysis. However, the same careful skills in analytic reasoning are needed by the qualitative researcher as those required by quantitative analysis.

The computer can make analysis of qualitative data much quicker and easier without the researcher losing touch with the data. The computer offers assistance in such activities as processing, storage, retrieval, cataloging, and sorting, and leaves the analysis activities up to the researcher. A number of computer programs have been developed specifically to perform qualitative analyses.

The credibility of qualitative data analysis has been seriously questioned in some cases by the larger scientific community. The concerns expressed are related to the inability to replicate the outcomes of a study. To respond to this concern, some qualitative researchers have attempted to develop strategies by which other researchers, using the same data, can follow the logic of the original researcher and

arrive at the same conclusions. This strategy is referred to as a decision trail.

Some studies are appearing in the literature in which the researchers have combined portions of various qualitative methodologies extracted from the philosophical bases for which the methodologies were developed. This violates the assumptions of the methodologies. It is essential that the researcher make the philosophical base of the study explicit and that methodologies used be compatible with the philosophical base.

Because data collection is occurring simultaneously with data analysis, the process is complex. The procedure of collecting data is not a mechanical process that can be carefully planned prior to initiation. The researcher as a whole person is totally involved. One of the important differences between quantitative and qualitative research is the nature of relationships between the researcher and the individuals being studied. The nature of these relationships has an impact on the data collected and their interpretation. In varying degrees, the researcher influences the individuals being studied and, in turn, is influenced by them.

In the initial phases of data analysis, the researcher needs to become very familiar with the data that are gathered. This may involve reading and rereading notes and transcripts,

continued

continued

recalling observations and experiences, listening to tapes, and viewing videotapes until the researcher becomes immersed in the data. Initial efforts at analysis focus on reducing the volume of data to facilitate examination. During data reduction, you begin attaching meaning to elements in the data. Coding is a means of categorizing. A code is a symbol or abbreviation used to classify words or phrases in the data. As the study progresses, relationships among categories, participants, actions, and events will begin to emerge.

Displays contain highly condensed versions of the outcomes of qualitative research. They are equivalent to the summary tables of statistical outcomes developed in quantitative research. The last stage of qualitative analysis is drawing and verifying conclusions. These steps result in a gradual move from empirical data to a conceptual overview of the findings.

The research methodologies of six approaches to qualitative research are discussed. A detailed presentation of a nursing study is used as an example of each approach. In addition, content analysis, an analysis strategy used by some of the qualitative methodologies, is described. Content analysis is designed to classify the words in a text into a few categories chosen because of their theoretical importance. The technique provides a systematic means of measuring the frequency, order, or intensity of occurrence of words, phrases, or sentences.

References

Allen, D. G. (1986). Professionalism, occupational segregation by gender and control of nursing. *Women and Politics, 6*(3), 1–24.

Anderson, N. L. R. (1987a). Computer applications for qualitative analysis. *Western Journal of Nursing Research, 9*(3), 408–411.

Anderson, N. L. R. (1987b). Computer-assisted analysis of textual field note data. *Western Journal of Nursing Research, 9*(4), 626–630.

Beck, C. T. (1994). Phenomenology: Its use in nursing research. *International Journal of Nursing Studies, 31*(6), 499–510.

Bell, S. E. (1988). Becoming a political woman: The reconstruction and interpretation of experience through stories. In A. D. Todd & S. Fisher (Eds.), *Gender and discourse: The power of talk* (pp. 97–123). Norwood, NJ: Ablex.

Benner, P. (1984). *From novice to expert: Excellence and power in clinical nursing practice.* Menlo Park, CA: Addison-Wesley.

Brennan, P. F., Moore, S. M., & Smyth, K. A. (1995). The effects of a special computer network on caregivers of persons with Alzheimer's disease. *Nursing Research, 44*(3), 166–172.

Briggs, C. L. (1986). *Learning how to ask: A socio-linguistic appraisal of the role of the interview in social science research.* Cambridge, MA: Cambridge University Press.

Brykczynski, K. (1989). An interpretive study describing the clinical judgement of nurse practitioners. *Scholarly Inquiry for Nursing Practice, 3*(2), 75–104.

Burns, N. (1989). Standards for qualitative research. *Nursing Science Quarterly, 2*(1), 44–52.

Carper, B. (1978). Fundamental patterns of knowing in nursing. *Advances in Nursing Science, 1*(1), 13–24.

Christy, T. E. (1975). The methodology of historical research: A brief introduction. *Nursing Research, 24*(3), 189–192.

Christy, T. E. (1978). The hope of history. In M. L. Fitzpatrick (Ed.), *Historical studies in nursing* (pp. 3–11). New York: Teachers College.

Cohen, M. Z., & Loomis, M. E. (1985). Linguistic analysis of questionnaire responses: Methods of coping with work stress. *Western Journal of Nursing Research, 7*(3), 357–366.

Colaizzi, P. (1978). Psychological research as the phenomenologist views it. In R. S. Valle & M. King (Eds.), *Existential phenomenological alternatives for psychology* (pp. 48–71). New York: Oxford University.

Connors, D. D. (1988). A continuum of researcher-participant relationships: An analysis and critique. *Advances in Nursing Science, 10*(4), 32–42.

Cooper, M. C. (1988). Covenantal relationships: Grounding for the nursing ethic. *Advances in Nursing Science, 10*(4), 48–59.

Cowles, K. V. (1988). Issues in qualitative research on sensitive topics. *Western Journal of Nursing Research, 10*(2), 163–179.

Drew, N. (1989). The interviewer's experience as data in phenomenological research. *Western Journal of Nursing Research, 11*(4), 431–439.

Dubos, R. L. (1980). *Man adapting.* New Haven, CT: Yale University Press.

Ellis, R. (1983). Philosophic inquiry. In H. H. Werley & J. J. Fitzpatrick (Eds.), *Annual review of nursing research* (Vol. I, pp. 211–228). New York: Springer.

Engel, G. L. (1977). The need for a new medical model: A challenge for biomedicine. *Science, 196*(4286), 129–136.

Fagerhaugh, S., & Strauss, A. (1977). *Politics of pain management: Staff-patient interaction.* Menlo Park, CA: Addison-Wesley.

Field, P. A., & Morse, J. M. (1985). *Nursing research: The application of qualitative approaches.* Rockville, MD: Aspen.

Fisher, S. (1986). *In the patient's best interest.* New Brunswick, NJ: Rutgers University Press.

Fisher, S., & Todd, A. D. (Eds.). (1983). *The social organization of doctor-patient communication.* Washington, DC: Center for Applied Linguistics.

Fowler, M. D. M. (1988). Issues in qualitative research. *Western Journal of Nursing Research, 10*(1), 109–111.

Germain, C. P. H. (1986). Ethnography: The method. In P. L. Munhall & C. J. Oiler (Eds.), *Nursing research: A qualitative perspective* (pp. 147–162). Norwalk, CT: Appleton-Century-Crofts.

Giorgi, A. (1970). *Psychology as a human science: A phenomenologically based approach.* New York: Harper & Row.

Glaser, B. G. (1973). *Ward four hundred two.* New York: George Braziller.

Glaser, B. G., & Strauss, A. (1965). *Awareness of dying.* Chicago: Aldine.

Glaser, B. G., & Strauss, A. (1968). *Time for dying.* Chicago: Aldine.

Guba, E. G., & Lincoln, Y. S. (1982). *Effective evaluation.* Washington, DC: Jossey-Bass.

Hall, J. M., & Stevens, P. E. (1991). Rigor in feminist research. *Advances in Nursing Science, 13*(3), 16–29.

Halliday, M. A. K., & Hasan, R. (1976). *Cohesion in English.* London: Longman.

Hedin, B. A. (1986). Nursing, education, and emancipation: Applying the critical theoretical approach to nursing research. In P. L. Chinn (Ed.), *Nursing research methodology: Issues and implementation* (pp. 133–146). Rockville, MD: Aspen.

Henderson, V. (1964). The nature of nursing. *American Journal of Nursing, 64,* 62–68.

Hitchcock, J. M., & Wilson, H. S. (1992). Personal risking: Lesbian self-disclosure of sexual orientation to professional health care providers. *Nursing Research, 41*(3), 178–183.

Holter, I. M. (1988). Critical theory: A foundation for the development of nursing theories. *Scholarly Inquiry for Nursing Practice: An International Journal, 2*(3), 223–232.

Jaggar, A. M. (1988). *Feminist politics and human nature.* Sussex, England: Rowman & Littlefield.

Johnson, R. (1993). Nurse practitioner-patient discourse: Uncovering the voice of nursing in primary care practice. *Scholarly Inquiry for Nursing Practice: An International Journal, 7*(3), 143–157.

Kalisch, B. J., & Kalisch, P. A. (1977). An analysis of the sources of physician-nurse conflict. *Journal of Nursing Administration, 7*(1), 50–57.

Kalisch, B. J., Kalisch, P. A., & Belcher, B. (1985). Forecasting for nursing policy: A news-based image approach. *Nursing Research, 34*(1), 44–49.

Kalisch, B. J., Kalisch, P. A., & Young, R. L. (1983). Television news coverage of nurse strikes: A resource management perspective. *Nursing Research, 32*(3), 175–180.

Kalisch, P. A., Kalisch, B. J., & Clinton, J. (1982). The world of nursing on prime time television, 1950 to 1980. *Nursing Research, 31*(6), 358–363.

Kauffman, K. S. (1994). The insider/outsider dilemma: Field experience of a white researcher "getting in" a poor black community. *Nursing Research, 43*(3), 179–183.

Kayser-Jones, J., Davis, A., Wiener, C. L., & Higgins, S. S. (1989). An ethical analysis of an elder's treatment. *Nursing Outlook, 37*(6), 267–270.

Kelly, A. W., & Sime, A. M. (1990). Language as research data: Application of computer content analysis in nursing research. *Advances in Nursing Science, 12*(3), 32–40.

Knafl, K. A., & Howard, M. J. (1984). Interpreting and reporting qualitative research. *Research in Nursing & Health, 7*(1), 17–24.

Knafl, K. A., & Webster, D. C. (1988). Managing and analyzing qualitative data: A description of tasks, techniques, and materials. *Western Journal of Nursing Research, 10*(2), 195–218.

Labov, W., & Waletzky, J. (1967). Narrative analysis: Oral versions of personal experience. In J. Helm (Ed.), *Essays on the verbal and visual arts: Proceedings of the 1966 annual spring meeting of the American Ethnological Society* (pp. 12–44). Seattle: University of Washington Press.

Lamb, G. S., & Huttlinger, K. (1989). Reflexivity in nursing research. *Western Journal of Nursing Research, 11*(6), 765–772.

Lynaugh, J., & Bates, B. (1973). The two languages of nursing and medicine. *American Journal of Nursing, 73*(1), 66–69.

Lynaugh, J., & Reverby, S. (1987). Thoughts on the nature of history. *Nursing Research, 36*(1), 4, 69.

Manchester, P. (1986). Analytic philosophy and foundational inquiry: The method. In P. L. Munhall & C. J. Oiler (Eds.), *Nursing research: A qualitative perspective* (pp. 229–249). Norwalk, CT: Appleton-Century-Crofts.

Marsh, G. W. (1990). Refining an emergent life-style—Change theory through matrix analysis. *Advances in Nursing Science, 12*(3), 41–52.

Marshall, C. (1984). Elites, bureaucrats, ostriches, and pussycats: Managing research in policy settings. *Anthropology and Education Quarterly, 15*(3), 235–251.

Marshall, C. (1985). Appropriate criteria of trustworthiness and goodness for qualitative research on education organizations. *Quality and Quantity, 19*(4), 353–373.

Marshall, C., & Rossman, G. B. (1989). *Designing qualitative research.* Newbury Park, CA: Sage.

Maslow, A. (1971). *The farther reaches of human nature.* New York: Viking Press.

Matejski, M. (1986). Historical research: The method. In P. L. Munhall & C. J. Oiler (Eds.), *Nursing research: A qualitative perspective* (pp. 175–193). Norwalk, CT: Appleton-Century-Crofts.

Miles, M. B., & Huberman, A. M. (1994). *Qualitative data analysis: A sourcebook of new methods.* (2nd ed.) Beverly Hills, CA: Sage.

Mishler, E. G. (1984). *The discourse of medicine: Dialectics of medical interviews.* Norwood, NJ: Ablex Publishing.

Mishler, E. G. (1986). *Research interviewing: Context and narrative.* Cambridge, MA: Harvard University Press.

Morse, J. M. (1989). Qualitative nursing research: A free-for-all? In J. M. Morse (Ed.), *Qualitative nursing research: A contemporary dialogue.* Rockville, MD: Aspen.

Morse, J. M., & Morse, R. M. (1989). QUAL: A mainframe program for qualitative data analysis. *Nursing Research, 38*(3), 188–189.

Munhall, P. L. (1988). Ethical considerations in qualitative research. *Western Journal of Nursing Research, 10*(2), 150–162.

Murdock, G. (1971). *Outline of cultural materials.* New Haven, CT: Human Relation Area Files Press.

Newton, M. E. (1965). The case for historical research. *Nursing Research, 14*(1), 20–26.

Nightingale, F. (1860). *Notes on nursing: What it is, what it is not.* New York: Appleton.

Oiler, C. (1982). The phenomenological approach in nursing research. *Nursing Research, 31*(3), 178–181.

Pallikkathayil, L., & Morgan, S. A. (1991). Phenomenology as a method for conducting clinical research. *Nursing Research, 4*(4), 195–200.

Parsons, J. (1964). *Social structure and personality.* New York: Free Press of Glencoe.

Parse, R. R. (1990). Health: A personal commitment. *Nursing Science Quarterly, 3*(3), 136–140.

Podolefsky, A., & McCarty, C. (1983). Topical sorting: A technique for computer assisted qualitative data analysis. *American Anthropologist, 85*(4), 886–890.

Polanyi, L. (1985). *Telling the American story: A structural and cultural analysis of conversational storytelling.* Norwood, NJ: Ablex.

Potter, J., & Wetherrell, M. (1987). *Discourse and social psychology: Beyond attitudes and behaviors.* Beverly Hills, CA: Sage.

Rich, A. (1980). Compulsory heterosexuality and lesbian existence. *Signs: Journal of Women in Culture and Society, 5*(4), 631–660.

Richardson, L. (1988). The collective story: Postmodernism and the writing of sociology. *Sociological Focus, 21*(3), 199–208.

Robinson, C. A., & Thorne, S. E. (1988). Dilemmas of ethics and validity in qualitative nursing research. *Canadian Journal of Nursing Research, 20*(1), 65–76.

Rodgers, B. L. (1989). Concepts, analysis and the development of nursing knowledge: The evolutionary cycle. *Journal of Advanced Nursing, 14*(4), 330–335.

Ruffing-Rahal, M. A. (1986). Personal documents and nursing theory development. *Advances in Nursing Science, 8*(3), 50–57.

Sandelowski, M. (1994). Notes on transcription. *Research in Nursing & Health, 17*(4), 311–314.

Sandelowski, M. (1995a). On the aesthetics of qualitative research. *Image: Journal of Nursing Scholarship, 27*(3), 205–209.

Sandelowski, M. (1995b). Qualitative analysis: What it is and how to begin. *Research in Nursing & Health, 18*(4), 371–375.

Smith, E. M., Johnson, S. R., & Guenther, S. M. (1985). Health care attitudes and experiences during gynecological care among lesbians and bisexuals. *American Journal of Public Health, 75*(9), 1085–1087.

Smith, J. A. (1986). The idea of health: Doing foundational inquiry. In P. L. Munhall & C. J. Oiler (Eds.), *Nursing research: A qualitative perspective* (pp. 251–262). Norwalk, CT: Appleton-Century-Crofts.

Stern, P. N. (1980). Grounded theory methodology: Its uses and processes. *Image: Journal of Nursing Scholarship, 12*(1), 20–23.

Stevens, P. E. (1992a). Lesbian health care research: A review of the literature from 1970 to 1990. *Health Care for Women International, 13,* 91–120.

Stevens, P. E. (1992b). Who gets care? Access to health care as an arena for nursing action. *Scholarly Inquiry for Nursing Practice: An International Journal, 6*(3), 185–200.

Stevens, P. E. (1995). Structural and interpersonal impact of heterosexual assumptions on lesbian health care clients. *Nursing Research, 44*(1), 25–30.

Stevens, P. E., & Hall, J. M. (1988). Stigma, health beliefs, and experiences with health care in lesbian women. *Image: Journal of Nursing Scholarship, 20*(2), 69–73.

Strauss, A. L. (1975). *Chronic illness and quality of life.* St. Louis: Mosby.

Strauss, A. L., Corbin, J., Fagerhaugh, S., Glaser, B. G., Maines, D., Suczek, B., & Wiener, C. L. (1984). *Chronic illness and the quality of life* (2nd ed.). St. Louis: Mosby.

Strauss, A. L., & Glaser, B. G. (1970). *Anguish.* Mill Valley, CA: Sociology Press.

Taft, L. B. (1993). Computer-assisted qualitative research. *Research in Nursing & Health, 16*(5), 379–383.

Thompson, J. L. (1987). Critical scholarship: The critique of domination in nursing. *Advances in Nursing Science, 10*(1), 27–38.

Todd, A. D. (1989). *Intimate adversaries: Cultural conflict between doctor and women patients.* Philadelphia: University of Pennsylvania Press.

Toseland, R. W., & Rossiter, C. M. (1989). Group interventions to support family caregivers: A review and analysis. *The Gerontologist, 29*(4), 438–477.

Turner, B. (1981). Some practical aspects of qualitative data analysis: One way of organizing the cognitive processes associated with the generation of grounded theory. *Quality and Quantity, 15*(3), 225–247.

Van Kaam, A. L. (1966). *Existential foundations of psychology* (Vol. 3). Pittsburgh: Duquesne University.

Watson, J. (1985). *Nursing: Human science & human care.* Norwalk, CT: Appleton.

Weitzman, E. A., & Miles, M. B. (1995). *A software sourcebook: Computer programs for qualitative data analysis.* Thousand Oaks, CA: Sage.

West, C. (1984). *Routine complications: Troubles with talk between doctors and patients.* Bloomington: Indiana University Press.

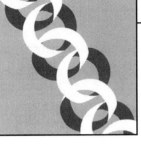

21

Outcomes Research

A new paradigm for research is emerging in health care called *outcomes research,* with a focus on the end-results of patient care. The momentum propelling outcomes research is coming from policymakers, insurers, and the public. There is a growing demand that providers justify interventions and systems of care in terms of improved patient lives and that costs of care be considered in evaluating treatment outcomes (Hinshaw, 1992). The strategies used in outcomes research are, to some extent, a departure from the accepted scientific methodology for health care research and incorporate evaluation methods, epidemiology, and economic theory.

This chapter includes a brief history of endeavors to examine outcomes, outcomes research and nursing practice, the theoretical basis of outcomes research, and methodologies used in outcomes research. A broad base of literature from a variety of disciplines was used to develop the content for this chapter, in keeping with the multidisciplinary perspective of outcomes research.

A BRIEF HISTORY OF OUTCOMES RESEARCH

PROMINENT FIGURES IN HISTORY

Sir William Petty (1623–1687) was the first physician to question the effectiveness of medical care (at least, in writing). Sir Petty was also a professor at Oxford and an economist. He is considered by many to be the father of economics and epidemiology. He influenced public policy through his writing and challenged the Royal College of Physi-

cians by asking the following questions about the medical practice of the time.

"Whether they take as much medicine and remedies as the like number of men of other societyes.

"Whether of 1,000 patients to the best physicians, aged of any decad, there do not dye as many as out (of) the inhabitants of places where there dwell no physicians.

"Whether of 100 sick of acute diseases who use physicians, as many dye and (in) misery, as where no art is used, or only chance." (Petty, as cited in White, 1993, p. 12) ∎

In the eighteenth century, French statisticians developed methods of examining the effectiveness of medical interventions. These statistical methods were applied by a French physician, Louis (1787–1872), to clinical data. Using his *numerical method,* Louis demonstrated the uselessness and often harmfulness of bloodletting. The following quote from his writing illustrates his approach to examining medical practice.

"In any epidemic . . . let us suppose 500 of the sick, *taken indiscriminately,* to be subjected to one kind of treatment, and 500 others, taken in the same manner, to be treated in a different mode; if the mortality is greater among the first, than among the second, must we not conclude that the treatment was less appropriate or less efficacious in the first class, than in the second? . . . (I)t is impossible to appreciate each case with mathematical exactness, and it is precisely on this account that enumeration becomes necessary; by so doing the errors (which are inevitable) being the same in both groups of patients subjected to different treatment, mutually compensate each other, and they may be disregarded without sensibly affecting the exactness of the results." (Louis, as cited in White, 1993, p. 12) ■

Louis's approach angered the physicians of his period, who believed that their own personal experience was sufficient to provide understanding of origins, diagnosis, treatment, and outcomes of disease. However, he continued to teach his medical students to critically appraise the effectiveness of their practice. A number of American physicians traveled to Paris for postgraduate studies with Louis, among them Oliver Wendell Holmes (1809–1894), who later made himself unpopular with practicing physicians in America with his observations on the causes of puerperal fever (White, 1993).

Semmelweiss, a Viennese physician of the eighteenth century, used hospital records to show that women in labor who were assisted by midwives had lower mortality rates than those attended by physicians in hospital wards. After prolonged efforts, he was able to identify the specific cause and demonstrate an effective prophylaxis (rigorous hand-washing). Many physicians scoffed at his ideas, which were not widely applied to medical practice for some period of time (Johnson & Granger, 1994).

Florence Nightingale (1823–1910), nurse, statistician, administrator, and health policy advocate, was also among the first to conduct outcomes studies. She developed the first Uniform Hospital Discharge Data Set and used the data to link mortality rates with diagnoses and treatments. Nightingale was a pioneer in statistical analysis and used graphical representations of her results to demonstrate that patient care outcomes could be changed. She was astute in disseminating her findings to those who formulated health policy, distributing them widely to members of Parliament, the government, and the army. She enraged the military and civilian medical establishment of

her day and it was several decades before the medical community began to apply her ideas (Mahrenholz, 1991; White, 1993).

Early in this century, Ernest A. Codman, a Boston surgeon, proposed a method of evaluating the effectiveness of care based on an examination of the patient one year after surgery or discharge from a hospital. He believed this process would speed up the time required for physicians to determine whether a particular operative procedure was worthwhile, ineffective, or even harmful. He also proposed that the information be used to identify the types of errors physicians made and serve as a basis for promotions in hospitals and medical schools. Results of the patient examinations could be recorded on end-result cards that could be used by patients in choosing where to obtain medical care. Codman asked questions such as: What was the patient's problem? Did the doctors diagnose it in time? Did the patient get entirely well? If not, why not? Was it the fault of the surgeon, the disease, or the patient? What could be done to prevent similar failures in the future? (Altman, 1993; Bloom, 1990; Neuhauser, 1990). Codman's ideas were very unpopular at Harvard, where he taught, and at Massachusetts General Hospital, where he practiced. He was roundly attacked by his colleagues and under pressure had to leave his position. He established his own private hospital, where he implemented his proposed end-result cards. However, with intense competition from the Boston medical establishment, he lost money and had to close the hospital. His ideas lay fallow for three decades before being reconsidered. Ultimately, his ideas were the basis for the formation of the Joint Commission for the Accreditation of Health Care Organizations (JCAHO).

Efforts of the Health Care Financing Administration and the New York State Health Department in the early 1990s sparked an even greater controversy than Codman by using a variation of his end-result cards to publish a ranking of outcomes of doctors and hospitals performing cardiac surgery in New York. Newspapers obtained information for this ranking—in spite of obstructionist efforts by physicians and hospitals—by appealing to the courts using the Freedom of Information

Act (Altman, 1993; Bloom, 1990; Neuhauser, 1990; White, 1993).

THE AGENCY FOR HEALTH SERVICES RESEARCH (AHSR)

In 1959, two National Institutes of Health study sections, the Hospital and Medical Facilities Study Section and the Nursing Study Section, met to discuss concerns with the adequacy and appropriateness of medical care, patient care, and hospital and medical facilities. As a result of their dialogue, a Health Services Research Study Section was initiated. This study section eventually became the Agency for Health Services Research and with small amounts of funding from Congress continued to study the effectiveness of health services, primarily supporting the research of economists, epidemiologists, and health policy analysts (White, 1993). Two projects that were to have the greatest impact were small area analyses and the Medical Outcomes Study.

Small Area Analyses

In the 1970s Wennberg, an epidemiologist, began a series of studies examining small area variations in medical practice across towns and counties. He found a wide variation in the tonsillectomy rate from one town to another in the New England area that could not be explained by differences such as health status, insurance, or demographics. These findings were replicated across a variety of medical procedures. Investigators began a search for the underlying causes of such variation and their implications for health status (O'Connor, Plume, & Wennberg, 1993; Wennberg, Barry, Fowler, & Mulley, 1993). Studies also revealed that many procedures, such as coronary artery bypass, were being performed on patients who did not have appropriate clinical indications of needing that surgery (Power, Tunis, & Wagner, 1994).

The Medical Outcomes Study (MOS)

MOS was the first large-scale study to examine factors influencing patient outcomes. The study was designed to identify elements of physician care associated with favorable patient outcomes. The conceptual framework for the MOS is shown in Figure 21–1 (on p. 572). Variations in use of resources, and physician technical and interpersonal styles were examined (Greenfield, et al., 1992; Kelly, Huber, Johnson, McClosky, & Maas, 1994; Riesenberg & Glass, 1989; Stewart, Greenfield, & Hays, 1989). However, Kelly and colleagues (1994) complained that the MOS study failed to control for the effect of nursing interventions, staffing patterns, or nursing practice delivery models on medical outcomes. Coordination of care, counseling, and referrals, activities more commonly performed by nurses than physicians, were considered by MOS to be components of medical practice.

THE AGENCY FOR HEALTH CARE POLICY AND RESEARCH (AHCPR)

AHCPR was created in 1989 by Congress and replaced the Agency for Health Services Research. The Congressional mandate for *AHCPR* was "to carry out research, demonstrations, guideline development, training, and dissemination activities with respect to health care services and systems of information regarding the following areas: the effectiveness, efficiency, quality, and outcomes of health services; clinical practice, including primary care; health care technologies, facilities, and equipment; health care costs, productivity, and market forces; health promotion and disease prevention; health statistics and epidemiology; and medical liability" (Gray, 1992, p. 40). A National Advisory Council for Health Care Policy, Research, and Evaluation was established by Congress and was required to include health care researchers; health professionals (specifically including nurses); individuals from business, law, ethics, economics, and public policy; and individuals representing the interests of consumers. The budget for outcomes research increased to $1.9 million in 1988, $5.9 million in 1989, and $37.5 million in 1990. With an increasing budget and strong political support, proponents of AHCPR were becoming a powerful force in demanding

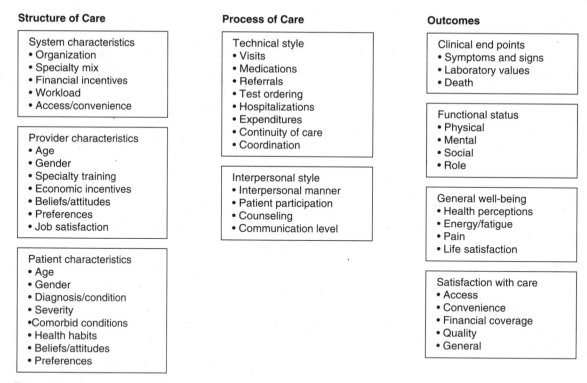

Structure of Care

System characteristics
• Organization
• Specialty mix
• Financial incentives
• Workload
• Access/convenience

Provider characteristics
• Age
• Gender
• Specialty training
• Economic incentives
• Beliefs/attitudes
• Preferences
• Job satisfaction

Patient characteristics
• Age
• Gender
• Diagnosis/condition
• Severity
• Comorbid conditions
• Health habits
• Beliefs/attitudes
• Preferences

Process of Care

Technical style
• Visits
• Medications
• Referrals
• Test ordering
• Hospitalizations
• Expenditures
• Continuity of care
• Coordination

Interpersonal style
• Interpersonal manner
• Patient participation
• Counseling
• Communication level

Outcomes

Clinical end points
• Symptoms and signs
• Laboratory values
• Death

Functional status
• Physical
• Mental
• Social
• Role

General well-being
• Health perceptions
• Energy/fatigue
• Pain
• Life satisfaction

Satisfaction with care
• Access
• Convenience
• Financial coverage
• Quality
• General

Figure 21–1
The MOS conceptual framework. (Reprinted with permission of the *Journal of the American Medical Association* [1989]. 262: 925–930. Copyright 1989, American Medical Association.)

change in health care due to the demand for health care reform throughout the government and the public. However, much controversy presently exists about the role of AHCPR. For example, orthopedic surgeons are upset about the guidelines on the treatment of back pain. AHCPR has been under attack by powerful forces and is in danger of being eliminated or having a greatly reduced budget. In the 1997 fiscal year budget, AHCPR funding was cut by $35 million. This will enable them to continue currently funded projects but seriously curtails the funding of new projects.

In the past few years, AHCPR has initiated several major research efforts to examine medical outcomes. Of these, two of the most significant, which are described below, are the Medical Treatment Effectiveness Program (MEDTEP), and a component of MEDTEP referred to as Patient Out-comes Research Teams (PORTs) (Greene, Bondy, & Maklan, 1994).

The Medical Treatment Effectiveness Program (MEDTEP)

MEDTEP was established by Congress in 1989 to be implemented by AHCPR. The purpose of the program was to improve the effectiveness and appropriateness of medical practice. The term *medical* was used by Congress when the program was mandated. However, it is being broadly interpreted to include health care in general, particularly—from our perspective—nursing care. The program was charged to develop and disseminate scientific information about the effects of health care services and procedures on patients' survival, health status, functional capacity, and quality of life, a remarkable shift from the narrow focus of traditional medical research. The three research areas funded through this program were (1) patient outcomes research (PORTs); (2) database development; and (3) research on effective methods of disseminating the information gathered. In 1993, studies were implemented to examine the effects of pharmaceuticals on patient outcomes and $19 million was provided to establish Research Centers on Minority Populations (Clinton, 1993).

Patient Outcomes Research Team (PORT) Projects

PORTs are large-scale, multifaceted, and multidisciplinary projects mandated by Congress to "identify and analyze the outcomes and costs of current alternative practice patterns in order to determine the best treatment strategy and to develop and test methods for reducing inappropriate variations." The PORTs are required to "conduct literature reviews and synthesis; analyze practice variations and associated patient outcomes, using available data augmented by primary data collection where desired; disseminate research findings; and evaluate the effects of dissemination" (U.S. Congress, 1994, p. 67). Questions which might be addressed by PORTs include: Do patients benefit from the care provided? What treatments work best? Has the patient's functional status improved? According to whose viewpoint? Are health care resources well spent? (Tanenbaum, 1994; Wood, 1990). PORTs have studied outcomes of treatment for hip fracture repair and osteoarthritis, prevention of low birthweight and its sequelae in minority and high-risk women, total knee replacements, therapies for benign prostatic hypertrophy and localized prostate cancer, pneumonia, back pain, biliary tract disease, ischemic heart disease, schizophrenia, stroke prevention, acute myocardial infarction, cataracts, childbirth, and diabetes (Goldberg & Cummings, 1994). Smaller projects are examining the management of peripheral vascular disease, cerebral vascular disease, hip dis-

ease, colon cancer, gall bladder disease, and coronary artery disease (Wood, 1990).

A major task of PORTs is to disseminate their findings and change the practice of health care providers to improve patient outcomes. A framework for dissemination has been developed that identifies the audiences for disseminated products, the media involved, and the strategies that foster assimilation and adoption of information (Goldberg, et al., 1994).

A Cost of Care Workgroup, including a representative from each PORT, has been convened with four goals: (1) to determine the best methods for estimating the cost of certain conditions using claims data; (2) to evalute methods for estimating the cost of care using billing information and patient interview data; (3) to examine methods for determining the indirect cost of care, and (4) to evaluate methods for comparing the cost of care internationally (Lave, et al., 1994).

Clinical guideline panels were developed to incorporate available evidence on health outcomes into sets of recommendations concerning appropriate management strategies for patients with the studied conditions (Wennberg et al. 1993). This information has been widely disseminated to providers and to patients. Current guidelines can be obtained on the World Wide Web at http://text.nlm.nih.gov/ahcpr/list.html or by contacting AHCPR.

AHCPR is no longer in the business of developing guidelines. They are, however, developing liaisons with other nongovernment groups, both national and international, who are currently developing clinical guidelines. AHCPR also plans to fund several centers whose mission will be clinical guideline development. Whether or not nursing will again be excluded from the group's developing guidelines is of concern.

Example: Guidelines for Management of Heart Failure

The process used in a guideline panel is illustrated by Hadorn and Baker (1994) and Hadorn,

Baker, Dracup, and Pitt (1994) in papers describing the development of heart failure guidelines. This project was led by two co-chairs, one a cardiologist and the other a doctorally prepared nurse. The decision of which health care outcomes are important and relevant in developing clinical practice guidelines and in evaluating patient response to treatment is critical. Rather than using biochemical, physiological, anatomical, or histological outcomes, this team focused on clinical outcomes such as reduced mortality, improved physical functioning, and lessened symptoms to study patients experiencing heart failure. Contrary to most medical studies, patient self-reports played an important role in determining symptoms and functional status. Clinical algorithms were used to develop practice guidelines. Algorithms are flow diagrams with branching-logic pathways, allowing carefully defined criteria to be used to develop appropriate management strategies as illustrated in Figure 21–2. Developing the algorithms assisted the Guideline Panel in identifying key clinical decision points, organizing the guideline, and being specific about recommendations (Hadorn & Baker, 1994).

The focus of outcome research has been medical practice, perhaps because the greatest problems in health care—from the perspective of both cost and quality—are seen as related to the actions of physicians (Wennberg, 1990). According to O'Conner and colleagues (1993, p. 45) "the individual clinician rarely knows with certainty the quality of care that he or she is providing." Unlike nurses, the practicing physician rarely has opportunities to compare his or her practice patterns with those of other clinicians. In addition, the existing evidence of the effect medical practice has on patients is of such poor quality that it is impossible to determine the most desirable approaches to care.

OUTCOMES RESEARCH AND NURSING PRACTICE

Outcome studies provide rich opportunities to build a stronger scientific underpinning for nursing practice (Rettig, 1990). "Nursing needs to be able to explain the impact of care provided by its prac-

titioners through measures of outcomes of patient care that reflect nursing practice" (Moritz, 1991, p. 113). We need to know how nurses make decisions. Most clinical judgment research focuses on medical practice and examines diagnostic judgments. Outcome studies by nurses examining nursing practice are in a very preliminary stage. Patient satisfaction surveys have been used for many years in nursing but the link to specific nursing care is vague. Nurses have conducted quality assurance or quality improvement studies, primarily in hospital settings, and critical pathways and care maps have stimulated interest in studying related outcomes.

Nurse case management lends itself well to evaluation using an outcome research focus. We need to know how case management is implemented in an organization, the roles of case managers, how high-risk patients are identified, who is most likely to benefit from case management, and the impact of case management on the quality of patient care and costs (Lamb, 1992; Marschke & Nolan, 1993). Issel (1995) designed an approach to evaluating obstetric case management programs which is illustrated in Table 21–1.

Nurse practitioners, an emerging force in the primary health care arena, need to be proactive in defining the uniqueness of interventions they provide and documenting their effectiveness. A flurry of studies in the 1970s documented the effectiveness of nurse practitioner outcomes compared to those of physicians. Few studies have been conducted since that time to define nursing practitioner interventions or examine the outcomes of nurse practitioner practice. Nurse practitioners, as a group, are as yet uncommitted to examining the outcomes of their practice. Given what is happening to reimbursement for medical interventions, this seems at least shortsighted. Molde and Diers (1985, p. 362) recommend studies examining questions related to outcomes of advanced nurse practitioner practice such as: "What explains when hypertensive patients cared for by nurse practitioners have better controlled blood pressures than those cared for by physicians (Ramsey, McKenzie, & Fish, 1982); why the suicide rate dropped in a jail staffed with nurse practitioners

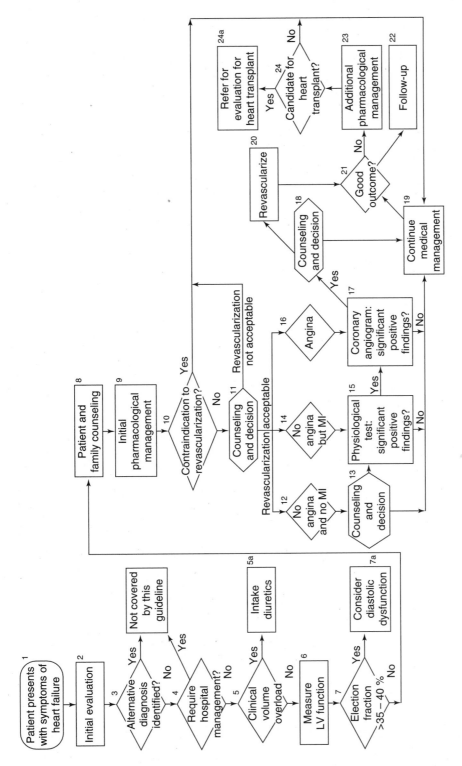

Figure 21–2

Management algorithm for patients with heart failure. Key: LV = left ventricles, MI = myocardial infarction. (From Hadorn, D. C., & Baker, D. [1994]. Development of the AHCPR-sponsored heart failure guideline: Methodological and procedural issues. *Joint Commission Journal of Quality Improvement, 20*[10], 543.)

Table 21–1
Health Outcomes Categories and Suggested Impact Indicators for Obstetric Case Management Programs

Outcome Category	Prepregnancy Antecedents	Baseline at Entry to Case Management	Outcomes at Delivery	Postpartum Outcomes
Physical status and morbidity	Race, age Prepregnancy weight Height Medical history Obstetrical history	Accurate weight Height Nutritional status Morbidity	Type of delivery Gestational weight gain Maternal morbidity Weeks' gestation at delivery Birth weight Newborn morbidity	Weight of mother Nutritional status of mother Maternal morbidity Using birth control method of choice Nutritional status of infant Weight of infant Infant morbidity
Psychological, behavioral, and developmental	History of substance abuse	Substance abuse Social support network Depression or anxiety Smoking pattern Readiness for parenthood	 Depression or anxiety Smoking pattern Readiness for parenthood Independently sought needed services Attachment to infant Satisfaction with care	Substance abuse Social support network Depression Smoking pattern Parenting confidence Parent-infant interactions Satisfaction with care
Knowledge	Educational level	Self-care behavior Nutritional behavior Labor and delivery knowledge	Self-care behavior Breast-feeding Infant-care behavior	Self-care behavior Nutritional behavior Breast-feeding Infant-care behavior Growth and development knowledge Family planning knowledge Knowledge of community resources
Family and role functioning	Occupation	Working status Marital status Family functioning History of domestic violence Size and composition of family Income	 Participation of significant others during pregnancy Infant caretaking	Working status Marital status Family functioning History of domestic violence Infant caretaking
Utilization and cost	 Previous health services utilization Previous social services	Health insurance type	Length of stay for mother Length of stay for infant Number/type of health services utilized during pregnancy Number/type of social services utilized during pregnancy	 Number/type of health services utilized Number/type of social services utilized

(From Issel, L. M. [1995]. Evaluating case management programs. *Maternal–Child Nursing, 20*[2], 67–70, 72–74.)

(Hastings et al., 1980), and how nurse practitioners are more effective in helping patients lose weight, keep appointments, and comply with recommendations (Watkins & Wagner, 1982). Clearly the style of practice that has evolved in nurse practitioner work is different than that of physicians. This style of practice needs to be described."

Community health is an area of practice that is expected to greatly expand in the future. Mittelmark, Hunt, Heath, and Schmid (1993, p. 442) point out that "it is clear that a community turns first to its medical leaders when questions about new health promotion programs arise. Very little is known about the potential for community change that rests with primary care providers who are not physicians. In many communities, nurse practitioners, physician assistants, chiropractors, podiatrists, dietitians, and others are in daily contact with patients and many are leaders of community organizations. . . . Most if not all of these professions are attracted to the idea that prevention is integral to primary care." Nursing needs to take the lead in conducting studies to examine the outcomes of programs designed to protect or improve the health of the community.

Hospitals are a major target of outcome research, and yet the outcomes are attributed either to the hospital as a whole or to physicians. Nursing practice in the hospital setting is invisible as a force influencing patient outcomes (Clark & Lang, 1992; Kelly, et al., 1994). In any practice setting, the physician sees the patient for only a fraction of the total time care is being provided, and generally does not personally deliver the medical interventions that he or she prescribes. In addition, not all health care is related to medical diagnosis and treatment (Kelly, et al., 1994). Other providers (e.g., nurses, pharmacists, therapists, social workers) impact treatment through their interventions and style of care delivery. When outcomes of care involving multiple disciplines are being studied, attributing outcomes to a single provider is not appropriate and raises questions of validity and reliability of the research findings. Hegyvary (1992) suggests that each group of practitioners define and measure their actions and the intended results, and then integrate those disparate views. The in-

terdependence of health care providers in producing health outcomes must be recognized (Holzemer, 1990; Kelly, et al., 1994). The momentum to make this happen must come from within nursing. We cannot rely on some benevolent force to do this for us.

In 1992, the National Center for Nursing Research (NCNR) sponsored a Conference on Patient Outcomes Research: Examining the Effectiveness of Nursing Practice. In the keynote speech, Hinshaw (1992, p. 9), then director of NCNR, suggested that "from a nursing perspective, particular clinical conditions need to be identified that are more specific to nursing's focus on prevention, health promotion, symptom management, and the amelioration of the effects of acute and chronic illnesses. We are all familiar with clinical conditions that are central to our practice, such as skin integrity, pain, urinary incontinence, nausea and vomiting, nutritional deficits, confusion, restricted mobility, depression, fatigue, and illness-related stress. It will be particularly important in our research programs that we begin to both define and refine the patient outcomes specific to interventions focused on such clinical conditions." Examining the impact of nursing on overall hospital outcomes will require inclusion of nursing data in the large databases used to analyze outcomes. The cost of adding new variables to these databases is high. Nursing is competing with other voices who wish to add other variables. Currently, adding nursing variables is considered a low priority. We must make our voice heard.

NCNR, now the National Institute for Nursing Research (NINR), developed a partnership with AHCPR to fund outcome studies of importance to nursing. Calls for proposals jointly supported by AHCPR and NINR are being announced each year. These calls for proposals can be found in NINR's home page on the World Wide Web: http://www.nih.gov/ninr/.

THE THEORETICAL BASIS OF OUTCOMES RESEARCH

The theory on which outcomes research is based emerged from evaluation research. The theorist,

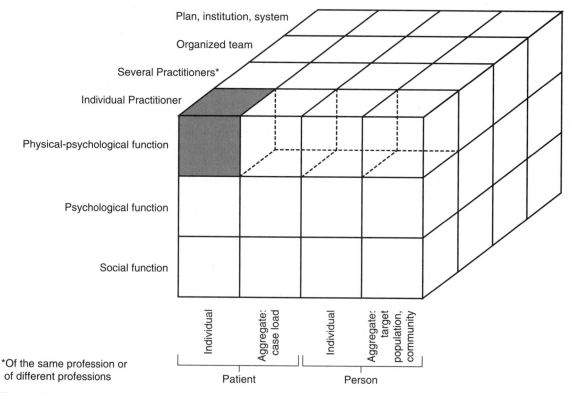

Plan, institution, system

Organized team

Several Practitioners*

Individual Practitioner

Physical-psychological function

Psychological function

Social function

Individual

Aggregate: case load

Individual

Aggregate: target population, community

*Of the same profession or
of different professions

Patient

Person

Figure 21–3

Level and scope of concern as factors in the definition of quality. (From Donabedian, A. [1987]. Some basic issues in evaluating the quality of health care. In L. K. Rinke [Ed.], *Outcome measures in home care* [vol. 1, pp. 3–28]. New York: National League for Nursing [original work published in 1976], with permission.)

Avedis Donabedian, MD, PhD (1987) proposed a theory of quality health care and the process of evaluating it. Quality is the overriding construct of the theory, although Donabedian never defines this concept (Mark, 1995). The cube shown in Figure 21–3 is used to explain the elements of quality health care. The three dimensions of the cube are health, subjects of care, and providers of care. The concept *health* has many aspects; three are shown on the cube: physical-physiological function, psychological function, and social function. Donabedian (1987) proposes that "the manner in which we conceive of health and of our responsibility for it, makes a fundamental difference to the concept of quality and, as a result, to the methods that we use to assess and assure the quality of care" (p. 4).

The concept *subjects of care* has two primary aspects: patient and person. A patient is defined

as someone who has already gained access to some care and a person as someone who may or may not have gained access to care. Each of these concepts are further categorized by the concepts of individual and aggregate. Within patient, the aggregate is a case load; within person, the aggregate is a target population or a community. The concept *providers of care* shows levels of aggregation and organization of providers. The first level is the individual practitioner. At this level, no consideration is given to anyone else who might be involved in the care of a subject of care, whether individual or aggregate.

As the levels progress, providers of care include several practitioners, who might be of the same profession or different professions and "who may be providing care concurrently, as individuals, or jointly, as a team" (p. 5). At higher levels of aggregation, the provider of care is institutions, programs, or the health care system as a whole. Donabedian indicates that the dimensions of health are defined by the subjects of care, not by the providers of care and are based on "what consumers expect, want, or are willing to accept" (p. 5). Thus, practitioners cannot unilaterally enlarge the definition of health to include other aspects; this action requires social consensus that "the scope of professional competence and responsibility embraces these areas of function" (p. 5). However, Donabedian indicates that providers of care may make efforts to persuade subjects of care to expand their definition of the dimensions of health.

The *primordial cell* of Donabedian's framework is the physical-physiological function of the individual patient being cared for by the individual practitioner. Examining quality at this level is relatively simple. As one moves outward to include more of the cubical structure, the notions of quality and its assessment become increasingly difficult. When more than one practitioner is involved, both individual and joint contributions to quality must be evaluated. Concepts such as coordination and teamwork must be conceptually and operationally defined. When *person* is the subject of care, an important attribute is access. When an aggregate is the subject of care, an important attribute is resource allocation. Access and resource allocation are interrelated, since they each define who gets care, the kind of care received, and how much care is received.

As more elements of the cube are included, conflicts among competing objectives emerge. The chief conflict is between the practitioner's responsibility to the individual and his or her responsibility to the aggregate. The practitioner is expected to have an exclusive commitment to each patient, and yet the aggregate demands a commitment to the well-being of the society, leading to ethical dilemmas for the practitioner. Investing more time with an individual patient means decreased access for other patients. Society's demand to reduce costs for an overall financing program may require increasing costs to the individual. Examining the cube, logic would suggest that one could build up

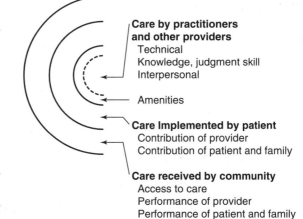

Care by practitioners and other providers
Technical
Knowledge, judgment skill
Interpersonal

Amenities

Care Implemented by patient
Contribution of provider
Contribution of patient and family

Care received by community
Access to care
Performance of provider
Performance of patient and family

Figure 21–4
Various levels at which the quality of health care can be assessed. (From Donabedian, A [1988]. The quality of care: How can it be assessed? *Journal of the American Medical Association, 260* [12], 1744. Copyright © 1988 American Medical Association. Used with permission.)

quality beginning with the primordial cell and increase by increments with the assumption that each increment would contribute positively to a greater total quality. However, the conflicts in competing objectives may preclude this possibility and lead instead to moral dilemmas.

Loegering, Reiter, and Gambone (1994) modified Donabedian's levels to include the patient and family, and the community as providers of care as well as recipients of care. They suggest that access to care is one dimension of the provision of care by the community. Figure 21–4 is a model of their modifications.

Donabedian identifies three objects of evaluation in appraising quality: structure, process, and outcome. A complete quality assessment program requires the simultaneous use of all three concepts and an examination of the relationships among the three. However, researchers have had little success in accomplishing this theoretical goal. Studies designed to examine all three concepts would require sufficiently large samples of various structures, each with the various processes being compared and large samples of subjects who have experienced the outcomes of those processes. The funding and the cooperation necessary to accomplish this goal are not yet available.

EVALUATING OUTCOMES

The goal of outcome research is the evaluation of outcomes as defined by Donabedian. However, this goal is not as simplistic as it might immediately appear. Donabedian's theory requires that identified outcomes be clearly linked with the process that caused the outcome. To accomplish this the researcher must define the process and justify the causal links with the selected outcomes. The identification of desirable outcomes requires dialogue between the subjects of care and the providers of care. Although the providers of care may delineate what is achievable, the subjects of care must clarify what is desirable. The outcomes must also be relevant to the goals of the health professionals, the health care system of which the professionals are a part, and society.

Outcomes are time-dependent. Some outcomes may not be apparent for some period of time after the process that is purported to cause them while others may be immediately apparent. Some outcomes are temporary while others are permanent. Thus, the selection of an appropriate time frame for determining the selected outcomes must be established.

A final obstacle to outcome evaluation is one of attribution. This requires assigning the place and degree of responsibility for the outcomes observed. There is often a multiplicity of factors influencing a particular outcome. Lewis (1995) points out that health care represents only one dimension of a complex situation. Patient factors, such as compliance, predisposition to disease, age, propensity to use resources, high risk behaviors such as smoking, and life style, must also be taken into account. Environmental factors such as air quality, public policies related to smoking, and occupational hazards must also be included. Responsibility for outcomes may be distributed among providers, patients, employers, insurers, and the community. There is as yet little scientific basis for judging the precise relationship between each factor and the selected outcome. Many of the influencing factors may be outside the jurisdiction or influence of the health care system or the providers within it. One solution to this problem is to define a set of proximate outcomes specific to the condition for which care is being provided. Critical pathways and care maps may be useful in defining at least proximate outcomes.

EVALUATING PROCESS

The process of clinical management has been, for most health professionals, an art rather than a science. Understanding the process sufficiently to study it must begin with much careful reflection, dialogue, and observation. There are multiple components of clinical management, many of which have not yet been clearly defined or tested. Bergmark and Oscarsson (1991, pp. 139–140) suggest the following questions as important to consider in evaluating process: (1) "What constitutes the 'therapeutic agent'?" (2) "Do practitioners actually do what they say they do?" (3) "Do practitioners always know what they do?" Current outcome studies are using process variables easy to identify. Answers to questions such as those posed by Bergmark and Oscarsson are more difficult to define and will initially require observation, interviews, and the use of qualitative research methodologies. Three components of process are of particular interest to Donabedian: standards of care, practice styles, and costs of care.

Standards of Care

A standard of care is a norm on which quality of care is judged. Clinical guidelines, critical paths, and care maps define standards of care. According to Donabedian, a practitioner has legitimate responsibility to apply available knowledge in the management of a dysfunctional state. This management includes the identification or diagnosis of the dysfunction, the decision of whether or not to intervene, the choice of intervention objectives, the choice of methods and techniques to achieve the objectives, and the skillful execution of the selected techniques. Donabedian recommends the development of criteria to be used as a basis for judging the quality of care. These criteria may take the form of clinical guidelines or care maps based on prior validation of the contribution of the care to outcomes. The clinical guidelines currently being published by AHCPR establish norms on which the validity of clinical management can be judged. However, the core of the problem, from Donabedian's perspective, is clinical judgment. Analyses of the process of making diagnoses and therapeutic decisions is critical to evaluating quality of care. The emergence of decision trees and algorithms are a response to Donabedian's concerns and provide a means of evaluating the adequacy of clinical judgments.

Practice Styles

The style of practice is another dimension of the process of care that influences quality; however, it is problematic to judge what constitutes "goodness" in style and provide justification for the decisions. Problem-solving styles identified by Donabedian include routine approaches to care versus flexibility, parsimony versus redundancy, variations in degree of tolerance of uncertainty, propensity to take risks, and preference for Type I errors versus Type II errors. There are also diverse styles of interpersonal relationships. Lowenberg (1994) has initiated a research program to examine practice styles of nurses. She has identified five dimensions of the nurse-patient relationship: affectivity, specificity, status differential, placebo salience, and trust. Previous nursing research in this area has focused on affectivity.

Costs of Care

A third dimension of the examination of quality of care is cost. There are cost consequences to maintaining a specified level of quality of care. More and better care are likely to increase costs. But this care is also likely to produce savings. Economic benefits can be obtained by preventing illness, preventing complications, maintaining a higher quality of life, or prolonging productive life. A related issue is who bears the costs of care. Some measures purported to reduce costs have instead simply shifted costs to another party. For example, a hospital might reduce their costs by discharging a particular type of patient early but total costs could increase if the necessary community-based health care raised costs above that incurred by keeping the patient hospitalized longer. In this case, the third-party provider could experience increased costs. In many cases, the costs are shifted from the health care system to the family as out-of-pocket costs. Studies examining changes in costs of care must consider total costs.

EVALUATING STRUCTURE

Structures of care are the elements of organization and administration that guide the processes of care. The first step in evaluating structure is to identify and describe the elements of the structure. Various administration and management theories could be used to identify the elements of structure to be studied. These elements might include leadership, tolerance of innovativeness, organizational hierarchy, decision-making processes, distribution of power, financial management, and administrative decision-making processes. The second step is to evaluate the impact of various structure elements on the process of care and upon outcomes. This requires comparing different structures providing the same processes of care. In evaluating structures, the unit of measure is the structure. The evaluation requires access to a sufficiently large sample of like structures with similar processes and outcomes which can then be compared to a sample of another structure providing the same processes and outcomes. For example, one might compare various structures providing primary health care such as the private physician office, the HMO, the rural health clinic, the community-oriented primary care clinic, and the nurse-managed center. One might examine surgical care provided within the structures of a private outpatient surgical clinic, a private hospital, a county hospital, and a teaching hospital associated with a health science center. Within each of these, the focus of study would be the impact of structure on processes of care and outcomes of care.

A number of frameworks for research have emerged from Donabedian's theory. Each includes

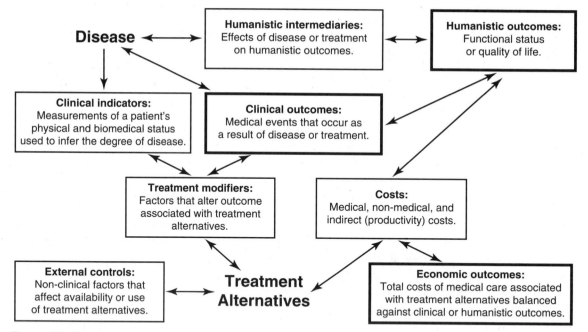

Figure 21–5

The conceptual model: Economic, clinical, and humanistic outcome (ECHO) model. (Reprinted by permission of the publisher from Kozma, C. M., Reeder, C. E., & Schulz, R. M. [1993]. Economic, clinical, and humanistic outcomes: A planning model for pharmacoeconomic research. *Clinical Therapeutics, 15*[6], 1125. Copyright © 1993 by Excerpta Medica, Inc.)

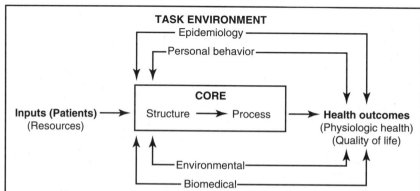

Figure 21–6

A systems perspective of health services research. (From Anderson, R. M., Davidson, P. L., & Ganz, P. A. [1994]. Symbiotic relationships of quality of life, health services research and other health research. *Quality of Life Research, 3*[5], 367.)

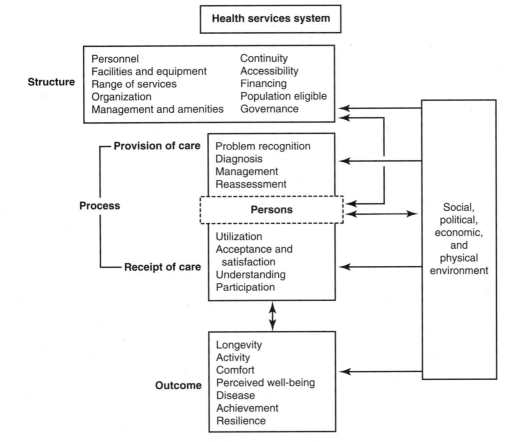

Figure 21–7

The health services system. (From Vivier, P. M., Bernier, J. A., & Starfield, B. [1994]. Current approaches to measuring health outcomes in pediatric research. *Current Opinions in Pediatrics, 6*[5], 531. Copyright © Rapid Science Publishers, with permission.)

Donabedian's basic concepts, adds more detail, and organizes the concepts somewhat differently. For examples, see Figures 21–5, 21–6, 21–7, and 21–8.

METHODOLOGIES FOR OUTCOME STUDIES

A research tradition for the outcome paradigm is still emerging. A research tradition defines acceptable research methodologies. The lack of an established set of methodologies should encourage increased creativity in seeking new strategies for studying the phenomena of concern. Small single

studies using untried methodologies may be useful. Research teams need to develop research programs with a planned sequence of studies focused on a particular outcome concern. The PORTs are beginning to define a research process for conducting programs of funded outcome studies. These programs are complex and may include multiple studies using a variety of research strategies whose findings must be merged in the process of forming conclusions. Although implementing a research program as extensive as a PORT would be unrealistic without the funding a PORT receives, ideas for developing outcome research programs on a smaller scale can be generated by examining these plans. The following steps were constructed

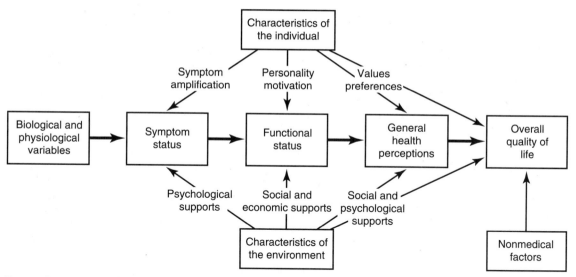

Figure 21–8

Relationships among measures of patient outcome in a health-related quality of life conceptual model. (From Wilson, I. B., & Cleary, P. D. [1995]. Linking clinical variables with health-related quality of life: A conceptual model of patient outcomes. *Journal of the American Medical Association, 273*[1], 60. Copyright © 1995 by the American Medical Association.)

combining PORT plans proposed by Freund, Dittus, Fitzgerald, and Heck (1990); Sledge (1993); and Turk and Rudy (1994).

1. Perform a critical review of the published literature or a meta-analysis.
2. Conduct large database analyses based on the results of the critical literature review.
3. Identify outcomes measures for use in the study and evaluate their sensitivity to change.
4. Identify variables that might affect the outcomes.
5. Achieve consensus on definitions for all variables to be used in the research program.
6. Develop assessment instruments or techniques.
7. Conduct patient surveys or focus groups to gain information on outcomes such as level of functional status and perceived pain and how these outcomes may improve or regress over time.
8. Determine patterns of care (who provides care at what points of time for what purposes?).
9. Perform a cohort analysis. Follow a cohort of patients, some of whom will receive one treatment and others of whom will not receive the treatment to assess changes in outcomes over time. Use a telephone survey at selected intervals to gather information. Evaluate the proportion of patients who improve as well as the group mean differences.
10. Determine, through follow-up studies, differences in patient selection or interventions that are associated with different outcomes. Evaluate the durability of change by conducting sufficiently long follow-up. Determine the percentage of patients dropping out from different treatments and, when possible, determine the reasons for dropping out.
11. Determine the clinical significance of improvement as well as the statistical significance.
12. Determine the cost-benefit and cost-effectiveness of the treatments under evaluation.
13. Use decision analyses to synthesize information regarding patients' outcomes and preferences for various types of outcomes.
14. Disseminate information to both patients and health care providers about which individuals

would and which would not benefit from the procedure.

15. Conduct a clinical trial to evaluate the effects of the intervention.
16. Incorporate findings into treatment guidelines.
17. Modify provider and patient behavior so that proven, effective treatment is applied to those who are most likely to benefit.

The PORTs have recognized the need to allow diversity in research strategies, measures, and analyses to facilitate methodologic advances (Fowler, Cleary, Magaziner, Patrick, & Benjamin, 1994). Creative flexibility is often necessary to develop ways to answer new questions. Finding ways to determine the impact of a condition on a person's life is difficult. Interpreting results can also be problematic since clinical significance is considered to be equally as important as statistical significance. This requires a judgment by the research team of what constitutes clinical significance in their particular area of study. Examples of published outcome studies from a variety of disciplines can be found in the appendices of the Student Study Guide.

The following section describes some of the sampling issues, research strategies, measurements, and statistical approaches being used by researchers in outcome studies. The descriptions provided are not sufficient to guide the researcher in using the approaches described but rather provide a broad overview of a variety of methodologies being used. For additional information, refer to the citations in each section. Outcome studies cross a variety of disciplines, thus the emerging methodologies are being enriched by a cross-pollination of ideas, some of which may be new to nursing research.

SAMPLES AND SAMPLING

The preferred methods of obtaining samples are different in outcome studies; random sampling is not considered desirable and is seldom used. Heterogeneous, rather than homogeneous, samples are obtained. Rather than using sampling criteria that restrict subjects that are included in the study in order to decrease possible biases, and that reduce the variance and increase the possibility of identifying a statistically significant difference, outcome researchers seek large heterogeneous samples that reflect as much as possible all patients who would be receiving care in the real world. Samples, then, need to include, for example, patients with various comorbidities and patients with varying levels of health status. In addition, persons need to be identified who do not receive treatment for their condition. Devising ways to evaluate the representativeness of such samples is problematic. Developing strategies to locate untreated individuals and include them in follow-up studies will be a challenge.

Traditional researchers and statisticians argue that when patients are not selected randomly, biases and confounding are more likely to occur and that this is a particular problem when the sample size is small. In nonexperimental studies, variation is likely to be greater, resulting in an increased risk of a Type II error. Traditional analysts consider nonrandomized studies to be based on observational data and therefore not credible (Orchard, 1994). Using this argument, traditionalists claim the findings of most outcome studies are not valid and should not be used as a basis for establishing guidelines for clinical practice or building a body of knowledge.

Large Databases as Sample Sources

One source of samples used for outcome studies is large databases. There are two broad categories of databases emerging from patient care encounters: clinical databases and administrative databases as illustrated by Figure 21–9. Clinical databases were created by providers such as hospitals, HMOs, and health care professionals. The clinical data are generated as a result of routine documentation of care, or in relation to a research protocol. Some are data registries that have been developed to gather data related to a particular disease, such as cancer (Lee & Goldman, 1989). Using a clinical database, it is possible to link observations made by many practitioners over long periods of time.

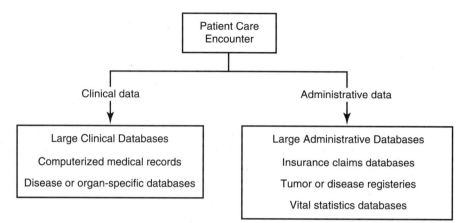

Figure 21-9

Types of databases emanating from patient care encounters. (From Lange, L. L., & Jacox, A. [1993]. Using large databases in nursing and health policy research. *Journal of Professional Nursing, 9*[4], 204, with permission.)

Links can be made between the process of care and outcomes (Mitchell, et al., 1994; Moses, 1995).

Administrative databases are created by insurance companies, government agencies, and others not directly involved in providing patient care. Administrative databases have standardized sets of data for enormous numbers of patients and providers (Deyo, et al., 1994; McDonald & Hui, 1991). An example is the Medicare database managed by the Health Care Financing Administration (HCFA). These large databases can be used to determine the incidence or prevalence of disease, geographic variations in medical care utilization, characteristics of medical care, outcomes of care, and complementarity with clinical trials. However, Wray and colleagues (1995) caution that analyses should be restricted to outcomes specific to a particular subgroup of patients, rather than one adverse outcome of all disease states.

There are problems with the quality of data in the large databases. The data have been gathered and entered by hundreds of individuals in a variety of settings. There are few quality checks on the data and within the same data sets records may have different lengths and structures. Missing data are common. Sampling and measurement error are inherent in all large databases. Sampling error is a result of the way in which cases are selected for inclusion in the database; measurement error emerges from problems related to the operational definition of concepts. Thus, reliability and validity of the data are a concern (Davis, 1990; Lange & Jacox, 1993).

Large databases are used in outcome studies to examine patient care outcomes. The outcomes that can be examined are limited to those recorded in the database and thus, tend to be rather general. Existing databases can be used for such analyses as assessment of nursing care delivery models, variation in nursing practices, evaluation of the patients' risk of hospital-acquired infection, hospital-acquired pressure ulcer, or of patient falls. Lange and Jacox (1993) identify the following important health policy questions related to nursing that should be examined using large databases.

1. What is standard nursing practice in various settings?
2. What is the relationship between variations in nursing practice and patient outcomes?
3. What are the effects of different nursing staff mixes on patient outcomes and costs?
4. What are the total costs for episodes of treatment of specific conditions, and what part of those are attributable to nursing care?
5. Who is being reimbursed for nursing care delivery? (Lange & Jacox, 1993, p. 207)

In order to examine these questions, nurses need to develop the statistical and methodological skills needed for working with large databases. Large databases contain patient and institutional information from huge numbers of patients. They exist in computer-readable form, require special statistical methods and computer techniques, and can be used by researchers who were not involved in the creation of the database.

Regrettably, nursing data are noticeably missing from these databases, and thus, from funded health policy studies using the large databases. A nursing minimum data set has been repeatedly recommended for inclusion in these databases (Werley, Devine, Zorm, Ryan, & Westra, 1991; Werley & Lang, 1988; Zielstorff, Hudgings, Grobe, & the National Commission on Nursing Implementation Project [NCNIP] Task Force on Nursing Information Systems, 1993). This minimum data set would comprise a set of variables necessary and sufficient to describe an episode of illness or the care given by a provider. The American Nurses Association has mandated the formation of a Steering Committee on Databases to Support Clinical Nursing Practice. Four nursing classification schemes have been recognized for use in national databases: the North American Nursing Diagnosis Association (NANDA), The Omaha System: Applications for Community Health Nursing, The Home Health Care Classification developed by Saba and colleagues, and The Nursing Interventions Classification (McCormick, Lang, Zielstorff, Milholland, Saba, & Jacox, 1994). McNeil (1993) indicates the following information which must be available to allow evaluation or monitoring of individual patient care: information about the patient such as disease severity, comorbidity, and types of outcomes; processes of care provided; patient status over time; and follow-up information. Because of the absence of this information, current databases are inadequate to judge the appropriateness of individual patient care.

Temple (1990, p. 211) expresses concerns regarding the use of large data sets rather than controlled trials to assess effectiveness of treatments. "We have traveled this route before with uncontrolled observations. It has always been hoped, and has often been asserted, that uncontrolled databases can be adjusted in some way that will allow valid comparisons of treatments. I know of no systematic attempt to document this." Outcome researchers counter these criticisms by saying that experimental studies lack external validity and are not useful for application in clinical settings. They claim the findings of clinical trials are not being used by clinicians because they are not representative of the patients seeking care.

RESEARCH STRATEGIES FOR OUTCOME STUDIES

Outcome research programs usually include studies with a mix of strategies carried out sequentially. Although these strategies could be referred to as designs, for some the term *design* as used in Chapters 10 and 11 is inconsistent with their use here. Research strategies for outcome studies have emerged from a variety of disciplines and innovative new strategies continue to appear in the literature. Strategies for outcome studies tend to have less control than traditional research designs and cannot be as easily categorized. The research strategies for outcome studies described below are only a sampling from the literature and include consensus knowledge building, practice pattern profiling, prospective cohort studies, retrospective cohort studies, population based studies, clinical decision analysis, studying the effectiveness of interdisciplinary teams, geographic studies, economic studies, ethical studies, and defining and testing interventions.

Consensus Knowledge Building

Consensus knowledge building is usually performed by a multidisciplinary group representing a variety of constituencies. Initially, an extensive international search of the literature on the topic of concern, including unpublished studies, studies in progress, dissertations, and theses is conducted. Several separate reviews may be conducted, focusing on specific questions about the outcomes of care, diagnosis, prevention, or prognosis. Because meta-analytic methods often cannot be applied to the literature pertinent to PORTs, systematic approaches to critique and synthesis have been developed to identify relevant studies and gather and analyze data abstracted from the studies (Powe, Turner, Maklan, & Ersek, 1994). The results are dispersed to researchers and clinical experts in the field, who are asked to carefully examine the material and then participate in a consensus conference. Emerging from the consensus conference are clinical guidelines, which are published and widely distributed to clinicians. The clinical guidelines are also used as practice norms to study process and outcomes in that field. Gaps in the knowledge base are identified and research priorities determined by the consensus group. Preliminary steps in this process might include conducting extensive integrative reviews and seeking consensus from a multidisciplinary research team and locally available clinicians. A review could be accomplished by establishing a World Wide Web site, and conducting dialogue with experts across the Internet. The review could be published in Sigma Theta Tau's online journal, *Knowledge Synthesis in Nursing,* and then dialogue related to the review could be conducted across the Internet. The Delphi method has also been used to seek consensus (Vermeulen, Ratko, Erstad, Brecher, & Matuszewski, 1995). An appendix in the Student Study Guide provides a list of published reviews from projects using consensus building.

Practice Pattern Profiling

Practice pattern profiling is an epidemiologic technique that focuses on patterns of care rather than individual occurrences of care. Large database analysis is used to identify a provider's pattern of practice and compare it with that of similar providers or with an accepted standard of practice. The technique has been used to determine over- and underutilization of services, to determine costs associated with a particular provider's care, to uncover problems related to efficiency and quality of care, and to assess provider performance. The provider being profiled could be an individual practitioner, a group of practitioners, or a health care organization such as a hospital or HMO. The provider's pattern is expressed as a rate aggregated across time for a defined population of patients under the provider's care. For example, the analysis might examine the number of sigmoidoscopy claims filed per 100 Medicare patients seen by the provider in a given year. Analyses might examine whether diabetic patients have had at least one annual glucose test and have received an ophthalmology exam or could examine the frequency of flu shots, pap smears, and mammograms for various target populations (Lasker, Shapiro, & Tucker, 1992; McNeil, Pedersen, & Gatsonis, 1992).

Profiling can be used when the data contain hierarchical groupings: patients could be grouped by nurse, nurse by unit, units by larger organizations. The analysis uses regression equations to examine the relation of an outcome to the characteristics of the various groupings. To be effective, the analysis needs to include data on the different sources of variability that might contribute to a given outcome. The structure of the analysis reflects the structure of the data. For example, patient characteristics might include data on disease severity, comorbidity, emergent status, behavioral characteristics, socioeconomic status, and demographics. Nurse characteristics might include level of education, specialty status, years of practice, age, gender, and certifications. Unit characteristics might include number of beds, nursing management style used on the unit, ratio of patients to nurses, and the proportion of staff who are RNs (McNeil et al., 1992).

Profiles are designed to generate some type of action, such as to inform the provider that their rates are too high or too low compared to the norm. By examining aggregate patterns of practice, profiling can be used to compare the care provided by different organizations or received by different populations of patients. Critical pathways or care maps could be used to determine the proportion of patients who diverged from the pathway for a particular nurse, group of nurses, or group of nursing units. Profiling can be used for quality improvement, assessment of provider performance, and utilization review. Methods of improving outcomes are not addressed by profiling al-

Table 21–2
Examples of Large Database Measures Used in Profiling

Quality of Care Issue	Measures	Example	Criteria
Access	Proportion of population receiving care during the year, classified by age and sex	% of children under age 2 seen for at least one well-care visit	National
		% of children seen in emergency rooms for any reason, for trauma, and for medical problems	Trends
Preventive	Proportion of population in specific age and sex groups receiving recommended tests or procedures	% of children by group having recommended immunizations in previous year	National recommendation
		% of women age 50 and over having mammography in past year	National recommendation
		% of deliveries with prenatal care beginning in first trimester	National recommendation
Diagnosis	% of population diagnosed (and under care) for specific chronic conditions by age and sex	% of adults diagnosed at one or more visits as having essential hypertension by age and sex	Epidemiologic data on prevalence of hypertension
Treatment	Medications		
	Average number of new prescriptions per person per year	Average number of new prescriptions for antibiotics per person per year	Trends and comparison data
	Surgery		
	Rate of surgical procedures per year; total, inpatient, and ambulatory (if applicable)	Cesarian section rate for all deliveries	Trends and comparison data
Outcomes	Hospital readmissions within 3 months of discharge	% of readmissions for same condition	Comparison data and trends
		% of readmissions identifying a complication	

(Table reproduced in part from: Steinwachs, D. M., et al. [1989]. Management Information Systems and Quality. In N. Goldfield and D. B. Nash. *Providing Quality Care: The Challenge to Clinicians.* Philadelphia: ACP, Chapter 6, 160–180.)

though it can identify problem areas. It can be used to determine how and by whom performance should be changed to improve outcome. Profiling can also identify outliers, allowing more detailed examination of these individuals. The databases currently being used for profiling are not ideal since they were developed for other purposes. Outcomes that can be examined are limited to broad outcomes such as morbidity and mortality, complications, readmissions, and frequency of utilization of various services (Lasker et al., 1992; McNeil et al., 1992). Table 21–2 provides examples of the large database measures that might be used in profiling.

Prospective Cohort Studies

A *prospective cohort study* is an epidemiologic study in which a group of people are identified who are at risk for experiencing a particular event. Sample sizes for these studies often must be very large, particularly if only a small portion of the at-risk group will experience the event. The entire group is followed across time to determine the point in time at which the event occurs, variables associated with the event, and outcomes for those experiencing the event compared to those who did not experience the event. The Harvard Nurses Health Study is an example of a prospective cohort study. One hundred thousand nurses were recruited into the study to determine the long-term consequences of birth control pills. Nurses are sent a questionnaire every two years to gather data about their health and health behaviors. The study has now been in progress for over twenty years. Multiple studies have been reported in the literature using the large data set from the study. Prospective nursing studies could be conducted on a smaller scale on such populations as patients identified as high risk for the development of pressure ulcers.

Retrospective Cohort Studies

A *retrospective cohort study* is an epidemiologic study in which a group of people are identified who have experienced a particular event. This is a common research technique used by epidemiology to study occupational exposure to chemicals. Events of interest to nursing might be a procedure, an episode of care, a nursing intervention, or a diagnosis. Nurses might use a retrospective cohort study to follow a cohort of women who had received a mastectomy for breast cancer, or patients who have had a urinary bladder catheter during and after surgery. The cohort is followed up after the event to determine the occurrence of changes in health status, usually the development of a particular disease or death. Nurses might be interested in the pattern of recovery after an event, or in the case of catheterization, the incidence of bladder infections in the months following surgery. Based on study findings, epidemiologists calculate the relative risk for the group of the identified change in health. For example, if death were the occurrence of interest, the expected number of deaths would be determined. The observed number of deaths, divided by the expected number of deaths and multiplied by 100 yields a standardized mortality ratio (SMR) that is regarded as a measure of the relative risk of the studied group to die of a particular condition. In nursing studies, patients might be followed across time after discharge from a health care facility (Swaen & Meijers, 1988).

In retrospective studies, researchers often ask patients to recall information relevant to their previous health status. This information is often used to determine the amount of change occurring before and after an intervention. However, recall can easily be distorted, misleading researchers, and thus, should be used with caution. Herrmann (1995) identified three sources of distortion in recall. (1) the question posed to the subject may be conceived or expressed incorrectly, (2) the recall process may be in error, and (3) the research design used to measure recall can result in the recall appearing to be different from what actually occurred. There are four bases of recall: (1) direct recall in which the subject "accesses the memory without having to think or search memory" resulting in correct information, (2) indirect recall in which the subject "accesses the memory after thinking or searching memory" resulting in correct information, (3) limited recall in which "access to the memory does not occur but information that suggests the contents of the memory is accessed" resulting in an educated guess, and (4) no recall in which "neither the memory nor information relevant to the memory may be accessed" resulting in a wild guess (Herrmann, 1995, p. AS90).

Population Based Studies

Population based studies are also important in outcomes research. Conditions need to be studied in the context of the community, rather than the context of the medical system. Using this method, all cases of a condition occurring in the defined population are included, rather than including only patients treated at a particular health care facility, since the latter could introduce a selection bias. Efforts might be made to include individuals with the condition who had not received treatment. Community based norms of tests and survey instruments obtained in this manner provide a clearer picture of range of values than the limited spectrum of patients seen in specialty clinics. Estimates of instrument sensitivity and specificity are more accurate. This method is useful in gaining understanding of the natural history of a condition, or of the long-term risks and benefits of a particular intervention (Guess, et al., 1995).

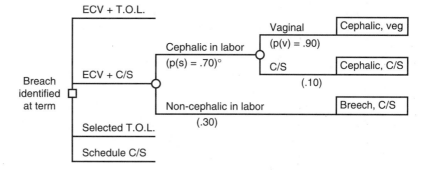

Figure 21-10
Simplified decision tree for breech delivery. (From Keeler, E. B. [1994]. Decision analysis and cost-effectiveness analysis in women's health care. *Clinical Obstetrics and Gynecology, 37*[1], 208, with permission.)

* Numbers in parentheses refer to estimated probability of event.

Clinical Decision Analysis

Clinical decision analysis is a systematic method of describing clinical problems, identifying possible diagnostic and management courses of action, assessing the probability and value of various outcomes, and then calculating the optimal course of action. Decision analysis is based on four assumptions: (1) decisions can be quantified; (2) all possible courses of action can be identified and evaluated; (3) the different values of outcomes, viewed from the perspective of the physician, patient, payer, and administrator can be examined; and (4) the analysis allows selection of an optimal course of therapy. To perform the analysis, the boundaries of the clinical problem must be defined in terms of a logical sequence of events over time. Then, all the possible courses of action are determined. These courses of action are usually represented in a decision tree consisting of a starting point, available alternatives, probable events, and outcomes. Then the goals and objectives of problem resolution are defined. The probability of occurrence of each path of the decision tree is calculated. For each potential path, there is an outcome. Each outcome is assigned a value. These values may be in terms of money, morbidity incidents, quality-of-life measures, or length of stay. A simplified decision tree for breech delivery in obstetrics is shown in Figure 21-10. An optimal course of action is identified based on which decision maximizes the chances of the most desirable outcomes (Crane, 1988; Keeler, 1994; Sonnenberg, Roberts, Tsevat, Wong, Barry, & Kent, 1994).

Nursing decisions have not reached the point of definition to allow decision analyses and little is known about how nurses make decisions regarding their nursing practice (Greiner, 1994).

Studies analyzing clinical decisions have primarily used questionnaires and interviews. However, determining the clinical decisions of practitioners is not an easy task. Much of patient care involves the clinician and the patient alone. The underlying theories of care and the processes of care are hidden from view. Thus it is difficult for clinicians to compare their approaches to care. Among physicians, care delivered by other physicians is rarely observed (O'Connor, Plume, & Wennberg, 1993). Studies have found that physicians have difficulty recalling their decisions and providing rationales for their decisions (Chaput de Saintonge & Hattersley, 1985; Kirwan, et al., 1986).

Chaput de Saintonge, Kirway, Evans, and Crane (1988) propose a strategy for analyzing clinical decisions using "paper patients." The techniques seem to parallel the decisions made by clinicians in the clinical setting. Ten common clinical variables used to evaluate the status of patients with rheumatoid arthritis were collected on 30 patients participating in a clinical trial, at the time of entry and one year later. Twenty of the patients were duplicated throughout the table to check the consistency of responses, making 50 responses in all. The variables were presented to rheumatologists on a single sheet of paper labeled "before" and "after a year." Physicians were asked to indicate the degree of change in each patient's condition using a visual analogue scale (VAS) with the ends labeled "greatest possible deterioration" and "greatest possible improvement." They were also asked whether they considered the change clinically important or not. Then they were asked to indicate the relative importance of each variable, rating the variables on a scale of 1 to 100. Regression analyses were performed using the VAS values as the dependent variable. With increasing VAS values, judgments of clinical importance changed from "not important" to "important." This change occurred over a 5 mm length of the scale or less. The researchers designated the midpoint of this transition zone as the "threshold value of clinical importance." Consistency of responses was tested using Spearman rank correlation to compare responses to the duplicate cases. Then a consensus model was developed by weighing each physician's responses based on the Spearman coefficient. The VAS scores were multiplied by the Spearman coefficient. These VAS scores were then used as the dependent variable in another regression analysis. This method is useful in identifying the important variables in making clinical decisions and the consistency of practitioners in their decisions.

Studying the Effectiveness of Interdisciplinary Teams

According to Schmitt, Farrell, and Heinemann (1988, p. 753), interdisciplinary teams have the following characteristics: (1) multiple health disciplines are involved in the care of the same patients, (2) the disciplines encompass a diversity of dissimilar knowledge and skills required by the patients, (3) the plan of care reflects an integrated set of goals shared by the providers of care, and (4) the team members share information and coordinate their services through a systematic communication process. Part of the communication process is regularly scheduled face-to-face meetings. The assumption is that collaborative team approaches provide more effective care than non-team approaches or than non-collaborative multidisciplinary approaches (parallel care). These

teams are becoming more common as health care changes. Examples are hospice care teams, home health teams, and psychiatric care teams. However, studying the effectiveness of interdisciplinary teams is difficult. The characteristics that makes team care more effective have not been identified. Studies usually focus on the evaluation of a single team, rather than conducting comparison studies. The outcomes of team care are also multidimensional, requiring multiple dependent variables to be used. Evaluation studies examining team care often examine only post-treatment data without baseline data. If groups are compared, there is no evidence that the groups were similar on important variables before the intervention. Involvement of family members with the team has not been examined. Clearly, this is an important focus of research requiring more rigorous designs than have previously been used.

GEOGRAPHIC STUDIES

Geographic analyses are used to examine variations in health status, health services, patterns of care, or patterns of use by geographic area and are sometimes referred to as small-area analyses. Variations may be associated with sociodemographic, economic, medical, cultural, and/or behavioral characteristics. Locality-specific health care system factors such as capacity, access, and convenience may also be important in explaining variations. The social setting, environment, living conditions, and community may also be important factors. There are complex interactions between the characteristics of a locality and of its inhabitants. The characteristics of the total community may transcend the characteristics of individuals within the community and may influence subgroup behavior. High education levels in the community are frequently associated with increased access to information and receptiveness to ideas from outside the community. Regression analyses are commonly used to develop models using all of the risk factors and the characteristics of the community. Results are often displayed using maps (Kieffer, Alexander, & Mor, 1992). After the analysis, the researcher must determine whether differences in rates are due to chance alone and whether high rates are too high. From a more theoretical perspective, the researcher must then explain the geographic variation uncovered by the analysis (Volinn, Diehr, Ciol, & Loeser, 1994).

Economic Studies

Many of the problems studied in health services research address concerns related to the efficient use of scarce resources, and thus, with economics. Economists are concerned with the costs and benefits of alternative treatments, or ways of identifying the most efficient means of care. The economist's definition of efficiency is the least cost method of achieving a desired end with the maximum benefit to be obtained from available resources. If available resources must be shared with other programs or other types of patients, the concern addressed is whether changing the distribution of resources will increase total benefit or welfare. To determine efficiency, the economist will conduct a *cost-effectiveness analysis*. This technique uses a single measure of outcomes and all other factors are expressed in monetary terms as net cost per unit of output (Ludbrook, 1990). Cost-effectiveness analyses compare different ways of accomplishing a clinical goal, such as diagnosing a condition, treating an illness, or providing a service. The alternative approaches are compared in terms of costs and benefits. The purpose is to identify the strategy that provides the most value for the money. There are always tradeoffs between costs and benefits (Oster, 1988).

To examine overall benefits, a *cost-benefit analysis* will be performed. Using this method, costs and benefits of alternative ways of using resources as assessed in monetary terms and the use that produces the greatest net benefit is chosen. The costs included in an economic study are defined in very exact ways. The actual costs associated with an activity, not prices, must be used. Costs are not the same as price. In most cases, price will be greater than cost. Costs are a measure of the actual use of resources, rather than the price charged. Charges are a poor reflection of actual

costs. Costs that might be included are costs to the provider, costs to third-party payers (e.g., insurance), out-of-pocket costs, and opportunity costs. Out-of-pocket costs are those expenses incurred by the patient and/or family that are not reimbursable. These costs might include supplies, dressings, special food, transportation expenses, medications, and unreinbursable care expenses. Opportunity costs are lost opportunities that the patient, family member, or others experience. A family member might have lost the opportunity to earn more if he or she had not had to stay home to care for the patient. The child might have been able to advance her education if she had not had to drop out of school for a semester to care for a parent. A husband might have been able to take a better job if the family could have moved to another town rather than stay in place in order to receive medical care. Opportunity costs are often not included in considering overall costs. This results in an underestimation of costs and an overestimation of benefit. For example, one can demonstrate that caring for an acutely ill patient at home is cost-effective if one does not consider out-of-pocket costs and opportunity costs. However, total costs of providing the activity, regardless of who pays or who receives the money, must be included. In performing such a study, it is important to state whose costs are being considered, and who is to weigh the benefits against consequences.

Ethical Studies

Outcomes studies often result in the development of policies for the allocation of scarce resources. Ethicists take the position that there are moral principles such as justice that must be considered as constraints on using costs and benefits to choose treatments in terms of maximizing the benefit per unit cost. Value commitments are inherent in choices about research methods and about the selection and interpretation of outcome variables which should be acknowledged by researchers. "The choices researchers make should be documented and the reasons for those choices should be given explicitly in publications and presentations so that readers and other users of the information are enabled and expected to bear more responsibility for interpreting and applying the findings appropriately" (Lynn & Virnig, 1995). Veatch (1993) proposes that analysis of the implications of rationing decisions in terms of the principles of justice and autonomy will provide more acceptable criteria than outcome predictors alone. As an example, Veatch performs an ethical analysis of the use of outcome predictors in decisions related to early withdrawal of life support. Ethical studies should play an important role in outcomes programs of research.

Defining and Testing Interventions

Second only to the interest in outcomes is the interest in interventions. Consistent with an outcomes research focus, it is important to consider different questions than have previously been asked about interventions, such as the following: What proportion of people experiencing a specific cluster of symptoms were diagnosed (correctly or not) as having a particular diagnosis, and of this group, who received what treatment? Should a treatment or procedure have been performed? Did persons with a particular diagnosis receive appropriate treatment? What proportion of people with the cluster of symptoms received no treatment? (Kane & Lurie, 1992). Intervention studies from an outcome perspective tend to be more varied than those of traditional research in which the ideal is the clinical trial. There are problems with the clinical trial that have led to the method being heavily criticized by outcome researchers. To be included in a clinical trial, subjects must meet rigorous sampling criteria. These criteria severely limit generalization, and physicians are often reluctant to apply the findings from clinical trials in their patient care, because their patients do not fit the sampling criteria used in the clinical trial. The outcomes studied in these trials tend to be biophysical and intermediate. Clinical trials are only beginning to examine issues related to quality of life (Orchard, 1994).

The following section describes a sample of the various research strategies that are being used to examine interventions in outcome studies.

These include defining an intervention, preference clinical trials, treatment matching, and probing the effects of multicomponent treatments.

Defining an Intervention

In many clinical intervention studies, the assumption has been made that the intervention was consistent across clinicians with no effort made to test this assumption. Medical protocols, the basis of many clinical trials, define specific tasks that are required components of treatment but do not specify who performs the task or by what means. Maynard (1990, p. 763) recommends that the description of interventions should indicate: (1) *Who does* (i.e., who is the decision maker in each alternative) (2) *what* (i.e., what is the alternative) (3) *to whom* (i.e., who are the recipients of treatment and do third parties [e.g., those who care]) (4) *how often* (i.e., what is the frequency and phasing of each intervention) and (5) *what are the effects* (i.e., what is the effect on length and quality of life). Determining these may require direct observation and queries to the clinicians regarding their reasoning and decisions. After defining an intervention, feedback should be obtained from the clinicians regarding accuracy of the description. Obtaining the patient's and family member's perspective of the treatment or intervention would add an important dimension to the description. Katz and Schroeder (1994) have begun the process of defining and categorizing nursing interventions by identifying generic functions that cross specialty areas in nursing.

Interventions are often multifaceted and complex. Identification of critical elements of interventions have lagged behind other areas of research. It is important to determine which facets of these interventions produce the desired outcome and to identify the alternative treatments (Donovan, et al., 1994). While some facets may work together to maximize the effect on outcomes, some may have no effect (except to increase costs), while others may actually diminish the desired effect. The factors actually causing the desired outcome may be very different from those expected by clinicians. There is also a possibility of an interaction effect, where some types of patients benefit from a treatment while others do not (Bergmark & Oscarsson, 1991). Nolan and Grant (1993) point out that treatments have both anticipated and unanticipated effects, that may be either beneficial or detrimental.

Preference Clinical Trials (PCT)

In the typical clinical trial, subjects are randomized into groups. However, in some cases patient preference is an important variable. The effect of active choice on outcomes is important to understand. Wennberg and colleagues (1993, p. 56) indicate that "when symptom reduction and improvement in the quality of life are the main effects of treatment and the proper decision involves the evaluation of risk aversion and degree of botheredness, then these topics cannot be ignored; they must be made the object of investigation." Thus, in *PCT*, rather than being randomized, patients choose among all treatments available. The Standard Gamble Method is used to measure individual's preferences under uncertainty (Gafni, 1994).

Treatment Matching

Treatment matching is performed to compare the relative effectiveness of various treatments. Treatment matching designs are used when the following conditions are met: (1) There is no clearly superior treatment for all individuals with a given problem; (2) there are a number of treatments with some proven efficacy that are relatively comparable in their effectiveness for undifferentiated groups of subjects; and (3) there is evidence of differential outcome either within or across treatments for defined subtypes of clients (Donovan, et al., 1994, p. 139). No control group is used. Sampling criteria are selected to promote heterogeneity rather than homogeneity. Randomization is used but stratification and other strategies to obtain balanced distribution, such as client matching, will also be used. Creative sampling methods may be required to fulfill sampling requirements (Carroll, Kadden, Donovan, Zweben,

& Rounsaville, 1994; Connors, et al., 1994; DiClemente, Carroll, Connors, & Kadden, 1994; Miller & Cooney, 1994; Zweben, et al., 1994).

Probing the Effects of Multicomponent Treatments

Multicomponent treatments occur when a set of treatments are combined to manage a patient problem. Although those studies have tended to be treatment programs for such problems as substance abuse and psychiatric treatment, there are a number of nursing situations in which a set of nursing activities have been combined to achieve the most desirable outcome that would lend themselves to these designs. The effects of multicomponent programs are difficult to assess. West, Aiken, and Todd (1993) have described a series of designs that can be used to test the effectiveness of various components of such a treatment.

1. **Treatment package strategy.** The total treatment package is compared with that of an appropriate comparison group.
2. **Comparative Treatment Strategy.** Two or more alternative interventions are directly compared. An additional no-treatment comparison group is often included. Using this strategy, the most effective treatment strategy can be selected from a set of alternative strategies.
3. **Dismantling Strategy (subtraction design).** The full version of the program is compared with a reduced version in which one or more components have been removed. Criteria for selecting components to delete vary but are often based on theory or information from review of the literature. Components that are expensive or difficult to provide may also be selected for deletion. Components are removed one at a time, and the reduced set tested against the full version until a single base component remains. When programs are complex and include many components, various mixes of components may be tested.
4. **Constructive Strategy.** A base intervention is identified. A component expected to increase the effectiveness of the base intervention is

added and the two interventions are tested. It is important that there be a theoretical rationale for the selection of components to add to the base intervention. Additional components are added, one at a time, and each set of components tested for effectiveness until the full set of possible combinations is studied. As with the dismantling strategy, with large programs, various mixes of components may be tested.

5. **Factorial ANOVA Designs.** These designs, commonly used in psychology, are potentially the most powerful way to examine all possible combinations of a program. Factorial designs used in intervention trials are usually limited to a 2 × 2 design examining the presence or absence of two intervention components. The complexity of using this method in multicomponent intervention leads to difficulties in acquiring sufficient sample sizes, achieving adequate statistical power, and in interpreting the results.

6. **Fractional Factorial Designs.** These designs are simplifications of the factorial design in which the researcher systematically selects a portion of all possible treatment combinations to implement. This requires that the researcher be willing to assume that the effects of higher order interactions (multiple combination effects) are negligible.

7. **Dose Response Designs.** This design requires that the researcher be able to provide varying doses of a component of a treatment. The strategy was developed for use in testing drug therapy; however, it is possible to apply it to any component in which degrees of application can be quantified. The duration of the program or the length of time for a treatment could be varied. This strategy is used to determine the amount of treatment that provides optimal strength in achieving the desired outcome.

8. **Response Surface Methodology.** This design allows the dose response to be applied to more than one dimension of a treatment. If several interventions are constructed representing a number of combinations of differing levels of strength of each component and the outcome

is plotted for each combination, the plotted figure is referred to as a response surface. This methodology can be used to determine the combination of components that produces the optimum outcome. Results from previous response surface analyses have shown that increasing the strength of a component does not always lead to increases in effectiveness. Combining two individually effective components can result in a program that is either more or less effective than each individual component. Programs can be improved sequentially by refining each individual component and then studying their combined effects. This suggests that developing an optimal program is an evolutionary process.

9. **Mediational Analysis.** This design is used to examine the processes through which each component of an intervention has its effect. This requires that the researcher be able to identify the processes through which each component effects the outcome. Reliable measures of each of the processes and each of the outcome variables are included in the design. Structural equation analysis is used to examine the contribution of each component to the outcome.

MEASUREMENT METHODS

The selection of appropriate outcome variables is critical to the success of a study (Bernstein & Hilborne, 1993). As in any study, evidence of validity and reliability of the methods of measurement need to be evaluated. Outcomes selected for nursing studies should be those most consistent with nursing practice and theory (Harris & Warren, 1995). In some studies, rather than selecting the final outcome of care which may not occur for months or years, measures of intermediate end points are used. Intermediate end points are events or markers that act as a precursor to the final outcome. However, it is important to document the validity of the intermediate end point in predicting the outcome (Freedman & Schatzkin, 1992). A selection of outcome measures that have been used in published studies are listed in Table 21–3. In

Table 21-3
Examples of Measures Commonly Used in Outcome Studies

Patient Characteristics
- age
- beliefs/attitudes
- comorbid conditions
- diagnosis/condition
- gender
- health habits
- laboratory values
- medical care utilization
- medications
- preferences
- prognosis
- resource use
- severity
- symptoms and signs
- understanding of a condition

Provider Personal Characteristics
- age
- beliefs/attitudes
- economic incentives
- gender
- job satisfaction
- preferences
- specialty training

Provider Technical Style
- continuity of care
- coordination
- expenditures
- hospitalizations
- medications
- referrals
- test ordering
- visits

Provider Interpersonal Style
- communication level
- counseling
- interpersonal manner
- patient participation

Institutional Characteristics
- avoidable deaths
- cancellation of an ambulatory procedure on the day of the procedure
- cases where a discrepancy between initial and final X-ray reports required an adjustment in patient management
- cesarean sections
- costs
- Council on Teaching Hospitals membership
- fetal death rate
- hospital-acquired infections
- iatrogenic problems
- incidence of complications
- inpatient mortality
- neonatal mortality
- number of technological services
- patients in the emergency department more than six hours
- patients who leave the emergency department prior to completion of treatment

- patient satisfaction
  - access
  - convenience
  - organization
  - specialty mix
  - financial incentives
- percentage of board-certified physicians
- perinatal death
- perinatal mortality rate
- perioperative death
- postneonatal mortality rate
- presence of discharge planning services
- provider mix
- ratio of registered nurses to beds
- readmission rates
- risk adjustment
- service mix
- surgical-wound infections
- unplanned admissions following ambulatory procedure
- unplanned readmissions
- unplanned returns to a special care unit
- unplanned returns to the operating room
- unplanned returns to the emergency department within 72 hours
- whether patients were dead or alive at the end of their hospital stay
- work load

Community Outcomes
- immunization rate
- incidence of infectious diseases (e.g., measles)
- infant mortality rate
- neonatal mortality rate

Process Characteristics
- appropriateness of care
- post-hospital care
- time

Functional Status
- amount of assistance needed
- disability
  - behavioral functioning
  - task performance
    - speed
    - pain
    - confidence
  - dependence
  - quality of performance
- functional changes in advanced dementia
- handicap
  - social roles
  - social expectations
- impairment
  - range of motion
  - strength
  - endurance
  - pain

continued

Table 21-3
Examples of Measures Commonly Used in Outcome Studies *Continued*

productive activity
  gainful employment
  homemaking
  school or training
  volunteer services
  leisure activities
skill indicators
  self-care
  mobility
  social behavior
  communication
  vocational activity
  homemaking

Physiologic Outcomes
  asthma symptoms
  complications
  health status
  survival

Social Outcomes
  school absence rates
  social support
  social investment
  status indicators
    employment
    income
    education
    family role
    living arrangements

Quality of Life
  Health-related quality of life
  Quality-adjusted life years (QALYs)
  quality of life

General Well-being
  energy/fatigue
  health perceptions
  life satisfaction
  living arrangements at discharge
  pain

Behavioral Outcomes
  activity pattern indicators
    percentage of time spent out of the residence
    time in travel
    diversity of activities
    time spent in inactivity
    time spent in passive recreation
  breast-feeding after hospital discharge
  self report of health behavior
  weight change

Mental Health Outcomes
  increased screening and early detection efforts
  reductions in the incidence or prevalence rates of diagnosable emotional and behavioral disorders
  reductions in the need for mental health services

early outcome studies, researchers selected outcome measures that could be easily obtained, rather than those most desirable for outcome studies. Characteristics important to evaluate in selecting methods of measuring outcomes are identified in Table 21–4. In evaluating a particular outcome measure, the literature should be consulted for previous studies that have used that particular method of measurement, including the publication describing development of the method of measurement. Information related to the measurement can be organized into a table such as Table 21–5 (on p. 600), allowing easy comparison of several methods of measuring a particular outcome.

Outcome researchers are moving away from classical measurement theory as a means of evaluating the reliability of measurement methods. They are interested in identifying change in measures across time in a subject and instruments developed using measurement theory are often not sensitive to these changes. The magnitude of change that can be detected is also important to determine. In addition, measures may detect change within a particular range of values but may not be sensitive to changes outside that range. The sensitivity to change of many frequently used outcome measures has not been examined (Deyo & Carter, 1992; Felson, Anderson, & Meenan, 1990). Studies need to be conducted specifically to determine the sensitivity of measures prior to their use in outcome studies. As sensitivity increases, statistical power increases, allowing smaller sample sizes to detect significant differences.

The Analysis of Measurement Reliability

Estimating the reliability of outcome measures using classical measurement theory may be problematic. The traditional concept of measurement reliability was developed to evaluate quantities that were not expected to change over time in an individual. This assessment of reliability is irrelevant or only partially relevant to assessing the suitability or precision of measures selected because of their sensitivity to change within the individual over time. Traditional evaluations of measurement

Table 21–4
Characteristics of Outcomes Assessment Instruments

Characteristic	Considerations in Patient Outcomes Evaluation	Reference

Applicability	Consider purpose of instruments
	  Discriminate between subjects at a point in time
	  Predict future outcomes
	  Evaluate changes within subjects over time
	  Screen for problems
	  Provide case-mix adjustment
	  Assess quality of care
	Consider whether
	  Norms are established for clinical population of interest
	  Instrument format is compatible with assessment approach (e.g., observer rated vs. self-administered)
	  Setting in which instrument was developed
		Deyo & Carter, 1992
		Stewart et al., 1989
		Guyatt, Walter, & Norman, 1987
		Feinstein, Josephy, & Wells, 1986
		Deyo, 1984

Practicality (clinical utility)	The instrument:
	  Includes outcomes important to the patient
	  Is short & easy to administer (low respondent burden)
	  Questions are easy to understand and acceptable to patients and interviewers
	  Scores reflect condition severity, condition-specific features, and discriminate those with condition from those without
	  Is easily scored and scores are readily understandable
	  Level of measurement allows a change score to be determined
	  Provides information that is clinically useful
	  Performance or capacity based
	  Includes patient rating of magnitude of effort and support needed for performance of physical tasks
		Leidy, 1991
		Nelson, Landgraf, Hays, Wasson, & Kirk, 1990
		Stewart et al., 1989
		Lohr, 1988
		Bombardier and Tugwell, 1987
		Feinstein et al., 1986
		Kirshner & Guyatt, 1985
		Deyo, 1984

Comprehensiveness	Generic measures are designed to summarize a spectrum of concepts applied to different impairments, illnesses, patients, and populations Disease-specific measures are designed to assess specific patients with specific conditions or diagnoses Dimensions of the instrument; a core set of physical, mental, and role functions desirable	Nelson et al., 1990 Patrick & Deyo, 1989 Deyo, 1984
Reliability	Can be influenced by day-to-day variations in patients, differences between observers, items in the scale, mode of administration This is the critical determinant of usefulness of an instrument designed for discriminative purpose	Nelson et al., 1990 Spitzer, 1987 Guyatt et al., 1987 Deyo, 1984
Validity	No consensus of what are scientifically admissible criteria for many indices No "gold standard" exists for establishing criterion validity for many indices	Spitzer, 1987 Deyo, 1984
Responsiveness	Not yet indexed for virtually any evaluative measures Coarse scale rating may not detect changes Aggregated scores may obscure changes in subscales Useful for determining sample size and statistical power Reliable instruments are likely to be responsive but reliability not adequate as sole index of consistent results over time Consider detail in scaling As baseline variability of score changes within stable subjects, may need larger treatment effects to demonstrate efficacy Consider temporal relationship between intervention and outcome	Stewart & Archbold, 1992 Leidy, 1991 Jaeschke, Singer, & Guyatt, 1989 Guyatt et al., 1989 Bombardier & Tugwell, 1987 Guyatt et al., 1987 Deyo & Centor, 1986 Deyo, 1984

(From Harris, M. R., & Warren, J. J. [1995]. Patient outcomes: Assessment issues for the CNS. *Clinical Nurse Specialist, 9*[2], 82, with permission.)

Table 21-5
Characteristics of the Katz ADL Scale, a Proposed Outcome Instrument

Characteristic	Reference
Applicability	
Purpose is to objectively evaluate results of treatment in chronically ill and aging populations	Katz, 1970
Predicts service utilization in elderly population	Wiener et al., 1990
Used in case-mix adjustments	Fries, 1990
Scale discriminates well on disability in elderly population, norms easily referenced	Spector, 1990
Ratings judgment based on direct observation and caregiver reports, known differences in observed vs. reported ratings	Spector, 1990 Burns, 1992
Practicality	
Brief, 6 items with 3 levels of dependency	Katz, 1970
Can be used by clinicians and nonclinicians	Spector, 1990
Measures performance (not ability)	Katz, 1970
Aggregate score represents increasing level of dependency	Spector, 1990
Comprehensiveness	
Includes bathing, dressing, toileting, transfer, continence, and eating	Katz, 1970
Does not explain etiology of level of performance	Kane & Bayer, 1991
Generic measure (not disease specific)	
Reliability	
Performance may be influenced by motivational, social, and environmental factors	Kane & Bayer, 1991
High internal consistency reported	Spector, 1990
Validity	
Content and construct validity assessments are acceptable	Spector, 1990
Responsiveness	
No published reports that quantify relationship of scale change to minimal clinically important change	

(From Harris, M. R., & Warren, J. J. [1995]. Patient outcomes: Assessment issues for the CNS. *Clinical Nurse Specialist, 9*[2], 85, with permission.)

methods assume that any change in group values is a result of variation between individuals. Patient change, however, results in changes within the individual. Using traditional measurement theory analysis, a measure that did not vary between individuals would have zero (or poor) reliability. This measure, however, may be an excellent measure of change over time if individuals change on that measure (even if group averages do not change much). Thus, it is inappropriate to assess the reliability of difference scores based on the internal consistency of measures (Collins & Johnston, 1995).

Multiple outcome measures are commonly used in outcome studies. Researchers want to evaluate all relevant effects of care. However, quantity of measures is not necessarily evidence of the quality of the measures. The measures most relevant to the treatment should be selected. Measures selected should not be closely correlated. Interpreting the results of studies in which multiple outcomes have been used can be problematic. For example, Felson and colleagues (1990, p. 141) ask "which is the better therapy, the one that shows a change in 6 outcome measures out of 12 tested or the one that shows a change in 4 of the 12 measures? What if the 4 that demonstrate change with one therapy are not the same as the 6 that show a change in another therapy?" If multiple comparisons are made, it is important to make statistical adjustments for them; the risk of a Type I error is greater when multiple comparisons are made. Some researchers recommend combining various measures into a single summary score (DesHarnais, McMahon, & Wroblewski, 1991; Felson et al., 1990). However, such global composite measures have not been widely used. The various measures used in such an index may not be equally weighted and may be difficult to combine. Also, the composite index value may not be readily interpretable by clinicians.

The focus of most measures developed for outcome studies has been the individual patient. However, a number of organizations are now developing measures of the quality of performance of systems of care. In 1990 the Consortium Research on Indicators of System Performance

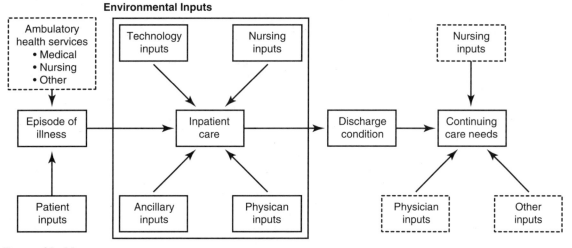

Figure 21-11
Framework for ANA Report Card. (From American Nurses Association. [1995]. *Nursing report card for acute care.* Washinton, DC: ANA, with permission.)

(CRISP) project began to develop indicators of the quality of performance of integrated delivery systems. From the perspective of CRISP, the success of a health system was associated with its ability to decrease the number of episodes of diseases in the population. Therefore, the impact of the delivery system on the community was considered an important measure of performance. CRISP has developed a number of indicators now in use by consortium members, who pay to participate in the studies (Bergman, 1994). The Joint Commission on Accreditation of Healthcare Organizations (JCAHO) is also applying outcomes data to quality management efforts in hospitals using the IMSytem (McCormick, 1990; Nadzam, Turpin, Hanold, & White, 1993). The National Committee for Quality Assurance, the organization that accredits managed care plans, has developed a tool (HEDIS) for comparing managed care plans. Comparisons involve more than 60 measures, including patient satisfaction, quality of care, and financial stability (Guadagnoli & McNeil, 1994). Researchers at the Henry Ford Health Systems' Center for Health System Studies in Detroit have developed 80 performance indicators to evaluate health systems (H. J. Anderson, 1991).

The American Nurses' Association has devel-

oped a Nursing Care Report Card for Acute Care (ANA, 1995). Their model identifying concepts critical to quality acute care and illustrating the relationships among them is shown in Figure 21–11. The Acute Care Nursing Quality Indicators developed through this project are listed in Figure 21–12 (on p. 602). The project is in the early stages of development. Pilot studies have been conducted using the indicators. Problems with use of the indicators and consistency of measurement across facilities were identified. Strategies for improving consistency in measurement have been developed and a second phase of study was implemented late in 1995.

STATISTICAL METHODS FOR OUTCOME STUDIES

Although outcome researchers test for statistical significance of their findings, this is not considered sufficient to judge the findings as important. The focus of their attention is on the clinical significance of study findings (see Chapter 16 for more information on clinical significance). In analyzing data, outcome researchers have moved away from statistical analyses, using the mean to test for

Patient-focused Outcome Indicators

- Mortality rate
- Length of stay
- Adverse incidents
  - Adverse incident rate (total)
  - Medication error rate
  - Patient injury rate
- Complications
  - Total complication rate
  - Decubitus ulcer rate
  - Nosocomial infection rate (total)
  - Nosocomial urinary tract infection rate
  - Nosocomial pneumonia rate
  - Nosocomial surgical wound infection rate

- Patient/family satisfaction with nursing care
  - Patient willingness to recommend hospital to others/use hospital again
- Patient adherence to discharge plan
  - Readmission rates
  - Emergency room visits post-discharge
  - Unscheduled physician visits post-discharge
  - Patient knowledge of disease/condition and care requirements

Process of Care Indicators

- Nurse satisfaction
- Assessment and implementation of patient care requirements
  - Assessment of patient care requirements
  - Development of a nursing care plan
  - Accurate and timely execution of therapeutic interventions and procedures
  - Documentation of nursing diagnoses, therapeutic objectives, and care given
- Pain management
- Maintenance of skin integrity

- Patient education
- Discharge planning
- Assurance of patient safety
  - Overall assurance of patient safety
  - Appropriate use of restraints (all)
  - Appropriate use of pharmaceutical restraints
  - Appropriate use of physical restraints
- Responsiveness to unplanned patient care needs

Structure of Care Indicators—Nurse Staffing Patterns

- Ratio of total nursing staff to patients
  - RN/patient ratio
  - LPN/patient ratio
  - Unlicensed workers/patient ratio
- Ratio of RNs to total nursing staff
  - RN staff experience
  - RN staff education (i.e., MSNs, BSNs)

- Total nursing care hours provided per patient (case mix, acuity adjusted)
  - RN hours per patient
  - LPN hours per patient
  - Unlicensed worker hours per patient
- Staff continuity
  - Use of agency nurses
  - Use of float nurses
  - Unsafe assignment rate
  - Nurse staff turnover rates
  - FT/PT RN ratio
- RN overtime
- Nursing staff injury rate

Figure 21–12

Acute care nursing quality indicators. (From American Nurses Association. [1995]. *Nursing report card for acute care.* Washington, DC: ANA, with permission.)

group differences. They place greater importance on analyzing change scores and use exploratory methods of examining the data to identify outliers.

The Analysis of Change

With the focus on outcome studies has come a renewed interest in methods of analyzing change. Gottman and Rushe (1993) report that the first book addressing change in research, *Problems in Measuring Change* edited by Harris (1967) is the basis for most current approaches to analyzing change. Since then, a number of new ideas have emerged regarding the analysis of change (e.g., Collins & Horn, 1991; Rovine & Von Eye, 1991; Von Eye, 1990a, 1990b). However, many researchers are unfamiliar with these new ideas and continue to base their reasoning on Harris's 1967 book. Gottman and Rushe (1993) suggest that many beliefs related to the analysis of change are based on little more than fallacies.

Fallacy 1: In change, regression toward the mean is an unavoidable law of nature.

Fallacy 2: The difference score between pre- and postmeasurement is unreliable.

Fallacy 3: Analysis of covariance (ANCOVA—or related methods such as path analysis) is the way to analyze change.

Fallacy 4: Two points (pre- and posttest) are adequate for the study of change.

Fallacy 5: The correlation between change and initial level is always negative.

The method of analysis of change is also being questioned by outcome researchers. Collins and Johnston (1995) suggest that the recommended analysis method of regressing pretest scores on outcome scores and basing the analysis of change on residual change scores is overly conservative and tends to understate the extent of real change. There are serious questions about the conceptual meaning of these residual change scores.

For some outcomes, the changes may be nonlinear or may go up and down rather than always increasing. Thus, it is as important to uncover patterns of change as it is to test for statistical differences across time. Some changes may occur in relation to stages of recovery or improvement. These changes may occur over weeks, months, or even years. A more complete picture of the process of recovery can be obtained by examining the process in greater detail and over a broader range. Using this approach, a recovery curve can be developed that provides a model of the recovery process that can then be tested (Collins & Johnston, 1995; Ottenbacher, Johnson, & Hojem, 1995).

The Analysis of Improvement

In addition to reporting the mean improvement score for all patients treated, it is important to report what percentage of patients improve. Do all patients improve slightly, or is there a divergence among patients, with some improving greatly while others do not improve at all? This may best be illustrated by plotting the data. Researchers studying a particular treatment or approach to care might develop a standard or index of varying degrees of improvement that might occur. This would allow better comparisons of the effectiveness of various treatments. Characteristics of patients who experience varying degrees of improvement should be described, and outliers should be carefully examined. This requires that the study design include baseline measures of patient status, such as demographic characteristics, functional status, and disease severity measures. This will allow better judgments of appropriate use of various treatments (Felson et al., 1990).

Variance Analysis

Variance analysis is used to track individual and group variance from a specific critical pathway. The goal is to decrease preventable variance in process, thus helping patients and their families achieve optimal outcomes. Some of the variance is due to comorbidities. Maintaining a patient with comorbidities on the desired pathway may require increased resource utilization early in their care. Thus, it is important to track both variance and comorbidities. Studies examining variations from pathways may facilitate tailoring of existing critical pathways for specific comorbidities. Variance

Table 21–6 Sample Data Using Longitudinal Guttman Scale			
	Functional Items		
	M1	*M2*	*M3*
Patient A			
Time 1	Fail	Fail	Fail
Time 2	Pass	Fail	Fail
Time 3	Pass	Pass	Fail
Patient B			
Time 1	Fail	Fail	Fail
Time 2	Pass	Pass	Fail
Time 3	Pass	Pass	Fail
Patient C			
Time 1	Pass	Fail	Fail
Time 2	Pass	Pass	Fail
Time 3	Pass	Pass	Pass

(From Collins, L. M., & Johnston, M. V. [1995]. Analysis of stage-sequential change in rehabilitation research. *American Journal of Physical Medicine and Rehabilitation, 74*[2], 167.)

analysis can also be used to identify at risk patients who might benefit from the services of a case manager. Variance analysis tracking is expressed using graphics, and the expected pathway is plotted on the graph. The care providers plot deviations (negative variance) on the graph, allowing immediate comparison with the expected pathway. Deviations may be related to the patient, the system, or the provider (Tidwell, 1993).

The Longitudinal Guttman Simplex (LGS) Model

The LGS is an extension of the Guttman scale that involves times as well as items and persons. For example, an LGS of mobility might involve the following items: (M1) moving unassisted from bed to chair; (M2) moving unassisted from bed to another room; (M3) moving unassisted up stairs. Table 21–6 shows hypothetical data using this measure on three patients at three time periods showing a pattern of increasing ability over time (Collins & Johnston, 1995).

Latent Transition Analysis (LTA)

LTA is used in situations where stages or categories of recovery have been defined and transitions across stages can be identified. To use the analysis method, each member of the population is placed in a single category or stage for a given point of time. However, stage membership changes across time. The analysis tests stage membership to provide a realistic picture of development. Collins and Johnston (1995) provide an example of this type of analysis with a hypothetical model of recovery from functional neglect following stroke.

"Let's assume that we can define a study subpopulation displaying four latent stages or types of functional neglect: sensory limitations (S), cognitive limitations (C), both (S and C) or patients may recover and adapt to the point that they are functional (F) . . . Membership in each category is inferred from several clinical symptoms or test items, which supposedly go together but in fact may not for some patients. The items have some error and are imperfect indicators of true (latent) stage membership. Our objective is to estimate in which category a patient probably falls at any point in time and the probability of movement between stages over time, conditional on previous stage membership. . . Suppose we use a large number of times periodically to monitor progress, testing the same group of patients at multiple points in time. We record which items the patient passes and which the patient does not." (p. 47) ■

Using a computerized program designed to perform LTA analysis, the results shown in Table 21–7 are obtained. Only two points of time are shown although the program will handle up to five points in time.

The first line of the table contains the estimate of the proportion of patients in each of the four stages at Time 1. In this example, 30% of the sample had both S and C limitations, 30% had S limitations, and 40% had C limitations, while none were functional. At Time 2, the proportion in each functional limitation appears to decline, except sensory limitations which is unchanged, and 27% are now in the functional stage. The bottom half of the table is a matrix of transition probabilities

Table 21–7
A Hypothetical Latent Transition Model of Recovery from Neglect Following Stroke

	Latent Status			
	F	*C*	*S*	*S and C*
Total Marginal Proportions				
Time 1 proportions	0.0	0.40	0.30	0.30
Time 2 proportions	0.27	0.25	0.30	0.18
	Time 2 Latent Status			
Time 1 Latent Status	*F*	*C*	*S*	*S and C*
Time 1 to Time 2 Transition				
Proportions within Rows				
Functional (F)	0	0	0	0
Cognitive Limitation (C)	0.46	0.54	0.0	0.0
Sensory Limitation (S)	0.30	0.0	0.70	0.0
S and C	0.0	0.10	0.30	0.60

>No patients were functional at time 1. (From Collins, L. M., & Johnston, M. V. [1995]. Analysis of stage-sequential change in rehabilitation research. *American Journal of Physical Medicine and Rehabilitation, 74*[2], 168.)

that reveals patterns of change. Of patients who started with S, 30% improved; however, the overall percentage at S remained the same because 30% of the patients who started at S & C transitioned to the S category. Of patients who initially had C problems alone, 46% moved to the functional category.

A third set of quantities estimated by the full LTA model but not shown in the table are the relationships between items and stage memberships. This relationship indicates the probability that when a subject moves from one category to another, each item will also change to reflect the new stage membership. Thus, this relationship is a determination of the effectiveness of the items as an indicator of stage membership.

Multilevel Analysis

Multilevel analysis is used in epidemiology to study how environmental factors (aggregate-level characteristics) and individual attributes and behaviors (individual-level characteristics) interact to influence individual-level health behaviors and disease risks. For example, the risk of an adolescent initiating smoking is associated with the fol-

lowing variables: attributes of the child (e.g., self-esteem, academic achievement, refusal skills); attributes of the child's family (e.g., parental attitudes toward smoking, smoking behavior of parents), general characteristics of the community (e.g., ease of minors' access to cigarettes, school policies regarding smoking, city smoking ordinances, social norms of students toward smoking); and general social factors (e.g., geographic region, economic policies that influence the price of cigarettes). The researcher might ask, "Does smoking status covary with the level of restriction of smoking in public places after controlling for the individual-level variables that influence smoking risks?" (Von Korff, Koepsell, Curry, & Diehr, 1992, p. 1078).

DISSEMINATING OUTCOMES RESEARCH FINDINGS

Including plans for the dissemination of findings as a component of a program of research is a new idea within nursing if one considers the process of dissemination to be greater than that of publishing the results in professional journals. The costs associated with dissemination are not included in funding for nursing studies beyond publishing the research findings. As discussed in Unit III of this text, strategies for the dissemination of research findings tend to be performed by groups other than the original researchers. The transfer of knowledge from nurse researchers to nurse clinicians has been for the most part ineffective. Nursing, as a discipline, has not yet addressed the various constituencies of nursing research knowledge. A research team conducting a program of outcomes research needs to identify their constituencies. These should include the clinicians who will apply the knowledge to practice, the public who may make health care decisions based on the information, health care institutions who need to evaluate care in their facilities based on the information, health policymakers who may set standards based on the information, and researchers who may use the information in designing new studies. Disseminating information to these various constituencies through presentations at meetings and publications in a wide diversity of journals and magazines, as well as releasing the information to the news media, will require careful planning. Mattson and Donovan (1994) suggest that dissemination involved strategies of debunking myths, addressing issues related to feasibility, effective communication, and identifying opinion leaders.

■ SUMMARY

Outcomes research was developed to examine the end results of patient care. The momentum propelling outcomes research today is coming from policymakers, insurers, and the public. The scientific approaches used in outcome studies differ in some important ways from those of traditional research. These differences have led traditional researchers and statisticians to criticize the credibility of outcomes research. Outcomes researchers counter these criticisms by saying that experimental studies lack external validity and are not useful for application in clinical settings.

A number of health care providers throughout history have attempted to examine the outcomes of patient care. Their efforts were not well received by the medical community. Because of growing concerns about the quality of medical care, the Agency for Health Services Research (AHSR) was developed in 1959. This agency supported small area analyses that examined variations in medical practice across towns and counties. The first large scale study of patient outcomes, the Medical Outcomes Study, was funded through this agency. In 1989, the Agency for Health Care Policy and Research (AHCPR) replaced the AHSR and, with much increased funding, was mandated to conduct studies of patient outcomes of health care. Patient Outcomes Research Teams (PORTs), large scale, multifaceted, and multidisciplinary projects, were designed to address this mandate. The focus of outcome research has been medical practice. However, nursing needs to become involved in examining the outcomes of nursing practice in hospital settings, in managed care, and in community settings such as nurse practitioners providing primary health care.

The theory on which outcome research is based was developed by Donabedian. Quality is the overriding construct of the theory although Donabedian never defines this concept. The three major concepts of the theory are health, subjects of care, and providers of care. Donabedian identifies three objects of evaluation in appraising quality: structure, process, and outcome. The goal of outcome research is the evaluation of outcomes as defined by Donabedian, whose theory requires that identified outcomes be clearly linked with the process that caused the outcome. Three compo-

continued

continued

nents of process are of interest to Donabedian: standards of care, practice styles, and costs of care. Structures of care are the elements of organization and administration that guide the processes of care.

Because outcomes research is relatively new, methods are still being developed that will provide answers to the questions posed. However, a research process for conducting outcome studies is being defined. Outcome research programs are complex and may include multiple studies using a variety of designs whose findings must be merged in the process of forming conclusions. Outcome designs tend to have less control than traditional research designs and, other than the clinical trial, seldom use random samples but rather use large representative samples. Outcomes selected for nursing studies should be those most consistent with nursing practice and theory. The researcher must consider the measure's sensitivity to change and the magnitude of change

that can be detected. Multiple outcome measures are commonly used in outcome studies. Although the focus of most measures developed for outcome studies has been the individual patient, a number of organizations are now developing measures of the quality of performance of systems of care.

Statistical approaches used in outcome studies include new approaches to examining measurement reliability, strategies to analyze change, and the analysis of improvement. A variety of techniques have been developed to address the analysis needs of outcomes researchers, including ways to use structural equation modeling, the longitudinal Guttman Simplex model, latent transition analysis, variance analysis, profiling, multilevel analysis, and geographic analyses. Strategies need to be developed in nursing to disseminate the findings from outcomes studies to the various constituences needing the information.

References

Altman, L. K. (1993). Bringing the news to the public: The role of the media. *Annals of the New York Academy of Sciences, 703,* 200–209.

American Nurses' Association. (1995). *Nursing report card for acute care.* Washington, DC: American Nurses' Publishing.

Anderson, C. (1994). Measuring what works in health care. *Science, 263*(5150), 1080, 1082.

Anderson, H. J. (1991). Sizing up systems: Researchers to test performance measures. *Hospitals, 65*(20), 33–34.

Bergman, R. (1994). Are my outcomes better than yours? *Hospital Health Network, 68*(15), 113–116.

Bergmark, A., & Oscarsson, L. (1991). Does anybody really know what they are doing? Some comments related to methodology of treatment service research. *British Journal of Addiction, 86*(2), 139–142.

Bernstein, S. J., & Hilborne, L. H. (1993). Clinical indicators: The road to quality care? *Joint Commission Journal on Quality Improvement, 19*(11), 501–509.

Bloom, B. S. (1990). Does it work? The outcomes of medical interventions. *International Journal of Technology Assessment in Health Care, 6*(2), 326–332.

Bombardier, C., & Tugwell, P. (1987). Methodological consid-

erations in functional assessment. *Journal of Rheumatology, 14*(Suppl. 15), 7–10.

Burns, R. B., Moskowitz, M. A., Ash, A., Kane, R. L., Finch, M. D., & Bak, S. M. (1992). Self-report *versus* medical record functional status. *Medical Care. 30*(Suppl. 5), MS85–MS95.

Carroll, K. M., Kadden, R. M., Donovan, D. M., Zweben, A., & Rounsaville, B. J. (1994). Implementing treatment and protecting the validity of the independent variable in treatment matching studies. *Journal on Studies of Alcohol, 12*(Suppl.), 149–155.

Chaput de Saintonge, D. M., & Hattersley, L. A. (1985). Antibiotics for otitis media: Can we help doctors agree? *Family Practice, 2,* 205–212.

Chaput de Saintonge, D. M., Kirway, J. R., Evans, S. J., & Crane, G. J. (1988). How can we design trials to detect clinically important changes in disease severity? *British Journal of Clinical Pharmacology, 26*(4), 355–362.

Clark, J., & Lang, N. (1992). Nursing's next advance: An internal classification for nursing practice. *International Nursing Review, 39*(4), 109–111, 128.

Clinton, J. J. (1993). Financing medical effectiveness research: Role of the agency for health care policy and research. *Annals of the New York Academy of Sciences, 703,* 295–297.

Collins, L. M., & Horn, J. L. (1991). *Best methods for the* analysis of change: Recent advances, unanswered questions, future directions. Washington, DC: American Psychological Association.

Collins, L. M., & Johnston, M. V. (1995). Analysis of stage-sequential change in rehabilitation research. *American Journal of Physical Medicine and Rehabilitation, 74*(2), 163–170.

Connors, G. J., Allen, J. P., Cooney, N. L., DiClemente, C. C., Tonigan, J. S., & Anton, R. F. (1994). Assessment issues and strategies in alcoholism treatment matching research. *Journal of Studies on Alcohol, 12*(Suppl.), 92–100.

Crane, V. S. (1988). Economic aspects of clinical decision making: Applications of clinical decision analysis. *American Journal of Hospital Pharmacy, 45*(3), 548–553.

Davis, K. (1990). Use of data registries to evaluate medical procedures: Coronary artery surgery study and the balloon valvuloplasty registry. *International Journal of Technology Assessment in Health Care, 6*(2), 203–210.

DesHarnais, S., McMahon, L. F., Jr., & Wroblewski, R. (1991). Measuring outcomes of hospital care using multiple risk-adjusted indexes. *HSR: Health Services Research, 26*(4), 425–445.

Deyo, R. A. (1984). Measuring functional outcomes in therapeutic trials for chronic disease. *Controlled Clinical Trials, 5,* 223–240.

Deyo, R. A., & Carter, W. B. (1992). Strategies for improving and expanding the application of health status measures in clinical settings. *Medical Care, 30*(5), MS176–MS186.

Deyo, R. A., & Centor, R. M. (1986). Assessing the responsiveness of functional scales to clinical change: An analogy to diagnostic test performance. *Journal of Chronic Disease, 39*(11), 897–906.

Deyo, R. A., Taylor, V. M., Diehr, P., Conrad, D., Cherkin, D. C., Ciol, M., & Kreuter, W. (1994). Analysis of automated administrative and survey databases to study patterns and outcomes of care. *Spine, 19*(18S), 2083S–2091S.

DiClemente, C. C., Carroll, K. M., Connors, G. J., & Kadden, R. M. (1994). Process assessment in treatment matching research. *Journal of Studies on Alcohol, 12*(Suppl), 156–162.

Donabedian, A. (1987). Some basic issues in evaluating the quality of health care. In L. T. Rinke (Ed.) *Outcome measures in home care* (Vol. I, pp. 3–28). New York: National League for Nursing. (Original work published in 1976.)

Donovan, D. M., Kadden, R. M., DiClemente, C. C., Carroll, K. M., Longabaugh, R., Zweben, A., & Rychtarik, R. (1994). Issues in the selection and development of therapies in alcoholism treatment matching research. *Journal of Studies on Alcohol, 12*(Suppl.), 138–148.

Feinstein, A. R., Josephy, B. R., & Wells, C. K. (1986). Scientific and clinical problems in indexes of functional disability. *Annals of Internal Medicine, 105*(3), 413–420.

Felson, D. T., Anderson, J. J., & Meenan, R. F. (1990). Time for changes in the design, analysis, and reporting of rheumatoid arthritis clinical trials. *Arthritis and Rheumatism, 33*(1), 140–149.

Fowler, F. J., Jr., Cleary, P. D., Magaziner, J., Patrick, D. L., & Benjamin, K. L. (1994). Methodological issues in measuring patient-reported outcomes: The agenda of the work group on outcomes assessment. *Medical Care, 32*(7 Supp), JS65–JS76.

Freedman, L. S., & Schatzkin, A. (1992). Sample size for studying intermediate endpoints within intervention trials or observational studies. *American Journal of Epidemiology, 136*(9), 1148–1159.

Freund, D. A., Dittus, R. S., Fitzgerald, J., & Heck, D. (1990). Assessing and improving outcomes: Total knee replacement. *HSR: Health Services Research, 25*(5), 723–726.

Fries, B. E. (1990). Comparing case-mix systems for nursing home payment. *Health Care Financing Review, 11*(4), 103–119.

Gafni, A. (1994). The standard gamble method: What is being measured and how it is interpreted. *HSR: Health Services Research, 29*(2), 207–224.

Goldberg, H. I., & Cummings, M. A. (1994). Conducting medical effectiveness research: A report from the Inter-PORT work groups. *Medical Care, 32*(7 Suppl.), JS1–JS12.

Goldberg, H. I., Cummings, M. A., Steinberg, E. P., Ricci, E. M., Shannon, T., Soumerai, S. B., Mittman, B. S., Eisenberg, J., Heck, D. A., Kaplan, S., Kenzora, J. E., Vargus, A. M., Mulley, A. G., Jr., & Rimer, B. K. (1994). Deliberations on the dissemination of PORT products: Translating research findings into improved patient outcomes. *Medical Care, 32*(7 Supp.), JS90–JS110.

Gottman, J. M., & Rushe, R. H. (1993). The analysis of change: Issues, fallacies, and new ideas. *Journal of Consulting and Clinical Psychology, 61*(6), 907–910.

Gray, B. H. (1992). The legislative battle over health services research. *Health Affairs, 11*(4), 38–66.

Greene, R., Bondy, P. K., & Maklan, C. W. (1994). The national medical effectiveness research initiative. *Diabetes Care, 17*(Suppl. 1), 45–49.

Greenfield, S., Nelson, E. C., Zubkoff, M., Manning, W., Rogers, W., Kravitz, R. L., Keller, A., Tarlov, A. R., & Ware, J. E., Jr. (1992). Variations in resource utilization among medical specialities and systems of care: Results from the Medical Outcomes study. *Journal of the American Medical Association, 267*(12), 1624–1630.

Greiner, J. E. (1994). Microlevel documentation: Relational database for critical path development. *Seminars for Nurse Managers, 2*(2), 72–78.

Guadagnoli, E., & McNeil, B. J. (1994). Outcomes research: Hope for the future or the latest rage? *Inquiry, 31*(1), 14–24.

Guess, H. A., Jacobsen, S. J., Girman, C. J., Oesterling, J. E., Chute, C. G., Panser, L. A., & Lieber, M. M. (1995). The role of community-based longitudinal studies in evaluating treatment effects: Example: Benign prostatic hyperplasia. *Medical Care, 33*(4 Suppl.), AS26–AS35.

Guyatt, G., Walter, S., & Norman, G. (1987). Measuring change over time: Assessing the usefulness of evaluative instruments. *Journal of Chronic Disease, 40*(2), 171–178.

Hadorn, D., Baker, D., Dracup, K., & Pitt, B. (1994). Making judgments about treatment effectiveness based on health outcomes: Theoretical and practical issues. *Joint Commission Journal of Quality Improvement, 20*(10), 547–554.

Hadorn, D. C., & Baker, D. (1994). Development of the AHCPR-sponsored heart failure guideline: Methodologic and procedural issues. *Joint Commission Journal of Quality Improvement, 20*(10), 539–547.

Harris, C. W. (Ed.). (1967). *Problems in measuring change.* Madison: University of Wisconsin Press.

Harris, M. R., & Warren, J. J. (1995). Patient outcomes: Assessment issues for the CNS. *Clinical Nurse Specialist, 9*(2), 82–86.

Hastings, G. E., Vick, L., Lee, G., Sasmor, L., Natiello,

T. A., & Sanders, J. H. (1980). Nurse practitioners in a jailhouse clinic. *Medical Care, 18*(7), 731–744.

Hegyvary, S. T. (1992). Outcomes research: Integrating nursing practice into the world view. In *Patient Outcomes Research: Examining the Effectiveness of Nursing Practice. Proceedings of a Conference Sponsored by the National Center for Nursing Research, September 11–13, 1991.* U.S. Department of Health and Human Services, Public Health Services, National Institutes of Health, NIH Publication No. 93–3411, October 1992.

Herrmann, D. (1995). Reporting current, past, and changed health status: What we know about distortion. *Medical Care, 33*(4 Suppl.), AS89–AS94.

Hinshaw, A. S. (1992). Welcome: Patient outcome research conference. In *Patient Outcomes Research: Examining the Effectiveness of Nursing Practice. Proceedings of a Conference Sponsored by the National Center for Nursing Research, September 11–13, 1991.* U.S. Department of Health and Human Services, Public Health Services, National Institutes of Health, NIH Publication No. 93–3411, October 1992.

Hirshfeld, E. (1993). Use of practice parameters as standards of care and in health care reform: A view from the American Medical Association. *The Joint Commission Journal on Quality Improvement, 19*(8), 322–329.

Holzemer, W. (1990). Quality and cost of nursing care. *Nursing and Health Care, 11*(8), 412–415.

Issel, L. M. (1995). Evaluating case management programs. *Maternal–Child Nursing, 20*(2), 67–70, 72–74.

Jaeschke, R., Singer, J., & Guyatt, G. H. (1989). Measurement of health status: Ascertaining the minimal clinically important difference. *Controlled Clinical Trials, 10*(4), 407–415.

Johnston, M. V., & Granger, C. V. (1994). Outcomes research in medical rehabilitation: A primer and introduction to a series. *American Journal of Physical and Medical Rehabilitation, 73*(4), 296–303.

Kane, R. A., & Bayer, A. J. (1991). Assessment of functional status. In M. S. J. Pathy (Ed.), *Principles and practices of geriatric medicine* (2nd ed.) (pp. 265–277). New York: John Wiley & Sons Ltd.

Kane, R. L., & Lurie, N. (1992). Appropriate effectiveness: A tale of carts and horses. *Quality Review Bulletin, 18*(10), 322–326.

Katz, S., Downs, T. D., Cash, H. R., & Grotz, R. C. (1970). Progress in the development of the Index of ADL. *The Gerontologist* (Spring), 20–30.

Katz, J., & Schroeder, P. (1994). Linking key functions and important aspects of care: Perspectives on perioperative, medical-surgical, and perinatal nursing. *Journal of Nursing Care Quality, 9*(1), 66–77.

Keeler, E. B. (1994). Decision analysis and cost-effectiveness analysis in women's health care. *Clinical Obstetrics and Gynecology, 37*(1), 207–215.

Kelly, K. C., Huber, D. G., Johnson, M., McCloskey, J. C., & Maas, M. (1994). The Medical Outcomes Study: A nursing perspective. *Journal of Professional Nursing, 10*(4), 209–216.

Kieffer, E., Alexander, G. R., & Mor, J. (1992). Area-level predictors of use of prenatal care in diverse populations. *Public Health Reports, 107*(6), 653–658.

Kirshner, B., & Guyatt, G. (1985). A methodological framework for assessing health indices. *Journal of Chronic Diseases, 38*(1), 27–36.

Kirwan, J. R., Chaput de Saintonge, D. M., Joyce, C. R. B., Holmes, J., & Currey, H. L. F. (1986). Inability of rheumatologists to describe their true policies for assessing rheumatoid arthritis. *Annals of Rheumatic Diseases, 45,* 156–161.

Lamb, G. S. (1992). Conceptual and methodological issues in nurse case management research. *Advances in Nursing Science, 15*(2), 16–24.

Lange, L. L., & Jacox, A. (1993). Using large data bases in nursing and health policy research. *Journal of Professional Nursing, 9*(4), 204–211.

Lasker, R. D., Shapiro, D. W., & Tucker, A. M. (1992). Realizing the potential of practice pattern profiling. *Inquiry, 29*(3), 287–297.

Lave, J. R., Pashos, C. L., Anderson, G. F., Brailer, D., Bubloz, T., Conrad, D., Freund, D. A., Fox, S. H., Keeler, E., Lipscomb, J., Luft, H. S., & Provenzano, G. (1994). Costing medical care: Using medicare administrative data. *Medical Care, 32*(7 Suppl.), JS77–JS89.

Lee, T. H., & Goldman, L. (1989). Development and analysis of observational data bases. *Journal of the American College of Cardiology, 14*(3, Suppl. A), 44A–47A.

Leidy, N. K. (1991). Survey measures of functional ability and disability of pulmonary patients. In B. L. Metzger (Ed.), *Synthesis conference on altered functioning: Impairment and disability* (pp. 52–79). Indianapolis. IN: Nursing Center Press of Sigma Theta Tau International.

Lewis, B. E. (1995). HMO outcomes research: Lessons from the field. *Journal of Ambulatory Care Management, 18*(1), 47–55.

Loegering, L., Reiter, R. C., & Gambone, J. C. (1994). Measuring the quality of health care. *Clinical Obstetrics and Gynecology, 37*(1), 122–136.

Lohr, K. N. (1988). Outcome measurement: Concepts and questions. *Inquiry, 25*(1), 37–50.

Lowenberg, J. S. (1994). The nurse-patient relationship reconsidered: An expanded research agenda. *Scholarly Inquiry for Nursing Practice: An International Journal, 8*(2), 167–190.

Ludbrook, A. (1990). Using economic appraisal in health services research. *Health Bulletin, 48*(2), 81–90.

Lynn, J., & Virnig, B. A. (1995). Assessing the significance of treatment effects: Comments from the perspective of ethics. *Medical Care, 33*(4 Suppl.), AS292–AS298.

Mahrenholz, D. M. (1991). Outcomes research and nurses. *Nursing Connections, 4*(1), 58–61.

Mark, B. A. (1995). The black box of patient outcomes research. *Image: Journal of Nursing Scholarship,*(1), 42.

Marschke, P., & Nolan, M. T. (1993). Research related to case management. *Nursing Administration Quarterly, 17*(3), 16–21.

Mattson, M. E., & Donovan, D. M. (1994). Clinical applications: The transition from research to practice. *Journal of Studies on Alcohol, 12*(Suppl.), 163–166.

Maynard, A. (1990). The design of future cost-benefit studies. *American Heart Journal, 119*(3 Pt. 2), 761–765.

McCormick, B. (1990). Outcomes in action: The JCAHO's clinical indicators. *Hospitals, 64*(19), 34–38.

McCormick, L. A., Lang, N., Zielstorff, R., Milholland, K., Saba, V., & Jacox, A. (1994). Toward standard classification schemes for nursing language: Recommendations of the American Nurses Association Steering Committee on Databases to Support Clinical Nursing Practice. *Journal of the Medical Informatics Association, 1*(6), 421–427.

McDonald, C. J., & Hui, S. L. (1991). The analysis of humongous databases: Problems and promises. *Statistics in Medicine, 10*(4), 511–518.

McNeil, B. (1993). Use of claims data to monitor patients over time: Acute myocardial infarction as a case study. *Annals of the New York Academy of Sciences, 703,* 63–73.

McNeil, B. J., Pedersen, S. H., & Gatsonis, C. (1992). Current issues in profiling quality of care. *Inquiry, 29*(3), 298–307.

Miller, W. R., & Cooney, N. L. (1994). Designing studies to investigate client-treatment matching. *Journal of Studies on Alcohol, 12*(Suppl.), 38–45.

Mitchell, J. B., Bubolz, T., Pail, J. E., Pashos, C. L., Escarce, J. J., Muhlbaier, L. H., Weisman, J. M., Young, W. W., Epstein, R. S., & Javitt, J. C. (1994). Using Medicare claims for outcomes research. *Medical Care, 32*(7 Suppl.), JS38–JS51.

Mittelmark, M. B., Hunt, M. K., Heath, G. W., & Schmid, T. L. (1993). Realistic outcomes: Lessons from community-based research and demonstration programs for the prevention of cardiovascular diseases. *Journal of Public Health Policy, 14*(4), 437–462.

Molde, S., & Diers, D. (1985). Nurse practitioner research: Selected literature review and research agenda. *Nursing Research, 34*(6), 362–367.

Moritz, P. (1991). Innovative nursing practice models and patient outcomes. *Nursing Outlook, 39*(3), 111–114.

Moses, L. E. (1995). Measuring effects without randomized trials? Options, problems, challenges. *Medical Care, 33*(4 Suppl.), AS8–AS14.

Nadzim, D. M., Turpin, R., Hanold, L. S., & White, R. E. (1993). Data-driven performance improvement in health care: The Joint Commission's Indicator Measurement System (IMSystem). *The Joint Commission Journal on Quality Improvement, 19*(11), 492–500.

Nelson, E. C., Landgraf, J. M., Hays, R. D., Wasson, J. H., & Kirk, J. W. (1990). The functional status of patients. How can it be measured in physicians' offices? *Medical Care, 28*(12), 1111–1126.

Neuhauser, D. (1990). Ernest Amory Codman, M.D., and end results of medical care. *International Journal of Technology Assessment in Health Care, 6*(2), 307–325.

Nolan, M., & Grant, G. (1993). Service evaluation: Time to open both eyes. *Journal of Advanced Nursing, 18*(9), 1434–1442.

O'Connor, G. T., Plume, S. K., & Wennberg, J. E. (1993). Regional organization for outcomes research. *Annals of the New York Academy of Sciences, 703,* 44–51.

Orchard, C. (1994). Comparing healthcare outcomes. *British Medical Journal, 308*(6942), 1493–1496.

Oster, G. (1988). Economic aspects of clinical decision making: Applications in patient care. *American Journal of Hospital Pharmacy, 45*(3), 543–547.

Ottenbacher, K. J., Johnson, M. B., & Hojem, M. (1995). The significance of clinical change and clinical change of significance: Issues and methods. *American Journal of Occupational Therapy, 42*(3), 156–163.

Patrick, D. L., & Deyo, R. A. (1989). Generic and disease-specific measures in assessing health status and quality of life. *Medical Care. 27*(3 Suppl.), S217–S232.

Pentz, M. A., & Chou, C. (1994). Measurement invariance in longitudinal clinical research assuming change from development and intervention. *Journal of Consulting and Clinical Psychology, 62*(3), 450–462.

Powe, N. R., Turner, J. A., Maklan, C. W., & Ersek, M. (1994). Alternative methods for formal literature review and meta-analysis in AHCPR Patient Outcomes Research Teams. *Medical Care, 32*(7), JS22–JS37.

Power, E. J., Tunis, S. R., & Wagner, J. L. (1994). Technology assessment and public health. *Annual Review of Public Health, 15,* 561–579.

Prior, D. B., & DeLong, E. R. (1994). Programmed Outcome Research Teams (PORTs) and implications for clinical practice. *The American Journal of Cardiology, 73*(6), 34B–38B.

Ramsey, J. A., McKenzie, J. K., & Fish, D. G. (1982). Physicians and nurse practitioners: Do they provide equivalent health care? *American Journal of Public Health, 72*(1), 55–57.

Rettig, R. (1990). History, development, and importance to nursing of outcomes research. *Journal of Nursing Quality Assurance, 5*(2), 13–17.

Riesenberg, D., & Glass, R. M. (1989). The Medical Outcomes Study. *Journal of the American Medical Association, 262*(7), 943.

Rovine, M. J., & Von Eye, A. (1991). *Applied computational statistics in longitudinal research.* San Diego, CA: Academic Press.

Schmitt, M. H., Farrell, M. P., & Heinemann, G. D. (1988). Conceptual and methodological problems in studying the effects of interdisciplinary geriatric teams. *The Gerontologist, 28*(6), 753–764.

Sledge, C. B. (1993). Why do outcomes research? *Orthopedics, 16*(10), 1093–1096.

Sonnenberg, F. A., Roberts, M. S., Tsevat, J., Wong, J. B., Barry, M., & Kent, D. L. (1994). Toward a peer review process for medical decision analysis models. *Medical Care, 32*(7 Suppl.), JS52–JS64.

Spector, W. D. (1990). Functional disability scales. In B. Spilker (Ed.), *Quality of life assessments in clinical trials* (pp. 115–129). New York: Raven Press.

Spitzer, W. O. (1987). State of science 1986: Quality of life and functional status as target variables for research. *Journal of Chronic Disease, 40*(6), 465–471.

Stewart, A. L., Greenfield, S., Hays, R. D., Wells, K., Rogers, W. H., Berry, S. D., McGlynn, E. A., & Ware, J. E. (1989). Functional status and well-being of patients with chronic conditions. *Journal of the American Medical Association. 262*(7), 907–913.

Stewart, B. J., & Archbold, P. G. (1992). Nursing intervention studies require outcome measures that are sensitive to change: Part two. *Research in Nursing & Health, 16*(1), 77–81.

Swaen, G. M. H., & Meijers, J. M. M. (1988). Influence of design characteristics on the outcomes of retrospective cohort studies. *British Journal of Industrial Medicine, 45*(9), 624–629.

Tanenbaum, S. J. (1994). Knowing and acting in medical practice: The epistemological politics of outcomes research. *Journal of Health Politics, Policy and Law, 19*(1), 27–44.

Temple, R. (1990). Problems in the use of large data sets to assess effectiveness. *International Journal of Technology Assessment in Health Care, 6*(2), 211–219.

Tidwell, S. L. (1993). A graphic tool for tracking variance & comorbidities in cardiac surgery case management. *Progress in Cardiovascular Nursing, 8*(2), 6–19.

Turk, D. C., & Rudy, T. E. (1994). Methods for evaluating treatment outcomes: Ways to overcome potential obstacles. *Spine, 19*(15), 1759–1763.

U.S. Congress, Office of Technology Assessment. (1994). *Identifying Health Technologies That Work: Searching for Evidence.* OTA-H-608, Washington, DC: U.S. Government Printing Office.

Veatch, R. M. (1993). Justice and outcomes research: The ethical limits. *The Journal of Clinical Ethics, 4*(3), 258–261.

Vermeulen, L. C., Jr., Ratko, T. A., Erstad, B. L., Brecher, M. E., & Matuszewski, K. A. (1995). A paradigm for consensus: The University Hospital Consortium Guidelines for the use of albumin, nonprotein colloid, and crystalloid solutions. *Archives of Internal Medicine, 155*(4), 373–379.

Volinn, E., Diehr, P., Ciol, M. A., & Loeser, J. D. (1994). Why does geographic variation in health care practices matter (And seven questions to ask in evaluating studies on geographic variation). *Spine, 19*(18S), 2092S–2100S.

Von Eye, A. (Ed.). (1990a). *Statistical methods in longitudinal research: Volume I—Principles and structuring change.* Boston: Academic Press.

Von Eye, A. (Ed.). (1990b). *Statistical methods in longitudinal research: Volume II—Time series and categorical longitudinal data.* Boston: Academic Press.

Von Korff, M., Koepsell, T., Curry, S., & Diehr, P. (1992). Multi-level analysis in epidemiologic research on health behaviors and outcomes. *American Journal of Epidemiology, 135*(10), 1077–1082.

Watkins, L., & Wagner, E. (1982). Nurse practitioner and physician adherence to standing orders: Criteria for consultation or referral. *American Journal of Public Health, 72*(1), 55–57.

Wennberg, J. E. (1990). Outcomes research, cost containment, and the fear of health care rationing. *The New England Journal of Medicine, 323*(17), 1202–1204.

Wennberg, J. E., Barry, M. J., Fowler, F. J., & Mulley, A. (1993). Outcomes Research, PORTs, and health care reform. *Annals of the New York Academy of Sciences, 703,* 52–62.

Werley, H., Devine, E., Zorn, C., Ryan, P., & Westra, B. (1991). The nursing minimum data set: Abstraction tool for standardized, comparable, essential data. *American Journal of Public Health, 81*(4), 421–426.

Werley, H., & Lang, N. (1988). *Identification of the nursing minimum data set.* New York: Springer.

West, S. G., Aiken, L. S., & Todd, M. (1993). Probing the effects of individual components in multiple component prevention programs. *American Journal of Community Psychology, 21*(5), 571–605.

White, K. L. (1993). Health care research: Old wine in new bottles. *The Pharos of Alpha Omega Alpha Honor Medical Society, 56*(3), 12–16.

Wiener, J. M., Hanley, R. J., Clark, R., & Van Norstrand, J. F. (1990). Measuring the activities of daily living: Comparisons across national surveys. *Journal of Gerontology, 45*(6), S229–S237.

Wilson, I. B., & Cleary, P. D. (1995). Linking clinical variables with health-related quality of life: A conceptual model of patient outcomes. *Journal of the American Medical Association, 273*(1), 60.

Wood, L. W. (1990). Medical treatment effectiveness research. *Journal of Occupational Medicine, 32*(12),1173–1174.

Wray, N. P., Ashton, C. M., Kuykendall, D. H., Petersen, N. J., Souchek, J., & Hollingsworth, J. C. (1995). Selecting disease-outcome pairs for monitoring the quality of hospital care. *Medical Care, 33*(1), 75–89.

Zielstorff, R., Hudgings, C., Grobe, S., & the National Commission on Nursing Implementation Project (NCNIP) Task Force on Nursing Information Systems. (1993). *Next generation nursing information systems: Essential characteristics for professional practice.* Washington, DC: ANA.

Zweben, A., Donovan, D. M., Randall, C. L., Barrett, D., Dermen, K., Kabela, E., McRee, B., Meyers, R., Rice, C., Rosengren, D., Schmidt, P., Show, M., Thevos, A. K., & Velasquez, M. (1994). Issues in the development of subject recruitment strategies and eligibility criteria in multisite trials of matching. *Journal of Studies on Alcohol, 12*(Suppl.), 62–69.

22

Interpreting
Research Outcomes

When data analysis is complete, there is a feeling that the answers are in and the study is finished. However, the results of statistical analysis, alone, are inadequate to complete the study. The researcher may know the results, but without careful intellectual examination, these results are of little use to others or to nursing's body of knowledge. To be useful, the evidence from data analysis needs to be carefully examined, organized, and given meaning, and both statistical and clinical significance need to be assessed. This process is referred to as *interpretation.*

Data collection and analysis are action-oriented activities that require concrete thinking. However, when the results of the study are being interpreted, abstract thinking is used, including the creative use of introspection, reasoning, and intuition. In some ways, these last steps in the research process are the most difficult. They require a synthesis of the logic used to develop the research plan, strategies used in the data collection phase, and the mathematical logic or insight and gestalt formation used in data analysis. Evaluating the research process used in the study, producing meaning from the results, and forecasting the usefulness of the findings, all of which are involved in interpretation, require high-level intellectual processes.

Translation is frequently thought of as being synonymous with interpretation. Abstract theoretical statements are sometimes referred to as being translated into more concrete meaning, as, for example, in the operationalization of a variable. Although the two words *translate* and *interpret* are similar, their meanings have subtle differences. *Translation* means to transform from one language to another or to use terms that can be more easily understood. *Interpreting* involves explaining the meaning of information. Interpretation seems to include translation and to go beyond it to explore and impart meaning. Thus, in this step of the research process, the researcher translates the results of analysis into findings and then interprets by attaching meaning to the findings.

Within the process of interpretation are several intellectual activities that can be isolated and explored. These activities include examining evidence, forming conclusions, exploring the significance of the findings, generalizing the findings, considering implications, and suggesting further studies. Each of these activities is discussed in this chapter. The final chapter of theses and dissertations and the final sections of research articles and presentations include interpretation of research outcomes.

EXAMINING EVIDENCE

The first step in interpretation is a consideration of all the evidence available that supports or contradicts the validity of results related to the research objectives, questions, or hypotheses. In order to consider the evidence, one needs first to determine what the evidence is and then gather it together. The impact of each bit of evidence on the validity of results needs to be carefully considered; then, the evidence as a whole needs to be synthesized for a final judgment. The process is somewhat like critiquing your own work. The temptation is to ignore flaws—certainly not to point them out. However, this process is essential to the building of a body of knowledge. It is a time not for confession, remorse, and apology, but rather for thoughtful reflection. Problems and strengths of the study need to be identified by the researcher and shared with colleagues at presentations and in publications. They affect the meaning of the results and can serve as guideposts for future researchers.

EVIDENCE FROM THE RESEARCH PLAN

The initial evidence for the validity of the study results is derived from a reexamination of the research plan. The reexamination requires a reexploration of the logic of the methodology. This exploration will involve analyzing the logical links among the problem statement, purpose, research questions, variables, design, methods of observation, methods of measurement, and types of analyses. These elements of the study logically link together and are consistent with the research problem. Remember the old adage, a chain is only as strong as its weakest link? This is also true of research. Therefore, the study needs to be examined to identify its weakest links.

These weak links then need to be examined in terms of their impact on the results. Could the results, or some of the results, be a consequence of a weak link in the methodology rather than a true test of the hypotheses? Can the research objectives, questions, or hypotheses be answered from the methodology used in the study? Could the results be a consequence of an inappropriate conceptual or operational definition of the variable? Do the research questions clearly emerge from the framework? Can the results be related back to the framework? Are the analyses logically planned to test the questions?

If the types of analyses are inappropriate to examine the research questions, what do the results of analyses mean? For example, if the design failed to control extraneous variables, could some of these variables explain the results rather than their being explained by the variables measured and examined through statistical analysis? Was the sample studied a logical group on which to test the hypotheses? Each link in the design needs to be carefully evaluated in this way to determine potential weaknesses. Every link is clearly related to the meaning given to the study results. If the researcher is reviewing a newly completed study and determines that the types of analyses were inappropriate, the analyses, of course, need to be redone. If the study is being critiqued, the findings may need to be seriously questioned.

EVIDENCE FROM MEASUREMENT

One of the assumptions often made in interpreting study results is that the study variables were adequately measured. This adequacy is determined through examination of the fit of operational definitions with the framework and through validity and reliability information. Although reliability and validity of measurement strategies should be determined prior to their use in the study, the measures need to be reexamined at this point to determine the strength of evidence available from results. For example, did the scale used to measure anxiety truly reflect the anxiety experienced in the study population? What was the effect size? Were validity and reliability of instruments examined in the present study? Can this information be used to interpret the results? The validity and reliability of measurement are critical to the validity of results. If the instruments used do not measure the variables as defined conceptually and operationally in the study, the results of analyzed measurement scores mean little.

Scores from measurement instruments without validity and reliability can be used for statistical analyses just as easily as those with validity and reliability. The mathematical formula or the computer cannot detect the difference. Results of the analyses give the same information regardless of the validity and reliability. The difference is in the meaning attributed to the results. This difference is detectable only by scientists, not by computers.

EVIDENCE FROM THE DATA COLLECTION PROCESS

Many activities that occur during data collection affect the meaning of results. Was the sample size sufficient? Did unforeseen events occur during the study that might have changed or had an impact on the data? Did strategies for acquiring a sample eliminate important groups whose data would have influenced results? Were measurement techniques consistent? What impact do inconsistencies have on interpreting results? Sometimes data collection does not proceed as planned. Unforeseen situations alter the collection of data. What were these variations in the study? What impact do they have on interpreting the results? Sometimes data collection forms are completed by someone other than the subject. Variations may occur in events surrounding the administration of scales. For example, an anxiety scale may be given to one subject immediately before a painful procedure and to another subject upon awakening in the morning. Values on these measures cannot be considered comparable. These types of differences are seldom reported and sometimes are not even recorded. To some extent, only the researcher knows how consistently the measurements were taken. Reporting this information is dependent on the integrity of the researcher.

EVIDENCE FROM THE DATA ANALYSIS PROCESS

The process of data analysis is an important factor in evaluating the meaning of results. One important part of this examination is to summarize the study weaknesses related to the data analysis process. A number of pertinent questions can be asked that are related to the meaning of results. How many errors were made in entering the data into the computer? How many subjects have missing data that could affect statistical analyses? Were the analyses accurately calculated? Were statistical assumptions violated? Were the statistics used appropriate to the data? These issues need to be addressed initially before analyses are performed, and again on completing the analyses prior to writing the final report. Prior to submitting a paper for publication, we recheck each analysis reported in the paper. We reexamine the analysis statements in the paper. Are we correctly interpreting the results of the analysis? Documentation on each statistical value or analysis statement reported in the paper is filed with a copy of the paper. The documentation includes the date of the analysis, page number of the computer printout showing the results (printout is stored in a file by date of analysis), the sample size for the analysis, and the number of missing values.

Except in simple studies, data analysis in quantitative studies is usually performed using a computer. Using prepared statistical analysis programs, multiple analyses can be performed on the data that are not well understood by the researcher. To the neophyte researcher, the computer spits out reams of paper with incomprehensible printed information and, in the end, gives a level of significance. The appropriateness of the data and the logic behind the program may remain unknown, but the level of significance may be considered by a new researcher as absolute "proof" of an important finding.

The analysis process in qualitative studies is, to some degree, subjective. The process itself, however, requires great skill and can seldom be learned by reading a journal article. Sorting, organizing, and developing theoretical formulations from the data require great care and experience, yet the meaning derived from the analysis is dependent on the skill of conducting the analysis.

In gathering evidence for the implications of the study results, it is critical to reexamine the data analysis process. The researcher needs to examine the sufficiency of personal knowledge of the statistics and proficiency in the analyses used. Data need to be reexamined for accuracy and completeness. Mathematical operations performed manually need to be rechecked for accuracy. Computer printouts need to be reexamined for meaningful information that may have been overlooked. Tables of data need to be rechecked for accuracy and clarity. In qualitative studies, another qualitative researcher validates the analysis process by following the decision trail initially used to analyze the data. In all studies, researchers need to have a high level of confidence in the results they report.

EVIDENCE FROM DATA ANALYSIS RESULTS

The outcomes of data analyses are the most direct evidence available of the results. The researcher has intimate knowledge of the research, and needs to carefully evaluate its flaws and strengths in judging the validity of the results. In descriptive and correlational studies, the validity of the results is dependent on how accurately the variables were measured in selected samples and settings. The value of evidence in any study is dependent on the amount of variance in the phenomenon explained within the study, a factor that is often not considered in interpreting the results (Tulman & Jacobsen, 1989). In quasi-experimental and experimental studies, in which hypothesized differences in groups are being examined, the differences or lack of differences do not indicate the amount of variance explained. This needs to be reported in all studies and should serve as a basis for interpreting the results. (See Chapters 17, 18, and 19 for discussions of methods of identifying the variance explained in an analysis.)

Interpretation of results from quasi-experimental and experimental studies is traditionally based on decision theory, with five possible results: (1) significant results that are in keeping with those predicted by the researcher, (2) nonsignificant results, (3) significant results that are opposite to those predicted by the researcher, (4) mixed results, and (5) unexpected results.

Significant and Predicted Results

Results that are in keeping with those predicted by the researcher are the easiest to explain and, unless weak links are present, validate the proposed logical links among the elements of the study. These results support the logical links developed by the researcher among the framework, questions, variables, and measurement tools. This is very satisfying to the researcher. However, in this situation, the researcher needs to consider alternative explanations for the positive findings. What other elements could possibly have led to the significant results?

Nonsignificant Results

Unpredicted nonsignificant or inconclusive results are the most difficult to explain. These results are often referred to as negative results. The negative results could be a true reflection of reality. In this case, the reasoning of the researcher or the theory used by the researcher to develop the hypothesis is in error. If so, the negative findings are an important addition to the body of knowledge. Any report of nonsignificant results needs to indicate the results of power analysis to indicate the risk of a Type II error in relation to the nonsignificant results.

The negative results could also be due to inappropriate methodology, a deviant sample, a small sample, problems with internal validity, inadequate measurement, use of weak statistical techniques, or faulty analysis. This result may be a Type II error, which may mean that in reality the findings are significant but, because of weaknesses in the methodology, the significance was not detected. Unless these weak links are detected, the reported results could lead to faulty information in the body of knowledge (Angell, 1989). It is easier for the researcher to blame faulty methodology for nonsignificant findings than to find failures in theoretical or logical reasoning. If faulty methodology is blamed, the researcher needs to explain exactly how the breakdown in methodology led to the negative results. Negative results, in any case, do not mean that there are no relationships among the variables; they indicate that the study failed to find any.

Significant and Not Predicted Results

Significant results opposite to those predicted, if the results are valid, are an important addition to the body of knowledge. An example would be a study in which social support and ego strength were proposed to be positively related. If the study showed that high social support was related to low ego strength, the result would be opposite to that predicted. Results such as this, when verified by other studies, indicate that we were headed in the wrong direction theoretically. Since these types of studies direct nursing practice, this is important information. In some of these cases, the researcher believes so strongly in the theory that the results are not believed. The researcher remains convinced that there was a problem in the methodology. Sometimes this belief remains entrenched in the minds of scientists for many years due to the bias that good research supports its hypotheses.

Mixed Results

Mixed results are probably the most common outcome of studies. In this case, one variable may uphold predicted characteristics while another does not, or two dependent measures of the same variable may show opposite results. These differences may be due to methodology problems, such as differing reliability or sensitivity of two methods of measuring variables. The mixed results may also indicate the need to modify existing theory.

Unexpected Results

Unexpected results are usually relationships found between variables that were not hypothesized and not predicted from the framework being used. These are serendipitous results. Most researchers examine as many elements of data as possible in addition to those directed by the questions. These findings can be useful in theory development or refinement and in the development of later studies. In addition, serendipitous results are important as evidence in developing the implications of the study. However, serendipitous results need to be dealt with carefully in considering meaning because the study was not designed to examine these results.

EVIDENCE FROM PREVIOUS STUDIES

The results of the present study should always be examined in light of previous findings. It is important to know whether results are consistent with past research. Consistency in findings across studies is important in theory development and scientific progress. Therefore, any inconsistencies need to be explored to determine reasons for the differences. The replication of studies and synthesis of findings of existing studies are critical to the building of a body of knowledge and theory development.

FINDINGS

Results in a study are translated and interpreted; then they become findings. *Findings* are a consequence of evaluating evidence. Although much of the process of developing findings from results occurs in the mind of the researcher, evidence of the thinking can be found in published research reports. The 1994 study of McMillan and Mahon examining the quality of life of hospice patients on admission and at week 3 of hospice care presents the following research questions, results, and findings.

Research Question 1

"Is there a significant improvement in quality of life from admission to week 3 of hospice care as perceived by the patient?"

Results. "Only 31 of the original 67 patients who had a primary caregiver survived and were able to complete the SQLI (Sendra Quality of Life Index) a second time. The mean score for this group was 49.2 on admission and 49.7 at 3 weeks; there was no significant difference. Although grouped (mean) scores did not suggest a trend toward improvement, individual SQLI scores showed that approximately half of the subjects reported an improved quality of life with an increase of 10 points or more, whereas the other half reported a decrease in perceived quality of life . . . Results of item analysis indicated that the greatest improvement in SQLI scores was in items related to support from nurses, worry about medical care, and sexual activity. The greatest decrease in SQLI scores was in items related to control over life and health, fun, being happy, and having a satisfying life . . . Three items showed an improvement of more than six points. These items were subjected to paired t test comparisons to determine whether these improvements were statistically significant. The improvement in items related to sexual activity ($t = 6.18$, $p < 0.001$), worry over cost of medical care ($t = 6.6$, $p < 0.001$), and feeling support from the nurse ($t = 14.4$, $p < 0.0001$) were all found to be statistically significant with the greatest improvement being in feeling support from the nurse. Perceptions of physician support remained constant at about 62. The first item on the SQLI asks the patient, 'How much pain are you feeling?' The mean pain score from admission to week 3 shows a slight increase in mean scores on the pain item (from 56.9 to 59.3, $t = 1.86$, $p < 0.05$), indicating a slight but significant decrease in level of reported pain." (p. 56)

Findings. "Earlier research has found that for the vast majority of patients, quality of life declines rapidly near the end of life. However, the mean quality of life scores for patients remaining in this study remained at ~49. This result might suggest that hospice services in this case were unusually effective. However, individual scores showed that scores improved for some patients and decreased for others. Although the patient sample did not report a significant increase in their overall mean level of quality of life, when looked at individually it is encouraging to note that half of these patients did report summed scores that suggest such an improvement. Taken in the context of hospice where the average length of life after admission is 40 days, it is possible that the patients who did not report an overall increase in quality of life were those who were closer to death and thus were in a rapid decline." (p. 58)

Research Question 2

"Is there a significant improvement in quality of life from admission to week 3 of hospice care as perceived by the caregiver?" (p. 54)

Results. "The 31 caregivers who remained in the study until the third week reported a significantly improved perception of the patient's quality of life from an admission mean of 48.2 to a week 3 mean of 53.3 ($t = 2.06$, $p < 0.05$)." (p. 56)

Findings. "It is also encouraging that caregivers reported a significant increase in their perceptions of the patient's quality of life. Although the increase was not large (5.3 points), it was statistically significant. There is more than one possible explanation for this finding. First, the patients' mean quality of life might really have improved. However, the patient data seem to refute this. Not only did patient scores not improve significantly, but the modest correlations between patient and caregiver scores suggest that patients' and caregivers' perceptions are not completely congruent. A second explanation for the overall increase in caregiver scores may be that the caregivers, after 3 weeks of involvement with the hospice team, want or need to believe that the patient quality of life has improved, regardless of the real situation. Or perhaps the support from the hospice team has improved the caregiver's quality of life in some way, causing a general improvement in caregiver attitude that was evident on the measure of the caregiver's perception of the patient's quality of life." (p. 58)

Research Question 3

"Is there a relationship between the patient's perceived quality of life and the demographic variables (age, gender, location of care)?" (p. 54)

Results. "At admission, there was a weak correlation between age and quality of life ($r = 0.30$). By week 3 there was no correlation. Using χ^2 analysis, there was no relationship found between gender and quality of life. Of the 80 subjects admitted to the study, data on location were available on 78. Sixty-five of these (83.3%) were being cared for in the home. The remaining subjects were receiving hospice care either in nursing homes ($n = 2$, 2.6%) or the hospital ($n = 11$, 14.1%)." (p. 57)

Findings. "No comparison was possible between location of care and perceived quality of life due to the small numbers of patients in nursing homes and hospitals." (p. 57)

Research Question 4

"Is there a relationship between functional status as measured by the Karnofsky Performance

Scale and quality of life as perceived by the patient?'' (p. 54)

Results. ''The mean Karnofsky Scale score at admission to hospice was 51.8. A weak relationship was found with SQLI scores at admission ($r = 0.25$). No Karnofsky scores were collected at week 3.''

Findings. ''The literature on quality of life included a number of studies that used the Karnofsky Performance Status Scale as a measure of quality of life. Although functional status is an important aspect of quality of life and may be correlated with it, functional status does not capture all of the aspects of quality of life that would be assessed by a multidimensional quality of life scale. The Karnofsky Performance Status Scale scores were available on these patients, so data were incorporated into the study. The correlations between the Karnofsky and SQLI scores were low ($r = 0.25$), as might be expected, providing evidence that the Karnofsky alone is not an adequate assessment of overall quality of life.'' (p. 58)

Research Question 5

''Is there a correlation between quality of life as perceived by the patient and as perceived by the caregiver?'' (p. 54)

Results. ''Results showed a moderately weak to weak relationship, with the correlation decreasing slightly from admission ($r = 0.45$) to week 3 ($r = 0.39$).'' (p. 57)

Findings. ''Although it was expected, based on earlier research, that patient and caregiver scores would be correlated, it was expected that the correlations would be weak to moderate, and they were weak. This seems to confirm that quality of life is a subjectively experienced phenomenon, and although caregivers are very 'tuned in' to the patients for whom they are providing care, the patients are the most reliable reporter of their own quality of life.'' (p. 58)

''It might be expected that although the correlation between patients and caregivers would be modest, the correlation would increase in magnitude from admission to week 3. That is, as the caregiver became increasingly involved in the patient's care, the ability to understand and report quality of life would increase. This was not the case. Although the correlations between patients and caregivers changed a little (from $r = 0.45$ to $r = 0.39$) from admission to week 3, it went

in a downward direction. The reason for this slight decrease is unclear.'' (p. 58) ∎

FORMING CONCLUSIONS

Conclusions are derived from the findings and are a synthesis of findings. Forming these conclusions requires a combination of logical reasoning, creative formation of a meaningful whole from pieces of information obtained through data analysis and findings from previous studies, receptivity to subtle clues in the data, and use of an open context in considering alternative explanations of the data.

In forming conclusions, it is important to remember that research never proves anything; rather, research offers support for a position. Proof is a logical part of deductive reasoning but not of the research process. Because of this, formulation of causal statements is risky. For example, the causal statement that A *causes* B (absolutely, in all situations) cannot be scientifically proved. It is more credible to state conclusions in the form of conditional probabilities that are qualified. For example, it would be more appropriate to state in the study that if A occurred, then B occurred under conditions x, y, and z (Kerlinger, 1986), or that B had an 80% probability of occurring. Thus, one could conclude that if preoperative teaching were given, postoperative anxiety was lowered as long as pain was controlled, complications did not occur, and family contacts were high.

McMillan and Mahon (1994) reached the following conclusions.

''Results of this study suggest that hospice services are successful in improving the overall quality of life of some but not all patients who remain in care for 3 weeks. This is a very positive finding in light of previous research that suggests a rapid decline as death nears. Hospice services seemed to have a greater effect in some areas than in others. Patients felt increasingly supported by nurses from admission to week 3 and felt a constant level of support from their physicians. Patients seemed to worry less about the cost of medical care after 3 weeks in hospice care and reported an increase in sexual activity. Although some increase was seen in pain relief, pain management in hospice patients appears to need continued attention and monitoring." (p. 59) ∎

The methodology of the study was examined in drawing conclusions from the findings. In spite of the researcher's higher motives to be objective, subjective judgments and biases will sometimes creep into the conclusions. The researcher needs to be alert and control subjectivity and biases. Students sometimes want positive findings so much that they will misinterpret statistical results on computer printouts as significant when they are clearly nonsignificant.

The researcher needs to identify the limitations of the study in forming conclusions about the findings. The limitations need to be included in the research report. McMillan and Mahon (1994) provided the following discussion of limitations.

∎ ─────────────────────────────

"A limitation of this study was the elimination of patients who were unable to self-report their quality of life. Thus, a large number of debilitated, comatose, or actively dying patients had to be eliminated. Although the quality of life of these patients could be reported by the caregivers, the data suggest that patient and caregiver reports are not completely congruent. Despite this lack of congruence, future studies should account for a wider sampling of all hospice patients even if the data source is less than ideal.

A second limitation of this study was the inclusion of persons with diagnoses other than cancer. It is possible that persons with AIDS or cardiovascular disease may respond differently than would persons with cancer or that some cancers have a different course, affecting quality of life.

A third limitation of the study was the lack of any quality of life tools designed especially for hospice patients. Because the SQLI is a fairly new instrument and has been validated for use with cancer patients rather than hospice patients per se, the appropriateness of the tool may be in

question. However, the majority of patients in this study (80%) were cancer patients." (p. 59) ∎

One of the risks in developing conclusions in research is going beyond the data. This means forming conclusions that are not warranted by the data. The most common example is a study that examines relationships between A and B by correlational analysis and then concludes that A causes B. Going beyond the data is due to faulty logic and occurs more frequently in published studies than one would like to believe. The researcher needs to check the validity of arguments related to conclusions before revealing findings.

EXPLORING THE SIGNIFICANCE OF FINDINGS

The word *significance* is used in two ways in research. Statistical significance is related to quantitative analyses of the results of the study. To be important, the results of quantitative studies that use statistical analysis must be statistically significant. *Statistical significance* means that the results are unlikely to be due to chance. However, statistically significant results are not necessarily important in clinical practice. The results can indicate a real difference that is not necessarily an important difference clinically. For example, Yonkman (1982, p. 356), in reporting results from her study of the effect of cool or heated aerosol on oral temperature, reported that "the statistical tests yielded small values which implied that differences were statistically significant. It is not clear that these differences in temperature are clinically significant."

The *practical significance of a study* is associated with its importance to nursing's body of knowledge. Significance is not a dichotomous characteristic, because studies contribute in varying degrees to the body of knowledge. Statistically nonsignificant results can have practical significance. Significance may be associated with the amount of variance explained, control in the study design to eliminate unexplained variance, or detection of statistically significant differences. The researcher is expected to clarify the significance as much as possible. The areas of significance may be obvious to the researcher who has been immersed in the study but not to the reader or listener. Therefore, the researcher needs to delineate the areas of significance. Determining clinical significance is a judgment based on the researcher's clinical expertise. It is often based, in part, on whether treatment decisions or outcomes would be different based on the study findings.

A few studies, referred to as landmark studies, become important referent points in the discipline; those by Johnson, 1972; Lindeman and Van Aernam, 1971; Passos and Brand, 1966; and Williams, 1972. The importance of a study may not become apparent for years after publication. However, some characteristics are associated with the significance of studies. Significant studies make an important difference in peoples' lives. The findings have external validity. Therefore, it is possible to generalize the findings far beyond the study sample so that the findings have the potential of affecting large numbers of people. The implications of significant studies go beyond concrete facts to abstractions and lead to the generation of theory or revisions in existing theory. A highly significant study has implications for one or more disciplines in addition to nursing. The study is accepted by others in the discipline and is frequently referenced in the literature. Over a period of time, the significance of a study is measured by the number of studies it generates.

GENERALIZING THE FINDINGS

Generalization extends the implications of the findings from the sample studied to a larger population or from the situation studied to a larger situation. For example, if the study were conducted on diabetic patients, it may be possible to generalize the findings to persons with other illnesses or to well individuals. Highly controlled experimental studies, which are high in internal validity, tend to be low in generalizability because they tend to have low external validity.

How far can generalizations be made? This is a debatable question. From a narrow perspective, one cannot really generalize from the sample on which the study was done. Any other sample is likely to be different in some way. The conservative position, represented by Kerlinger (1986), recommends caution in considering the extent of generalization. Generalization is considered particularly risky by conservatives if the sample was not randomly selected. According to Kerlinger (1986, p. 301), "Unless special precautions are taken and special efforts made, the results of research are frequently not representative, and hence not generalizable." This is the classic sampling theory position. However, as discussed in Chapter 17, generalizations are often made to abstract or theoretical populations. Thus, conclusions need to address applications to theory. Judgments about the reasonableness of generalizing need to address issues related to external validity, discussed in Chapter 10.

Generalizations based on accumulated evidence from many studies are called *empirical generalizations*. These generalizations are important for the verification of theoretical statements or the development of new theory. Empirical generalizations are the base of a science and contribute to scientific conceptualization. Nursing currently has few empirical generalizations.

CONSIDERING IMPLICATIONS

Implications are the meanings of conclusions for the body of knowledge, theory, and practice. Implications are based on the conclusions and are more specific than conclusions. They provide specific suggestions for implementing the findings. The researcher needs to consider the areas of nursing for which the study findings would be useful. For example, suggestions could be made about how nursing practice should be modified. If a study indicated that a specific solution was effective in decreasing stomatitis, the implications would state that the findings had implications for caring for patients with stomatitis. It would not be sufficient to state that the study had implications for nurses practicing in oncology.

McMillan and Mahon (1994) suggested the following implications.

■

"One important goal of hospice care is pain relief. Although pain is a symptom that can be brought under control in hours or days, there was only limited improvement in pain after 3 weeks of hospice care. Although a statistically significant decrease in pain intensity was reported, a decrease of only 2.4 points on a 100-point scale is not clinically significant. This finding of lack of improvement in pain is consistent with results of earlier studies. This finding would seem to suggest that greater attention needs to be paid to pain relief among these patients . . . Even patients who are greatly debilitated and very near death should expect their level of pain to decrease." (p. 58) ■

SUGGESTING FURTHER STUDIES

Completing a study and examining its implications should culminate in recommendations for future studies that emerge from the present study and from previous studies in the same area of interest. Suggested studies or recommendations for further study may include replications or repeating the design with a different or larger sample. In every study, the researcher gains knowledge and experi-

ence that can be used to design "a better study next time." Formulating recommendations for future studies stimulates the researcher to define more clearly how to improve the study. From a logical or theoretical point of view, the findings should lead directly to more hypotheses to further test the framework in use.

McMillan and Mahon (1994) provide the following suggestions for future research.

■

"Subsequent hospice quality of life studies should include number of days from death as part of the investigation . . . Future studies might focus on what is actually done to assess and manage pain or might ask patients and caregivers whether they believe that everything possible was being done to relieve pain." (p. 58)

"The data suggest that patient and caregiver reports are not completely congruent. Despite this lack of congruence, future studies should account for a wider sampling of all hospice patients even if the data source is less than ideal." (p. 59)

"Future studies should control the diagnoses of hospice patients admitted to the study." (p. 59)

"Future studies should use an instrument that is specifically designed for hospice patients. In addition, a method should be formed to collect data from patients who are very debilitated when they are admitted to hospice so that the sample may be more representative of the population of interest." (p. 59)

(From McMillan, S. C., & Mahon, M. [1994]. A study of quality of life of hospice patients on admission and at week 3. *Cancer Nursing, 17*[1], 52–60, with permission.) ■

■ SUMMARY

To be useful, the evidence from data analysis needs to be carefully examined, organized, and given meaning. This process is referred to as interpretation. Data collection and analysis are action-oriented activities that are concrete. However, when the results of the study have been obtained, more abstract thinking is used to interpret results. Within the process of inter-

pretation, several intellectual activities can be isolated and explored. These include examining evidence, forming conclusions, exploring the significance of the findings, generalizing the findings, considering implications, and suggesting further studies.

The first step in interpretation is consideration of all evidence available that supports or

continued

continued

contradicts the validity of results. Strengths and weaknesses of the study are explored. The evidence is obtained from a variety of sources, including the research plan, measurement validity and reliability, data collection process, data analysis process, data analysis results, and previous studies. Evidence of the validity of the results is derived from a reexamination of the research plan. The reliability and validity of measurement strategies need to be determined prior to their use, and these measures need to be reexamined to determine the strength of evidence available from results. Many factors can occur during the data collection process that affect the meaning of results, such as insufficient sample size, inappropriate sampling strategies, or unforeseen events. The evidence from data analysis is dependent on the researcher's knowledge of statistics and the proficiency of the analysis methods used.

The outcomes of data analyses are the most direct evidence available of the results related to the research objectives, questions, or hypotheses. Five possible results include: (1) significant results that are in keeping with those predicted by the researcher, (2) nonsignificant results, (3) significant results that are opposite to those predicted by the researcher, (4) mixed results, and (5) unexpected results. The results of a study should always be examined in light of previous findings.

The results of a study are translated and interpreted and then become findings. Findings are a consequence of evaluating evidence. Conclusions are derived from the findings and are a synthesis of findings. Forming conclusions requires a combination of logical reasoning, creative formation of a meaningful whole from pieces of information obtained through data analysis and findings from previous studies, receptivity to subtle clues in the data, and utilization of an open context in considering alternative explanations of the data.

Implications are the meanings of study conclusions for the body of knowledge, theory, and practice. The significance of a study is associated with its importance to the body of knowledge. A study needs to be clinically significant as well as statistically significant. Significance is not a dichotomous characteristic, because studies contribute in varying degrees to the body of knowledge. Generalization extends the implications of the findings from the sample studied to a larger population. Completion of a study and examination of implications should culminate in recommending future studies that emerge from the present study and previous studies. Suggested studies or recommendations for further study may include replications or repeating the design with a different or larger sample.

References

Angell, M. (1989). Negative studies. *New England Journal of Medicine, 321*(7), 464–466.

Johnson, J. E. (1972). Effects of structuring patients' expectations on their reactions to threatening events. *Nursing Research, 21*(6), 499–503.

Kerlinger, F. N. (1986). *Foundations of behavioral research* (3rd ed.). New York: Holt, Rinehart and Winston.

Lindeman, C. A., & Van Aernam, B. (1971). Nursing intervention with the presurgical patient—The effects of structured and unstructured preoperative teaching. *Nursing Research, 20*(4), 319–332.

McMillan, S. C., & Mahon, M. (1994). A study of quality of life of hospice patients on admission and at week 3. *Cancer Nursing, 17*(1), 52–60.

Passos, J. Y., & Brand, L. M. (1966). Effects of agents used for oral hygiene. *Nursing Research, 15*(3), 196–202.

Tulman, L. R., & Jacobsen, B. S. (1989). Goldilocks and variability. *Nursing Research, 38*(6), 377–379.

Williams, A. (1972). A study of factors contributing to skin breakdown. *Nursing Research, 21*(3), 238–243.

Yonkman, C. A. (1982). Cool and heated aerosol and the measurement of oral temperature. *Nursing Research, 31*(6), 354–357.

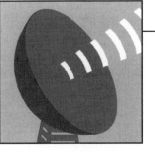

23

Communicating Research Findings

Imagine a nurse researcher conducting a study in which a unique phenomenon is described, a previously unrecognized relationship is detected, or the effectiveness of an intervention is determined. This information might make a difference in nursing practice; however, the nurse feels unskilled in presenting the information and overwhelmed by the idea of publishing. She places the study in a bottom drawer with an intent to communicate the findings "some day." This type of response results in many valuable nursing studies not being communicated and the information being lost.

Communicating research findings, the final step in the research process, involves developing a research report and disseminating it through presentations and publications to audiences of nurses, health care professionals, policymakers, and health care consumers. Disseminating research findings provides many advantages for the researcher, the nursing profession, and the consumer of nursing services. By presenting and publishing their findings, researchers are able to advance the knowledge of a discipline and to receive personal recognition, professional advancement, and other psychological and financial compensations for their work. These rewards are essential for the continuation of research in a discipline. Communicating research findings also promotes the critique and replication of studies, the identification of additional research problems, and the use of findings in practice. Using research findings in practice promotes improved patient outcomes. To promote the communication of research findings in nursing, this chapter describes the content of a research report, the audiences for communication of findings,

and the processes for presenting and publishing research findings.

CONTENT OF A RESEARCH REPORT

Both quantitative and qualitative research reports include similar sections. The report usually has four major sections: (1) introduction, (2) methods, (3) results, and (4) discussion of the findings (Field & Morse, 1985; Tornquist, Funk, & Champagne, 1989). The type and depth of information included in these sections depend on the type of study conducted, intended audiences, and mechanisms for disseminating the report. For example, theses and dissertations are research reports that are usually developed in-depth to demonstrate the student's understanding of the research problem and process to faculty members. Research articles for publication in journals are concisely written to communicate research findings efficiently and effectively to nurses and health professionals. The methods, results, and discussion sections of qualitative studies are usually more detailed than those of quantitative studies due to the complex data collection and analysis procedures and the comprehensive findings (Knafl & Howard, 1984).

QUANTITATIVE RESEARCH REPORT

An outline of the content covered in the four major sections of a quantitative research report is presented in Table 23–1.

Table 23-1
Outline for a Quantitative Research Report

INTRODUCTION
    Statement of the problem and significance
    Statement of the purpose
    Brief literature review
    Identification of the framework
    Identification of research objectives, questions, or hypotheses (if applicable)

METHODS
    Identification of the research design
    Description of the sample and setting
    Description of the methods of measurement
    Discussion of the data collection process

RESULTS
    Description of the data analysis procedures
    Presentation of results

DISCUSSION
    Discussion of major findings
    Identification of the limitations
    Presentation of conclusions
    Identification of the implications for nursing
    Recommendations for further research

REFERENCES

Introduction

The introduction of a research report briefly identifies the problem that was studied, provides a rationale for studying that problem, and presents an empirical and theoretical basis for the study. An introduction includes the following content: a problem statement; significance of the problem; study purpose; a review of relevant literature; framework; and research objectives, questions, or hypotheses (if applicable). This content is developed for the research proposal and is then summarized in the final report. Depending on the type of research report, the review of literature and framework might be separate sections or even separate chapters.

Review of Literature

The review of literature documents the current knowledge of the problem investigated. The sources included in the literature review are those that were used to develop the study and to interpret the findings. A review of literature can be two or three paragraphs or several pages in length. In journal articles, the review of literature is concise and usually includes 10 to 15 sources. Theses and dissertations frequently include an extensive literature review to document the student's knowledge of the research problem.

Framework

A research report needs to include an explicitly identified framework. The major concepts in the framework need to be defined and the relationships among the concepts described. A map or model can be developed to clarify the logic within the framework. If a particular proposition is being tested, that proposition should be clearly stated. Developing a framework map and identifying the proposition(s) examined in a study provide a clear connection between the framework and the research objectives, questions, or hypotheses.

Methods

The methods section of a research report describes how the study was conducted. This section needs to be concise, yet provide sufficient information for nurses to critique or replicate the study procedures. The study design, sample, setting, methods of measurement or instruments, and the data collection process are described in this section. If the research project included a pilot study, the planning, implementation, and results obtained from the pilot study are presented briefly. Any changes made in the research project based on the pilot study are described.

Design

The study design and level of significance (.05, .01, or .001) selected are identified in the research report. If the design included a treatment, the report needs to describe the treatment, including the protocol for implementing the treatment, training of people to implement the protocol, and a discussion of the consistency of the treatment administration (Egan, Snyder, & Burns, 1992; Kirchhoff & Dille, 1994). A complex study design might be presented using a table or figure, such as the examples that are provided in Chapter 11, Selecting a Research Design.

Sample and Setting

The research report usually includes the criteria for selecting the sample, the sample size, and sample characteristics. The use of power analysis to determine sample size needs to be discussed. If the subjects were divided into groups (experimental and comparison groups), the method for assigning subjects to groups, and the number of subjects in each group need to be identified. The protection of subjects' rights and the process of informed consent is also covered briefly. The setting of the study is often described in one or two sentences, and agencies are not identified by name unless permission has been obtained. The sample and setting for a study are often presented in narrative format; however, some researchers present the characteristics of their sample in a table.

Methods of Measurements

The variables of the study are operationalized by identifying the method of measurement for each. The details about methods of measurement or instruments used in the data collection process are critical in order for nurses to critique and replicate a study. The report needs to describe what information is collected by each instrument, the frequency with which the instrument has been used in previous research, and any reliability and validity information previously published on the instrument. In addition, the report needs to include the reliability and any further validity development for the current study. If psychologic measures are used, their accuracy, precision, selectivity, sensitivity, and sources of error need to be addressed.

Data Collection Process

The description of the data collection process in the research report details who collected the data, the procedure for collecting data, and the type and frequency of measurements obtained. In describing who collected the data, the report needs to indicate the experience of the data collector and any training provided. If more than one person collected data, the precautions taken to ensure consistency in data collection need to be described.

Results

The results section reveals what was found by conducting the study and includes the data analysis procedures, the results generated from these analyses, and sometimes the effect size achieved (Kraemer & Thiemann, 1987). For example, Lander and colleagues (1996) compared the effect of 5% lidocaine ointment to that of the eutectic mixture of local anesthetics (EMILA) cream on dermal anesthesia. The authors analyzed the data by a within-subject analysis of variance and found: "Significantly more pain was reported for 5% lidocaine ($M = 9.6$) than for EMILA ($M = 2.4$, $F = 11.5$, $p = .02$). The observed power was determined to be .77. The effect size for the study was .70" (Lander et al., 1996, p. 52).

The results section is best organized by the research objectives, questions, or hypotheses if stated in the study and if not, then by the study purpose. Research results can be presented in narrative format and organized into figures and tables. The methods used to present the results depend on the end product of data analyses and the researcher's preference. When reporting results in a narrative format, the value of the calculated statistic, the number of degrees of freedom, and probability or *p* value are identified. When insignificant results are reported, the power level for that analysis should also be reported in order to evaluate the risk of a Type II error. The *Publication Manual for the American Psychological Association* (APA) (1994) provides direction for citing a variety of statistical results in a research report. For example, the format for reporting chi-square results are: χ^2 (degrees of freedom, sample size) = statistical value, *p* value. Wikblad and Anderson (1995) compared three wound dressings—conventional absorbent, semiocclusive hydroactive, and occlusive hydrocolloid—in patients undergoing heart surgery and expressed their results in narrative format according to the APA (1994) guidelines.

"Patients in the hydroactive dressing group had significantly poorer wound healing (27% of the wounds were well healed, and 25% were partially healed), compared with patients treated with the absorbent dressing (57% of the wounds were well healed, and 33% were partially healed); χ^2 (2, *n* = 153) = 23.1, *p* < .0001; and with patients in the hydrocolloid dressing groups (50% of the wounds were well healed and 27% were partially healed); χ^2 (2, *n* = 129) = 7.6, *p* < .02. The differences in wound healing between the hydrocolloid and the absorbent dressing groups were not significant; χ^2 (2, *n* = 150) = 5.3, *p* > .05." (p. 314) ■

Presentation of Results in Figures and Tables

Figures and tables are used to present concisely and clearly a large amount of detailed in-

formation. Researchers use figures and tables to demonstrate relationships, document change over time, and reduce the amount of discussion needed in the text of the report (Mirin, 1981). However, figures and tables are useful only if they are appropriate for the results generated and are well constructed (Wainer, 1984). Table 23–2 provides guidelines for the development of accurate and clear figures and tables for a research report.

FIGURES. Figures or illustrations provide the reader with a picture of the results. Researchers often use computer programs to generate a variety of sophisticated black-and-white and color figures. Some common figures included in nursing research reports are bar-and-line graphs. Bar graphs can have horizontal or vertical bars, which represent the size or amount of the group or variable studied. The bar graph is also a means of comparing one item with another. McFarlane, Parker, and Soeken (1996) studied abuse during pregnancy and the associations with maternal health and infant birth weight. The ethnic-specific birth weights by abuse status were presented in a figure (see Figure 23–1 on p. 630). The researchers' discussion of this figure was: "Mean birth weights were lowest for women abused during pregnancy, followed by women abused within the last year but not during pregnancy. The highest mean birth weight infants were born to women reporting no abuse. Specific to ethnicity, abused African American women delivered infants weighing 127 g (grams) less, Hispanic 40 g less, and White 151 g less" (McFarlane et al., 1996, p. 39).

A line graph is developed by joining a series of points with a line, and shows how something varies over time. In this type of graph, the horizontal scale is used to measure time, and the vertical scale is used to measure number and quantity (Shurter et al., 1965). Figure 23–2 (on p. 631) is a line graph developed by Swain and Steckel (1981, p. 219) to demonstrate the effects of three treatments (routine clinical care, health education, and contingency contracting) upon patients' blood pressure over four visits. The discussion of this graph indicated that the blood pressures for the three groups were significantly different (*F* =

Table 23-2
Guidelines for Developing Tables and Figures in Research Reports

1. Examine the results obtained from a study and determine what results are essential to include in the report. Determine which results are best conveyed in figure and table format.
2. Use figures and tables to explain or support only the major points of the report. Using too many figures and tables can overwhelm the rest of the report, but a few receive attention and are effective in conveying the main results. Statistically nonsignificant findings are usually not presented in tables.
3. Keep the figures and tables simple; do not try to convey too much information in a single table. Two simple tables are better than one complex one.
4. Tables and figures should be complete and clear to the reader without referring to the text.
5. Each table and figure needs a clear, brief title.
6. Tables and figures are numbered separately and sequentially in a report. Thus, a report might have a Table 1 and Table 2 and a Figure 1 and Figure 2.
7. The headings, labels, symbols, and abbreviations used in figures and tables need to be appropriate, clear, and easy to read. Any symbols and abbreviations used need to be explained in a note included with the table or figure.
8. Probability values need to be identified with actual p values or with asterisks. If asterisks are used, a single asterisk is used for the least stringent significance level and two asterisks for more stringent significance, such as $* p < .05$ and $** p < .01$.
9. Figures and tables need to be referred to in the written text, such as "Table 3 presents . . ." or "(see Figure 1)." Figures and tables also need to be placed as close as possible to the section of the text where they are discussed (APA, 1994; Shurter, Williamson, & Broehl, 1965; Wainer, 1984).

3.39, $p < 0.05$) with the contingency contracting group demonstrating the greatest drop in diastolic blood pressure.

TABLES. Tables are used more frequently in research reports than figures and can be developed to present results from numerous statistical analyses. In tables, the results are presented in columns and rows for easy review by the reader. The sample tables included in this section present means, standard deviations, t values, chi-square values, and correlations. The means and standard deviations for study variables should be included in the published study. These values provide a basis for comparison across studies and are important for future meta-analyses. When replicating a study, the means and standard deviations are used to calculate the effect size when performing a power analysis to determine sample size (Tulman & Jacobsen, 1989).

McKenna, Maas, and McEniery (1995) examined coronary risk factors pre- and post-percutane-

ous transluminal coronary angioplasty (PTCA). Table 23-3 (on p. 631) presents the results of this study including descriptive (means, standard deviations, and frequencies) and inferential statistics (t test and chi-square). The t test was used to analyze ratio level data (serum cholesterol, body mass index, and number of cigarettes per day) and the chi-square to analyze nominal data (exercising and smoking habits). McKenna and colleagues (1995, p. 209) noted that "at post-PTCA follow-up, significant improvements had occurred in mean serum cholesterol levels, mean body mass index, and the number of subjects engaging in regular exercise ($p < .001$). . . . But the frequency of patients smoking after PTCA increased significantly ($p < .001$)."

Tables are used to identify correlations among variables, and often the table presents the correlation matrix generated from the data analysis. The significance of each correlation value needs to be indicated in the table. Reece (1995) studied the intercorrelations among dimensions of maternal

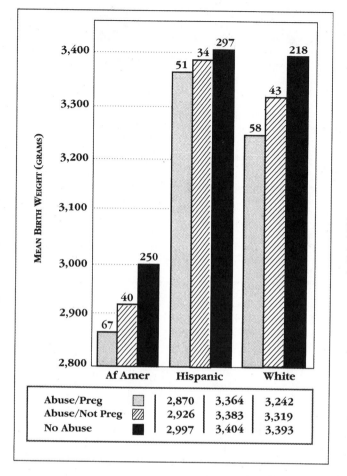

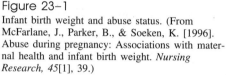

Figure 23–1
Infant birth weight and abuse status. (From McFarlane, J., Parker, B., & Soeken, K. [1996]. Abuse during pregnancy: Associations with maternal health and infant birth weight. *Nursing Research, 45*[1], 39.)

adaptation and stress at one year after delivery. The correlation matrix for the eight study variables is presented in Table 23–4 (on p. 632) and the significance of each correlation is indicated by the use of asterisks. The discussion of this table was, "in addition to associations with stress, gratification with the labor and delivery experience were correlated additionally with spouse/partner relationship and satisfaction with the infant" (Reece, 1995, p. 65).

Discussion

The discussion section ties the other sections of the research report together and gives them meaning. This section includes the major findings, limi-

tations of the study, conclusions drawn from the findings, implications of the findings for nursing, and recommendations for further research. The major findings, which are generated through an interpretation of the results, should be discussed in relationship to the research problem; purpose; and objectives, questions, or hypotheses (if applicable). Frequently, a study's findings are compared with the findings from previous research and are linked to the study's framework and the existing theoretical knowledge base. The discussion of the findings also includes the limitations that were identified in the proposal and during the conduct of the study. For example, a study might have limitations related to sample size, design, or in-

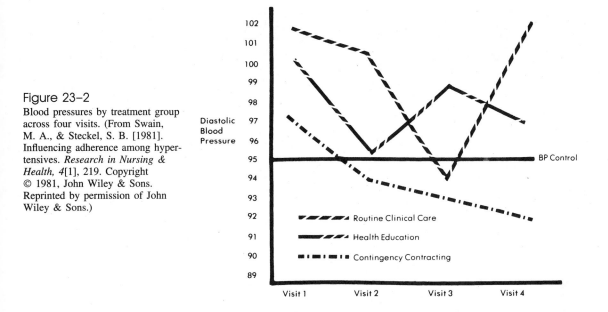

Figure 23–2
Blood pressures by treatment group across four visits. (From Swain, M. A., & Steckel, S. B. [1981]. Influencing adherence among hypertensives. *Research in Nursing & Health, 4*[1], 219. Copyright © 1981, John Wiley & Sons. Reprinted by permission of John Wiley & Sons.)

Table 23–3
Central Tendency, Variability, and Frequencies with Corresponding Statistics for Risk Factors at Pre-PTCA and Follow-up

| | Descriptive Statistics | | | |
Risk Factor	*Pre-PTCA*	*Follow-up*	*n*	*Statistic (test)*
Serum cholesterol	Mean = 240 SD = 47.5	Mean = 222 SD = 39.4	198	$t = 6.24$*
Body mass index	Mean = 26.58 SD = 3.65	Mean = 26.17 SD = 3.61	208	$t = 3.93$*
Currently exercising	f = 66 (31.7%)	f = 135 (64.9%)	208	$\chi^2 = 38.06$*
Currently smoking	f = 10 (4.8%)	f = 27 (13.0%)	208	$\chi^2 = 13.80$*
Cigarettes/day	Mean = 9.8 SD = 6.6	Mean = 20.4 SD = 11.9	208	$t = 2.38$†

* $p < 0.001$.
† $p < 0.05$.
(From McKenna, K. T., Maas, F., & McEniery, P. T. [1995]. Coronary risk factor status after percutaneous transluminal coronary angioplasty. *Heart & Lung, 24*[3], 210, with permission.)

Table 23–4
Intercorrelations Among Dimensions of Maternal Adaptation and Stress at 1 Year After Delivery (*N* = 82)

Outcome Variables	1	2	3	4	5	6	7	8
Dimensions of maternal adaptation								
1. Quality of relationship with husband		.63**	.24*	.12	.09	.25*	.30*	.35**
2. Father's participation in infant care			.09	−.02	.11	.08	.07	.06
3. Gratification with delivery				.09	.24	.37**	.12	.32**
4. Satisfaction with life situation and life circumstance					.30**	.23	.22	.50**
5. Confidence in motherhood						.44**	.32**	.42**
6. Satisfaction with the infant and infant care tasks							.40**	.55**
7. Support for the parental role								.33**
Stress								
8. Global perceived stress								

Low scores on the PSQ indicate maternal satisfaction and adaptation, and high scores indicate maladaptation, difficulty coping, and dissatisfaction.
* *p* < .05.
** *p* < .01.
(From Reece, S. M. [1995]. Stress and maternal adaptation in first-time mothers more than 35 years old. *Applied Nursing Research, 8*[2], 61–66, with permission.)

struments. The generalizability of the findings is influenced by these limitations.

The research report includes the conclusions or the knowledge that was generated from the findings. Conclusions are frequently stated in tentative or speculative terms, because one study does not produce conclusive findings (Tornquist et al., 1989). The researcher might provide a brief rationale for accepting certain conclusions and rejecting others. The conclusions need to be discussed in terms of their implications for nursing knowledge, theory, and practice. The researcher often describes how the findings and conclusions might be implemented in specific practice areas. The research report concludes with recommendations for further research. Specific problems that require investigation are identified, and the procedures for replicating the study are described. The discussion section of the research report demonstrates the value of conducting the study and stimulates the reader to use the findings in practice or to conduct additional research.

QUALITATIVE RESEARCH REPORT

The reports for qualitative research are as diverse as the different types of qualitative studies. (The different types of qualitative research are presented in Chapter 4 and the results from specific qualitative studies are presented in Chapter 20.) The intent of a qualitative research report is to describe the flexible, dynamic implementation of the research project and the unique, creative findings obtained. Like the quantitative report, a qualitative research report usually includes the four sections of introduction, methods, results, and discussion (see Table 23–5).

Introduction

The introduction section of the report identifies the phenomenon under investigation and indicates the type of qualitative study that was conducted. The study purpose and specific research aims or questions flow from the phenomenon, clarify the study focus, and identify expected outcomes of the investigation. The significance of the study topic to nursing knowledge and practice is described, with documentation from the literature. Qualitative studies are based on a variety of assumptions and philosophies that are identified in the report to provide a basis for the methodology, results, and discussion sections. In a sense, the philosophy provides a theoretical perspective for the study (Burns, 1989). Some qualitative studies include a

Table 23-5
Outline for a Qualitative Research Report

INTRODUCTION
  Identification of the phenomenon
  Identification of the study purpose and type of qualitative study
  Identification of the study questions or aims
  Discussion of the significance of the study
  Identification of assumptions
  Identification of philosophy
  Literature reviewed as appropriate for the qualitative study planned

METHODS
  Demonstration of researcher's credentials for conducting a particular type of qualitative
    study
  Identification of a site and population
  Description of the researcher's role
    1. Entry into the site
    2. Selection of a sample
    3. Ethical considerations
  Description of the data collection process

RESULTS
  Description of the data analysis procedures
  Presentation of results (such as development of a theory or model, description of a culture
    or historical event)

DISCUSSION
  Presentation of conclusions
  Discussion of the implications for nursing
  Recommendations for further research

REFERENCES

brief literature review in the introduction or as a separate section of the report. Other studies include a review of literature only in the discussion of findings.

Methods

In the methods section, the researcher documents his or her credentials for conducting the study. This documentation is valuable in determining the worth of the study, since the researcher serves as a primary data-gathering instrument and the data analyses occur within the reasoning processes of the researcher (Burns, 1989). The site and population selected for the study are described. The unique role of the researcher is also detailed, including training of project staff, entry into the setting, selection of subjects, and ethical considerations extended to the subjects during data collection and analysis.

The data collection process is time-consuming and complex. The research report includes a description of the variety of data collection tools used, such as observation guides, open-ended interviews, direct participation, documents, life histories, audiovisual media (photographs, videotapes), biographies, and diaries (Knafl & Howard, 1984; Leininger, 1985). The flexible, dynamic way in which the researcher collects data is described, including the time spent collecting data, how data were recorded, and the amount of data collected. For example, if the data collection involved participant-observation, the number, length, structure, and focus of the observation and participation periods need to be described. In addition, the tools (such as audio- or videotapes) for recording the information gained from these periods of observation and participation are identified.

Packard, Haberman, Woods, and Yates (1991,

p. 439) conducted a qualitative longitudinal investigation of "the stressful illness-related experiences reported by women living with one of three different diseases: nonmetastatic breast cancer, diabetes, and fibrocystic breast disease." The data were gathered through interviews conducted in the subjects' homes on "five occasions at 4-month intervals over a 17- to 18-month period" (p. 440). The subjects' responses to questions were recorded verbatim.

Results

The results section of the research report includes data analysis procedures and presentation of the findings. The data, in the form of notes, tapes, and other materials from observations and interviews, must be synthesized into meaningful categories or organized using common themes by the researcher. The data analysis procedures (content, symbolic, structural, interactional, philosophical, ethnographic, phenomenological, semantic, historical, inferential, grounded theory, perceptual, and reflexive) are performed during and after the data collection process (Leininger, 1985). These analysis procedures and the process for implementing them are described in the report. Packard and colleagues (1991) used content analysis to analyze the verbatim reports from their subjects. They summarized their data analysis procedures in Table 23–6, which identifies the number of cycles of data analysis, the analysis procedures, and the number of categories identified.

The results are presented in a manner that clarifies the phenomenon under investigation for the reader. These results include gestalts, patterns, and theories that are developed to describe life experiences, cultures, and historical events, which are frequently expressed in narrative format. Sometimes these theoretical ideas are organized into conceptual maps, models, or tables. Researchers often gather additional data or reexamine existing data to verify their theoretical conclusions and this process is described in the report (Burns, 1989). Some of the results from the study of Packard and colleagues (1991) are presented in Table 23–7. The discussion of Table 23–7 indicated that 22 categories were identified and organized into seven domains of illness demands, and these "domains were grouped into three overriding or core

Table 23–6
Data Analysis Procedure

Cycle	Sample Size	Occasion	Procedure	Results
1	66	1	Unitize data Group data by category Label categories	41 categories
2	49	1	Unitize data Classify data Revise schema Revise labels	35 categories
3	115	2, 3	Repeat cycle 2 procedure Reclassify data; Cycles 1 and 2 Interrater reliability Develop domains Develop core constructs	22 categories 85% 7 domains 3 constructs
4	115	1, 2, 3	Determine prevalence rates	(see Figure 1)

(From Packard, N. J., Haberman, M. R., Woods, N. F., & Yates, B. C. [1991]. Demands of illness among chronically ill women. *Western Journal of Nursing Research, 13*[4], 442. © 1991. Reprinted by permission of Sage Publications, Inc.)

Table 23–7
Core Constructs, Conceptual Domains, and Categories

Core Construct	Conceptual Domain	Category
Direct disease effects	Direct disease effects	1. Direct disease effects
Personal disruption	Disruption of continuity	2. Vulnerability
		3. Uncertainty
		4. Unmet expectations
		5. Future concerns
		6. Confrontation with time
		7. Reminders
	Disruption of integrity	8. Self-image
		9. Social comparisons
		10. Social-emotional disturbances
	Disruption of normality	11. Monitoring symptoms
		12. Monitoring coping (self and others)
Environmental transactions	Social response	13. Social network
		14. Role compensation
		15. Marital dynamics
	Treatment process	16. Financial costs
		17. Treatment effects
		18. Accommodation
		19. Waiting for results
		20. Additional treatment
	Patient provider interaction	21. Information exchange
		22. Negative relationships

(From Packard, N. J., Haberman, M. R., Woods, N. F., & Yates, B. C. [1991]. Demands of illness among chronically ill women. *Western Journal of Nursing Research, 13*[4], 443. © 1991. Reprinted by permission of Sage Publications, Inc.)

constructs of illness demands: (1) direct disease effects, (2) personal disruption, and (3) environmental transactions" (p. 442).

Discussion

The discussion section includes conclusions, implications for nursing, and recommendations for further research. The conclusions are a summary of the findings and indicate what was and was not accomplished during the study. Each research question is answered, and the findings are linked to relevant theoretical and empirical literature. The implications of the findings for nursing practice and theory development are explored, and suggestions are provided for further research.

THESES AND DISSERTATIONS

Theses and dissertations are research reports that are developed in-depth by students as part of the requirements for a degree. The content included in a thesis or dissertation depends on the members of the student's research committee, but the organization of the content usually follows the outline presented in Table 23–8 (on p. 636). The introduction, review of relevant literature, framework, and the methods and procedures sections of this outline are described in Chapter 26. The content of the results and discussion sections is similar to that just described for a research report.

AUDIENCES FOR COMMUNICATION OF RESEARCH FINDINGS

Before developing a research report, the investigator needs to determine *who* will benefit from knowing the findings. The greatest impact on nursing practice can be achieved by communicating

Table 23-8
Outline for Theses and Dissertations

Chapter I　INTRODUCTION
　　　　　Statement of the problem
　　　　　Background and significance of the problem
　　　　　Statement of the purpose
Chapter II　REVIEW OF RELEVANT LITERATURE
　　　　　Review of relevant theoretical literature
　　　　　Review of relevant research
　　　　　Summary
Chapter III　FRAMEWORK
　　　　　Development of a framework
　　　　　Formulation of objectives, questions, or hypotheses
　　　　　Definition of research variables
　　　　　Definition of relevant terms
　　　　　Identification of assumptions
Chapter IV　METHODS AND PROCEDURES
　　　　　Identification of the research design
　　　　　Description of the population and sample
　　　　　Identification of the setting
　　　　　Presentation of ethical considerations
　　　　　Description of measurement methods
　　　　　Description of the data collection process
Chapter V　RESULTS
　　　　　Description of data analysis procedures
　　　　　Presentation of results
Chapter VI　DISCUSSION
　　　　　Presentation of major findings
　　　　　Identification of limitations
　　　　　Identification of conclusions
　　　　　Discussion of the implications for nursing
　　　　　Recommendations for further research
References
Appendices

nursing research findings to a variety of audiences, including nurses, other health professionals, health care consumers, and policymakers. Nurses, including educators, practitioners, and researchers, must be aware of research findings for communication in academic programs, for use in practice, and as a basis for conducting additional studies. Other health professionals need to be aware of the knowledge generated by nurse researchers and facilitate the use of that knowledge in the health care industry. Consumers are interested in the outcomes produced by nursing interventions that have been tested through research. Policymakers at the local, state, and federal levels are using research findings to generate health policy that will impact individual practitioners and the health care industry.

STRATEGIES FOR COMMUNICATING RESEARCH TO DIFFERENT AUDIENCES

Research findings can be communicated through written reports and oral and visual presentations. The different strategies for communicating findings to nurses, health care professionals, policymakers, and consumers are outlined in Table 23–9.

Audience of Nurses

The most common mechanisms used by nurses to communicate research findings to their peers are presentations at conferences and meetings. An increasing number of nursing organizations and in-

Table 23-9
Audiences and Strategies for Communicating Research

Audience	Strategies for Communicating Research

Nurses—Practitioners, researchers, and educators	Oral and visual presentations
	    Nursing research conferences
	    Professional nursing meetings and conferences
	    Collaborative nursing groups
	    Thesis and dissertation defenses
	    Videotaped and audiotaped presentations
	Written reports
	    Nursing referred journals
	    Nursing books
	    Monographs
	    Research newsletter
	    Theses and dissertations
	    Foundation reports
	    Electronic databases

Other health care professionals	Oral and visual presentations
	    Professional conferences and meetings
	    Interdisciplinary collaboration
	    Taped presentations
	Written reports
	    Professional journals and books
	    Newsletters
	    Foundational reports
	    Electronic databases

Policymakers	Oral and visual presentations
	    Testifying on health problems to state and federal legislators
	Written reports
	    Research reports to legislators
	    Research reports to funding agencies
	    Electronic databases
	    AHCPR reports and presentations to policymakers, practitioners, and consumers

Health care consumers	Oral and visual presentations
	    Television and radio
	    Community meetings
	    Patient and family teaching
	Written reports
	    Newspaper
	    News and popular magazines
	    Electronic databases

stitutions are sponsoring research conferences. The American Nurses' Association and many of its state associations sponsor annual nursing research conferences. The Western Council of Higher Education for Nursing has been sponsoring annual research conferences since 1968, and the proceedings from these conferences are published in a volume entitled *Communicating Nursing Research Findings.* The members of Sigma Theta Tau, the international honor society for nursing, sponsor international, national, regional, and local research conferences. Specialty organizations, such as the American Association of Critical Care Nurses, Oncology Nurses' Society, and Maternal-Child Health Nursing Association sponsor research meetings and conferences. Many universities and some health care agencies sponsor or cosponsor research conferences. For a variety of reasons, many nurses are unable to attend research conferences. To increase the communication of research findings, conference sponsors provide audio- or videotapes of the research presentations. Some sponsors publish abstracts of studies with the conference proceedings or in a specialty journal or make them available electronically, such as on the World Wide Web (WWW).

The publishing opportunities in nursing continue to escalate—the number of nursing journals published in the United States has increased from 22 in 1977 (McCloskey, 1977) to 92 in 1991 (Swanson, McCloskey, & Bodensteiner, 1991). Opportunities to publish research have expanded with the growth of research journals (*Advances in Nursing Science, Applied Nursing Research, Clinical Nursing Research, Nursing Research, Research in Nursing & Health, Scholarly Inquiry for Nursing Practice: An International Journal,* and *Western Journal of Nursing Research*) and with specialty journals publishing more studies. *Heart & Lung* is now 70% research publications; *Maternal-Child Nursing (MCN)* is 75% research; and *Journal of Nursing Education* is 80% research (Swanson et al., 1991). An increasing number of researchers are also communicating their findings by publishing books or chapters in books.

Many universities and hospitals publish regular newsletters or monographs, which include abstracts or articles about the research conducted by their members. The American Nurses' Association Council of Nurse Researchers publishes a newsletter, which reports studies that have been presented at conferences and identifies the ongoing studies of the council members. Foundations and federal government agencies publish reports of studies that have been conducted or are in progress. The American Nurses' Foundation publishes a newsletter, *Nursing Research Report,* that identifies the studies funded and includes abstracts of these studies. The National Institute for Nursing Research (NINR) publishes reports on their grants, including research project titles, names and addresses of researchers, period of support, a brief description of each project, and publication citations.

Audience of Health Care Professionals and Policymakers

Nurse researchers communicate their research to other health professionals at meetings and conferences sponsored by such organizations as the American Heart Association, American Public Health Association, American Cancer Society, American Lung Association, National Hospice Organization, and National Rural Health Association. Nurses must believe in the value of their research and present their findings at conferences that attract a variety of health care professionals. Nurse researchers and other health professionals conducting research on the same or similar problems might publish a journal article, series of articles, book chapter, or even a book together. This type of interdisciplinary collaboration might increase the communication of research findings and the impact of the findings on health care.

In 1989, the Agency for Health Care Policy and Research (AHCPR) was established to enhance the quality, appropriateness, and effectiveness of health care services and access to these services. This agency has promoted the conduct of patient outcomes research and facilitated the dissemination and use of research findings in practice. To promote the communication of research findings, AHCPR formed a work group for the dissemination of patient outcomes research. This work group included a variety of researchers and health practitioners, including nurses and physicians. The purpose of this group was to develop a plan for the dissemination of research findings that identified the audiences and strategies for communication of research. The audiences identified included consumers, health care practitioners, health care industry, policymakers, researchers, and journalists. Strategies for the dissemination of research included printed materials provided through direct mail, technical journals, health journals, the popular press, and electronic media, with communication by radio, television, and WWW. This group would review research and determine the knowledge that was ready for dissemination to practice. Other bodies within AHCPR, such as the Forum for Effectiveness and Quality in Health Care and the Center for Research Dissemination, would then create and disseminate research-based clinical guidelines for use in practice (Goldberg et al., 1994). The clinical practice guidelines are discussed in more depth in Chapter 25, Utilization of Research in Nursing Practice.

Nurse researchers also need to communicate their findings to legislators through written reports and personal presentations, so that their findings have an impact on health policies. Expert nurse researchers are being asked to testify in their areas of expertise, such as the prevention of pressure ulcers and the treatment of incontinence, to members of Congress as policies related to health care have been developed.

Audience of Health Care Consumers

An audience that is frequently neglected by nurse researchers is the health care consumer. The findings from nursing studies can be communicated to the public through news releases. A nursing research article published in a local paper has the potential of being picked up by the National Wire Service and published in other papers across the country. Thus, the study findings can reach many potential health care consumers. Nurse researchers also need to make their findings available through electronic databases. An increasing amount of health care information is being made available electronically on the WWW and consumers can access current research information from their home using their personal computer.

Nursing research findings could be communicated to consumers by being published in news magazines, such as *Time* and *Newsweek,* or popular women's and health magazines, such as *American Baby* and *Health.* Health articles published for consumer magazines can reach from 20,000 to 24,000,000 readers at a time (Jimenez, 1991). Television and radio are other valuable sources for communicating research findings. Currently, the findings from many medical studies are covered through these media. Another important method of communicating research findings to consumers is through patient and family teaching. Nursing interventions and practice protocols based on research are more credible to consumers than are unresearched actions.

PRESENTING RESEARCH FINDINGS

Research findings are communicated at conferences and meetings through verbal and poster presentations. With presentations, researchers have an opportunity to share their findings, answer questions about their studies, interact with other interested researchers, and receive immediate feedback on their study. There is frequently little delay between the completion of the research project and the presentation of the findings. When research findings are published, there is usually a 1- to 3-year delay in the communication process.

VERBAL PRESENTATIONS

Researchers communicate their findings through verbal presentations at local, national, and international nursing and health care conferences. Presenting findings at a conference requires receiving acceptance as a presenter, developing a research report, delivering the report, and responding to questions.

Receiving Acceptance as a Presenter

Most research conferences require the submission of an abstract, and acceptance as a presenter is based on the quality of the abstract. An *abstract* is a clear, concise summary of a study that is usually limited to 100 to 250 words (Crosby, 1990; Juhl & Norman, 1989). Nine months to a year before a research conference, the sponsors circulate a call

Table 23-10
Outline for an Abstract

I.   TITLE OF THE STUDY

II. INTRODUCTION OF THE SCIENTIFIC PROBLEM
    A. Statement of the problem and purpose
    B. Identification of the framework

III. METHODOLOGY
    A. Design
    B. Sample size
    C. Identification of data analysis methods

IV. RESULTS
    A. Major findings
    B. Conclusions
    C. Implications for nursing
    D. Recommendations for further research

The title of an abstract must create interest, while the body of the abstract "sells" the study to the reviewers. An example of an abstract is presented in Figure 23–3. Writing an abstract requires practice; frequently, a researcher will rewrite an abstract many times until it meets all the criteria outlined by the conference sponsors. Cason, Cason, and Redland (1988) identified six criteria that are often used in rating the quality of an abstract: (1) acceptability of a study for a specific program; (2) overall quality of the work; (3) contribution to nursing scholarship; (4) contribution to nursing theory and practice; (5) originality of the work; and (6) clarity and completeness of the abstract, according to the content outlined in Table 23–10. These criteria might assist you in critiquing and refining your abstract.

for abstracts. Many research journals and newsletters publish these calls for abstracts and they are also available electronically. In addition, conference sponsors will mail the calls for abstracts to universities, major health care agencies, and known nursing researchers.

The call for abstracts will indicate the format for the development of the abstract. Frequently, abstracts are limited to one page, single-spaced, and include the content outlined in Table 23–10.

Developing a Research Report

The report developed depends on the focus of the conference, the audience, and the time designated for each presentation. Some conferences focus on certain sections of the research report, such as tool development, data collection and analyses, findings, or implications of the findings for nursing

Title: Symptoms of Female Survivors of Child Sexual Abuse

Investigator: Polly A. Hulme

Research indicates that at least 20% of all women have been victims of serious sexual abuse involving unwanted or coerced sexual contact up to the age of 17 years. Women who suffered sexual abuse as children often experience a variety of physical and psychosocial symptoms as adults. Identifying this pattern of symptoms might assist health professionals in recognizing and treating nonreporting survivors of child sexual abuse. The framework for this study is Finkelhor and Browne's (1986) theory of traumagenic dynamics in the impact of child sexual abuse. This theory indicates that child sexual abuse is at the center of the adult survivor's existence and results in four trauma-causing dynamics: traumatic sexualization, betrayal, powerlessness, and stigmatization. These traumagenic dynamics lead to behavioral manifestations that collectively indicate a history of child sexual abuse. The severity of the behavioral manifestations are influenced by the contributing factors or characteristics of the abuse that affect the survivor's life.

The study design was descriptive correlation and the Adult Survivors of Incest (ASI) Questionnaire (Brown & Garrison, 1990) was used to determine the symptoms and contributing factors for 22 adult survivors of child sexual abuse. Six physical symptoms were experienced by 50% of the subjects, and over 75% of the subjects experienced 11 psychosocial symptoms. The number of physical symptoms correlated significantly with other victimizations ($r = .59$) and number of psychosocial symptoms ($r = .56$). The number of psychosocial symptoms also correlated significantly with other victimizations ($r = .40$) and duration of abuse ($r = .40$).

The findings suggest that the ASI Questionnaire was effective in identifying patterns of symptoms and contributing factors of adult survivors of child sexual abuse. Additional study is needed to determine the usefulness of this questionnaire in identifying nonreporting survivors in clinical situations (Hulme & Grove, 1994).

Figure 23–3

Example of an abstract.

practice. However, it is usually important to address the major sections of a research report (introduction, methods, results, and discussion) in a presentation. The content of a presentation varies depending on whether the audience consists of mainly researchers or clinical nurses (Jackle, 1989). If you do not know who your audience is, ask the sponsors of the conference.

Time is probably the most important factor in developing a presentation, since many presenters are limited to 12 to 15 minutes with 5 minutes for questions (Selby, Tornquist, & Finerty, 1989a). As a guideline, you might spend 10% of your time on the introduction, 20% on the methodology, 35% on the results, and 35% on the discussion. The introduction might include reasons for the study, a brief review of the literature, a simple discussion of the framework, and the research questions or hypotheses. The methodology content includes a brief identification of the design, sampling method, and measurement techniques. The content covered in the results section includes a simple rationale for analysis methods used and the major statistical results. The presentation concludes with a brief discussion of findings, implications of the findings for nursing practice, and recommendations for future research (Miracle & King, 1994). Most researchers find that the shorter the presentation time, the greater the preparation time that is needed.

Many researchers develop a typed script of their study for presentation and include visuals, such as slides or transparencies. The script for the presentation needs to indicate when a visual is to be shown. The information presented on each visual should be limited to eight lines or less, with six or less words per line. Thus, a single visual contains information that can be easily read and examined in 30 seconds or a minute (Selby, Tornquist, & Finerty, 1989b). Only major points are presented on visuals; thus, single words or short phrases are used to convey ideas, not complete sentences. Figures such as bar-and-line graphs usually convey ideas more clearly than tables. Slides of the research setting, equipment, and researcher collecting data are effective in helping the audience visualize the research project. The use of color on a visual can increase the clarity of the information presented and can be appealing to the audience.

Preparing the script and visuals for a presentation is difficult; thus, the assistance of an experienced researcher and audiovisual expert can be valuable. Rehearse your presentation with an experienced researcher and use his or her comments to refine your script, visuals, and presentation style. If your presentation is too long, you need to synthesize your script and possibly provide handouts for important content. Audiovisual experts will ensure that your materials are clear and properly constructed, with the print large enough and dark enough to be easily read.

Delivering a Research Report and Responding to Questions

A novice researcher might attend conferences and examine the presentation style of other researchers. Even though researchers need to develop their own presentation style, observing others can promote the development of an effective style. The research report can be read from a script, given from an outline, or delivered using slides or transparencies. An effective presentation requires practice. You need to rehearse your presentation several times, using the script, until you are comfortable with the timing, content, and your presentation style. In practicing a presentation, use the visuals so that you are comfortable with the audiovisual equipment. The presentation must be within the time frame designated by conference sponsors.

Some conferences include a presentation by the researcher, a critique of the study by another researcher, and a question period. When preparing for a presentation, you should try to anticipate the questions that might be asked and rehearse your answers. The presentation could be given to colleagues, who might be asked to raise questions. If you practice making clear, concise responses to specific questions, this will decrease your anxiety during the actual presentation. When giving a presentation, make notes of questions, suggestions, or comments made by the audience. These are often useful in preparing a manuscript for publication or developing the next study.

POSTER SESSIONS

Sometimes your research will be accepted at a conference not as a presentation but as a poster session. A *poster session* is a visual presentation of your study. Before developing a poster, contact the conference sponsors regarding (1) size limitations or format restrictions for the poster, (2) the size of the poster display area, and (3) the background and potential number of conference participants (Lippman & Ponton, 1989). A poster usually includes the following content: the title of the study; investigator and institution names; brief abstract; purpose; research objectives, questions, or hypotheses (if applicable); framework; design; sample; instruments; essential data collection procedures; results; conclusions; implications for nursing; and recommendations for further research. For clarity and conciseness, a poster often includes pictures, tables, or figures to communicate the study. Often one color is used for most of the poster and one or two additional colors are used for accents (McDaniel, Bach, & Poole, 1993). The structure for a poster is provided in Figure 23-4.

A poster can be developed from sturdy cardboard, or a special display board can be purchased. Your budget will determine the type of poster you develop, but it should be easy to transport and assemble at the conference setting. A quality poster is complete in the presentation of a study, yet easily comprehended in five minutes or less (Ryan, 1989). Bold headings are used for the different parts of the research report, followed by clear, concise narratives. The size of the print on a poster needs to be large enough to be read easily at four to six feet (McDaniel et al., 1993). Poster sessions usually last from one to two hours; the researcher should remain with the poster during this time. Most researchers provide conference participants with a copy of their abstracts and other relevant handouts and offer to answer any questions.

An advantage of a poster session is the opportunity for one-to-one interaction between the researcher and those viewing the poster. At the end of the poster session, individuals interested in a study will frequently stay to speak to the re-

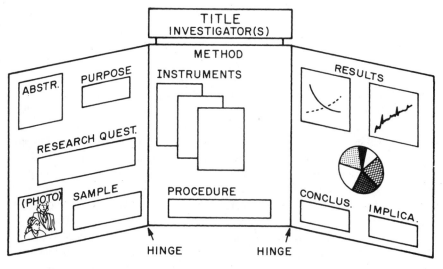

Figure 23-4
Three-part hinged poster. (From Ryan, N. M. [1989]. Developing and presenting a research poster. *Applied Nursing Research*, 2[1], 53, with permission.)

searcher. A notepad is often needed to record comments and the names and addresses of those conducting similar research. This is an excellent opportunity to begin networking with other researchers involved in the same area of research. Sometimes conference participants will want study instruments or other items to be mailed, faxed, or e-mailed to them, so a record of their names, addresses, fax numbers, and requests must be kept.

PUBLISHING RESEARCH FINDINGS

Presentations are valuable means to rapidly communicate findings, but their impact is limited. Published research findings are permanently recorded in a journal or book and usually reach a larger audience than presentations (Diers, 1981). However, the research report developed for a presentation can provide a basis for writing an article for publication. Regrettably, many researchers present their findings at a conference and never submit the paper for publication. Hicks (1995) studied the publishing activities of 500 randomly selected nurses and found only 10% submitted their studies for publication. Studies with negative findings, such as no significant differences or relationships, are frequently not submitted for presentation or publication. These negative findings can be as important to the development of knowledge as the positive findings (Angell, 1989).

Publishing research findings is a rewarding experience but the process demands a great deal of time and energy. The manuscript rejections or requests for major revisions that most authors receive can be discouraging. However, one can take certain steps to increase the probability of having a manuscript accepted for publication. Plans for publishing a study should be outlined during proposal development. At this time, investigators should discuss and, if possible, determine authorship credit. This becomes complex when the research is a collaborative project among individuals from different disciplines. Some researchers de-

velop the entire manuscript and are then faced with the decision of who will be first, second, or third author. There are many ways to determine authorship credit, but the decision should be one that is acceptable to all investigators involved (Hanson, 1988). Authorship credit should be given only to those who made substantial contributions toward developing and implementing a study and in writing the final report (Shapiro, Wenger, & Shapiro, 1994).

PUBLISHING JOURNAL ARTICLES

Developing a manuscript for publication includes the following steps: (1) selecting a journal, (2) developing a query letter, (3) preparing a manuscript, (4) submitting the manuscript for review, and (5) responding to requests for revision of the manuscript.

Selecting a Journal

Selecting a journal for publication of a study requires knowledge of the basic requirements of the journal, the journal's refereed status (see next paragraph), and the recent articles published in the journal. Swanson et al. (1991) studied the publishing opportunities for nurses by surveying 92 U.S. nursing journals. The authors provided, in table format, the following basic information on each journal: circulation; number of issues published each year; article length; number of copies of the manuscript submitted; format for the manuscript; query letter; free reprints; and the percentage of staff-written, unsolicited, and research manuscripts published. Other information in the article of interest to potential authors is number of unsolicited manuscripts received, number of unsolicited manuscripts published, number of manuscripts rejected, percentage of manuscripts accepted, refereed status, review process, time for acceptance, and time until publication (Swanson et al., 1991, p. 35). Table 23–11 presents some essential publishing information for five research journals included in this survey.

A *refereed journal* uses referees or expert re-

Table 23–11
Publishing Information for Selected Research Journals

Journal	Number of Issues	Query Letter	Referred Status	Article Length	Format	Copies Required	Acceptance Rate (%)
Advances in Nursing Science	4	Optional	Yes	15–30 pages	APA*	3	13
Applied Nursing Research	4	Optional	Yes	8–12 pages	APA*	5	48
Nursing Research	6	Preferred	Yes	14–16 pages	APA*	3	15
Research in Nursing & Health	6	Optional	Yes	10–15 pages	APA*	4	22
Western Journal of Nursing Research	6	Optional	Yes	15 pages	APA*	4	20

* APA, American Psychological Association.
(Adapted from Swanson, E. A., McCloskey, J. C., & Bodensteiner, A. [1991]. Publishing opportunities for nurses: A comparison of 92 U.S. journals. *Image: Journal of Nursing Scholarship, 23*[1], 33–38.)

viewers to determine whether a manuscript is accepted for publication. In nonrefereed journals, the editor makes the decisions for acceptance or rejection of manuscripts, but these decisions are usually made after consultation with a nursing expert (Carnegie, 1975). Most refereed journals require manuscripts to be reviewed anonymously by two or three reviewers. The reviewers are asked to determine the strengths and weaknesses of a manuscript, and their comments or a summary of the comments is sent to the author. Most academic institutions support the refereed system and will recognize only those publications that are in refereed journals. The five research journals presented in Table 23–11 are refereed and have the following review process: "Editor receives manuscripts, reviews, and distributes them to experts selected from an established group of reviewers. Decision on the manuscript is based on reviews and mediated by editor" (Swanson et al., 1991, p. 35).

Researchers often review the articles recently published in the journal to which they plan to submit a manuscript. This review will indicate whether a research topic has been recently covered and whether the research findings would be of interest to the journal's readers. This selection process enables researchers to identify a few journals that would be appropriate for publishing their findings.

Developing a Query Letter

A *query letter* is developed to determine an editor's interest in reviewing a manuscript. This letter should be no more than one or two pages and usually includes the research problem, a brief discussion of the major findings, the significance of the findings, and the researcher's qualifications for writing the article (Mirin, 1981). A query letter is addressed to the current editor of a journal; frequently, three or four letters are sent to different journals at the same time. Of the five journals presented in Table 23–11, only *Nursing Research* prefers a query letter; the other research journals indicated these letters were optional. Some researchers send query letters because the response (positive or negative) enables them to make the final selection of a journal for submission of a manuscript. An example of a query letter is presented in Figure 23–5.

Preparing a Manuscript

A manuscript is written according to the format outlined by the journal. The guidelines for developing a manuscript are usually published in an issue of the journal; however, some journals require that you write and request the author guidelines. These guidelines should be followed explicitly to increase the probability of your manuscript being published. The information provided for authors include (1) directions for manuscript preparation, (2) discussion of copyright, and (3) guidelines for submission of the manuscript.

Writing research reports for publication requires skills in technical writing that are not used in other types of publication. Technical writing

January 31, 1997

Joyce J. Fitzpatrick, PhD, FAAN
Editor
Applied Nursing Research

Case Western Reserve University
Frances Payne Bolton School of Nursing
10900 Euclid Avenue
Cleveland, OH 44106

Dear Dr. Fitzpatrick:

An increasing number of nursing studies are focused on clinical problems and specifically on the outcomes of nursing interventions. Currently, many nursing interventions are implemented without adequate research, such as the treatments for pain. I have just completed a study to examine the effects of ice therapy versus heat therapy on patients who are experiencing chronic low back pain.

The framework for this study was the Melzack and Wall gate-control theory of pain. The independent variables, ice and heat therapies, were consistently implemented with structured protocols by nurses in a pain clinic. The dependent variable, perception of pain, was measured with a visual analogue scale. The sample included 90 clinic patients with low back pain. The subjects were randomly assigned to three groups: a comparison group that received no treatment, an experimental group that received ice therapy, and an experimental group that received heat therapy.

An analysis of variance (ANOVA) with post hoc analyses indicated that patients in the comparison group and heat therapy group perceived their pain to be significantly greater than the perception of pain by the patients receiving ice therapy. The findings suggest that ice therapy is more effective than heat in reducing chronic low back pain. Ice therapy is an intervention that can be prescribed and implemented by nurses to reduce patients' perception of pain.

I hope you will consider reviewing this manuscript for possible publication. I look forward to receiving a response from you.

Sincerely,

Susan K. Grove, PhD, R.N.
Professor, School of Nursing
The University of Texas at Arlington

Figure 23–5
Example of a query letter.

condenses information and is stylistic. The *Publication Manual for the APA* (APA, 1994) and the *Chicago Manual of Style* (University of Chicago Press, 1993) are considered useful sources for quality technical writing. A quality research report has no punctuation, spelling, or sentence structure errors; confusing words; cliches; jargon; or wordiness (Camilleri, 1987, 1988). Computer programs have been developed with the capacity to proof manuscripts for grammar, punctuation, spelling, and sentence structure errors. However, the writer still needs to respond and correct the sentences that are identified as problematic by the computer.

Knowledge about the author guidelines provided by the journal and a background in technical writing facilitate developing an outline for a proposed manuscript. The initial brief outlines presented in Tables 23–1 and 23–5 must be developed in detail to guide the writing of a manuscript. A rough draft of the article is developed from the outline and is revised numerous times. The content

of an article should be logically and concisely developed under clear headings, and the title selected for the manuscript needs to create interest and reflect the content.

Developing a clear, concise manuscript is difficult. Often, universities and other agencies offer writing seminars to assist students and other researchers in preparing a research report for publication. Some faculty members who chair thesis and dissertation committees will also assist their students in developing an article for publication. In this situation, the faculty member is almost always the second author for the article.

When researchers are satisfied with their manuscripts, they usually ask one or two colleagues to review it for organization, completeness of content, and writing style. Colleagues' comments can be used to make the final revisions in the manuscript (Hagemaster & Kerrins, 1984). The manuscript should be expertly typed according to the journal's specifications; most research journals require the APA (1994) format. The reference list for the manuscript needs to be in a complete and correct format. Computer programs are available with bibliography systems that enable you to develop a complete, consistently formatted reference list using any format you desire. Using these programs, you can maintain a permanent collection of reference citations. When you need a reference list for a manuscript, you can select the appropriate references from the collection and use the program to print the list. Computer programs can also be used to scan your manuscript and create a reference list based on the citations in the manuscript.

Submitting a Manuscript for Review

Guidelines in each journal indicate the name of the editor and the address for manuscript submission. A manuscript must be submitted to only one journal at a time. The researcher should submit the number of copies of the manuscript requested and the original manuscript, if required. Research journal editors require from three to five copies of a manuscript (see Table 23–11) and some also request a disk of the manuscript. When submitting the manuscript, the researcher identifies his or her complete mailing address, phone number, fax number, and e-mail address. An author usually receives notification of receipt of the manuscript within one to two weeks.

Responding to Requests to Revise a Manuscript

The review of a manuscript results in one of four possible decisions: (1) acceptance of the manuscript as submitted, (2) acceptance of the manuscript pending minor revisions, (3) tentative acceptance of the manuscript pending major revisions, and (4) rejection of the manuscript. Accepting a manuscript as submitted is extremely rare. The editor will send the author a letter that indicates the acceptance of the manuscript and a possible issue of publication.

Most manuscripts are returned for minor or major revisions before they are published. It is regrettable that many of these returned manuscripts are never revised. The author incorrectly interprets the request for revision as a rejection and assumes that the revised manuscript will also be rejected. This is usually not true, since revising a manuscript based on reviewers' comments improves the quality of the manuscript. When editors return a manuscript for revision, they include the reviewers' actual comments or a summary of the comments to direct the revision. The researcher must carefully review the comments and make those revisions that improve the quality of the research report without making inaccurate statements about the study. Sometimes a paper must be revised more than once before it is published. Frequently, editors request that the final manuscript be submitted on disk.

The author who receives a rejection feels devastated, but he or she is not alone. All authors, even famous ones, have had their manuscripts rejected (Gay & Edgil, 1989). Manuscripts are rejected for a variety of reasons. Swanson and colleagues (1991, p. 38) asked journal editors to rate the frequency of 14 reasons for manuscript rejection. Table 23–12 identifies these reasons and their mean frequencies. "Poorly written" and "poorly developed idea" were the most frequent reasons for rejecting manuscripts. If you receive a rejection notice, give yourself a cooling-off period, then determine why the manuscript was rejected. Most manuscripts, especially those that are poorly written, can be revised and submitted to another journal.

PUBLISHING RESEARCH FINDINGS IN BOOKS

Some qualitative studies and large, complex quantitative studies are published in books or chapters of books. Publishing a book requires extensive

Table 23–12
Reasons for Manuscript Rejection

Factor	Mean (1 = rarely; 5 = very frequently)
Poorly written	3.72
Poorly developed idea	3.62
Not consistent with purpose	3.37
Term paper style	3.28
Methodology problems	3.13
Content undocumented	2.98
Content inaccurate	2.94
Content not important	2.84
Clinically not applicable	2.83
Statistical problems	2.82
Data interpretation problems	2.80
Subject covered recently	2.39
Content scheduled for future	2.11
Too technical	1.66

(From Swanson, E. A., McCloskey, J. C., & Bodensteiner, A. [1991]. Publishing opportunities for nurses: A comparison of 92 U.S. journals. *Image: Journal of Nursing Scholarship, 23*[1], 38, with permission.)

commitment on the part of the researcher. In addition, the researcher must select a publisher and convince the publisher to support the book project. A prospectus must be developed that identifies the proposed content of the book, describes the market for the book, and includes a rationale for publishing the book. The publisher and researcher must negotiate a contract that is mutually acceptable regarding (1) the content and length of the book, (2) the time required to complete the book, (3) the percentage of royalties to be received, and (4) the advances to be offered. The researcher must fulfill the obligations of the contract by producing the proposed book within the time frame agreed upon. Publishing a book is a significant accomplishment and an effective but sometimes slow means of communicating research findings.

DUPLICATE PUBLICATION IN THE NURSING LITERATURE

Duplicate publication is the practice of publishing the same article or major portions of the article in two or more print or electronic media without notifying the editors or referencing the other publication in the reference list (Blancett, Flanagin, & Young, 1995). Duplicate publications of studies are a poor practice because this limits the opportunities for publishing new knowledge, artificially inflates the importance of a study topic, clutters the literature with redundant information, rewards researchers for publishing the same content, and may violate the copyright law. Blancett and colleagues (1995) studied the incidence of duplicate publications in the nursing literature. In a sample of 642 articles published by 77 authors over five years, 181 of the articles were classified as duplicate publications. Forty-one of the 77 authors published at least one form of duplicate article and 59 of the duplicate articles did not include a reference of the primary article. Thus, duplicate publications are a serious concern in the nursing literature.

Journals require the submission of an original manuscript or one that has not been previously published. Thus, submitting a manuscript that has been previously published without referencing the duplicate work or notifying the editor of the previous publication is unethical and probably violates the copyright law. In 1994, the International Academy of Nursing Editors developed guidelines for nurse authors and editors regarding duplicate publications. Both authors and editors have the responsibility to inform readers and reviewers of duplicate publications. Authors must avoid unethical duplication by submitting original manuscripts or by providing full disclosure if portions or the entire manuscript has been previously published. Previous publications must be cited in the text of the manuscript and the reference list. Editors have the responsibility for developing a policy on duplicate publications and informing all authors, reviewers, and readers of this policy. In addition, editors must ensure that readers are informed of duplicate materials by adequate citations of the materials in the article's text and reference list (Yarbro, 1995).

SUMMARY

Communicating research findings, the final step in the research process, involves developing a research report and disseminating it through presentations and publications to audiences of nurses, health care professionals, policymakers, and health care consumers. Both quantitative and qualitative research reports include four basic sections: (1) introduction, (2) methods, (3) results, and (4) discussion. In a quantitative research report, the introduction briefly identifies the problem that was studied, provides a rationale for studying that problem and presents an empirical and theoretical basis for the study. The methods section of the report describes how the study was conducted and includes the design, setting, sample, methods of measurement, and the data collection process. The results section reveals what was found by conducting the study and includes the data analysis procedures, the results generated from these analyses, and the effect size determined for each analysis procedure. The discussion section ties the other sections of the research report together and gives them meaning. This section includes the major findings, limitations of the study, conclusions, implications of the findings for nursing, and recommendations for further research.

Research reports developed for qualitative research are as diverse as the different types of qualitative studies. However, qualitative research reports, like quantitative reports, usually include introduction, methods, results, and discussion sections. The introduction section identifies the phenomenon under investigation and indicates the type of qualitative study that was conducted. In the methods section, the researcher documents his or her credentials for conducting the study, identifies the site and sample, describes the researcher's role, and details the data collection process. The results section of the research report includes the data analysis procedures and presentation of the findings. The discussion section includes conclusions, limitations, implications for nursing, and recommendations for further research.

Before writing a research report, the investigator needs to determine who will benefit from knowing the findings. The greatest impact on nursing practice can be achieved by communicating nursing research findings to nurses, other health professionals, policymakers, and health care consumers. A variety of strategies for communicating to these audiences, such as oral and visual presentations and publications, are discussed in this chapter.

Research findings are presented at conferences and meetings through verbal and poster presentations. Presenting findings at a conference requires receiving acceptance as a presenter, developing a research report, delivering the report, and responding to questions. Most research conferences require the submission of an abstract, and acceptance as a presenter is based on the quality of the abstract. The report developed depends on the focus of the conference, the audience, and the time designated for each presentation. Delivering a research report and responding to questions involves practice to improve timing, content, and presentation style.

Sometimes a research project will be accepted at a conference not as a presentation but as a poster session. A poster session is a visual presentation of a study. The conference sponsors can guide the development of a poster by providing the following information: (1) size limitations or format restrictions for the poster, (2) the size of the poster display area, and (3) the background and potential number of conference participants.

Presentations are valuable means to rapidly communicate findings, but their impact is limited. Published research findings are perma-

continued

continued

nently recorded in a journal or book and usually reach a larger audience than presentations. Developing a manuscript for publication includes the following steps: (1) selecting a journal, (2) developing a query letter, (3) preparing a manuscript, (4) submitting the manuscript for review, and (5) responding to requests for revision of the manuscript. Selecting a journal for publication of a study requires knowledge of the basic requirements of the journal, the journal's refereed status, and the recent articles published in the journal. A query letter is developed to determine an editor's interest in reviewing a manuscript. A manuscript is then written according to the format outlined by the journal and submitted to the journal editor. The manuscript is then reviewed and usually requires revisions before it is accepted for publication.

A concern that was recently identified in the nursing literature is the publication of duplicate articles. Duplicate publication is the practice of publishing the same article or major portions of the article in two or more print or electronic media without notifying the editors or referencing the other publication in the reference list. In 1994, the International Academy of Nursing Editors developed guidelines for nurse authors and editors regarding duplicate publications. Publishing research findings is a rewarding experience, but the process of publishing demands a great deal of time and energy. We hope that this information will stimulate researchers to present and publish their findings.

References

American Psychological Association. (1994). *Publication manual of the American Psychological Association* (4th ed.). Washington, DC: American Psychological Association.

Angell, M. (1989). Negative studies. *New England Journal of Medicine, 321*(7), 464–466.

Blancett, S. S., Flanagin, A., & Young, R. K. (1995). Duplicate publication in the nursing literature. *Image: Journal of Nursing Scholarship, 27*(1), 51–56.

Brown, B. E., & Garrison, C. J. (1990). Patterns of symptomatology of adult women incest survivors. *Western Journal of Nursing Research, 12*(5), 587–600.

Burns, N. (1989). Standards for qualitative research. *Nursing Science Quarterly, 2*(1), 44–52.

Camilleri, R. (1987). Six ways to write right. *Image: Journal of Nursing Scholarship, 19*(4), 210–212.

Camilleri, R. (1988). On elegant writing. *Image: Journal of Nursing Scholarship, 20*(3), 169–171.

Carnegie, M. E. (1975). The referee system. *Nursing Research, 24*(4), 243.

Cason, C. L., Cason, G. J., & Redland, A. R. (1988). Peer review of research abstracts. *Image: Journal of Nursing Scholarship, 20*(2), 102–105.

Crosby, L. J. (1990). The abstract: An important first impression. *Journal of Neuroscience Nursing, 22*(3), 192–194.

Diers, D. (1981). Why write? Why publish? *Image: Journal of Nursing Scholarship, 13*(1), 3–8.

Egan, E. C., Snyder, M., & Burns, K. R. (1992). Intervention studies in nursing: Is the effect due to the independent variable? *Nursing Outlook, 40*(4), 187–190.

Field, P. A., & Morse, J. M. (1985). *Nursing research: The application of qualitative approaches.* Rockville, MD: Aspen.

Finkelhor, D., & Browne, A. (1986). Initial and long term effects: A conceptual framework. In D. Finkelhor (Ed.), *A source book on child sexual abuse* (pp. 180–198). Beverly Hills, CA: Sage.

Gay, J. T., & Edgil, A. E. (1989). When your manuscript is rejected. *Nursing & Health Care, 10*(8), 459–461.

Goldberg, H. I., Cummings, M. A., Steinberg, E. P., Ricci, E. M., Shannon, T., Soumerai, S. B., Mittman, B. S., Eisenberg, J., Heck, D. A., Kaplan, S., Kenzora, J. E., Vargus, A. M., Mulley, A. G., & Rimer, B. K. (1994). Deliberations on the dissemination of PORT products: Translating research findings into improved patient outcomes. *Medical Care, 32*(7), JS90–JS110.

Hagemaster, J. N., & Kerrins, K. M. (1984). Six easy steps to publishing. *Nurse Educator, 9*(4), 32–34.

Hanson, S. M. (1988). Collaborative research and authorship credit: Beginning guidelines. *Nursing Research, 37*(1), 49–52.

Hicks, C. (1995). The shortfall in published research: A study of nurses' research publication activities. *Journal of Advanced Nursing, 21*(3), 594–604.

Hulme, P. A., & Grove, S. K. (1994). Symptoms of female survivors of child sexual abuse. *Issues in Mental Health Nursing, 15*(5), 519–532.

Jackle, M. (1989). Presenting research to nurses in clinical practice. *Applied Nursing Research, 2*(4), 191–193.

Jimenez, S. L. M. (1991). Consumer journalism: A unique nursing opportunity. *Image: Journal of Nursing Scholarship, 23*(1), 47–49.

Juhl, N., & Norman, V. L. (1989). Writing an effective abstract. *Applied Nursing Research, 2*(4), 189–191.

Kirchhoff, K. T., & Dille, C. A. (1994). Issues in intervention research: Maintaining integrity. *Applied Nursing Research, 7*(1), 32–38.

Knafl, K. A., & Howard, M. J. (1984). Interpreting and reporting qualitative research. *Research in Nursing & Health, 7*(1), 17–24.

Kraemer, H. C., & Thiemann, S. (1987). *How many subjects? Statistical power analysis in research.* Newbury Park, CA: Sage.

Lander, J., Nazarali, S., Hodgins, M., Friesen, E., McTavish, J., Ouellette, J., & Abel, R. (1996). Evaluation of a new topical anesthetic agent: A pilot study. *Nursing Research, 45*(1), 50–53.

Leininger, M. M. (1985). *Qualitative research methods in nursing.* New York: Grune & Stratton.

Lippman, D. T., & Ponton, K. S. (1989). Designing a research poster with impact. *Western Journal of Nursing Research, 11*(4), 477–485.

McCloskey, J. C. (1977). Publishing opportunities for nurses: A comparison of 65 journals. *Nurse Educator, 11*(4), 4–13.

McDaniel, R. W., Bach, C. A., & Poole, M. J. (1993). Poster update: Getting their attention. *Nursing Research, 42*(5), 302–304.

McFarlane, J., Parker, B., & Soeken, K. (1996). Abuse during pregnancy: Associations with maternal health and infant birth weight. *Nursing Research, 45*(1), 37–42.

McKenna, K. T., Maas, F., & McEniery, P. T. (1995). Coronary risk factor status after percutaneous transluminal coronary angioplasty. *Heart & Lung, 24*(3), 207–212.

Miracle, V. A., & King, K. C. (1994). Presenting research: Effective paper presentations and impressive poster presentations. *Applied Nursing Research, 7*(3), 147–157.

Mirin, S. K. (1981). *The nurse's guide to writing for publication.* Wakefield, MA: Nursing Resources.

Packard, N. J., Haberman, M. R., Woods, N. F., & Yates, B. C. (1991). Demands of illness among chronically ill women. *Western Journal of Nursing Research, 13*(4), 434–457.

Reece, S. M. (1995). Stress and maternal adaptation in first-time mothers more than 35 years old. *Applied Nursing Research, 8*(2), 61–66.

Ryan, N. M. (1989). Developing and presenting a research poster. *Applied Nursing Research, 2*(1), 52–54.

Selby, M. L., Tornquist, E. M., & Finerty, E. J. (1989a). How to present your research. Part I: What they didn't teach you in nursing school about planning and organizing the content of your speech. *Nursing Outlook, 37*(4), 172–175.

Selby, M. L., Tornquist, E. M., & Finerty, E. J. (1989b). How to present your research. Part II: The ABCs of creating and using visual aids to enhance your research presentation. *Nursing Outlook, 37*(5), 236–238.

Shapiro, D. W., Wenger, N. S., & Shapiro, M. F. (1994). The contributions of authors to multiauthored biomedical research papers. *JAMA, 271*(6), 438–442.

Shurter, R. L., Williamson, J. P., & Broehl, W. G. (1965). *Business research and report writing.* New York: McGraw-Hill.

Swain, M. A., & Steckel, S. B. (1981). Influencing adherence among hypertensives. *Research in Nursing & Health, 4*(1), 213–222.

Swanson, E. A., McCloskey, J. C., & Bodensteiner, A. (1991). Publishing opportunities for nurses: A comparison of 92 U.S. journals. *Image: Journal of Nursing Scholarship, 23*(1), 33–38.

Tornquist, E. M., Funk, S. G., & Champagne, M. T. (1989). Writing research reports for clinical audiences. *Western Journal of Nursing Research, 11*(5), 576–582.

Tulman, L. R., & Jacobsen, B. S. (1989). Goldilocks and variability. *Nursing Research, 38*(6), 377–379.

University of Chicago Press. (1993). *The Chicago manual of style* (14th ed.). Chicago: University of Chicago Press.

Wainer, H. (1984). How to display data badly. *American Statistician, 38*(2), 137–147.

Wikblad, K., & Anderson, B. (1995). A comparison of three wound dressings in patients undergoing heart surgery. *Nursing Research, 44*(5), 312–316.

Yarbro, C. H. (1995). Duplicate publication: Guidelines for nurse authors and editors. *Image: Journal of Nursing Scholarship, 27*(1), 57.

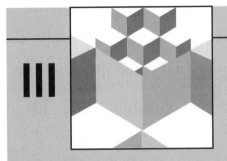

III

Strategies for Using Research in Practice

24 Critical Analysis of Nursing Studies

The critique of studies is an essential process in the development of a body of knowledge, yet this process is poorly understood by many nurses. The word *critique* is often linked with the word *criticize,* which has negative connotations and is often considered untherapeutic in nursing. However, in the arts and sciences, critique takes on another meaning. It is associated with critical thinking and appraisal and requires carefully developed intellectual skills. This type of critique is sometimes referred to as intellectual critique. An intellectual critique is directed not at the person who created but at the product of creation. For example, one might critique an art object, an architectural design, a ballet performance, a theory, or a study. One can even critique a critique, such as a faculty member critiquing a student's critique of a study.

An *intellectual critique of research* involves a careful examination of all aspects of a study to judge the merits, limitations, meaning, and significance, based on previous research experience and knowledge of the topic. Conducting a research critique requires a background in critical analysis and skills in logical reasoning to examine the credibility and integrity of a study. The intent of this chapter is to provide a background for critiquing studies. The evolution of the research critique in nursing and the different types of research critiques conducted by nurses are discussed. The critique processes for both quantitative and qualitative research are described, including the unique skills, guidelines, and standards for critiquing different types of studies.

EVOLUTION OF THE RESEARCH CRITIQUE IN NURSING

The process for critiquing research has evolved gradually in nursing because until recently only a few nurses have been prepared to conduct comprehensive, scholarly critiques. During the 1940s and 1950s, the presentations of nursing research were followed by critiques of the research. These critiques often focused on the faults or limitations of the studies and tended to be harsh and traumatic for the researcher (Meleis, 1991). As a consequence of these early unpleasant experiences, nurse researchers moved to a strategy of protecting and sheltering their nurse scientists from the threat of criticism. Public critiques, written or verbal, were rare in the 1960s and 1970s. Those responding to research presentations focused on the strengths of studies, and the limitations were either not mentioned or minimized. Thus, the impact of the limitations on the meaning and significance of the study was often lost.

Incomplete critiques or the absence of critiques may have served a purpose as nurses gained basic skills in the conduct of research. However, the discipline of nursing has moved past this point, and intellectual critiques are essential to strengthen scientific investigation and utilization of research findings in practice. Many nurses now have the preparation and expertise for conducting intellectual critiques owing to advances in the nursing profession during the 1980s and 1990s. Nursing research textbooks provide detailed information on the critique process. Nursing research skills, including critique, are introduced at the baccalaureate level of nursing education and are expanded at the master's and doctoral levels. Specialty organizations provide workshops on the critique process to promote the use of research findings in practice.

Intellectual critiques of studies are essential for the development and refinement of nursing knowledge. Nurses need the skills to examine the meaning of study findings and to ask searching questions. Are the findings an accurate reflection of reality? Do they lead to increased understanding of the nature of phenomena that are important in nursing? Are the findings from the present study consistent with those from previous studies? Can the study be replicated? Are the findings ready for use in nursing practice? The answers to these questions require a careful examination of the research problem, the theoretical basis of the study, and the study's methodology. Not only must the mechanics for conducting the study be examined, but also the abstract and logical reasoning used by the researcher in planning and implementing the study. If there are flaws in the reasoning processes used to develop the study, there are probably flaws in interpreting the meaning of the findings.

All studies have flaws. If all flawed studies were discarded, there would be no scientific base for practice (Oberst, 1992). In fact, science itself is flawed. Science does not completely or perfectly describe, explain, predict, and control reality. However, improved understanding and increased ability to predict and control phenomena depend on recognizing the flaws in studies and in science. New studies can then be planned to minimize the flaws or limitations of earlier studies. Thus, a researcher must critique previous studies to determine their limitations, and the study findings need to be interpreted in light of the limitations. These limitations can lead to inaccurate data, inaccurate outcomes of analyses, and decreased ability to generalize the findings. When using study findings in practice, one recognizes that knowledge is not absolute; however, confidence in empirical knowledge grows as the number of quality studies conducted increases.

All studies have strengths as well as limitations. Recognition of these strengths is also critical to the generation of scientific knowledge and utilization of findings in practice. If only weaknesses are identified, nurses might discount the value of the study and refuse to invest time in examining research (Oberst, 1992). The continued work of the researcher also depends on the recognition of the study's strengths. If no study is good enough, why invest time conducting research? Points of strength in a study, added to points of strength from multiple other studies, slowly build a solid knowledge base.

TYPES OF RESEARCH CRITIQUES CONDUCTED IN NURSING

In general, research is critiqued to broaden understanding, summarize knowledge for use in practice, and provide a base for the conduct of a study. Formal research critiques are often conducted after verbal presentations of studies, after a published research report, for abstract or article selection, and for evaluating research proposals. Thus, nursing students, practicing nurses, nurse educators, and nurse researchers are all involved in critiquing research.

Student Critiques

In nursing education, a critique is often seen as a first step in learning the research process. And it is true that part of learning the research process is being able to read and comprehend published research reports. However, comprehension of the research report is dependent upon understanding the research process. Thus, conducting a critique is not a basic skill, and the content presented in previous chapters is essential for implementing the critique process. Basic knowledge of the research process and critique process is usually provided early in professional nursing education. More advanced critique skills are often taught at the master's and doctoral level. Students' skills in the steps of critique (comprehension, comparison, analysis, evaluation, and conceptual clustering) increase as their knowledge of the research process expands. By conducting research critiques, students strengthen their knowledge base and increase their use of research findings in practice.

Critiques by the Practicing Nurse

Critiques of studies by practicing nurses are essential for use of research findings in practice (Stetler, 1994; Titler et al., 1994). Nursing actions require updating in response to the current body of knowledge that is derived from current research and theory development. Practicing nurses need to design methods for remaining current in their practice areas. A bulletin board for posting current studies can be helpful but is not sufficient for critique to occur. However, a research journal club might be formed where studies are presented and critiqued by members of the group (Tibbles & Sanford, 1994).

Critiques by Nursing Educators

Educators conduct research critiques to expand their knowledge base and to develop and refine the educational process. The careful critique of current nursing studies provides a basis for updating curricular content taught in clinical and classroom settings. Educators act as role models for their students by examining new studies, valuing the information obtained from research, and using research knowledge as a basis for practice. In addition, educators have a responsibility to generate and conduct research which requires the critique of previous studies.

Critiques by Nurse Researchers

Researchers conduct critiques to plan and implement a study. Many researchers focus their studies in one area, and they update their knowledge base by critiquing new studies in this area. The outcome of the critique influences the selection of research problems, development of methodology, and interpretation of findings in future studies.

Critiques of previous studies are presented in the review of literature for a research proposal or report.

Critiques After Verbal Presentations of Studies

Verbal critiques need to be considered part of a research presentation. Through verbal critique, researchers can gain increased understanding of the strengths and weaknesses of their studies and generate ideas for further research. Participants listening to critiques might gain insight into the conduct of research. Experiencing the critique process can increase the participants' ability to critique studies and to judge the usefulness of the findings for nursing practice.

Critiques After Published Research Reports

Currently, at least two nursing research journals, *Scholarly Inquiry for Nursing Practice: An International Journal* and *Western Journal of Nursing Research,* include commentaries (a partial critique) after a published research report. In these journals, authors receive feedback on their work and have an opportunity to respond to the critiques. Published critiques increase readers' understanding of the study and their abilities to critique research. Another more informal critique of a published study might appear in a letter to the editor. Readers have the opportunity to comment on the strengths and weaknesses of published studies by writing to the editor.

Critique for Abstract Selection

One of the most difficult types of critique to perform is that of examining abstracts. The amount of information available is usually limited, since many abstracts are restricted to 100 to 250 words (Crosby, 1990). Despite this, reviewers must select the best-designed studies with the most significant outcomes for presentation at nursing meetings. This process requires an experienced researcher who requires few cues to determine the quality of a study. The critique of an abstract usually addresses the following criteria: (1) appropriateness of the study for the program, (2) completeness of the research project, (3) overall quality of the work, (4) contribution of the study to nursing scholarship, (5) contribution of the study to nursing theory, (6) originality of the work (not previously published), and (7) clarity and completeness of the abstract (Cason, Cason, & Redland, 1988; Morse, Dellasega, & Doberneck, 1993).

Critique of an Article for Publication

Nurse researchers serve as reviewers for professional journals to evaluate the quality of research papers submitted for publication. The role of these scientists is to examine the quality of the studies submitted to ensure that those accepted for publication are well designed and contribute to the body of knowledge. Most of these reviews are conducted anonymously so that friendships or reputations do not interfere with the selection process. In most refereed journals (82%), the research report is examined by experts selected from an established group of reviewers (Swanson, McCloskey, & Bodensteiner, 1991). The reviewers' comments or a summary of these comments is sent to the researcher. These comments are also used by the editor in making selections for publication. The process for publishing research is described in Chapter 23.

Critique of Research Proposals

Critiques of research proposals are conducted to approve student research projects, to permit data collection in an institution, and to select the best studies for funding. Seeking approval to conduct a study is presented in Chapter 26. The peer review process in federal funding agencies involves an extremely complex critique. Nurses are involved in this level of research review through the National Institute of Nursing Research (NINR) and the Agency for Health Care Policy and Research (AHCPR). Kim and Felton (1993) identified some of the criteria that are used to evaluate the quality

of a proposal for possible funding, such as the (1) appropriate use of measurement for the types of questions the research is designed to answer, (2) appropriate use and interpretation of statistical procedures, (3) the evaluation of clinical practice and forecasting of the need for nursing or other appropriate interventions, and (4) construction of models to direct the research and interpret the findings.

CRITIQUE PROCESS FOR QUANTITATIVE STUDIES

The critique process for quantitative research includes five steps: (1) comprehension, (2) comparison, (3) analysis, (4) evaluation, and (5) conceptual clustering. Conducting a critique is a complex mental process that is stimulated by raising questions. The level of critique conducted is influenced by the level of sophistication of the individual doing the critique (see Table 24–1). The initial critique of an undergraduate student often involves only the comprehension step of the critique process. The critique of a master's student usually involves the steps of comprehension, comparison, analysis, and evaluation. Conceptual clustering is a complex process that is usually perfected by doctoral students or experienced researchers as they develop integrated reviews of research for publication.

The conduct of an intellectual critique of quan-

Table 24–1
Educational Level and Expected Level of Expertise in the Critique Process

Educational Level	Expected Level of Expertise in the Critique Process
Baccalaureate	Step I—Comprehension
	Step II—Comparison
Master's	Step III—Analysis
	Step IV—Evaluation
Doctorate and/or experienced researcher	Step V—Conceptual Clustering

Table 24–2
Guidelines for Conducting a Quantitative Research Critique

1. **Read and critique the entire study.** A research critique requires identifying and examining all steps of the research process. (Comprehension)
2. **Examine the research and clinical expertise of the authors.** The authors need a clinical and scientific background that is appropriate for the study conducted. (Comprehension)
3. **Examine the organization and presentation of the research report.** The report usually includes an abstract, main body of the report, and references. The abstract of the study needs to clearly present the purpose of the study and the major study findings. The body of the report needs to be complete, concise, clearly presented, and logically organized. The references need to be complete and presented in a consistent format. (Comparison)
4. **Identify the strengths and weaknesses of a study.** All studies have strengths and weaknesses and you can use the questions in this chapter to facilitate identifying these. Address the quality of the steps of the research process and the logical links among the steps of the process. (Comparison and Analysis)
5. **Provide specific examples of the strengths and weaknesses of a study.** These examples provide rationale and documentation for your critique of the study. (Comparison and Analysis)
6. **Be objective and realistic in identifying the study's strengths and weaknesses.** Try not to be overly critical when identifying a study's weaknesses or overly flattering when identifying the strengths.
7. **Suggest modifications for future studies** to increase the strengths and decrease the weaknesses in the study.
8. **Evaluate the study.** Indicate the overall quality of the study and its contribution to nursing knowledge. Discuss the consistency of the findings of this study with those of previous research. Discuss the need for further research and the potential to use the findings in practice. (Evaluation)

titative research involves applying some basic guidelines that are outlined in Table 24–2. These guidelines stress the importance of examining the expertise of the authors; critiquing the entire study; addressing the study's strengths, weaknesses, and logical links; and evaluating the contribution of the study to nursing knowledge. These guidelines are linked to the steps of the critique process, comprehension, comparison, analysis, and evaluation. These steps occur in sequence, vary in depth, and presume accomplishment of the preceding steps. However, an individual with critique experience frequently performs several steps of this process simultaneously.

This section includes the steps of the critique process and provides relevant questions for each step. These questions are not comprehensive but have been selected as a means for stimulating the abstract reasoning necessary for conducting a critique. Persons experienced in critique formulate additional questions as part of their reasoning processes. The comprehension step is covered separately, since those new to critique start with this step. The comparison and analysis steps are covered together because these steps often occur simultaneously in the mind of the person conducting the critique. Evaluation and conceptual clustering are covered separately because of the increased expertise needed to perform each step.

STEP I—COMPREHENSION

Initial attempts to comprehend research articles are often frustrating because the terminology and stylized manner of the report are unfamiliar. *Comprehension* is the first step in the critique process and involves understanding the terms and concepts in the report as well as identifying study elements and grasping the nature, significance, and meaning of these elements. Comprehension is demonstrated as the reviewer identifies each element or step of the study.

Guidelines for Comprehension

The first step involves reviewing the abstract and reading the study from the beginning to the end. As you read, address the following questions about the presentation of the study: Does the title of the research report clearly identify the focus of the study? Was the abstract clear? Was the writing style of the report clear and concise? Were the different parts of the research report clearly identified? Were relevant terms clearly defined? (Phillips, 1986; Ryan-Wenger, 1992). You might underline the terms you do not understand and determine their meaning using the Glossary at the end of this text. Read the article a second time and highlight or underline each step of the quantitative research process. An overview of these steps is presented in Chapter 3. To write a research critique, you need to identify each step of the research process concisely and respond briefly to the following questions:

1. State the problem.
2. State the purpose.
3. Examine the literature review.
   a. Are relevant previous studies and theories described?
   b. Are the references current?
   c. Is the current knowledge about the research problem described, including what is known and not known?
4. Examine the study framework.
   a. Is the framework explicitly expressed or must the reviewer extract the framework from implicit statements in the literature review?
   b. Is the framework based on substantive theory or a tentative theory?
   c. Does the framework describe and define the concepts of interest, show relationships among the concepts, and relate them to the variables of the study?
   d. Is a map of the framework provided for clarity? If a map is not presented, develop a map that represents the study's framework and describe the map.
5. List any research objectives, questions, or hypotheses.

6. Identify and define (conceptually and operationally) the study variables or concepts.
   a. Independent variables
   b. Dependent variables
   c. Research variables or concepts
7. Identify attributes and extraneous variables.
8. Identify the research design.
   a. Identify the specific design of the study and draw a model of the design using the sample designs presented in Chapter 11.
   b. Identify the treatment or intervention if appropriate for the study conducted.
   c. Were pilot study findings used to design this study? If yes, briefly discuss the pilot and the changes made in this study based on the pilot.
9. Describe the sample.
   a. Sampling criteria
   b. Sample size (indicate if a power analysis was conducted)
   c. Characteristics of the sample
   d. Sample mortality
   e. Method used to obtain the sample
   f. Type of consent obtained
10. Describe the measurement strategies.
    a. Describe the methods of measurement, including the author of each instrument, how the instrument was developed, how the instrument was used in the study, and the level of measurement achieved with the instrument.
    b. Describe the validity and reliability of each instrument.
11. Describe the procedures for data collection.
12. Describe the statistical analyses used.
    a. What are the purposes of the analyses, description, and/or examination of differences or relationships?
    b. Are the statistics descriptive and/or inferential?
    c. List the statistical procedures conducted and their results for each research objective, question, or hypothesis.
13. Describe the researcher's interpretation of findings.
    a. Are the findings related back to the study framework?

b. Which findings are in keeping with those expected? Which findings were not expected? Are serendipitous findings described?

c. Are the findings consistent with previous research findings?

14. What study limitations were identified by the researcher?
15. How did the researchers generalize the findings?
16. What were the implications of the findings for nursing?
17. What suggestions for further study were identified?
18. Is the description of the study sufficiently clear to allow replication?

STEP II—COMPARISON

The next step, *comparison,* requires knowledge of what each step of the research process should be like. The ideal is compared with the real. During the comparison step, you examine the extent to which the researcher followed the rules for an ideal study. You also need to gain a sense of how clearly the researcher grasped the study situation and expressed it. The clarity of the researcher's explanation of the elements of research demonstrates the researcher's skill in using and expressing ideas that require abstract reasoning.

STEP III—ANALYSIS

The *analysis step* involves a critique of the logical links connecting one study element with another. For example, the problem needs to provide background and direction for the statement of the purpose. In addition, the overall flow of logic in the study must be examined (Liehr & Houston, 1993). The variables identified in the study purpose need to be consistent with the variables identified in the research objectives, questions, or hypotheses. The variables identified in the research objectives, questions, or hypotheses need to be conceptually defined in light of the study framework. The con-

ceptual definitions provide the basis for the development of the operational definitions. The study design and analyses need to be appropriate for the investigation of the study purpose, as well as for the specific objectives, questions, or hypotheses (Ryan-Wenger, 1992).

Most of the limitations in a study result from breaks in logical reasoning. For example, the biases due to sampling and design impair the logical flow from design to interpretation of findings. The previous levels of critique have addressed concrete aspects of the study. During analysis, the process moves into examining abstract dimensions of the study, thus requiring a greater familiarity with the logic behind the research process and increased skills in abstract reasoning.

Guidelines for Comparison and Analysis

To conduct the steps of comparison and analysis, you need to review Unit II of this text on the research process and other sources on the steps of the research process (Kerlinger, 1986; Liehr & Houston, 1993; LoBiondo-Wood & Haber, 1994; Phillips, 1986; Polit & Hungler, 1995; Ryan-Wenger, 1992; Shelley, 1984; Woods & Catanzaro, 1988). Then compare the elements in the study you are critiquing with the criteria established for each element in this textbook or in other sources (Step II—Comparison). Then analyze the logical links among the steps of the study by examining how each step provides a basis for and links with the following steps of the research process (Step III—Analysis). The following guidelines will assist you in implementing the steps of comparison and analysis for each step of the research process. Those questions relevant to analysis are identified; all other questions direct the comparison of the steps of the study with the ideal. The written critique will be a summary of the strengths and weaknesses that you noted in the study.

1. Research problem and purpose
   a. Is the problem sufficiently delimited in scope without being trivial?

b. Is the problem significant to nursing?

c. Does the problem have a gender bias and only addresses the health needs of men to the exclusion of women's health needs? (Yam, 1994)

d. Does the purpose narrow and clarify the aim of the study?

2. Review of literature

a. Is the literature review organized to demonstrate the progressive development of ideas through previous research? (Analysis)

b. Is a theoretical knowledge base developed for the problem and purpose? (Analysis)

c. Does the literature review provide rationale and direction for the study? (Analysis)

d. Is a clear, concise summary presented of the current empirical and theoretical knowledge in the area of the study?

3. Study framework

a. Is the framework presented with clarity? If a model or conceptual map of the framework is present, is it adequate to explain the phenomenon of concern?

b. Is the framework linked to the research purpose? Would another framework fit more logically with the study? (Analysis)

c. Is the framework related to nursing's body of knowledge? (Analysis)

d. If a proposition from a theory is to be tested, is the proposition clearly identified and linked to the study hypotheses?

4. Research objectives, questions, or hypotheses

a. Are the objectives, questions, or hypotheses expressed clearly?

b. Are the objectives, questions, or hypotheses logically linked to the research purpose and framework? (Analysis)

5. Variables

a. Are the variables reflective of the concepts identified in the framework? (Analysis)

b. Are the variables clearly defined (conceptually and operationally), based on previous research or theories?

c. Is the conceptual definition of a variable consistent with the operational definition? (Analysis)

6. Design

a. Is the design used in the study the most appropriate design to obtain the needed data?

b. Does the design provide a means to examine all of the objectives, questions, or hypotheses? (Analysis)

c. Is the treatment clearly described? Was a protocol developed to promote consistent implementation of the treatment? Did the researcher monitor the implementation of the treatment to ensure consistency? If the treatment was not consistently implemented, what might be the impact on the findings? (Analysis) (Egan, Snyder, & Burns, 1992)

d. Have the threats to design validity been minimized?

e. Is the design logically linked to the sampling method and statistical analyses? (Analysis)

7. Sample, population, and setting

a. Is the sampling method adequate to produce a representative sample?

b. What are the potential biases in the sampling method? Are any subjects excluded from the study based on age, socioeconomic status, or race without a sound rationale? (Larson, 1994)

c. Were the sampling criteria appropriate for the type of study conducted?

d. Is the sample size sufficient to avoid a Type II error?

e. If more than one group is used, do the groups appear equivalent?

f. Are the rights of human subjects protected?

g. Is the setting used in the study typical of clinical settings?

h. Was sample mortality a problem? If so, how might this influence the findings?

8. Measurements

a. Do the instruments adequately measure the study variables? (Analysis)

b. Are the instruments sufficiently sensitive to detect small differences between subjects? (Analysis)

c. Does the instrument have adequate validity and reliability for use in a study?

d. Respond to the following questions, which are relevant to the measurement approaches used in the study:

Scales and Questionnaires

(1) Are the instruments clearly described?

(2) Are techniques to complete and score the instruments provided?

(3) Are validity and reliability of the instruments described?

(4) Did the researcher reexamine the validity and reliability of instruments for the present sample?

(5) If the instrument was developed for the study, is the instrument development process described?

Observation

(1) Is what is to be observed clearly identified and defined?

(2) Is interrater reliability described?

(3) Are the techniques for recording observations described?

Interviews

(1) Do the interview questions address concerns expressed in the research problem? (Analysis)

(2) Are the interview questions relevant for the research purpose and objectives, questions, or hypotheses? (Analysis)

(3) Does the design of the questions tend to bias subjects' responses?

(4) Does the sequence of questions tend to bias subjects' responses?

Physiologic Measures

(1) Are the physiologic measures or instruments clearly described? If appropriate, are the brand names, such as Space Labs or Hewlett-Packard, of the instruments identified?

(2) Are the accuracy, selectivity, precision, sensitivity, and error of the instruments discussed?

(3) Are the physiologic measures appropriate for the research purpose and objectives, questions, or hypotheses? (Analysis)

(4) Are the methods for recording data from the physiologic measures clearly described? Is the recording of data consistent?

9. Data collection

a. Is the data collection process clearly described?

b. Are the forms used to collect data organized to facilitate computerizing the data?

c. Is the training of data collectors clearly described and adequate?

d. Is the data collection process conducted in a consistent manner?

e. Are the data collection methods ethical?

f. Do the data collected address the research objectives, questions, or hypotheses? (Analysis)

10. Data analysis

a. Are data analysis procedures appropriate to the type of data collected?

b. Are data analysis procedures clearly described?

c. Are the results presented in an understandable way?

d. Are the statistical analyses logically linked to the design? (Analysis)

e. Is the sample size sufficient to detect significant differences if they are present? Was power analysis used to determine sample size? (Analysis)

f. Do data analyses address each research objective, question, or hypothesis? (Analysis)

g. Are the analyses interpreted appropriately?

11. Interpretation of findings

a. Are findings discussed in relation to each objective, question, or hypothesis?

b. Are various explanations for significant and nonsignificant findings examined?

c. Are the findings clinically significant? (LeFort, 1993)

d. Do the conclusions fit the findings from the analyses? Are the conclusions based on statistically significant and clinically significant results? (Analysis)

e. Are there limitations the researcher did not identify? (Analysis)

STEP IV—EVALUATION

Evaluation involves determining the meaning and significance of the study by examining the links between the study process, study findings, and previous studies. The steps of the study are evaluated based on previous studies, such as an evaluation of present hypotheses based on previous hypotheses, present design based on previous designs, and present methods of putting variables into operation based on previous approaches. The findings of the present study are also examined in light of findings of previous studies. Evaluation builds upon conclusions reached during the first three stages of the critique and provides the basis for conceptual clustering.

Guidelines for Evaluation

You need to reexamine the findings, conclusions, and implications sections of the study and the researcher's suggestions for further study. Using the following questions as a guide, summarize the strengths and weaknesses of the study.

1. What rival hypotheses can be suggested for the findings?
2. How much confidence can be placed in the study findings?
3. To what populations can the findings be generalized?
4. What questions emerge from the findings and are these identified by the researcher?
5. What future research can be envisioned?
6. Could the limitations of the study have been corrected?
7. When the findings are examined based on previous studies, what is now known and not known about the phenomenon under study?

You need to read previous studies conducted in the area of the research being examined and summarize your responses to the following questions.

1. Are the findings of previous studies used to generate the research problem and purpose?
2. Is the design an advancement over previous designs?
3. Do sampling strategies show an improvement over previous studies? Does the sample selection have the potential for adding diversity to samples previously studied? (Larson, 1994)
4. Does the current research build upon previous measurement strategies so that measurement is more precise or more reflective of the variables?
5. How do statistical analyses compare with those used in previous studies?
6. Do the findings build upon findings of previous studies?
7. Is the current knowledge in this area identified?
8. Does the author indicate the implication of the findings for practice?

STEP V—CONCEPTUAL CLUSTERING

The last step of the critique process is *conceptual clustering,* which involves the synthesis of study findings to determine the current body of knowledge in an area (Pinch, 1995). Until the 1980s, conceptual clustering was seldom addressed in the nursing literature. However, in 1983, the initial volume of the *Annual Review of Nursing Research* was published to provide conceptual clustering of specific phenomena of interest to nursing in the areas of nursing practice, nursing care delivery, nursing education, and the profession of nursing (Werley & Fitzpatrick, 1983). Conceptual clustering is also evident in the publication of several integrative reviews of research in the clinical and research journals (Ganong, 1987). A list of integrative reviews is provided in the Student Study Guide that accompanies this text. These reviews are organized by relevant nursing topics.

Guidelines for Conceptual Clustering

Through conceptual clustering, current knowledge in an area of study is carefully analyzed, relationships are examined, and the knowledge is summarized and organized theoretically. Conceptual clustering maximizes the meaning attached to research findings, highlights gaps in knowledge, generates new research questions, and provides knowledge to be used in practice.

1. Process for clustering findings and developing the current knowledge base:
   a. Is the purpose for reviewing the literature clearly identified?
   b. Are the criteria for including studies in the review clearly identified and used appropriately?
   c. Is the process for clustering study findings clearly described?
   d. Is the current knowledge base clearly expressed? What is known and not known?
2. Theoretical organization of the knowledge base. Draw a map showing the concepts and relationships found in the studies reviewed in the previous criteria (1) to detect the gaps in understanding relationships. The map can also be compared with current theory in the area of study using the following questions:
   a. Is the map consistent with current theory?
   b. Are there differences in the map that are upheld by well-designed research? If so, modification of existing theory should be considered.
   c. Are there concepts and relationships in existing theory that have not been examined in the studies diagrammed in the map? If so, studies should be developed to examine these gaps.
   d. Are there conflicting theories within the field of study? Do existing study findings tend to support one of the theories?
   e. Are there no existing theories to explain the phenomenon under consideration?
   f. Can current research findings be used to begin the development of nursing theory to explain the phenomenon more completely?
3. Utilization of research findings in practice.
   a. Is there sufficient confidence in the findings to use them in nursing practice? If so, de-

velop a protocol to promote the use of this knowledge in practice.
   b. If the confidence is not sufficient, what further knowledge is needed before the findings can be utilized?
   c. What are the benefits and risks of using the findings for the patients and health care agencies?
   d. How will patient outcomes be affected by utilization of the findings?
   e. Would the changes in outcomes make a significant difference in the health of the client?

Meta-analysis is another form of conceptual clustering that goes beyond critique and integration of research findings to conducting statistical analyses on the outcomes of similar studies (Pillemer & Light, 1980). Meta-analysis is used to integrate and synthesize findings from completed studies to determine what is currently known about a phenomenon (Massey & Loomis, 1988). Chapter 25 discusses the use of meta-analysis to synthesize research for use in practice.

CRITIQUE PROCESS FOR QUALITATIVE STUDIES

Critique in qualitative research also requires comprehension, comparison, analysis, and evaluation; however, the skills and standards for critique are different (Burns, 1989). The skills and standards for critiquing qualitative research are described in the following sections.

SKILLS NEEDED TO CRITIQUE QUALITATIVE STUDIES

The skills needed to critique qualitative studies include (1) context flexibility; (2) inductive reasoning; (3) conceptualization, theoretical modeling, and theory analysis; and (4) transforming ideas across levels of abstraction (Burns, 1989).

Context Flexibility

Context flexibility is the capacity to switch from one context or world view to another, to shift perception in order to see things from a different perspective. Each world view is based on a set of assumptions through which reality is defined. Developing skills in the critique of qualitative studies requires that the individual be willing to move from the assumptions of quantitative research to those of qualitative research. This skill is not new in nursing, since beginning students are encouraged to see things from the patient's perspective. However, accomplishing this switch of context requires investing time and energy to learn more about the patient and setting aside personal, sometimes strongly held, views. It is not necessary for one to become committed to a perspective in order to follow or apply its logical structure. In fact, all scholarly work requires a willingness and ability to examine and evaluate works from diverse perspectives. For example, analysis of the internal structure of a theory requires this same process.

Inductive Reasoning Skills

Although all research requires skills in both deductive and inductive reasoning, the transformation process used during data analysis in qualitative research is based on inductive reasoning. The individual conducting a critique of a qualitative study must be able to exercise skills in inductive reasoning in order to follow the logic of the researcher. This logic is revealed in the systematic move from the concrete descriptions in a particular study to the abstract level of science.

Conceptualization, Theoretical Modeling, and Theory Analysis Skills

Qualitative research is oriented toward theory construction. Therefore, an effective reviewer of qualitative research needs to have skills in conceptualization, theoretical modeling, and theory analysis. The theoretical structure in a qualitative study is developed inductively and is expected to emerge from the data. The reviewer must be able to follow

the logical flow of thought of the researcher and be able to analyze and evaluate the adequacy of the resulting theoretical schema as well as its connection to theory development within the discipline.

Transforming Ideas Across Levels of Abstraction

Closely associated with the necessity of having skills in theory analysis is the ability to follow the transformation of ideas across several levels of abstraction and to judge the adequacy of the transformation. Whenever one reviews the literature, organizes ideas from the review, and then again modifies those ideas in the process of developing a summary of the existing body of knowledge, one is involved in the *transformation of ideas*. Developing a research proposal requires transforming ideas across levels of abstraction. Those critiquing the proposal evaluate the adequacy of this transformation process.

STANDARDS FOR CRITIQUE OF QUALITATIVE STUDIES

Multiple problems can occur in qualitative studies as in quantitative studies. However, the problems are likely to be different. Reviewers need not only to know the problems that are likely to occur but also must be able to determine the probability that the problem may have occurred in a study being critiqued. A scholarly critique includes a balanced evaluation of study strengths and limitations. The following five standards have been proposed to evaluate qualitative studies: descriptive vividness, methodological congruence, analytical preciseness, theoretical connectedness, and heuristic relevance (Burns, 1989). The next sections describe these standards and the threats to them.

Standard I: Descriptive Vividness

The description of the site, the subjects, the experience of collecting the data, and the thinking of the researcher during the process needs to be presented so clearly that the reader has the sense of personally experiencing the event. Glaser and Strauss (1965) say that the researcher should "describe the social world studied so vividly that the reader can almost literally see and hear its people" (p. 9). Since one of the assumptions of qualitative research is that all data are context specific, the evaluator of a study must understand the context of that study. From this description, the reader gets a sense of the data as a whole as they are collected and the reactions of the researcher during the data collection and analysis processes. A contextual understanding of the whole is essential and prerequisite to the capability of the reviewer to evaluate the study in light of the other four standards.

Threats to Descriptive Vividness (Burns, 1989; Kahn, 1993)

1. Failure to include essential descriptive information.
2. Lack of clarity and/or depth of the description.
3. Lack of credibility of description (Beck, 1993).
4. Inadequate skills in writing descriptive narrative.
5. Reluctance to reveal self in the written material.

Standard II: Methodological Congruence

Evaluation of *methodological congruence* requires that the reviewer have knowledge of the philosophy and the methodological approach that was used by the researcher. The researcher needs to identify the philosophy and methodological approach and cite sources where the reviewer can obtain further information (Beck, 1994; Munhall, 1989). Methodological excellence has four dimensions: rigor in documentation, procedural rigor, ethical rigor, and auditability.

Rigor in Documentation

Rigor in documentation requires the clear, concise presentation by the researcher of the study elements: phenomenon, purpose, research question, justification of the significance of the phenomenon, identification of assumptions, identification of philosophy, researcher credentials, the context, the role of the researcher, ethical implications, sampling and subjects, data-gathering strategies, data-analysis strategies, theoretical development, conclusions, implications and suggestions for further study and practice, and a literature review. The reviewer examines the study elements or steps for completeness and clarity and identifies any threats to rigor in documentation.

Threats to Rigor in Documentation

1. Failure to present all elements or steps of the study.
2. Failure to present all elements or steps of the study accurately or clearly.

Procedural Rigor

Another dimension of methodological congruence is the rigor of the researcher in applying selected procedures for the study. To the extent possible, the researcher needs to make clear the steps taken to ensure that data were accurately recorded and that the data obtained are representative of the data as a whole (Beck, 1993; Knafl & Howard, 1984). When critiquing a qualitative study, the reviewer examines the description of the data collection process and the study findings for threats to procedural rigor.

Threats to Procedural Rigor

1. The researcher asked the wrong questions. The questions need to tap the subjects' experiences, not their theoretical knowledge of the phenomenon.
2. The questions included terminology from the theoretical orientation of the researcher (Kirk & Miller, 1986; Knaack, 1984).
3. The informant might have misinformed the researcher and this can occur for several reasons. The informant might have had an ulterior motive for deceiving the researcher. Some indi-

viduals might have been present who inhibit free expression by the informant. The informant might have wanted to impress the researcher by giving the response that seemed the most desirable (Dean & Whyte, 1958).

4. The informant did not observe the details requested or was not able to recall the event and substituted instead what he or she supposed happened (Dean & Whyte, 1958).

5. The researcher placed more weight on data obtained from well-informed, articulate, high-status individuals (an elite bias) than on data from those who were less articulate, obstinate, or of low status (Miles & Huberman, 1994).

6. The presence of the researcher distorted the event being observed.

7. The researcher's involvement with the subject-participants distorted the data (LeCompte & Goetz, 1982).

8. Atypical events were interpreted as typical.

9. The informants lacked credibility (Beck, 1993; Becker, 1958).

10. An insufficient amount of data were gathered.

11. An insufficient length of time was spent in data gathering.

12. The approaches for gaining access to the site and/or the subjects were inappropriate.

13. Researcher failed to keep in-depth field notes.

Ethical Rigor

Ethical rigor requires recognition and discussion by the researcher of the ethical implications related to the conduct of the study. Consent is obtained from subjects and documented. The report must indicate that the researcher took action to ensure that the rights of subjects were protected during the study. The reviewer examines the data-gathering process and identifies potential threats to ethical rigor.

Threats to Ethical Rigor

1. The researcher failed to inform the subjects of their rights.

2. The researcher failed to obtain consent from the subjects.

3. The researcher failed to ensure the protection of the subjects' rights.

Auditability

A fourth dimension of methodological congruence is the rigorous development of a decision trail (Beck, 1993; Miles & Huberman, 1994). Guba and Lincoln (1982) refer to this dimension as *auditability*. To achieve this, the researcher must report all the decisions involved in the transformation of data to the theoretical schema. This reporting should be in sufficient detail to allow a second researcher, using the original data and the decision trail, to arrive at conclusions similar to those of the original researcher. When critiquing the study, the reviewer examines the decision trail for threats to auditability.

Threats to Auditability

1. The description of the data collection process was inadequate.

2. The researcher failed to develop or identify the decision rules for arriving at ratings or judgments.

3. The researcher failed to record the nature of the decisions, data upon which they were based, and reasoning that entered into the decisions.

4. The evidence for conclusions was not presented (Becker, 1958).

5. Other researchers were unable to arrive at similar conclusions after applying the decision rules to the data (Beck, 1993).

Standard III: Analytical Preciseness

The analytical process in qualitative research involves a series of transformations during which concrete data are transformed across several levels of abstractions. The outcome of the analysis is a theoretical schema that imparts meaning to the phenomenon under study. The analytical process occurs primarily within the reasoning of the researcher and is frequently poorly reported in published reports. Some transformations may occur intuitively. However, *analytical preciseness* requires that the researcher make intense efforts to identify and record the decision-making processes through which the transformations are made. The processes by which the theoretical schema are cross-checked with data also need to be reported in detail.

Premature patterning may occur before the researcher can logically fit all of the data within the emerging schema. Nisbett and Ross (1980) have shown that patterning happens rapidly and is the way individuals habitually process information. The consequence may be a poor fit between data and theoretical schema (LeCompte & Goetz, 1982; Sandelowski, 1986). Miles and Huberman (1994) suggest that plausibility is the opiate of the intellectual. If the emerging schema makes sense and fits with other theorists' explanations of the phenomenon, the researcher locks into it. This is why it is critical to test the schema by rechecking the fit between the schema and the original data. Beck (1993, p. 265) recommends the researcher have the "data analysis procedures reviewed by a judge panel to prevent researcher bias and selective inattention." When critiquing a study, the reviewer examines the decision-making processes and the theoretical schema to detect threats to analytical preciseness.

Threats to Analytical Preciseness

1. The interpretive statements do not correspond with findings (Parse, Coyne, & Smith, 1985).
2. The categories, themes, or common elements are not logical.
3. The samples are not representative of the class of joint acts referred to by the researcher (Denzin, 1989).
4. The set of categories, themes, or common elements fails to set forth a whole picture.
5. The set of categories, themes, or common elements is not inclusive of data that exist.

6. The data are inappropriately assigned to categories, themes, or common elements.
7. The inclusion and exclusion criteria for categories, themes, or common elements are not consistently followed.
8. The working hypotheses or propositions are not identified or cannot be verified by data.
9. Various sources of evidence fail to provide convergence.
10. There is incongruence of evidence.
11. The subject-participants fail to validate findings when appropriate.
12. The conclusions are not data-based or do not encompass all of the data.
13. The data are made to appear more patterned, regular, or congruent than they are (Beck, 1993; Sandelowski, 1986).

Standard IV: Theoretical Connectedness

Theoretical connectedness requires that the theoretical schema developed from the study be clearly expressed, logically consistent, reflective of the data, and compatible with the knowledge base of nursing.

Threats to Theoretical Connectedness

1. The findings are trivialized (Goetz & LeCompte, 1981).
2. The concepts are inadequately refined.
3. The concepts are not validated by data.
4. The set of concepts lacks commonality.
5. The relationships between concepts are not clearly expressed.
6. The proposed relationships between concepts are not validated by data.
7. The working propositions are not validated by data.
8. Data are distorted during the development of the theoretical schema (Bruyn, 1966).
9. The theoretical schema fails to yield a meaningful picture of the phenomenon studied.
10. A conceptual framework or map is not derived from the data.

Standard V: Heuristic Relevance

To be of value, the results of a study need *heuristic relevance* for the readers. This value is reflected in the reader's capacity to recognize the phenomenon described in the study, its theoretical significance, its applicability to nursing practice situations, and its influence on future research activities. The dimensions of heuristic relevance include intuitive recognition, relationship to existing body of knowledge, and applicability.

Intuitive Recognition

Intuitive recognition indicates that when individuals are confronted with the theoretical schema derived from the data, it has meaning within their personal knowledge base. They immediately recognize the phenomenon being described by the researcher and its relationship to a theoretical perspective in nursing.

Threats to Intuitive Recognition

1. The reader is unable to recognize the phenomenon.
2. The description is not consistent with common meanings.
3. The theoretical connectedness is lacking.

Relationship to Existing Body of Knowledge

The existing *body of knowledge,* particularly the nursing theoretical perspective from which the phenomenon was approached, must be reviewed by the researcher and compared with the findings of the study. There should be intersubjectivity with existing theoretical knowledge in nursing and previous research. Reasons for differences with the existing body of knowledge should be explored by the researcher. When critiquing a study, the reviewer examines the strength of the link of study findings to the existing knowledge.

Threats to Relationship to Existing Body of Knowledge

1. The researcher failed to examine the existing body of knowledge.
2. The process studied was not related to nursing and health.
3. There is a lack of correspondence with the existing knowledge base in nursing (Parse et al., 1985).

Applicability

Nurses need to be able to integrate the findings into their knowledge base and apply them to nursing practice situations. The findings also need to contribute to theory development. The reviewer examines the discussion section of the research report for threats to applicability.

Threats to Applicability

1. The findings are not significant for the discipline of nursing.
2. There is a failure to achieve methodological congruence.
3. There is a failure to achieve analytical preciseness.
4. There is a failure to achieve theoretical connectedness.

Application of these five standards in critiquing qualitative studies determines the strengths and weaknesses of a study. A summary of the strengths will indicate the adherence to the standards, and a summary of weaknesses will indicate the potential threats to the integrity of the study.

SUMMARY

An intellectual critique of research involves the careful examination of all aspects of a study to judge the merits, limitations, meaning, and significance of the study based on previous research experience and knowledge of the topic. Intellectual critiques of studies are essential for the development and refinement of nursing knowledge. In nursing, a critique is often seen as a first step in learning the research process. However, conducting a critique is not a basic skill, and the content presented in previous chapters is necessary for implementing the critique process.

Research is critiqued to improve practice, broaden understanding, and provide a base for the conduct of a study. Nursing students, practicing nurses, nurse educators, and nurse researchers perform research critiques. These critiques are often conducted after verbal presentations of studies, after a published research report, for abstract or article selection, and for evaluating research proposals. A critique process is described for both quantitative and qualitative research. The steps in the critique process include comprehension, comparison, analysis, evaluation, and conceptual clustering. These steps occur in sequence, vary in depth, and presume accomplishment of the preceding steps. However, the person with critique experience frequently performs several steps of this process simultaneously.

The first step, comprehension, involves understanding the terms and concepts in the report as well as identifying study elements and grasping the nature, significance, and meaning of these elements. The next step, comparison, requires knowledge of what each step of the research process should be like. The ideal is compared with the real. The analysis step involves a critique of the logical links connecting one study element with another. The fourth step, evaluation, involves examining the meaning and significance of the study according to set criteria. During this step of the critique, the internal and external validity of the study are examined. The last step of the critique process is the clustering of present knowledge within a given area of study. Conceptual clustering is a means of generating new research questions, developing and refining theory, and synthesizing research for use in practice. Each step of the critique process is described and questions are provided to direct the critique of quantitative studies.

Critique in qualitative research requires the same steps as those of quantitative research. However, the skills and standards for critique of qualitative research are different. The skills needed to critique qualitative studies include (1) context flexibility; (2) inductive reasoning; (3) conceptualization, theoretical modeling, and theory analysis; and (4) transforming ideas across levels of abstraction.

The standards proposed to evaluate qualitative studies include descriptive vividness, methodological congruence, analytical preciseness, theoretical connectedness, and heuristic relevance. Descriptive vividness means that the site, subjects, experience of collecting data, and the thinking of the researcher during the process are presented so clearly that the reader has the sense of personally experiencing the event. Methodological congruence has four dimensions: rigor in documentation, procedural rigor, ethical rigor, and auditability. Analytical preciseness is essential to perform a series of transformations in which concrete data are transformed across several levels of abstractions.

The outcome of the analysis is a theoretical schema that imparts meaning to the phenomenon under study. Theoretical connectedness requires that the theoretical schema developed from the study be clearly expressed, logically consistent, reflective of the data, and compatible with the knowledge base of nursing. Heuristic relevance includes intuitive recognition, a relationship to the existing body of knowledge, and applicability. These standards and the threats to these standards are presented to guide the critique of qualitative studies.

References

Beck, C. T. (1993). Qualitative research: The evaluation of its credibility, fittingness, and auditability. *Western Journal of Nursing Research, 15*(2), 263–266.

Beck, C. T. (1994). Reliability and validity issues in phenomenological research. *Western Journal of Nursing Research, 16*(3), 254–267.

Becker, H. S. (1958). Problems of inference and proof in participant observation. *American Sociological Review, 23*(6), 652–660.

Bruyn, S. T. (1966). *The human perspective in sociology.* Englewood Cliffs, NJ: Prentice-Hall.

Burns, N. (1989). Standards for qualitative research. *Nursing Science Quarterly, 2*(1), 44–52.

Cason, C. L., Cason, G. J., & Redland, A. R. (1988). Peer review of research abstracts. *Image: Journal of Nursing Scholarship, 20*(2), 102–105.

Crosby, L. J. (1990). The abstract: An important first impression. *Journal of Neuroscience Nursing, 22*(3), 192–194.

Dean, J. P., & Whyte, W. F. (1958). How do you know if the informant is telling the truth? *Human Organization, 17*(2), 34–38.

Denzin, N. K. (1989). *The research act* (3rd ed.). New York: McGraw-Hill.

Egan, E. C., Snyder, M., & Burns, K. R. (1992). Intervention studies in nursing: Is the effect due to the independent variable? *Nursing Outlook, 40*(4), 187–190.

Ganong, L. H. (1987). Integrative reviews of nursing research. *Research in Nursing & Health, 10*(1), 1–11.

Glaser, B., & Strauss, A. L. (1965). Discovery of substantive theory: A basic strategy underlying qualitative research. *American Behavioral Scientist, 8*(1), 5–12.

Goetz, J. P., & LeCompte, M. D. (1981). Ethnographic research and the problem of data reduction. *Anthropology and Education Quarterly, 12*(1), 51–70.

Guba, E. G., & Lincoln, Y. S. (1982). *Effective evaluation.* Washington, DC: Jossey-Bass.

Kahn, D. L. (1993). Ways of discussing validity in qualitative nursing research. *Western Journal of Nursing Research, 15*(1), 122–126.

Kerlinger, F. N. (1986). *Foundations of behavioral research* (3rd ed.). New York: Holt, Rinehart, and Winston.

Kim, M. J., & Felton, F. (1993). The current generation of research proposals: Reviewers' viewpoints. *Nursing Research, 42*(2), 118–119.

Kirk, J., & Miller, M. L. (1986). *Reliability and validity in qualitative research.* Beverly Hills, CA: Sage.

Knaack, P. (1984). Phenomenological research. *Western Journal of Nursing Research, 6*(1), 107–114.

Knafl, K. A., & Howard, M. J. (1984). Interpreting and reporting qualitative research. *Research in Nursing & Health, 7*(1), 17–24.

Larson, E. (1994). Exclusion of certain groups from clinical research. *Image: Journal of Nursing Scholarship, 26*(3), 185–190.

LeCompte, M. D., & Goetz, J. P. (1982). Problems of reliability and validity in ethnographic research. *Review of Educational Research, 52*(1), 31–60.

LeFort, S. M. (1993). The statistical versus clinical significance debate. *Image: Journal of Nursing Scholarship, 25*(1), 57–62.

Liehr, P., & Houston, S. (1993). Critique and using nursing research: Guidelines for the critical care nurse. *American Journal of Critical Care, 2*(5), 407–412.

LoBiondo-Wood, G. L., & Haber, J. (1994). *Nursing research: Methods, critical appraisal, and utilization* (3rd ed.). St. Louis: Mosby.

Massey, J., & Loomis, M. (1988). When should nurses use research findings? *Applied Nursing Research, 1*(1), 32–40.

Meleis, A. I. (1991). *Theoretical nursing: Development and progress* (2nd ed.). Philadelphia: Lippincott.

Miles, M. B., & Huberman, A. M. (1994). *Qualitative data analysis: A source book of new methods* (2nd ed.). Beverly Hills, CA: Sage.

Morse, J. M., Dellasega, C., & Dobernck, B. (1993). Evaluating abstracts: Preparing a research conference. *Nursing Research, 42*(5), 308–310.

Munhall, P. L. (1989). Philosophical ponderings on qualitative research methods in nursing. *Nursing Science Quarterly, 2*(1), 20–28.

Nisbett, R., & Ross, L. (1980). *Human inference: Strategies and shortcomings of social judgment.* Englewood Cliffs, NJ: Prentice-Hall.

Oberst, M. T. (1992). Warning: Believing this report may be hazardous . . . *Research in Nursing & Health, 15*(2), 91–92.

Parse, R. R., Coyne, A. B., & Smith, M. J. (1985). *Nursing research: Qualitative methods.* Bowie, MD: Brady.

Phillips, L. R. F. (1986). *A clinician's guide to the critique and utilization of nursing research.* Norwalk, CT: Appleton-Century-Crofts.

Pillemer, D. B., & Light, R. J. (1980). Synthesizing outcomes: How to use research evidence from many studies. *Harvard Educational Review, 50*(2), 176–195.

Pinch, W. J. (1995). Synthesis: Implementing a complex process. *Nurse Educator, 20*(1), 34–40.

Polit, D. F., & Hungler, B. P. (1995). *Nursing research: Principles and methods* (5th ed.). Philadelphia: Lippincott.

Ryan-Wenger, N. (1992). Guidelines for critique of a research report. *Heart & Lung, 21*(4), 394–401.

Sandelowski, M. (1986). The problem of rigor in qualitative research. *Advances in Nursing Science, 8*(3), 27–37.

Shelley, S. I. (1984). *Research methods in nursing and health.* Boston: Little, Brown.

Stetler, C. B. (1994). Refinement of the Stetler/Marram Model for application of research findings to practice. *Nursing Outlook, 42*(1), 15–25.

Swanson, E. A., McCloskey, J. C., & Bodensteiner, A. (1991). Publishing opportunities for nurses: A comparison of 92 U.S. journals. *Image: Journal of Nursing Scholarship, 23*(1), 33–38.

Tibbles, L., & Sanford, R. (1994). The research journal club: A mechanism for research utilization. *Clinical Nurse Specialist, 8*(1), 23–26.

Titler, M. G., Kleiber, C., Steelman, V., Goode, C., Rakel, B., Barry-Walker, J., Small, S., & Buckwalter, K. (1994). Infusing research into practice to promote quality care. *Nursing Research, 43*(5), 307–313.

Werley, H. H., & Fitzpatrick, J. J. (1983). *Annual review of nursing research* (Vol. 1). New York: Springer.

Woods, N. F., & Catanzaro, M. (1988). *Nursing research: Theory and practice.* St. Louis: Mosby.

Yam, M. (1994). Strategies for teaching nursing research: Teaching nursing students to critique research for gender bias. *Western Journal of Nursing Research, 16*(6), 724–727.

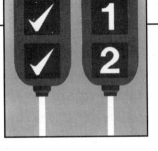

25

Utilization of Research in Nursing Practice

The preceding chapters of this book describe what nursing research is; the critical thinking processes associated with research; the techniques for developing, implementing, and communicating research; and the skills needed for critiquing studies. Implicit in all these chapters is the belief that the expected outcome of nursing research activities is to improve nursing practice. In order for research to have an impact on practice, the findings of studies must be utilized by practitioners. However, much of our current nursing practice is not based on research.

The generation of empirical knowledge to improve clinical practice was the major focus of researchers in the 1980s and continues to be the emphasis for the 1990s. During the last 15 years, many quality clinical studies and an increasing number of replications have been conducted. In addition, dissemination of research findings has increased through presentations at conferences, communication through electronic media (radio, television, and World Wide Web), and publications in research and clinical journals. Thus, the generation and diffusion of empirical knowledge are expanding; but a limited amount of this knowledge is being used in practice (Coyle & Sokop, 1990; Michel & Sneed, 1995).

With the current changes in the health care system, society is demanding more of nurses than ever before. Nurses now have the attention of the health policymakers and can influence the future health care delivery system (Jones, 1993; Maurin, 1990). Meeting these policymakers' expectations will require increased scientific productivity for all

nurses, including the conduct of high-quality research and the use of those findings in practice. In addition, the utilization of nursing research knowledge needs to produce measurable, quality patient outcomes in a variety of clinical settings (Davies et al., 1994). This chapter was developed to promote an understanding of the research utilization process. Some of the problems or barriers related to knowledge utilization are identified and the theories relevant to research utilization are introduced. The chapter concludes with a presentation of strategies to promote the use of research findings in practice.

PROBLEMS RELATED TO KNOWLEDGE UTILIZATION

Knowledge utilization is the process of disseminating and using research-generated information to make an impact on or change in the existing practices in society. The time lag between generating and using knowledge by society has been a concern for numerous years. For example, the time lag between the discovery of citrus juice as a preventive measure for scurvy and its use on British ships was 264 years. The span of time between the first conception of 10 important ideas and initial utilization of them are presented in Table 25–1 (Glaser, Abelson, & Garrison, 1983). The table suggests that the average length of time between discovery and utilization is almost 20 years. Lynn (cited in Glaser et al., 1983) reports a decrease in

Table 25-1
Time Span Between Idea and Utilization

Innovation	Year of First Conception	Year of First Realization	Duration in Years
Heart pacemaker	1928	1960	32
Input-output economic analysis	1936	1964	28
Hybrid corn	1908	1933	25
Electrophotography	1937	1959	22
Magnetic ferrites	1933	1955	22
Hybrid small grains	1937	1956	19
Green revolution: wheat	1950	1966	16
Organophosphorus insecticides	1934	1947	13
Oral contraceptive	1951	1960	9
Videotape record	1950	1956	6
Average duration			19.2

(From Glaser, E. M., Abelson, H. H., & Garrison, K. N. *Putting knowledge to use,* p. 8 [Table 1]. © 1983 by Jossey-Bass, Inc., Publishers.)

time for utilization of discoveries made in the period between 1885 and 1965 from 30 years (1885 to 1919) to nine years (1945 to 1965). Why some findings require much longer to implement than others is not clearly understood. Historical events, attitudes toward researchers and research in general, and the necessity with some innovations to change attitudes before the findings can be accepted and utilized seem to influence the time required.

PROBLEMS RELATED TO THE USE OF RESEARCH FINDINGS IN NURSING

Most people believe that a good idea will sell itself—the word will spread rapidly and the idea will quickly be used. Unfortunately, this is seldom true. Even today, research findings that clearly warrant utilization are not being used in nursing practice. Brett (1987) studied the extent to which 14 nursing research findings, which met the Conduct and Utilization of Research in Nursing (CURN) Project's (1982) criteria for use in practice, were being used by practicing nurses. A stratified sample of 216 nurses was obtained from small, medium, and large hospitals. One of the findings (innovations) examined was the following

technique for giving intramuscular injections: "Internal rotation of the femur during injection into the dorsogluteal site, in either the prone or the side-lying position, results in reduced discomfort from the injection" (Brett, 1987, p. 346). Forty-four percent of the nurses were aware of the finding, 34% were persuaded that the finding was useful for practice, 29% were implementing this finding in practice sometimes, but only 10% were implementing it always. Coyle and Sokop (1990) replicated Brett's (1987) study with a sample of 113 nurses in North Carolina. Thirty-four percent of these nurses were aware of this finding, 21% were persuaded that the finding was useful, but only 4% used the intervention sometimes and 22% used it always. This indicates a limited increase in the use of this innovation from 1987 to 1990.

The findings regarding intramuscular injections would be comparatively simple to implement. The decision could be made by the nurse alone; no physician's order would be needed. Administrative personnel would not have to give approval. No additional cost or nursing time would be involved. At the time of Brett's (1987) and Coyle and Sokop's (1990) studies, the findings on intramuscular injections (Kruszewski, Lang, & Johnson, 1979) had been available in the literature over 10 years. Why were over 56 to 66% of the nurses unaware of the findings? Had the nurses not read the information? Was it not taught in nursing schools? Or was the suggested change in nursing practice not considered important by those who did read the information? Did those nurses who implemented the findings sometimes in practice not perceive a positive impact on patient care? What are the barriers that interfere with the use of research findings in practice? These are questions nursing must address to increase the utilization of research in practice.

Barriers to Knowledge Utilization in Nursing

A common barrier to research utilization is the communication gap between the university-based researcher and the institutional-based practitioner. This concern is not unique to nursing; it was a major topic of discussion at the think tanks convened by the federal government to promote utilization of research. Criticisms included the following: (1) Researcher-originated studies do not solve pressing clinical problems, (2) findings from researcher-originated studies often cannot be utilized in practice, (3) the studies conducted lack replication, (4) findings are communicated primarily to other researchers, (5) findings are not expressed in terms understood by practitioners, (6) practitioners do not value research, (7) practitioners are unaware of or unwilling to read research reports, (8) practitioners have inadequate education related to the research process, (9) practitioners do not believe the research findings, and (10) practitioners do not know how to apply research findings or are not allowed to apply them (Bock, 1990; MacGuire, 1990; Phillips, 1986; Rogers, 1983; Tibbles & Sanford, 1994). Every effort needs to be made to bridge the gap between researchers and practitioners by enhancing the communication of research, synthesis of findings, and generation of protocols for use in practice.

Several sources have identified the barriers to using research in practice, but the specific barriers need to be identified for different settings and situations. Funk, Champagne, Wiese, and Tornquist (1991) developed a scale to measure the barriers to research utilization. The BARRIERS Scale includes 29 items that were developed from the utilization literature, the CURN Project Research Utilization Questionnaire, and informal data gathered from nurses. The items were refined based on the input from research utilization consultants, nursing researchers, practicing nurses, and a psychometrician. The items on the scale cover four areas: (1) characteristics of the adopter, the nurse's research values, skills, and awareness; (2) characteristics of the organization, setting barriers and limitations; (3) characteristics of the innovation, qualities of the research; and (4) characteristics of the communication, presentation, and accessibility of the research. The BARRIERS Scale provides a way to identify the different problems in varied clinical settings and groups of practicing nurses or administrators. Some of the most common barriers identified by practicing nurses included time, limited support of nursing administrators and others, and lack of knowledge of research findings (Pettengill, Gillies, & Clark, 1994). The greatest barriers to research utilization identified by administrators include nurses not aware of research findings, insufficient time, and research reports are not understandable (Funk, Champagne, Tornquist, & Wiese, 1995). Identifying barriers to research utilization can promote communication between researchers and practitioners and can facilitate problem solving, with the goal of using research findings in practice.

THEORIES OF UTILIZATION

The problems related to knowledge utilization became a major concern in the early 1970s when it was discovered that many of the findings from research funded by the federal government were not being used by society. A think tank of experts in the area of research utilization was convened by the government to examine reasons for the lack of utilization and to propose strategies to improve it. From the work done by this group, a field of study evolved that examines the process of utilization. With the increased focus on knowledge utilization, two prominent theories about diffusion and adoption of innovations were developed: Rogers's theory of diffusion of innovations and Havelock's theory of linker systems. These theories have provided frameworks for most of the studies in the area of utilization. In addition, these theories provide direction for implementing strategies to increase the use of research findings in nursing practice.

ROGERS'S THEORY OF DIFFUSION OF INNOVATIONS

E. M. Rogers is an expert and noted theorist in the field of knowledge diffusion and utilization. Rogers has conducted research related to knowledge diffusion and utilization for 25 years and his theory is a synthesis of the findings from his and other scientists' research in this field. In his theory, Rogers (1983) defines knowledge diffusion and identifies a process to promote the diffusion of innovations or new knowledge.

Knowledge Diffusion

According to Rogers (1983), "*Diffusion* is the process by which an innovation is communicated through certain channels over time among the members of a social system" (p. 5). The word dissemination is considered synonymous with diffusion. The main elements of diffusion include (1) an innovation, (2) communication channels, (3) time, and (4) a social system. He defines an *innovation* as "an idea, practice, or object that is perceived as new by an individual or other unit of adoption" (p. 11). The idea might not necessarily be new, but must be perceived as new by those considering adoption.

Communication channels may include one-to-one communication; one individual communicating to several others; or mass media such as books, journals, newspapers, television, and computer networks like the World Wide Web (WWW). Mass media is effective for achieving diffusion; however, interpersonal channels involving face-to-face exchange have been found to be more effective in facilitating adoption of an inno-

vation. The communication is most effective when the two interacting individuals are similar in such characteristics as beliefs, values, education, social status, and profession. Rogers refers to these individuals as near-peers.

Time is another important element in understanding the diffusion-adoption process. The three time-related elements of interest in this process are (1) the time span from the point at which an individual first hears about an innovation to the point at which a decision is made to accept or reject the innovation, (2) the innovativeness of the individual or agency that determines the time needed to achieve adoption, and (3) the number of individuals within a social system who adopt an innovation within a given time period.

Rogers (1983) defines a *social system* as "a set of interrelated units that is engaged in joint problem-solving to accomplish a common goal" (p. 24). Diffusion occurs within a social system, and the social structure of the system affects the diffusion of the innovation. A social system has both formal and informal structure. Formal structure is related to authority and power. Informal structure is related to who interacts with whom under what circumstances. Every social system has *opinion leaders* who are in favor of innovations and those who oppose change. Opinion leaders are at the center of the system's interpersonal communication networks and tend to reflect the norms of the system. In seeking adoption of an innovation within a social system, one must identify the opinion leaders and seek their acceptance.

Innovation-Decision Process

Rogers (1983) conceptualizes that the diffusion of knowledge could be achieved by an *innovation-decision process* that consists of five stages: (1) knowledge, (2) persuasion, (3) decision, (4) implementation, and (5) confirmation (see Figure 25–1). The *knowledge stage* is the first awareness of the existence of the innovation, and the *persuasion stage* occurs when the individual forms an attitude toward the innovation. A *decision stage* occurs when the individual chooses to adopt or reject the innovation. The *implementation stage* is

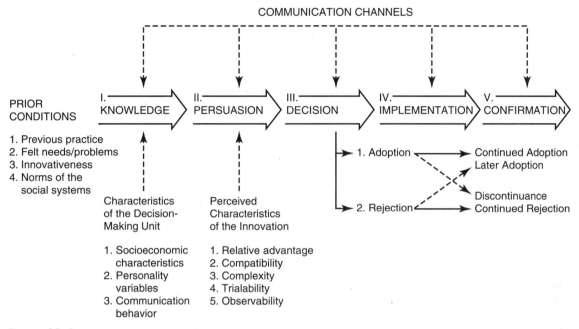

COMMUNICATION CHANNELS

PRIOR CONDITIONS

1. Previous practice
2. Felt needs/problems
3. Innovativeness
4. Norms of the
   social systems

I. KNOWLEDGE II. PERSUASION III. DECISION IV. IMPLEMENTATION V. CONFIRMATION

1. Adoption → Continued Adoption / Later Adoption

2. Rejection → Discontinuance / Continued Rejection

Characteristics of the Decision-Making Unit

1. Socioeconomic characteristics
2. Personality variables
3. Communication behavior

Perceived Characteristics of the Innovation

1. Relative advantage
2. Compatibility
3. Complexity
4. Trialability
5. Observability

Figure 25–1

A model of stages of the innovation-decision process. (Reprinted with the permission of The Free Press, a division of Simon & Schuster, from *Diffusion of innovations,* 3rd ed., by Everett M. Rogers. Copyright © 1962, 1971, 1983 by The Free Press.)

when the individual uses the innovation. The *confirmation stage* occurs when the individual evaluates the effectiveness of the innovation and decides to either continue or discontinue it.

Knowledge Stage

Knowledge of an innovation in nursing can be achieved by formal communication through media such as television, newspapers, computer networks, publications, or seminars. In addition, informal communication within an agency from one nurse to another can be effective in increasing awareness of an innovation. Certain prior conditions influence the knowledge stage, such as previous practice, felt needs/problems, innovativeness, and norms of the social system. Dissatisfaction with previous practice can lead to recognizing the needs or problems that require change. A need might create a search for an innovation to improve practice, but also knowledge of a new innovation might create a need for change. For example,

knowledge of a new treatment for pressure sores might create the need to change the existing treatment policy.

Innovativeness is the "degree to which an individual or other unit of adoption is relatively earlier in adopting new ideas than are the other members of a system" (Rogers, 1983, p. 22). Rogers uses five categories to describe adopters, based on their degree of innovativeness: (1) innovators, (2) early adopters, (3) early majority, (4) late majority, and (5) laggards.

Innovators are active information seekers of new ideas. They have a high level of mass media exposure and interpersonal networks that are widely extended, reaching beyond their local social system. From these sources, they receive early information about innovations. Innovators usually function outside the existing social structures and tend to have cosmopolitan relationships. They are the change agents an agency might hire to implement an innovation. Their social support system is diverse and not tightly linked. Innovators can cope with higher levels of uncertainty related to an innovation than can other adopters and are the first to adopt a new idea. They do not rely on subjective evaluations of the innovation by other system members. Because innovators are less closely linked with the local social system, they have less influence on adoption of an innovation within the system than do early adopters.

Early adopters tend to be opinion leaders in existing social systems. They learn about new ideas rapidly, utilize them, and then serve as role models in their use. In the hospital, early adopters might be nurses in advanced roles such as administrators, acute care nurse practitioners, clinical nurse specialists, and inservice educators. The *early majority* rarely are leaders but are active followers and will readily follow in the use of a new idea. The *late majority* are skeptical about new ideas and will adopt them only if group pressure is great. The *laggards* are security-oriented, tend to cling to the past, and are often isolates without a strong support system. By the time they adopt a new idea, it is considered by most to be an old idea.

Research has shown that the adopter distribution over time approaches a bell-shaped curve (see Figure 25–2). The innovators (2.5%) and the early adopters (13.5%) are comparable in numbers to the laggards (16%). This distribution can assist agencies in realistically identifying the number of individuals who will and will not support a

change. The early adopters and early majority can form a powerful group to promote change of the late majority. All groups (innovators, early adopters, and early and late majority) can apply pressure to persuade the laggards to change, but many of the laggards will continue to resist change and some might leave the agency.

Norms, the expected behavior patterns within a social system, affect diffusion of innovations. Norms can serve as barriers to change or can facilitate change. When the norms of the social system are oriented toward change, the opinion leaders tend to be innovative (early adopters), and change is facilitated. When the norms are opposed to change, so are the opinion leaders, thus creating barriers to change. When innovations are diffused and adopted or rejected within a social system, social change occurs, affecting the norms of the system.

During the knowledge stage, the characteristics of the individual, organization, or institution that is considering the adoption of an innovation need to be examined (see Figure 25–1). The characteristics requiring examination include socioeconomic elements, personality variables, and communication behavior of the decision-making unit. The socioeconomic characteristics include social status, interactional patterns, and economic level of those involved in adopting an innovation. Examination of personality variables will indicate individuals' innovativeness (early adopter or lag-

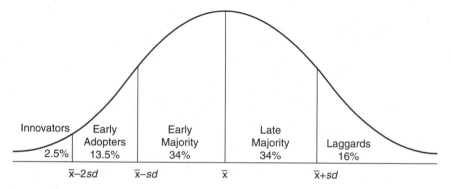

Figure 25–2

Adopter categorization on the basis of innovativeness. (Reprinted with the permission of The Free Press, a division of Simon & Schuster, from *Diffusion of innovations,* 3rd ed., by Everett M. Rogers. Copyright © 1962, 1971, 1983 by The Free Press.)

gard), and whether they will facilitate or obstruct change. Communication behavior, whether it is open and honest or closed and subversive, has a strong impact on the diffusion process.

Persuasion Stage

During the persuasion stage, an individual or other decision-making unit develops a favorable or unfavorable attitude toward the change or innovation (Rogers, 1983). Characteristics of an innovation that determine the probability and speed of an adoption include (1) relative advantage, (2) compatibility, (3) complexity, (4) trialability, and (5) observability (see Figure 25–1). *Relative advantage* is the extent to which the innovation is perceived to be better than current practice. *Compatibility* is the degree to which the innovation is perceived to be consistent with current values, past experience, and priority of needs. *Complexity* is the degree to which the innovation is perceived to be difficult to understand or use. If the innovation requires the development of new skills, complexity increases. *Trialability* is the extent to which an individual or agency can try out the idea on a limited basis with the option of returning to previous practices. *Observability* is the extent to which the results of an innovation are visible to others. An innovation with highly visible, beneficial results is more rapidly diffused. In conclusion, innovations that have great relative advantage, are compatible, have trialability, are not complex, and are observable will be adopted more quickly than innovations that do not meet these criteria.

Effective communication can occur through mass media at the knowledge stage, because the individual seeks information in order to reduce uncertainty. However, at the persuasion stage and throughout the rest of the innovation-decision process, mass media are less effective than informal communication. Rather than information, the individual seeks evaluative statements related to the innovation. Have you used it? How do you feel about it? What are the consequences of using it? What are the advantages and disadvantages of using it in my situation? Would you advise me to use it? Will I still be approved of and accepted if I use it? Interpersonal networks with near-peers are much more likely to influence individuals during the persuasion stage and subsequent stages.

Decision Stage

At the decision stage, the individual either adopts or rejects the innovation (see Figure 25–1). *Adoption* involves full acceptance of the innovation and the implementation of the ideas in practice. Adoption can be continued infinitely or can be discontinued based on evaluation of the effectiveness in the social system. *Rejection* is a decision not to use an innovation, which can be active or passive. *Active rejection* indicates that the innovation was examined and a decision was made not to adopt it. With *passive rejection,* the innovation was never seriously considered. Over time, the social system might continue with the decision to reject or might initiate a later adoption.

Implementation Stage

In the implementation stage, the innovation is put to use by an individual (or other decision-making unit). A detailed plan for implementation that addresses the risks and benefits of the innovation will facilitate diffusion. The three types of implementation are (1) direct application, (2) reinvention, and (3) indirect effects.

Direct application occurs when an innovation is used exactly as it was developed. In fact, some scientists would not consider the innovation to have been adopted unless its original form has been kept intact. For example, if a study demonstrated that a particular intervention, conducted in specifically defined steps, was effective in achieving an outcome, adoption would require that the nurse perform the steps of the intervention in exactly the same way in which they were described in the study. This expectation reflects the narrow, precise definition of an innovation that is necessary to the scientific endeavor. However, this preciseness is not compatible with typical practice behavior, and research has indicated that maintenance of the original innovation does not always occur.

With *reinvention,* adopters modify the innovation to meet their own needs. Using this strategy, the steps of a procedure might be changed, or some of the steps might be combined with care activities emerging from previous experience. To some researchers, adding, deleting, altering, or rearranging steps in a procedure means that it is no longer the same innovation. Thus, adoption has not occurred. However, from the practitioner's viewpoint, the innovation has been adopted.

The expectation is that the new knowledge will directly modify the actions of the individual, either in the original suggested way or as a reinvention. However, individuals usually incorporate the knowledge and use it in diffuse ways. Thus, the implementation of knowledge can be indirect. For example, practitioners and researchers might discuss the findings, cite them in clinical papers and textbooks, and use them to provide strength to arguments. Thus, the knowledge would be incorporated into the individual's thinking and combined with past experience, previous education, and current values. In this instance, determining that the innovation was being utilized would be more difficult. Thus, the use of certain nursing research findings may be underestimated.

Weiss (1980), another theorist in the field of knowledge utilization, suggests considering utilization as a continuum. One extreme of the continuum is that findings have a direct effect on decisions and activities, and the other extreme is that findings have a diffuse or indirect effect. This indirect effect involves awareness, insight, or cumulative understanding that may lead to subtle, gradual changes in behavior. The middle of the continuum reflects a modified impact in which the findings are combined with other types of information for problem solving and decision making.

Confirmation Stage

During the confirmation stage, the individual evaluates the effectiveness of the innovation and decides either to continue or to discontinue it. If an innovation is evaluated positively by those involved, the decision might be to continue the innovation and expand its use throughout an agency

or a corporation. *Discontinuance* can be of at least two types: (1) replacement and (2) disenchantment. With *replacement discontinuance,* the innovation is rejected in order to adopt a better idea. Thus, innovations can occur in waves as new ideas replace outdated, impractical innovations. The computer is an excellent example, since users can constantly upgrade their systems with new, more powerful interactive innovations in hardware and software. *Disenchantment discontinuance* occurs when an idea is rejected because the user is dissatisfied with its outcome.

Rogers's theory has been used to facilitate the utilization of research findings in nursing practice. His innovation-decision process has provided the framework for the implementation of some major research utilization projects that are discussed later in this chapter. The innovation-decision process could be very helpful in assisting individual nurses or groups of nurses within an agency to implement research findings to directly influence practice or to merge findings with other knowledge to indirectly affect nursing practice.

HAVELOCK'S LINKER SYSTEMS

Havelock (1970, 1974) added a new dimension to the current knowledge of utilization theory by proposing the development of a linker system. This linker system is used to transfer new knowledge, skills, or products (innovations) from resource systems (researchers and their publications) to user systems (practitioners) for utilization. Havelock's model (see Figure 25–3) illustrates the link of the user-client system to the resources and the interaction with a change agent (outside process consultant) (Havelock & Havelock, 1973). The change process using the linker system is depicted as a six-step process: (1) need felt, (2) problem diagnosis, (3) search for resources, (4) retrieval of ideas and information, (5) fabrication of a solution, and (6) application.

Change Process Using the Linker System

Step 1 is the identification of a need by a client, who might be an individual, organization, or insti-

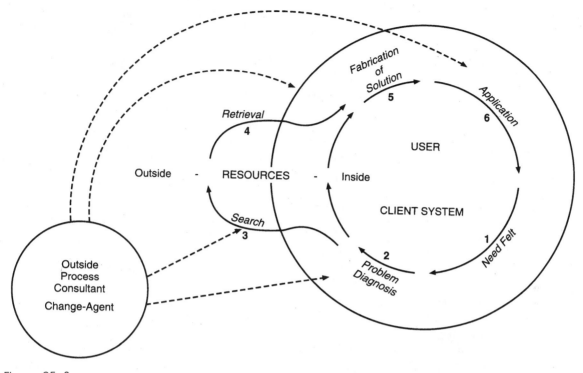

Figure 25–3

The problem-solver view of the change process. (From Havelock, R. G., & Havelock, M. C. [1973]. *Training for change agents: A guide to the design of training programs in education and other fields* [p. 9]. Ann Arbor, MI: Litho Crafters, with permission.)

tution. The need is then translated into a diagnosis in Step 2. The diagnosis represents a set of problems to be solved and should be based on the values of the user-client system. At this point, the change agent shares diagnostic skills with the client system and facilitates the diagnostic process. Step 3 is the initiation of a link to resources outside the agency (including research publications and researchers' ideas) and inside the agency (administration, personnel, and financial support). Change is frequently more effective when initiated from inside, rather than outside, a client system. Step 4 completes the link with the resource system, in which ideas and information are retrieved to solve the identified problem(s). Step 5 is the fabrication of a solution that involves selecting or formulating an innovation. The change agent assists in the evaluation of the information and determination of the knowledge that is ready for use

in practice. Step 6 is application of the innovation, which includes adapting the innovation as needed, implementing it, and evaluating its effectiveness.

The change agent clearly identifies the desired outcome, and actions are selected to achieve this outcome. Persons, groups, or factors that will facilitate or resist change are identified. Careful plans are made to strengthen and promote those factors facilitating the change. Strategies are designed to counter factors resisting the change. When the change has been adopted by the majority of the members, the agent leaves the system. Unfortunately, in some cases, when the change agent is withdrawn, use of the innovation gradually declines. As indicated in Figure 25–3, the change process is continuous with the identification of additional problems, the search and retrieval of information from resources, formulation of additional innovations, and the application of innovations by the user.

Linker

Havelock (1970, 1973) also suggests the establishment of a *linker,* an individual who could serve as a connection between the user system and the resource system. The linker would have extensive knowledge of research findings and strategies for implementing them and could serve as an advisor to the user system in implementing new ideas. The linker could package the innovation in a form that would increase its acceptability to the user system and, thus, increase utilization. The idea of packaging comes from the research and development (R & D) programs of technology in which researchers make a discovery; then another group (the linker system) takes the new idea and develops practical ways to use it (Havelock & Lingwood, 1973). The linker can also be involved in the transmission of user needs to the resource systems, thus increasing the probability of new studies addressing practitioner concerns.

The idea of using a linker and packaging innovations for practice is evident in the clinical practice guidelines that are being developed by U.S. Department of Health and Human Services. The Agency for Health Care Policy and Research (AHCPR) has facilitated the organization of panels of expert clinicians (linkers) to summarize the research in selected areas and to develop protocols for use in practices. These practice guidelines (packaged innovations) are available in formats that are suitable for health care practitioners, the scientific community, educators, and consumers. More details on these guidelines are presented later in this chapter.

RESEARCH UTILIZATION PROJECTS AND MODELS FOR NURSING

During the last three decades, nursing has focused increased energy on the utilization of research in nursing practice. Two major projects that were undertaken to promote the adoption of innovations in nursing included: (1) the Western Interstate Commission for Higher Education (WICHE) regional nursing research development project and (2) the Conduct and Utilization of Research in Nursing (CURN) project. In these projects, nurse researchers, with the assistance of federal funding, designed and implemented strategies for using research in practice. The works of Rogers (1983) and Havelock (1970) were used as the frameworks for these projects. Two models have also been developed by nurses to promote the utilization of research findings in practice, the WICHE Project Model and the Stetler Model for Research Utilization. These research utilization projects and models are presented in this section.

WICHE

The WICHE project, initiated in the mid-1970s, was the first major nursing project to address research utilization in nursing. The 6-year project was directed by Krueger and colleagues (Krueger, 1978; Krueger, Nelson, & Wolanin, 1978) and was funded by the Division of Nursing. The initial goal of the project was to increase nursing research activities within the western region of the United States.

The WICHE project involved the development of the first model for the utilization of nursing research, the Five-Phase Resources Linkage Model (see Figure 25–4). This model was based on Havelock's linker system theory and focused on linking nursing resources with the users of research findings in practice. Phase 1 involved using resources, as outlined in Figure 25–4, to recruit members for the project and to prepare research-based materials. Phase 2 consisted of a workshop, where participants were organized into dyads composed of a nurse educator and clinician. The objective of the workshop was to help participants develop skills in critiquing research and applying utilization theory. Each dyad selected a research-based intervention they were willing to implement within an institution. The dyad was to function as

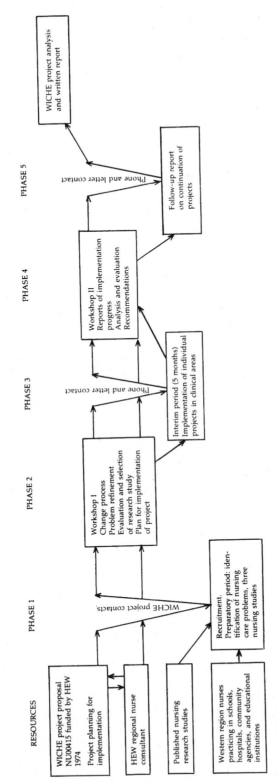

Figure 25–4

The five-phase resources linkage model. (Reprinted with permission from *Nursing Research: Development, Collaboration, and Utilization*, by J. C. Krueger, A. H. Nelson, and M. A. Wolanin, © 1978, Aspen Publishers, Inc.)

a change agent in Phase 3, when the utilization projects were implemented in the participants' agencies for 5 months. Phase 4 was a second workshop for reports, analysis, and evaluation of the project. Phase 5 was the follow-up report on continuation of the utilization projects 3 and 6 months later.

The project staff and participants had difficulty identifying clinical studies with findings appropriate to implement in practice. Findings that were identified tended to be merged with other activities by the dyad and then implemented as a package. Since the project staff expected the findings to be implemented in pure form, this strategy was viewed with disfavor. Three reports from this project were published: (1) Axford and Cutchen (1977) developed a preoperative teaching program; (2) Dracup and Breu (1978) devised a care plan for grieving spouses and tested its effectiveness; and (3) Wichita (1977) developed a program to treat and prevent constipation in nursing home residents by increasing the fiber in their diets.

CURN

The CURN project, directed by Horsley (Horsley, Crane, & Bingle, 1978; Horsley, Crane, Crabtree, & Wood, 1983), was awarded to the Michigan Nurses Association by the Division of Nursing. The 5-year (1975 to 1980) project was developed to increase the utilization of research findings by (1) disseminating findings, (2) facilitating organizational modifications necessary to implementation, and (3) encouraging collaborative research that was directly transferable to clinical practice. The theoretical base for this project included Rogers's theory of diffusion of innovations. Research utilization was seen as an organizational process rather than as a process to be implemented by an individual practitioner. The activities of the utilization process include: (1) the identification and synthesis of multiple research studies in a common conceptual area (research base); (2) the transformation of the knowledge derived from a research base into a solution or clinical protocol; (3) the transformation of the clinical

protocol into specific nursing actions (innovations) that are administered to patients; and (4) a clinical evaluation of the new practice to ascertain whether it produced the predicted result (Horsley et al., 1983, p. 2).

During this project, published clinical studies were critiqued for scientific merit, replication, and relevance to practice. The relevance of the research for practice involved examining (1) clinical merit or significance in addressing patient problems, (2) the extent to which the clinical control belonged to nursing, (3) feasibility of implementing a change in an agency, and (4) an analysis of the cost-benefit ratio. The following 10 areas were considered to have sufficient quality research to warrant implementation: (1) structured preoperative teaching, (2) reducing diarrhea in tube-fed patients, (3) preoperative sensory preparation to promote recovery, (4) preventing decubitus ulcers, (5) intravenous cannula change, (6) closed urinary drainage systems, (7) distress reduction through sensory preparation, (8) mutual goal setting in patient care, (9) clean intermittent catheterization, and (10) pain: deliberative nursing interventions (CURN Project, 1981, 1982).

Protocol Development and Implementation

The CURN project involved the development of protocols from research findings to implement and evaluate a change in practice (Horsley et al., 1983). Each protocol contained the following content: (1) identification of the practice problem and the need for change; (2) summary of the research base, including the limitations of the research; (3) design of the nursing practice innovation or intervention; (4) description of the research-based principle to guide the innovation; (5) description of the implementation of the innovation, the clinical trial; (6) evaluation of the effects of the innovation, including evaluation procedures and recording forms; and (7) summary and references. The protocols were implemented in clinical trials and evaluated for effectiveness. Based on the evaluations, a decision was made to reject, modify, or adopt the intervention (innovation). Strategies could then be developed to extend the innovation to other appropriate nursing practice settings (Horsley et al., 1983).

The CURN project was implemented on a test unit within a hospital. Outcomes from the implementation were evaluated using baseline data and comparison groups. Follow-up questionnaires were sent to the 17 participating hospitals for a 4-year period to determine the long-term impact of the implementation on the organization. Pelz and Horsley (1981) reported that prior to the project, research utilization was low in both comparison and experimental groups. One year after the intervention, significant differences were found, with experimental organizations having higher levels of utilization. The second year after the intervention, there were still differences between the groups, but differences were not significant for all 10 utilization activities. The third year, experimental units continued to perform the protocols. The rate of diffusion of the innovations to other units was not reported. The clinical protocols developed during the project were published (CURN Project, 1981, 1982). Today, the CURN project is a valuable strategy for teaching baccalaureate and master's students about using research findings in practice and for encouraging practicing nurses to use findings in practice.

STETLER MODEL OF RESEARCH UTILIZATION

An initial model of research utilization was developed by Stetler and Marram in 1976 and expanded by Stetler in 1994. The Stetler Model for Research Utilization (see Figure 25-5 on pp. 684-685) provides a comprehensive framework to enhance the use of research findings by nurses. The use of research findings can be at the institutional or individual level. At the institutional level, study findings are synthesized and the knowledge generated is used to develop or refine policy, procedures, protocols, or other formal programs implemented in the institution. Individual nurses, such as practitioners, educators, and policymakers, summarize

research and use the knowledge to influence educational programs, make practice decisions, and impact political decision making. The Stetler Model of Research Utilization is included in this text to promote the use of research findings by individuals and institutions. The phases of the Stetler model presented below include (1) preparation, (2) validation, (3) comparative evaluation, (4) decision making, (5) translation/application, and (6) evaluation.

Phase I: Preparation

The intent of Stetler's model is to make using research findings in practice a conscious, critical thinking process that is initiated by the user. Thus, the first phase involves determination of the purpose and focus of the research review. The research literature might be reviewed to solve a difficult clinical, managerial, or educational problem; to provide the basis for a policy, standard, or protocol; or to prepare for an in-service program or other type of professional presentation. Sometimes the literature is reviewed just so the nurse is kept current with the new content in a specialty area.

Phase II: Validation

In the validation phase, the research reports are critiqued to determine their scientific soundness. If the studies are limited in number and/or are weak, then findings and conclusions are considered inadequate and the utilization process stops. If the research knowledge base is strong in the selected area, the decision must be made if the findings are applicable or useful for the institution or individual conducting the utilization project. Thus, the purpose of the utilization project is examined in light of the research findings and a decision made either to or not to proceed to Phase III.

Phase III: Comparative Evaluation

Comparative evaluation includes four parts: substantiating evidence, fit of setting, feasibility, and

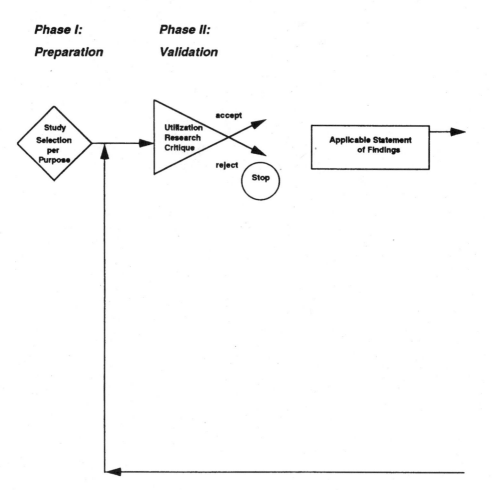

Figure 25-5
Stetler Model for Research Utilization. (From Stetler, C. B. [1994]. Refinement of the Stetler/Marram Model for application of research findings to practice. *Nursing Outlook 42*[1], 18–19, with permission.)

current practice. Substantiating evidence exists with replication, in which consistent findings are obtained from studies in similar settings. In addition, substantial knowledge for change can be obtained from clinical articles, textbooks, theories, and standards and guidelines from professional organizations (Stetler, 1994). To determine the fit with the setting, the characteristics of the setting are examined to determine the forces that will facilitate or inhibit the implementation of the research findings. The feasibility of using research findings in practice involves examining the three

Rs related to making changes in practice: (1) potential risks, (2) resources needed, and (3) readiness of those involved. The final comparison involves determining if the research information provides a basis for making changes in the current practice. Thus, the research knowledge needs to promote increased quality in the current practice by solving practice problems and improving patient outcomes. By conducting Phase III, the overall benefits and risks of using the research base in a practice setting can be assessed. If the benefits are much greater than the risks for the organiza-

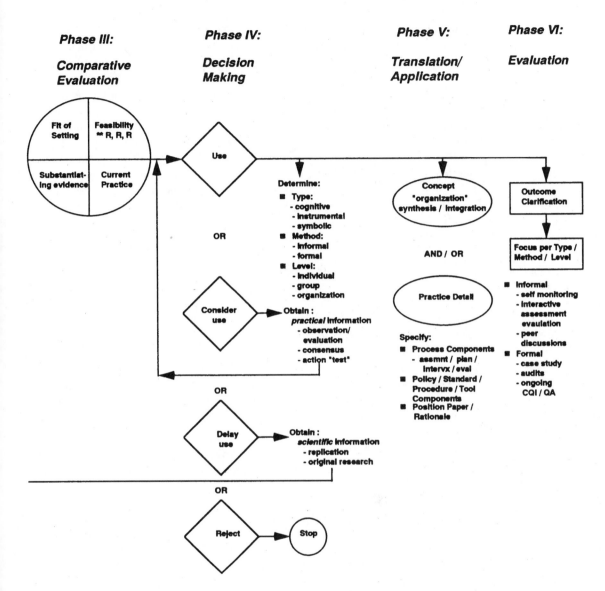

tion and/or the individual nurse, then using the research findings to change practice is feasible.

Phase IV: Decision Making

Four types of decisions are possible during this phase: to use the findings, to consider using the findings, to delay using the findings, and to reject or not use the findings. The use of the research findings can be cognitive, instrumental, or symbolic (see Figure 25–5). With cognitive application, the research base is a means of modifying a way of thinking or one's appreciation of an issue (Stetler, 1994). Thus, cognitive application may improve the nurse's understanding of a situation, allow analysis of practice dynamics, or improve problem-solving skills for clinical problems. Instrument application involves using study findings to support the need for change in nursing interventions or practice protocols. For example, the findings from research on the use of self-regulatory interventions to decrease blood pressure might be implemented to change the care provided hypertensive patients (Massey & Loomis, 1988). Patients could be taught self-regulatory interventions such as progressive muscle relaxation (PMR), biofeedback, or transcendental meditation and then monitored for changes in their blood pressure. Symbolic or political utilization occurs when information is used to support or change a current policy.

Another decision might be to consider the use of available findings in practice. When a change is complex and involves multiple disciplines, additional time is often needed to determine how findings might be used and what measures will be taken to coordinate the involvement of different health professionals in the change. The use of findings can also be delayed until additional research is conducted or until agency personnel are ready to make changes in practice. A final option might be to reject or not use the findings in practice because the findings are not strong or the risks or costs of change to the current practice are too high.

Phase V: Translation/Application

The translation/application phase involves planning for and the actual implementation of the findings in practice. The translation phase involves determining exactly what knowledge will be used and how that knowledge will be applied to practice. The application phase includes the following steps for planned change: (1) assess the situation to be changed, (2) develop a plan for change, and (3) implement the plan. During the application phase, the protocols, policies, or procedures developed with research knowledge are implemented in practice (Stetler, 1994).

Phase VI: Evaluation

The final stage in the research utilization process is to evaluate the impact of the research-based change on the health care agency, personnel, and patients. The evaluation process can include both formal and informal activities that are conducted by administrators, nurse clinicians, and other health professionals. The informal evaluations might include self-monitoring or discussions with patients, families, peers, and other professionals. The formal evaluations can include case study, audits, or quality assurance projects (Stetler, 1994).

Since utilization is an essential component of professional nursing practice, nurses need to seek the outcomes of current research, evaluate the research for use in practice, and modify practice based on this research. Utilization of research findings in practice needs to be continuous and considered the norm in an institution. Professional nurses could be viewed as knowledge-oriented rather than rule-oriented and could function as critical thinkers, using research to "more scientifically provide care, teach, and/or manage" (Stetler, 1985, p. 42). The Stetler Model for Research Utilization can provide direction to the practicing nurse and an organization to make the essential changes in practice based on research.

PROMOTING RESEARCH UTILIZATION IN NURSING

An examination of barriers to knowledge utilization and utilization theory provides a basis for encouraging you to summarize research and use the knowledge to change your practice. To assist you in conducting your first research utilization project, some strategies to facilitate research utilization are identified and an example research utilization project is presented using the steps in Rogers's (1983) Innovation-Decision Model.

STRATEGIES TO FACILITATE RESEARCH UTILIZATION

The lack of diffusion of research-based knowledge is a serious problem in nursing that has a number of facets and possible solutions. Educators, researchers, practitioners, and administrators need to collaborate in the application of a variety of strategies to increase the use of research knowledge to make essential changes in practice. Currently, many theses and dissertations are not being published and educators could provide more assistance to new graduates in publishing their works. The graduate receives first author and the chair of the thesis or dissertation committee receives second author credit. Educators might also encourage students to synthesize research in an area of interest and develop a protocol for implementation in practice. Doctorate students might be encouraged to conduct meta-analyses to synthesize research in selected areas of their dissertation.

Educating students about the research process and the use of findings in practice has expanded since an increasing number of faculty are doctorally prepared and involved in research. In addition, the conduct of research and the publication of studies have increasing support in academic settings, which has facilitated faculty research activities. However, not all nursing educators are providing sufficient research information to nursing students to allow them to make intelligent judgments about using research in practice. Students need a stronger background in utilization theory and guidance in developing and implementing research utilization projects.

Some researchers view the utilization problem as due to the inability of practitioners to read and comprehend research reports. Thus, a strategy to increase utilization is to translate research findings into a more popular form for publication in clinical practice journals. Although this idea has appeal, it also has some drawbacks. The clinician would have to accept the validity of the findings with little or no opportunity to evaluate the quality of the research or the degree of similarity between the study setting, the study sample, and the clinician's clinical situation. Another solution provided by some clinical practice journals is to have a special section for reporting recent research findings. These news items generally cite the research journal in which the original research report can be found; thus, the clinician can identify research that seems relevant and obtain the study for additional information. A publication, *Nursing Scan in Research: Application for Clinical Practice,* was developed to summarize findings for use in practice. The publication includes several studies from a variety of research and clinical journals. For each study, there is a complete citation, a synopsis of the study findings, a critique of the study, and ideas for clinical application of the findings.

Another effort to increase the communication between researcher and practitioner was the development of research journals for clinicians, such as *Applied Nursing Research* in 1988 and *Clinical Nursing Research* in 1992. The studies in these journals are presented in a format to promote the interest and understanding of practitioners. Some articles focus on summarizing research findings for use in practice. For example, Beyea and Nicoll (1995) conducted an integrative review of the literature and developed a research-based protocol for the administration of medications via the intramuscular route. This protocol is included in Appendix 25-A at the end of this chapter.

Practicing nurses could increase their use of research knowledge to improve patient outcomes. For example, practicing nurses might use research as a basis for evaluating products for purchase in an agency. Janken, Rudisill, and Benfield (1992) used research in evaluating a new product, a closed-system catheter for endotracheal suctioning of mechanically ventilated patients, for possible purchase. Practicing nurses could also evaluate and revise agency procedure manuals, standards of care, and nursing care plans so they are reflective of current nursing research-based knowledge. In the future, accrediting agencies for health care institutions will require that nursing care measures be documented with research. Many progressive nursing executives realize the importance of research and are hiring nurse researchers to increase the use of research findings in practice and to promote the conduct of relevant studies. Another helpful strategy is the publication of papers by clinicians reporting effective clinical use of research findings.

Administrators can facilitate the use of research in agencies by showing support for and rewarding activities to base nursing care on research. Champion and Leach (1989) studied three variables related to research utilization in nursing: (1) availability of research findings, (2) attitude toward use of findings in practice, and (3) the perceived support for using findings. Attitude ($r = 0.55$) and availability ($r = 0.52$) were strongly correlated with research utilization. In addition, key administrative persons such as the unit director ($r = 0.35$, $p = 0.004$), chairperson ($r = 0.32$, $p = 0.02$), and director of nursing ($r = 0.44$, $p = 0.001$) can significantly influence research utilization. Additional research is needed to determine the variables that motivate nurses to use research findings in practice and those that facilitate the utilization process.

UTILIZATION STRATEGIES FROM THE NATIONAL INSTITUTE FOR NURSING RESEARCH (NINR)

The NINR has identified research utilization as one of its main priorities. National and regional conferences are being held and a variety of utilization projects are being funded to promote research utilization. The NINR funded a project to "facilitate the use of research in clinical settings by providing findings that are relevant and ready to use, in a form that maintains the richness of full research reports yet is still understandable to the general reader, and that provides suggestions for implementation and further clinical evaluation, opportunities for dialogue between researcher and clinician, and support and consultation during implementation" (Funk, Tornquist, & Champagne, 1989a, p. 363). Three mechanisms were used for research dissemination: "(1) topic-focused, practice-oriented research conferences; (2) related, broadly distributed, carefully edited volumes based on the conference presentations; and (3) an information center to provide ongoing dialogue, support, and consultation" (Funk, Tornquist, & Champagne, 1989b, p. 486).

CLINICAL PRACTICE GUIDELINES

The federal government has long recognized the importance of research utilization and has been concerned about the delay between the discovery of new knowledge and the use of that knowledge by society. In 1989, the Agency for Health Care Policy and Research (AHCPR), within the U.S. Department of Health and Human Services (DHHS), convened panels of expert health care providers and researchers to summarize research and develop clinical practice guidelines. These panels summarized research findings and developed guidelines for practice in the following areas:

1. *Acute pain management in infants, children, and adolescents: Operative and medical procedures*
2. *Pressure ulcers in adults: Predication and prevention*
3. *Urinary incontinence in adults*
4. *Cataracts in adults: Management of functional impairment*
5. *Depression in primary care:* Volume 1. *Detection and diagnosis* and Volume 2. *Treatment of major depression*
6. *Sickle cell disease: Screening, diagnosis, management, and counseling in newborns and infants*
7. *Evaluation and management of early HIV infection*
8. *Benign prostatic hyperplasia: Diagnosis and treatment*
9. *Management of cancer-related pain*
10. *Diagnosis and treatment of heart failure*
11. *Low back problems*
12. *Otitis media in children*
13. *Post-stroke rehabilitation*
14. *Screening for Alzheimer's and related dementias*
15. *Chest pain due to unstable angina*
16. *Treatment of pressure ulcers in adults*
17. *Quality determinants of mammography*
18. *Cardiac rehabilitation services*

These clinical practice guidelines provide clear directives to practitioners in managing a variety of acute and chronic conditions. The intent of the guidelines is to promote quality health care that will improve patient outcomes. The clinical practice guidelines are published in documents that are free on request from the DHHS. For each practice guideline, there is also a quick reference guide for clinicians and a patient guide. These documents can be obtained by calling (800) 358–9295 or by writing to the following address:

AHCPR Clearinghouse
P. O. Box 8547
Silver Spring, MD 20907

EXAMPLE RESEARCH UTILIZATION PROJECT

Preparing to conduct a utilization project usually raises some important questions. Which research findings are ready for use in clinical practice? How can you use these findings to improve your practice? What are the most effective strategies for implementing findings in practice? We suggest that effective strategies for using research findings will require a multifaceted approach, taking into consideration research findings, practicing nurses, and the organizations within which nursing functions. In this section, an example of research utilization is presented using Rogers's (1983) five-stage process: (1) knowledge, (2) persuasion, (3) decision, (4) implementation, and (5) confirmation (see Figure 25–1). Research knowledge about the effects of heparin flush versus saline flush for irrigating peripheral heparin locks is evaluated for use in nursing practice. Using this research knowledge, a protocol is developed to promote the use of these findings in practice.

Knowledge

The body of nursing research must be evaluated for scientific merit and clinical relevance; then the current findings need to be integrated in preparation for use in practice (Massey & Loomis, 1988; Mateo & Kirchhoff, 1991; Stetler, 1985; Tanner, 1987). The integration of findings from scientifically sound research is referred to as *cognitive clustering*.

Evaluation for Scientific Merit

The scientific merit of nursing studies is evaluated by criteria such as (1) conceptualization and internal consistency or logical links of a study; (2) methodological rigor or the strength of the design, sample, instruments, and data collection and analysis processes; (3) generalizability of the findings or the representativeness of the sample and setting; and (4) the number of replications of the study (Tanner & Lindeman, 1989). The critique steps in Chapter 24 can be used to evaluate the scientific merit of quantitative and qualitative research.

Evaluation of Clinical Relevance

The nature and scope of research utilization are evaluated by determining clinical relevance. Research-based knowledge might be used to solve practice problems, to enhance clinical judgment, or to measure phenomena in clinical practice. The scope of utilization might be a single patient care unit, a hospital, or all hospitals in a corporation. A risk-benefit analysis is needed to determine the impact of the proposed change on the clinical setting. The practitioner desiring to implement an innovation must be able to assure the agency that the cost in time, energy, and money, and any real or potential risks are outweighed by the benefits of the innovation (Tanner & Lindeman, 1989).

Cognitive Clustering

The research on a topic needs to be examined and clustered to determine what is currently known. These activities of cognitive clustering are accomplished through integrative reviews and meta-analyses of nursing research. The importance of cognitive clustering is evident by the increasing number of integrative reviews of nursing research that are being published. Ganong (1987) proposed that "integrative reviews should be held to the same standards of clarity, rigor, and replication as primary research" (p. 1). He compared 17 reviews from nursing journals and proposed the following steps for the review process: "(1) Formulate the purpose of the review and develop related questions to be answered by the review or hypotheses to be tested, (2) establish tentative criteria for inclusion of studies in the review such that as data are gathered criteria may be changed on substantive or methodological grounds, (3) conduct a literature search making sampling decisions if the number of studies located is large, (4) develop a questionnaire with which to gather data from studies, (5) identify rules of inference to be used in data analyses and interpretation, (6) revise criteria for inclusion in the questionnaire as needed, (7) read the studies using the questionnaire to gather data, (8) analyze data in a systematic fashion, (9) discuss and interpret data, and (10) report the review as clearly and completely as possible" (pp. 10–11).

Pillemer and Light (1980) suggest that nursing must go beyond critique and integration of research findings to conducting statistical analyses on the outcomes of similar studies. This type of analysis is referred to as *meta-analysis*. Meta-analysis can be used "to integrate and synthesize findings from completed studies to determine what is known about a particular subject area" (Massey & Loomis, 1988, p. 32). This approach allows the application of scientific criteria to such factors as sample size, level of significance, and variables examined. Through the use of meta-analysis, the following can be generated:

1. the determination of the overall significance of probability of pooled data from confirmed studies;
2. the average of the effect size indicating the degree to which the null hypothesis is false, or the degree to which the phenomenon is present in the population; and
3. the relationship between variables (Hunt, 1987, pp. 104–105).

Meta-analyses make it possible to be objective rather than subjective in evaluating research findings. This objectivity makes it possible to determine the usefulness of findings for practice. Massey and Loomis (1988) developed a coding form to be used in gathering data for a meta-analysis

(see Table 25–2). This form could be used to conduct a meta-analysis on research findings to determine their usefulness for practice. Several integrative reviews and meta-analyses conducted on nursing research are listed in the Student Study Guide that accompanies this textbook.

Goode et al. (1991, p. 324) conducted a meta-analysis "to estimate the effects of heparin flush and saline flush solutions on maintaining patency, preventing phlebitis, and increasing duration of peripheral heparin locks." The meta-analysis was conducted on 17 quality studies that are described in Table 25–3 (on p. 692). The total sample size of the 17 studies was 4,153 and the settings of these studies was a variety of medical-surgical and critical care units. The small effect size values (most are less than .20) for clotting, phlebitis, and duration indicate that saline flush is as effective as heparin flush in maintaining peripheral heparin locks. Goode et al. (1991) summarized the current knowledge on the use of saline versus heparin.

"It can be concluded that saline is as effective as heparin in maintaining patency, preventing phlebitis, and increasing duration in peripheral intravenous locks. Quality of care can be enhanced by using saline as the flush solution, thereby eliminating problems associated with anticoagulant effects and drug incompatibilities. In addition, an estimated yearly savings of $109,100,000 to $218,200,000 U.S. health care dollars could be attained." (p. 324) ∎

The meta-analysis provides a sound scientific basis for making a change in practice. The clinical relevance is evident since the use of saline to flush heparin locks promotes quality of care and extensive cost savings.

If you plan on making this change in your practice setting, you need to examine the following prior conditions: (1) previous practice, (2) felt/needs or problems, (3) innovativeness, and (4) norms of the social system (Rogers, 1983). Does your institution currently use heparin, not saline, to irrigate their heparin locks? Do the nurses be-

Table 25–2
Coding Form for a Meta-Analysis

I. Description
Topic area
Study ID number
Publication date _____
Source
    Journal, nursing
    Journal, non-nursing (area)
    Thesis, doctoral; master's nursing
    Thesis, doctoral; master's non-nursing (area)
    Other (specify)
Highest level of preparation of primary author
    Doctoral   Master's
    Baccalaureate   Other (specify)
Area of interest
    Nursing   Education
    Psychology   Social work
    Medicine   Psychiatry
    Health education   Religion
    Other (specify)

II. Study characteristics
Design
    Descriptive   Correlational
    Experimental   Quasi-experimental
Appears representative of population?
    Yes   No
Medical diagnosis or treatment (ICDA)
Sample size (N)
Treatment group size (n)
Control group size (n)
Sex of subjects
    Male   Female
    Both
Age range of subjects
Mean age of subjects
Developmental level of subjects
    Infant   Child
    Adolescent   Young adult
    Middle-aged adult
    Geriatric   Mixed (specify)
    Other (specify)
Subject assignment to treatment
    Random   Matching
    Nonrandom

III. Intervention
Type of treatment (specify)
Special equipment with treatment condition (specify)
Treatment provider
    Nurse   Psychiatrist
    Educator   Health educator
    Psychologist   Religious
    Physician   Other (specify)
Treatment provider assignment
    Random   Single provider
    Matched   Other (specify)
    Nonrandom
Treatment duration
Number of treatments

Type of control
    Usual care   Other (specify)
    Placebo

IV. Validity
Internal
    High
    Medium
    Low
External
    High
    Medium
    Low
Number of threats
Percentage subject mortality treatment group
Percentage subject mortality control group

V. Reliability of Dependent Variables
Reliability (specify type)
    High
    Medium
    Low
Number of comparisons in study
Dependent variables (list)
Dependent variable of concern (name and code)
Type of measure
    Physiological   Psychological
Standardized
    Yes   No
Independent variables (other than treatment)
    of concern (name and code)
Reactivity of measure
    Very low   High
    Low   Very high
    Medium

VI. Overall Quality of Study
Significance of treatment effect
    $p < .01$ Nonsignificant
    $0.01 < p < .05$ $-0.01 < p < -0.5$
    $0.5 < p < .10$
Control group mean ($\bar{X}_c$)
Control group standard deviation: (S_c)
Treatment group mean ($\bar{X}_e$)
Treatment group standard deviation: (S_e)
Effect size calculation:

$$ES = \frac{\bar{X}_e - \bar{X}_c}{S}$$

$$S = \sqrt{\frac{(n^e - 1)(S^e)^2 + (n^c - 1)(S^c)^2}{n^e + n^c - 2}}$$

(From Massey, J., & Loomis, M. [1988]. When should nurses use research findings? *Applied Nursing Research, 1*[1], 34–35, with permission.)

Table 25-3
Studies Included in the Meta-Analysis

Study	N	Subjects	Assignment	Heparin Dose	Clotting Effect size (d_c)	Phlebitis Effect size (d_p)	Duration Effect size (d_d)
Ashton et al., 1990	16 exp$_c$ 16 con$_c$ 13 exp$_p$ 14 con$_p$	Adult critical care	Random double blind	10/u/cc	.3590	−.1230	
Barrett et al., 1990	59 experimental 50 control	Adult Med-Surg patients	Nonrandom double blind crossover	10/u/cc	−.1068	−.4718	
Craig & Anderson, 1991	129 exp 145 con	Adult Med-Surg patients	Random double blind crossover	10/u/cc	.0095	−.0586	
Cyganski et al., 1987	225 exp 196 con	Adult Med-Surg patients	Nonrandom	100/u/cc	.2510		
Donhan & Denning, 1987	8 exp$_c$ 4 con$_c$ 7 exp$_p$ 5 con$_p$	Adult critical care	Random double blind	10/u/cc	.0000	.0548	
Dunn & Lenihan, 1987	61 experimental 51 control	Adult patients	Nonrandom	50/u/cc	−.2057	−.2258	
Epperson, 1984	138 exp 120 con 138 exp 154 con	Adult Med-Surg patients	Random double blind	10/u/cc 100/u/cc			−.1176 −.1232
Garrelts et al., 1989	131 exp 173 con	Adult Med-Surg patients	Random double blind	10/u/cc	−.1773	.1057	.2753
Hamilton et al., 1988	137 exp 170 con	Adult patients	Random double blind	100/u/cc	.0850	−.1819	−.0604
Holford et al., 1977	39 experimental 140 control	Young adult volunteers	Nonrandom double blind	3.3, 10, 16.5 100, 132/u/cc	.6545		
Kasparek et al., 1988	49 exp 50 con	Adult Med patients	Random double blind	10/u/cc	.3670	−.5430	
Lombardi et al., 1988	34 experimental 40 control	Pediatric patients (4 wks to 18 yrs)	Nonrandom sequential double blind	10/u/cc		−.2324	.0000
Miracle et al., 1989	167 exp 441 con	Adult Med-Surg patients	Nonrandom	100/u/cc	−.0042		
Shearer, 1987	87 exp 73 con	Med-Surg patients	Nonrandom	10/u/cc	−.1170	−.0977	
Spann, 1988	15 experimental 19 control	Adult telemetry step down	Nonrandom double blind	10/u/cc	−.3163	−.3252	
Taylor et al., 1989	369 exp 356 con	Adult Med-Surg patients	Nonrandom time series	10/u/cc	.0308	.0288	−.1472
Tuten & Gueldner, 1991	43 exp 71 con	Adult Med-Surg patients	Nonrandom	100/u/cc	.0000	.1662	

(From Goode, C. J., et al. [1991]. A meta-analysis of effects of heparin flush and saline flush: Quality and cost implications. *Nursing Research, 40*[6], 325.)

lieve this is a problem? You need to highlight the problems with heparin that have been identified in the research literature. Are the nurses innovative and willing to change or are they very resistant to change? Which nurses might be most helpful in assisting with the change? You also need to talk with your administrator about the change. Is the administration in your agency open or resistant to change?

Persuasion

During the persuasion stage of the research utilization process, you want to encourage the adminis-

tration and other nurses to change current practice. Persuasion might be accomplished by demonstrating the relative advantage, compatibility, complexity, trialability, and observability of changing from heparin to saline as a flush solution (see Figure 25–1). The relative advantages of using saline are the improved quality of care and cost savings that are clearly documented in the research literature (Goode et al., 1991; Shoaf & Oliver, 1992). The cost savings for different sizes of hospitals is summarized in Table 25–4. The compatibility of the change can be determined by identifying the changes that will need to occur in your agency. What changes will the nurses have to make in irri-

Table 25–4
Annual Cost Savings from Changing to Saline

Study	Cost Savings	Hospital
Craig & Anderson, 1991	$40,000/yr	525-bed tertiary care hospital
Dunn & Lenihan, 1987	$19,000/yr	530-bed private hospital
Goode et al., 1991 (this study)	$38,000/yr	879-bed tertiary care hospital
Kasparek et al., 1988	$19,000/yr	350-bed private hospital
Lombardi et al., 1988	$20,000–$25,000/yr	52-bed pediatric unit
Schustek, 1984	$20,000/yr	391-bed private hospital
Taylor et al., 1989	$30,000–$40,000/yr	216-bed private hospital

(From Goode, C. J., et al. [1991]. A meta-analysis of effects of heparin flush and saline flush: Quality and cost implications. *Nursing Research, 40*[6], 328.)

gating heparin locks with saline? What changes will have to occur in the pharmacy to provide the saline flush? Are the physicians aware of the research in this area? Are the physicians willing to order the use of saline to flush the heparin locks?

The change of peripheral heparin lock irrigant from heparin flush to saline flush has minimal complexity. The only thing changed is the flush, so no additional skills, expertise, or time is required by the nurse to make the change. Since saline flush, unlike heparin flush, is compatible with any drug that might be administered through the heparin lock, the number of potential complications are decreased. The change might be started on one unit as a clinical trial and then evaluated. Once the quality of care and cost savings become observable to the nurses, physicians, and hospital administrators, the change will probably spread rapidly throughout the institution. Persuasion is strong to change irrigants from heparin flush to saline flush, because the advantages are extensive and there are no identified disadvantages. This change is also compatible with existing nursing care and would be relatively simple to implement on a trial basis to demonstrate the positive outcomes for patients, nurses, and the health care agency.

Decision

The decision to use saline flush versus heparin flush as an irrigant requires institutional approval, physician approval, and approval of the nurses managing patients' heparin locks. When a change requires institutional approval, decision making may be distributed through several levels of the organization. Thus, a decision at one level may lead to contact with another official who must approve the action. In keeping with the guidelines of planned change, institutional changes are more likely to be effective if all those affected by the change have a voice in the decision. In your institution, who needs to approve the change? What steps do you need to take to get the change approved within your institution? Do the physicians support the change? Do the nurses on the units support the change? Who are the leaders in the institution and can you get them to support the change? Try to get the nurses to make a commitment and take a public stand to make the change, because this increases the probability that they will make the change. Contact the appropriate administrative people and physicians and detail the pros and cons of making the change to saline flush for irrigating heparin locks. You need to clearly indicate to the physicians and administrators that the change is based on extensive research findings. Most physicians are positively influenced by research-based knowledge.

Implementation

Implementing a research-based change can be simple or complex, depending on the change. The change might be implemented as indicated in the research literature or may be modified to meet the agency's needs. In some cases, a long time might be spent in planning the implementation after the decision is made. In other cases, implementation can begin immediately. Usually, a great deal of support is needed during initial implementation of a change. As with any new activity, unexpected events often occur. The nurse adopter frequently does not know how to interpret these events. Contact with a person experienced in the change can make the difference between continuation and rejection of the innovation.

The change from heparin flush to saline flush will involve the physicians ordering saline for flushing heparin locks. You will need to speak with the physicians to gain their support for the change. You might convince some key physicians to support the change and they will convince others to make the change. The pharmacy will have to package saline for use as an irrigant. The nurses will also be provided information about the change and the rationale for the change. It might be best to implement the change on one nursing unit and give the nurses on this unit an opportunity to design the protocol and plan for implementing the change. The nurses might develop a protocol similar to the one in Figure 25–6. This protocol

directs you in preparing for irrigating a heparin lock, irrigating the heparin lock, and documenting your actions.

Confirmation

After a change has been implemented in practice, the nurses who implemented the change need to confirm or document the effectiveness of the change. They need to document that the change improved quality of care, decreased the cost of care, and/or saved nursing time. If the outcomes from the change in practice are positive, nurses, administrators, and physicians will often want to continue the change. Nurses usually seek feedback from those around them. Their peers' reactions to the change in nursing practice will influence the continuation of the change. If the peers approve, the nurses will often adopt the change and even encourage others to do the same. If the peers disapprove or provide negative feedback, the nurses will often abandon the change.

You can confirm the effectiveness of the saline flush for peripheral heparin lock irrigation by ex-

1. Obtain the saline flush for irrigation from the pharmacy.
2. Wash hands, collect equipment for irrigating the heparin lock, and put on gloves.
3. Cleanse the heparin lock with alcohol prior to injection with saline solution.
4. Flush the peripheral heparin lock with 1 mL of normal saline every 8 hours (Goode et al., 1991; Shoaf & Oliver, 1992).
5. If a patient is on IV medication, administer 1 mL of saline, administer the medication, and follow with 1 mL of saline (Shoaf & Oliver, 1992).
6. Check the peripheral heparin lock site for complications of phlebitis or loss of patency. The symptoms of phlebitis include presence of erythema, tenderness, warmth, and tender or palpable cord. Loss of patency is indicated by resistance to flushing, "as evidenced by inability to administer 1 mL of flushing solution within 30 seconds" (Shoaf & Oliver, 1992).
7. Chart the time the peripheral heparin lock was irrigated with saline and any complications of phlebitis or loss of patency.

FIGURE 25–6

Protocol for irrigating peripheral heparin locks. (From Goode, C. J., Titler, M., Rakel, B., Ones, D. S., Kleiber, C., Small, S., & Triolo, P. K. [1991]. A meta-analysis of effects of heparin flush and saline flush: Quality and cost implications. *Nursing Research, 40*[6], 324–330 and Shoaf, J., & Oliver, S. [1992]. Efficacy of normal saline injection with and without heparin for maintaining intermittent intravenous site. *Applied Nursing Research, 5*[1], 9–12.)

amining patient care outcomes and cost benefits. Patient care outcomes can be examined by determining the number of clotting and phlebitis complications with peripheral heparin locks one month before the change and one month after the change. If there is no significant difference, this supports the use of saline flush. The cost saving can be calculated for one month by determining the cost difference between heparin flush and saline flush. This cost difference can then be multiplied by the number of saline flushes conducted in one month. This cost savings can then be multiplied by 12 months and compared with the cost savings summarized in Table 25–4. If positive patient outcomes and cost savings are demonstrated,

the adoption of saline flush for irrigating peripheral heparin locks will probably continue and be used by all nurses in the agency.

In the future, accrediting agencies for health care organizations will require protocols for nursing interventions to be documented with research. The procedure manuals, standards of care, and nursing care plans will need to reflect current nursing research. Many progressive nurse executives realize the importance of research and are encouraging their nursing staff to use research findings in their practice. However, to effectively improve nursing practice with research knowledge, research utilization must become a priority for all nurses.

SUMMARY

Most people believe that a good idea will sell itself. Unfortunately, this is seldom true. Even today, research findings that clearly warrant utilization are not being used. Nurses need to understand the process of research utilization and develop strategies to achieve this process. Two important theories in the area of research utilization are Rogers's theory of diffusion of innovations and Havelock's theory of linker systems. Rogers is an expert and noted theorist in the field of knowledge diffusion and utilization. He has conducted research related to diffusion for 25 years, and his theory is a synthesis of the findings from his research. The main elements of diffusion are innovation, communication channels, time, and social system. Rogers conceptualized the innovation-decision process as consisting of five stages: (1) knowledge, (2) persuasion, (3) decision, (4) implementation, and (5) confirmation. The types of utilization identified by Rogers include direct application, reinvention, and indirect effects.

Havelock added a new dimension to utilization theory by proposing the development of a linker system. This linker system is used to

transfer new knowledge, skills, or products (innovations) from resource systems (researchers and their publications) to user systems (practitioners) for dissemination. Both theories focus on change and describe the use of a change agent external to the system to initiate and facilitate the change process.

Two federally funded projects that were developed to increase utilization of nursing research findings include the WICHE Regional Program for Nursing Research Development and the Conduct and Utilization of Research in Nursing (CURN) Project. Rogers's and Havelock's theories were used as the theoretical frameworks for these projects. The WICHE project was the first major nursing project to address research utilization. This project focused on critiquing research, using change theory, and diffusing innovations. The CURN Project was developed to increase the utilization of research findings in the following ways: dissemination of findings, facilitating organizational modifications necessary to implementation, and encouraging collaborative research that was directly transferable to clin-

continued

continued

ical practice. Clinical studies were critiqued, protocols were developed from the findings, and implementation was initiated on test units within hospitals.

The Stetler/Marram model was developed in 1976 and refined by Stetler in 1994 to direct utilization of nursing research. In this model, utilization includes critical thinking and a series of judgmental activities that occur in phases. The phases of the revised Stetler Model for Research Utilization are: (1) preparation, (2) validation, (3) comparative evaluation, (4) decision making, (5) translation/application, and (6) evaluation. The activities of each phase are identified in the model and can be used to critique and cluster findings for use in practice; direct the use of findings in practice; and evaluate the impact of the research knowledge on the practice setting, personnel, and patients.

Strategies are identified for educators, researchers, practitioners, and administrators to promote research utilization. Educators might encourage students to synthesize research in an area of interest and develop a protocol for implementation in practice. Researchers might publish findings in a way that facilitate the understanding of practitioners. The practicing nurse needs to seek outcomes of current research, evaluate their potential for practice, and modify practice with new knowledge. Administrators can facilitate the use of research in agencies by showing support for and rewarding activities to base nursing care on research. The NINR has identified research utilization as one of its main priorities. The AHCPR organized panels of expert health care providers and researchers to summarize research and develop clinical practice guidelines. For each topic, a clinical practice guideline book, quick reference guide for clinicians, and patient guide have been developed. These clinical practice guidelines provide clear directives to practitioners in managing a variety of acute and chronic conditions. The chapter concludes with an example research utilization project that is presented using Rogers's five decision-making steps: knowledge, persuasion, decision, implementation, and confirmation.

References

Ashton, J., Gibson, V., & Summers, S. (1990). Effects of heparin versus saline solution on intermittent infusion device irrigation. *Heart & Lung, 19*(6), 608–612.

Axford, R., & Cutchen, L. (1977). Using nursing research to improve preoperative care. *Journal of Nursing Administration, 7*(10), 16–20.

Barrett, P. J., & Lester, R. L. (1990). Heparin versus saline flush solutions in a small community hospital. *Hospital Pharmacy, 25,* 115–118.

Beecroft, P. C., & Redick, S. A. (1989). Possible complications of intramuscular injections on the pediatric unit. *Pediatric Nursing, 15,* 333–336, 376.

Beecroft, P. C., & Redick, S. A. (1990). Intramuscular injection practices of pediatric nurses: Site selection. *Nurse Educator, 15*(4), 23–28.

Belanger-Annable, M. C. (1985). Long acting neuroleptics: Technique for intramuscular injection. *The Canadian Nurse, 81*(8), 41–44.

Berger, K. J., & Williams, M. B. (1992). *Fundamentals of nursing: Collaborating for optimal health.* Norwalk, CT: Appleton & Lange.

Beyea, S. C., & Nicoll, L. H. (1995). Administration of medications via the intramuscular route: An integrative review of the literature and research-based protocol for the procedure. *Applied Nursing Research, 8*(1), 23–33.

Bock, L. R. (1990). From research to utilization: Bridging the gap. *Nursing Management, 21*(3), 50–51.

Brandt, P. A., Smith, M. E., Ashburn, S. S., & Graves, J. (1972). IM injections in children. *American Journal of Nursing, 72*(7), 1402–1406.

Brett, J. L. (1987). Use of nursing practice research findings. *Nursing Research, 36*(6), 344–349.

Centers for Disease Control. (1985). Recommendation of the Immunization Practices Advisory Committee. Diphtheria, Tetanus and Pertussis: Guidelines for vaccine prophylaxis and other preventive measures. *Morbidity and Mortality Weekly Report, 34*(27), 405–426.

Champion, V. L., & Leach, A. (1989). Variables related to research utilization in nursing: An empirical investigation. *Journal of Advanced Nursing, 14*(9), 705–710.

Chaplin, G., Shull, H., & Welk, P. C. (1985). How safe is the air-bubble technique for I.M. injections? *Nursing85,* 6–7.

Conduct and Utilization of Research in Nursing (CURN) Project. (1981–1982). *Using research to improve nursing practice.* New York: Grune & Stratton. [Series of clinical protocols: *Clean intermittent catheterization* (1982),

Closed urinary drainage systems (1981), *Distress reduction through sensory preparation* (1981), *Intravenous cannula change* (1981), *Mutual goal setting in patient care* (1982), *Pain: Deliberative nursing interventions* (1982), *Preventing decubitus ulcers* (1981), *Reducing diarrhea in tube-fed patients* (1981), *Structured preoperative teaching* (1981).]

Coyle, L. A., & Sokop, A. G. (1990). Innovation adoption behavior among nurses. *Nursing Research, 39*(3), 176–180.

Craig, F. D., & Anderson, S. R. (1991). *A comparison of normal saline versus heparinized normal saline in the maintenance of intermittent infusion devices.* Manuscript submitted for publication.

Cyganski, J. M., Donahue, J. M., & Heaton, J. S. (1987). The case for the heparin flush. *American Journal of Nursing, 86*(6), 796–797.

Daly, J. M., Johnston, W., & Chung, Y. (1992). Injection sites utilized for DPT immunizations in infants. *Journal of Community Health Nursing, 9*(2), 87–94.

Davies, A. R., Doyle, M. A. T., Lansky, D., Rutt, W., Stevic, M. O., & Doyle, J. B. (1994). Outcome assessments in clinical settings: A consensus statement on principles and best practices in project management. *The Joint Commission Journal on Quality Improvement, 20*(1), 6–16.

Donham, J., & Denning, V. (1987). Heparin vs. saline in maintaining patency intermittent infusion devices: Pilot study. *The Kansas Nurse, 62*(11), 6–7.

Dracup, K. A., & Breu, C. S. (1978). Using nursing research findings to meet the needs of grieving spouses. *Nursing Research, 27*(4), 212–216.

Dunn, D. L., & Lenihan, S. F. (1987). The case for the saline flush. *American Journal of Nursing, 87*(6), 798–799.

Epperson, E. L. (1984). Efficacy of 0.9% sodium chloride injection with and without heparin for maintaining indwelling intermittent injection sites. *Clinical Pharmacy, 3,* 626–629.

Farley, F., Joyce, N., Long, B., & Roberts, R. (1986). Will that IM needle reach the muscle? *American Journal of Nursing, 86*(12), 1327–1328.

Funk, S. G., Champagne, M. T., Tornquist, E. M., & Wiese, R. A. (1995). Administrators' views on barriers to research utilization. *Applied Nursing Research, 8*(1), 44–49.

Funk, S. G., Champagne, M. T., Wiese, R. A., & Tornquist, E. M. (1991). BARRIERS: The barriers research utilization scale. *Applied Nursing Research, 4*(1), 39–45.

Funk, S. G., Tornquist, E. M., & Champagne, M. T. (1989a). A model for improving the dissemination of nursing research. *Western Journal of Nursing Research, 11*(3), 361–367.

Funk, S. G., Tornquist, E. M., & Champagne, M. T. (1989b). Application and evaluation of the dissemination model. *Western Journal of Nursing Research, 11*(4), 486–491.

Ganong, L. H. (1987). Integrative reviews of nursing research. *Research in Nursing & Health, 10*(1), 1–11.

Garrelts, J., LaRocca, J., Ast, D., Smith, D. F., & Sweet, D. E. (1989). Comparison of heparin and 0.9% sodium chloride injection in the maintenance of indwelling intermittent I.V. devices. *Clinical Pharmacy, 8*(1), 34–39.

Glaser, E. M., Abelson, H. H., & Garrison, K. N. (1983). *Putting knowledge to use.* San Francisco: Jossey-Bass.

Goode, C. J., Titler, M., Rakel, B., Ones, D. S., Kleiber, C., Small, S., & Triolo, P. K. (1991). A meta-analysis of effects of heparin flush and saline flush: Quality and cost implications. *Nursing Research, 40*(6), 324–330.

Hahn, K. (1990). Brush up on your injection technique. *Nursing90, 20*(9), 54–58.

Hahn, K. (1991). Extra points on injections (letter). *Nursing91, 21*(1), 6.

Hamilton, R. A., Plis, J. M., Clay, C., & Sylvan, L. (1988). Heparin sodium versus 0.9% sodium chloride injection for maintaining patency of indwelling intermittent infusion devices. *Clinical Pharmacy, 7*(6), 439–443.

Havelock, R. G. (1970). *A guide to innovation in education.* Ann Arbor, MI: Center for Research on Utilization of Scientific Knowledge, Institute for Social Research, University of Michigan.

Havelock, R. G. (1973). *The change agent's guide to innovation in education.* Englewood Cliffs, NJ: Educational Technology Publications.

Havelock, R. G. (1974). *Ideal systems for research utilization: Four alternatives.* Washington, DC: Social and Rehabilitation Service, U.S. Department of Health, Education & Welfare.

Havelock, R. G., & Havelock, M. C. (1973). *Training for change agents: A guide to the design of training programs in education and other fields.* Ann Arbor, MI: Center for Research on Utilization of Scientific Knowledge, Institute for Social Research, University of Michigan.

Havelock, R. G., & Lingwood, D. A. (1973). *R&D utilization strategies and functions: An analytical comparison of four systems.* Ann Arbor, MI: Center for Research on Utilization of Scientific Knowledge, Institute for Social Research, University of Michigan.

Hays, D. (1974). Do it yourself the Z-track way. *American Journal of Nursing, 74*(6), 1070–1071.

Hick, J. F., Charboneau, J. W., Brakke, D. M., & Goergen, B. (1989). Optimum needle length for DPT inoculation of infants. *Pediatrics, 84*(1), 136–137.

Hochstetter, V. A. V. (1954). Über die intraglutäale Injektion, ihre Komplikationen und deren Verhütung. *Schweizerische Medizinische Wochenschrift, 84,* 1226–1227.

Hochstetter, V. A. V. (1955). Über Probleme und Technik der intraglutäalen injektion, Teil I. Der Einfluß des Medikamentes und der Individualität des Patienten auf die Entstehung von Spritzenschäden. *Schweizerische Medizinische Wochenschrift, 85,* 1138–1144.

Hochstetter, V. A. V. (1956). Über probleme und Technik der intraglutäalen Injektion, Teil II. Der Einfluß der Injektionstechnick auf die Entstehung von Spritzenschäden. *Schweizerische Medizinische Wochenschrift, 86,* 69–76.

Holford, N. H. G., Vozeh, S., Coates, P., Porvell, J. R., Thiercelin, J. F., & Upton, R. (1977). More on heparin lock. *The New England Journal of Medicine, 296,* 1300–1301.

Horsley, J. A., Crane, J., & Bingle, J. D. (1978). Research utilization as an organizational process. *Journal of Nursing Administration, 8*(7), 4–6.

Horsley, J. A., Crane, J., Crabtree, M. K., & Wood, D. J. (1983). *Using research to improve nursing practice: A guide* [CURN Project]. New York: Grune & Stratton.

Howard-Jones, N. (1971). The origins of hypodermic medication. *Scientific American, 224,* 96–102.

Hunt, M. (1987). The process of translating research findings into nursing practice. *Journal of Advanced Nursing, 12*(1), 101–110.

Janken, J. K., Rudisill, P., & Benfield, L. (1992). Product evaluation as a research utilization strategy. *Applied Nursing Research, 5*(4), 188–201.

Johnson, E. W., & Raptou, A. D. (1965). A study of intragluteal injections, *Archives of Physical Medicine and Rehabilitation, 46,* 167–177.

Jones, K. R. (1993). Outcomes analysis: Methods and issues. *Nursing Economics, 11*(3), 145–152.

Kasparek, A., Wenger, J., & Feldt, R. (1988). *Comparison of normal versus heparinized saline for flushing or intermittent intravenous infusion devices.* Unpublished manuscript. Mercy Medical Center, Cedar Rapids, IA, pp. 1–18.

Keen, M. F. (1981). Comparison of two intramuscular injection techniques on the incidence and severity of discomfort and lesions at the injection site. *Dissertation Abstracts International, 42*(4), 1394B. (University Microfilms No. 8120152).

Keen, M. F. (1986). Comparison of intramuscular injection techniques to reduce site discomfort and lesions. *Nursing Research, 35*(4), 207–210.

Keen, M. F. (1990). Get on the right track with Z-track injections. *Nursing90, 20*(8), 59.

King, D., Barnard, K. E., & Hoehn, R. (1981). Disseminating the results of nursing research. *Nursing Outlook, 29*(3), 164–169.

Krueger, J. C. (1978). Utilization of nursing research: The planning process. *Journal of Nursing Administration, 8*(1), 6–9.

Krueger, J. C., Nelson, A. H., & Wolanin, M. O. (1978). *Nursing research: Development, collaboration, and utilization.* Germantown, MD: Aspen.

Kruszewski, A., Lang, S., & Johnson, J. (1979). Effect of positioning on discomfort from intramuscular injections in the dorsogluteal site. *Nursing Research, 28*(2), 103–105.

Lachman, E. (1963). Applied anatomy of intragluteal injections. *The American Surgeon, 29,* 236–241.

Lombardi, T. P., Gunderson, B., Zammett, L. O., Walters, J. K., & Morris, B. A. (1988). Efficacy of 0.9% sodium chloride injection with or without heparin sodium for maintaining patency of intravenous catheters in children. *Children Pharmacy, 7*(11), 832–836.

Losek, J. D., & Gyuro, J. (1992). Pediatric intramuscular injections: Do you know the procedure and complications? *Pediatric Emergency Care, 8*(2), 79–81.

MacGuire, J. M. (1990). Putting nursing research findings into practice: Research utilization as an aspect of the management of change. *Journal of Advanced Nursing, 15*(5), 614–620.

Massey, J., & Loomis, M. (1988). When should nurses use research findings? *Applied Nursing Research, 1*(1), 32–40.

Mateo, M. A., & Kirchhoff, K. T. (1991). *Conducting and using nursing research in the clinical setting.* Baltimore: Williams & Wilkins.

Maurin, J. T. (1990). Research utilization in the social-political arena. *Applied Nursing Research, 3*(2), 48–51.

McConnell, E. A. (1982). The subtle art of really good injections. *RN, 45*(2), 25–35.

Michaels, L., & Poole, R. W. (1970). Injection granuloma of the buttock. *Canadian Medical Association Journal, 102,* 626–628.

Michel, Y., & Sneed, N. V. (1995). Dissemination and use of research findings in nursing practice. *Journal of Professional Nursing, 11*(5), 306–311.

Miracle, V., Fangman, B., Kayrouz, P., Kederis, K., & Pursell, L. (1989). Normal saline vs. heparin lock flush solution: One institution's findings. *The Kentucky Nurse, 37*(4), 1, 6–7.

Murphy, J. I. (1991). Reducing the pain of intramuscular (IM) injections. *Advancing Clinical Care, 6*(4), 35.

Newton, M., Newton, D., & Fudin, J. (1992). Reviewing the "big three" injection techniques. *Nursing92, 22*(2), 34–41.

Pelz, D., & Horsley, J. (1981). Measuring utilization of nursing research. In J. Ciarlo (Ed.), *Utilizing evaluation.* Beverly Hills, CA: Sage.

Pettengill, M. M., Gillies, D. A., & Clark, C. C. (1994). Factors encouraging and discouraging the use of nursing research findings. *Image: Journal of Nursing Scholarship, 26*(2), 143–147.

Phillips, L. R. F. (1986). *A clinician's guide to the critique and utilization of nursing research.* Norwalk, CT: Appleton-Century-Crofts.

Pillemer, D. B., & Light, R. J. (1980). Synthesizing outcomes: How to use research evidence from many studies. *Harvard Educational Review, 50*(2), 176–195.

Pitel, M., & Wemett, M. (1964). The intramuscular injection. *American Journal of Nursing, 64*(4), 104–109.

Rettig, F. M., & Southby, J. R. (1982). Using different body positions to reduce discomfort from dorsogluteal injection. *Nursing Research, 31*(4), 219–221.

Rogers, E. M. (1983). *Diffusion of innovations* (3rd ed.). New York: Free Press.

Shearer, J. (1987). Normal saline flush versus dilute heparin flush. *National Intravenous Therapy Association, 10*(6), 425–427.

Shoaf, J., & Oliver, S. (1992). Efficacy of normal saline injection with and without heparin for maintaining intermittent intravenous site. *Applied Nursing Research, 5*(1), 9–12.

Spann, J. M. (1988). Efficacy of two flush solutions to maintain catheter patency in heparin locks. *Dissertation Abstracts, 28*(1) 1337125, 1–58.

Stetler, C. B. (1985). Research utilization: Defining the concept. *Image: Journal of Nursing Scholarship, 17*(2), 40–44.

Stetler, C. B. (1994). Refinement of the Stetler/Marram model for application of research findings to practice. *Nursing Outlook, 42*(1), 15–25.

Stetler, C. B., & Marram, G. (1976). Evaluating research findings for applicability in practice. *Nursing Outlook, 24*(9), 559–563.

Stokes, J. H., Beerman, H., & Ingraham, N. R. (1944). *Modern clinical syphilology: Diagnosis, treatment, case study* (3rd ed.). Philadelphia: Saunders.

Talbert, J. L., Haslam, R. H. A., & Haller, J. A. (1967). Gangrene of the foot following intramuscular injection in the lateral thigh: A case report with recommendations for prevention. *Journal of Pediatrics, 70,* 110–117.

Tanner, C. A. (1987). Evaluating research for use in practice: Guidelines for the clinician. *Heart & Lung, 16*(4), 424–431.

Tanner, C. A., & Lindeman, C. A. (1989). *Using nursing research.* New York: National League for Nursing.

Taylor, N., Hutchison, E., Milliken, W., & Larson, E. (1989). Comparison of normal versus heparinized saline for flushing infusion devices. *Journal of Nursing Quality Assurance, 3*(4), 49–55.

Tibbles, L., & Sanford, R. (1994). The research journal club: A mechanism for research utilization. *Clinical Nurse Specialist, 8*(1), 23–26.

Weiss, C. J. (1980). Knowledge creep and decision accretion.

Knowledge: Creation, Diffusion, Utilization, 1(3), 381–404.

Wichita, C. (1977). Treating and preventing constipation in nursing home residents. *Journal of Gerontological Nursing, 3*(6), 35–39.

Zelman, S. (1961). Notes on the techniques of intramuscular injection. *The American Journal of Medical Science, 241*(5), 47–58.

Zenk, K. E. (1982). Improving the accuracy of mini-volume injections. *Infusion, 6*(1), 7–12.

Zenk, K. E. (1993). Beware of overdose. *Nursing93, 23*(3), 28–29.

Appendix 25–A
Procedure for Administration of IM Injections

Procedure	Rationale	References
1. For adults, select a 1.5-in needle. For children, select a 1-in needle. Use a needle of 21–23 gauge.	The needle must be long enough to reach the muscle. Injections into the subcutaneous tissue cause pain to the patient. The VG site provides the most consistent depth of subcutaneous tissue; in adults, the adipose tissue layer over the VG muscle is less than 3.75 cm (1.47 in) in depth. Using a smaller gauge needle minimizes tissue injury and subcutaneous leakage.	Hick, Charboneau, Brakke, & Goergen, 1989; Johnson & Raptou, 1965; Michaels & Poole, 1970; Shaffer, 1929; Talbert, Haslam, & Haller, 1967
2. The maximum volume to be administered in one injection should not exceed 4 mL in adults with well-developed muscles such as the ventrogluteal. Children and individuals with less well developed muscles should receive no more than 1 to 2 mL. Children under the age of 2 years should not receive more than 1 mL. If using the deltoid, do not exceed a volume of 0.5 to 1 mL. The size of the syringe is determined by the volume to be administered and the size of the syringe should correspond as closely as possible to the amount to be administered. Volumes less than 0.5 mL require a low-dose syringe such as a tuberculin syringe.	High volume injections cause more pain. Finely graduated syringes such as tuberculin syringes ensure administration of the correct dose.	Farley, Joyce, Long, & Roberts, 1986; Losek & Gyuro, 1992; Zenk, 1982
3. Use a filter needle to draw up medication from a glass ampule or vial. Hold the vial or ampule down and do not draw up the last drop in the container. After drawing the medication into the syringe, change the needle prior to administration. If using a pre-filled syringe, such as Tubex® or Carpuject®, and drawing from a vial or ampule, instill the medication into another syringe and ensure the use of a clean needle prior to injection. If using a pre-filled unit-dose medication, take caution to avoid dripping medication on the needle prior to injection. If this does occur, wipe the medication off the needle with a sterile gauze.	Glass and rubber particulate has been found in medications withdrawn with a regular needle. Holding the vial or ampule down will allow particulate matter to precipitate out of the solution, and leaving the last drops reduces the chance of withdrawing foreign particles. Changing the needle will prevent tracking the medication through the subcutaneous tissue during insertion of the needle, which can cause pain. Similarly, medication should be wiped from the needle as this can also cause pain when it is tracked through the subcutaneous tissue.	Hahn, 1990; Keen, 1986; McConnell, 1982
4. Do not use an air bubble.	An air bubble affects the dose administered, causing an overdose of medication of at least 5% and as great as 100%, depending on the dose administered.	Chaplin, Shull, & Welk, 1985; Zenk, 1982, 1993
5. Select the ventrogluteal (VG) site as the injection site for children over seven months and adults unless there is a strict contraindication. Strict contraindications would include pre-existing tissue injury and administration of hepatitis-B vaccine, which should only be administered in the deltoid. In infants less than 7 mo, the vastus lateralis should be used for administration of hepatitis-B vaccine.	The VG site is free of nerves and blood vessels. There are no documented reports of complications from IM injections administered at this site. The VG muscle is a well-developed muscle in infants, children, and adults.	Beecroft & Redick, 1990; Brandt, Smith, Ashburn, & Graves, 1972; Centers for Disease Control, 1990; Daly, Johnston, & Chung, 1992; Hochstetter, 1954, 1955, 1956

Appendix 25–A
Procedure for Administration of IM Injections *Continued*

Procedure	Rationale	References
6. Prior to the administration of any IM injection, carefully assess the site for evidence of induration, abscesses or other contraindications for use of the site.	Injections are contraindicated in previously injured muscles or tissues.	Stokes, Beerman, & Ingraham, 1944
7. Position the patient to relax the muscle. Prone: Have the patient "toe in" to internally rotate the femur. Side-lying: Have the patient flex upper leg at 20°. Supine: Have the patient flex both knees, if possible, or if not possible, flex the knee on the side where the medication will be administered.	There is reduced pain with a relaxed muscle.	Keen, 1986; Kruszewski, Lang, & Johnson, 1979; Rettig & Southby, 1982
8. Identify the site by placing the palm of the hand on the greater trochanter, with the index finger toward the anterior superior iliac spine and the middle finger spread away to form a "V." Use the right hand on the left VG site; left hand on the right VG site.	The landmarks are described by Hochstetter.	Hochstetter, 1954, 1955, 1956; Zelman, 1961
9. Pull the skin down so as to administer the injection in a Z-track manner at a 90 degree angle to the iliac crest in the middle of the "V."	Z-track technique reduces discomfort and incidence of lesions.	Keen, 1981, 1986, 1990
10. Cleanse the skin in a circular fashion in an area of approximately 5–8 cm (2–3 in) and allow the alcohol to dry.	Deep tissues can be infected with skin contaminants injected via the needle; the skin is the first line of defense. Alcohol is irritating to the subcutaneous tissue and causes pain.	Berger & Williams, 1992; Murphy, 1991
11. Insert the needle with a steady pressure and then aspirate for at least 5–10 s. Inject the medication slowly at a rate of approximately 10 s/mL.	Aspirating for 5–10 s is adequate to ensure the needle is not in a small, low-flow blood vessel. A slow, steady injection rate promotes comfort and minimizes tissue damage.	Stokes, Beerman, & Ingraham, 1944; Zelman, 1961
12. Wait 10 seconds after injecting the medication before withdrawing the needle.	Waiting 10 s allows the medication to be deposited in the muscle and begin to diffuse through the muscle.	Belanger-Annable, 1985; Hahn, 1990, 1991; Keen, 1990
13. Smoothly and steadily withdraw the needle and apply gentle pressure at the site with a dry sponge.	This minimizes tissue injury. Massaging the site can result in tissue irritation.	Newton, Newton, & Fudin, 1992
14. Encourage leg exercises.	Leg exercises will promote the absorption of the medication.	Stokes, Beerman, & Ingraham, 1944
15. Whenever possible, assess the site 2–4 h after injection and as needed to identify any side effects.	Given the number of complications reported in the literature, it is important to assess the site for any signs of redness, swelling, pain, or other iatrogenic effects from the injection.	Beecroft & Redick, 1989, 1990

(From Beyea, S. C., & Nicoll, L. H. [1995]. Administration of medication via the intramuscular route: An integrative review of the literature and research-based protocol for the procedure, *Applied Nursing Research, 8*[1], 23–33.)

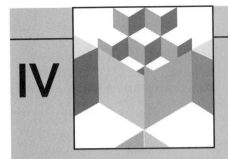

IV Seeking Support for Research Activities

26

Proposal Writing for Research Approval

With a background in critique and utilization of research, you are ready to propose a study for implementation. A *research proposal* is a written plan that identifies the major elements of a study, such as the research problem, purpose, and framework, and outlines the methods and procedures to conduct the study. A proposal is a formal way to communicate ideas about a proposed study to receive approval to conduct the study and to seek funding. Seeking approval for the conduct or funding of a study involves submission of a research proposal to a selected group for review and, in many situations, verbally defending that proposal. Receiving approval to conduct research has become more complicated over the past few years because of the increasing complexity of nursing studies and the rising concern over legal and ethical issues. In many large hospitals, research proposals are reviewed by the lawyer in addition to the institutional research review committee. This chapter focuses on writing a research proposal and seeking approval to conduct a study. Chapter 27 presents the process of seeking funding for a study.

WRITING A RESEARCH PROPOSAL

A well-written proposal communicates a significant, carefully planned research project; demon-

strates the qualifications of the researcher; and generates support for the project. Conducting research requires precision and rigorous attention to details. Thus, reviewers often judge a researcher's ability to conduct a study by the quality of the proposal. A quality proposal is concise, clear, and complete (Cook, 1985; Tornquist, 1986). Writing a quality proposal involves (1) developing ideas logically, (2) determining the depth or detail of the proposal content, (3) identifying critical points in the proposal, and (4) developing an esthetically appealing copy.

DEVELOPING IDEAS LOGICALLY

The ideas in a research proposal must logically build upon each other to justify or defend a study, just as a lawyer would logically organize information in the defense of a client. A case is built for why a problem should be studied, and appropriate methodology for conducting the study is proposed. Each step in the research proposal builds on the problem statement to give a clear picture of the study and its merit (Barnard, 1986; Rogers, 1987). A variety of resources have been developed to assist individuals in improving their writing skills (American Psychological Association [APA], 1994; Krathwohl, 1977; University of Chicago Press, 1993).

DETERMINING THE DEPTH OF A PROPOSAL

The depth of a proposal is determined by the guidelines developed by schools of nursing, funding agencies, and institutions where research is conducted. Guidelines provide specific directions for the development of a proposal and should be followed explicitly. The omission or misinterpretation of a guideline is frequently the basis for rejection of a proposal. In addition to following the guidelines, you must determine the amount of information necessary to describe clearly each step of your study. The content in a proposal needs to be detailed enough to inform the reader, yet concise enough to be interesting and easily reviewed. Often the guidelines will stipulate a page limitation that determines the depth of the proposal. Relevant content of a research proposal is discussed later in this chapter.

IDENTIFYING CRITICAL POINTS

The key or critical points in a proposal must be clear, even to the hasty reader. Critical points might be highlighted with bold type or underlined. Sometimes headings are created to highlight critical content, or the content is organized into tables or graphs. The research problem, significance of the problem, purpose, framework, research objectives, questions, or hypotheses, and methodological procedures are considered critical content in a proposal (Tornquist, 1986).

DEVELOPING AN ESTHETICALLY APPEALING COPY

An esthetically appealing copy is well typed on quality paper without spelling, punctuation, or grammatical errors. Even a proposal with excellent content that is poorly typed or formatted will probably not receive the full attention or respect of the reviewer. The format used in typing the proposal should follow the guidelines developed by the reviewer. If no particular format is requested, the APA (1994) format is commonly used. An appealing copy is legible (print is dark enough to be read) and is neatly organized in a folder for easy examination by the reviewer.

CONTENT OF A RESEARCH PROPOSAL

The content of a proposal is written with the interest and expertise of the reviewers in mind. Proposals are frequently reviewed by faculty, clinical agency members, and representatives of funding institutions. The content of a proposal varies depending on the reviewer, the guidelines developed for the review, and the type of study (quantitative or qualitative) proposed. This section addresses the content of (1) a student proposal for both quantitative and qualitative studies, (2) condensed research proposals, and (3) preproposals.

CONTENT OF A STUDENT PROPOSAL

Student researchers develop proposals to communicate their research projects to the faculty and members of university and agency research review committees. Student proposals are written to satisfy requirements for a degree and are usually developed according to guidelines outlined by faculty. These guidelines are usually reviewed with the faculty member (the chair of the student's thesis or dissertation committee), who will be assisting with the research project. Each faculty member has a unique way of interpreting and emphasizing aspects of the guidelines. In addition, a student needs to evaluate the faculty member's background regarding a research topic of interest and determine whether a productive working relationship can be developed. Faculty members who are actively involved in their own research have extensive knowledge and expertise that can be helpful to a novice researcher. Both the student and the faculty member benefit when a student becomes involved in an aspect of the faculty's research.

The content of a student proposal usually requires greater detail than the proposal developed for review by agency personnel or funding organizations. The proposal is often the first three or four chapters of the student's thesis or dissertation, and the proposed study is discussed in the future tense of what *will be* done in conducting the research. A title page, which includes the title of the proposal, name of the investigator, and the date the proposal is submitted, and a table of contents often precedes the proposal content.

Content of a Quantitative Research Proposal

A quantitative research proposal usually includes the following chapters or sections: (1) introduction, (2) review of relevant literature, (3) framework, and (4) methods and procedures. Some graduate schools require an in-depth development of these sections, whereas others require a condensed version of the same content. Another approach is that proposals for theses and dissertations are written in a form that can ultimately be submitted for publication. The content often covered in the chapters of a quantitative research proposal is outlined in Table 26–1 (on p. 708).

Introduction

The introductory chapter identifies the research topic and problem and provides the background and significance of this problem. The background of a problem describes how the problem was identified and historically links the problem to nursing. The background information might also include one or two major studies conducted to resolve the problem, some key theoretical ideas related to the problem, and possible solutions to the problem. The significance of the problem addresses the importance of this problem in nursing practice and the expected generalizability of the findings. The interests of nurses, other health care professionals, policymakers, and health care consumers in the problem at the local, state, national, or international level are part of determining the problem significance. This interest can usually be documented with sources from the literature. The background and significance of the problem indicate the need for further research and are followed by a clear, concise statement of the research purpose.

Review of Relevant Literature

The review of relevant literature provides an overview of the essential information that will guide the development of a study and includes relevant theoretical and empirical literature. The theoretical literature provides a background for defining and interrelating relevant study concepts, while the empirical literature includes a summary and critique of previous studies. The recommendations, such as changing or expanding a study made by other researchers, are discussed related to the proposed study. The depth of the literature review varies and might include only recent studies and theorists' works, or it might be extensive and include a description and critique of a number of past and current studies and an in-depth discussion of theorists' works. The literature review demonstrates that the researcher has command of the current empirical and theoretical knowledge regarding the proposed problem.

This chapter concludes with a summary. The summary includes a synthesis of the theoretical literature and the findings from previous research that describes the current knowledge of a problem (Pinch, 1995). The gaps in the knowledge base are also identified, with a description of how the proposed study is expected to contribute to nursing's body of knowledge.

Framework

A framework provides the basis for generating and refining the research problem and purpose and linking them to the relevant theoretical knowledge in nursing or related fields. The framework includes concepts and relationships among concepts, which are sometimes represented in a model or map. The concepts to be studied are conceptually defined and linked to the study variables. If a theorist's or researcher's model from a journal article

---

Table 26–1
Quantitative Research Proposal Guidelines for Students

CHAPTER I   Introduction
    A. Statement of the problem
    B. Background and significance of the problem
    C. Statement of the purpose
CHAPTER II   Review of Relevant Literature
    A. Review of relevant theoretical literature
    B. Review of relevant research
    C. Summary
CHAPTER III   Framework
    A. Development of a framework
       (Define concepts, identify relationships among concepts, and develop a
         model of the framework)
    B. Formulation of objectives, questions, or hypotheses
    C. Definition of research variables
    D. Definition of relevant terms
    E. Identification of assumptions
CHAPTER IV   Methods and Procedures
    A. Description of the research design
       (Model of design, strengths and weaknesses of design, and description
         of treatment if appropriate)
    B. Identification of the population and sample
       (Sample size; use of power analysis; sampling criteria; and sampling
         method, including strengths and weaknesses)
    C. Selection of a setting
       (Strengths and weaknesses of the setting)
    D. Presentation of ethical considerations
       (Protection of subjects' rights and review process)
    E. Selection of measurement methods
       (Reliability, validity, scoring, and level of measurement of instruments,
         and plans for examining reliability and validity of the instruments,
         in the present study)
    F. Plan for data collection
       (Data collection process, data collector(s), training of data collectors if
         appropriate, schedule, data collection forms, and management of
         data)
    G. Plan for data analysis
       (Analysis of demographic data; analyses for research objectives, ques-
         tions, or hypotheses; level of significance if appropriate; and other
         analysis techniques)
    H. Identification of limitations
       (Methodological and theoretical limitations)
    I. Discussion of communication of findings
    J. Presentation of a study budget and timetable
REFERENCES
APPENDICES

---

or book is used in a proposal, letters documenting permission to use this model from the publisher and the theorist or researcher must be included in the proposal appendices.

In some studies, research objectives, questions, or hypotheses are developed to direct the study. The objectives, questions, or hypotheses evolve from the research purpose and study framework and identify the study variables. The variables are conceptually defined to show the link to the framework and operationally defined to indicate the procedures for measurement. Other terms relevant to the study are defined; and assumptions that provide a basis for the study are identified.

Methods and Procedures

The design or general strategy for conducting the study is described, and sometimes a diagram of the design is included. The designs for descriptive and correlational studies are flexible and can be unique to the study being conducted. Because of this uniqueness, the designs need to be clearly described, including their strengths and weaknesses. Presenting a design for quasi-experimental and experimental studies involves (1) describing how the research situation will be structured; (2) detailing the treatment to be implemented; (3) describing how the effect of the treatment will be measured; (4) indicating the variables to be controlled and the methods for controlling them; (5) identifying uncontrolled extraneous variables and determining their impact on the findings; (6) describing the methods for assigning subjects to the treatment and control groups; and (7) describing the strengths and weaknesses of a design. The design needs to account for all the objectives, questions, or hypotheses identified in the proposal. If a pilot study is planned, the design should include the procedure for conducting the pilot and for incorporating the results into the proposed study.

The proposal identifies the population to which the study findings will be generalized and the target population from which the sample will be selected. The criteria for selecting a subject and the rationale for these criteria are presented. For example, a subject might be selected according to the following criteria: female, aged 20 to 50 years, hospitalized for three days, and two days postoperative from abdominal surgery. The rationale for these criteria might be that the researcher wants to examine the effects of preoperative teaching about pain management on adult females who have recently experienced hospitalization and abdominal surgery. The sampling method and the approximate sample size are discussed in terms of their adequacy and limitations in investigating the research purpose. Usually a power analysis is conducted to determine an adequate sample size.

A proposal includes a description of the study setting, which often includes the name of the agency and the structure of the units or sites where the study is to be conducted. The setting is often identified in the proposal but not in the final research report. The agency selected should have the potential to generate the type and size of sample required for the study. Thus, the proposal usually includes the number of individuals who meet the sample criteria who are cared for by the agency in a given period of time. In addition, the structure and activities in the agency need to be able to accommodate the proposed design of the study.

The ethical considerations in a proposal include the rights of the subjects and the rights of the agency where the study is to be conducted. The protection of the subjects' rights and the risks and potential benefits of the study are described. The steps taken to reduce the study risks also need to be addressed. Many agencies require a written consent form, and that form is often included in the appendices of the proposal. The risks and potential benefits of the study for the institution also need to be addressed. If risks exist for the agency, the steps that will be taken to reduce or eliminate these risks are outlined. The researcher also indicates that the proposal will be reviewed by the thesis or dissertation committee, university human rights review committee, and agency research review committee.

The methods for measuring study variables are described, including each instrument's reliability, validity, methods of scoring, and level of measurement. A plan for examining the reliability and validity of the instruments in the present study needs to be addressed. If an instrument has no reported reliability and validity, a pilot study is usually conducted to examine its reliability and validity. If the intent of the proposed study is to develop an instrument, the process of instrument development is described. A copy of the interview questions, questionnaires, scales, physiological instruments, or other tools to be used in the study is usually included in the proposal appendices. Permission to use copyrighted instruments must be obtained from the authors, and letters documenting that permission has been obtained are included in the proposal appendices.

The data collection plan clarifies what data are to be collected and the process for collecting the data. In this plan, the data collectors are identified, data collection procedures are described, and a schedule is presented for data collection activities. If more than one person will be involved in data collection, the training of data collectors to ensure consistency is described. A method for recording data is often described, and example data recording sheets are placed in the proposal appendices. Any special equipment that will be used or developed to collect data for the study is also discussed, and data security is usually addressed, including the methods of data storage.

The plan for data analysis identifies the analysis techniques to be used in summarizing the demographic data and in answering the research objectives, questions, or hypotheses. The analysis section is often organized using the study objectives, questions, or hypotheses. The analysis techniques identified need to be appropriate for the type of data collected. For example, if an associative hypothesis is developed, correlational analysis must be planned. If a researcher plans to determine the differences among groups, the analysis techniques might include a *t* test or analysis of variance (ANOVA). A level of significance (α = .05, .01, or .001) is also identified. Often a researcher projects the type of results that will be generated from data analyses. Then dummy tables, graphs, and charts can be developed for the presentation of these results and included in the proposal appendices. The investigator might also project the possible findings for a study. For example, the researcher might consider what support or nonsupport of a proposed hypothesis would mean in light of the study framework and previous research findings. Projecting a study's findings facilitates logical examination of the findings when the study is complete.

The methods and procedures' chapter of a proposal usually concludes with a discussion of study limitations and a plan for communication of the findings. Both methodological and theoretical limitations are addressed. The methodological limitations might include areas of weakness in the design, sampling method, sample size, measurement tools, data collection procedures, or data analysis techniques, while theoretical limitations set boundaries for the generalization of study findings. For example, the accuracy with which the conceptual definitions and relational statements in a theory reflect reality has a direct impact on the generalization of findings. Theory that has withstood frequent testing provides a stronger framework for the interpretation and generalization of findings. A plan is included for the communication of the research through presentations and publications to audiences of nurses, other health professionals, policymakers, and health care consumers.

Frequently, a budget and timetable are included in the proposal appendices. The budget projects the expenses for the study, which might include costs for data collection tools and procedures; special equipment; consultants for data analysis; computer time; travel related to data collection and analysis; typing; copying; and developing, presenting, and publishing the final report. Funded study budgets frequently include investigators' salaries and secretarial costs. A timetable is needed to direct the steps of the research project and to facilitate the completion of the project on schedule. A timetable identifies the tasks to be done, who will accomplish these tasks, and when these tasks will be completed.

Content of a Qualitative Research Proposal

A qualitative research proposal might include some content similar to that of a quantitative proposal, but the guidelines are usually more flexible and abstract to accommodate the emergent design of the study. A qualitative proposal usually includes the following sections or chapters: (1) introduction, (2) literature review, and (3) methods (Burns, 1989; Marshall & Rossman, 1989; Sandelowski, Davis, & Harris, 1989). The quality of the proposal is determined based on the potential scientific contribution of the research; conceptual framework guiding the study; research methods; and knowledge, skills, and resources available to the researchers (Cohen, Knafl, & Dzurec, 1993). Guidelines for a qualitative research proposal are outlined in Table 26–2.

Table 26-2
Qualitative Research Proposal Guidelines for Students

I. Introduction
  A. Identification of the phenomenon
  B. Identification of the study purpose and type of qualitative study
  C. Identification of study questions or aims
  D. Significance of the study
  E. Identification of assumptions and philosophy
II. Review of Literature
  A. Relevant literature reviewed as appropriate for the qualitative study planned
III. Methods
  A. Demonstration of researcher's credentials for conducting a particular type of qualitative study
  B. Selection of a site and population
  C. Description of the researcher's role
    1. Entry into the site
    2. Selection of a sample
    3. Ethical considerations
  D. Data collection process
  E. Data analysis techniques
  F. Communication of findings
  G. Presentation of a study budget and timetable
REFERENCES
APPENDICES

Introduction

The introduction usually provides a general background for the proposed study by identifying the phenomenon to be investigated and linking this phenomenon to nursing knowledge. The general purpose of the study is identified and indicates the type of qualitative study to be conducted. The purpose is often followed by research questions or aims that direct the investigation (Parse, Coyne, & Smith, 1985). These questions or aims focus on real-world problems and dilemmas, such as: How do people cope with a new diagnosis of chronic illness? What is it like to live with a chronic illness for five or more years? What type of support exists for a person with a chronic illness? What is the impact on the family? An aim might be to describe the burden of the caregiver role in a family with a chronically ill member.

The introduction also includes the significance of the proposed study to practice and policy, and the potential contribution the study will make to

nursing knowledge. The discussion of the study's significance often includes how the problem developed, who or what is affected by the problem, and how costly the problem is. Whenever possible, the significance of a study needs to be documented from the literature. Marshall and Rossman (1989) identified the following questions to assess the significance of a study.

"**1.** Who has an interest in this domain of inquiry?
2. What do we already know about the topic?
3. What has not been answered adequately in previous research and practice?
4. How will this research add to knowledge, practice, and policy in this area?" (p. 31) ∎

The researchers' assumptions or preconceptions about the phenomenon they plan to study are addressed in the introduction. These assumptions, as well as the philosophy that influences a researcher's thinking, are identified, because the assumptions and philosophy influence the focus of the study, data collection and analysis, and the articulation of the findings. The philosophy in a sense provides the theoretical perspective for the study.

Literature Review

Some qualitative studies involve a literature review prior to conducting the study. For example, ethnographic research requires a literature review to provide a background for conducting the study as in quantitative research. Historical research involves a literature review to develop research questions, as does philosophical inquiry to raise philosophical questions. The literature review needs to provide a basis for the aims of the study and clearly indicate how this study will expand nursing knowledge (Cohen et al., 1993).

In phenomenological research, grounded theory research, and critical social theory, the literature review is usually conducted at the end of the research project. The findings from a phenomenological study are compared and combined with the literature to determine the current knowledge of the phenomenon. In grounded theory research, the literature is used to explain, support, and extend the theory generated in the study. The study findings obtained through critical social theory are examined using existing literature to determine the current knowledge of a social situation. The literature review of qualitative research is discussed in Chapter 6.

Methods

Developing and implementing the methodology of qualitative research requires a certain expertise that some believe can only be obtained through a mentorship with an experienced qualitative researcher. The role of the researcher and the intricate techniques of data collection and analysis are thought to be best communicated through a one-to-one relationship. Thus, planning the methods of a qualitative study requires knowledge of relevant sources that describe the different qualitative research techniques and procedures (Chenitz & Swanson, 1986; Leininger, 1985; Marshall & Rossman, 1989; Miles & Huberman, 1994; Munhall & Oiler, 1986; Parse et al., 1985) and interaction with a qualitative researcher.

Identifying the methods for conducting a qualitative study is a difficult task because the design of the study is emergent. Unlike quantitative research in which the design is a fixed blueprint for a study, the design in qualitative research emerges or evolves as the study is conducted. Thus, the researcher must document the logic and appropriateness of the qualitative method and develop a tentative plan for conducting the study. This plan is tentative and the researcher reserves the right to modify or change that plan at any point during the conduct of the study (Sandelowski et al., 1989). However, the design or plan must be consistent with the study aims, well conceived, and address prior criticism, as appropriate (Cohen et al., 1993). The tentative plan describes the process for selecting a site and sample. The site will allow the researcher entry and include the subjects that are necessary to answer the research questions or aims. For the research question "How do individuals cope with a new diagnosis of chronic illness?" the subjects might be identified in hospitals, clin-

ics, practitioners' offices, home care organizations, or in rehabilitation facilities, and the data collection might be conducted in the subjects' homes.

The methods section includes a detailed description of the proposed researcher's role. The researcher must gain entry into the setting, develop a rapport with the subjects that will facilitate the detailed data collection process, and protect the rights of the subjects (Marshall & Rossman, 1989; Sandelowski et al., 1989). The following questions are addressed in describing the researcher's role: (1) What is the best setting for the study? (2) How will the researcher ease his or her entry into the research site? (3) How will the researcher gain access to the subjects? (4) What actions will the researcher take to facilitate the participation and cooperation of the subjects? and (5) What precautions will be taken to protect the rights of the subjects and to prevent the setting and the subjects from being harmed? The process of obtaining informed consent and the actions planned by the researcher to decrease study risks need to be described. The sensitive nature of some qualitative studies increases the risks for the subjects, which makes ethical concerns and decisions a major focus of the study.

The primary data collection techniques used in qualitative research are observation and in-depth interviewing. The observations can range from highly detailed, structured notations of behavior to ambiguous descriptions of behaviors or events. The interview can also have a range from structured, closed-ended questions to unstructured open-ended questions (Marshall & Rossman, 1989). The following questions are addressed in developing a description of the proposed data collection process: (1) Who will collect data and provide any training required for the data collectors? (2) What data will be collected? (3) What techniques or procedures will be used to collect the data? and (4) What is the anticipated length of time needed to collect data? In some qualitative studies, data are collected through an exhaustive review of published and unpublished literature.

The methods section of the proposal also includes the analysis techniques and the steps for conducting these techniques. In qualitative research, often data collection and analysis occur simultaneously. The data are in the form of notes, tapes, and other materials that are obtained from observation and interviews. Through qualitative analysis techniques, these data are structured and reduced to determine meaning (Burns, 1989). Strategies to ensure the credibility, fittingness, and auditability of the findings need to be addressed (Beck, 1993). These qualitative terms are related to the concepts of reliability and validity used in quantitative research and are addressed in Chapter 24, Critical Analysis of Nursing Studies. Qualitative analysis techniques are the focus of Chapter 20.

The proposal describes how findings will be communicated to a variety of audiences through presentations and publications, and a realistic budget and timetable are developed to provide direction for the investigation. A qualitative study budget is similar to a quantitative study budget, including costs for data collection tools and procedures; consultants for data analysis; travel related to data collection and analysis; typing; copying; and developing, presenting, and publishing the final report. However, the greatest expenditure in qualitative research is usually the researcher's time. A timetable is developed to project how long the study will take, and often two or more years are designated for data collection and analysis (Marshall & Rossman, 1989). The budget and timetable can be used to make decisions regarding funding, since funding is essential for many qualitative studies.

CONTENT OF A CONDENSED PROPOSAL

The content of proposals developed for review by clinical agencies and funding institutions is usually a condensed version of the student proposal. However, even though these proposals are condensed, the logical links between components of the study need to be clearly demonstrated. A condensed proposal often includes a statement of the problem and purpose, previous research that has been conducted in the area (usually limited to no more than three to five studies), the framework, variables, design, sample, ethical considerations, plans for data collection and analysis, and plans for dissemination of findings.

A proposal submitted to a clinical agency needs to identify clearly the specific setting, such as the emergency room or intensive care unit, and the projected time span for the study. Members of clinical agencies are particularly interested in the data collection process and the involvement of institutional personnel in the study. Any expected disruptions in institutional functioning need to be identified, with plans for preventing these disruptions when possible. The researcher must recognize that anything that slows down or disrupts employee functioning costs the agency money and can interfere with the quality of patient care. Indications in the proposal that the researcher is aware of these concerns and has addressed ways to minimize their effect will increase the probability of obtaining approval to conduct the study.

A variety of companies, corporations, and organizations provide funding for research projects. A proposal developed for these types of funding institutions frequently includes a brief description of the study, the study significance to the institution, a timetable, and budget. Most of these proposals are brief and might contain a one-page summary sheet or abstract at the beginning of the proposal, which summarizes the steps of the study. The salient points of the study are included on this page in simple, easy-to-read, nontechnical terminology. Some proposal reviewers for funding institutions are lay persons with no background in research or nursing. Inability to understand the terminology might put the reviewer on the defensive or create a negative reaction, which could lead to disapproval of the study. When multiple studies are examined by funding institutions, the summary sheet is often the basis for final decisions about the study. The summary should be concise, informative, and designed to sell the study.

In proposals for both clinical and funding agencies, the investigators need to document their research background and supply a curriculum vitae if requested. The research review committee for approval or funding will be interested in previous research, research publications, and clinical expertise, especially if a clinical study is proposed. If the researcher is a graduate student, the committee may request the names of the university committee members and verification that the proposal has been approved by the student's thesis or dissertation committee and the university human subjects review committee.

CONTENT OF A PREPROPOSAL

Sometimes a researcher will send a preproposal or query letter rather than a proposal to a funding institution. A *preproposal* is a short document of four to five pages plus appendices that is written to explore the funding possibilities for a research project. The parts of the preproposal are logically ordered as follows: "(1) letter of transmittal, (2) proposal for research, (3) personnel, (4) facilities, and (5) budget" (Malasanos, 1976, p. 223). The proposal provides a brief overview of the proposed project, including the research problem; purpose; methodology (brief description); and, most important, a statement of the significance of the work to knowledge in general and the funding institution in particular. By developing a preproposal, researchers are able to determine the agencies interested in funding their study and limit the submission of their proposals to only those institutions that indicate an interest.

SEEKING APPROVAL FOR A STUDY

Initially, proposal reviews were limited to graduate students developing theses or dissertations and researchers seeking grant money. However, as a consequence of stricter rules related to the protection of human subjects, most nursing studies will be reviewed by at least one research committee. *Seeking approval to conduct a study* is an action that should be based in knowledge and guided by purpose. Obtaining approval for a study from a research committee requires understanding the approval process, writing a research proposal for review, and, in many cases, verbally defending the proposal. Little has been written providing guidance to the researcher who is going through the labyrinth of approval mechanisms. The intent of

this section is to provide a background for obtaining approval to conduct a study.

Clinical agencies and health care corporations review studies for the following reasons: (1) to evaluate the quality of the study, (2) to ensure that adequate measures are being taken to protect human subjects, and (3) to evaluate the impact of conducting the study on the reviewing institution. The desired outcomes from a review by an institution are to receive approval to collect data at the reviewing institution and to obtain support for the proposed study.

APPROVAL PROCESS

An initial step in seeking approval is to determine exactly what committees in which agencies must grant approval before the study can be conducted. Researchers need to take the initiative to determine the formal approval process rather than assume that they will be told if a formal review system exists. Information on the formal research review system might be obtained from administrative personnel, special projects or grant officers, chairs of the research review committees in clinical agencies, clinicians who have previously conducted research, and university faculty who are involved in research.

Graduate students usually require approval from their thesis or dissertation committee, the university human subjects review committee, and the research committee in the agency where the data are to be collected. University faculty conducting research seek approval through the latter two committees. Nurses conducting research in an agency where they are employed must seek approval only at that agency. If outside funding is sought, additional review committees are involved. Not all studies require full review by the human subjects review committee; the types of studies that qualify for exempt or expedited review are discussed in Chapter 9.

When multiple committees must review a study, sometimes an agreement is made, by the respective committees, that review for the protection of human subjects will be done by only one of the committees, with the findings of that committee generally being accepted by other committees. For example, if the university human subjects review committee reviewed and approved a proposal for the protection of human subjects, funding agencies usually recognize that review as sufficient. Reviews in other committees are then focused on approval to conduct the study within the institution or decisions to provide study funding.

As part of the approval process, the researcher must determine the agency's policy regarding (1) the use of the clinical facility's name in reporting findings, (2) presentation and publication of the study, and (3) authorship of publications. The facility's name is used when presenting or publishing a study only with prior written administrative approval. The researcher may feel more free to report findings that could be interpreted negatively in terms of the institution if the agency is not identified. Some institutions have rules about presenting and publishing a study that limit what is presented or published, where it is presented or published, and who is the presenter or author. Prior to conducting a study, researchers, especially employees of agencies, must clarify the rules and regulations of an agency regarding authorship, presentations, and publications. In some cases, recognition of these rules must be included in the proposal if it is to be approved.

PREPARING PROPOSALS FOR REVIEW COMMITTEES

The initial proposals for thesis and dissertation are often developed as part of a formal class. The faculty provide specific proposal guidelines and assist students in developing their proposals. The student then selects a chair and committee members, who work together to refine the final proposal. This proposal requires approval by the thesis or dissertation committee and by the university human rights review committee.

Conducting research in a clinical agency requires approval by the institutional research committee. This committee has the responsibility to (1) provide researchers with copies of institutional policies and requirements, (2) screen proposals for scientific merit and consistency with the institu-

tion's goals, and (3) assist the researcher with the institutional review board (IRB) process (Vessey & Campos, 1992). The approval process policy and proposal guidelines are usually available from the chair of the research committee. Guidelines established by the committee should be followed carefully, particularly page limitations. Some committees refuse to review proposals that exceed these limitations. Reviewers in these committees are usually evaluating proposals in addition to other full-time responsibilities, and reading lengthy proposals uses the scarce time of the reviewer.

Investigators also need to be familiar with the research committee's process for screening proposals. Most agency research committees screen proposals for (1) scientific merit, (2) protection of human rights, (3) study congruence with the agency research agenda, and (4) impact of the study on patient care (Vessey & Campos, 1992). Researchers need to develop their proposal with these ideas in mind. They also need to determine whether the committee requires specific forms to be completed and submitted with the research proposal. Other important information can be gathered by addressing these questions: (1) How often does the committee meet? (2) How long before the next meeting? (3) What materials should be submitted prior to the meeting? (4) When should these materials be submitted? (5) How many copies of the proposal are required? and (6) What period of time is usually involved in committee review?

SOCIAL AND POLITICAL FACTORS

Social and political factors play an important role in obtaining approval to conduct a study. The researcher needs to treat the review process with as much care as the development of the study. The dynamics of the relationships among committee members are important to assess. This is especially important in the selection of a thesis or dissertation committee, so that the selected members are willing to work productively together.

A thorough assessment of the social and political situation in which the study will be reviewed and implemented may be crucial to the success of the study. Agency research committees may include nurse clinicians who have never conducted research, nurse researchers, and researchers in other disciplines. The reactions of each of these groups to a study could be very different. Sometimes the committees are made up primarily of physicians, which is often the case in health science centers. Physicians often are not oriented to nursing research methods. The lack of control in nursing studies concerns them, and some believe that the topics of these studies are not important. Sometimes they do not see the nurse researcher as credible because of educational differences, lack of previous experience in research, and few published studies. However, not all physicians view nursing research negatively. Many are strong supporters of nursing research, helpful in suggesting changes in design to strengthen the study, and eager to facilitate access to subjects.

The researcher needs to anticipate potential responses of committee members, prepare the proposal to elicit a favorable response, and consider means of minimizing negative responses. It is wise to meet with the chair of the agency research committee early in the development of a proposal. This meeting could facilitate proposal development, rapport between the researcher and agency personnel, and approval of the research proposal.

In addition to the formal committee approval mechanisms, the researcher will need the tacit approval of administrative personnel and staff who will be affected in some way by the study. Obtaining informal approval and support often depends on the way in which a person is approached. The researcher needs to demonstrate interest in the institution and the personnel as well as interest in the research project. The relationships formed with agency personnel should be equal, sharing ones, because these people often can provide ideas and strategies for conducting the study that never occurred to the researcher. Support of agency personnel during data collection can also make the difference between a successful or unsuccessful study.

Conducting nursing research can provide benefits to the institution as well as to the researcher. Clinicians have an opportunity to see nursing research in action, which can influence their thinking and clinical practice if the relationship with the researcher is positive. These clinicians may be having their first close contact with a researcher, and interpretation of the researcher's role and the study may be necessary. In addition, clinicians tend to be more oriented in the present than are researchers, and they need to see the possible immediate impact that the study findings can have on nursing practice in their institution. Thus, utilization of research findings may be enhanced, and clinicians may even become involved in research activities. All these activities can add prestige to an institution.

VERBAL DEFENSE OF A PROPOSAL

Graduate students conducting theses or dissertations are frequently required to defend their proposal verbally to their university committee members. Some institutions also require the researcher to meet with the research committee or a subcommittee to defend a proposal. In a verbal defense, the reviewers can evaluate the researcher as a person, the researcher's knowledge and understanding of the content of the proposal, and his or her ability to reason and provide logical explanations related to the study. The researcher also has the opportunity to persuade reluctant committee members to approve the study.

Appearance is important in a personal presentation, because it can give an impression of competence or incompetence. Since these presentations are business-like, with logical and rational interactions, one should dress in a business-like manner. Individuals who are casually dressed might be perceived by the committee as not valuing the review process.

Nonverbal behavior is important during the meeting as well, so appearing calm, in control, and confident projects a positive image. Planning and rehearsing a presentation can reduce anxiety. Obtaining information on the personalities of committee members, their relationships with each other, vested interests of each member, and their areas of expertise can increase confidence and provide a sense of control. It is important to arrive at the meeting early, assess the environment for the meeting, and carefully select a seat. As the presenter, all members of the committee need to be able to see you. However, selecting a seat on one side of a table with all the committee members on the other side could feel uncomfortable and simulate an atmosphere similar to that of an interrogation rather than a scholarly interaction. Sitting at the side of a table rather than at the head of the table might be a strategic move to elicit support.

The verbal defense usually begins with a brief presentation of the study. The presentation needs to be carefully planned, timed, and rehearsed. Salient points should be highlighted, which can be accomplished by the use of audiovisuals. The presentation is followed by questions from the reviewers, and the researcher needs to be prepared to defend or justify the methods and procedures of the study. Sometimes it is helpful to practice responding to questions related to the study with a friend as a means of determining the best ways to defend ideas without appearing defensive. When the meeting has ended, the researcher should thank the members of the committee for their time. If a decision regarding the study has not been made during the meeting, ask when the committee will make a decision.

REVISING A PROPOSAL

Reviewers sometimes suggest changes in a proposal; however, some of these changes may be of benefit to the institution but not to the study. In these situations, try to remain receptive to the suggestions, explore with the committee the impact of the changes on the proposed study, and try to resolve the conflict. If the conflict cannot be resolved, the researcher might need to find another setting.

Many times reviewers make valuable suggestions that might improve the quality of a study or facilitate the data collection process. The proposal is often revised based on these suggestions before the study is implemented. Sometimes a study requires revisions while it is being conducted because of problems with data collection tools or subjects' participation. However, if a proposal has been approved by clinical agency personnel or representatives of funding institutions, the researcher needs to examine the situation seriously before making major changes in the study.

Before revising a proposal, a researcher needs to address three questions: (1) What needs to be changed? (2) Why is the change necessary? and (3) How will the change affect the implementation of the study and the study findings? (Diers, 1979). Students need to seek advice from the faculty before revising their studies. Sometimes it is beneficial for seasoned researchers to discuss their proposed study changes with other researchers or agency personnel for suggestions and additional viewpoints.

If a revision is necessary, the researcher should revise the proposal and discuss the change with the members of the research committee in the agency where the study is being conducted. The committee members might indicate that the investigators can proceed with the study or that they will have to seek approval for the revised proposal. If a study is funded, the study changes must be discussed with the representatives of the funding agency. The funding agency has the power to approve or disapprove the changes. However, realistic changes that are clearly described and backed with a rationale will probably be approved.

SAMPLE QUANTITATIVE RESEARCH PROPOSAL

A proposal of a quantitative study is provided to direct students in the development of their first research proposal. The proposal was developed by a thesis student to conduct a quasi-experimental study (Ulbrich, 1995). The content of this proposal is very brief and does not include the detail normally presented in a thesis or dissertation.

Title: The Effect of Operator Technique on Tympanic Membrane Thermometry
Investigator: Sherri L. Ulbrich

Chapter 1

Introduction

Temperatures are used to monitor and diagnose infection, inflammation, neoplasia, neurological insults, hypothermia, hyperthermia, and metabolic disorders (Wolff, 1988). Accurate assessment of the body's thermal responses can provide information that results in prompt treatment and may prevent further injury, especially in acute care settings. The tympanic thermometer assesses body temperature by measuring the infrared radiation emitted from the tympanic membrane. Clinical studies have shown the tympanic thermometer to be extremely useful when compared with oral and rectal thermometers (Terndrup, 1992). However, some experts doubt the thermometer's ability to detect fever and others note cases of large differences between tympanic and other core temperature routes (Zinder & Holtel, 1995). Consequently, some health care providers are skeptical about tympanic measurements and adoption in the clinical setting has been delayed.

Some of the skepticism arises from inconsistent measurements and unanswered questions about the technique to be used with tympanic thermometers. Though technique is critical in producing accurate measurements of all vital signs including temperature, little is known about how to best use the tympanic thermometer. Information regarding the operation of this device from the manufacturer and clinical studies is conflicting. In addition, many sources fail to give specific descriptions of operator techniques or only make limited comparisons of these techniques. Currently, few tympanic thermometer technique studies have been conducted on adults (Erickson & Meyer, 1994). If a single, accurate technique for taking tympanic temperatures could be determined, patients and health care providers might benefit from the many advantages of this safe, efficient, and less invasive temperature device. Thus, the purpose of this study is to examine the effects of operator techniques on the measurement of tympanic temperatures in adult critical care patients. This information can be used to develop a research-based protocol, expand the knowledge base about tympanic thermometry, and help meet the demand for better assessment of temperature in critically ill patients.

Chapter 2

Review of Relevant Literature

Temperature measurement is an important nursing assessment, especially in critically ill patients.

Changes in temperature are physiological cues, when accurately assessed, that can lead to prompt, effective treatment (Bruce & Grove, 1991; Holtzclaw, 1992). Temperature can be measured by many routes and instruments. The specifications for the development of tympanic thermometers were congruent with the principles and theories in physics, engineering (Fraden, 1991), and physiology.

Research has shown that tympanic thermometers are accurate in healthy and ill patients of all ages in a variety of clinical and hospital settings, except in the cases of inconsistent or poor operator technique (Terndrup, 1992), exposure to low or high ambient temperatures within 20 minutes of measurement (Doyle, Zehner, & Terndrup, 1992; Zehner & Terndrup, 1991), and near complete occlusion of the tympanic membrane by cerumen or severe scarring (Pransky, 1991). Having otitis media, small or moderate amounts of cerumen, and small ear canals in children do not cause significant differences in temperature. Studies have shown tympanic temperatures to be at least as accurate as oral and rectal temperatures and much more accurate than axillary temperatures (Erickson & Yount, 1991; Schmitz, Bair, Falk, & Levine, 1995). However, tympanic temperatures are not as accurate as bladder or pulmonary artery temperatures (Erickson & Meyer, 1994; Milewski, Ferguson, & Terndrup, 1991; Nierman, 1991; Summers, 1991), especially in detecting fever (Zinder & Holtel, 1995). Tympanic thermometers are also less invasive and more time and cost efficient (Alexander & Kelly, 1991a); do not transmit infectious agents among patients (Livornese, Dias, & Samuel, 1992); preserve the patient's modesty; and produce minimal discomfort (Alexander & Kelly, 1991b).

The effect of operator technique on tympanic measurements needs to be investigated carefully. Determining the optimal technique could reduce erroneous and inconsistent measurements in future research and clinical practice (Erickson & Meyer, 1994; Erickson & Woo, 1994; Guthrie & Keunke, 1992; Pransky, 1991). Three elements in tympanic measurement technique have been identified: (1) an eartug to straighten the auditory canal; (2) aiming at the tympanic membrane; and (3) making a snug seal. Additional research is needed that provides control of extraneous variables, use of a core reference temperature, and use of consistent and meaningful analyses for comparison. Multiple techniques have not been previously studied to identify the aspects of technique or combination of techniques that are essential for obtaining the most accurate tympanic temperature measurement. The current study is proposed to increase the knowledge about the effects of operator technique on tympanic temperature measurements in critically ill adults. The information obtained from this study can assist nurses in comparing tympanic temperatures with those obtained through bladder or other core temperature routes. (To promote concise coverage of this proposal, only a summary of the theoretical and empirical literature was provided.)

Chapter 3

Framework

Thermometry is the science of temperature measurement (Schooley, 1986) and provides the framework for this study. As shown in Figure 26–1, a linear path of unimpeded heat transfer between the heat source and the thermometer system response results in a temperature measurement under ideal conditions of thermometry.

However, in reality, physiological, mechanical, and environmental factors, as well as instrumental error must be controlled or manipulated to facilitate the transfer of heat and ensure accuracy of the measurement. The extent to which each of these complex factors affects the transfer of heat and temperature measurement has not yet been fully determined. The extent to which operator technique can effectively manipulate or control these factors and influence the transfer of heat to promote optimal accuracy of the thermometer is also unknown.

In this study, the heat sources are the tympanic membrane and urinary bladder. Bladder temperature will be used as the reference core temperature and represents the ideal, accurate temperature measurement. The difference between tympanic temperatures measured using different operator techniques and the accepted standard of measured bladder temperature is the dependent variable in this study. Heat transfer between the heat sources and the thermometer system response occurred by radiation with the tympanic thermometer and conduction with the bladder thermometer. Operator technique is shown in bold face type because it is the

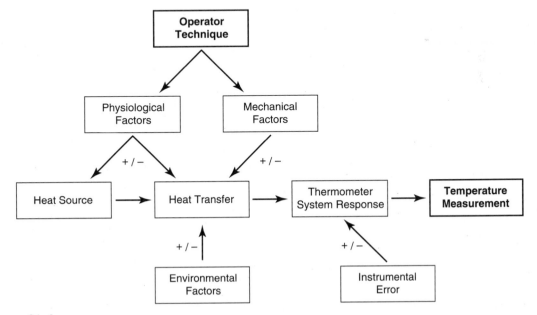

Figure 26–1
Thermometry framework. (From Ulbrich, S. L. [1995]. *The effect of operator technique on tympanic membrane thermometry.* Unpublished master's thesis. The University of Texas at Arlington, with permission.)

concept that represents the independent variables in this study. The three components of operator technique are otoscopic eartug, aim, and seal when using tympanic thermometers. Combinations of these components are the independent variables and will be used to provide additional control over physiological and mechanical factors and thus influence the transfer of heat and subsequently, the temperature measurement.

Hypothesis

There is no clinically important difference in tympanic temperature measurements using four operator techniques: (1) an otoscopic eartug with aim and seal; (2) an otoscopic eartug and seal without aim; (3) aim and seal without otoscopic eartug; and (4) seal without otoscopic eartug or aim when compared with bladder temperatures taken in critically ill adults.

Definitions of Independent Variables

Operator techniques for tympanic temperatures

Conceptual definition—Operator techniques are actions used by persons when taking temperatures that affect the physiological and mechanical factors and subsequently influence heat transfer and tympanic temperature measurement.

Operational definition—Each of the combined techniques for taking tympanic temperatures listed in the hypotheses is considered to be a single independent variable. The separate elements of each technique are operationally defined as follows:

Otoscopic eartug is the manipulation of the cartilaginous outer portion of the ear by grasping the auricle firmly but gently, pulling it upward, back, and slightly out in order to straighten the elliptical S-shaped outer canal and improve the view of the lower ear canal and tympanic membrane (Bates, 1983; Erickson & Meyer, 1994).

Aim is aligning the warmest area of the tympanic membrane, the anterior, inferior third, with the tympanic thermometer sensor tip by holding the device level while directing the tip of the probe at the midpoint between the ear and the outer canthus of the eye on the opposite side (Terndrup, 1992).

Seal is leaving no space between the walls of the auditory canal and the covered probe tip by placing the probe tip in the opening of the ear canal and applying gentle but firm pressure to seal the canal from ambient air (Erickson & Yount, 1991).

Definitions of the Dependent Variables

Bladder Temperature

Conceptual definition—Bladder temperature is the approximation of core body heat reflected in the amount of heat in the bladder (Erickson & Meyer, 1994).

Operational definition—Bladder temperature is the numerical measurement of heat in the bladder as detected by Bard thermocath and displayed by Bard and Hewlett Packard monitors using a Fahrenheit scale to the nearest tenth of a degree.

Tympanic Temperature

Conceptual definition—Tympanic temperature is the amount of heat from the tympanic membrane as detected in the auditory canal. This temperature is used as an indicator of core temperature because of its proximity and shared common blood supply with the hypothalamic thermoregulatory center (Fraden, 1991).

Operational definition—Tympanic temperature is the numerical measurement of temperature as determined and displayed by the infrared tympanic thermometer Genius 3000A Model using the Fahrenheit scale to the nearest tenth of a degree.

Attribute Variables

The attribute or demographic variables of this study are age; race; gender; admitting diagnosis to the intensive care unit (ICU); other significant diagnoses or complications; temperature changes in the previous four hours; history of carotid artery disease, stroke, head trauma, or cranial surgery; cranial turban dressing; and type of supplemental oxygenation.

Relevant Terms

Adult is a person over the age of 18 years.
Intensive care is a part of the hospital which deals specifically with life-threatening health

problems (American Association of Critical Care Nurses, 1984).

Assumptions

1. Temperature measurement is important in patient care.
2. Accurately measuring temperature is an important nursing responsibility.
3. The optimal thermometer is accurate, precise, safe, efficient, and noninvasive.

Chapter 4

Methods and Procedures

this chapter identifies the design, setting, sample, methods of measurement, data collection and analysis plan, and limitations for this proposed study. For conciseness, the key ideas of these sections are presented but not in the detail that usually is included in a thesis.

Design

This study's design is quasi-experimental and includes multiple treatments with nonequivalent dependent variables (see Figure 26–2). An attempt will be made to control the carryover effect of the treatments by changing treatment order for each subject (Burns & Grove, 1993). Efforts will be made to control the extraneous variables of environmental temperature, condition of the ear and tympanic membrane, age, activity level, and diurnal effects. A plan was developed for controlling and/or recording essential infor-

mation regarding each of these extraneous variables . . .

A protocol was developed to ensure the consistent implementation of the four treatments: tug with aim, tug without aim, aim without tug, and no tug and no aim (see Appendix 26–A). The seal is considered essential and will be achieved with all four treatments. The investigator will implement all treatments and obtain and record all measurements according to protocol to ensure consistency. A pilot study will be conducted on five subjects to assess the technique administration, determine the adequacy of the treatment protocol, and discover problems in data collection . . . Any problems noted in the design and data collection process for the study will be examined and modified as needed.

Setting and Sample

The data will be collected in the ICU of two recently merged, fully accredited, and licensed metropolitan hospitals in north central Texas. The strengths and weaknesses of these units are described. The target population is adult ICU patients who meet the sample criteria and consent to participate in the study. The sample criteria are nonexclusive to gender, ethnic background, diagnosis, or hospital treatment plan. The sample inclusion criteria consist of: (1) being a patient in the ICU, (2) being an adult over 18 years of age, (3) having a Bard Urotrack thermocatheter in place and functioning, (4) having no significant scarring or inflammation of the tympanic membrane, (5) having no bleeding or drainage from

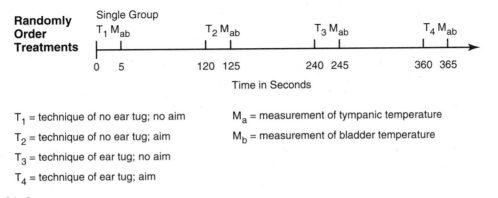

Figure 26–2

Multiple treatments with nonequivalent dependent variables design. (From Ulbrich, S. L. [1995]. *The effect of operator technique on tympanic membrane thermometry.* Unpublished master's thesis. The University of Texas at Arlington, with permission.)

the tympanic membrane or ear canal, (6) having no obvious occlusion of the ear canal with cerumen, (7) having not been given antipyretics within the previous three hours, (8) having no exposure to extreme temperatures of $< -5.0°C$ or $> 35.0°C$ within the past two hours, (9) having not been on a heating or cooling blanket within the past two hours, and (10) having a bladder temperature in the range of $96.0–102.0°F$ or $15.6–43.3°C$. The sample size was calculated using a power analysis with a standard power of .8, effect size of .4, and alpha of .05. It was determined that a minimum of 73 subjects will be needed for this study. A nonprobability sample of convenience will be used. However, the design is strengthened by a random selection of right or left ear and a random ordering of treatments. The strengths and weaknesses of this sampling method are described.

Measurement Methods

The tympanic temperatures will be measured using the single First Temp Genius Model 3000A thermometer. This thermometer is equipped with a unique "Peak Select System" that internally records and analyzes 32 separate measurements from the incoming radiation, and displays the average of the highest two readings . . . The precision, accuracy, sensitivity, and potential error of this thermometer are described.

Bladder temperatures will be measured using Bard Urotrack Foley Catheters, model number 890216/18 sizes 16–18 French, manufactured by Bard Urologic Division of Covington, Georgia. These modified transurethral indwelling Foley catheters, like standard catheters, are made from hydrogel-coated latex tubes with a five milliliter balloon encircling the catheter just below the tip to anchor the catheter in place within the bladder . . . The precision, accuracy, sensitivity, and potential error for this catheter are described.

Plan for Data Collection

The treatments will be implemented and data will be collected by the investigator using the protocol outlined in Appendix 26–A. Data will be recorded on the data collection form developed for this study (see Appendix 26–B). The investigator will note the consistency of the treatment implementation and the data collection process. When the protocol is not followed consistently, this will be recorded (Egan, Snyder, &

Burns, 1992). A complete plan for the data collection process is outlined in Appendix 26–C. Raw data and consent forms will be stored in a locked file drawer in the investigator's house for five years.

Ethical Considerations

Permission to conduct this study will be obtained from the investigator's thesis committee, the Human Rights Review Committee for The University of Texas at Arlington, and the hospital's Institutional Review Board. In addition, verbal approval will be obtained from the ICU managers and the primary physicians of the subjects. Subjects will be provided essential information for informed consent and will sign a consent form (see Appendix 26–D). The benefit-risk ratio was assessed for this study, indicating minimal risk and important benefits.

Data Analysis

Data will be input and analyzed by the researcher using Mystat, a software package developed by Munro and Page (1993). All raw data entered in the computer will be checked for errors. Demographic data will be analyzed with frequencies, percents, means, standard deviations, and ranges and presented in a table (see Appendix 26–E). The hypothesis will provide direction for the analysis of study data. Means, standard deviations, and ranges will be calculated on the bladder and tympanic temperatures for the four treatments of tug with aim, tug without aim, aim without tug, and no tug and no aim. The Bland-Altman method will be used to compare bladder and tympanic temperatures for each operator technique. Researchers have begun to use this method rather than conventional statistics such as Pearson's product-moment correlations or tests of statistical differences. Bland and Altman (1986) have suggested that conventional statistics are inappropriate when an established method of measurement, such as bladder temperature, is compared to a new method of measurement, such as tympanic temperature. . . . The results will be presented in graphs.

Methodological Limitations

The limitations of this study include that (1) the extraneous variables of environmental and core body temperatures will not be completely con-

Table 26–3
Study Timetable

Task to Be Performed	Performer of Task	Completion of Task
1. Complete proposal and forms	Researcher	First through sixth months
2. Defend and revise proposal	Researcher	Seventh month
3. Review board approvals	Researcher	Eighth month
4. Equipment gathering and training	Researcher	Eighth month
5. Assemble data collection packets	Researcher	Eighth month
6. Establish potential subject notification with personnel at clinical agency	Researcher	Eighth month
7. Pilot study	Researcher	Ninth month
8. Analyze pilot data and revise	Researcher	Ninth month
9. Data collection	Researcher	Tenth & eleventh months
10. Analyze data	Researcher	Twelfth month
11. Interpret results	Researcher	Twelfth month
12. Final defense	Researcher	Thirteenth month
13. Communicate findings	Researcher	2–3 years

(From Ulbrich, S. L. [1995]. *The effect of operator technique on tympanic membrane thermometry.* Unpublished master's thesis. The University of Texas at Arlington, with permission.)

trolled; (2) nonrandom sample will limit generalizability; and (3) estimation of core body temperature by the bladder thermometer is not quite as accurate as the pulmonary artery catheter, although they correlate at $r = .99$ (Erickson & Meyer, 1994).

Communication of Findings

The study findings will be presented to the thesis committee, hospital research committee, ICU nurses and managers, and the manufacturer of the equipment. In addition, an abstract of the study will be submitted for possible presentation of the research at a national critical care meeting. The study will be submitted for publication in a clinical journal such as *Heart & Lung* or *American Journal of Critical Care.* A study timetable and budget have been developed to direct this project and are presented in Tables 26–3 and 26–4. ∎

Table 26–4
Study Budget

Budget Items	Cost per Item	Total Cost
1. Printing costs	1,500 pages @ .05/page	75.00
2. Consultant costs	Provided by the Center for Nursing Research	.00
3. Statistical software		50.00
4. Genius II tympanic thermometer and probe covers	Provided by Sherwood Medical	.00
5. Bard calibration plug	Provided by Bard Urologic Division	.00
6. Travel costs		150.00
7. Supplies		80.00
8. Communication costs		100.00
	Total	**455.00**

(From Ulbrich, S. L. [1995]. *The effect of operator technique on tympanic membrane thermometry.* Unpublished master's thesis. The University of Texas at Arlington, with permission.)

Appendix 26–A

Data Collection Protocol

1. After consent is signed, the data collection form with the corresponding ID No. will be taken to the nursing station.
2. Place the room thermometer in the subject's room.
3. Questions one through ten will be answered by the researcher from information contained within the chart. All demographic questions will be completed prior to experimental data collection.
4. Enter the subject's room, ask any additional questions, and review the procedure if this is appropriate.
5. Record the room temperature from the thermometer left earlier.
6. Place the data collection form, otoscope, tympanic thermometer, and stopwatch on the same side of the patient as the ear selected for intervention.
7. Perform the brief otoscopic examination by gently retracting the subject's ear and inserting the otoscope into the external canal.
8. Note on the data collection form any large amount of cerumen, presence of any trauma, drainage, significant scarring, or severe inflammation. If any of these conditions are present, explain to the subject reasons for exclusion from the study and notify the nursing staff of the findings.
9. Insert the Bard calibration plug into the Urotrack monitor for calibration if applicable.
10. Record the time of day when data collection began.
11. Review the selected treatment order.
12. Remove the tympanic thermometer from its base and place a disposable cover on the probe tip.
13. Manipulate the ear and insert the probe in the *exact* manner outlined below for the first technique.
    T1 (tug: aim)—Gently grasp the superior aspect of the pinna and retract the ear in an upward, outward, and backward motion. Maintain this position and insert the covered tip of the probe, aiming at the point between the bridge of the nose and outer canthus of the eye on the opposite side of the head. Apply gentle pressure with the probe tip to seal the canal.
    T2 (tug: no aim)—Gently grasp the superior aspect of the pinna and retract the ear in an upward, outward, and backward motion. Maintain this position and insert the covered tip of the probe, directing it toward the opposite ear or along the mid-frontal plane of the head. Apply gentle pressure with the probe tip to seal the ear canal.
    T3 (no tug: aim)—Steady the subject's head by placing a hand over the temporal area. Insert the covered probe tip, aiming at the point between the bridge of the nose and outer canthus of the eye on the opposite side of the head. Apply gentle pressure with the probe tip to seal the ear canal.
    T4 (no tug: no aim)—Steady the subject's head by placing a hand over the temporal area. Insert the covered tip of the probe, directing it at the opposite ear or the probe along the mid-frontal plane of the head. Apply gentle pressure with the probe tip to seal the ear canal.
14. Press the SCAN button on the thermometer.
15. Remove the thermometer, release the ear, and dispose of the probe tip cover.
16. Begin the 2-minute interval timer on the stopwatch.
17. Record the temperature in the appropriate blank on the data collection form.
18. Immediately read the bladder temperature from the thermocath monitor.
19. Record the bladder temperature in the appropriate blank on the data collection form.
20. Allow the 2 minutes to pass.
21. Repeat steps 12–20 for each of the remaining techniques in the order on the data collection form.
22. Record the time that data collection ended.
23. Thank the subject (if appropriate) for participation in the study. Answer any questions or address any concerns.
24. Review the data collection sheet for completeness.
25. Gather the equipment and leave the data collection area.

(From Ulbrich, S. L. [1995]. *The effect of operator technique on tympanic membrane thermometry.* Unpublished master's thesis. The University of Texas at Arlington, with permission.) ∎

Appendix 26–B

Data Collection Form

ID No. _____   Date _____

Demographic Data

A. Age _____
                                      B. Gender _____ (1) female _____ (2) male
C. Race _____ (1) Caucasian   _____ (2) Asian   _____ (3) American Indian
       _____ (4) African American _____ (5) Hispanic _____ (6) Other
D. Unit _____ (1) CCU   _____ (2) MICU   _____ (3) SICU   _____ (4) NICU
E. Campus   _____ (1) East   _____ (2) West
F. Admitting/Major diagnosis: _____
G. Other significant diagnoses: _____
H. Supplemental oxygen   _____ (1) NC   _____ (2) vent   _____ (3) FM
                                    _____ (4) FT   _____ (5) other   _____ (6) none
I. Turban cranial dressing   _____ (1) yes   _____ (2) no
J. Hx _____ (1) carotid artery disease   _____ (2) cerebral vascular accident
      _____ (3) major head trauma   _____ (4) cranial surgery
      _____ (5) none
K. Most recent temperature _____ F   Time taken _____
L. Room temperature   _____ F

Experimental Data

M. Ear _____ (1) right   _____ (2) left
N. Noted upon aural exam   _____ (1) large amount of cerumen   _____ (2) trauma
                                  _____ (3) significant scarring   _____ (4) drainage
                                  _____ (5) significant inflammation   _____ (6) hair
                                  _____ (7) other

Time data collection began _____

Treatment Order	Tympanic Temp.	Bladder Temp.

Time data collection ended _____

O. Data collection & treatments followed the protocol _____ (1) yes _____ (2) no _____ (3) partial
   Explain, if partial _____

Comments:

(From Ulbrich, S. L. [1995]. *The effect of operator technique on tympanic membrane thermometry.* Unpublished master's thesis. The University of Texas at Arlington, with permission.)

Appendix 26–C

Data Collection Plan

1. Locate potential subjects by making a daily phone call or visit to the intensive care units. Potential subjects might also be located by asking staff to notify the researcher by telephone of patients with bladder thermocatheters. The phone number of the researcher is already in the list of numbers in each unit.

2. Assess potential subjects in person using the sample criteria. This information can be gathered from the chart or staff. Timing should be considered in this step to avoid the hours near midnight to 3:00 a.m. and 6:00 a.m. to 8:00 a.m. or when nursing activities can be anticipated (timed dressing changes, scheduled procedures, etc.).

3. If all sample criteria are met, pursue consent to participate from the patient or legal representative.

4. Place the signed consent form in a folder to be kept with the researcher until it can be secured in the safe. Give one copy to the subject and place another in the chart.

5. Gather and record the demographic data from the chart or staff.

6. Follow the specific procedures outlined in the protocol (see Appendix 26–B) to implement the procedures and gather the experimental data.

7. Review forms for completeness.

8. Thank the staff and patient (if appropriate) for their participation and assistance.

9. Initiate the entire process with any additional subjects.

10. Gather equipment and return to the office.

11. File and secure all consent and data collection forms.

12. Repeat steps 1–11 until at least 30 subjects are recruited and data is collected.

(From Ulbrich, S. L. [1995]. *The effect of operator technique on tympanic membrane thermometry.* Unpublished master's thesis. The University of Texas at Arlington, with permission.) ∎

Appendix 26–D

Consent Form

Study Title: The Effect of Operator Technique on Tympanic Membrane Thermometry
Investigator: Sherri L. Ulbrich R.N., B.S.N., CCRN
Subject ID No. _____   **Hospital No.** _____   **Protocol No.** _____

You are invited to be in a research study to determine how different techniques used by nurses in taking tympanic temperatures affect the accuracy of these thermometers in adult patients in the intensive care unit. Over the next four months about 70 participants will be chosen in this nontherapeutic study without regard for race, gender, or socioeconomic status. Since you are already a patient in the intensive care unit and have a special bladder catheter to monitor your temperature you have been selected as a possible participant. As a benefit, your temperature will be monitored closely and will provide information that might enable nurses to better assess the temperatures of their patients in the future.

The study and its procedures have been approved by the appropriate people and review boards at The University of Texas at Arlington and the hospital. If you were to participate in the study the specially trained researcher would (1) complete a demographic data sheet, (2) perform a brief ear (otoscopic) examination, (3) take a series of tympanic temperatures using different techniques to straighten the ear canal (similar to an ear examination) and aim the instrument, and (4) record the temperature from the special catheter you already have in place. The risk associated with this study is the possibility of injury to the ear canal and/or tympanic membrane. Neither have ever occurred in previous studies. Also, this risk is no greater than with the routine measurement of your temperature with the thermometer that is currently used throughout the hospital. You will be excluded from the study if any abnormalities are found during the ear examination to avoid this risk. Participation in this study will take approximately 10 minutes. You are free to ask any questions about the study or about being a subject and you may call the investigator at (817) 273-2776 if you have further questions.

Your participation in this study is voluntary: You are under no obligation to participate. You have the right to withdraw at any time and the care you receive and your relationship with the health care team will not be affected. Neither you nor the hospital will be charged or incur any expense or compensation for your participation. Although your physician is not an investigator, he or she will be informed of your participation.

The study data will be coded so they will not be linked to your name. Your identity will not be revealed while the study is being conducted, except to the doctors and nurses caring for you, or when the study is reported or published. All study data will be collected by the researcher, stored in a secure place, and will not be shared without your permission. A copy of the consent form will be given to you.

I have read this consent form and voluntarily consent to participate in this study. I understand that I am to rely on the investigator for information regarding the nature and purpose of the research study, the risks involved in the research study, and the possibility of complications, and I have been given an opportunity to discuss these with the investigator.

_____   Date   _____   Date
Subject's Signature   Legally Authorized Representative

I have explained this study to the above subject and have sought his/her understanding for informed consent.

_____   Date
Investigator's Signature

(From Ulbrich, S. L. [1995]. *The effect of operator technique on tympanic membrane thermometry*. Unpublished master's thesis. The University of Texas at Arlington, with permission.) ∎

Appendix 26–E

Dummy Table to Present Sample Characteristics

Demographic Variables	Sample Statistics* N = 60	
	M (SD)	range
Age Most Recent Temperature Room Temperature		
	Frequency	Percent

Gender
  male
  female		

Race
  Caucasian
  African American
  Asian
  Hispanic
  American Indian
  Other		

Unit
  CCU
  MICU
  SICU
  NICU		

Primary Diagnosis
  XXXXXXXX
  XXXXXXXX
  XXXXXXXX
  XXXXXXXX		

Other Significant Diagnoses
  XXXXXXXX
  XXXXXXXX
  XXXXXXXX
  XXXXXXXX		

Mechanically Ventilated		
Turban-Type Cranial Dressing		

History of:
  carotid artery disease
  cerebral vascular accident
  major head trauma
  cranial surgery		

Note: *Only selected statistics are used to analyze each variable.

(From Ulbrich, S. L. [1995]. *The effect of operator technique on tympanic membrane thermometry.* Unpublished master's thesis. The University of Texas at Arlington, with permission.) ■

SUMMARY

This chapter focuses on writing a research proposal and seeking approval to conduct a study. A research proposal is a written plan that identifies the major elements of a study, such as the research problem, purpose, and framework, and outlines the methods and procedures to conduct a study. A well-written proposal communicates a significant, carefully planned research project; demonstrates the qualifications of the researcher; and generates support for the project. Writing a quality proposal involves (1) developing the ideas logically, (2) determining the depth or detail of the proposal content, (3) identifying the critical points in the proposal, and (4) developing an esthetically appealing copy.

The content of a proposal needs to be written with the interest and expertise of the reviewers in mind. Proposals are frequently reviewed by faculty, clinical agency members, and representatives of funding institutions. The content of a proposal varies depending on the reviewers, the guidelines developed for the review, and the type of study (quantitative or qualitative) proposed. There are usually four chapters or sections in a quantitative research proposal: (1) introduction, (2) review of relevant literature, (3) framework, and (4) methods and procedures. A qualitative research proposal usually includes the following chapters or sections: (1) introduction, (2) literature review, and (3) methods.

The content of a student proposal usually requires greater detail than a proposal developed for review by clinical agency personnel or funding organizations. Most clinical agencies and funding institutions require a condensed proposal. However, even though these proposals are condensed, the logical links between the components of the study need to be clearly demonstrated. The proposal usually includes a problem, a purpose, previous research conducted in the area, a framework, variables, design, sample, ethical considerations, plan for data collection and analysis, and plan for dissemination of findings.

Sometimes a researcher will send a preproposal or query letter to a funding institution rather than a proposal. A preproposal is a short document of four to five pages plus appendices that is written to explore the funding possibilities for a research project. The parts of the preproposal are logically ordered as follows: (1) letter of transmittal, (2) proposal for research, (3) personnel, (4) facilities, and (5) budget. Using the preproposal, researchers can submit their proposals only to those institutions that indicate an interest in their projects.

A research proposal is a formal way to communicate ideas about a proposed study to receive approval to conduct the study or to seek funding. Seeking approval for the conduct or funding of a study is a process that involves submission of a proposal to a selected group for review and, in many situations, verbally defending that proposal. Research proposals are reviewed to (1) evaluate the quality of the study, (2) ensure that adequate measures are being taken to protect human subjects, and (3) evaluate the impact of the conduct of the study on the reviewing institution. An initial step in seeking approval to conduct a study is to determine what committees in which agencies must grant approval before the study can be conducted. Receiving approval to conduct a study requires preparing a scholarly proposal, examining the social and political factors in the review committee, and defending the proposal to the committee.

Proposals often require some revisions before or during the implementation of a study. Before revising a proposal, a researcher needs to address these questions: (1) What needs to be changed? (2) Why is the change necessary? and (3) How will the change affect the implementation of the study and the study findings? If a change is necessary, the researcher needs to discuss the change with the members of the clinical agency research review committee or the funding agency. The chapter concludes with an example of a brief quantitative research proposal of a quasi-experimental study (Ulbrich, 1995).

References

Alexander, D., & Kelly, B. (1991a). Cost effectiveness of tympanic thermometry in the pediatric office setting. *Clinical Pediatrics* (Suppl.), *30*(4), 57–59.

Alexander, D., & Kelly, B. (1991b). Responses of children, parents, and nurses to tympanic thermometry in the pediatric office. *Clinical Pediatrics* (Suppl.), *30*(4), 53–56.

American Association of Critical Care Nurses. (1984). *Definition of critical care nursing.* Newport Beach, CA: AACCN.

American Psychological Association. (1994). *Publication manual of the American Psychological Association* (4th ed.). Washington, DC: American Psychological Association.

Barnard, K. E. (1986). MCN keys to research: Writing a research proposal. *Maternal Child Nursing, 11*(1), 76.

Bates, B. (1983). *A guide to physical examination* (3rd ed.). Philadelphia: Lippincott.

Beck, C. T. (1993). Qualitative research: The evaluation of its credibility, fittingness, and auditability. *Western Journal of Nursing Research, 15*(2), 263–266.

Bland, J. M., & Altman, D. G. (1986). Statistical methods for assessing agreement between two methods of clinical measurement. *Lancet, 1*(8476), 307–310.

Bruce, J. L., & Grove, S. K. (1991). Fever: Pathology and treatment. *Critical Care Nurse, 12*(1), 40–49.

Burns, N. (1989). Standards for qualitative research. *Nursing Science Quarterly, 2*(1), 44–52.

Burns, N., & Grove, S. K. (1993). *The practice of nursing research: Conduct, critique, and utilization* (2nd ed.). Philadelphia: Saunders.

Chenitz, W. C., & Swanson, J. M. (1986). *From practice to grounded theory: Qualitative research in nursing.* Menlo Park, CA: Addison-Wesley.

Cohen, M. Z., Knafl, K., & Dzurec, L. C. (1993). Grant writing for qualitative research. *Image: Journal of Nursing Scholarship, 25*(2), 151–156.

Cook, C. K. (1985). *Line by line: How to edit your own writing.* Boston: Houghton Mifflin.

Diers, D. (1979). *Research in nursing practice.* Philadelphia: Lippincott.

Doyle, F., Zehner, W. J., & Terndrup, T. E. (1992). The effect of ambient temperature on tympanic and oral temperatures. *American Journal of Emergency Medicine, 10*(4), 285–289.

Egan, E. C., Snyder, M., & Burns, K. R. (1992). Intervention studies in nursing: Is the effect due to the independent variable. *Nursing Outlook, 40*(4), 187–190.

Erickson, R. S., & Meyer, L. T. (1994). Accuracy of infrared ear thermometry and other temperature methods in adults. *American Journal of Critical Care, 3*(1), 40–54.

Erickson, R. S., & Woo, T. M. (1994). Accuracy of ear thermometry and traditional temperature methods in young children. *Heart & Lung, 23*(3), 181–195.

Erickson, R. S., & Yount, S. T. (1991). Comparison of tympanic and oral temperatures in surgical patients. *Nursing Research, 40*(2), 90–93.

Fraden, J. (1991). Noncontact temperature measurements in medicine. In D. L. Wise (Ed.), *Bioinstrumentation and biosensors* (pp. 511–549). New York: Marcel Dekker.

Guthrie, K. A., & Keunke, N. E. (1992). *Tympanic-based core temperature measurement in relation to thermometer and technique.* Unpublished master's thesis, Oregon Health Sciences University, Portland, OR.

Holtzclaw, B. J. (1992). The febrile response in critical care: State of the science. *Heart & Lung, 21*(5), 482–501.

Krathwohl, D. R. (1977). *How to prepare a research proposal* (2nd ed.). Syracuse: Syracuse University Bookstore.

Leininger, M. M. (1985). *Qualitative research methods in nursing.* Orlando, FL: Grune & Stratton.

Livornese, L. L., Dias, S., & Samuel, C. (1992). Hospital acquired infection with vancomycin-resistant *Enterococcus faectium* transmitted by electronic thermometers. *Annals of Internal Medicine, 117*(2), 112–116.

Malasanos, L. J. (1976). What is the preproposal? What are its component parts? Is it an effective instrument in assessing funding potential of research ideas? *Nursing Research, 25*(3), 223–224.

Marshall, C., & Rossman, G. B. (1989). *Designing qualitative research.* Newbury Park, CA: Sage.

Miles, M. B., & Huberman, A. M. (1994). *Qualitative data analysis* (2nd ed). Thousand Oaks, CA: Sage.

Milewski, A., Ferguson, K. L., & Terndrup, T. E. (1991). Comparison of pulmonary artery, rectal, and tympanic membrane temperatures in adult intensive care patients. *Clinical Pediatrics* (Suppl.), *30*(4), 13–16.

Munhall, P. L., & Oiler, C. J. (1986). *Nursing research: A qualitative perspective.* Norwalk, CT: Appleton-Century-Crofts.

Munro, B. H., & Page, E. B. (1993). *Statistical methods for health care research* (2nd ed.). Philadelphia: Lippincott.

Nierman, D. M. (1991). Core temperature measurement in the intensive care unit. *Critical Care Medicine, 19*(6), 818–823.

Parse, R. R., Coyne, A. B., & Smith, M. J. (1985). *Nursing research: Qualitative methods.* Bowie, MD: Brady.

Pinch, W. J. (1995). Synthesis: Implementing a complex process. *Nurse Educator, 20*(1), 34–40.

Pransky, S. M. (1991). The impact of technique and conditions of the tympanic membrane upon infrared tympanic thermometry. *Clinical Pediatrics* (Suppl.), *30*(4), 50–51.

Rogers, B. (1987). Research proposals: The significance of the study. *AAOHN Journal, 35*(4), 190.

Sandelowski, M., Davis, D. H., & Harris, B. G. (1989). Artful design: Writing the proposal for research in the naturalist paradigm. *Research in Nursing & Health, 12*(2), 77–84.

Schmitz, T., Bair, N., Falk, M., & Levine, C. (1995). A comparison of five methods of temperature measurement in febrile intensive care patients. *American Journal of Critical Care, 4*(4), 286–292.

Schooley, J. F. (1986). *Thermometry.* Boca Raton, FL: CRC Press.

Summers, S. (1991). Axillary, tympanic, and esophageal measurement: Descriptive comparisons in postanesthesia patients. *Journal of Post Anesthesia Nursing, 6*(6), 420–425.

Terndrup, T. E. (1992). An appraisal of temperature assessment by infrared emission detection tympanic thermometry. *Annals of Emergency Medicine, 21*(12), 92–101.

Tornquist, E. M. (1986). *From proposal to publication: An informal guide to writing about nursing research.* Menlo Park, CA: Addison-Wesley.

Ulbrich, S. L. (1995). *The effect of operator technique on tympanic membrane thermometry.* Unpublished master's thesis. The University of Texas at Arlington, Arlington, TX.

University of Chicago Press. (1993). *The Chicago manual of style* (14th ed.). Chicago: University of Chicago Press.

Vessey, J. A., & Campos, R. G. (1992). Commentary: The role of nursing research committee. *Nursing Research, 41*(4), 247–249.

Wolff, S. M. (1988). The febrile patient. In J. B. Wyngaarden, & L. H. Smith, (Eds.), *Cecil textbook of medicine* (18th ed., Vol. 2, pp. 1524–1525). Philadelphia: Saunders.

Zehner, W. J., & Terndrup, T. E. (1991). The impact of moderate temperature variance on the relationship between oral, rectal, and tympanic membrane temperatures. *Clinical Pediatrics* (Suppl.), *30*(4), 61–64.

Zinder, D. J., & Holtel, M. (1995). Fever detection in intensive care unit patients using infrared tympanic thermometry. *Critical Care Medicine, 23*(1), A28.

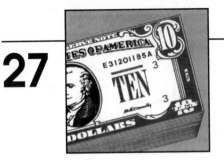

27

Seeking Funding for Research

Seeking funding for research is important, both for the researcher and for the profession. Well-designed studies cost money. As the control of variance and the complexity of the design increase, the cost of the study tends to increase. By obtaining funding, the researcher can conduct a complex, well-designed study. Funding also indicates that the study has been reviewed by others who have recognized its scientific and social merit. In fact, the scientific credibility of the profession is related to the quality of studies conducted by its researchers. Thus, scientific credibility and funding for research are interrelated.

The profession of nursing has invested a great deal of energy in increasing the sources of funding and amount of money available for nursing research. Each incidence of funding enhances the status of the researcher and increases possibilities of greater funding for later studies. In addition, funding provides some practical advantages. For example, funding may reimburse part or all of the researcher's salary, releasing the researcher from other responsibilities to devote time to conducting the study. The availability of research assistants facilitates careful data collection and allows the researcher to use time productively. Thus, skills in seeking funding for research are as important as skills in the conduct of research.

PURPOSES FOR SEEKING RESEARCH FUNDING

Two general types of grants are sought in nursing: developmental (or program) grants and research grants. Developmental grant proposals are written to obtain funding for the development of new programs in nursing, such as a program designed to teach nurses to provide a new type of nursing care or to implement a new approach to patient care. Although these programs may involve evaluation, they seldom involve research. For example, the effectiveness of a new approach to patient care may be evaluated, but the findings can seldom be generalized beyond the unit or institution in which the patient care was provided. The emphasis is on implementing the new approach to care, not on research. Research grants provide funding specifically to conduct a study. Although there are similarities between the two types of grant proposals, there are also important differences in writing techniques and flow of ideas, as well as content. This chapter focuses on seeking funding for research.

The researcher may have one of two purposes for seeking research funding. First, the funding may allow the researcher to conduct a single study that is of immediate concern or interest. This is most common among nursing students who are preparing theses and dissertations. However, nurses in clinical practice may also develop an interest in a single study that has emerged from their clinical situation. Except in unusual circumstances, the person seeking funding for a single study, such as a master's thesis, needs to consider sources of small amounts of money. In most cases, this type of funding will not reimburse for salary and will pay only a portion of the costs of the study. Sources of funding are likely to be those described in the section entitled "Conducting Research on a Shoestring." These funds may pay for the costs of purchasing or printing instruments, postage, research assistants' salaries, travel to data collection sites, costs of computer analyses, and/ or the services of a statistician. If the researcher's experience is a positive one, further studies may be conducted later in his or her career. Thus, these small grants can be stepping-stones to larger grants.

Another purpose for seeking funding is to initiate or maintain a career of conducting research. This is most common among nursing faculty and nurses employed in research positions in health care agencies. The individual planning to continue research activities throughout a career needs to plan a strategy for progressively more extensive funding of research activities. It is unrealistic, even in a university setting, to expect the time and money needed to conduct full-time research without external funding. An aspiring career researcher needs to be willing to invest the time and energy to develop grantsmanship skills. The researcher must also develop a goal to obtain funding for that portion of time that it seems desirable to commit to research activities. This goal is discussed with administrative personnel.

An aspiring career researcher needs to initiate a program of research in a specific area of study, and funding is sought in this area. For example, if the research interest is health promotion in rural areas, a series of studies focusing on rural health promotion needs to be planned. Even more desirable is an interdisciplinary team committed to a research program. Funding agencies are usually more supportive of researchers who focus their efforts in one area of study. Each study conducted within this area will increase the researcher's database and familiarity with the area. Research designs can be built on previous studies. This base of previous research and knowledge greatly increases the probability of receiving further funding. Publications of the studies will also increase the credibility of the researcher.

WAYS TO LEARN GRANTSMANSHIP

Grantsmanship is not an innate skill; it must be learned. Learning the process requires a commitment of both time and energy. However, the re-

wards can be great. Strategies used to learn grantsmanship are described in the following section and are listed in order of increasing time commitment, involvement, and level of expertise needed. The strategies are attending grantsmanship courses, developing a reference group, joining research organizations, participating on research committees or review panels, networking, assisting a researcher, and obtaining a mentor.

ATTENDING GRANTSMANSHIP COURSES

Some universities offer elective courses on grantsmanship. Continuing education programs or professional conferences sometimes offer topics related to grantsmanship. The content of these sessions may include the process of grant writing, techniques for obtaining grant funds, and sources of grant funds. In some cases, representatives of funding agencies will be invited to explain funding procedures. This information is useful for developing skills in writing proposals.

DEVELOPING A REFERENCE GROUP

A reference group consists of individuals who share common values, ways of thinking, and/or activities. These individuals become a reference group when a person identifies with the group, takes on group values and behaviors, and evaluates his or her own values and behaviors in relation to those of the group (Cartwright & Zander, 1968). For the new researcher moving into grantsmanship, this may mean switching from a reference group that views research and grant writing to be either over their heads or not worth their time to a group that values this activity. From this group will come the support and feedback necessary to develop grant-writing skills.

JOINING RESEARCH ORGANIZATIONS

Research organizations are another source of support and new information for grant writing. Membership in the Council of Nurse Researchers provides an excellent source of information and support related to grant funding for research. To be a member, one must belong to the American Nurses' Association (ANA) and either be involved in nursing research or be supervising others who are conducting research. The council is an important reference group for researchers. Communication is maintained through annual meetings and a newsletter. The council also provides opportunities for interaction with other nurse researchers on international and national levels and facilitates the development of networks of researchers conducting studies within similar areas of interest. Regional nursing research associations, not affiliated with ANA, are also located across the United States. Many specialty nursing organizations have research groups for members interested in conducting studies related to a particular nursing specialty.

SERVING ON RESEARCH COMMITTEES

Research committees and institutional review boards exist in many work and professional organizations. Through membership on these committees, contacts with researchers can be made. Also, many research committees are involved in reviewing proposals for funding of small grants or granting approval to collect data in an institution. Reviewing proposals and making decisions about funding helps researchers become better able to critique their own proposals and revise them before submitting them for review.

NETWORKING

Networking is a process of developing channels of communication among people with common interests throughout the country. Contacts may be made by computer networks, mail, telephone, or arrangements to meet in groups. Through this process, nurses interested in a particular area of study can maintain contacts made at meetings by exchanging addresses and telephone numbers. These contacts provide opportunities for brainstorming, sharing ideas and problems, and discussing grant-writing opportunities. In some cases, it is possible to write a grant to include members of a network in various parts of the country. When a proposal is being developed, the network, which may become a reference group, can provide feedback at various stages of the proposal development.

ASSISTING A RESEARCHER

Volunteering to assist with the activities of another researcher is an excellent way to learn research and grantsmanship. Graduate students can gain this experience by becoming graduate research assistants. Assisting in grant writing and reading proposals that have been funded can be particularly helpful. Examination of proposals that have been rejected can also be useful if the comments of the review committee are available. The criticisms of the review committee point out the weaknesses of the study and therefore clarify the reasons why the proposal was rejected. Examining these comments within the proposal can increase the insight of the new grant writer and also prepare him or her for similar experiences. However, some researchers are sensitive about these criticisms and may be reluctant to share them. If the experienced researcher is willing, it is enlightening to hear his or her perceptions and opinions about the criticisms.

OBTAINING A MENTOR

Learning effective means of acquiring funding is difficult. Much of the information needed is transmitted verbally, requires actual participation in grant-writing activities, and is best learned in a mentor relationship. A mentor is a person who is more experienced professionally and who is willing to "teach the ropes" to a less-experienced professional. Modeling is an important part of the mentoring process. This type of relationship requires a willingness to invest time and energy by both professionals. A mentor relationship has characteristics of both a teacher-learner relationship and a close friendship. Each must have an affinity for the other, from which a close working relationship can be developed. The relationship usually continues for a long period. However, mentorship is not well developed in nursing, and nurses who have this opportunity should consider themselves fortunate.

BECOMING A FUNDED RESEARCHER

Many of us, as neophyte researchers, have had the fantasy of writing a grant proposal to the federal government or a large foundation for our first study and suddenly achieving "stardom" (100 percent of our salary and everything needed to conduct the ultimate study, including a microcomputer, a secretary, and multiple graduate research assistants). Unfortunately, in reality, this seldom occurs for an inexperienced researcher. The new researcher is usually caught in a "Catch-22" situation. One needs to be an experienced researcher in order to get funded; however, one needs funding in order to get release time to conduct research. One way of resolving this dilemma is to design initial studies that can realistically be done without release time and with little or no funding. This approach requires a commitment to putting in extra hours of work, which are often unrewarded, monetarily or socially. However, these types of studies, well carried out and published, will provide the credibility one needs to begin the process toward major grant funding.

CONDUCTING RESEARCH ON A SHOESTRING

Ideas for studies often begin in grandiose ways. You envision the ideal study and follow all the rules in the textbooks and in research courses. Then when you begin to determine what is needed in time and money in order to conduct this wonderful study, you find your resources sadly lacking. This discovery should not lead you to give up the idea of conducting research. Rather, you need to take stock of your resources and determine exactly what realistically can be done. Then modify your study to meet existing constraints. The modified study must remain good research but be scaled down to an achievable level. This might involve studying only one aspect of the original study, decreasing the number of variables examined, or limiting the study to a single site. In many cases, a minimum amount of money is needed to conduct small studies. This project can be the pilot study that is essential to attracting larger amounts of research funding.

The next step is to determine potential sources of this small amount of money. In some cases, management in the employing institution can supply limited funding for research activities if a good case is presented for the usefulness of the study to the institution. In many universities, funds are available for intramural grants, which are obtained competitively by submitting a brief proposal to a university committee. Some nursing organizations also have money available for research activities. For example, Sigma Theta Tau, the honor society for nurses, provides small grants for nursing research that can be obtained through submission to international, national, regional, or local review committees. Another source is local agencies, such as the American Cancer Society and the American Heart Association. Although grants from the national offices of these organizations require sophistication in research, local or state levels of the organization may have small amounts of funds available for studies in the area of interest of the organization.

Private individuals who are locally active in philanthropy may be willing to provide financial assistance for a small study in an area appealing to them. One needs to know who to approach and how and when to make the approach in order to increase the probability of successful funding. Sometimes this requires knowing someone who knows someone who might be willing to provide financial support. Acquiring funds from private individuals also requires more assertiveness than the other approaches to funding (Holmstrom & Burgess, 1982).

Requests for funding need not be limited to a single source. If a larger amount of money is needed than can be supplied by one source, funds can be sought from one source for a specific research need and from another source for another research need. Also, one source may be able to provide funds for a small segment of time, and another source can then be approached to provide funding to continue another phase of the study. A combination of these two strategies can also be used.

Seeking funding from local sources is less demanding in terms of formality and length of proposal than are other grants. Often the process is informal and may require only a two- or three-page description of the study. The important thing is knowing what funds are available and how to apply for them. Some of these funds go unused each year because nurses are not aware of their existence or think that they are unlikely to be successful in obtaining the money. This unused money leads granting agencies or potential granting agencies to conclude that nurses do not need more money for research.

Small grants are also available nationally. The American Nurses' Foundation and Sigma Theta Tau award a number of grants for less than $5,000 on a yearly basis. The grants are competitive and are awarded to new investigators with promising ideas, and receiving funding from these organizations is held in high regard. Information regarding these grants is available from the American Nurses' Foundation, Inc. Several federal granting agencies also provide small grants through the Public Health Service. These grants usually limit the amount of money requested to $50,000 to $75,000. Information regarding small grants can be obtained from the Federal Register, which is available in local libraries.

Small grants do more than just provide necessary funds to conduct the research. They are the first step in being recognized as a credible researcher and in being considered for more substantial grants for later studies. Receipt of these grants and your role in the grant need to be listed on curricula vitae or biographical sketches as an indication of first-level recognition as a researcher.

OBTAINING FOUNDATION GRANTS

Identifying Potentially Interested Foundations

Many foundations in the United States provide funding for research. The problem is to determine which foundations have interests in a particular field of study. Priorities for funding tend to change annually. When these foundations have been identified, the characteristics of the foundation need to be determined, appropriate foundations selected, query letters sent, a proposal prepared, and, if possible, a personal visit made to the foundation. Several publications list foundations and their interests. Bauer and American Association of Colleges of Nursing (1988) have compiled a list of those of particular interest to nursing. A computerized information system, the Sponsored Programs Information Network (SPIN), can also assist researchers in locating the most appropriate funding sources to support their research interests. The database contains approximately 2,000 programs that provide information on federal agencies, private foundations, and corporate foundations. Many universities and research institutions have access to SPIN.

Determining Foundation Characteristics

When these foundations have been identified, funding information needs to be gathered from each foundation. A foundation might fund only studies by female researchers, or it may be interested only in studies of low-income groups. A foundation may fund only studies being conducted in a specific geographic region. The average amount of money awarded for a single grant and the ranges of awards need to be determined for each foundation. If the average award of a particular foundation was $2,500 and if $30,000 was needed, that foundation is not the most desirable source of funds. However, if the researcher has never been funded previously and the project could be conducted with less money, an application to that foundation could be combined with applications to other foundations to obtain needed funds. The book most useful in determining this information is *The Foundation Directory,* which is available from The Foundation Center, 888 Seventh Avenue, New York, New York 10106.

Verifying Institutional Support

Grant awards are most commonly made to institutions rather than to individuals. Therefore, it is important to determine the willingness of the institution to receive the grant and support the study. This willingness needs to be documented in the proposal. Supporting the study involves appropriateness of the study topic; adequacy of facilities and services; availability of space needed for the study; contributions that the institution is willing to make to the study such as staff time, equipment, or data processing; and provision for overseeing the rights of human subjects.

Sending Query Letters

The next step is to send a query letter to foundations that might be interested in the planned study. The letter is addressed to the person who is director or head of the appropriate office rather than addressed to an impersonal title such as "Dear Director." Names of directors are available in a number of reference books or can be obtained by calling the organization's switchboard. The letter needs to reflect spontaneity and enthusiasm for the study, with the opening paragraph providing a reason why the letter is being sent to that particular foundation. The query letter should include a succinct description of the proposed study, an explanation of why the study is important, an indication of who will conduct the study, a description of required facilities, and the estimated duration and cost of the study. The qualifications of the researchers to conduct the study need to be made clear. This is no time to be modest about credentials or past achievements. The letter should inquire about the foundation's interest in the topic and information regarding how to apply for funds. If a personal visit is possible, the letter should close with a request for an appointment.

Preparing Proposals

In preparing the proposal, the foundation's guidelines for an application need to be followed carefully. In some cases, funding is sought from several sources. For example, funding requests may be submitted to an agency of the federal government, a nonprofit volunteer agency, and several private foundations. The temptation is to send each source the same proposal, rather than retyping it to meet specific guidelines. This can be counterproductive, since the proposal will not focus on the interests of each foundation and will not be in the format requested by the foundation, which may lead to rejection of the proposal. Developing a proposal is described in Chapter 26.

Making a Personal Visit

A personal visit to the foundation can be helpful if this is feasible and permitted by the foundation. Some foundations wish to see only the written application, whereas others prefer personal contact. A visit should not be made without an appointment. Preparations need to begin for the visit as soon as the appointment has been made, and a fully developed proposal needs to be written before the visit. This allows the researcher to have carefully thought through the study and have ideas well developed and organized when he or she goes to the foundation. Friedman suggested the following behaviors when visiting foundations: "One, be businesslike; two, be honest; three, know what you mean to do; four, ask questions; and finally, never, never argue with a foundation about the relevance of your proposed project to their program . . . If they say it doesn't fit, it doesn't" (White, 1975, pp. 219–220).

Although the visit may be informal in a social context, foundation representatives will tend to ask hard, searching questions about the study and the planned use of funding. In a way, this is similar to talking to a banker about a loan. Questions will be geared to help the foundation determine the following: Is the study feasible? Is the institution willing to provide sufficient support to permit the study to be completed? Is the researcher using all available resources? Have other sources of funding been sought? Has the researcher examined anticipated costs in detail and been realistic? What are the benefits of conducting the study? Who will benefit, and how? Is the researcher likely to complete the study? Are the findings likely to be published? If the written proposal has not been submitted, the visit is an appropriate time to submit it. Additional information or notes prepared for the visit can be left with foundation representatives for consideration as the decision is made.

OBTAINING FEDERAL GRANTS

The largest source of grant monies is the federal government—so much so that, in effect, the federal government influences what is studied and what is not. Funding can be requested from multiple divisions of the government. Information on funding agencies can be obtained from a document compiled by the federal government, *The Catalog of Federal Domestic Assistance*. This document is available from the U.S. Government Printing Office, Washington, DC 20402. Each agency has areas of focus and priorities for funding that change yearly. It is important to know these and prepare proposals within these areas in order to obtain funding. Therefore, calling or writing the agency for the most recent list of priorities is essential.

Two approaches can be used to seek federal funding for research. The researcher can identify a significant problem, develop a study to examine it, and submit a proposal for the study to the appropriate federal funding agency. Or an agency within the federal government can identify a significant problem, develop a plan through which the problem can be studied, and publish a Request for Proposals (RFP) or a Request for Applications (RFA) from researchers.

Researcher-Initiated Proposals

If the study is researcher-initiated, it is useful for the researcher to contact an official within the government agency early in the planning process to inform the agency of the intent to submit a proposal. Each agency has established dates, usually three times a year, when proposals are reviewed. Preparation of the proposal needs to begin months ahead of this deadline. Some agencies are willing to provide assistance and feedback to the researcher during the development of the proposal. This may occur through telephone conversation or feedback on a draft of the proposal.

Reviewing proposals that have been funded by that agency can be helpful. Although the agency cannot provide these proposals, they can often be obtained by contacting the principal investigator of the study personally. In some cases, the researcher may travel to Washington to meet with an agency representative. This allows modification of the proposal to fit more closely within agency guidelines, thus increasing the probability of funding. In many cases, proposals will fit within the interests of more than one government agency at the time of submission. It is permissible and perhaps desirable to request that the proposal be assigned to two agencies within the Public Health Service.

Requests for Proposals (RFP)

An RFP is published in the Federal Register and usually has a deadline date that is only a few weeks after the publication. This means that the researcher needs to have a good background in the field of study and be able to write a proposal quickly. Since a number of researchers will be responding to the same RFP and only one or a few proposals will be approved, these proposals are competitive. The agency staff will not be able to provide the same type of feedback as occurs in researcher-initiated proposals. The agency needs to be informed that a proposal is being submitted. Some questions that require clarification about elements of the RFP can be answered; however, other questions cannot be answered because the proposals are competitive and answering might give one researcher an advantage over others. The RFP allows a wide range of creativity in developing a study design to examine the problem of concern.

Requests for Applications (RFA)

An RFA is similar to an RFP except that with an RFA, the government agency not only identifies the problem of concern but also describes the design of the study. The RFA is a contract for which researchers bid. A carefully written proposal is still required and needs to follow the RFA in detail. After funding, federal agency staff maintain much more control and supervision of the process of the study than is the case with an RFP.

Developing a Proposal

Several excellent sources are available that provide detailed guidelines for the development of grant proposals. For a brief but excellent discussion of this topic, see Tornquist and Funk (1990). A number of books provide more detailed directions for grant proposal development. For example, Bauer (1988, 1989), who has led a number of proposal development workshops in coordination with the American Association of Colleges of Nursing, has developed a grants manual, a series of videotapes, a computer program to guide proposal development, and a proposal development workbook that can be used to develop skills in proposal writing. The videotapes can be purchased from the American Council on Education, Publications Department, One Dupont Circle, Washington, DC 20036. Grant development materials can be ordered from Bauer Associates, 3357 Stadium Court, San Diego, California 92122; (619) 452–9011.

It is helpful to examine proposals that have been funded as a guide in developing a new proposal. Two proposals have been published to serve as guides in proposal development. Sandelowski, Davis, and Harris (1989) have provided an example of a qualitative proposal, and Naylor (1990) has provided an example of a quantitative proposal.

Set aside sufficient time for careful development of the proposal, including rewriting the text several times. Writing your first proposal on a tight deadline is not wise. We recommend that you plan for 6 to 12 months for proposal development from the point of early development of your research ideas. Contact the agency to obtain written guidelines for development of the proposal and follow them rigidly. Page limitations and type sizes need to be strictly adhered to.

Input from colleagues can be invaluable in refining your ideas. You need individuals whose opinions you trust and who will go beyond telling you globally how magnificent your proposal is. Seek individuals who have experience in grant writing who are willing to critique your proposal thoroughly. After you have revised the proposal based on their feedback, contact a nationally known expert in your research field who will agree to examine your proposal critically. Be prepared to pay a consultant fee for this service.

After revising the proposal again, you are ready to submit it for funding. A number of federal funding agencies are willing to provide feedback on a preliminary draft of a proposal after initial interaction with the researcher by phone. Traveling to make a personal contact with agency staff for this feedback is even more helpful. Before making personal contact, the researcher needs to contact a staff member by phone, make an appointment, and send the draft by mail or fax in time for the staff member to review it before the meeting.

Neophytes are least willing to request a critique by colleagues and experts. There is almost a desire to write the proposal in secrecy, submit it quietly, and wait for the letter from the funding agency. That way, if you fail, no one will know about it. If others do know about the proposal development, another strategy is often used. The author furiously writes up to the very last possible deadline and then, in exhaustion, proclaims that there is no time for review before it is submitted. Both of these strategies almost guarantee rejection of the proposal. Remember, the critiques of your friends and the expert you have sought are unlikely to be as devastating as that of reviewers at the funding agency. And you have a chance to make changes after your friends review it.

The Federal Grant Review Process

After submission, a grant is assigned to one of 90 study sections for scientific evaluation. The study sections have no alignment with the funding agency. Thus, staff in the agencies have no influence on the committee's work of judging the scientific merit of the proposal. The proposal is sent to two or more researchers from the study section who are considered qualified to evaluate the proposal. These scientists prepare a written critique of the study. The proposal is then sent to all the members of the study section. Each member may have 50 to 100 proposals to read in a 1- to 2-month period. Then, a meeting of the full study section is held. Each application is discussed by those who critiqued the proposal, and other members comment or ask questions. A majority vote determines whether the proposal is approved, disapproved, or deferred.

Approved proposals are assigned a numerical score used to develop a priority rating (White, 1975). A study that is approved is not necessarily funded. The principal investigator (PI) will be notified at this point whether or not the study was approved. At a later time, approved studies are further examined to determine actual funding. Funding begins with the proposal that has the highest rank order. Funding of proposals will continue until available funds are depleted. This process can take 6 months or longer. Because of this process, receipt of the money to initiate a grant may not occur for up to a year after submission of the proposal.

Often, researcher-initiated proposals are rejected (or approved but not funded) after the first submission. The critique of the scientific committee is sent to the researcher on a *pink sheet.* Often the agency staff will encourage the researcher to rewrite the proposal using the comments on the pink sheet and resubmit it to the same agency. The probability of funding is often greater the second time if suggestions are followed.

Review of RFPs or RFAs is slightly different. These applications first go through a technical (scientific) evaluation. Those proposals that pass the technical review are then evaluated from the standpoint of cost. After the financial review, the contracting officer may negotiate levels of funding with the proposal writers. Funding decisions are made based on identification of well-designed proposals that offer the best financial advantage to the government (White, 1975).

Pink Sheets

The reaction of a researcher to a pink sheet is usually anger and then depression. The proposal is rejected by the researcher, stuffed in a bottom drawer somewhere, and forgotten. There really seems to be no way to avoid the anger and depression after a rejection because of the amount of emotional and time investment required to write a proposal. However, after a few weeks, it is advisable to examine the pink sheet again. The comments can be useful in rewriting the proposal for resubmission. The learning experience of rewriting the proposal and evaluating the comments will also provide a background for seeking funding for another study.

A skilled grant writer will have approximately one proposal funded for every five submitted. The average is far less than this. Thus, the researcher needs to be committed to repeated efforts of proposal submission in order to achieve grant funding.

RECEIVING A GRANT

Receiving notice that a grant proposal has been funded is one of the highlights in a researcher's career and warrants a celebration. However, when the euphoria begins to fade and reality sets in, careful plans need to be made for implementing the study. To avoid problems, consideration needs to be given to managing the budget, hiring and training research personnel, maintaining the promised timetable, and coordinating activities of the study.

Managing the Budget

Although the supporting institution has ultimate responsibility for dispensing and controlling grant monies, the principal investigator (PI) is also responsible for keeping track of budget expenditures and making decisions about how the money is to be spent. If this is the first grant received, the PI who has no previous administrative experience may need some initial guidance in how to keep records and make reasonable budget decisions. If funding is through a federal agency, interim reports will include reports on the budget as well as on the progress of the study.

Training Research Personnel

When a new grant is initiated, time needs to be set aside for interviewing, hiring, and training grant personnel. Personnel who will be involved in data collection need to learn the process, and then data collection needs to be refined to ensure that each data collector is consistent with the other data collectors. This process helps ensure *interrater reliability*. The PI needs to set aside time to oversee the work of personnel hired for the grant.

Maintaining the Study Schedule

The timetable submitted with the proposal needs to be adhered to whenever possible. This requires some careful planning. Otherwise, other work activities are likely to take precedence, delaying the grant work. Unexpected events do happen; however, careful planning can minimize their impact. The PI needs to constantly refer back to the timetable to evaluate progress. If the project falls behind schedule, actions need to be taken to return to the original schedule or to readjust the timetable. Keeping on schedule will be a plus when it is time to apply for the next grant.

Coordinating Activities

During a large study, with several investigators and other grant personnel, coordinating activities can be a problem. It is useful to arrange meetings of all grant workers at intervals to facilitate sharing of ideas and problem solving. Records need to be kept of discussions at these meetings. These actions can lead to a smoother functioning team.

Submitting Reports

Federal grants require the submission of interim reports according to preset deadlines. The federal agency involved will send written guidelines for the content of the reports, which will consist of a description of grant activities and expenditures of grant monies. Time needs to be set aside to prepare the report, which usually requires compiling figures and tables. In addition to the written reports, it is often useful to maintain phone contact with the appropriate staff at the federal agency.

PLANNING YOUR NEXT GRANT

The researcher should not wait until funding from the first grant has ended to begin seeking funds for a second study because of the length of time required to obtain funding. In fact, it may be wise to have several ongoing studies in various stages of implementation. For example, one could be planning a study, collecting data on a second study, analyzing data on a third study, and writing papers for publication on a fourth study. A full-time researcher could have completed one funded study, be in the last year of funding for a second study, be in the first year of funding for a third study, and be seeking funding for a fourth study. This may sound unrealistic, but with planning, it is not. This strategy not only provides continuous funding for research activities but also facilitates a rhythm of research that prevents time pressures and makes use of lulls in activities in a particular study. To increase the ease in obtaining funding, the studies need to be within the same area of research, each building on the previous studies.

SUMMARY

Seeking funding for research is important, both for the researcher and for the profession. Researchers may have one of two purposes for seeking research funding. First, the funding may allow the researcher to conduct a single study that is of concern or interest. The second purpose is to initiate or maintain a career of conducting research. To receive funding, grantsmanship skills need to be learned. Strategies used to learn grantsmanship are attending grantsmanship courses, developing a reference group, joining research organizations, participating on research committees or review panels, networking, assisting a researcher, and obtaining a mentor.

Writing a grant proposal for funding requires a commitment to putting in extra hours of work, which are often unrewarded, monetarily and socially, at first. The first studies are usually conducted on a shoestring budget. A small amount of money might be obtained from a variety of sources, such as management in employing institutions, universities (intramural grants), or nursing organizations. A study that is well carried out and published using limited funds will often give the credibility one needs to achieve major grant funding.

Larger sums of money can be sought by writing for foundation grants. The researcher needs initially to identify potentially interested foundations and determine the characteristics of those foundations. Foundation grant awards are most commonly made to institutions rather than to individuals. Therefore, it is important to determine the willingness of the institution to receive the grant and support the study. The institution's willingness needs to be documented in the proposal. Query letters are sent to all foundations that might be interested in the planned study. If a foundation is interested, a personal visit, if possible, needs to be made. The grant proposal is developed according to the guidelines of the foundation.

The largest source of grant monies is the federal government. Two approaches can be used to seek federal funding for research. The researcher can identify a significant problem, develop a study to examine it, and submit a proposal for the study to an appropriate federal funding agency. Or, someone within the federal government can identify a significant problem, develop a plan through which the problem can be studied, and publish a Request for Proposals (RFP) or a Request for Applications (RFA) from researchers.

After submission, grant requests are initially reviewed by staff members of the agency. Researchers who are writing their first federal grant request frequently receive rejection notices or approval-but-not-funded notices. The critique of the scientific committee is sent to the researcher on a pink sheet. Often the agency staff will encourage the researcher to rewrite and resubmit the proposal using the comments on the pink sheet.

When a grant proposal is funded, it is a time of celebration for the researcher. However, then the researcher needs to make careful plans for implementing the study. The principal investigator (PI) is responsible for keeping up with the budget, training research personnel, keeping up the schedule, and coordinating activities. Federal grants also require the submission of interim reports. A researcher should not wait until funding from the first grant has ended to begin seeking funds for a second study and then a third and then a fourth. An example grant proposal is presented for use as a guide in developing proposals.

References

Bauer, D. G. (1988). *The "how to" grants manual: Successful grantseeking techniques for obtaining public and private grants* (2nd ed.). New York: American Council on Education/Macmillan.

Bauer, D. G. (1989). *Administering grants, contracts, and funds: Evaluating and improving your grants system.* New York: American Council on Education/Macmillan.

Bauer, D. G., & American Association of Colleges of Nursing (1988). *The complete grants sourcebook for nursing and health.* (B. K. Redman, ed.; R. Lamothe; managing ed.). New York: American Council on Education/Macmillan.

Cartwright, D., & Zander, A. (1968). *Group dynamics: Research and theory.* New York: Harper & Row.

Holmstrom, L. L., & Burgess, A. W. (1982). Low-cost research: A project on a shoestring. *Nursing Research, 31*(2), 123–125.

Naylor, M. D. (1990). An example of a research grant application: Comprehensive discharge planning for the elderly. *Research in Nursing & Health, 13*(5), 327–348.

Sandelowski, M., Davis, D., & Harris, B. (1989). Artful design: Writing the proposal for research in the naturalist paradigm. *Research in Nursing & Health, 12*(2), 77–84.

Tornquist, E. M., & Funk, S. G. (1990). How to write a research grant proposal. *Image: Journal of Nursing Scholarship, 22*(1), 44–51.

White, V. P. (1975). *Grants: How to find out about them and what to do next.* New York: Plenum.

Appendices

APPENDIX A

Table of Random Numbers

71510	68311	48214	99929	64650	13229
36921	58733	13459	93488	21949	30920
23288	89515	58503	46185	00368	82604
02668	37444	50640	54968	11409	36148
82091	87298	41397	71112	00076	60029
47837	76717	09653	54466	87988	82363
17934	52793	17641	19502	31735	36901
92296	19293	57583	86043	69502	12601
00535	82698	04174	32342	66533	07875
54446	08795	63563	42296	74647	73120
96981	68729	21154	56182	71840	66135
52397	89724	96436	17871	21823	04027
76403	04655	87277	32593	17097	06913
05136	05115	25922	07123	31485	52166
07645	85123	20945	06370	70255	22806
32530	98883	19105	01769	20276	59402
60427	03316	41439	22012	00159	08461
51811	14651	45119	97921	08063	70820
01832	53295	66575	21384	75357	55888
83430	96917	73978	87884	13249	28870
00995	28829	15048	49573	65278	61493
44032	88720	73058	66010	55115	79227
27929	23392	06432	50201	39055	15529
53484	33973	10614	25190	52647	62580
51184	31339	60009	66595	64358	14985
31359	77470	58126	59192	23371	25190
37842	44387	92421	42965	09736	51873
94596	61368	82091	63835	86859	10678
58210	59820	24710	23225	45788	21426
63354	29875	51058	29958	61221	61200
79958	67599	74103	49824	39306	15069
56328	26905	34454	53965	66617	22137
72806	64421	58711	68436	60301	28620
91920	96081	01413	27281	19397	36231
05010	42003	99866	20924	76152	54090
88239	80732	20778	45726	41481	48277
45705	96458	13918	52375	57457	87884
64274	26236	61096	01309	48632	00431
63731	18917	21614	06412	71008	20255
39891	75337	89452	88092	61012	38072
26466	03735	39891	26362	86817	48193
33492	70485	77323	01016	97315	03944
04509	46144	88909	55261	73434	62538
63187	57352	91208	33555	75943	41669
64651	38741	86190	38197	99113	59694
46792	78975	01999	78892	16177	95747
78076	75002	51309	18791	34162	32258
05345	79268	75608	29916	37005	09213
10991	50452	02376	40372	45077	73706

APPENDIX B

Cumulative Normal Distribution (Z)

Z	X	Area	Z	X	Area
−3.25	μ − 3.25σ	.0006	−1.00	μ − 1.00σ	.1587
−3.20	μ − 3.20σ	.0007	− .95	μ − .95σ	.1711
−3.15	μ − 3.15σ	.0008	− .90	μ − .90σ	.1841
−3.10	μ − 3.10σ	.0010	− .85	μ − .85σ	.1977
−3.05	μ − 3.05σ	.0011	− .80	μ − .80σ	.2119
−3.00	μ − 3.00σ	.0013	− .75	μ − .75σ	.2266
−2.95	μ − 2.95σ	.0016	− .70	μ − .70σ	.2420
−2.90	μ − 2.90σ	.0019	− .65	μ − .65σ	.2578
−2.85	μ − 2.85σ	.0022	− .60	μ − .60σ	.2743
−2.80	μ − 2.80σ	.0026	− .55	μ − .55σ	.2912
−2.75	μ − 2.75σ	.0030	− .50	μ − .50σ	.3085
−2.70	μ − 2.70σ	.0035	− .45	μ − .45σ	.3264
−2.65	μ − 2.65σ	.0040	− .40	μ − .40σ	.3446
−2.60	μ − 2.60σ	.0047	− .35	μ − .35σ	.3632
−2.55	μ − 2.55σ	.0054	− .30	μ − .30σ	.3821
−2.50	μ − 2.50σ	.0062	− .25	μ − .25σ	.4013
−2.45	μ − 2.45σ	.0071	− .20	μ − .20σ	.4207
−2.40	μ − 2.40σ	.0082	− .15	μ − .15σ	.4404
−2.35	μ − 2.35σ	.0094	− .10	μ − .10σ	.4602
−2.30	μ − 2.30σ	.0107	− .05	μ − .05σ	.4801
−2.25	μ − 2.25σ	.0122			
−2.20	μ − 2.20σ	.0139			
−2.15	μ − 2.15σ	.0158	.00	μ	.5000
−2.10	μ − 2.10σ	.0179			
−2.05	μ − 2.05σ	.0202			
−2.00	μ − 2.00σ	.0228	.05	μ + .05σ	.5199
−1.95	μ − 1.95σ	.0256	.10	μ + .10σ	.5398
−1.90	μ − 1.90σ	.0287	.15	μ + .15σ	.5596
−1.85	μ − 1.85σ	.0322	.20	μ + .20σ	.5793
−1.80	μ − 1.80σ	.0359	.25	μ + .25σ	.5987
−1.75	μ − 1.75σ	.0401	.30	μ + .30σ	.6179
−1.70	μ − 1.70σ	.0446	.35	μ + .35σ	.6368
−1.65	μ − 1.65σ	.0495	.40	μ + .40σ	.6554
−1.60	μ − 1.60σ	.0548	.45	μ + .45σ	.6736
−1.55	μ − 1.55σ	.0606	.50	μ + .50σ	.6915
−1.50	μ − 1.50σ	.0668	.55	μ + .55σ	.7088
−1.45	μ − 1.45σ	.0735	.60	μ + .60σ	.7257
−1.40	μ − 1.40σ	.0808	.65	μ + .65σ	.7422
−1.35	μ − 1.35σ	.0885	.70	μ + .70σ	.7580
−1.30	μ − 1.30σ	.0968	.75	μ + .75σ	.7734
−1.25	μ − 1.25σ	.1056	.80	μ + .80σ	.7881
−1.20	μ − 1.20σ	.1151	.85	μ + .85σ	.8023
−1.15	μ − 1.15σ	.1251	.90	μ + .90σ	.8159
−1.10	μ − 1.10σ	.1357	.95	μ + .95σ	.8289
−1.05	μ − 1.05σ	.1469	1.00	μ + 1.00σ	.8413

Table continued on following page

APPENDIX B (*Continued*)

Z	X	Area	Z	X	Area
1.05	$\mu+1.05\sigma$	.8531	−4.265	$\mu-4.265\sigma$	.00001
1.10	$\mu+1.10\sigma$	.8643	−3.719	$\mu-3.719\sigma$	.0001
1.15	$\mu+1.15\sigma$	.8749	−3.090	$\mu-3.090\sigma$	.001
1.20	$\mu+1.20\sigma$	.8849	−2.576	$\mu-2.576\sigma$	.005
1.25	$\mu+1.25\sigma$	.8944	−2.326	$\mu-2.326\sigma$	.01
1.30	$\mu+1.30\sigma$	.9032	−2.054	$\mu-2.054\sigma$	.02
1.35	$\mu+1.35\sigma$	.9115	−1.960	$\mu-1.960\sigma$	.025
1.40	$\mu+1.40\sigma$	.9192	−1.881	$\mu-1.881\sigma$	.03
1.45	$\mu+1.45\sigma$	.9265	−1.751	$\mu-1.751\sigma$	.04
1.50	$\mu+1.50\sigma$	.9332	−1.645	$\mu-1.645\sigma$	.05
1.55	$\mu+1.55\sigma$	.9394	−1.555	$\mu-1.555\sigma$	.06
1.60	$\mu+1.60\sigma$	.9452	−1.476	$\mu-1.476\sigma$	.07
1.65	$\mu+1.65\sigma$	.9505	−1.405	$\mu-1.405\sigma$	.08
1.70	$\mu+1.70\sigma$	.9554	−1.341	$\mu-1.341\sigma$	.09
1.75	$\mu+1.75\sigma$	.9599	−1.282	$\mu-1.282\sigma$	.10
1.80	$\mu+1.80\sigma$	.9641	−1.036	$\mu-1.036\sigma$	.15
1.85	$\mu+1.85\sigma$	.9678	−.842	$\mu-.842\sigma$	.20
1.90	$\mu+1.90\sigma$	.9713	−.674	$\mu-.674\sigma$	.25
1.95	$\mu+1.95\sigma$	.9744	−.524	$\mu-.524\sigma$	.30
2.00	$\mu+2.00\sigma$	.9772	−.385	$\mu-.385\sigma$	.35
2.05	$\mu+2.05\sigma$	.9798	−.253	$\mu-.253\sigma$	.40
2.10	$\mu+2.10\sigma$	.9821	−.126	$\mu-.126\sigma$	.45
2.15	$\mu+2.15\sigma$	.9842	0	μ	.50
2.20	$\mu+2.20\sigma$	.9861	.126	$\mu+.126\sigma$	.55
2.25	$\mu+2.25\sigma$	.9878	.253	$\mu+.253\sigma$	.60
2.30	$\mu+2.30\sigma$	.9893	.385	$\mu+.385\sigma$	.65
2.35	$\mu+2.35\sigma$	.9906	.524	$\mu+.524\sigma$	.70
2.40	$\mu+2.40\sigma$	.9918	.674	$\mu+.674\sigma$	.75
2.45	$\mu+2.45\sigma$	.9929	.842	$\mu+.842\sigma$	.80
2.50	$\mu+2.50\sigma$	.9938	1.036	$\mu+1.036\sigma$	.85
2.55	$\mu+2.55\sigma$	.9946	1.282	$\mu+1.282\sigma$	.90
2.60	$\mu+2.60\sigma$	.9953	1.341	$\mu+1.341\sigma$	.91
2.65	$\mu+2.65\sigma$	.9960	1.405	$\mu+1.405\sigma$	.92
2.70	$\mu+2.70\sigma$	.9965	1.476	$\mu+1.476\sigma$	.93
2.75	$\mu+2.75\sigma$	.9970	1.555	$\mu+1.555\sigma$	.94
2.80	$\mu+2.80\sigma$	.9974	1.645	$\mu+1.645\sigma$	.95
2.85	$\mu+2.85\sigma$	.9978	1.751	$\mu+1.751\sigma$	.96
2.90	$\mu+2.90\sigma$	.9981	1.881	$\mu+1.881\sigma$	.97
2.95	$\mu+2.95\sigma$	.9984	1.960	$\mu+1.960\sigma$	.975
3.00	$\mu+3.00\sigma$	.9987	2.054	$\mu+2.054\sigma$	.98
3.05	$\mu+3.05\sigma$	.9989	2.326	$\mu+2.326\sigma$	.99
3.10	$\mu+3.10\sigma$	.9990	2.576	$\mu+2.576\sigma$	.995
3.15	$\mu+3.15\sigma$	.9992	3.090	$\mu+3.090\sigma$	.999
3.20	$\mu+3.20\sigma$	.9993	3.719	$\mu+3.719\sigma$	.9999
3.25	$\mu+3.25\sigma$	.9994	4.265	$\mu+4.265\sigma$	.99999

(From Dixon, W. J. and Massey, F. J. Jr.: *Introduction to statistical analysis* (3rd ed). New York: McGraw-Hill Book Company, 1969; with permission.)

APPENDIX C

Percentage Points of Student's *t* Distribution

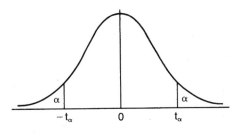

df	α .25 2α .50	.20 .40	.15 .30	.10 .20	.05 .10	.025 .05	.01 .02	.005 .01	.0005 .001
1	1.000	1.376	1.963	3.078	6.314	12.706	31.821	63.657	636.619
2	.816	1.061	1.386	1.886	2.920	4.303	6.965	9.925	31.598
3	.765	.978	1.250	1.638	2.353	3.182	4.541	5.841	12.924
4	.741	.941	1.190	1.533	2.132	2.776	3.747	4.604	8.610
5	.727	.920	1.156	1.476	2.015	2.571	3.365	4.032	6.869
6	.718	.906	1.134	1.440	1.943	2.447	3.143	3.707	5.959
7	.711	.896	1.119	1.415	1.895	2.365	2.998	3.499	5.408
8	.706	.889	1.108	1.397	1.860	2.306	2.896	3.355	5.041
9	.703	.883	1.100	1.383	1.833	2.262	2.821	3.250	4.781
10	.700	.879	1.093	1.372	1.812	2.228	2.764	3.169	4.587
11	.697	.876	1.088	1.363	1.796	2.201	2.718	3.106	4.437
12	.695	.873	1.083	1.356	1.782	2.179	2.681	3.055	4.318
13	.694	.870	1.079	1.350	1.771	2.160	2.650	3.012	4.221
14	.692	.868	1.076	1.345	1.761	2.145	2.624	2.977	4.140
15	.691	.866	1.074	1.341	1.753	2.131	2.602	2.947	4.073
16	.690	.865	1.071	1.337	1.746	2.120	2.583	2.921	4.015
17	.689	.863	1.069	1.333	1.740	2.110	2.567	2.898	3.965
18	.688	.862	1.067	1.330	1.734	2.101	2.552	2.878	3.922
19	.688	.861	1.066	1.328	1.729	2.093	2.539	2.861	3.883
20	.687	.860	1.064	1.325	1.725	2.086	2.528	2.845	3.850
21	.686	.859	1.063	1.323	1.721	2.080	2.518	2.831	3.819
22	.686	.858	1.061	1.321	1.717	2.074	2.508	2.819	3.792
23	.685	.858	1.060	1.319	1.714	2.069	2.500	2.807	3.767
24	.685	.857	1.059	1.318	1.711	2.064	2.492	2.797	3.745
25	.684	.856	1.058	1.316	1.708	2.060	2.485	2.787	3.725
26	.684	.856	1.058	1.315	1.706	2.056	2.479	2.779	3.707
27	.684	.855	1.057	1.314	1.703	2.052	2.473	2.771	3.690
28	.683	.855	1.056	1.313	1.701	2.048	2.467	2.763	3.674
29	.683	.854	1.055	1.311	1.699	2.045	2.462	2.756	3.659
30	.683	.854	1.055	1.310	1.697	2.042	2.457	2.750	3.646
40	.681	.851	1.050	1.303	1.684	2.021	2.423	2.704	3.551
60	.679	.848	1.046	1.296	1.671	2.000	2.390	2.660	3.460
120	.677	.845	1.041	1.289	1.658	1.980	2.358	2.617	3.373
∞	.674	.842	1.036	1.282	1.645	1.960	2.326	2.576	3.291

(This table is taken from Table III p 46 of Fisher, R. A. and Yates, F.: *Statistical tables for biological, agricultural, and medical research* (6th ed.). Published by Longman Group UK Ltd., 1974. By permission of the authors and publishers.)

APPENDIX D

Percentage Points of the *F* Distribution

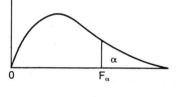

$\alpha = .05$

Degrees of Freedom

V_1

v_2	1	2	3	4	5	6	7	8	9
1	161.4	199.5	215.7	224.6	230.2	234.0	236.8	238.9	240.5
2	18.51	19.00	19.16	19.25	19.30	19.33	19.35	19.37	19.38
3	10.13	9.55	9.28	9.12	9.01	8.94	8.89	8.85	8.81
4	7.71	6.94	6.59	6.39	6.26	6.16	6.09	6.04	6.00
5	6.61	5.79	5.41	5.19	5.05	4.95	4.88	4.82	4.77
6	5.99	5.14	4.76	4.53	4.39	4.28	4.21	4.15	4.10
7	5.59	4.74	4.35	4.12	3.97	3.87	3.79	3.73	3.68
8	5.32	4.46	4.07	3.84	3.69	3.58	3.50	3.44	3.39
9	5.12	4.26	3.86	3.63	3.48	3.37	3.29	3.23	3.18
10	4.96	4.10	3.71	3.48	3.33	3.22	3.14	3.07	3.02
11	4.84	3.98	3.59	3.36	3.20	3.09	3.01	2.95	2.90
12	4.75	3.89	3.49	3.26	3.11	3.00	2.91	2.85	2.80
13	4.67	3.81	3.41	3.18	3.03	2.92	2.83	2.77	2.71
14	4.60	3.74	3.34	3.11	2.96	2.85	2.76	2.70	2.65
15	4.54	3.68	3.29	3.06	2.90	2.79	2.71	2.64	2.59
16	4.49	3.63	3.24	3.01	2.85	2.74	2.66	2.59	2.54
17	4.45	3.59	3.20	2.96	2.81	2.70	2.61	2.55	2.49
18	4.41	3.55	3.16	2.93	2.77	2.66	2.58	2.51	2.46
19	4.38	3.52	3.13	2.90	2.74	2.63	2.54	2.48	2.42
20	4.35	3.49	3.10	2.87	2.71	2.60	2.51	2.45	2.39
21	4.32	3.47	3.07	2.84	2.68	2.57	2.49	2.42	2.37
22	4.30	3.44	3.05	2.82	2.66	2.55	2.46	2.40	2.34
23	4.28	3.42	3.03	2.80	2.64	2.53	2.44	2.37	2.32
24	4.26	3.40	3.01	2.78	2.62	2.51	2.42	2.36	2.30
25	4.24	3.39	2.99	2.76	2.60	2.49	2.40	2.34	2.28
26	4.23	3.37	2.98	2.74	2.59	2.47	2.39	2.32	2.27
27	4.21	3.35	2.96	2.73	2.57	2.46	2.37	2.31	2.25
28	4.20	3.34	2.95	2.71	2.56	2.45	2.36	2.29	2.24
29	4.18	3.33	2.93	2.70	2.55	2.43	2.35	2.28	2.22
30	4.17	3.32	2.92	2.69	2.53	2.42	2.33	2.27	2.21
40	4.08	3.23	2.84	2.61	2.45	2.34	2.25	2.18	2.12
60	4.00	3.15	2.76	2.53	2.37	2.25	2.17	2.10	2.04
120	3.92	3.07	2.68	2.45	2.29	2.17	2.09	2.02	1.96
∞	3.84	3.00	2.60	2.37	2.21	2.10	2.01	1.94	1.88

Table continued on opposite page

APPENDIX D (*Continued*)

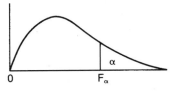

$$\alpha = .05$$

V_1

10	12	15	20	24	30	40	60	120	∞	v_2
241.9	243.9	245.9	248.0	249.1	250.1	251.1	252.2	253.3	254.3	1
19.40	19.41	19.43	19.45	19.45	19.46	19.47	19.48	19.49	19.50	2
8.79	8.74	8.70	8.66	8.64	8.62	8.59	8.57	8.55	8.53	3
5.96	5.91	5.86	5.80	5.77	5.75	5.72	5.69	5.66	5.63	4
4.74	4.68	4.62	4.56	4.53	4.50	4.46	4.43	4.40	4.36	5
4.06	4.00	3.94	3.87	3.84	3.81	3.77	3.74	3.70	3.67	6
3.64	3.57	3.51	3.44	3.41	3.38	3.34	3.30	3.27	3.23	7
3.35	3.28	3.22	3.15	3.12	3.08	3.04	3.01	2.97	2.93	8
3.14	3.07	3.01	2.94	2.90	2.86	2.83	2.79	2.75	2.71	9
2.98	2.91	2.85	2.77	2.74	2.70	2.66	2.62	2.58	2.54	10
2.85	2.79	2.72	2.65	2.61	2.57	2.53	2.49	2.45	2.40	11
2.75	2.69	2.62	2.54	2.51	2.47	2.43	2.38	2.34	2.30	12
2.67	2.60	2.53	2.46	2.42	2.38	2.34	2.30	2.25	2.21	13
2.60	2.53	2.46	2.39	2.35	2.31	2.27	2.22	2.18	2.13	14
2.54	2.48	2.40	2.33	2.29	2.25	2.20	2.16	2.11	2.07	15
2.49	2.42	2.35	2.28	2.24	2.19	2.15	2.11	2.06	2.01	16
2.45	2.38	2.31	2.23	2.19	2.15	2.10	2.06	2.01	1.96	17
2.41	2.34	2.27	2.19	2.15	2.11	2.06	2.02	1.97	1.92	18
2.38	2.31	2.23	2.16	2.11	2.07	2.03	1.98	1.93	1.88	19
2.35	2.28	2.20	2.12	2.08	2.04	1.99	1.95	1.90	1.84	20
2.32	2.25	2.18	2.10	2.05	2.01	1.96	1.92	1.87	1.81	21
2.30	2.23	2.15	2.07	2.03	1.98	1.94	1.89	1.84	1.78	22
2.27	2.20	2.13	2.05	2.01	1.96	1.91	1.86	1.81	1.76	23
2.25	2.18	2.11	2.03	1.98	1.94	1.89	1.84	1.79	1.73	24
2.24	2.16	2.09	2.01	1.96	1.92	1.87	1.82	1.77	1.71	25
2.22	2.15	2.07	1.99	1.95	1.90	1.85	1.80	1.75	1.69	26
2.20	2.13	2.06	1.97	1.93	1.88	1.84	1.79	1.73	1.67	27
2.19	2.12	2.04	1.96	1.91	1.87	1.82	1.77	1.71	1.65	28
2.18	2.10	2.03	1.94	1.90	1.85	1.81	1.75	1.70	1.64	29
2.16	2.09	2.01	1.93	1.89	1.84	1.79	1.74	1.68	1.62	30
2.08	2.00	1.92	1.84	1.79	1.74	1.69	1.64	1.58	1.51	40
1.99	1.92	1.84	1.75	1.70	1.65	1.59	1.53	1.47	1.39	60
1.91	1.83	1.75	1.66	1.61	1.55	1.50	1.43	1.35	1.25	120
1.83	1.75	1.67	1.57	1.52	1.46	1.39	1.32	1.22	1.00	∞

Table continued on following page

APPENDIX D (*Continued*)

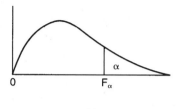

$$\alpha = .01$$

Degrees of Freedom

v_1

v_2	1	2	3	4	5	6	7	8	9
1	4052	4999.5	5403	5625	5764	5859	5928	5982	6022
2	98.50	99.00	99.17	99.25	99.30	99.33	99.36	99.37	99.39
3	34.12	30.82	29.46	28.71	28.24	27.91	27.67	27.49	27.35
4	21.20	18.00	16.69	15.98	15.52	15.21	14.98	14.80	14.66
5	16.26	13.27	12.06	11.39	10.97	10.67	10.46	10.29	10.16
6	13.75	10.92	9.78	9.15	8.75	8.47	8.26	8.10	7.98
7	12.25	9.55	8.45	7.85	7.46	7.19	6.99	6.84	6.72
8	11.26	8.65	7.59	7.01	6.63	6.37	6.18	6.03	5.91
9	10.56	8.02	6.99	6.42	6.06	5.80	5.61	5.47	5.35
10	10.04	7.56	6.55	5.99	5.64	5.39	5.20	5.06	4.94
11	9.65	7.21	6.22	5.67	5.32	5.07	4.89	4.74	4.63
12	9.33	6.93	5.95	5.41	5.06	4.82	4.64	4.50	4.39
13	9.07	6.70	5.74	5.21	4.86	4.62	4.44	4.30	4.19
14	8.86	6.51	5.56	5.04	4.69	4.46	4.28	4.14	4.03
15	8.68	6.36	5.42	4.89	4.56	4.32	4.14	4.00	3.89
16	8.53	6.23	5.29	4.77	4.44	4.20	4.03	3.89	3.78
17	8.40	6.11	5.18	4.67	4.34	4.10	3.93	3.79	3.68
18	8.29	6.01	5.09	4.58	4.25	4.01	3.84	3.71	3.60
19	8.18	5.93	5.01	4.50	4.17	3.94	3.77	3.63	3.52
20	8.10	5.85	4.94	4.43	4.10	3.87	3.70	3.56	3.46
21	8.02	5.78	4.87	4.37	4.04	3.81	3.64	3.51	3.40
22	7.95	5.72	4.82	4.31	3.99	3.76	3.59	3.45	3.35
23	7.88	5.66	4.76	4.26	3.94	3.71	3.54	3.41	3.30
24	7.82	5.61	4.72	4.22	3.90	3.67	3.50	3.36	3.26
25	7.77	5.57	4.68	4.18	3.85	3.63	3.46	3.32	3.22
26	7.72	5.53	4.64	4.14	3.82	3.59	3.42	3.29	3.18
27	7.68	5.49	4.60	4.11	3.78	3.56	3.39	3.26	3.15
28	7.64	5.45	4.57	4.07	3.75	3.53	3.36	3.23	3.12
29	7.60	5.42	4.54	4.04	3.73	3.50	3.33	3.20	3.09
30	7.56	5.39	4.51	4.02	3.70	3.47	3.30	3.17	3.07
40	7.31	5.18	4.31	3.83	3.51	3.29	3.12	2.99	2.89
60	7.08	4.98	4.13	3.65	3.34	3.12	2.95	2.82	2.72
120	6.85	4.79	3.95	3.48	3.17	2.96	2.79	2.66	2.56
∞	6.63	4.61	3.78	3.32	3.02	2.80	2.64	2.51	2.41

Table continued on opposite page

APPENDIX D (*Continued*)

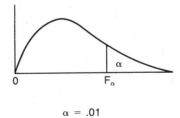

$\alpha = .01$

v_1

10	12	15	20	24	30	40	60	120	∞		v_2
6056	6106	6157	6209	6235	6261	6287	6313	6339	6366		1
99.40	99.42	99.43	99.45	99.46	99.47	99.47	99.48	99.49	99.50		2
27.23	27.05	26.87	26.69	26.60	26.50	26.41	26.32	26.22	26.13		3
14.55	14.37	14.20	14.02	13.93	13.84	13.75	13.65	13.56	13.46		4
10.05	9.89	9.72	9.55	9.47	9.38	9.29	9.20	9.11	9.02		5
7.87	7.72	7.56	7.40	7.31	7.23	7.14	7.06	6.97	6.88		6
6.62	6.47	6.31	6.16	6.07	5.99	5.91	5.82	5.74	5.65		7
5.81	5.67	5.52	5.36	5.28	5.20	5.12	5.03	4.95	4.86		8
5.26	5.11	4.96	4.81	4.73	4.65	4.57	4.48	4.40	4.31		9
4.85	4.71	4.56	4.41	4.33	4.25	4.17	4.08	4.00	3.91		10
4.54	4.40	4.25	4.10	4.02	3.94	3.86	3.78	3.69	3.60		11
4.30	4.16	4.01	3.86	3.78	3.70	3.62	3.54	3.45	3.36		12
4.10	3.96	3.82	3.66	3.59	3.51	3.43	3.34	3.25	3.17		13
3.94	3.80	3.66	3.51	3.43	3.35	3.27	3.18	3.09	3.00		14
3.80	3.67	3.52	3.37	3.29	3.21	3.13	3.05	2.96	2.87		15
3.69	3.55	3.41	3.26	3.18	3.10	3.02	2.93	2.84	2.75		16
3.59	3.46	3.31	3.16	3.08	3.00	2.92	2.83	2.75	2.65		17
3.51	3.37	3.23	3.08	3.00	2.92	2.84	2.75	2.66	2.57		18
3.43	3.30	3.15	3.00	2.92	2.84	2.76	2.67	2.58	2.49		19
3.37	3.23	3.09	2.94	2.86	2.78	2.69	2.61	2.52	2.42		20
3.31	3.17	3.03	2.88	2.80	2.72	2.64	2.55	2.46	2.36		21
3.26	3.12	2.98	2.83	2.75	2.67	2.58	2.50	2.40	2.31		22
3.21	3.07	2.93	2.78	2.70	2.62	2.54	2.45	2.35	2.26		23
3.17	3.03	2.89	2.74	2.66	2.58	2.49	2.40	2.31	2.21		24
3.13	2.99	2.85	2.70	2.62	2.54	2.45	2.36	2.27	2.17		25
3.09	2.96	2.81	2.66	2.58	2.50	2.42	2.33	2.23	2.13		26
3.06	2.93	2.78	2.63	2.55	2.47	2.38	2.29	2.20	2.10		27
3.03	2.90	2,75	2.60	2.52	2.44	2.35	2.26	2.17	2.06		28
3.00	2.87	2.73	2.57	2.49	2.41	2.33	2.23	2.14	2.03		29
2.98	2.84	2.70	2.55	2.47	2.39	2.30	2.21	2.11	2.01		30
2.80	2.66	2.52	2.37	2.29	2.20	2.11	2.02	1.92	1.80		40
2.63	2.50	2.35	2.20	2.12	2.03	1.94	1.84	1.73	1.60		60
2.47	2.34	2.19	2.03	1.95	1.86	1.76	1.66	1.53	1.38		120
2.32	2.18	2.04	1.88	1.79	1.70	1.59	1.47	1.32	1.00		∞

(From Merrington, M. and Thompson, C. M.: Biometrika, *33*:73–78, 1943; with permission.)

APPENDIX E

Critical Values of the χ^2 Distribution

df	$P_{0.5}$	P_{01}	$P_{02.5}$	P_{05}	P_{10}	P_{90}	P_{95}	$P_{97.5}$	P_{99}	$P_{99.5}$
1	.000039	.00016	.00098	.0039	.0158	2.71	3.84	5.02	6.63	7.88
2	.0100	.0201	.0506	.1026	.2107	4.61	5.99	7.38	9.21	10.60
3	.0717	.115	.216	.352	.584	6.25	7.81	9.35	11.34	12.84
4	.207	.297	.484	.711	1.064	7.78	9.49	11.14	13.28	14.86
5	.412	.554	.831	1.15	1.61	9.24	11.07	12.83	15.09	16.75
6	.676	.872	1.24	1.64	2.20	10.64	12.59	14.45	16.81	18.55
7	.989	1.24	1.69	2.17	2.83	12.02	14.07	16.01	18.48	20.28
8	1.34	1.65	2.18	2.73	3.49	13.36	15.51	17.53	20.09	21.96
9	1.73	2.09	2.70	3.33	4.17	14.68	16.92	19.02	21.67	23.59
10	2.16	2.56	3.25	3.94	4.87	15.99	18.31	20.48	23.21	25.19
11	2.60	3.05	3.82	4.57	5.58	17.28	19.68	21.92	24.73	26.76
12	3.07	3.57	4.40	5.23	6.30	18.55	21.03	23.34	26.22	28.30
13	3.57	4.11	5.01	5.89	7.04	19.81	22.36	24.74	27.69	29.82
14	4.07	4.66	5.63	6.57	7.79	21.06	23.68	26.12	29.14	31.32
15	4.60	5.23	6.26	7.26	8.55	22.31	25.00	27.49	30.58	32.80
16	5.14	5.81	6.91	7.96	9.31	23.54	26.30	28.85	32.00	34.27
18	6.26	7.01	8.23	9.39	10.86	25.99	28.87	31.53	34.81	37.16
20	7.43	8.26	9.59	10.85	12.44	28.41	31.41	34.17	37.57	40.00
24	9.89	10.86	12.40	13.85	15.66	33.20	36.42	39.36	42.98	45.56
30	13.79	14.95	16.79	18.49	20.60	40.26	43.77	46.98	50.98	53.67
40	20.71	22.16	24.43	26.51	29.05	51.81	55.76	59.34	63.69	66.77
60	35.53	37.48	40.48	43.19	46.46	74.40	79.08	83.30	88.38	91.95
120	83.85	86.92	91.58	95.70	100.62	140.23	146.57	152.21	158.95	163.64

(From Dixon, W. J. and Massey, F. J. Jr.: *Introduction to statistical analysis* (3rd ed.). New York: McGraw-Hill Book Company, 1969; with permission.)

APPENDIX F

Table of Probabilities Associated with Values as Small as Observed Values of U in the Mann–Whitney Test

$n_2 = 3$			
U \ n_1	1	2	3
0	.250	.100	.050
1	.500	.200	.100
2	.750	.400	.200
3		.600	.350
4			.500
5			.650

$n_2 = 4$				
U \ n_1	1	2	3	4
0	.200	.067	.028	.014
1	.400	.133	.057	.029
2	.600	.267	.114	.057
3		.400	.200	.100
4		.600	.314	.171
5			.429	.243
6			.571	.343
7				.443
8				.557

$n_2 = 5$					
U \ n_1	1	2	3	4	5
0	.167	.047	.018	.008	.004
1	.333	.095	.036	.016	.008
2	.500	.190	.071	.032	.016
3	.667	.286	.125	.056	.028
4		.429	.196	.095	.048
5		.571	.286	.143	.075
6			.393	.206	.111
7			.500	.278	.155
8			.607	.365	.210
9				.452	.274
10				.548	.345
11					.421
12					.500
13					.579

$n_2 = 6$						
U \ n_1	1	2	3	4	5	6
0	.143	.036	.012	.005	.002	.001
1	.286	.071	.024	.010	.004	.002
2	.428	.143	.048	.019	.009	.004
3	.571	.214	.083	.033	.015	.008
4		.321	.131	.057	.026	.013
5		.429	.190	.086	.041	.021
6		.571	.274	.129	.063	.032
7			.357	.176	.089	.047
8			.452	.238	.123	.066
9			.548	.305	.165	.090
10				.381	.214	.120
11				.457	.268	.155
12				.545	.331	.197
13					.396	.242
14					.465	.294
15					.535	.350
16						.409
17						.469
18						.531

Table continued on following page

APPENDIX F *(Continued)*

U	$n_2 = 7$						
	1	**2**	**3**	**4**	**5**	**6**	**7**
0	.125	.028	.008	.003	.001	.001	.000
1	.250	.056	.017	.006	.003	.001	.001
2	.375	.111	.033	.012	.005	.002	.001
3	.500	.167	.058	.021	.009	.004	.002
4	.625	.250	.092	.036	.015	.007	.003
5		.333	.133	.055	.024	.011	.006
6		.444	.192	.082	.037	.017	.009
7		.556	.258	.115	.053	.026	.013
8			.333	.158	.074	.037	.019
9			.417	.206	.101	.051	.027
10			.500	.264	.134	.069	.036
11			.583	.324	.172	.090	.049
12				.394	.216	.117	.064
13				.464	.265	.147	.082
14				.538	.319	.183	.104
15					.378	.223	.130
16					.438	.267	.159
17					.500	.314	.191
18					.562	.365	.228
19						.418	.267
20						.473	.310
21						.527	.355
22							.402
23							.451
24							.500
25							.549

Table continued on opposite page

APPENDIX F (*Continued*)

U	$n_2 = 8$									
n_1	1	2	3	4	5	6	7	8	t	**Normal**
0	.111	.022	.006	.002	.001	.000	.000	.000	3.308	.001
1	.222	.044	.012	.004	.002	.001	.000	.000	3.203	.001
2	.333	.089	.024	.008	.003	.001	.001	.000	3.098	.001
3	.444	.133	.042	.014	.005	.002	.001	.001	2.993	.001
4	.556	.200	.067	.024	.009	.004	.002	.001	2.888	.002
5		.267	.097	.036	.015	.006	.003	.001	2.783	.003
6		.356	.139	.055	.023	.010	.005	.002	2.678	.004
7		.444	.188	.077	.033	.015	.007	.003	2.573	.005
8		.556	.248	.107	.047	.021	.010	.005	2.468	.007
9			.315	.141	.064	.030	.014	.007	2.363	.009
10			.387	.184	.085	.041	.020	.010	2.258	.012
11			.461	.230	.111	.054	.027	.014	2.153	.016
12			.539	.285	.142	.071	.036	.019	2.048	.020
13				.341	.177	.091	.047	.025	1.943	.026
14				.404	.217	.114	.060	.032	1.838	.033
15				.467	.262	.141	.076	.041	1.733	.041
16				.533	.311	.172	.095	.052	1.628	.052
17					.362	.207	.116	.065	1.523	.064
18					.416	.245	.140	.080	1.418	.078
19					.472	.286	.168	.097	1.313	.094
20					.528	.331	.198	.117	1.208	.113
21						.377	.232	.139	1.102	.135
22						.426	.268	.164	.998	.159
23						.475	.306	.191	.893	.185
24						.525	.347	.221	.788	.215
25							.389	.253	.683	.247
26							.433	.287	.578	.282
27							.478	.323	.473	.318
28							.522	.360	.368	.356
29								.399	.263	.396
30								.439	.158	.437
31								.480	.052	.481
32								.520		

(From Mann, H. B. and Whitney, D. R.: Ann. Math. Statist., *18*:52–54, 1947; with permission.)

Table of Critical Values of *U* in the Mann-Whitney Test

TABLE G–1
Critical Values of *U* for a One-Tailed Test at $\alpha = .001$ or for a Two-Tailed Test at $\alpha = .002$

n_1 \ n_2	9	10	11	12	13	14	15	16	17	18	19	20
1												
2												
3									0	0	0	0
4		0	0	0	1	1	1	2	2	3	3	3
5	1	1	2	2	3	3	4	5	5	6	7	7
6	2	3	4	4	5	6	7	8	9	10	11	12
7	3	5	6	7	8	9	10	11	13	14	15	16
8	5	6	8	9	11	12	14	15	17	18	20	21
9	7	8	10	12	14	15	17	19	21	23	25	26
10	8	10	12	14	17	19	21	23	25	27	29	32
11	10	12	15	17	20	22	24	27	29	32	34	37
12	12	14	17	20	23	25	28	31	34	37	40	42
13	14	17	20	23	26	29	32	35	38	42	45	48
14	15	19	22	25	29	32	36	39	43	46	50	54
15	17	21	24	28	32	36	40	43	47	51	55	59
16	19	23	27	31	35	39	43	48	52	56	60	65
17	21	25	29	34	38	43	47	52	57	61	66	70
18	23	27	32	37	42	46	51	56	61	66	71	76
19	25	29	34	40	45	50	55	60	66	71	77	82
20	26	32	37	42	48	54	59	65	70	76	82	88

TABLE G–2
Critical Values of *U* for a One-Tailed Test at $\alpha = .01$ or for a Two-Tailed Test at $\alpha = .02$

n_1 \ n_2	9	10	11	12	13	14	15	16	17	18	19	20
1												
2					0	0	0	0	0	0	1	1
3	1	1	1	2	2	2	3	3	4	4	4	5
4	3	3	4	5	5	6	7	7	8	9	9	10
5	5	6	7	8	9	10	11	12	13	14	15	16
6	7	8	9	11	12	13	15	16	18	19	20	22
7	9	11	12	14	16	17	19	21	23	24	26	28
8	11	13	15	17	20	22	24	26	28	30	32	34
9	14	16	18	21	23	26	28	31	33	36	38	40
10	16	19	22	24	27	30	33	36	38	41	44	47
11	18	22	25	28	31	34	37	41	44	47	50	53
12	21	24	28	31	35	38	42	46	49	53	56	60
13	23	27	31	35	39	43	47	51	55	59	63	67
14	26	30	34	38	43	47	51	56	60	65	69	73
15	28	33	37	42	47	51	56	61	66	70	75	80
16	31	36	41	46	51	56	61	66	71	76	82	87
17	33	38	44	49	55	60	66	71	77	82	88	93
18	36	41	47	53	59	65	70	76	82	88	94	100
19	38	44	50	56	63	69	75	82	88	94	101	107
20	40	47	53	60	67	73	80	87	93	100	107	114

TABLE G–3
Critical Values of *U* for a One-Tailed Test at α = .025 or for a Two-Tailed Test at α = .05

n_1 \ n_2	9	10	11	12	13	14	15	16	17	18	19	20
1												
2	0	0	0	1	1	1	1	1	2	2	2	2
3	2	3	3	4	4	5	5	6	6	7	7	8
4	4	5	6	7	8	9	10	11	11	12	13	13
5	7	8	9	11	12	13	14	15	17	18	19	20
6	10	11	13	14	16	17	19	21	22	24	25	27
7	12	14	16	18	20	22	24	26	28	30	32	34
8	15	17	19	22	24	26	29	31	34	36	38	41
9	17	20	23	26	28	31	34	37	39	42	45	48
10	20	23	26	29	33	36	39	42	45	48	52	55
11	23	26	30	33	37	40	44	47	51	55	58	62
12	26	29	33	37	41	45	49	53	57	61	65	69
13	28	33	37	41	45	50	54	59	63	67	72	76
14	31	36	40	45	50	55	59	64	67	74	78	83
15	34	39	44	49	54	59	64	70	75	80	85	90
16	37	42	47	53	59	64	70	75	81	86	92	98
17	39	45	51	57	63	67	75	81	87	93	99	105
18	42	48	55	61	67	74	80	86	93	99	106	112
19	45	52	58	65	72	78	85	92	99	106	113	119
20	48	55	62	69	76	83	90	98	105	112	119	127

TABLE G–4
Critical Values of *U* for a One-Tailed Test at α = .05 or for a Two-Tailed Test at α = .10

n_1 \ n_2	9	10	11	12	13	14	15	16	17	18	19	20
1											0	0
2	1	1	1	2	2	2	3	3	3	4	4	4
3	3	4	5	5	6	7	7	8	9	9	10	11
4	6	7	8	9	10	11	12	14	15	16	17	18
5	9	11	12	13	15	16	18	19	20	22	23	25
6	12	14	16	17	19	21	23	25	26	28	30	32
7	15	17	19	21	24	26	28	30	33	35	37	39
8	18	20	23	26	28	31	33	36	39	41	44	47
9	21	24	27	30	33	36	39	42	45	48	51	54
10	24	27	31	34	37	41	44	48	51	55	58	62
11	27	31	34	38	42	46	50	54	57	61	65	69
12	30	34	38	42	47	51	55	60	64	68	72	77
13	33	37	42	47	51	56	61	65	70	75	80	84
14	36	41	46	51	56	61	66	71	77	82	87	92
15	39	44	50	55	61	66	72	77	83	88	94	100
16	42	48	54	60	65	71	77	83	89	95	101	107
17	45	51	57	64	70	77	83	89	96	102	109	115
18	48	55	61	68	75	82	88	95	102	109	116	123
19	51	58	65	72	80	87	94	101	109	116	123	130
20	54	62	69	77	84	92	100	107	115	123	130	138

(From Siegel, S.: *Nonparametric statistics for the behavioral sciences.* New York: McGraw-Hill Book Company, 1956, as adapted from Auble, D.: Bulletin of Institute of Educational Research at Indiana University, Vol. 1, No. 2, 1953; with permission.)

Percentiles of the Kolmogorov–Smirnov Test Statistic

		One-Sided Test: $\alpha =$				
		.90	.95	.975	.99	.995
		Two-Sided Test: $\alpha =$				
		.80	.90	.95	.98	.99
n_1	n_2					
3	3	.667	.667			
3	4	.750	.750			
3	5	.667	.800	.800		
3	6	.667	.667	.833		
3	7	.667	.714	.857	.857	
3	8	.625	.750	.750	.875	
3	9	.667	.667	.778	.889	.889
3	10	.600	.700	.800	.900	.900
3	12	.583	.667	.750	.833	.917
4	4	.750	.750	.750		
4	5	.600	.750	.800	.800	
4	6	.583	.667	.750	.833	.833
4	7	.607	.714	.750	.857	.857
4	8	.625	.625	.750	.875	.875
4	9	.556	.667	.750	.778	.889
4	10	.550	.650	.700	.800	.800
4	12	.583	.667	.667	.750	.833
4	16	.563	.625	.688	.750	.812
5	5	.600	.600	.800	.800	.800
5	6	.600	.667	.667	.833	.833
5	7	.571	.657	.714	.829	.857
5	8	.550	.625	.675	.800	.800
5	9	.556	.600	.689	.778	.800
5	10	.500	.600	.700	.700	.800
5	15	.533	.600	.667	.733	.733
5	20	.500	.550	.600	.700	.750
6	6	.500	.667	.667	.833	.833
6	7	.548	.571	.690	.714	.833
6	8	.500	.583	.667	.750	.750
6	9	.500	.556	.667	.722	.778
6	10	.500	.567	.633	.700	.733
6	12	.500	.583	.583	.667	.750
6	18	.444	.556	.611	.667	.722
6	24	.458	.500	.583	.625	.667
7	7	.571	.571	.714	.714	.714
7	8	.482	.589	.625	.732	.750
7	9	.492	.556	.635	.714	.746
7	10	.471	.557	.614	.700	.714
7	14	.429	.500	.571	.643	.714
7	28	.429	.464	.536	.607	.643
8	8	.500	.500	.625	.625	.750
8	9	.444	.542	.625	.667	.750
8	10	.475	.525	.575	.675	.700
8	12	.458	.500	.583	.625	.667

Table continued on opposite page

APPENDIX H (Continued)

		One-Sided Test: $\alpha =$				
		.90	.95	.975	.99	.995
		Two-Sided Test: $\alpha =$				
		.80	.90	.95	.98	.99
n_1	n_2					
8	16	.438	.500	.563	.625	.625
8	32	.406	.438	.500	.563	.594
9	9	.444	.556	.556	.667	.667
9	10	.467	.500	.578	.667	.689
9	12	.444	.500	.556	.611	.667
9	15	.422	.489	.533	.600	.644
9	18	.389	.444	.500	.556	.611
9	36	.361	.417	.472	.528	.556
10	10	.400	.500	.600	.600	.700
10	15	.400	.467	.500	.567	.633
10	20	.400	.450	.500	.550	.600
10	40	.350	.400	.450	.500	.576
11	11	.454	.454	.545	.636	.636
12	12	.417	.417	.500	.583	.583
12	15	.383	.450	.500	.550	.583
12	16	.375	.438	.479	.542	.583
12	18	.361	.417	.472	.528	.556
12	20	.367	.417	.467	.517	.567
13	13	.385	.462	.462	.538	.615
14	14	.357	.429	.500	.500	.571
15	15	.333	.400	.467	.467	.533
16	16	.375	.375	.438	.500	.563
17	17	.353	.412	.412	.471	.529
18	18	.333	.389	.444	.500	.500
19	19	.316	.368	.421	.473	.473
20	20	.300	.350	.400	.450	.500
21	21	.286	.333	.381	.429	.476
22	22	.318	.364	.364	.454	.454
23	23	.304	.348	.391	.435	.435
24	24	.292	.333	.375	.417	.458
25	25	.280	.320	.360	.400	.440

For other sample sizes, let $C = \sqrt{\dfrac{n_1 + n_2}{n_1 n_2}}$, and use as an approximation:

		.90	.95	.975	.99	.995
		$1.07C$	$1.22\,C$	$1.36\,C$	$1.52\,C$	$1.63\,C$

(From Marascuilo, L. A. and McSweeney, M.: *Nonparametric and distribution-free methods for the social sciences.* Monterey, California: Brooks/Cole Publishing Company, as adapted from Massey, F. J. Jr: Ann. Math. Statist., *23:* 435–441, 1952; with permission.)

APPENDIX I

Table of Critical Values of *r* in the Runs Test

Given in the bodies of Table I–1 and Table I–2 are various critical values of *r* for various values of n_1 and n_2. For the one-sample runs test, any value of *r* that is equal to or smaller than that shown in Table I–1 or equal to or larger than that shown in Table I–2 is significant at the .05 level. For the Wald-Wolfowitz two-sample runs test, any value of *r* that is equal to or smaller than that shown in Table I–1 is significant at the .05 level.

TABLE I–1

n_2 \ n_1	2	3	4	5	6	7	8	9	10	11	12	13	14	15	16	17	18	19	20
2											2	2	2	2	2	2	2	2	2
3					2	2	2	2	2	2	2	2	2	3	3	3	3	3	3
4				2	2	2	3	3	3	3	3	3	3	3	4	4	4	4	4
5			2	2	3	3	3	3	3	4	4	4	4	4	4	4	5	5	5
6		2	2	3	3	3	3	4	4	4	4	5	5	5	5	5	5	6	6
7		2	2	3	3	3	4	4	5	5	5	5	5	6	6	6	6	6	6
8		2	3	3	3	4	4	5	5	5	6	6	6	6	6	7	7	7	7
9		2	3	3	4	4	5	5	5	6	6	6	7	7	7	7	8	8	8
10		2	3	3	4	5	5	5	6	6	7	7	7	7	8	8	8	8	9
11		2	3	4	4	5	5	6	6	7	7	7	8	8	8	9	9	9	9
12	2	2	3	4	4	5	6	6	7	7	7	8	8	8	9	9	9	10	10
13	2	2	3	4	5	5	6	6	7	7	8	8	9	9	9	10	10	10	10
14	2	2	3	4	5	5	6	7	7	8	8	9	9	9	10	10	10	11	11
15	2	3	3	4	5	6	6	7	7	8	8	9	9	10	10	11	11	11	12
16	2	3	4	4	5	6	6	7	8	8	9	9	10	10	11	11	11	12	12
17	2	3	4	4	5	6	7	7	8	9	9	10	10	11	11	11	12	12	13
18	2	3	4	5	5	6	7	8	8	9	9	10	10	11	11	12	12	13	13
19	2	3	4	5	6	6	7	8	8	9	10	10	11	11	12	12	13	13	13
20	2	3	4	5	6	6	7	8	9	9	10	10	11	12	12	13	13	13	14

Table continued on opposite page

APPENDIX I (Continued)

TABLE I-2

n_2 \ n_1	2	3	4	5	6	7	8	9	10	11	12	13	14	15	16	17	18	19	20
2																			
3																			
4				9	9														
5			9	10	10	11	11												
6			9	10	11	12	12	13	13	13	13								
7				11	12	13	13	14	14	14	14	15	15	15					
8				11	12	13	14	14	15	15	16	16	16	16	17	17	17	17	17
9					13	14	14	15	16	16	16	17	17	18	18	18	18	18	18
10					13	14	15	16	16	17	17	18	18	18	19	19	19	20	20
11					13	14	15	16	17	17	18	19	19	19	20	20	20	21	21
12					13	14	16	16	17	18	19	19	20	20	21	21	21	22	22
13						15	16	17	18	19	19	20	20	21	21	22	22	23	23
14						15	16	17	18	19	20	20	21	22	22	23	23	23	24
15						15	16	18	18	19	20	21	22	22	23	23	24	24	25
16							17	18	19	20	21	21	22	23	23	24	25	25	25
17							17	18	19	20	21	22	23	23	24	25	25	26	26
18							17	18	19	20	21	22	23	24	25	25	26	26	27
19							17	18	20	21	22	23	23	24	25	25	26	27	27
20							17	18	20	21	22	23	24	25	25	26	27	27	28

(From Siegel, S.: *Nonparametric statistics for the behavioral sciences.* New York: McGraw-Hill Book Company, 1956, as adapted from Swed, F. S. and Eisenhart, C.: Ann. Math. Statist., *14*:83–86, 1943; with permission.)

APPENDIX J

Critical Values for the Wilcoxon Signed-Ranks Test
(N = 5(1)50)

One-sided	Two-sided	N=5	N=6	N=7	N=8	N=9	N=10	N=11	N=12	N=13	N=14	N=15	N=16
P = .05	P = .10	1	2	4	6	8	11	14	17	21	26	30	36
P = .025	P = .05		1	2	4	6	8	11	14	17	21	25	30
P = .01	P = .02			0	2	3	5	7	10	13	16	20	24
P = .005	P = .01				0	2	3	5	7	10	13	16	19

One-sided	Two-sided	N=17	N=18	N=19	N=20	N=21	N=22	N=23	N=24	N=25	N=26	N=27	N=28
P = .05	P = .10	41	47	54	60	68	75	83	92	101	110	120	130
P = .025	P = .05	35	40	46	52	59	66	73	81	90	98	107	117
P = .01	P = .02	28	33	38	43	49	56	62	69	77	85	93	102
P = .005	P = .01	23	28	32	37	43	49	55	61	68	76	84	92

One-sided	Two-sided	N=29	N=30	N=31	N=32	N=33	N=34	N=35	N=36	N=37	N=38	N=39
P = .05	P = .10	141	152	163	175	188	201	214	228	242	256	271
P = .025	P = .05	127	137	148	159	171	183	195	208	222	235	250
P = .01	P = .02	111	120	130	141	151	162	174	186	198	211	224
P = .005	P = .01	100	109	118	128	138	149	160	171	183	195	208

One-sided	Two-sided	N=40	N=41	N=42	N=43	N=44	N=45	N=46	N=47	N=48	N=49	N=50
P = .05	P = .10	287	303	319	336	353	371	389	408	427	446	466
P = .025	P = .05	264	279	295	311	327	344	361	379	397	415	434
P = .01	P = .02	238	252	267	281	297	313	329	345	362	380	398
P = .005	P = .01	221	234	248	262	277	292	307	323	339	356	373

(From Wilcoxon, F. and Wilcox, R. A.: Some rapid approximate statistical procedures [revised edition]. Pearl River, New York: Lederle Laboratories, 1964; with permission.)

APPENDIX K

Table of Probabilities Associated with Values as Large as Observed Values of *H* in the Kruskal–Wallis One-Way Analysis of Variance by Ranks

Sample Sizes					Sample Sizes				
n_1	n_2	n_3	*H*	*p*	n_1	n_2	n_3	*H*	*p*
2	1	1	2.7000	.500	4	3	2	6.4444	.008
								6.3000	.011
2	2	1	3.6000	.200				5.4444	.046
								5.4000	.051
2	2	2	4.5714	.067				4.5111	.098
			3.7143	.200				4.4444	.102
3	1	1	3.2000	.300	4	3	3	6.7455	.010
3	2	1	4.2857	.100				6.7091	.013
			3.8571	.133				5.7909	.046
								5.7273	.050
3	2	2	5.3572	.029				4.7091	.092
			4.7143	.048				4.7000	.101
			4.5000	.067					
			4.4643	.105	4	4	1	6.6667	.010
								6.1667	.022
3	3	1	5.1429	.043				4.9667	.048
			4.5714	.100				4.8667	.054
			4.0000	.129				4.1667	.082
								4.0667	.102
3	3	2	6.2500	.011					
			5.3611	.032	4	4	2	7.0364	.006
			5.1389	.061				6.8727	.011
			4.5556	.100				5.4545	.046
			4.2500	.121				5.2364	.052
								4.5545	.098
3	3	3	7.2000	004				4.4455	.103
			6.4889	.011					
			5.6889	.029					
			5.6000	.050	4	4	3	7.1439	.010
			5.0667	.086				7.1364	.011
			4.6222	.100				5.5985	.049
								5.5758	.051

Table continued on opposite page

APPENDIX K (*Continued*)

Sample Sizes			H	p	Sample Sizes			H	p
n_1	n_2	n_3			n_1	n_2	n_3		
4	1	1	3.5714	.200				4.5455	.099
								4.4773	.102
4	2	1	4.8214	.057					
			4.5000	.076	4	4	4	7.6538	.008
			4.0179	.114				7.5385	.011
								5.6923	.049
4	2	2	6.0000	.014				5.6538	.054
			5.3333	.033				4.6539	.097
			5.1250	.052				4.5001	.104
			4.4583	.100					
			4.1667	.105	5	1	1	3.8571	.143
4	3	1	5.8333	.021	5	2	1	5.2500	.036
			5.2083	.050				5.0000	.048
			5.0000	.057				4.4500	.071
			4.0556	.093				4.2000	.095
			3.8889	.129				4.0500	.119
								5.6308	.050
5	2	2	6.5333	.008				4.5487	.099
			6.1333	.013				4.5231	.103
			6.1600	.034					
			5.0400	.056	5	4	4	7.7604	.009
			4.3733	.090				7.7440	.011
			4.2933	.122				5.6571	.049
								5.6176	.050
5	3	1	6.4000	.012				4.6187	.100
			4.9600	.048				4.5527	.102
			4.8711	.052					
			4.0178	.095	5	5	1	7.3091	.009
			3.8400	.123				6.8364	.011
								5.1273	.046
5	3	2	6.9091	.009				4.9091	.053
			6.8218	.010				4.1091	.086
			5.2509	.049				4.0364	.105
			5.1055	.052					
			4.6509	.091	5	5	2	7.3385	.010
			4.4945	.101				7.2692	.010
								5.3385	.047

Table continued on following page

APPENDIX K (*Continued*)

Sample Sizes			H	p	Sample Sizes			H	p
n_1	n_2	n_3			n_1	n_2	n_3		
5	3	3	7.0788	.009				5.2462	.051
			6.9818	.011				4.6231	.097
			5.6485	.049				4.5077	.100
			5.5152	.051					
			4.5333	.097	5	5	3	7.5780	.010
			4.4121	.109				7.5429	.010
								5.7055	.046
5	4	1	6.9545	.008				5.6264	.051
			6.8400	.011				4.5451	.100
			4.9855	.044				4.5363	.102
			4.8600	.056					
			3.9873	.098	5	5	4	7.8229	.010
			3.9600	.102				7.7914	.010
								5.6657	.049
5	4	2	7.2045	.009				5.6429	.050
			7.1182	.010				4.5229	.099
			5.2727	.049				4.5200	.101
			5.2682	.050					
			4.5409	.098	5	5	5	8.0000	.009
			4.5182	.101				7.9800	.010
								5.7800	.049
5	4	3	7.4449	.010				5.6600	.051
			7.3949	.011				4.5600	.100
			5.6564	.049				4.5000	.102

(From Siegel, S.: *Nonparametric statistics for the behavioral sciences.* New York: McGraw-Hill Book Company, 1956, as adapted from Kruskal, W. H. and Wallis, W. A.: J. Am. Statist. Assoc., *47*:614–617, 1952; with permission.)

Table of Probabilities Associated with Values as Large as Observed Values of χ_r^2 in the Friedman Two-Way Analysis of Variance by Ranks

TABLE L–1. $k = 3$

N = 2		N = 3		N = 4		N = 5	
χ_r^2	p	χ_r^2	p	χ_r^2	p	χ_r^2	p
0	1.000	.000	1.000	.0	1.000	.0	1.00
1	.833	.667	.944	.5	.931	.4	.954
3	.500	2.000	.528	1.5	.653	1.2	.691
4	.167	2.667	.361	2.0	.431	1.6	.522
		4.667	.194	3.5	.273	2.8	.367
		6.000	.028	4.5	.125	3.6	.182
				6.0	.069	4.8	.124
				6.5	.042	5.2	.093
				8.0	.0046	6.4	.039
						7.6	.024
						8.4	.0085
						10.0	.00077

N = 6		N = 7		N = 8		N = 9	
χ_r^2	p	χ_r^2	p	χ_r^2	p	χ_r^2	p
.00	1.000	.000	1.000	.00	1.000	.000	1.000
.33	.956	.286	.964	.25	.967	.222	.971
1.00	.740	.857	.768	.75	.794	.667	.814
1.33	.570	1.143	.620	1.00	.654	.889	.865
2.33	.430	2.000	.486	1.75	.531	1.556	.569
3.00	.252	2.571	.305	2.25	.355	2.000	.398
4.00	.184	3.429	.237	3.00	.285	2.667	.328
4.33	.142	3.714	.192	3.25	.236	2.889	.278
5.33	.072	4.571	.112	4.00	.149	3.556	.187
6.33	.052	5.429	.085	4.75	.120	4.222	.154
7.00	.029	6.000	.052	5.25	.079	4.667	.107
8.33	.012	7.143	.027	6.25	.047	5.556	.069
9.00	.0081	7.714	.021	6.75	.038	6.000	.057
9.33	.0055	8.000	.016	7.00	.030	6.222	.048
10.33	.0017	8.857	.0084	7.75	.018	6.889	.031
12.00	.00013	10.286	.0036	9.00	.0099	8.000	.019
		10.571	.0027	9.25	.0080	8.222	.016
		11.143	.0012	9.75	.0048	8.667	.010
		12.286	.00032	10.75	.0024	9.556	.0060
		14.000	.000021	12.00	.0011	10.667	.0035
				12.25	.00086	10.889	.0029
				13.00	.00026	11.556	.0013
				14.25	.000061	12.667	.00066
				16.00	.0000036	13.556	.00035
						14.000	.00020
						14.222	.000097
						14.889	.000054
						16.222	.000011
						18.000	.0000006

Table continued on following page

APPENDIX L (*Continued*)

TABLE L–2. $k = 4$

N = 2		N = 3		N = 4			
χ_r^2	p	χ_r^2	p	χ_r^2	p	χ_r^2	p
.0	1.000	.2	1.000	.0	1.000	5.7	.141
.6	.958	.6	.958	.3	.992	6.0	.105
1.2	.834	1.0	.910	.6	.928	6.3	.094
1.8	.792	1.8	.727	.9	.900	6.6	.077
2.4	.625	2.2	.608	1.2	.800	6.9	.068
3.0	.542	2.6	.524	1.5	.754	7.2	.054
3.6	.458	3.4	.446	1.8	.677	7.5	.052
4.2	.375	3.8	.342	2.1	.649	7.8	.036
4.8	.208	4.2	.300	2.4	.524	8.1	.033
5.4	.167	5.0	.207	2.7	.508	8.4	.019
6.0	.042	5.4	.175	3.0	.432	8.7	.014
		5.8	.148	3.3	.389	9.3	.012
		6.6	.075	3.6	.355	9.6	.0069
		7.0	.054	3.9	.324	9.9	.0062
		7.4	.033	4.5	.242	10.2	.0027
		8.2	.017	4.8	.200	10.8	.0016
		9.0	.0017	5.1	.190	11.1	.00094
				5.4	.158	12.0	.000072

(From Siegel, S.: *Nonparametric statistics for the behavioral sciences.* New York: McGraw-Hill Book Company, 1956, as adapted from Friedman, M.: J. Am. Statist. Assoc., *32*:688–689, 1937; with permission.)

APPENDIX M

Statistical Power Tables
(Δ = Effect Size)

MASTER TABLE

5% Level, One-Tailed Test

					Power						
Δ	99	95	90	80	70	60	50	40	30	20	10
0.01	157695	108215	85634	61823	47055	36031	27055	19363	12555	6453	1321
0.02	39417	27050	21405	15454	11763	9007	6764	4841	3139	1614	331
0.03	17514	12019	9511	6867	5227	4003	3006	2152	1396	718	148
0.04	9848	6758	5348	3861	2939	2251	1691	1210	785	404	84
0.05	6299	4323	3421	2470	1881	1440	1082	775	503	259	54
0.06	4372	3000	2375	1715	1305	1000	751	538	349	180	38
0.07	3209	2203	1744	1259	959	734	552	395	257	133	29
0.08	2455	1685	1334	963	734	562	422	303	197	102	23
0.09	1938	1330	1053	761	579	444	334	239	156	81	18
0.10	1568	1076	852	616	469	359	270	194	126	66	15
0.11	1294	889	704	508	387	297	223	160	104	54	13
0.12	1086	746	590	427	325	249	188	135	88	46	11
0.13	924	635	503	363	277	212	160	115	75	39	10
0.14	796	546	433	313	238	183	138	99	65	34	•
0.15	692	475	376	272	207	159	120	86	56	30	•
0.16	607	417	330	239	182	140	105	76	50	27	•
0.17	537	369	292	211	161	124	93	67	44	24	•
0.18	478	328	260	188	144	110	83	60	39	21	•
0.19	428	294	233	169	129	99	75	54	35	19	•
0.20	385	265	210	152	116	89	67	49	32	17	•
0.22	317	218	173	125	96	74	56	40	27	15	•
0.24	265	182	144	105	80	62	47	34	23	12	•
0.26	224	154	122	89	68	52	40	29	19	11	•
0.28	192	132	105	76	58	45	34	25	17	10	•
0.30	166	114	91	66	51	39	30	22	15	•	•
0.32	145	100	79	58	44	34	26	19	13	•	•
0.34	127	88	70	51	39	30	23	17	12	•	•
0.36	113	78	62	45	35	27	20	15	10	•	•
0.38	100	69	55	40	31	24	18	14	•	•	•
0.40	89	62	49	36	28	21	16	12	•	•	•
0.45	69	48	38	28	21	17	13	10	•	•	•
0.50	54	37	30	22	17	13	10	•	•	•	•
0.55	43	30	24	17	14	11	•	•	•	•	•
0.60	34	24	19	14	11	•	•	•	•	•	•
0.65	28	19	16	12	•	•	•	•	•	•	•
0.70	23	16	13	10	•	•	•	•	•	•	•
0.75	18	13	10	•	•	•	•	•	•	•	•
0.80	15	10	•	•	•	•	•	•	•	•	•
0.85	12	•	•	•	•	•	•	•	•	•	•
0.90	•	•	•	•	•	•	•	•	•	•	•

Table continued on following page

MASTER TABLE

1% Level, One-Tailed Test

					Power						
Δ	*99*	*95*	*90*	*80*	*70*	*60*	*50*	*40*	*30*	*20*	*10*
0.01	216463	157695	130162	100355	81264	66545	54117	42972	32469	22044	10917
0.02	54106	39417	32535	25085	20313	16634	13528	10742	8117	5511	2730
0.03	24040	17514	14456	11146	9026	7391	6011	4773	3607	2449	1214
0.04	13517	9848	8128	6267	5075	4156	3380	2684	2029	1378	683
0.05	8646	6299	5200	4009	3247	2659	2163	1718	1298	882	437
0.06	6000	4372	3609	2783	2254	1846	1501	1192	901	612	304
0.07	4405	3209	2649	2043	1655	1355	1102	876	662	450	224
0.08	3369	2455	2027	1563	1266	1037	843	670	507	344	171
0.09	2660	1938	1600	1234	999	819	666	529	400	272	136
0.10	2152	1568	1295	998	809	663	539	428	324	220	110
0.11	1776	1294	1069	824	668	547	445	354	268	182	91
0.12	1490	1086	897	692	560	459	374	297	225	153	77
0.13	1268	924	763	589	477	391	318	253	191	130	65
0.14	1092	796	657	507	411	337	274	218	165	112	56
0.15	949	692	571	441	357	293	238	190	144	98	49
0.16	833	607	501	387	314	257	209	166	126	86	43
0.17	736	537	443	342	277	277	185	147	112	76	39
0.18	655	478	395	305	247	202	165	131	100	68	34
0.19	587	428	353	273	221	181	148	118	89	61	31
0.20	528	385	318	246	199	163	133	106	81	55	29
0.22	434	317	262	202	164	135	110	87	66	46	24
0.24	363	265	219	169	137	113	92	73	56	38	21
0.26	307	224	185	143	116	95	78	62	47	33	18
0.28	263	192	159	123	100	82	67	53	41	29	16
0.30	227	166	137	106	86	71	58	46	35	25	14
0.32	198	145	120	93	75	62	51	41	31	22	12
0.34	174	127	105	82	66	55	45	36	28	20	11
0.36	154	113	93	72	59	48	40	32	25	18	10
0.38	137	100	83	64	52	43	35	29	22	16	•
0.40	122	89	74	57	47	39	32	26	20	15	•
0.45	94	69	57	44	36	30	25	20	16	12	•
0.50	73	54	45	35	29	24	20	16	13	•	•
0.55	58	43	36	28	23	19	16	13	11	•	•
0.60	47	34	29	23	19	16	13	11	•	•	•
0.65	38	28	23	18	15	13	11	•	•	•	•
0.70	30	23	19	15	12	11	•	•	•	•	•
0.75	25	18	15	12	10	•	•	•	•	•	•
0.80	20	15	12	10	•	•	•	•	•	•	•
0.85	16	12	10	•	•	•	•	•	•	•	•
0.90	12	•	•	•	•	•	•	•	•	•	•

Table continued on opposite page

APPENDIX M (*Continued*)

MASTER TABLE

5% Level, Two-Tailed Test

Δ	99	95	90	80	Power 70	60	50	40	30	20	10
0.01	183714	129940	105069	78485	61718	48986	38414	29125	20609	12508	4604
0.02	45920	32480	26263	19618	15428	12245	9603	7281	5152	3127	1152
0.03	20403	14431	11669	8717	6855	5441	4267	3236	2290	1390	513
0.04	11472	8115	6562	4902	3855	3060	2400	1820	1288	782	289
0.05	7338	5191	4197	3136	2466	1958	1536	1165	824	501	185
0.06	5093	3602	2913	2177	1712	1359	1066	809	573	348	129
0.07	3739	2645	2139	1598	1257	998	783	594	421	256	95
0.08	2860	2023	1636	1223	962	764	599	455	322	196	73
0.09	2257	1597	1292	965	759	603	473	359	255	155	58
0.10	1826	1292	1045	781	615	488	383	291	206	126	47
0.11	1508	1067	863	645	507	403	316	240	170	104	39
0.12	1265	895	724	541	426	338	266	202	143	88	33
0.13	1076	762	616	461	363	288	226	172	122	75	29
0.14	927	656	531	397	312	248	195	148	105	64	25
0.15	806	570	461	345	272	216	170	129	92	56	22
0.16	707	500	405	303	238	190	149	113	81	50	20
0.17	625	442	358	268	211	168	132	100	71	44	18
0.18	556	394	319	238	188	149	117	89	64	39	16
0.19	498	353	286	214	168	134	105	80	57	35	15
0.20	449	318	257	192	152	121	95	72	52	32	13
0.22	369	261	212	158	125	99	78	60	43	27	11
0.24	308	218	177	133	105	83	66	50	36	23	10
0.26	261	185	150	112	89	71	56	43	31	20	•
0.28	223	159	128	96	76	61	48	37	27	17	•
0.30	193	137	111	83	66	53	42	32	23	15	•
0.32	169	120	97	73	58	46	36	28	21	13	•
0.34	148	105	85	64	51	41	32	25	18	12	•
0.36	131	93	75	57	45	36	29	22	16	11	•
0.38	116	83	67	51	40	32	26	20	15	10	•
0.40	104	74	60	45	36	29	23	18	13	•	•
0.45	80	57	46	35	28	22	18	14	11	•	•
0.50	62	45	36	27	22	18	14	11	•	•	•
0.55	50	35	29	22	18	14	12	•	•	•	•
0.60	40	29	23	18	14	12	10	•	•	•	•
0.65	32	23	19	15	12	10	•	•	•	•	•
0.70	26	19	15	12	10	•	•	•	•	•	•
0.75	21	15	13	10	•	•	•	•	•	•	•
0.80	17	12	10	•	•	•	•	•	•	•	•
0.85	13	10	•	•	•	•	•	•	•	•	•
0.90	10	•	•	•	•	•	•	•	•	•	•

Table continued on following page

APPENDIX M (*Continued*)

MASTER TABLE

1% Level, Two-Tailed Test

					Power						
Δ	99	95	90	80	70	60	50	40	30	20	10
0.01	240299	178131	148785	116783	96109	80039	66346	53937	42082	30074	16752
0.02	60064	44525	37190	29191	24024	20007	16584	13483	10520	7518	4188
0.03	26687	19783	16524	12970	10674	8890	7369	5991	4675	3341	1862
0.04	15005	11123	9291	7293	6002	4999	4144	3369	2629	1879	1047
0.05	9598	7115	5943	4665	3840	3198	2651	2155	1682	1202	670
0.06	6661	4938	4125	3238	2665	2220	1840	1496	1168	835	466
0.07	4890	3625	3028	2377	1957	1630	1351	1099	858	613	342
0.08	3740	2773	2316	1819	1497	1247	1034	841	656	469	262
0.09	2952	2189	1829	1436	1182	984	816	664	518	371	207
0.10	2389	1771	1480	1162	956	797	661	537	420	300	168
0.11	1972	1462	1221	959	789	658	545	444	346	248	139
0.12	1654	1227	1025	805	663	552	458	372	291	208	117
0.13	1407	1044	872	685	564	470	390	317	248	177	100
0.14	1212	898	751	590	485	405	336	273	213	153	86
0.15	1054	781	653	513	422	352	292	238	186	133	75
0.16	924	685	573	450	371	309	256	209	163	117	66
0.17	817	606	506	398	328	273	227	185	144	104	58
0.18	727	539	451	354	292	243	202	164	129	92	52
0.19	651	483	404	317	261	218	181	147	115	83	47
0.20	586	435	364	286	235	196	163	133	104	75	42
0.22	482	358	299	235	194	162	134	109	86	62	35
0.24	403	299	250	196	162	135	112	92	72	52	30
0.26	341	253	212	166	137	115	95	78	61	44	26
0.28	292	217	181	143	118	98	82	67	52	38	23
0.30	252	187	157	123	102	85	71	58	45	33	20
0.32	220	163	137	108	89	74	62	51	40	30	18
0.34	193	144	120	95	78	65	54	45	35	26	15
0.36	171	127	106	84	69	58	48	39	31	24	15
0.38	152	113	94	74	62	52	43	35	29	21	13
0.40	135	101	84	67	55	46	38	32	26	19	12
0.45	104	77	65	51	42	36	30	25	20	15	10
0.50	81	61	51	40	33	28	24	20	16	12	•
0.55	64	48	40	32	27	23	19	16	13	10	•
0.60	52	39	32	26	22	19	16	15	11	•	•
0.65	41	31	27	21	18	15	13	11	•	•	•
0.70	33	25	22	17	15	13	11	•	•	•	•
0.75	27	21	17	14	12	10	•	•	•	•	•
0.80	22	17	14	11	•	•	•	•	•	•	•
0.85	17	13	11	•	•	•	•	•	•	•	•
0.90	13	10	•	•	•	•	•	•	•	•	•

(From Kraemer, H. C., & Theimann, S. [1987]. *How many subjects: Statistical power analysis in research.* Newbury Park, California: Sage. Reprinted by permission of Sage Publications, Inc.)

Glossary

abstract. Clear, concise summary of a study, usually limited to 100–250 words.

abstract thinking. Oriented toward the development of an idea without application to, or association with, a particular instance and is independent of time and space. Abstract thinkers tend to look for meaning, patterns, relationships, and philosophical implications.

academic library. Located within institutions of higher learning and contain numerous resources for researchers.

accessible population. Portion of the target population to which the researcher has reasonable access.

accidental or convenience sampling. Subjects are included in the study because they happened to be in the right place at the right time; available subjects are simply entered into the study until the desired sample size is reached.

accuracy in physiological measures. Comparable to validity in that it addresses the extent to which the instrument measured the domain that is defined in the study.

across-method triangulation. Combining research methods or strategies from two or more research traditions in the same study.

action application of research. Using research findings to support the need for change, as impetus for evaluation of services, and/or a model for practice.

active rejection. An innovation is examined and a decision is made not to adopt it.

adoption. Full acceptance of the innovation and the implementation of the ideas in practice.

Agency for Health Care Policy and Research (AHCPR). Federal government agency created in 1989 to carry out research, demonstration projects, guideline development, training, and dissemination activities with respect to health care services and systems of information regarding the following areas: the effectiveness, efficiency, quality, and outcomes of health services; clinical practice, including primary care; health care technologies, facilities, and equipment; health care costs, productivity, and market forces; health promotion and disease prevention; health statistics and epidemiology; and medical liability.

alpha (α). Level of significance or cutoff point used to determine whether the samples being tested are members of the same population or of different populations; alpha is commonly set at .05, .01, or .001.

alternated forms reliability. Comparing the equivalence of two versions of the same paper-and-pencil instruments.

analysis of covariance (ANCOVA). Statistical procedure designed to reduce the error term (or variance within groups) by partialing out the variance due to a confounding variable by performing regression analysis prior to performing ANOVA.

analysis of variance (ANOVA). Statistical technique used to examine differences among two or more groups by comparing the variability between the groups to the variability within the groups.

analysis step of critique. Determining the strengths and limitations of the logical links connecting one study element with another.

analysis triangulation. Using two or more analysis techniques to analyze the same set of data for the purpose of validation.

analytic induction. Qualitative research technique that includes enumerative induction, in which a number and variety of instances are collected that verify the model, and eliminative induction, which requires that the hypothesis be tested against alternatives.

analytical preciseness. Performing a series of transformations during which concrete data are transformed across several levels of abstractions to develop a theoretical schema that imparts meaning to the phenomenon under study.

anonymity. Subject's identity cannot be linked, even by the researcher, with his or her individual responses.

applied research. Scientific investigations conducted to generate knowledge that will directly influence or improve practice.

ascendance to an open context. Ability to see depth and complexity within the phenomenon examined and a greater capacity for insight than with the sedimented view. Requires deconstructing sedimented views and reconstructing another view.

assent. A child's affirmative agreement to participate in research.

associative relationship. Identifies variables or concepts that occur or exist together in the real world; thus, when one variable changes, the other variable changes.

assumptions. Statements taken for granted or considered true, even though they have not been scientifically tested.

asymmetrical relationship. If A occurs (or changes), then B will occur (or change), but there may be no indication that if B occurs (or changes), A will occur (or change); $A \rightarrow B$.

auditability. Rigorous development of a decision trail that is reported in sufficient detail to allow a second researcher, using the original data and the decision trail, to arrive at conclusions similar to those of the original researcher.

authority. Person with expertise and power who is able to influence opinion and behavior.

autonomous agents. Prospective subjects informed about a proposed study can voluntarily choose to participate or not participate.

autoregressive integrated moving average (AR-IMA) model. This model is an equation or series of equations that explains a naturally occurring process and is the most commonly used time-series analysis model in nursing.

backward stepwise regression analysis. Type of stepwise regression analysis where all the independent variables are initially included in the analysis. Then, one variable at a time is removed from the equation and the effect of that removal on R^2 is evaluated.

basic research. Scientific investigations for the pursuit of knowledge for knowledge's sake or for the pleasure of learning and finding truth.

beneficence, principle of. Encourages the researcher to do good and above all, do no harm.

benefit-risk ratio. Researchers and reviewers of research weigh potential benefits and risks in a study to promote the conduct of ethical research.

between-group variance. The variance of the group means around the grand mean (the mean of the total sample) that is examined in analysis of variance (ANOVA).

between-method triangulation. *See* across-method triangulation.

bias. Any influence or action in a study that distorts the findings or slants them away from the true or expected.

bivariate analysis. Statistical procedures that involve the comparison of summary values from two groups of the same variable or of two variables within a group.

bivariate correlation. Analysis techniques that measure the extent of the linear relationship between two variables.

Bland and Altman plot. Analysis technique for examining the extent of agreement between two measurement techniques. Generally used to compare a new technique to an established one.

blocking. Design where the researcher includes subjects with various levels of an extraneous variable in the sample but controls the numbers of subjects at each level of the variable and their random assignment to groups within the study.

body of knowledge. Information, principles,

and theories that are organized by the beliefs accepted in a discipline at a given time.

Bonferroni's procedure. Parametric analysis technique that controls for escalation of significance and can be used if various *t* tests must be performed on different aspects of the same data.

borrowing. Appropriation and use of knowledge from other disciplines to guide nursing practice.

box-and-whisker plots. Exploratory data analysis technique to provide fast visualization of some of the major characteristics of the data, such as the spread, symmetry, and outliers.

bracketing. Qualitative research technique of suspending or laying aside what is known about an experience being studied.

breach of confidentiality. Accidental or direct action that allows an unauthorized person to have access to raw study data.

canonical correlation. Extension of multiple regression with more than one dependent variable.

carryover effect. Application of one treatment can influence the response to following treatments.

case study design. Intensive exploration of a single unit of study, such as a person, family, group, community, or institution.

catalog. Identifies what is available in the library.

causal hypothesis or relationship. Identifies a cause-and-effect interaction between two or more variables, which are referred to as independent and dependent variables.

causal relationship. Relationship between two variables where one variable (independent variable) is thought to cause or determine the presence of the other variable (dependent variable).

causality. Includes three conditions: (1) must be a strong correlation between the proposed cause and effect, (2) proposed cause must precede the effect in time, and (3) cause has to be present whenever the effect occurs.

cell. Intersection between the row and column in a table where a specific numerical value is inserted.

central limit theorem. States that even when statistics, such as means, come from a population with a skewed (asymmetrical) distribution, the sampling distribution developed from multiple means obtained from that skewed population will tend to fit the pattern of the normal curve.

change agent. Professional outside a system who enters the system to promote adoption of an innovation.

checklists. Techniques of indicating whether or not a behavior occurred.

chi-square test. Used to analyze nominal data to determine significant differences between observed frequencies within the data and frequencies that were expected.

chronology. A type of unstructured observation that provides a detailed description of an individual's behavior in a natural environment.

cleaning data. Checking raw data to determine errors in data recording, coding, or entry.

clinical decision analysis. A systematic method of describing clinical problems, identifying possible diagnostic and management courses of action, assessing the probability and value of the various outcomes, and then calculating the optimal course of action.

cluster sampling. A sampling frame is developed that includes a list of all the states, cities, institutions, or organizations (clusters) that could be used in a study and a randomized sample is drawn from this list.

Cochran Q test. Nonparametric test that is an extension of the McNemar test for two related samples.

codebook. Identifies and defines each variable in your study and includes an abbreviated variable name (limited to 6–8 characters), a descriptive variable label, and the range of possible numerical values of every variable entered into a computer file.

coding. Process of transforming qualitative data into numerical symbols that can be computerized.

coercion. An overt threat of harm or excessive reward intentionally presented by one person to another in order to obtain compliance, such as offering subjects a large sum of money to participate in a dangerous research project.

coefficient of determination (R^2). Computed from a matrix of correlation coefficients and provides important information on multicollinearity. This value indicates the degree of linear dependencies among the variables.

cognitive application of research. Research-based knowledge is used to affect a person's way of thinking, approaching, and/or observing situations.

cognitive clustering. Comprehensive, scholarly synthesis of scientifically sound research that is evident in integrative reviews of research and meta-analyses.

cohorts. Samples in time-dimensional studies within the field of epidemiology.

co-investigators. Two or more professionals conducting a study, whose salaries might be paid partially or in full by grant funding.

communicating research findings. Developing a research report and disseminating it through presentations and publications to a variety of audiences.

communication channels. Include one-to-one exchange of information; one individual communicating to several others; or mass media such as books, journals, newspapers, television, and computer networks.

comparative descriptive design. Used to describe differences in variables in two or more groups in a natural setting.

comparison group. The group not receiving a treatment or receiving the usual treatment (standard care) when nonrandom sampling methods are used.

comparison step of critique. The ideal for each step of the research process is compared to the real steps in a study.

complete observer. The researcher is passive and has no direct social interaction in the setting.

compatibility. The degree to which the innovation is perceived to be consistent with current values, past experience, and priority of needs.

complete participation. The researcher becomes a member of the group and conceals the researcher role.

complete review. Extensive review by an institutional review board (IRB) for studies with greater than minimal risks.

complex hypothesis. Predicts the relationship (associative or causal) among three or more variables; thus, the hypothesis could include two (or more) independent and/or two (or more) dependent variables.

complexity. The degree to which the innovation is perceived to be difficult to understand or use.

comprehension step of critique. Understanding the terms in a research report; identifying study elements; and grasping the nature, significance, and meaning of these elements.

computerized database. A structured compilation of information that can be scanned, retrieved, and analyzed by computer and can be used for decisions, reports, and research.

computer searches. Conducted to scan the citations in different databases and identify sources relevant to a research problem.

concept. A term that abstractly describes and names an object or phenomenon, thus providing it with a separate identity or meaning.

concept analysis. A strategy through which a set of attributes or characteristics essential to the connotative meaning or conceptual definition of a concept are identified.

concept derivation. Process of extracting and defining concepts from theories in other disciplines.

concept synthesis. Process of describing and naming a previously unrecognized concept.

conceptual clustering step of critique. Current knowledge in an area of study is carefully analyzed, summarized, and organized theoretically to maximize the meaning attached to research findings, highlight gaps in the knowledge base, generate research questions, and provide knowledge for use in practice.

conceptual definition. Provides a variable or concept with connotative (abstract, comprehensive, theoretical) meaning and is established through concept analysis, concept derivation, or concept synthesis.

conceptual map. Strategy for expressing a framework of a study that diagrammatically shows the interrelationships of the concepts and statements.

conceptual model. A set of highly abstract, related constructs that broadly explains phenomena of interest, expresses assumptions, and reflects a philosophical stance.

conclusions. Synthesis and clarification of the meaning of study findings.

concrete thinking. Thinking that is oriented toward and limited by tangible things or events observed and experienced in reality.

concurrent relationship. A relationship where both variables or concepts occur simultaneously.

confidence interval. A range where the value of the parameter is estimated to be.

confidentiality. Management of private data in research so subjects' identities are not linked with their responses.

confirmation stage. Stage of the innovation-decision process where the effectiveness of the innovation is evaluated and a decision is made to either continue or discontinue the innovation.

confirmatory data analysis. Performed to confirm expectations regarding the data that are expressed as hypotheses, questions, or objectives.

confirmatory factor analysis. Closely related to ordinary least squares regression analysis or path analysis and is based on theory and tests a hypothesis about the existing factor structure.

confirmatory regression analysis. Regression analysis procedures designed to confirm or support a theoretically proposed set of variables.

confounding variables. Variables recognized before the study is initiated but cannot be controlled or variables not recognized until the study is in process.

consensus knowledge building. Outcomes design that requires critique and synthesis of an extensive international search of the literature on the topic of concern, including unpublished studies, studies in progress, dissertations, and theses.

consent form. A written form, tape-recording, or videotape used to document a subject's agreement to participate in a study.

consent rate. The percentage of people that indicate a willingness to participate in a study based on the total number of people approached.

constructs. Concepts at very high levels of abstraction that have general meanings.

construct validity. Examines the fit between conceptual and operational definitions of variables and determines if the instrument actually measures the theoretical construct it purports to measure.

consultants. People hired for specific tasks during a study.

content analysis. Qualitative analysis technique to classify words in a text into a few categories chosen because of their theoretical importance.

content-related validity. Examines the extent to which the method of measurement includes all the major elements relevant to the construct being measured.

context. The body, the world, and the concerns unique to each person within which that person can be understood. Philosophical element of qualitative research.

context flexibility. Capacity to switch from one context or world view to another, to shift perception in order to see things from a different perspective.

contingency coefficient. A statistical test that is used with two nominal variables and is the most commonly used of the chi-square–based measures of association.

contingency tables. Cross-tabulation tables that allow visual comparison of summary data output related to two variables within a sample.

contingent relationship. Occurs only if a third variable or concept is present.

control. Imposing of rules by the researcher to decrease the possibility of error and increase the probability that the study's findings are an accurate reflection of reality.

control group. The group of elements or subjects not exposed to the experimental treatment. The term control group is used in studies with random sampling methods.

convenience sampling. See accidental or convenience sampling.

correlational analysis. Statistical procedure conducted to determine the direction (positive or negative) and magnitude (or strength) of the relationship between two variables.

correlational coefficient. Indicates the degree of relationship between two variables; the coefficients range in value from +1.00 (perfect positive relationship) to 0.00 (no relationship) to −1.00 (perfect negative or inverse relationship).

correlational research. Systematic investigation of relationships between two or more variables to explain the nature of relationships in the world and not to examine cause and effect.

cost-benefit analysis. Analysis technique used in outcomes research that examines costs and benefits of alternative ways of using resources as assessed in monetary terms and the use that produces the greatest net benefit.

cost-effectiveness analyses. Type of outcomes research where the costs and benefits are compared for different ways of accomplishing a clinical goal, such as diagnosing a condition, treating an illness, or providing a service. Goal of cost-effectiveness analyses is to identify the strategy that provides the most value for the money.

covert data collection. Occurs when subjects are unaware that research data are being collected.

Cramer's V. Analysis technique for nominal data that is a modification of phi for contingency tables larger than 2 × 2.

criterion-referenced testing. Comparison of a subject's score with a criterion of achievement that includes the definition of target behaviors. When the behaviors are mastered, the subject is considered proficient in these behaviors.

critical analysis of studies. Examination of the merits, faults, meaning, and significance of nursing studies using five steps: comprehension, comparison, analysis, evaluation, and conceptual clustering.

critical social theory. Qualitative research methodology guided by critical social theory; the researcher seeks to understand how people communicate and develop symbolic meanings in a society.

crossover or counterbalanced design. Includes the administration of more than one treatment to each subject and the treatments are provided sequentially, rather than concurrently, and comparisons are then made of the effects of the different treatments on the same subjects.

cross-sectional designs. Used to examine groups of subjects in various stages of development simultaneously with the intent of inferring trends over time.

cultural immersion. Used in ethnographic research for gaining increased familiarity with such things as language, sociocultural norms, and traditions in a culture.

curvilinear relationship. The relationship between two variables varies depending on the relative values of the variables. The graph of the relationship is a curved line rather than a straight one.

data. Pieces of information that are collected during a study.

database. See computerized databases.

data analysis. Conducted to reduce, organize, and give meaning to data.

data coding sheet. A sheet for organizing and recording data for rapid entry into a computer.

data collection. Precise, systematic gathering of information relevant to the research purpose or the specific objectives, questions, or hypotheses of a study.

data collection plan. Details how a study will be implemented.

data reduction. Technique for analyzing qualitative data that focuses on decreasing the volume of data to facilitate examination.

data storage and retrieval. The computer's ability to store vast amounts of data and rapidly retrieve these data for examination and analyses.

data triangulation. Collection of data from multiple sources in the same study.

debriefing. Complete disclosure of the study purpose and results at the end of a study.

debugging. Identifying and replacing errors in a computer program with accurate information.

deception. Misinforming subjects for research purposes.

decision stage. Stage in the innovation-decision process when an individual or group chooses to adopt or reject an innovation.

decision theory. Theory that is inductive in nature and is based on assumptions associated with the theoretical normal curve. The theory is applied when testing for differences between groups with the expectation that all of the groups are members of the same population.

decision trail. *See* auditability.

Declaration of Helsinki. Ethical code based on the Nuremberg code that differentiated therapeutic from nontherapeutic research.

deconstructing the sedimented views. Rigorous qualitative research requires that the researcher ascend to an open context and be willing to continue to let go of sedimented views, which involves the process of remaining open to new views.

deductive reasoning. Reasoning from the general to the specific or from a general premise to a particular situation.

degrees of freedom (*df*). The freedom of a score's value to vary given the other existing scores' values and the established sum of these scores ($df = N - 1$).

delphi technique. A method of measuring the judgments of a group of experts for assessing priorities or making forecasts.

demographic variables. Characteristics or attributes of the subjects that are collected to describe the sample.

dependent groups. Groups where the subjects or observations selected for data collection are in some way related to the selection of other subjects or observations. For example, if subjects serve as their own control by using the pretest as a control, the observations (and therefore the groups) are dependent. Use of twins in a study or matching subjects on a selected variable results in dependent groups.

dependent variable. The response, behavior, or outcome that is predicted or explained in research; changes in the dependent variable are presumed to be caused by the independent variable.

description. Involves identifying the nature and attributes of nursing phenomena and sometimes the relationships among these phenomena.

descriptive codes. Terms used to organize and classify qualitative data.

descriptive correlational design. Used to describe variables and examine relationships that exist in a situation.

descriptive design. Used to identify phenomenon of interest, identify variables within the phenomenon, develop conceptual and operational definitions of variables, and describe variables.

descriptive research. Provides an accurate portrayal or account of characteristics of a particular individual, event, or group in real-life situations for the purpose of discovering new meaning, describing what exists, determining the frequency with which something occurs, and categorizing information.

descriptive statistics. Statistics that allow the researcher to organize the data in ways that give meaning and facilitate insight, such as frequency distributions and measures of central tendency and dispersion.

descriptive vividness. Description of the site, subjects, experience of collecting data, and the researcher's thoughts during the qualitative research process presented so clearly the reader has the sense of personally experiencing the event.

design. Blueprint for conducting a study that maximizes control over factors that could interfere with the validity of the findings.

deterministic relationships. Statements of what always occurs in a particular situation, such as a scientific law.

developmental grant proposals. Proposals written to obtain funding for the development of a new program in a discipline.

dialectic reasoning. Involves the holistic perspective, where the whole is greater than the sum of the parts, and examining factors that are opposites and making sense of them by merging them into a single unit or idea, greater than either alone.

diary. Record of events kept by a subject over time that is collected and analyzed by a researcher.

difference scores. Deviation scores obtained by subtracting the mean from each raw score.

diffusion. Process of communicating research findings (innovations) through certain channels over time among the members of a discipline.

diminished autonomy. Subjects with decreased ability to voluntarily give informed consent because of legal or mental incompetence, terminal illness, or confinement to an institution.

directional hypothesis. States the specific nature of the interaction or relationship between two or more variables.

direct application. Occurs when an innovation is used exactly as it was developed.

direct measurement. The measurement object and measurement strategies are specific and straightforward, such as those for measuring the concrete variables of height, weight, or temperature.

discontinuance of an innovation. When using new ideas from research in practice, the individual or organization can decide to not use or discontinue the use of the idea or innovation at any point in time. Discontinuance can be of at least two types: replacement discontinuance or disenchantment discontinuance. Discontinuance is a possibility outlined in the confirmation stage of the innovation-decision process.

discriminant analysis. Designed to allow the researcher to identify characteristics associated with group membership and to predict group membership.

disenchantment discontinuance in utilization of innovations. Discontinuation of a new idea or innovation because the user is dissatisfied with its outcome.

dissemination of research findings. The diffusion or communication of research findings.

dummy variables. Categorical or dichotomous variables used in regression analysis.

duplicate publication. The practice of publishing the same article or major portions of the article in two or more print or electronic media without notifying the editors or referencing the other publication in the reference list.

early adopters of innovations. Opinion leaders in a social system who learn about new ideas rapidly, utilize them, and serve as role models for their use in nursing practice.

early majority in the use of innovations. Individuals who are rarely leaders but are active followers and will readily follow in the use of a new idea in nursing practice.

effect size. The degree to which the phenomenon is present in the population or to which the null hypothesis is false.

eigenvalues. Numerical values generated with factor analysis that are the sum of the squared weights for each factor.

electronic mail. Allows a computer user to rapidly exchange messages, computer files, data, and research reports using satellite networks.

element of a study. A person (subject), event, behavior, or any other single unit of a study.

eliminative induction. Qualitative data analysis technique that is part of a process referred to as analytic induction and requires that the hypothesis generated from the analysis be tested against alternatives.

emic approach. Anthropological research approach of studying behaviors from within the culture.

empirical generalization. Statements that have been repeatedly tested through research and have not been disproved. Scientific theories have empirical generalizations.

empirical literature. Includes relevant studies published in journals and books as well as unpublished studies, such as master's theses and doctoral dissertations.

empirical world. Experienced through our senses and is the concrete portion of our existence.

enumerative induction. Qualitative data analysis technique that is part of a process referred to as analytic induction and requires that a number and variety of instances are collected that verify a model that was developed from the research process.

environmental variable. Type of extraneous variable composing the setting where a study is conducted.

equivalence. Type of reliability testing that involves comparing two versions of the same paper-and-pencil instrument or two observers measuring the same event.

error score. Amount of random error in the measurement process.

errors in physiologic measures. Sources of erroneous measurement with physiological instruments that include environment, user, subject, machine, and interpretation error.

ethical inquiry. Intellectual analysis of ethical problems related to obligation, rights, duty, right and wrong, conscience, choice, intention, and responsibility to obtain desirable, rational ends.

ethical principles. Principles of respect for persons, beneficence, and justice relevant to the conduct of research.

ethical rigor. Requires recognition and discussion by the researcher of the ethical implications related to the conduct of the study.

ethnographic research. A qualitative research methodology for investigating cultures that involves collection, description, and analysis of data to develop a theory of cultural behavior.

ethnonursing research. Emerged from Leininger's theory of transcultural nursing and focuses mainly on observing and documenting interactions with people to determine how daily life conditions and patterns are influencing human care, health, and nursing care practices.

etic approach. Anthropological research approach of studying behavior from outside the culture and examining similarities and differences across cultures.

evaluation step of a critique. Examining the meaning and significance of a study according to set criteria and comparing it with previous studies conducted in the area.

event-partitioning designs. Merger of the longitudinal and trend designs to increase sample size and avoid the effects of history on the validity of findings.

event-time matrix. Qualitative analysis technique that can facilitate comparisons of the events occurring in different sites during particular time periods.

exclusion criteria. Sampling requirements identified by the researcher that eliminate or exclude an element or subject from being in a sample. Exclusion criteria are exceptions to the inclusion sampling criteria.

execution errors. Errors that occur because of a defect in the data collection procedure.

exempt studies. Studies that have no apparent risks for the research subjects are often designated as exempt from or not requiring institutional review.

existence statement. Declares that a given concept exists or that a given relationship occurs.

expedited review. Review process for studies that have some risks, but the risks are minimal or no greater than those ordinarily encountered in daily life or during the performance of routine physical or psychological exams.

experimental designs. Designs that provide the greatest amount of control possible in order to more closely examine causality.

experimental group. The subjects who are exposed to the experimental treatment.

experimental research. Objective, systematic, controlled investigation to examine probability and causality among selected variables for the purpose of predicting and controlling phenomena.

explanation. Achieved when research clarifies the relationships among phenomena and identifies why certain events occur.

explanatory codes. Developed late in the data collection process after theoretical ideas from the qualitative study have begun to emerge.

explanatory effects matrix. Qualitative analysis technique that can assist in answering questions, such as why an outcome was achieved or what caused the outcome.

exploratory data analysis. Examining the data descriptively, to become as familiar as possible with the nature of the data.

exploratory factor analysis. Similar to stepwise regression in which the variance of the first factor is partialed out before analysis is begun on the second factor. It is performed when the researcher has few prior expectations about the factor structure.

exploratory regression analysis. Used when the researcher may not have sufficient information to determine which independent variables are effective predictors of the dependent variable; thus, many variables may be entered into the analysis simultaneously. This is the most commonly used regression analysis strategy in nursing studies.

external criticism. A method of determining the validity of source materials in historical research and involves knowing where, when, why, and by whom a document was written.

external validity. The extent to which study findings can be generalized beyond the sample used in the study.

extraneous variables. Exist in all studies and can affect the measurement of study variables and the relationships among these variables.

face validity. Verify that the instrument looked like or gave the appearance of measuring the content.

factor analysis. Analysis that examines interrelationships among large numbers of variables and disentangles those relationships to identify clusters of variables that are most closely linked together. Two types of factor analysis are exploratory and confirmatory factor analysis.

factor rotation. An aspect of factor analysis where the factors are mathematically adjusted or rotated to reduce the factor structure and clarify the meaning.

factorial analysis of variance. Mathematically the analysis technique is simply a specialized version of multiple regression; a number of types of factorial ANOVAs have been developed to analyze data from specific experimental designs.

factorial design. Study design that includes two or more different characteristics, treatments, or events that are independently varied within a study.

fair treatment. Ethical principle that promotes fair selection and treatment of subjects during the course of a study.

fatigue effect. When a subject becomes tired or bored with a study.

feasibility of a study. Determined by examining the time and money commitment; the researcher's expertise; availability of subjects, facility, and equipment; cooperation of others; and the study's ethical considerations.

field research. The activity of collecting the data that requires taking extensive notes in ethnographic research.

findings. The translated and interpreted results from a study.

forced choice. Response set for items in a scale that have an even number of choices, such as four or six, where the respondents cannot choose an uncertain or neutral response and must indicate support for or against the topic measured.

forward stepwise regression analysis. Type of stepwise regression analysis where the independent variables are entered into the analysis one at a time and an analysis is made of the effect of including that variable on R^2.

foundational inquiry. Research examining the foundations for a science, such as studies that provide analyses of the structure of a science and the process of thinking about and valuing certain phenomena held in common by the science. Debates related to quantitative and qualitative research methods emerged from foundational inquiries.

framework. The abstract, logical structure of meaning that guides the development of the study and enables the researcher to link the findings to nursing's body of knowledge.

fraudulent publications. There is documentation or testimony from coauthors that the publication did not reflect what had actually been done.

frequency distribution. A statistical procedure that involves listing all possible measures of a variable and tallying each datum on the listing. There are two types of frequency distributions, ungrouped and grouped.

Friedman two-way analysis of variance by ranks. Nonparametric test used with matched samples or in repeated measures.

generalization. Extends the implications of the findings from the sample that was studied to the larger population or from the situation studied to a larger situation.

geographic analyses. Used to examine variations in health status, health services, patterns of care, or patterns of use by geographic area and are sometimes referred to as small area analyses.

gestalt. Organization of knowledge about a particular phenomenon into a cluster of linked ideas. The clustering and interrelatedness enhances the meaning of the ideas.

going native. In ethnographic research, when the researcher becomes a part of the culture and loses all objectivity, and, with it, the ability to observe clearly.

grant. A proposal developed to seek research funding from private or public institutions.

grounded theory research. An inductive research technique based on symbolic interaction theory, which is conducted to discover what problems exist in a social scene and the process persons use to handle them. The research process involves formulation, testing, and redevelopment of propositions until a theory is developed.

Hawthorne effect. A psychological response in which subjects change their behavior simply because they are subjects in a study, not because of the research treatment.

heterogeneity. The researcher's attempt to obtain subjects with a wide variety of characteristics to reduce the risk of bias in studies not using random sampling.

heuristic relevance. A standard for evaluating a qualitative study, where the study's intuitive

recognition, relationship to existing body of knowledge, and applicability are examined.

hierarchical statement sets. Composed of a specific proposition and an hypothesis or research question. If a conceptual model is included in the framework, the set may also include a general proposition.

highly controlled settings. Artificially constructed environments that are developed for the sole purpose of conducting research, such as laboratories, experimental centers, and test units.

historical research. A narrative description or analysis of events that occurred in the remote or recent past.

history effect. An event that is not related to the planned study but occurs during the time of the study and could influence the responses of subjects to the treatment.

homogeneity. The degree to which objects are similar or a form of equivalence, such as limiting subjects to only one level of an extraneous variable to reduce its impact on the study findings.

homogeneity reliability. Type of reliability testing used with paper-and-pencil tests and addresses the correlation of various items within the instrument.

homoscedastic. Data are evenly dispersed both above and below the regression line, which indicates a linear relationship on a scatter diagram (plot).

human rights. Claims and demands that have been justified in the eyes of an individual or by the consensus of a group of individuals and are protected in research.

hypothesis. Formal statement of the expected relationship between two or more variables in a specified population.

immersed in the culture. Involves gaining increasing familiarity with such things as language, sociocultural norms, traditions, communication patterns, religion, work patterns, and expression of emotion in a selected culture.

implementation stage. Stage in the innovation-decision process when an innovation is used by an individual or group.

implications. The meaning of research conclusions for the body of knowledge, theory, and practice.

inclusion criteria. Sampling requirements identified by the researcher that must be present for the element or subject to be included in the sample.

incomplete disclosure. Subjects are not completely informed about the purpose of a study because that knowledge might alter the subjects' actions. Following the study, the subjects must be debriefed.

independent groups. Groups where the selection of one subject is totally unrelated to the selection of other subjects. An example is when subjects are randomly assigned to the treatment and control groups.

independent variable. The treatment or experimental activity that is manipulated or varied by the researcher to create an effect on the dependent variable.

index. Provides assistance in identifying journal articles and other publications relevant to a topic of interest.

indirect measurement. Used with abstract concepts, when the concepts are not measured directly but, rather, indicators or attributes of the concepts are used to represent the abstraction.

inductive reasoning. Reasoning from the specific to the general where particular instances are observed and then combined into a larger whole or general statement.

inferential statistics. Statistics designed to allow inference from a sample statistic to a population parameter; commonly used to test hypotheses of similarities and differences in subsets of the sample under study.

inferred causality. A cause-and-effect relationship is identified from numerous studies conducted over time to determine risk factors or causal factors in selected situations.

informed consent. The prospective subject's agreement to voluntarily participate in a study, which is reached after assimilation of essential information about the study.

inherent variability. Data can be naturally expected to have a few random observations to be in the extreme ends of the tail.

innovation. An idea, practice, or object that is perceived as new by an individual or other unit of adoption.

innovation-decision process. Includes the steps of knowledge, persuasion, decision, implementation, and confirmation to promote diffusion or communication of research findings to members of a discipline for use in practice.

innovativeness. The degree to which an individual or other unit of adoption is more willing to adopt new ideas than are the other members of a system.

innovators. Individuals who actively seek out new ideas.

institutional review. A process of examining studies for ethical concerns by a committee of peers.

instrumentation. A component of measurement that involves the application of specific rules to develop a measurement device or instrument.

integrative review of research. Conducted to identify, analyze, and synthesize the results from independent studies to determine the current knowledge (what is known and not known) in a particular area.

intellectual critique of research. Involves a careful examination of all aspects of a study to judge the merits, limitations, meaning, and significance of the study based on previous research experience and knowledge of the topic.

interlibrary loan department. Department that locates books and articles in other libraries and provides the sources within a designated time.

internal criticism. Involves examination of the reliability of historical documents.

internal validity. The extent to which the effects detected in the study are a true reflection of reality, rather than being the result of the effects of extraneous variables.

interpretation of research outcomes. Involves examining the results from data analysis, forming conclusions, considering the implications for nursing, exploring the significance of the findings, generalizing the findings, and suggesting further studies.

interpretative codes. Organizational system developed late in the qualitative data collection and analysis process as the researcher gains some insight into the processes occurring.

interpretive reliability. Assesses the extent to which each judge assigns the same category to a given unit of data.

interrater reliability. The degree of consistency between two raters who are independently assigning ratings to a variable or attribute being investigated.

interrupted time-series designs. These designs are similar to descriptive time designs except that a treatment is applied at some point in the observations.

interval estimate. Researcher identifies a range of values on a number line where the population parameter is thought to be.

interval-scale measurement. Interval scales have equal numerical distances between intervals of the scale in addition to following rules of mutually exclusive categories, exhaustive categories, and rank ordering, such as temperature.

interviews. Structured or unstructured verbal communication between the researcher and subject, during which information is obtained for a study.

introspection. A process of turning your attention inward toward your own thoughts which provides an increased awareness and understanding of the flow and interplay of feelings and ideas.

intuiting. Process of actually looking at the phenomenon in qualitative research; the individual focuses all awareness and energy on the subject of interest.

intuition. An insight or understanding of a situation or event as a whole that usually cannot be logically explained.

intuitive recognition. When individuals are confronted with the theoretical schema derived from the data of a qualitative study, it has meaning within their personal knowledge base.

invasion of privacy. When private information is shared without an individual's knowledge or against his or her will.

inverse linear relationship. Indicates that as one variable or concept changes, the other variable or concept changes in the opposite direction. Also referred to as a negative linear relationship.

investigator triangulation. Exists when two or more research-trained investigators with divergent backgrounds explore the same phenomenon.

justice, principle of. States that human subjects should be treated fairly.

Kendall's tau. Nonparametric test to determine correlation used when both variables have been measured at the ordinal level.

knowledge stage. The stage in the innovation-decision process when the first awareness of the existence of the innovation occurs.

knowledge utilization. The process of disseminating and using research-generated information to make an impact on or change in the existing practices in society.

Kolmogorov-Smirnov two-sample test. Nonparametric test used to determine whether two independent samples have been drawn from the same population.

Kruskal-Wallis test. Most powerful nonparametric analysis technique for examining three independent groups for differences.

kurtosis. The degree of peakedness (platykurtic, mesokurtic, or leptokurtic) of the curve shape that is related to the spread or variance of scores.

laggards. Individuals who are security-oriented, tend to cling to the past, and are often isolates without a strong support system. Term used in the innovation-decision process to describe persons who are reluctant or refuse to adopt innovations.

lambda. Analysis technique that measures the degree of association (or relationship) between two nominal level variables.

landmark studies. Major projects that generate knowledge that influences a discipline and sometimes society in general.

late majority. Individuals who are skeptical about new ideas and will adopt them only if group pressure is great. Term used in the innovation-decision process to describe persons who are reluctant to adopt innovations.

latent transition analysis (LTA). Outcomes research strategy used in situations where stages or categories of recovery have been defined and transitions across stages can be identified. To use this analysis method, each member of the population is placed in a single category or stage for a given point of time.

least squares principle. The fact that when deviations from the mean are squared, the sum is smaller than the sum of squared deviations from any other value in a sample distribution.

level of significance. *See* alpha.

library resources. Includes library personnel, interlibrary loan department, circulation department, reference department, audiovisual department, computer search department, and photocopy services.

Likert scale. An instrument designed to determine the opinion or attitude of a subject; it contains a number of declarative statements with a scale after each statement.

limitations. Theoretical and methodological restrictions in a study that may decrease the generalizability of the findings.

linear relationship. The relationship between two variables or concepts will remain consistent regardless of the values of each of the variables or concepts.

linker. An individual who could serve as a connection between the user system and the resource system when research findings are being used in practice.

logic. A science that involves valid ways of relating ideas to promote human understanding and includes abstract and concrete thinking and logistic, inductive, and deductive reasoning.

logistic reasoning. Used to break the whole into parts that can be carefully examined, as can the relationships among the parts.

longitudinal designs. Panel designs used to examine changes in the same subjects over an extended period of time.

manipulate. Means to move around or to control the movement of, such as the manipulation of a treatment.

Mann-Whitney *U* test. Used to analyze ordinal data with 95% of the power of the *t* test to detect differences between groups of normally distributed populations.

manual search. Involves examining the catalog, indexes, abstracts, and bibliographies for relevant sources.

map. *See* conceptual map.

matching. This technique is used when an experimental subject is randomly selected and a subject similar in relation to important extraneous variables is randomly selected for inclusion in the control group.

maturation effect. Unplanned and unrecognized changes experienced during a study, such as growing older, wiser, stronger, hungrier, or more tired, that can influence the findings of a study.

McNemar test. Nonparametric test to analyze the changes that occur in dichotomous variables using a 2×2 table.

mean. The value obtained by summing all the scores and dividing that total by the number of scores being summed.

mean of means. Statistical value or mean obtained by analyzing the means from many samples obtained from the same population.

measurement. The process of assigning numbers to objects, events, or situations in accord with some rule.

measurement error. The difference between what exists in reality and what is measured by a research instrument.

measures of central tendency. Statistical procedures (mode, median, and mean) for determining the center of a distribution of scores.

measures of dispersion. Statistical procedures (range, difference scores, sum of squares, variance, and standard deviation) for examining how scores vary or are dispersed around the mean.

median. The score at the exact center of the ungrouped frequency distribution.

Medical Treatment Effectiveness Program (MEDTEP). Major research effort initiated by the Agency for Health Care Policy and Research that was implemented to improve the effectiveness and appropriateness of medical practice.

memo. Developed by the researcher to record insights or ideas related to notes, transcripts, or codes during qualitative data analysis.

mentor. Someone who provides information, advice, and emotional support to a mentee or protégé.

mentorship. An intense form of role-modeling where an expert nurse serves as a teacher, sponsor, guide, exemplar, and counselor for the novice nurse.

meta-analysis design. Merging of findings from several completed studies to determine what is known about a particular phenomenon.

method of least squares. Procedure in regression analysis for developing the line of best fit.

methodological congruence. A standard for evaluating qualitative research, where documentation rigor, procedural rigor, ethical rigor, and auditability of the study are examined.

methodological designs. Used to develop the validity and reliability of instruments to measure research concepts and variables.

methodological limitations. Restrictions in the study design that limit the credibility of the findings and the population to which the findings can be generalized.

methodological triangulation. The use of two or more research methods or procedures, such as different designs, instruments, and data collection procedures, in a study.

minimal risk. The risks of harm anticipated in the proposed research are not greater, considering probability and magnitude, than those ordinarily encountered in daily life or during the performance of routine physical or psychological examinations.

modal percentage. Appropriate for nominal data and indicates the relationship of the number of data scores represented by the mode to the total number of data scores.

mode. The numerical value or score that occurs with the greatest frequency in a distribution; but it does not necessarily indicate the center of the data set.

model testing designs. Used to test the accuracy of an hypothesized causal model or map.

mono-method bias. More than one measure of a variable is used in a study, but all measures use the same method of recording.

mono-operation bias. Occurs when only one method of measurement is used to measure a construct.

mortality. Subjects drop out of a study before completion, which creates a threat to the internal validity.

multicausality. The recognition that a number of interrelating variables can be involved in causing a particular effect.

multicollinearity. Occurs when the independent variables in a regression equation are strongly correlated.

multicomponent treatments, effects of. Occur when a set of treatments are combined to manage a patient problem. Outcomes research designs have been developed to examine the effects of these treatment programs and some of these designs include: treatment package strategy, comparative treatment strategy, dismantling strategy, constructive strategy, factorial ANOVA design, fractional factorial designs, dose-response designs, response surface methodology, and mediational analysis.

multilevel analysis. Used in epidemiology to study how environmental factors and individual attributes and behaviors interact to influence individual-level health behaviors and disease risks.

multimethod-multitrait technique. When a variety of data collection methods, such as interview and observation, are used and different measurement methods are used for each concept in a study.

multiple regression analysis. Extension of simple linear regression with more than one independent variable entered into the analysis.

multiple triangulation. The use of two or more types of triangulation (theoretical, data, methodological, investigator, and analysis) in a study.

multivariate analysis techniques. Used to analyze data from complex research projects. Techniques included in text: multiple regression, factorial analysis of variance, analysis of covariance, factor analysis, discriminant analysis, canonical correlation, structural equation modeling, time-series analysis, clinical trials, and survival analysis.

natural settings. Field settings or uncontrolled, real-life situations examined in research.

necessary relationship. One variable or concept must occur for the second variable or concept to occur.

negative linear relationship. See inverse linear relationship.

nested design. Design that allows the researcher to consider the effect of variables that are found only at some levels of the independent variables being studied.

nested variables. Variables found only at certain levels of the independent variable, such as gender, race, socioeconomic status, and education.

networking. A process of developing channels of communication between people with common interests throughout the country.

network sampling. Snowballing technique that takes advantage of social networks and the fact that friends tend to hold characteristics in common. Subjects meeting the sample criteria are asked to assist in locating others with similar characteristics.

nominal-scale measurement. Lowest level of measurement that is used when data can be organized into categories that are exclusive and exhaustive, but the categories cannot be compared, such as gender, race, marital status, and nursing diagnoses.

nondirectional hypothesis. States that a relationship exists but does not predict the exact nature of the relationship.

nonequivalent control group designs. Designs in which the control group is not selected by random means, such as the one-group post-test-only design, post-test-only design with nonequivalent groups, and one-group pretest–post-test design.

nonparametric statistics. Statistical techniques used when the assumptions of parametric statistics are not met and most commonly used to analyze nominal- and ordinal-level data.

nonprobability sampling. Not every element of the population has an opportunity for selection in the sample, such as convenience (accidental) sampling, quota sampling, purposive sampling, and network sampling.

nonrandom sampling. See nonprobability sampling.

nonsignificant results. Negative results or results contrary to the researcher's hypotheses that can be an accurate reflection of reality or can be caused by study weaknesses.

nontherapeutic research. Research conducted to generate knowledge for a discipline, and the results from the study might benefit future patients but will probably not benefit those acting as research subjects.

normal curve. A symmetrical, unimodal bell-shaped curve that is a theoretical distribution of all possible scores, but no real distribution exactly fits the normal curve.

norm-referenced testing. Test performance standards that have been carefully developed over years with large, representative samples using standardized tests with extensive reliability and validity.

norms. The expected behavior patterns within a social system that affect diffusion of innovations.

null hypothesis. States that there is no relationship between the variables being studied; a statistical hypothesis used for statistical testing and interpreting statistical outcomes.

Nuremberg Code. Ethical code of conduct to guide investigators in conducting research.

nursing process. A subset of the problem-solving process that includes assessment, diagnosis, plan, implementation, evaluation, and modification.

nursing research. A scientific process that validates and refines existing knowledge and generates new knowledge that directly and indirectly influences clinical nursing practice.

oblique rotation. A type of rotation in factor analysis used to accomplish the best fit (best factor solution) and the factors are allowed to be correlated.

observability. The extent to which the results of an innovation are visible to others.

observational measurement. The use of structured and unstructured observation to measure study variables.

observed score. The actual score or value obtained for a subject on a measurement tool.

observer-as-participant. The researcher's time is spent observing and interviewing subjects and less in the participation role.

one-tailed test of significance. An analysis used with directional hypotheses where extreme statistical values of interest are thought to occur in a single tail of the curve.

open context. Requires deconstructing a sedimented view, allowing one to see the depth and complexity within the phenomenon being examined in qualitative research.

operational definition. Description of how variables or concepts will be measured or manipulated in a study.

operational reasoning. Involves the identification and discrimination between many alternatives or viewpoints and focuses on the process of debating alternatives.

opinion leaders. Those who are in favor of innovations and support change.

ordinal-scale measurement. Yields data that can be ranked but the intervals between the ranked data are not necessarily equal, such as levels of coping.

outcomes research. Important scientific methodology that was developed to examine the end results of patient care. The strategies used in outcomes research are a departure from the traditional scientific endeavors and incorporate evaluation research, epidemiology, and economic theory perspectives.

outliers. The extreme scores or values in a set of data.

parallel-forms reliability. *See* alternated forms reliability.

parameter. A measure or numerical value of a population.

parametric statistical analyses. Statistical techniques used when three assumptions are met: (1) the sample was drawn from a population for which the variance can be calculated, the distribution is expected to be normal or approximately normal; (2) the level of measurement should be interval or ordinal with an approximately normal distribution; and (3) the data can be treated as random samples.

paraphrasing. Involves expressing clearly and concisely the ideas of an author in your own words.

partially controlled setting. An environment that is manipulated or modified in some way by the researcher.

participant-as-observer. A special form of observation where researchers immerse themselves in the setting so they can hear, see, and experience the reality as the participants do. But the participants are aware of the dual roles of the researcher (participant and observer).

passive rejection. Occurs when an innovation was never seriously considered for use in practice.

path coefficient. The effect of the independent variable on the dependent variable that is determined through path analysis.

patient outcomes research teams (PORTs). Large-scale, multifaceted, and multidisciplinary projects initiated by the Agency for Health Care Policy and Research designed to examine the outcomes and costs of current practice patterns, identify the best treatment strategy, and test methods for reducing inappropriate variations.

Pearson's product-moment correlation coefficient. Parametric test used to determine the relationship between variables.

percent of variance. The value obtained by squaring the Pearson's correlation coefficient (r) and that is the amount of variability explained by the linear relationship.

permission to participate in a study. The agreement of parents or guardian to the participation of their child or ward in research.

personal experience. Gaining knowledge by being personally involved in an event, situation, or circumstance. Benner described five levels of experience in the development of clinical knowledge and expertise: (1) novice, (2) advanced beginner, (3) competent, (4) proficient, and (5) expert.

persuasion stage. Stage in the innovation-decision process when an individual or group forms an attitude toward the innovation.

phenomenological research. Inductive, descriptive qualitative methodology developed from phenomenological philosophy for the purpose of describing experiences as they are lived by the study participants.

phi coefficient. Analysis technique to determine relationships in dichotomous, nominal data.

philosophical analysis. The use of concept or linguistic analyses to examine meaning and develop theories of meaning in philosophical inquiry.

philosophical inquiry. Research using intellectual analyses to clarify meanings, make values manifest, identify ethics, and study the nature of knowledge. Types of philosophical inquiry covered in this text are foundational inquiry, philosophical analyses, and ethical analyses.

philosophy. A broad, global explanation of the world.

physiologic measurement. Techniques used to measure physiologic variables either directly or indirectly, such as techniques to measure heart rate or mean arterial pressure.

pilot study. A smaller version of a proposed study conducted to develop and/or refine the methodology, such as the treatment, instrument, or data collection process.

pink sheet. A letter indicating the rejection of a research grant proposal and a critique by the scientific committee that reviewed the proposal.

point estimate. A single figure that estimates a related figure in the population of interest.

population. All elements (individuals, objects, events, or substances) that meet sample criteria for inclusion in a study. Sometimes referred to as a target population.

population-based studies. Important type of outcomes research that involves studying health conditions in the context of the community, rather than the context of the medical system.

population studies. Studies that target the entire population.

positive linear relationship. Indicates that as one variable changes (value of the variable increases or decreases), the second variable will also change in the same direction.

poster session. Visual presentation of a study, using pictures, tables, and illustrations on a display board.

post hoc analyses. Statistical tests developed specifically to determine the location of differences after ANOVA. Frequently used post hoc tests are Bonferroni's procedure, the Newman-Keuls test, the Tukey HSD test, the Scheffé test, and Dunnett's test.

power. The probability that a statistical test will detect a significant difference that exists; power analysis is used to determine the power of a study.

power analysis. Used to determine the risk of a Type II error, so the study can be modified to decrease the risk if necessary.

practical significance of a study. Associated with its importance to nursing's body of knowledge.

practice effect. Occurs when subjects improve as they become more familiar with the experimental protocol.

practice pattern profiling. An epidemiologic technique that focuses on patterns of care rather than individual occurrences of care that is used in outcomes research.

precision. The accuracy with which the population parameters have been estimated within a study. Also used to describe the degree of consistency or reproducibility of measurements using physiological instruments.

prediction. The ability to estimate the probability of a specific outcome in a given situation that can be achieved through research.

prediction equation. Outcome of regression analysis.

predictive design. Developed to predict the value of the dependent variable based on values obtained from the independent variables; one approach to examining causal relationships between variables.

preference clinical trials (PCTs). Studies where patients choose among all treatments available rather than being randomized into a study group.

preproposal. Short document (four to five pages plus appendices) written to explore the funding possibilities for a research project.

primary source. A source that is written by the person who originated or is responsible for generating the ideas published.

principal component analysis. The second step in exploratory factor analysis that provides preliminary information needed by the researcher in order for decisions to be made prior to the final factoring.

principal investigator (PI). In a research grant, the individual who will have primary responsibility for administering the grant and interacting with the funding agency.

privacy. The freedom an individual has to determine the time, extent, and general circumstances under which private information will be shared with or withheld from others.

probability sampling. Random sampling techniques in which each member (element) in the population should have a greater than zero opportunity to be selected for the sample; examples include simple random sampling, stratified random sampling, cluster sampling, and systematic sampling.

probability statement. Expresses the likelihood that something will happen in a given situation and addresses relative rather than absolute causality.

probability theory. Addresses statistical analysis from the perspective of the extent of a relationship or the probability of accurately predicting an event.

probing. Technique used by the interviewer to obtain more information in a specific area of the interview.

problematic reasoning. Involves identifying a problem, selecting solutions to the problem, and resolving the problem.

problem-solving process. Systematic identification of a problem, determination of goals related to the problem, identification of possible approaches to achieve those goals, implementation of selected approaches, and evaluation of goal achievement.

process-outcome matrix. Qualitative analysis technique that allows the researcher to trace the processes that led to differing outcomes.

projective techniques. A method of measuring individuals' responses to unstructured or ambiguous situations as a means of describing attitudes, personality characteristics, and motives of the individuals. An example is the Rorschach inkblot test.

proposal, research. Written plan identifying the major elements of a study, such as the problem, purpose, and framework, and outlining the methods to conduct the study. A formal way to communicate ideas about a proposed study to receive approval to conduct the study and to seek funding.

proposition. An abstract statement that further clarifies the relationship between two concepts.

prospective cohort study. An epidemiologic study in which a group of people are identified who are at risk for experiencing a particular event.

purposive sampling. Judgmental sampling that involves the conscious selection by the researcher of certain subjects or elements to include in a study.

Q-plot display. Exploratory data analysis technique, where the scores or data are displayed in a distribution by quantile.

Q-sort methodology. A technique of comparative rating where a subject sorts cards with statements on them into designated piles (usually 7 to 10 piles in the distribution of a normal curve) that might range from best to worst.

qualitative research. A systematic, interactive, subjective approach used to describe life experiences and give them meaning.

quantitative research. A formal, objective, systematic process to describe, test relationships, and examine cause and effect interactions among variables.

quasi-experimental designs. Designs with limited control that were developed to provide alternate means for examining causality in situations not conducive to experimental controls.

quasi-experimental research. A type of quantitative research conducted to explain relationships, clarify why certain events happen, and examine causality between selected independent and dependent variables.

query letter.   A letter sent to an editor of a journal to determine interest in publishing an article, or a letter sent to a funding agency to determine interest in funding a study.

questionable publication.   Publication in which no co-author could produce the original data or no co-author had personally observed or performed each phase of the research or participated in the research publication.

questionnaire.   A printed self-report form designed to elicit information that can be obtained through written responses of the subject.

quota sampling.   A convenience sampling technique with an added strategy to ensure the inclusion of subject types that are likely to be underrepresented in the convenience sample, such as women, minority groups, and the undereducated.

random assignment to groups.   A procedure used to assign subjects to the treatment or control groups, where the subjects have an equal opportunity to be assigned to either group.

random error.   An error that causes individuals' observed scores to vary haphazardly around their true score.

randomized clinical trials.   Classic means of examining the effects of various treatments where the effects of a treatment are examined by comparing the treatment group with the no-treatment group.

random sampling.   See probability sampling.

random variation.   The expected difference in values that occurs when one examines different subjects from the same sample.

range.   The simplest measure of dispersion obtained by subtracting the lowest score from the highest score.

rating scales.   Crudest form of measure using scaling techniques that include a list of an ordered series of categories of a variable, assumed to be based on an underlying continuum.

ratio-level measurement.   Highest measurement form that meets all the rules of other forms of measure: mutually exclusive categories, exhaustive categories, rank ordering, equal spacing between intervals, and a continuum of values and also has an absolute zero, such as weight.

reasoning.   Processing and organizing ideas in order to reach conclusions; examples include problematic, operational, dialectic, and logistic.

reconstructing new ideas or views.   In qualitative research, researchers examine many dimensions of the area being studied and form new ideas, while recognizing that the present reconstructing of ideas is only one of many possible ways of organizing data.

referencing.   Comparing a subject's score against a standard, used in norm-referenced and criterion-referenced testing.

refereed journal.   Uses referees or expert reviewers to determine whether a manuscript will be accepted for publication.

reflexive thought.   Critically thinking through the dynamic interaction between the self and the data occurring during analysis of qualitative data. During this process, the researcher explores personal feelings and experiences that may influence the study and integrates this understanding into the study.

regression line.   The line that best represents the values of the raw scores plotted on a scatter diagram and the procedure for developing the line of best fit is the method of least squares.

reinvention.   Adopters modify the innovation to meet their own needs.

rejection.   An active or passive decision not to use an innovation.

relational statement.   Declares that a relationship of some kind exists between two or more concepts.

relative advantage.   The extent to which the innovation is perceived to be better than current practice.

relevant literature.   Those sources that are pertinent or highly important in providing the in-depth knowledge needed to make changes in practice or to study a selected problem.

reliability.   Represents the consistency of the measure obtained.

reliability testing.   A measure of the amount of random error in the measurement technique.

replacement discontinuance in the utilization of innovations. Rejection of an innovation identified through research in order to adopt a better idea.

replication. Reproducing or repeating a study to determine whether similar findings will be obtained.

replication, approximate. An operational replication that involves repeating the original study under similar conditions, following the methods as closely as possible.

replication, concurrent. Involves the collection of data for the original study and its replication simultaneously to provide a check of the reliability of the original study. The confirmation, through replication, of the original study findings is part of the original study's design.

replication, exact. Involves the precise or exact duplication of the initial researcher's study to confirm the original findings.

replication, systematic. A constructive replication that is done under distinctly new conditions where the researchers conducting the replication do not follow the design or methods of the original researchers; rather, the second investigative team begins with a similar problem statement but formulates new means to verify the first investigator's findings.

representativeness of sample. A sample must be like the population in as many ways as possible.

research. Diligent, systematic inquiry or investigation to validate and refine existing knowledge and generate new knowledge.

research grant. Funding specifically for conducting a study.

research hypothesis. The alternative hypothesis to the null hypothesis that states there is a relationship between two or more variables.

research objectives. Clear, concise, declarative statements that are expressed to direct a study and are focused on identification and description of variables and/or determination of the relationships among variables.

research problem. A situation in need of a solution, improvement, or alteration, or a discrepancy between the way things are and the way they ought to be.

research proposal. *See* proposal, research.

research purpose. A concise, clear statement of the specific goal or aim of the study that is generated from the problem.

research questions. Concise, interrogative statements developed to direct studies that are focused on description of variables, examination of relationships among variables, and determination of differences between two or more groups.

research topics. Concepts or broad problem areas that provide the basis for generating numerous questions and research problems.

research tradition. A program of research that is important for building a body of knowledge related to the phenomena explained by a particular conceptual model.

respect for persons, principle of. Indicates that persons have the right to self-determination and the freedom to participate or not participate in research.

response set. The parameters within which the question or item is to be answered in a questionnaire.

results. The outcomes from data analysis that are generated for each research objective, question, or hypothesis.

retrospective cohort study. An epidemiologic study in which a group of people are identified who have experienced a particular event; for example, studying occupational exposure to chemicals.

review of relevant literature. An analysis and synthesis of research sources to generate a picture of what is known about a particular situation and the knowledge gaps that exist in the situation.

rigor. The striving for excellence in research through the use of discipline, scrupulous adherence to detail, and strict accuracy.

rigor in documentation. Standard for critiquing qualitative research that involves the clear, concise presentation of the study elements by the researcher.

robust. Analysis procedure that will yield accurate results even if some of the assumptions are violated by the data being analyzed.

role-modeling. Learning by imitating the behaviors of an exemplar or role model.

sample. A subset of the population that is selected for a study.

sample characteristics. Description of the research subjects obtained by analyzing the data obtained from the demographic variables.

sampling. Includes selecting groups of people, events, behaviors, or other elements with which to conduct a study.

sampling criteria. A list of the characteristics essential for membership in the target population.

sampling distribution. Developed using statistical values (such as means) of many samples obtained from the same population.

sampling error. The difference between a sample statistic used to estimate a parameter and the actual but unknown value of the parameter.

sampling frame. Listing of every member of the population using the sampling criteria to define membership.

sampling method. The process of selecting a group of people, events, behaviors, or other elements that are representative of the population being studied.

sampling plan. Describes the strategies that will be used to obtain a sample for a study and may include either probability or nonprobability sampling methods.

scale. A self-report form of measurement that is composed of several items that are thought to measure the construct being studied and the subject responds to each item on the continuum or scale provided.

science. A coherent body of knowledge composed of research findings, tested theories, scientific principles, and laws for a discipline.

scientific community. A cohesive group of scholars within a discipline who stimulate the creation of new research ideas and the development of innovative methodologies to conduct research.

scientific method. Incorporates all procedures that scientists have used, currently use, or may use in the future to pursue knowledge, such as quantitative research, qualitative research, and outcomes research.

scientific misconduct. Involves such practices as fabrication, falsification, or forging of data;

dishonest manipulation of the study design or methods; and plagiarism.

scientific theory. Theory with valid and reliable methods of measuring each concept and relational statements that have been repeatedly tested through research and demonstrated to be valid.

secondary analysis design. Involves studying data previously collected in another study; data are reexamined using different organizations of the data and different statistical analyses.

secondary source. A source that summarizes or quotes content from primary sources.

sedimented view. Seeing things from the perspective of a specific frame of reference, world view, or theory, which gives a sense of certainty, security, and control.

seeking approval to conduct a study. A process involving submission of a research proposal to a selected group for review and often verbally defending that proposal.

selectivity in physiological measures. An element of accuracy that involves the ability to identify correctly the signal under study to distinguish it from other signals.

self-determination. Based on the ethical principle of respect for persons, which states that humans are capable of controlling their own destiny. Right to self-determination is violated through the use of coercion, covert data collection, and deception.

semantic differential scale. An instrument that consists of two opposite adjectives with a seven-point scale between them. The subject selects one point on the scale that best describes his or her view of the concept being examined.

sensitivity of physiological measures. Related to the amount of change of a parameter than can be measured precisely.

sequential relationship. A relationship where one concept occurs later than the other.

serendipity. The accidental discovery of something valuable or useful during the conduct of a study.

setting. Location for conducting research, such as a natural, partially controlled, or highly controlled setting.

sign test. A nonparametric analysis technique developed for data that it is difficult to assign numerical values to, but the data can be ranked on some dimension.

significant results. Results that are in keeping with those identified by the researcher.

simple hypothesis. States the relationship (associative or causal) between two variables.

simple linear regression. Parametric analysis technique that provides a means to estimate the value of a dependent variable based on the value of an independent variable.

simple random sampling. Elements are selected at random from the sampling frame for inclusion in a study. Each study element has a probability greater than zero of being selected for inclusion in the study.

skewness. A curve that is asymmetrical (positively or negatively skewed) that is developed from an asymmetrical distribution of scores.

skimming. A quick review of a source to gain a broad overview of the content.

slope. Determines the direction and angle of the regression line within the graph. The value is represented by the letter b.

social system. A set of interrelated units that is engaged in joint problem-solving to accomplish a common goal.

Spearman rank-order correlation coefficient. A nonparametric analysis technique for ordinal data that is an adaptation of the Pearson's product-moment correlation used to examine relationships among variables in a study.

special library. Contains a collection of materials on a selected topic or for a specialty area, such as nursing or medicine.

split-half reliability. Used to determine the homogeneity of an instrument's items, where the items are split in half, and a correlational procedure is performed between the two halves.

stability. Aspect of reliability testing that is concerned with the consistency of repeated measures.

standard deviation. A measure of dispersion that is calculated by taking the square root of the variance.

standard scores. Used to express deviations from the mean (difference scores) in terms of standard deviation units, such as Z scores where the mean is zero and the standard deviation is 1.

statement synthesis. The researcher develops statements proposing specific relationships among the concepts being studied. This is a part of developing a framework for a study.

statistic. A numerical value obtained from a sample used to estimate the parameters of a population.

statistical conclusion validity. Concerned with whether the conclusions about relationships and differences drawn from statistical analyses are an accurate reflection of reality.

statistical regression. The movement or regression of extreme scores toward the mean in studies using a pretest–post-test design.

statistical significance. The results are unlikely to be due to chance.

stem-and-leaf displays. Type of exploratory data analysis where the scores are visually presented to obtain insights.

stepwise regression analysis. Type of exploratory regression analysis where the independent variables are entered into or removed from the analysis one at a time.

stratified random sampling. Used when the researcher knows some of the variables in the population that are critical to achieving representativeness. The sample is divided into strata or groups using these identified variables.

stratification. Used in a design so subjects are distributed throughout the sample using sampling techniques similar to those used in blocking but the purpose of the procedure is even distribution throughout the sample.

strength of relationship. The amount of variation that is explained by the relationship.

structural equation modeling. Analysis technique designed to test theories.

structured interviews. Use of strategies that provide increasing amount of control by the researcher over the content of the interview.

structured observation. Clearly identifying what is to be observed and precisely defining how the observations are to be made, recorded, and coded.

study validity. A measure of the truth or accuracy of a claim that is an important concern throughout the research process.

subjects.   Individuals participating in a study.

substantive theory.   A theory recognized within the discipline as useful for explaining important phenomenon.

substitutable relationship.   Relationship where a similar concept can be substituted for the first concept and the second concept will occur.

sufficient relationship.   States that when the first variable or concept occurs, the second will occur, regardless of the presence or absence of other factors.

sum of squares.   Mathematical manipulation that involves summing the squares of the difference scores and that is part of the analysis process for calculating the standard deviation.

summary statistics.   See descriptive statistics.

survey.   Technique of data collection using questionnaires or personal interviews to gather data about an identified population.

survey design.   A design to describe a phenomenon by collecting data using questionnaires or personal interviews.

survival analysis.   A set of techniques designed to analyze repeated measures from a given time (e.g., the beginning of the study, onset of a disease, the beginning of a treatment) until a certain attribute (e.g., death, treatment failure, recurrence of the phenomenon) occurs.

symmetrical relationship.   Complex relationship that consists of two statements: If A occurs (or changes), B will occur (or change); if B occurs (or changes), A will occur (or change); $A \leftrightarrow B$.

symmetry plot.   Exploratory data analysis technique designed to determine the presence of skewness in the data.

synthesis of sources.   Clustering and interrelating ideas from several sources to form a gestalt or new, complete picture of what is known and not known in an area.

systematic bias or variation.   A consequence of selecting subjects whose measurement values are different or vary in some way from the population.

systematic error.   Measurement error that is not random but occurs consistently, such as a scale that inaccurately weighs subjects three pounds heavy.

systematic sampling.   Conducted when an ordered list of all members of the population is available and involves selecting every kth individual on the list, using a starting point that is selected randomly.

tails.   Extremes of the normal curve where the significant statistical values exist.

target population.   A group of individuals who meet the sampling criteria.

tendency statement.   Deterministic relationship that describes what always happens if there are no interfering conditions.

tentative theory.   Theory that is newly proposed, has had minimal exposure to critique by the discipline, and has had little testing.

testable hypothesis.   Contains variables that are measurable or manipulatable in the real world.

test-retest reliability.   Determination of the stability or consistency of a measurement technique by correlating the scores obtained from repeated measures.

theoretical connectedness.   Theoretical schema developed from a qualitative study is clearly expressed, logically consistent, reflective of the data, and compatible with nursing's knowledge base.

theoretical limitations.   Weaknesses in the study framework and conceptual and operational definitions that restrict the abstract generalization of the findings.

theoretical literature.   Includes concept analyses, maps, theories, and conceptual frameworks that support a selected research problem and purpose.

theoretical substruction.   A process where the framework of a published study is separated into component parts to evaluate the logical consistency of the theoretical system and the interaction of the framework with the study methodology.

theoretical triangulation.   The use of two or more frameworks or theoretical perspectives in the same study, and the hypotheses are developed based on the different theoretical perspectives and tested using the same data set.

theory. Consists of an integrated set of defined concepts, existence statements, and relational statements that present a view of a phenomenon and can be used to describe, explain, predict, and/or control that phenomenon.

therapeutic research. Research that provides the patient an opportunity to receive an experimental treatment that might have beneficial results.

time-dimensional designs. Designs used to examine sequence and patterns of change, growth, or trends across time.

time-lag. The span of time between the generation of new knowledge through research and the use of this knowledge in practice.

time-series analysis. A technique designed to analyze changes in a variable across time and thus to uncover pattern in the data.

traditions. Truths or beliefs that are based on customs and past trends and provide a way of acquiring knowledge.

transformation of ideas. Movement of ideas across levels of abstraction to determine the existing knowledge base in an area of study.

translation. Involves transforming from one language to another to facilitate understanding and is part of the process of interpreting research outcomes where results are translated and interpreted into findings.

treatment. The independent variable that is manipulated in a study to produce an effect on the dependent variable. The treatment or independent variable is usually detailed in a protocol to ensure consistent implementation in the study.

treatment matching designs. Outcomes research design to compare the relative effectiveness of various treatments.

trend designs. Designs used to examine changes in the general population in relation to a particular phenomenon.

trialability. The extent to which an individual or agency can try out the idea on a limited basis with the option of returning to previous practices.

trial and error. An approach with unknown outcomes used in a situation of uncertainty, where other sources of knowledge are unavailable.

triangulation. The use of two or more theories, methods, data sources, investigators, or analysis methods in a study.

true score. Score that would be obtained if there were no error in measurement but there is always some measurement error.

t **test.** A parametric analysis technique used to determine significant differences between measures of two samples; *t* test analysis techniques exist for dependent and independent groups.

two-tailed test of significance. The analysis used for a nondirectional hypothesis where the researcher assumes that an extreme score can occur in either tail.

Type I error. Occurs when the researcher concludes that the samples tested are from different populations (there is a significant difference between groups) when, in fact, the samples are from the same population (there is no significant difference between groups). The null hypothesis is rejected when it is true.

Type II error. Occurs when the researcher concludes that there is no significant difference between the samples examined when, in fact, a difference exists. The null hypothesis is regarded as true when it is false.

unitizing reliability. The extent to which each judge (data collector, coder, researcher) consistently identifies the same units within the data as appropriate for coding.

unstructured interviews. Initiated with a broad question and subjects are usually encouraged to further elaborate on particular dimensions of a topic.

unstructured observations. Involve spontaneously observing and recording what is seen with a minimum of prior planning.

utilization of research findings. The use of knowledge generated through research to guide nursing practice.

validity, design. The strength of a design to produce accurate results which is determined by examining statistical conclusion validity, internal validity, construct validity, and external validity.

validity, instrument. Determining the extent to which the instrument actually reflects the abstract construct being examined.

validity, study. A measure of the truth or accuracy of a claim; an important concern throughout the research process.

variables. Qualities, properties, or characteristics of persons, things, or situations that change or vary and are manipulated or measured in research.

variance analysis. Outcomes research strategy to track individual and group variance from a specific critical pathway. The goal is to decrease preventable variance in process, thus helping patients and their families achieve optimal outcomes.

varimax rotation. A type of rotation in factor analysis used to accomplish the best fit (best factor solution) and the factors are uncorrelated.

visual analogue scale. A line of 100 mm in length with right angle stops at each end, where subjects are asked to record their response to a study variable.

voluntary consent. The prospective subject has decided to take part in a study of his or her own volition without coercion or any undue influence.

Wald-Wolfowitz runs test. Nonparametric analysis technique used to determine differences between two populations.

Wilcoxon matched-pairs signed-ranks test. Nonparametric analysis technique used to examine changes that occur in pretest/post-test measures or matched-pairs measures.

within-method triangulation. The use of both quantitative and qualitative research strategies in conducting a study but within one method, such as using only data triangulation in the study or using only theoretical triangulation in the study.

y-intercept. The point where the regression line crosses (or intercepts) the y axis. At this point on the regression line, $x = 0$.

z-scores. The standardized scores developed based on the normal curve.

Author Index

Subject Index

Note: Page numbers in *italics* refer to illustrations; page numbers followed by t refer to tables.

Abstract(s), critique of, 655–656
  in literature review, 125–126
  of verbal presentation, 639–640, *640*, 640t
Abstract thinking, 6, 7–10, 150. See also *Theory.*
  introspection in, 7
  intuition in, 7–8
  reasoning in, 8–10
Academic committees, support of, 401
Academic library, in literature review, 122
Accessible population, 293–294
Accidental sampling, 302–304
Accuracy, of measurement, 336
Acquired immunodeficiency syndrome (AIDS), grieving during, 72–73, 74t
  nursing care of, 332, 333t
Across-method triangulation, 243
Actualization, correlates of, 177–178, *177*
Acute Care Nursing Quality Indicators, 601, *602*
Adaptive model of health, 559
Adolescents, pregnancy in, 254
Adopters, of innovations, 675–676, *676*
Advanced beginner nurse, 13
Advances in Nursing Science, 22
Agency for Health Care Policy and Research, 25, 571–574, 638–639
  research priorities for, 102
Agency for Health Services Research, 571
Alzheimer's disease, behavior in, 265
  caregivers for, 564–565
  computer-assisted caregiving for, 305–306
  informed consent in, 202–203
American Journal of Nursing, 21
Analysis. See *Data analysis; Statistical analysis.*
Analysis of covariance (ANCOVA), 494–495
Analysis of variance (ANOVA), 467–470
  calculation of, 468–469
  interpretation of, 469–470
  post hoc tests in, 470
  statistical power and, 311
Animals, as research subjects, 220
Annual Review of Nursing Research, 23
Anonymity, right to, 204–205
Anxiety, of surgical patient's family, 186–187
  preparatory patient education for, 179
Applicability, in qualitative research critique, 668
Applied research, 40–41
Approximate replication, of research findings, 97–98
Arthritis, exercise in, 511–512, *513*
Associative hypotheses, 178–179
Assumptions, in quantitative research, 48–49
Asymmetrical relationship, 143
Audiences, for research findings, 635–639, 637t
Auditability, of qualitative research, 528–529
  of qualitative research critique, 666
Authority, knowledge from, 12
Autocorrelation function, in time-series analysis, 515–516

Autoregressive integrated moving average (ARIMA) model, in time-series analysis, 514–516, *514*
Average, statistical, 430
AVLINE (AudioVisual catalog OnLINE), for literature review, 127

BARRIERS Scale, in research utilization evaluation, 672
Basic research, 39–40
Being-in-time, 71
Beneficence, principle of, 199, 206
Benefit, of research, 208–209, *208*
Benefit-risk ratio, of study, 209
Best fit line, 442, *442, 443*
Between-method triangulation, 243
Bias, in quantitative research, 44
  in research design, 228
  mono-method, 232–233
  mono-operation, 232–233
Biased coin design, for random assignment, 305
BIOETHICSLINE database, for literature review, 127–128
Biography, 83
Biorhythms, in infant, 348, 349t
Bipolar disorders, grounded theory research on, 75–76, *76*
Bivariate inferential statistical analysis, 453–476
  for interval data—independent groups, 462–473, 462t, 464t, 466t, 469t, *471*, 472t, *473*
  for interval data—two dependent groups, 475–476
  for nominal data—independent groups, 453–458, 453t, 454t, 455t, 456t
  for nominal data—three or more dependent groups, 477
  for nominal data—three or more independent groups, 476
  for nominal data—two dependent groups, 473–474, *473, 474*
  for ordinal data—independent groups, 458–462, 458t, 460t, 461t, 462t
  for ordinal data—three or more dependent groups, 477–478
  for ordinal data—three or more independent groups, 476–477
  for ordinal data—two dependent groups, 474–475
Bland and Altman plot, 445–446
Blocking, subject, 240, 240t
Blood glucose, 351t
Blood pressure, 351t
  electronic monitoring of, 347
Bonferroni's procedure, 463
Books, research communication through, 647
Box-and-whisker plots, 443–444, *444*
Bracketing, 532
Breast cancer, care seeking for, 282
  chemotherapy for, 40
  screening for, 99–100, *100*
Breast self-examination, 276
Breast-feeding, 347–348
Breech delivery, 591, *591*
Bruising, postinjection, 181–182

Cancer, Jewish Chronic Disease Hospital study of, 198–199
  nutrition research and, 40
CANCERLIT, for literature review, 128

Methods of Statistical Data Analysis for Quantitative Nursing Research: Quick Access Chart

		Bivariate Data Analysis	
		Two Samples	**Three or More Samples**
Independent Groups	**Nominal Data**	Chi-square p. 454	Chi-square p. 454
		Phi p. 456	
		Cramer's *V* p. 457	
		Contingency Coefficient p. 457	
		Lambda p. 458	
Two Variables	**Ordinal Data**	Mann-Whitney *U* p. 458	
		Kolmogorov-Smirnov Two Sample Test p. 459	
		Wald-Wolfowitz Runs Test p. 460	Kruskal-Wallis One-Way Analysis of Variance by Ranks p. 476
		Spearman Rank Order Correlation p. 460	
		Kendall's Tau p. 461	
	Interval or Ratio Data	*t* Test for Independent Samples p. 463	Analysis of Variance p. 467
		Pearson's Correlation p. 465	Multiple Regression Analysis p. 481
		Analysis of Variance p. 467	
		Simple Regression p. 470	

Table continued on opposite page